NON-HODGKIN LYMPHOMAS

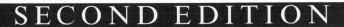

SECOND EDITION

NON-HODGKIN LYMPHOMAS

Editors

James O. Armitage, MD
The Joe Shapiro Professor of Medicine
Department of Internal Medicine
University of Nebraska Medical Center
Omaha, Nebraska

Peter M. Mauch, MD
Professor of Radiation Oncology
Harvard Medical School
Department of Radiation Oncology
Brigham and Women's Hospital
Dana-Farber Cancer Institute
Boston, Massachesetts

Nancy Lee Harris, MD
Professor of Pathology
Department of Pathology
Harvard Medical School
Massachusetts General Hospital
Boston, Massachusetts

Bertrand Coiffier, MD, PhD
Professor of Medicine
Department of Hematology
Hospices Civils de Lyon
Universite Claude Bernard
Lyon, France

Riccardo Dalla-Favera, MD
Uris Professor of Pathology and
Professor of Genetics and Development
Institute for Cancer Genetics
Columbia University College of Physicians and Surgeons
New York, New York

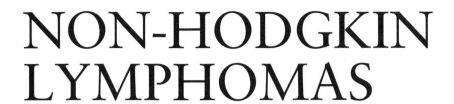

Wolters Kluwer | Lippincott Williams & Wilkins
Health

Philadelphia · Baltimore · New York · London
Buenos Aires · Hong Kong · Sydney · Tokyo

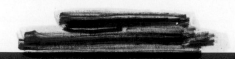

Senior Executive Editor: Jonathan W. Pine, Jr.
Senior Product Manager: Emilie Moyer
Senior Manufacturing Manager: Benjamin Rivera
Senior Marketing Manager: Angela Panetta
Design Coordinator: Terry Mallon
Production Services: Cadmus Communications

© 2010 by Lippincott Williams & Wilkins, a Wolters Kluwer business
530 Walnut Street
Philadelphia, PA 19106 USA
LWW.com

Library of Congress Cataloging-in-Publication Data
Non-Hodgkin lymphomas / editors, James O. Armitage ... [et al.]. – 2nd ed.
     p. ; cm.
  Rev. ed. of: Non-Hodgkin's lymphomas / editors, Peter M. Mauch ... [et al.]. c2004.
  Includes bibliographical references and index.
  ISBN 978-0-7817-9116-8
  1. Lymphomas. I. Armitage, James O., 1946- II. Non-Hodgkin's lymphomas.
  [DNLM: 1. Lymphoma, Non-Hodgkin. WH 525 N81185 2009]
  RC280.L9N6592 2009
  616.99'446–dc22

                                    2009022313

■ CONTRIBUTORS

Ranjana Advani, MD
Associate Professor
Department of Medicine
Stanford University
Stanford, California

Richard F. Ambinder, MD, PhD
James B. Murphy Professor of Oncology
Director, Hematologic Malignancies Division
Kimmel Comprehensive Cancer Center
Johns Hopkins School of Medicine
Bunting-Blaustein Cancer Research Building
Baltimore, Maryland

Marc P. E. André, MD
Chief, Department Hematologie et Oncologie
Grand Hôpital de Charleroi
Charleroi, Belgium

James O. Armitage, MD
The Joe Shapiro Professor of Medicine
Department of Internal Medicine
University of Nebraska Medical Center
Omaha, Nebraska

Herve Avet-Loiseau, MD, PhD
Professor of Hematology
Laboratoire d'Hematologie
Institut de Biologie
Nantes, France

Robert A. Baiocchi, MD, PhD
Assistant Professor of Internal Medicine
Hematology and Oncology
Department of Internal Medicine
The Ohio State University School of Medicine
Columbus, Ohio

Françoise Berger, MD, PhD
Professor of Pathology
Department of Pathology
Centre Hospitalier Lyon Sud.
Pierre-Bénite, France

Joseph R. Bertino, MD
Professor of Medicine and Pharmacology
The Cancer Institute of New Jersey
University Professor of Medicine & Pharmacology
UMDNJ—Robert Wood Johnson Medical School
New Brunswick, New Jersey

Françesco Bertoni, MD
Vice-Director
Laboratory of Experimental Oncology
Lymphoma Research Unit
Oncology Institute of Southern Switzerland
Bellinzona, Switzerland

Govind Bhagat, MBBS
Associate Professor of Clinical Pathology
New York-Presbyterian/Columbia
New York, New York

Philip J. Bierman, MD
Professor of Medicine
Department of Internal Medicine
Section of Oncology and Hematology
University of Nebraska Medical Center
Omaha, Nebraska

Michael J. Borowitz, MD, PhD
Professor of Pathology and Oncology
Department of Pathology
Johns Hopkins Medical Institutions
Baltimore, Maryland

Evelyne Callet-Bauchu, MD
Laboratory of Hematology
Centre Hospitalier Lyon Sud.
Pierre-Bénite, France

Daniel Catovsky, MD, DSc(Med)
Emeritus Professor of Haematology
Department of Academic Haematology
The Institute of Cancer Research
Sutton, Surrey, United Kingdom

Bruce D. Cheson, MD
Professor of Medicine
Head of Hematology
Georgetown University Hospital
Lombardi Comprehensive Cancer Center
Washington, D.C.

Bertrand Coiffier, MD, PhD
Professor of Medicine
Department of Hematology
Hospices Civils de Lyon
Universite Claude Bernard
Lyon, France

Riccardo Dalla-Favera, MD
Uris Professor of Pathology and Genetics
Director, Herbert Irving Comprehensive Cancer Center
Institute for Cancer Genetics
Columbia University
New York, New York

Lisa M. DeAngelis, MD
Professor and Chairwoman
Department of Neurology
Cornell University School of Medical Sciences
Memorial Sloan-Kettering Cancer Center
New York, New York

Claire Dearden, MD, FRCP, FRCPath
Consultant Haematologist and Head of the CLL Unit
Royal Marsden Hospital and Institute of Cancer Research
Sutton, Surrey, United Kingdom

Angela Dispenzieri, MD
Associate Professor of Medicine
Division of Hematology
Mayo Clinic
Rochester, Minnesota

Fabio Facchetti, MD, PhD
Director, Department of Pathology
Spedali Civili-University of Brescia
Brescia, Italy

Brunangelo Falini, MD
Professor of Hematology
Department of Clinical and Experimental Medicine
Section of Hematology and Clinical Immunology
University of Perugia
Perugia, Italy

Pascale Felman, MD
Laboratory of Hematology
Centre Hospitalier Lyon Sud.
Pierre-Bénite, France

Jean Feuillard, MD, PhD
Laboratoire d'Hématologie
Hospital University Campus of Limoges
Limoges, France

Kathryn Foucar, MD
Professor of Pathology
Department of Pathology
University of New Mexico Health Sciences Center
Albuquerque, New Mexico

Arnold S. Freedman, MD
Associate Professor of Medicine
Department of Medical Oncology
Harvard Medical School
Dana-Farber Cancer Institute
Boston, Massachusetts

Jonathan W. Friedberg, MD
Assistant Professor of Medicine
James P. Wilmore Cancer Center
University of Rochester School of Medicine
Rochester, New York

Randy D. Gascoyne, MD
Clinical Professor of Pathology
Department of Pathology & Laboratory Medicine
University of British Columbia
British Columbia Cancer Agency
Vancouver, British Columbia
Canada

Christian Gisselbrecht, MD
Professor of Hematology
Institut d'Hématologie–Hôpital Saint Louis
Paris, France

David J. Good, MD
Department of Pathology & Laboratory Medicine
British Columbia Cancer Agency
Vancouver, Bristish Columbia
Canada

Mary K. Gospodarowicz, MD, FRCPC, FRCR(Hon)
Professor Faculty of Medicine
Chair, Department of Radiation Oncology
University of Toronto School of Medicine
Princess Margaret Hospital
Toronto, Ontario
Canada

John G. Gribben, MD, DSc, FMedSci
Professor of Medicine
Institute of Cancer
Barts and The London School of Medicine
London, United Kingdom

Thomas G. Gross, MD, PhD
Associate Professor of Pediatrics
Department of Pediatrics
The Ohio State School of Medicine
Chief, Division of Hematology/Oncology/BMT
Nationwide Children's Hospital
Columbus, Ohio

Joan Guitart, MD
Professor of Dermatology and Pathology
Unit Director, Department of Dermatology
Robert H. Lurie Comprehensive
    Cancer Center
Northwestern University
Chicago, Illinois

Thomas M. Habermann, MD
Professor of Medicine
Department of Medicine
Division of Hematology
Mayo Clinic
Rochester, Minnesota

Jean-Luc Harousseau, MD
Professor
Department of Hematology
University of Nantes
Hotel Dieu Hospital
Nantes, France

Nancy Lee Harris, MD
Austin L. Vickery Professor of Pathology
Harvard Medical School
Massachusetts General Hospital
Boston, Massachusetts

Patricia Hartge, ScD
Deputy Director, Epidemiology and Biostatistics Program
Division of Cancer Epidemiology and Genetics
National Cancer Institute
Bethesda, Maryland

Jeff D. Harvell, MD
Department of Pathology
Stanford University
Stanford, California

Richard T. Hoppe, MD
Henry S. Kaplan-Harry Lebeson Professor of Cancer Biology
Department of Radiation Oncology
Stanford University School of Medicine
Stanford, California

Peter G. Isaacson, DM, DSc, FRCPath
Professor
Department of Histopathology
Royal Free and University College Medical School
London, United Kingdom

Elaine S. Jaffe, MD
Chief, Hematopathology Section and
    Laboratory of Pathology
Center for Cancer Research
National Cancer Institute
Bethesda, Maryland

Paul A. Jimenez, MD
Staff Physician
Department of Internal Medicine
United States Naval Hospital
Pensacola, Florida

Youn H. Kim, MD
Professor of Dermatology
Director, Multidisciplinary Cutaneous Lymphoma Program
Stanford Cancer Center
Stanford, California

Ralf Küppers, PhD
Professor of Molecular Genetics
Institute for Cell Biology (Tumor Research)
University of Duisburg-Essen Medical School
Essen, Germany

Anton W. Langerak, PhD
Molecular Immunologist
Medical Immunology
Department of Immunology
Erasmus MC, University Medical Center
Rotterdam, The Netherlands

Alexandra M. Levine, MD
Professor of Medicine
City of Hope National Medical Center
Duarte, California

Raymond H. S. Liang, MD, FRCP, FRACP
Dean of Medicine
Li Ka Shing Faculty of Medicine
University of Hong Kong
Queen Mary Hospital
Hong Kong

Ian T. Magrath, DSc(Med), FRCP
Professor of Pediatrics
International Network for Cancer Treatment and
    Research
Institut Pasteur
Brussels, Belgium

Karen J. Marcus, MD
Professor of Radiation Oncology
Harvard Medical School
Division Chief, Radiation Oncology
Children's Hospital
Dana-Farber Cancer Institute
Boston, Massachusetts

Estella Matutes, MD, PhD, FRCPath
Reader of Haematological Malignancies
Haemato-Oncology Unit
Institute of Cancer Research
Royal Marsden Hospital
London, United Kingdom

Peter M. Mauch, MD
Professor of Radiation Oncology
Harvard Medical School
Department of Radiation Oncology
Brigham and Women's Hospital
Dana-Farber Cancer Institute
Boston, Massachesetts

Giampaolo Merlini, MD
Professor of Clinical Biochemistry
Department of Biochemistry and Biotechnology Research
    Laboratories
University of Pavia
University Hospital Policlinico San Matteo
Pavia, Italy

Philippe Moreau, MD
Lecturer in Chemistry
University of Nantes
Institut des Materiaux Jean Rouxel
Nantes, France

Sujaatha Narayanan, MRCP, FRCPath
Attending Physician
Leukemia/Bone Marrow Transplant Program of British
    Columbia
Vancouver, British Columbia, Canada

Douglas E. Ney, MD
Fellow in Neuro-oncology
Department of Neurology
Memorial Sloan-Kettering Cancer Center
New York, New York

Andrea K. Ng, MD, MPH
Associate Professor of Radiation Oncology
Department of Radiation Oncology
Harvard Medical School
Brigham and Women's Hospital
Dana-Farber Cancer Institute
Boston, Massachuettes

Owen A. O' Connor, MD, PhD
Director, Lymphoid Development and Malignant
  Program
Herbert Irving Comprehensive Cancer Center
Chief, Lymphoma Service
College of Physicians and Surgeons
The New York Presbyterian Hospital
Columbia University
New York, New York

Mihaela Onciu, MD
Associate Member
Department of Pathology
Director, Hematology and Special Hematology
  Laboratories
St. Jude Children's Research Hospital
Memphis, Tennessee

Nnenna Osuji, MBChB, MD
Honorary Consultant
Section of Haemato-Oncology
Institute of Cancer Research/Royal Marsden
NHS Foundation Trust
Sutton, Surrey, United Kingdom

Laura Pasqualucci, MD
Assistant Professor of Clinical Pathology
Institute for Cancer Genetics
Columbia University
New York, New York

Stefania Pittaluga, MD, PhD
Staff Clinician
Hematopathology Section
Laboratory of Pathology
National Cancer Institute, NIH
Bethesda, Maryland

Pierluigi Porcu, MD
Associate Professor of Internal Medicine
Hematology and Oncology
Department of Internal Medicine
The Ohio State University School of Medicine
Columbus, Ohio

Christiane Querfeld, MD, PhD
Research Assistant Professor
Section of Dermatology
University of Chicago
Robert H. Lurie Comprehensive Cancer Center
Northwestern University
Chicago, Illinois

Mark Raffeld, MD
Chief, Specialized Diagnostics
Laboratory of Pathology
National Cancer Institute
National Institute of Health
Bethesda, Maryland

Steven T. Rosen, MD, FACP
Professor of Medicine
Department of Medicine
Division of Hematology/Oncology
Director, Robert H. Lurie Comprehensive Cancer Center
Northwestern University
Chicago, Illinois

Jonathan W. Said, MD
Professor of Pathology
Department of Pathology and Laboratory Medicine
University of California-Los Angeles
David Geffen School of Medicine
UCLA Center for Health Sciences
Los Angeles, California

Gilles Salles, MD, PhD
Professor of Medicine
Department of Hematology
Universite Claude Bernard
Hospices Civile de Lyon
Pierre Bénite Cédex, France

John T. Sandlund, MD
Member, Department of Oncology
St. Jude Children's Research Hospital
Professor, Department of Pediatrics
University of Tennessee College of Medicine
Memphis, Tennessee

Kerry J. Savage, MSc, FRCP(C), FACP
Assistant Professor of Medicine
University of British Columbia
Division of Medical Oncology
British Columbia Cancer Agency
Vancouver, British Columbia
Canada

Laurie Sehn, MD, MPH
Clinical Assistant Professor
Department of Medical Oncology
British Columbia Cancer Agency
Vancouver, British Columbia
Canada

Lena Specht, MD, PhD
Chief Oncologist and Professor of Oncology
Department of Oncology and Hematology
The Finsen Centre
Rigshospitalet, Copenhagen University Hospital
Copenhagen, Denmark

Frank J. T. Staal, MSc, PhD
Professor
Department of Immunology
Erasmus MC, University Medical Center
Rotterdam, The Netherlands

John W. Sweetenham, MD, FRCP
Professor of Medicine
Department of Medical Oncology
Cleveland Clinic Taussing Cancer Institute
Cleveland Clinic Lerner College of Medicine
Cleveland, Ohio

Catherine Thieblemont, MD, PhD
Professor
Department of Hemato-Oncology
Hôpital Saint-Louis
Institut Universitaire d'Hématologie
Paris, France

Kensei Tobinai, MD, PhD
Chief, Hematology Division
National Cancer Center Hospital
Tokyo, Japan

Alexandra Traverse-Glehen, MD
Service d'Anatomie Pathologique
Centre Hospitalier Lyon-Sud.
Pierre Bénite Cédex, France

Steven P. Treon, MD, PhD
Bing Center for Waldenstrom's Macroglobulinemia
Dana Farber Cancer Institute
Harvard Medical School
Boston, Massachusetts

Jacques J. M. van Dongen, MD, PhD
Professor of Immunology
Department of Immunology
Erasmus MC, University Medical Center
Rotterdam, The Netherlands

Flora van Leeuwen, PhD
Head, Department of Epidemiology
Netherlands Cancer Institute
Amsterdam, The Netherlands

Sophia S. Wang, PhD
Investigator, Hormonal and Reproductive
Epidemiology Branch
Division of Cancer Epidemiology and Genetics
National Cancer Institute
Bethesda, Maryland

Toshiki Watanabe, MD, PhD
Associate Professor
Department of Cancer Biology
Division of Pathology
University of Tokyo
The Institute of Medical Science
Tokyo, Japan

Thomas E. Witzig, MD
Professor of Medicine
Department of Medicine
Division of Hematology
Mayo Clinic
Rochester, Minnesota

Joachim Yahalom, MD
Professor of Radiation Oncology in Medicine
Department of Radiation Oncology
Memorial Sloan-Kettering Cancer Center
New York, New York

Jasmine Zain, MD
Assistant Clinical Professor
Medical Oncology
New York-Presbyterian/Columbia
New York, New York

Pier Luigi Zinzani, MD, PhD
Professor of Hematology
Institute of Hematology and Medical Oncology
"L. & A. Seràgnoli"
University of Bologna
Bologna, Italy

Emanuele Zucca, MD
Head of the Lymphoma Unit
Oncology Institute of Southern Switzerland
Ospedale San Giovanni
Bellinzona, Switzerland

■ PREFACE

The first edition of *Non-Hodgkin Lymphomas* was published in 2004. In only 5 years, the field has changed dramatically. The new World Health Organization classification, which is used in this edition of the book, has added new categories, clarified others, and even removed one from being considered as a lymphoid malignancy. The importance of genetic studies has expanded considerably, and is now affecting not just diagnosis and classification but also beginning to impact treatment and prognosis. Several new therapeutic agents have become available and are finding a valuable place in managing patients with these malignancies.

In the current text, we have attempted to be as inclusive as possible. We wanted broad representation of knowledge in the biology and treatment of the non-Hodgkin lymphomas, and we wished to credit those who have made important contributions to our understanding of these diseases. As a result, the editors and authors represent the disciplines of radiation oncology, medical oncology, molecular biology, and pathology with 87 contributors from all parts of the world.

Each chapter of the book has been designed to stand alone and to comprehensively cover a topic. One consequence of this approach is that portions of a topic may be addressed in more than one chapter. Chapters address the historical aspects of these disorders, the new methods of classification, the principles of biology that guide diagnosis and therapy, the techniques of staging and treatment, the approach to specific illnesses, and special problems common to the management of patients with these disorders.

In presenting this book, we wanted to provide a reference text for training programs and researchers. We also wanted to produce a text that would be useful for practicing physicians. Finally, we hope to provide a foundation for new ideas in laboratory and clinical investigation.

Non-Hodgkin lymphomas were almost uniformly fatal diseases only one-half century ago. The new insights into their biology, methods of diagnosis, classification and staging, and the development of combination chemotherapy and modern radiation therapy have made a cure for many of these patients possible. The outgrowth of the successful treatment of these disorders has provided a prototype for strategies for the curative treatment of other cancers. We look forward to further advances that will enable us to better understand the pathophysiology and etiology of the non-Hodgkin lymphomas that should translate into better treatments and better treatment outcomes.

James O. Armitage, Peter M. Mauch, Nancy Lee Harris,
Bertrand Coiffier, Riccardo Dalla-Favera

■ ACKNOWLEDGMENTS

We are deeply indebted to all of the authors whose expertise and promptness have eased the preparation of this text. We would like to thank our families, who endured our efforts in the preparation of this work, and our colleagues, who provided support and made numerous valuable suggestions.

We also want to thank Jonathan W. Pine, Jr., Senior Executive Editor at Lippincott Williams & Wilkins, whose guidance helped shape the book; RedAct Group, who handled all the preproduction; and Elaine Ryan (Omaha, Nebraska), whose assistance was vital to both the editors and the authors in preparing the book.

CONTENTS

SECTION I ■ HISTORICAL ASPECTS

SECTION II ■ ETIOLOGY, EPIDEMIOLOGY, AND BIOLOGY

SECTION III ■ DIAGNOSIS, STAGING, AND RESPONSE CRITERIA

SECTION V ■ LATE EFFECTS

SECTION VI ■ SPECIAL CLINICAL SITUATIONS

INTODUCTION ■ HISTORY AND CLASSIFICATION OF LYMPHOID NEOPLASMS

NANCY LEE HARRIS

Classification is the language of medicine. Diseases need to be defined and named before they can be diagnosed and treated. Classification has two aspects: disease definition (class discovery) and disease diagnosis (class prediction). Disease definition or class discovery is the process of determining what diseases exist and how to define them: when applied to a large group of diseases, this can be called developing a classification. Disease diagnosis, or class prediction, is the act of deciding which category of disease a given patient has. A wide variety of parameters may be combined to define a given disease; a smaller number of parameters may be required to assign a given specimen or patient to a particular category.

Lymphomas are a model for the progress that has been achieved in the diagnosis, classification, and treatment of malignant tumors. The process begins with recognition by an astute clinician or pathologist of a clinical syndrome or a morphologic pattern; the disease is then refined and redefined as new information (now often immunophenotypic or genetic) becomes available, and the new information is then translated into to a better understanding of the morphologic or clinical spectrum of the disease. The accurate description and definition of these distinct diseases is essential for understanding their pathogenesis and for developing specific targeted therapies.

HISTORY OF LYMPHOMA CLASSIFICATIONS

Controversy in lymphoma classification dates back to the first attempts to organize the variety of described neoplasms into a comprehensive scheme (1–15). This controversy stems from several factors, among them, the large variety of tumors that arise from cells of the lymphoid system, the relative insensitivity of the techniques of routine histopathology that are useful in other organ systems in recognizing defining features of lymphoid cells and their tumors, and the assumption of many authorities that there had to be a single guiding principle, a "gold standard," for lymphoma classification. Many classifications were based purely on morphology; others utilized primarily clinical features and still others were based primarily on cell lineage and differentiation, in the belief that each neoplasm corresponded to a recognizable normal cell or differentiation stage.

A review of the history of lymphoma classifications provides a useful perspective from which to view the currently accepted World Organization (WHO) classification.

Early Lymphoma Classifications

The first century of lymphoma classification consisted of the sequential recognition of different diseases characterized by distinctive morphology and clinical behavior [reviewed in Refs. (13), (16), and (17)]. Although mycosis fungoides had been described as a clinical syndrome by 1806 (18), the earliest description of what later proved to be a lymphoma is generally attributed to Thomas Hodgkin (19), who in 1832 described six patients with "disorders of the absorbent glands." Hodgkin believed that this disease was inflammatory, and indeed, later review of the original histologic material revealed that several of the cases were examples of tuberculosis (20). Other cases were examples of what in 1865 came to be called "Hodgkin's disease" (21), whereas at least one case appears to be a non-Hodgkin lymphoma. The first use of the term lymphosarcoma is attributed to Rudolf Virchow, who in 1863 distinguished it from leukemia, which he had described in 1845; the term malignant lymphoma was proposed by Theodore Billroth in 1871 [reviewed in Ref. (16)]. The first clear description of the pathology of lymphosarcoma is attributed to Kundrat (22,23). In 1898 and 1902, Carl Sternberg (24) and Dorothy Reed (25) independently described the characteristic binucleate cell that came to be called the Reed-Sternberg or Sternberg-Reed cell, and gave a more precise histologic definition of Hodgkin disease. In 1908, Sternberg described an aggressive mediastinal tumor in young males (26), initially known as Sternberg sarcoma; this was later recognized as lymphoblastic lymphoma (27).

Jackson and Parker (23) credit Ewing with proposing in 1913 that tumors of lymphoid tissues could arise from reticulum cells. In their paper discussing most of the malignant lymphomas that were distinguished at the time (1916), Gohn and Roman (16) also described cases of lymphosarcoma in which reticulum cells apparently took part in the proliferative process (28). The term was adopted by Roulet (29) (retothelsarkom) and others (30). The term reticulum cell had been applied to a large cell found within the supporting fibrous reticulum of lymphoid tissues. Some observers considered it to be related to an endothelial cell, some believed it to be an immature lymphoid cell, some a pluripotential stem cell, whereas others believed it was identical to the histiocyte or macrophage, also known as the "clasmatocyte" (3). The term reticulum cell sarcoma was generally applied to large cell neoplasms; this uncertainty about the lineage of large cell neoplasms of lymphoid tissues persisted well into the latter half of the 20th century, whereas terms such as lymphosarcoma or lymphoblastoma were applied to those composed of smaller cells recognized as lymphocytes. However, these terms were very inconsistently applied, causing Gall to comment that "when such variation of opinion exists it seems probable that the individual authors...cannot be describing the same tumor" (3).

Multiple myeloma was described in the late 19th century, beginning in 1848 with the recognition by Henry Bence Jones of abnormal protein in the urine of patients with softening of the bones (31). Von Rustizky (32) in 1873 recognized that multiple tumors he had found in the bones of a patient originated from the bone marrow, and introduced the term *multiple myeloma*; and in 1933, James Homer Wright (33) recognized it as a neoplasm of plasma cells, with the application of the Wright stain.

In 1925, Brill et al. (34) described an enlargement of lymph nodes characterized by a proliferation of lymphoid follicles; additional cases were reported by Symmers (35,36). As with Hodgkin disease, there was initial confusion about whether this represented a neoplasm or a progressive reactive process, and it is likely that initial reports contained, in addition to examples of what we would now call follicular lymphoma, cases of florid reactive follicular hyperplasia. By 1941, however, follicular lymphoma, or giant follicle lymphoma, was recognized and confirmed by Gall et al. (37) to be a distinctive form of lymphoid neoplasm, with frequent disseminated disease and a long natural history.

Sézary syndrome (38) and Waldenström macroglobulinemia (39) were recognized as distinct entities by the mid-1940s. In 1958, Burkitt (40) described a tumor of African children, which was rapidly recognized as a new and distinctive type of lymphoma (41–43), which also occurred in Western countries (44). The peculiar geographic distribution of this lymphoma led to the suspicion that it might be caused by a virus, and led to the discovery of the Epstein-Barr virus (45).

Gall and Mallory; Jackson and Parker

In the first half of the 20th century, the existing terms lymphoma, lymphosarcoma, giant follicle or follicular lymphoma, lymphocytoma, lymphoblastoma, reticulum cell sarcoma, and even Hodgkin disease were used heterogeneously by different pathologists and understood variably by clinicians. In the 1930s and 1940s, several attempts were made to develop a comprehensive list of the lymphomas that had been recognized, into what might be called a classification, and these were published in both the United States and Europe. Although those nostalgic for what they believe to have been a simpler past are fond of suggesting that early classifications contained only three diseases: lymphosarcoma, reticulum cell sarcoma, and Hodgkin disease; review of these early classifications actually reveals a far different picture. In fact, as early as 1948, Willis complained that "nowhere in pathology has a chaos of names so clouded clear concepts than in the subject of lymphoid tumors (46); cited in (16)." One of the earliest American attempts at a lymphoma classification came in 1934 from Callendar (1), at the ARP, the predecessor to the Armed Forces Institute of Pathology. This classification incorporated morphologic and clinical information into a scheme that included multiple categories for each morphologic type, depending on its clinical presentation and

---

TABLE 1.

THE ARP CLASSIFICATION OF LYMPHATIC AND RETICULAR TUMORS (1934)

Lymphocyte
  Leukemic lymphocytoma
    Chronic
    Acute
  Aleukemic lymphocytoma
    Diffuse
    Nodular
  Lymphosarcoma (lymphatic leukosarcoma)
    Aleukemic
    Leukemic
Reticulum cell
  Reticulocyte monocyte
    Leukemic reticulocytoma (monocytic leukemia)
    Aleukemic reticulocytoma
    Reticulum cell sarcoma
  Hodgkin disease
    Localized (sclerosing)
    Generalized (cellular)
    Sarcomatous

From Callendar GR. Tumors and tumor-like conditions of the lymphocyte, the myelocyte, the erythrocyte, and the reticulum cell. Am J Pathol 1934;10:443–465, with permission.

---

extent of disease (Table 1). A reading of this paper is instructive, in that it illustrates the complexity that can come from attempts to categorize with insufficient data. In 1938, Robb-Smith (2) published a classification of benign and malignant disorders of lymph nodes, based on the concept of the reticuloendothelial system and the relationship of neoplasms to these normal counterparts, which escalated the complexity even further.

In 1942, Gall and Mallory (3), at Massachusetts General Hospital, reviewed their own extensive material (618 cases) and concluded that the ARP proposal was not a practical approach; they proposed a classification based predominantly on morphology but showed that the different categories described had distinctive clinical behavior. In addition, the morphologic features of the different subtypes were carefully described and illustrated, so that pathologists could learn and use the classification. The classification included both what have come to be known as non-Hodgkin lymphomas and Hodgkin disease; the classification of the non-Hodgkin lymphomas appears to have been the first generally accepted classification of these disorders in the United States (Table 2). In 1947, Jackson and Parker (23,47–49), at Boston University Hospital, also published a comprehensive lymphoma classification, with a primary focus on Hodgkin disease. Their classification of Hodgkin disease rapidly became the standard in the United States and was not challenged until 1966.

The Rappaport Classification

In the mid-1950, Edward Gall and Henry Rappaport (50) comoderated a workshop on lymphoma at the American Society of Clinical Pathology; out of this collaboration,

TABLE 2.

GALL AND MALLORY CLASSIFICATION

Stem cell lymphoma
Clasmatocytic lymphoma
Lymphoblastic lymphoma
Lymphocytic lymphoma
Hodgkin lymphoma
Hodgkin sarcoma
Follicular lymphoma

From Gall EA, Mallory TB. Malignant lymphoma. A clinicopathologic survey of 618 cases. *Am J Pathol* 1942;18:381–395, with permission.

TABLE 3.

THE RAPPAPORT CLASSIFICATION (1956, 1966)

Nodular lymphomas	Diffuse lymphomas
Well-differentiated lymphocytic	Well-differentiated lymphocytic
PDL	PDL
Mixed lymphocytic and histiocytic	Mixed lymphocytic and histiocytic
Histiocytic	Histiocytic
Undifferentiated	Undifferentiated
Hodgkin disease	Hodgkin disease

From Rappaport H. Tumors of the hematopoietic system. In: *Atlas of tumor pathology. Series I.* Washington, DC: Armed Forces Institute of Pathology, 1966; and Rappaport H, Winter W, Hicks E. Follicular lymphoma. A re-evaluation of its position in the scheme of malignant lymphoma, based on a survey of 253 cases. *Cancer* 1956;9:792–821, with permission.

Rappaport developed a new classification proposal, based on the principles of the Gall and Mallory classification (Table 3) (4,5). Rappaport was concerned by the tendency of the day for pathologists and clinicians to believe that follicular hyperplasia was a precursor lesion or that it formed a continuum with follicular lymphoma. He recognized that there was no evidence that reactive follicles actually progressed to neoplastic ones but also questioned whether the nodules of follicular lymphoma were in any way related to normal lymphoid follicles. To avoid this confusion, he proposed the term *nodular* to replace *follicular*, when it describes the pattern of the lymphoma. The Rappaport classification, initially published in 1956 in a report primarily focused on follicular lymphoma (4) and fully developed in the Armed Forces Institute of Pathology fascicle of 1966 (5) took as its primary stratification the pattern of the lymphoma, and assumed that all lymphomas, including Hodgkin disease, could be either nodular or diffuse. Within each tumor type, those with a nodular pattern in general had a better prognosis than those with a diffuse pattern. In comparison with the Gall and Mallory classification, that of Rappaport provided some simplification; the unfortunate term, clasmatocytic, was dropped, and this classification was also characterized by clearly defined and well-illustrated categories, which made it accessible to pathologists.

Unfortunately, the concept of "nodularity" represented a step backwards from the recognition of distinct biologic entities. The previously well-defined follicular lymphoma of Gall and Mallory became lost amid four categories of nodular lymphoma (well-differentiated lymphocytic, poorly differentiated lymphocytic [PDL], mixed lymphocytic and histiocytic, and histiocytic), and its histologically obvious relationship to lymphoid follicles was denied. By 1966, when the classification was published in full, the phenomenon of lymphocyte transformation had been described (51), and it was known that large cells could be lymphoid in origin; despite this, the erroneous designation of "histiocytic" was retained for large cell neoplasms. Finally, the entity of lymphoblastic lymphoma was subsumed under diffuse PDL, thus mingling the distinctive "Sternberg sarcoma" and nodal infiltrates of acute lymphoblastic leukemia (ALL) with diffuse variants of follicle center lymphomas. In 1973, a large scale study of patients from Stanford confirmed the clinical predictive value of the Rappaport classification for adult patients in the United States, and ensured its adoption as the American standard (52,53).

The Rappaport classification was a paradox. It was concise but comprehensive, describing most of the entities known at the time, with clear morphologic criteria that made it possible for pathologists to learn and use the classification. It proved useful in stratifying patients for treatment and in predicting clinical outcome. However, it ignored much of what was currently known about lymphocyte biology, that is the morphologically obvious relationship of neoplastic follicles to germinal centers and the understanding that lymphoid cells could be large. Despite its many attractive features, it actually represented a step backwards in our understanding of the lymphomas.

If it was biologically incorrect, why was the Rappaport classification so successful in predicting patient outcome? The reason lies in the frequency distribution of lymphomas in the United States and Western Europe. Follicular lymphoma, which accounts for the vast majority of lymphomas with a nodular pattern, comprises almost 40% of adult non-Hodgkin lymphomas in the United States (14,52). Because the vast majority of these behave in an indolent manner, simply recognition of a nodular or follicular pattern would identify a large number of patients with an indolent disease. Diffuse large B-cell lymphoma, which comprises about 70% of diffuse lymphomas, is roughly equal in frequency to follicular lymphoma; because this is an aggressive disease, simply recognition of a diffuse pattern will identify an aggressive lymphoma in the majority of the cases. Because pattern alone identifies the two most common types of lymphoma, which have different clinical behavior, this simple approach to classification proved to have "clinical relevance" even though it was biologically incorrect. It was not, however, useful for childhood lymphomas because follicular lymphoma is rare in children, and the category of lymphoblastic lymphoma was not recognized (54). It was also less useful in parts of the world in which follicular lymphoma is less common.

Advances of the 1960s and 1970s: the Kiel and Lukes-Collins Classifications

In the 1960s, two discoveries revolutionized the understanding of the immune system and its neoplasms. These were: (a) the potential of lymphocytes, which had been thought to be end-stage, terminally differentiated cells, to transform into large, proliferating cells in response to mitogens or antigens

(51); and (b) the existence of several distinct lymphocyte lineages (T cells and B cells) that could not be predicted by morphology but that had different functions and physiology (55,56). In the early 1970s, lymphoid cells were found to have surface antigens or receptors that could be exploited to identify the lineage of both normal and neoplastic cells (57). A third development during the 1970s that had a major impact on classification was the development of effective therapies for some types of lymphomas (58): classification takes on new urgency when treatment can affect patients' survival. In response to the new information, pathologists quite appropriately began to try to apply it to the classification of lymphomas.

The Kiel Classification

The first of these efforts was led by Karl Lennert, in Kiel, Germany, who first recognized that many lymphomas resembled germinal center cells and produced immunoglobulin, consistent with an origin from germinal center B cells (59,60). These studies led to the Kiel classification, published in final form in 1974 (9), and updated in 1988 (61). In this approach (Table 4), lymphomas were classified according to a hypothetical scheme of lymphocyte differentiation, and the

---

TABLE 4.

THE KIEL CLASSIFICATION (1974, 1988)

B cell	T cell
Low-grade malignancy	Low-grade malignancy
Lymphocytic:	Lymphocytic:
CLL	CLL
Prolymphocytic leukemia	Prolymphocytic leukemia
Hairy cell leukemia	Small, cerebriform cell— mycosis fungoides, Sézary syndrome
Lymphoplasmacytic/ cytoid (immunocytoma)	Lymphoepithelioid (Lennert lymphoma)
Plasmacytic	Angioimmunoblastic (AILD, LgX)
Centroblastic/centrocytic –Follicular ± diffuse –Diffuse	T zone
Centrocytic	Pleomorphic, small cell (HTLV-1±)
High-grade malignancy	High-grade malignancy
Centroblastic	Pleomorphic, medium and large cell (HTLV-1 ±)
	Immunoblastic (HTLV-1±)
Immunoblastic	
Large cell anaplastic (Ki-1 +)	Large cell anaplastic (Ki-1 +)
Burkitt lymphoma	
Lymphoblastic	Lymphoblastic
Rare types	Rare types

AILD, angioimmunoblastic lymphadenopathy with dysproteinemia; HTLV-1, human T-cell leukemia virus type I; LgX, lymphogranulomatosis X.
From Gerard-Marchant R, Hamlin I, Lennert K, et al. Classification of non-Hodgkin's lymphomas. *Lancet* 1974;ii:406–408; and Stansfeld A, Diebold J, Kapanci Y, et al. Updated Kiel classification for lymphomas. *Lancet* 1988;i:292–293, with permission.

---

nomenclature reflected the putative normal counterpart of the neoplastic cells. Although the majority of the neoplasms described were B cell, several well-defined types of T-cell lymphomas were included. The neoplasms were grouped according to histologic features into low-grade malignancy (predominance of small cells or "-cytes") and high-grade malignancy (predominance of "-blasts"). After its initial reporting in the form of a letter to the *Lancet*, a comprehensive description accompanied by many color illustrations was later published by Lennert et al. (13), and this classification became widely used in Europe. After the updated version of the Kiel classification was published in 1988, revised definitions and illustrations were provided in 1992 (15). Large clinical studies in Europe demonstrated the clinical value of the classification in predicting patient outcomes (62).

The Kiel classification never achieved general acceptance in the United States. Possible reasons include the terminology, which included new names for most cell types and disease categories, the lack of inclusion of pattern as a major defining feature, and the lack of subclassification (grading) of nodular (follicular) lymphoma, which was perceived as having prognostic importance in the United States. Interestingly, follicular lymphoma was reported at the time to be less common in Europe than North America (13), a fact that probably influenced the attention paid by the two classifications to this disease. In fact, these problems were more a matter of perception than reality. The terminology was not particularly difficult and reflected usage adopted by immunologists (such as the term, immunoblast); newly described cell types had to be named, and the convention of hematologists was used: small resting cells were named "-cytes"; and large, transformed, or proliferating cells were named "-blasts." Follicular lymphoma was indeed recognized as an entity, given the cumbersome name "centroblastic/centrocytic (CB/CC)" lymphoma, and subclassified as follicular, follicular and diffuse, or diffuse. It was also graded, in the sense that this category included only the low-grade categories of "poorly differentiated lymphocytic" and "mixed lymphocytic and histiocytic" in the Rappaport scheme; cases composed of predominantly large cells (Rappaport "nodular histiocytic") were classified as centroblastic, follicular, a category of high-grade lymphoma. Thus, although cell type rather than pattern was the primary method of classification, the importance of pattern within this category was indeed recognized.

There is no question in retrospect that the Kiel classification represented the first major advance in classification since Gall and Mallory: it recognized and defined important disease entities and correctly predicted their relationship to normal cellular counterparts. It recognized that the majority of lymphomas were of B-lymphocyte origin, and included most of the entities that are diagnosed today. It was the first to recognize what we now know mantle cell lymphoma as a distinct entity (centrocytic lymphoma). The failure of American pathologists and oncologists to recognize the importance of this approach impeded progress in understanding the biology of lymphomas for the next 20 years.

The Lukes-Collins Classification

In 1974, Robert Lukes and Robert Collins (8) published an immunologically based classification of lymphomas (Table 5). Although it was based on essentially the same observations and immunologic data as the Kiel classification, the

TABLE 5.

THE LUKES-COLLINS CLASSIFICATION (1974)

I. U-cell (undefined cell) type
II. T-cell types
    Mycosis fungoides and Sézary syndrome
    Convoluted lymphocyte
    ? Immunoblastic sarcoma (of T cells)
    ? Hodgkin disease
III. B-cell types
    Small lymphocyte (CLL)
    Plasmacytoid lymphocyte
    Follicular center cell types (follicular, diffuse, follicular and
        diffuse, and sclerotic)
      Small cleaved
      Large cleaved
      Small noncleaved
      Large noncleaved
    Immunoblastic sarcoma of B cells
IV. Histiocytic type
V. Unclassifiable

From Lukes R, Collins R. Immunologic characterization of human malignant lymphomas. *Cancer* 1974;34:1488–1503, with permission.

approach to defining diseases was quite different. First, this scheme required primary division into T and B-cell lineage, despite the fact that methods for doing this were not widely available at the time, and no data existed to indicate whether this was either possible or clinically important. Second, it did not recognize pattern at all, taking the extreme view that pattern was unimportant, and that cell type alone would predict clinical behavior, again, without data to support this contention. Third, one category, follicular center cell lymphoma, contained the vast majority of all neoplasms, from follicular lymphoma (small-cleaved follicular center cell, large-cleaved follicular center cell) to diffuse large cell lymphoma (large-cleaved follicular center cell, large-noncleaved follicular center cell) to Burkitt lymphoma (small-noncleaved follicular center cell). The requirement for assigning lineage based on morphology, the lack of good illustrations, and the difficulty in relating the disease categories to the familiar categories of the Rappaport scheme resulted in resistance on the part of both pathologists and oncologists to this classification. A final problem was that neither in its original description, nor in subsequent publications, were clear criteria for diagnosis presented and illustrated; thus, it was difficult for pathologists to learn and apply the classification. It is unfortunate that, in some respects, the Lukes-Collins classification, because of its perceived impracticality, may have contributed to a degree of cynicism among American oncologists and pathologists about immunologic approaches to the classification of lymphomas.

Dorfman, British National Lymphoma Investigation, and World Health Organization Classifications

Shortly after the publication of the Kiel and Lukes-Collins classifications, several other proposals appeared: the "working classification" of Dorfman (6); the proposal of Bennett et al.

(7), which became the British National Lymphoma Investigation classification; and the WHO classification of Mathe et al. (11) . To varying extents, these classifications attempted to apply terminology that reflected immunologic advances, that is the recognition that large cell lymphomas were lymphoid, rather than histiocytic, to the basic framework of the Rappaport classification. The British National Lymphoma Investigation classification was used for many years in Britain, but the other two never achieved widespread use.

The International Working Formulation for Clinical Usage

By the mid-1970s, at least five new proposals for lymphoma classification had been made, in addition to the standard Rappaport classification. This situation was the subject of much humor (Table 6) (10) but also a cause for consternation among oncologists, who were concerned that the results of clinical trials from different institutions would be impossible to interpret. Several meetings were organized by oncologists in both the United States and Europe in the mid-1970s, in an attempt to produce a consensus among the expert pathologists on a unified approach to lymphoma classification; unfortunately, these were unsuccessful.

In response to this unacceptable situation, the American National Cancer Institute, under the leadership of Dr. Vincent de Vita, undertook a large-scale project in which histologic slides and clinical data from patients enrolled in clinical trials at centers around the world would be reviewed, in an attempt to develop data that could be used to determine which of the classifications was most effective in predicting the clinical behavior of lymphomas. Proponents of each of the six classifications traveled to the different sites and reviewed histologic sections from 1,245 patients with non-Hodgkin

TABLE 6.

CLASSIFICATION OF CLASSIFICATIONS (1974)

Well-defined, high-grade, oligosyllabic
Poorly differentiated, polysyllabic
    Diffuse
    Circumlocutory
    With dyslexogenesis
Unicentric
    Derivative
    Neologistic
Multicentric, cytophilic (Greek κμκνοω = swan).[a]
Cleaved and convoluted types
    Rappaport (non-Lukes)
    Lukes (non-Rappaport)

Note: This system makes no claim to be comprehensive or even comprehensible, so there may well be scope for other classifications of classifications and, ultimately, one hopes, a classification of classifications of classifications. At that point, we shall need a conference in the Caribbean.
[a]A former colleague of Dr. Kay's commented that this term was derived from the tendency of pathologists who had proposed lymphoma classifications to be found "swanning about" from one conference on classification to another.
From Kay HE. Letter: classification of non-Hodgkin's lymphomas. *Lancet* 1974;2:586, with permission.

lymphomas, each classifying them according to his or her own scheme. In addition, six other pathologists reviewed all cases and attempted to classify each case according to all six schemes. Several end points were used as markers of the validity of each classification; the most important was the overall actuarial survival of patients whose slides were reviewed, but both interobserver and intraobserver reproducibility were also evaluated.

After analysis of all the data, the survival curves showed that each of the classifications identified tumors with a broad spread of survival curves, and the statisticians were unable to identify any one classification as being superior to the others in this respect. Intraobserver and interobserver reproducibility was relatively poor for all of the classifications. In the end, none of the classifications could be agreed upon as the standard, and the "International Working Formulation for Clinical Usage" was developed to "translate" between the various classifications (Table 7) (14).

The WF essentially used the Rappaport categories of lymphomas but substituted terminology, primarily from the Lukes and Collins classification, that was believed to be biologically more correct, for example "small lymphocytic" instead of "well differentiated lymphocytic," "small cleaved cell" instead of "poorly differentiated lymphocytic," "large cell" instead of "histiocytic," and "follicular" rather than "nodular." It also recognized that not all lymphomas could have a truly follicular pattern. Unfortunately, in adapting the Lukes-Collins terminology, important modifying terms were left out, which led to a lack of specificity and clarity in the WF terminology. In the Lukes-Collins scheme, a "small cleaved follicular center cell" was a distinctive cell of the germinal center; this term did not apply to any cell with nuclear irregularity, in contrast to the term, "small cleaved cell." Similarly, a "small noncleaved follicular center cell" was a distinctive blastic cell (corresponding to Burkitt lymphoma cells), which was small only in comparison to "large noncleaved follicular center cells." The term "small noncleaved cell," however, could be confusing because a small lymphocyte is also small and "noncleaved."

The WF categories were deliberately broad, so that: (a) all lymphomas could be classified; and (b) all categories of all existing classifications could be accommodated, thus fulfilling its function as a sort of pathologic "lingua franca." Thus, the category of "diffuse mixed small and large cell" included both diffuse follicle center lymphomas and peripheral T-cell lymphomas, and the category of "large cell immunoblastic" included both B and T-cell cases. To further de-emphasize the idea of disease entities, each category was given a letter designation (A through J), which could be used instead of the category name.

An important and novel feature of the WF was the separation of the lymphomas into clinical prognostic groups, or "clinical grades," as they came to be called. These groupings differed from the "histologic grades" of the Kiel classification, in that they were based on the actuarial survival curves of the patients in the international study, and not on morphologic features such as cell size, nuclear immaturity, or proliferative activity. The oncologists involved in the study believed that these groupings were necessary to help clinicians deal with the large number of morphologic categories, by combining them into groups that could be used to suggest appropriate treatment. Thus, "low grade" lymphomas were treated palliatively, with an expectation of long survival

TABLE 7.

THE INTERNATIONAL WF FOR CLINICAL USAGE (1982)

Low grade
  A. Malignant lymphoma, small lymphocytic
     Consistent with CLL
     Plasmacytoid
  B. Malignant lymphoma, follicular, predominantly small-cleaved cell
     Diffuse areas
     Sclerosis
  C. Malignant lymphoma, follicular, mixed, small cleaved and large cell
     Diffuse areas
     Sclerosis
Intermediate grade
  D. Malignant lymphoma, follicular, predominantly large cell
     Diffuse areas
     Sclerosis
  E. Malignant lymphoma, diffuse, small-cleaved cell
     Sclerosis
  F. Malignant lymphoma, diffuse, mixed, small and large cell
     Sclerosis
     Epithelioid cell component
  G. Malignant lymphoma, diffuse, large cell
     Cleaved cell
     Noncleaved cell
     Sclerosis
High grade
  H. Malignant lymphoma, large cell, immunoblastic
     Plasmacytoid
     Clear cell
     Polymorphous
     Epithelioid cell component
  I. Malignant lymphoma, lymphoblastic
     Convoluted cell
     Nonconvoluted cell
  J. Malignant lymphoma, small noncleaved cell
     Burkitt
     Follicular areas
Miscellaneous
  Composite
  Mycosis fungoides
  Histiocytic
  Extramedullary plasmacytoma
  Unclassifiable
  Other

From National Cancer Institute sponsored study of classifications of non-Hodgkin's lymphomas: summary and description of a working formulation for clinical usage. The Non-Hodgkin's Lymphoma Pathologic Classification Project. *Cancer* 1982;49:2112–2135, with permission.

unaffected by treatment; "intermediate grade" lymphomas were treated aggressively with an expectation of cure, and "high grade" lymphomas were treated intensively, often with central nervous system prophylaxis.

In the mid-1970s, clinical studies had begun to show that some aggressive lymphomas (diffuse "histiocytic") could be cured with combination chemotherapy (63). At least one study appeared to show that histologic subclassification of large cell lymphomas (large-cleaved or noncleaved follicular center cell vs. immunoblastic types) could predict which cases could be cured with this treatment (64). Thus, there was considerable optimism that morphologic features could be used to predict the outcome of patients with large cell lymphomas. This hypothesis was tested in the National Cancer Institute study; unfortunately, the pathologists were unable to agree on subclassification of many of the cases. Nonetheless, in a subset of the cases that could be classified as immunoblastic, there was a small but statistically significant decrease in survival compared with the large-cleaved and noncleaved types (14). The WF thus divided large cell lymphomas into two categories: large cell (cleaved or noncleaved), and immunoblastic. The immunoblastic category was placed in the "high grade" clinical group, with Burkitt and lymphoblastic lymphomas, whereas the large cell category was considered "intermediate" grade. Unfortunately, clear and reproducible criteria for separating large cell and large cell immunoblastic lymphomas were not given in the paper, and pathologists found this distinction difficult to make. Thus, although the distinction could theoretically lead to important differences in treatment, it proved impossible for pathologists to make reliably (65).

Although it was not intended to be a freestanding classification, but rather a means of translating between classifications, the WF rapidly became the principal American classification, and by the late 1980s and early 1990s, it was the most commonly used classification worldwide. However, despite the fact that it was based largely on clinical survival data, clinicians typically modified its categories in practice. Reflecting the fact that the prognostic groups defined by the WF did not accurately predict the behavior of the tumors, many clinical trials of "low grade" lymphoma included diffuse small-cleaved cell lymphoma and follicular large cell lymphoma, although these are considered intermediate grade in the WF (66). Trials of aggressive lymphoma usually included some but not all intermediate (diffuse mixed and large cell, but not diffuse small-cleaved and follicular large cell) and some but not all high-grade (immunoblastic and sometimes small-noncleaved cell, but not usually lymphoblastic) lymphomas (67,68). Some entities, which were already recognized to have distinctive features, such as Burkitt lymphoma, lymphoblastic lymphoma, hairy cell leukemia, and B-cell chronic lymphocytic leukemia (CLL), were typically treated according to disease-specific protocols.

Because of the demographics of non-Hodgkin lymphoma in the United States, clinical trials of treatment of "WF low grade lymphoma" were essentially trials of follicular lymphoma, contaminated by a small number of cases of mantle cell, small lymphocytic, and marginal zone lymphoma of mucosa-associated lymphoid tissue (MALT), and trials of "WF intermediate/high grade lymphoma" were trials of diffuse large B-cell lymphoma, contaminated by small numbers of peripheral T-cell lymphomas and other rare diseases. Lumping diverse entities into these broad prognostic groups had the effect of distorting the data on the common entities, and obscuring the distinctive features of rare entities.

An additional result of the adoption of the WF, with its letter designations of categories and its clinical "grades," was a growing disregard among oncologists for the pathologic classification of lymphomas. Thus, instead of "follicular lymphoma," the terms "WF B-D" would be used, and rather than asking for a histologic diagnosis, many practicing oncologists simply wanted to know whether a tumor was low, intermediate, or high grade in the WF. The "crutch" of the WF prognostic groups gave oncologists a sense of security, but it delayed the recognition and development of new therapies for diseases such as extranodal low-grade B-cell lymphoma of MALT, mantle cell lymphoma, and peripheral T-cell lymphomas.

Although the WF represented a consensus among the participating pathologists, both Robert Lukes and Karl Lennert had published critical commentaries along with its initial publication (14), and many American and European pathologists continued to use the Lukes-Collins or Kiel classifications, respectively. Thus, the lack of consensus on lymphoma classification and terminology persisted, with the WF being the standard in the United States and several other countries, and the Kiel classification being the standard in many European countries. This situation caused continued problems for both pathologists and clinicians, and created difficulty in interpreting published studies. In addition, in the 1980s and 1990s, many new disease entities were described, which were not included in either classification, leading to confusion among both pathologists and oncologists about which were "real" diseases that they should be recognizing in daily practice. Finally, the introduction of the new techniques of immunophenotyping and molecular genetic analysis led to confusion about what, if anything, should be the modern "gold standard" for defining disease entities.

Most experienced hematopathologists began in the late 1980s and early 1990s to modify both the WF and the Kiel classification to address these issues. This led to even more confusion because not only were there differences between American and European classifications, but each institution was developing idiosyncratic internal classification schemes.

In the United States, consideration was given to updating the WF, and in Europe, the Kiel classification had been updated in 1988; there were discussions about adopting one or the other as the new international standard. However, both classifications had limitations that made this impractical. The WF was not intended to be a freestanding classification, and its categories were intentionally broad and imprecise. In addition, the clinical data that were thought to give it validity were based on the original study patients; thus, a similar large-scale clinical study would theoretically be required to provide an updated version with similar clinical relevance. The Kiel classification was intended for use on primary nodal lymphomas only; thus, the issue of extranodal lymphomas of MALT and their relationship to other lymphomas was not clarified, and other primary extranodal lymphomas other than mycosis fungoides were not addressed. In addition, classification of T-cell lymphomas was based on morphologic criteria that were difficult to reproduce, and the histologic grades did not appear to correlate well with clinical behavior (69,70).

THE REVISED EUROPEAN-AMERICAN CLASSIFICATION OF LYMPHOID NEOPLASMS

The International Lymphoma Study Group (ILSG) was formed in 1991 by Drs. Peter Isaacson of University College Hospital, London, and Harald Stein of the Free University of

Berlin to promote better communication between American and European hematopathologists. This informal group included 19 hematopathologists from the United States, Europe, and Asia, and began meeting annually to review interesting cases, present unpublished research data, and discuss issues in classification and diagnosis of lymphomas. It very soon became clear that there was general agreement among the members on diseases they were recognizing in their daily practice with a combination of morphology, immunophenotyping, and genetic techniques, and which appeared to be distinct clinical entities. However, it was also clear that there was no uniform approach to defining and diagnosing these entities at different centers around the world, and that a consensus was needed on the definitions and criteria for diagnosis, as well as nomenclature for these diseases.

In the first 2 years of its existence, the group published consensus papers on definitions, diagnostic criteria, and nomenclature for two diseases that were either controversial or poorly understood: mantle cell lymphoma and nodular lymphocyte predominant Hodgkin lymphoma (71,72). By the time of the third meeting, in 1993, the group was ready to approach the idea of a new lymphoma classification. This consensus approach represented a major departure from previous classifications, most of which represented the work of one or a few individuals. The ILSG recognized that the complexity of the field in the 1990s made it impossible for a single person or small group to be completely authoritative, and also that broad agreement is necessary if the result is to be used by multiple pathologists, even if it requires compromise.

Given the difficulty of defining an overarching principle for the classification of all lymphoid neoplasms, the group agreed that the best approach for the present was to try to reach a consensus on a list of distinct disease entities, including defining criteria, diagnostic criteria, and nomenclature, that its members recognized in daily practice, and that appeared to be distinct clinical entities. The diseases could then be grouped according to a variety of principles, depending on the needs of the user, but each disease could stand alone as an entity to be understood, diagnosed, and treated using currently available methods. As one of the group members, David Mason, said: the classification should reflect what pathologists *do*, not what they *should* do.

The ILSG approach to lymphoma classification was novel. In this approach, *all* available information, that is morphology, immunophenotype, genetic features, and clinical features, is used to define a disease entity. The relative importance of each of these features varies among diseases, and there is no one "gold standard." Morphology is always important, and some diseases are primarily defined by morphology, for example follicular lymphoma, angioimmunoblastic T-cell lymphoma, nodular sclerosis Hodgkin lymphoma with immunophenotype as backup in difficult cases. Some diseases have a virtually specific immunophenotype, for example mantle cell lymphoma, small lymphocytic lymphoma, anaplastic large cell lymphoma, such that one would hesitate to make the diagnosis in the absence of the immunophenotype. In a few lymphomas, a specific genetic abnormality is an important defining criterion, for example t(11;14) in mantle cell lymphoma, t(8;14) in Burkitt lymphoma, t(14;18) in follicular lymphoma, whereas others lack specific genetic abnormalities, for example MALT lymphoma and most types of diffuse large B-cell lymphoma. Still others require a knowledge of clinical features as well, for example nodal versus extranodal presentation in marginal zone lymphoma and peripheral T-cell lymphomas, and mediastinal location in mediastinal large B-cell lymphoma. The inclusion of clinical criteria was one of the most novel aspects of the ILSG approach. The emphasis on defining "real" disease entities, rather than focusing on subtleties of morphology or immunophenotype or primarily on patient survival, represented a new paradigm in lymphoma classification.

After a 3-day meeting in Berlin, a list of diseases on which a consensus had been reached was developed. The group held a joint meeting with an international group of hematologic oncologists at the National Cancer Institute in Bethesda, MD, in the spring of 1994, to get input from clinicians on the proposal, and a number of changes were made at their suggestions. The ILSG consensus list of well-defined, "real" diseases was published in 1994 (Table 8) (73). Because it represented a revision of current or prior European and American lymphoma classifications (Table 1), it was called the "Revised European-American Classification of Lymphoid Neoplasms" (REAL).

Although its initial publication incited considerable controversy, experience over the intervening years showed that it could be used by most pathologists, and that the entities it describes had distinctive clinical features, making it a useful and practical classification, despite its apparent complexity (74–77).

Clinical Implications of the Revised European-American Classification of Lymphoid Neoplasms Classification

An initial criticism of the REAL classification was that it had not been tested in a clinical study (78), although it only included diseases that had been previously published and for which the clinical features were known (79). To address this issue, an international group of oncologists and pathologists devised a clinical study of the classification, in which five expert pathologists reviewed >1,300 cases of non-Hodgkin lymphoma at centers around the world (76,77). The aims of the study were to: (a) see whether the classification could be used in practice, (b) test its interobserver reproducibility, (c) determine the need for immunophenotyping in diagnosis, (d) determine whether the categories of disease identified in the classification were clinically distinctive either at presentation or in outcome, and (e) determine the relative frequency of these diseases in the populations studied.

This study demonstrated that the classification could be used by expert hematopathologists: >95% of the cases with adequate material could be classified into one or another of the categories. The interobserver reproducibility was better than that for other classifications, >85% for most diseases (Table 9). Immunophenotyping was helpful in some diseases, such as mantle cell lymphoma and diffuse large B-cell lymphoma, where it improved accuracy by 10% to 15%, and was essential for all types of T-cell lymphoma, improving reproducibility from around 50% to >90%. It was not required for many diseases, such as follicular lymphoma, B-cell small lymphocytic lymphoma, and MALT lymphoma (76).

TABLE 8.

THE REAL CLASSIFICATION (1994)

B-CELL NEOPLASMS
I. Precursor B-cell neoplasm
Precursor B-lymphoblastic leukemia/lymphoma
II. Peripheral B-cell neoplasms
  1. B-cell CLL/prolymphocytic leukemia/ small lymphocytic lymphoma
  2. Lymphoplasmacytoid lymphoma/Immunocytoma
  3. Mantle cell lymphoma
  4. Follicle center lymphoma, follicular
     <u>Provisional cytologic grades:</u> I (small cell), II (mixed small and large cell), III (large cell)
     <u>Provisional subtype:</u> diffuse, predominantly small cell type
  5. Marginal zone B-cell lymphoma, extranodal MALT type (± monocytoid B cells)
     <u>Provisional subtype:</u> Nodal marginal zone lymphoma (± monocytoid B cells)
     <u>Provisional entity:</u> Splenic marginal zone lymphoma (± villous lymphocytes)
  6. Hairy cell leukemia
  7. Plasmacytoma/plasma cell myeloma
  8. Diffuse large B-cell lymphoma[a]
     Subtype: primary mediastinal (thymic) B-cell lymphoma
  9. Burkitt lymphoma
  10. <u>Provisional entity:</u> High-grade B-cell lymphoma, Burkitt-like[a]

T-CELL and PUTATIVE NK-CELL NEOPLASMS
I. Precursor T-cell neoplasm
Precursor T-lymphoblastic lymphoma/leukemia
II. Peripheral T-cell and NK-cell neoplasms
  1. T-cell CLL/prolymphocytic leukemia
  2. Large granular lymphocyte leukemia (LGL)
     T-cell type
     NK cell type
  3. Mycosis fungoides/Sézary syndrome
  4. Peripheral T-cell lymphomas, unspecified[a]
     <u>Provisional cytologic categories:</u> medium-sized cell, mixed medium and large cell, large cell, lymphoepithelioid cell
     <u>Provisional subtype:</u> Hepatosplenic γδ T-cell lymphoma
     <u>Provisional subtype:</u> Subcutaneous panniculitic T-cell lymphoma
  5. Angioimmunoblastic T-cell lymphoma (AILD)
  6. Angiocentric lymphoma
  7. Intestinal T-cell lymphoma (± enteropathy associated)
  8. Adult T-cell lymphoma/leukemia (ATL/L)
  9. Anaplastic large cell lymphoma (ALCL), CD30+, T- and null-cell types
  10. <u>Provisional entity:</u> Anaplastic large cell lymphoma, Hodgkin-like

[a]These categories are thought likely to include more than one disease entity.
Adapted from Harris NL, Jaffe ES, Stein H, et al. A revised European-American classification of lymphoid neoplasms: a proposal from the International Lymphoma Study Group. *Blood* 1994;84:1361–1392, with permission.

TABLE 9.

FREQUENCY OF LYMPHOMA TYPES IN THE REAL CLASSIFICATION

Diagnosis	Total cases (%)
Diffuse large B-cell lymphoma	31
Follicular lymphoma	22
MALT lymphoma	8
Mature T-cell lymphomas (except ALCL)	8
CLL/small lymphocytic lymphoma	7
Mantle cell lymphoma	6
Mediastinal large B-cell lymphoma	2
Anaplastic large cell lymphoma (ALCL)	2
Burkitt lymphoma	2
Nodal marginal zone lymphoma	2
Precursor T lymphoblastic	2
Lymphoplasmacytic lymphoma	1
Other types	7

Adapted from A clinical evaluation of the International Lymphoma Study Group classification of non-Hodgkin's lymphoma. The Non-Hodgkin's Lymphoma Classification Project. *Blood* 1997;89:3909–3918, with permission.

similar to previous patterns reported in the literature (Table 10). The most common lymphoma was diffuse large B-cell lymphoma, followed by follicular lymphoma; together, these comprised 50% of the lymphomas in the study. New entities not specifically recognized in the WF accounted for 27% of the cases: MALT lymphoma 8%, mantle cell 7%, peripheral T cell

TABLE 10.

REPRODUCIBILITY OF LYMPHOMA DIAGNOSIS IN THE REAL CLASSIFICATION

Reproducibility >85% (86–96%)	Contribution of immunophenotype (%)
B-CLL/SLL	3
Mantle cell lymphoma	10
Follicular lymphoma	0
Marginal zone/MALT	2
Diffuse large B-cell lymphoma	15
T-Lymphoblastic lymphoma	40
Anaplastic large cell lymphoma	39
Peripheral T-cell lymphoma, unspecified	41
Mycosis fungoides	
Reproducibility 80%	
Angioimmunoblastic T-cell lymphoma	
Extranodal NK/T-cell lymphoma	
Reproducibility <50%	
Burkitt-like lymphoma	6
Lymphoplasmacytic lymphoma	

Data from A clinical evaluation of the International Lymphoma Study Group classification of non-Hodgkin's lymphoma. The Non-Hodgkin's Lymphoma Classification Project. *Blood* 1997;89:3909–3918; and Armitage JO, Weisenburger DD. New Approach to classifying non-Hodgkin's lymphomas: clinical features of the major histologic subtypes. *J Clin Oncol* 1998;16:2780–2795, with permission.

The relative frequency of the different B and T/natural killer (NK)-cell lymphomas in the study population was

6%, nodal marginal zone 2%, mediastinal large B cell 2%, and anaplastic large T/null cell 2%. These results were reassuring, confirming that the majority of the cases that would be encountered by oncologists and pathologists would be only a few subtypes, with which they are already familiar. However, they also underscored the need for recognizing the more recently described entities, which, although less common, have important clinical differences. The study also found differences in geographic distribution of the lymphoma types, with follicular lymphoma being more common in North America and Western Europe, T-cell lymphomas more common in Hong Kong, and both mediastinal large B-cell lymphoma and mantle cell lymphoma more common in Ticino (the Italian-speaking canton), Switzerland (80).

The different diseases had significantly different clinical presentations and survivals. For example, diffuse aggressive lymphomas, which would be lumped as intermediate/high grade in the WF, include diffuse large B-cell lymphoma, mediastinal large B-cell lymphoma, peripheral T-cell lymphoma, and anaplastic large T/null-cell lymphoma. The clinical features at presentation were strikingly different, with a younger age group for mediastinal large T-cell lymphoma and anaplastic large T/null lymphoma, and striking differences in male-female ratios, suggesting that these are distinctive biologic entities (Table 11). When overall survivals were analyzed, entities that would have been lumped together as "low grade" or "intermediate/high grade" in the WF showed marked differences in survival, confirming that they need to be recognized and treated as distinct entities.

A critical finding was that classification is not the only predictor of clinical outcome. Patients with any of these diseases could be stratified into better and worse prognostic groups according to the International Prognostic Index (81). For example, although patients with follicular lymphoma typically have International Prognostic Index scores of one through three, those patients with scores of four or five had a predicted median overall survival of only 18 months. Thus, to plan treatment for an individual patient, the oncologist must know not only the diagnosis, but also the clinical prognostic factors that will influence that patient's course.

THE WORLD HEALTH ORGANIZATION CLASSIFICATION OF NEOPLASMS OF HEMATOPOIETIC AND LYMPHOID TISSUES

In 1993, the WHO decided to update the "blue book" on neoplasms of hematopoietic and lymphoid tissues, which had last been published in 1975, and which was seldom used (11). This was undertaken as a joint project of the Society for Hematopathology, which is based largely in the United States, and the European Association of Hematopathologists. The project, which began in earnest in 1995, was an opportunity to update and obtain a broader consensus on the REAL classification for lymphomas and to apply the principles of the REAL classification to the classification of myeloid and histiocytic neoplasms (82,83). It included >50 pathologists from around the world. In addition, building on the experience of the ILSG and the REAL classification, the Steering Committee of the WHO project formed a Clinical Advisory Committee of >30 international expert hematologists and oncologists, to advise the pathologists on clinical issues related to the classification (84,85). The final classification was published in 2001 (Table 11) (86). Proponents of all existing classifications, that is WF, Kiel, REAL, and French-American-British, agreed that the final WHO consensus would replace existing classifications. Thus, it represented the first true international consensus on the classification of hematologic malignancies.

Beginning in 2006, joint committees of the Society for Hematopathology and European Haematopathology Association collaborated on an update of the classification, which was published in September, 2008 (87). The project was led by an eight-member steering committee, involved two clinical advisory committees (one for myeloid neoplasms and acute leukemias, and one for lymphoid neoplasms), ultimately involving >130 pathologists and clinicians.

Principles of the World Health Organization Classification of Lymphoid Neoplasms

Like the REAL classification, on which it is based, the WHO classification is a list of distinct disease entities, which are defined by a combination of morphology, immunophenotype, and genetic features, and which have distinct clinical features. The classification includes all lymphoid neoplasms: Hodgkin disease, non-Hodgkin lymphomas, lymphoid leukemias, and plasma cell neoplasms. Both lymphomas and lymphoid leukemias are included because both solid and circulating phases are present in many lymphoid neoplasms, and distinction between them is artificial. Thus, B-cell CLL and B-cell small lymphocytic lymphoma are simply different manifestations of the same neoplasm, as are lymphoblastic lymphomas and ALLs. In addition, Hodgkin lymphoma and plasma cell myeloma are now recognized as lymphoid neoplasms of B lineage, and, therefore, belong in a compilation of lymphoid neoplasms. Immunodeficiency associated lymphomas are classified according to the basic lymphoma classification; a separate classification of the posttransplant lymphoid proliferations that do not fulfill criteria for lymphoma is also given.

Morphology, immunophenotype, and genetic and clinical features are understood to be surrogates or approximations for whatever the true, defining abnormality of a disease may be. Because we do not understand the basic pathophysiology of most malignancies, continued research and experience will be needed to continue to improve the definition of these diseases. Furthermore, the important "defining" criteria may vary depending on what preventive or therapeutic measures exist. In current clinical practice, morphology remains the first and most basic approach for classification of lymphoid neoplasms, and is sufficient for both diagnosis and classification in many typical cases of lymphoma. Immunophenotyping and, particularly, molecular genetic studies are not needed in all cases; however, they are an important part of the definition of a disease entity, are useful in the diagnosis of difficult cases, and improve interobserver reproducibility. It is the availability of these more objective methods that makes a consensus on lymphoma classification possible now,

TABLE 11.

WHO CLASSIFICATION OF LYMPHOID NEOPLASMS (2008)

Precursor lymphoid neoplasms
B-lymphoblastic leukaemia/lymphoma
   B-lymphoblastic leukaemia/lymphoma, not otherwise specified
   B-lymphoblastic leukaemia/lymphoma with t(9:22) (q34;q11.2); BCR/ABL
   B-lymphoblastic leukaemia/lymphoma with t(v;11q23); MLL rearranged
   B-lymphoblastic leukaemia/lymphoma with t(12;21) (p13;q22); TEL/AML1 (ETV6-RUNX1)
   B-lymphoblastic leukaemia/lymphoma with hyperdiploidy
   B-lymphoblastic leukaemia/lymphoma with hypodiploidy (Hypodiploid ALL)
   B-lymphoblastic leukaemia/lymphoma with t(5;14)(q31;q32)(IL3-IGH)
   B-lymphoblastic leukaemia/lymphoma with t(1;19)(Q23;P13.3); (E2A-PBX1; TCF3/PBX1)
T-lymphoblastic leukaemia/lymphoma

Mature B-cell neoplasms
Chronic lymphocytic leukaemia/small lymphocytic lymphoma
B-cell prolymphocytic leukaemia
Splenic marginal zone lymphoma
Hairy cell leukaemia
Splenic lymphoma/leukaemia, unclassifiable[a]
Splenic diffuse red pulp small B-cell lymphoma
Hairy cell leukaemia variant
Lymphoplasmacytic lymphoma
Waldenström macroglobulinemia
Heavy chain diseases
   α Heavy chain disease
   γ Heavy chain disease
   μ Heavy chain disease
Plasma cell myeloma
Solitary plasmacytoma of bone
Extraosseous plasmacytoma
Extranodal marginal zone lymphoma of MALT (lymphoma)
Nodal marginal zone lymphoma
Paediatric nodal marginal zone lymphoma
Follicular lymphoma
Paediatric follicular lymphoma
Primary cutaneous follicle centre lymphoma
Mantle cell lymphoma
Diffuse large B-cell lymphoma (DLBCL), NOS
   T-cell/histiocyte rich large B-cell lymphoma
   Primary DLBCL of the CNS
   Primary cutaneous DLBCL, leg type
   EBV positive DLBCL of the elderly
DLBCL associated with chronic inflammation
Lymphomatoid granulomatosis
Primary mediastinal (thymic) large B-cell lymphoma
Intravascular large B-cell lymphoma
ALK positive large B-cell lymphoma
Plasmablastic lymphoma
Large B-cell lymphoma arising in HHV8-associated multicentric Castleman disease
Primary effusion lymphoma
Burkitt lymphoma
B-cell lymphoma, unclassifiable, with features intermediate between diffuse large B-cell lymphoma and Burkitt lymphoma
B-cell lymphoma, unclassifiable, with features intermediate between diffuse large B-cell lymphoma and classic Hodgkin lymphoma

Mature T-cell and NK-cell neoplasms
T-cell prolymphocytic leukaemia
T-cell large granular lymphocytic leukaemia
Chronic lymphoproliferative disorder of NK-cells
Aggressive NK cell leukaemia
Systemic EBV positive T-cell lymphoproliferative disease of childhood
Hydroa vacciniforme-like lymphoma
Adult T-cell leukaemia/lymphoma
Extranodal NK/T cell lymphoma, nasal type
Enteropathy associated T-cell lymphoma

(Continued)

TABLE 11. (CONTINUED)

Hepatosplenic T-cell lymphoma
Subcutaneous panniculitis-like T-cell lymphoma
Mycosis fungoides
Sézary syndrome
Primary cutaneous CD30 positive T-cell lymphoproliferative disorders
   Lymphomatoid papulosis
   Primary cutaneous anaplastic large cell lymphoma
Primary cutaneous gamma-delta T-cell lymphoma
Primary cutaneous CD8 positive aggressive epidermotropic cytotoxic T-cell lymphoma
Primary cutaneous CD4 positive small/medium T-cell lymphoma
Peripheral T-cell lymphoma, NOS
Angioimmunoblastic T-cell lymphoma
Anaplastic large cell lymphoma, *ALK* positive
Anaplastic large cell lymphoma, ALK negative

AML1, acute myeloid leukemia 1; BCR, B-cell receptor; CNS, central nervous system; DLBCL, diffuse large B-cell lymphoma; EBV, Epstein-Barr virus; HHV8, human herpesvirus 8; IGH, immunoglobulin H; IL3, interleukin 3; NOS, not otherwise specified.
*a*Those in italics are provisional entities.
Adapted from Swerdlow SH, Campo E, Harris NL, et al. *WHO classification of tumours of haematopoietic and lymphoid tissues*, 4th ed. Lyon, France: International Agency for Research on Cancer, 2008, with permission.

whereas it was impossible in the 1970s, when classification was based purely on subjective morphologic features.

Normal Counterparts of Neoplastic Cells

Attempting to understand the normal counterpart of the neoplastic cell is an important component of any tumor classification. At present, the normal counterpart, both lineage and differentiation stage, of many hematologic malignancies can be postulated with reasonable certainty. However, our understanding of the immune system is insufficient to permit this to be done in all cases, and, therefore, rigid adherence to classification by normal counterpart is not feasible at this time. Diseases must be defined, diagnosed, and treated, even if the normal counterpart is not known or is controversial. Three major lineages of lymphoid malignancies can be defined, corresponding to normal lymphocyte subsets: B-cell neoplasms, T-cell neoplasms, and NK-cell neoplasms. However, it is sometimes difficult to distinguish between T-cell and NK-cell neoplasms, and some well-defined clinical entities, such as nasal-type lymphoma, appear to be of T-cell lineage in some cases and NK cell in others. For this reason, T- and NK-cell neoplasms are lumped into one category in the REAL and WHO classifications. Hodgkin disease, or as we now prefer to call it, Hodgkin lymphoma, is now known to be a B-cell neoplasm in virtually all the cases, but both types (nodular lymphocyte predominant and classic Hodgkin lymphoma) differ both morphologically and clinically from other B-cell lymphomas, and have both morphologic and clinical similarities with one another; for these reasons, Hodgkin lymphoma is still considered a distinct category. Within the B and T/NK-cell neoplasms, two major categories are recognized: precursor neoplasms, corresponding to the earliest, lymphoblastic, stages of differentiation (lymphoblastic lymphomas and ALLs); and peripheral or mature neoplasms, corresponding to more differentiated B- and T-cell stages.

Classification according to the normal counterpart of the malignant cell has limitations. For example, a clinically identical neoplasm may in some cases be composed of γ/δ T cells and in others of α/β T cells (hepatosplenic T-cell lymphoma and subcutaneous T-cell lymphoma are two examples). Conversely, neoplasms of the same apparent cell type or differentiation stage may be clinically very different depending on their site of origin. For example, marginal zone B-cell lymphomas of extranodal, nodal, and splenic types appear to be distinct, unrelated diseases, as are anaplastic large T-cell lymphomas of cutaneous and systemic types and diffuse large B-cell lymphomas of cutaneous and systemic origin. This fact should not be surprising when we consider that nonlymphoid neoplasms of similar cell types have distinctive clinical behavior in different sites, for example, squamous cell carcinomas of cutaneous versus pulmonary versus uterine cervical origin, or adenocarcinomas of various sites.

Finally, it has been recognized in recent years that a surprising amount of lineage plasticity exists in hematopoietic neoplasms, with genetic abnormalities such as *FGFR1*, *PDGFA*, and *PDGFB* rearrangements, giving rise to tumors having both lymphoid and myeloid features, and rare cases of histiocytic neoplasms arising from lymphoblastic or follicular lymphomas (88,89).

Grading and Prognostic Groups

The WHO classification of 2008 includes >50 distinct categories of "non-Hodgkins" lymphomas. These diseases are in most cases unrelated to one another, that is, we can no longer talk about "lymphoma" or "non-Hodgkin lymphoma" as a single disease with a range of histologic grade and clinical aggressiveness. Now that lymphomas can be defined more precisely with the aid of immunophenotype and genetic features, we find that many malignant lymphomas have, within the same disease entity, a spectrum of morphologic features and clinical aggressiveness. Thus, histologic grade is just one of many prognostic factors that should be applied *within* a disease entity, not across the whole range of lymphoid neoplasms. Another corollary of defining distinct lymphoma entities is that it is neither possible nor helpful to sort them broadly according to histologic grade or clinical aggressiveness. For example, although it is true that many lymphomas composed of relatively small cells with a low proliferation fraction have a generally indolent course, at least one of them, mantle cell lymphoma, is rather aggressive. In addition, they each have a distinctive set of presenting features and, often, different treatments. Thus, both the pathologist and the oncologist must "get to know" each disease entity, its spectrum of morphology and clinical behavior, and its peculiarities of occurrence and response to therapy.

The WHO Clinical Advisory Committee agreed that clinical groupings of lymphoid neoplasms are of no practical value and may be misleading (85). In practice, treatment of a specific patient should be determined not by which broad prognostic group the patient's neoplasm falls into, but by the specific *type* of neoplasm, with the addition of grade *within* the tumor type, if applicable, and *clinical prognostic factors* such as stage, age, performance status, and/or the International Prognostic Index (81).

Provisional Entities and Borderline Categories

Most of the diseases described in the WHO classification are considered to be distinct entities; however, some are not as clearly defined, and these are listed as provisional entities. In addition, borderline categories have been created in this edition for cases that do not clearly fit into one category, so that well-defined categories can be kept homogenous, and the borderline cases can be studied further. The two important borderline categories are: (a) B-cell lymphoma with features intermediate between diffuse large B-cell lymphoma and Burkitt lymphoma, and (b) B-cell lymphoma with features intermediate between diffuse large B-cell lymphoma and classical Hodgkin lymphoma. Provisional entities include some rare types of cutaneous T-cell lymphomas, and anaplastic large cell lymphoma, anaplastic lymphoma kinase (ALK) negative.

Clonal Lymphoid Populations that May Not Be "Malignant"

The increased use of immunophenotyping and molecular genetic studies has led to the recognition of small clonal cell populations (usually B cell) in apparently healthy individuals, which appear to have little potential to evolve into progressive malignant tumors. Examples include: clonal populations of memory B cells with the t(14;18)(q32;q21), characteristic of follicular lymphoma, found in up to 70% of adults (90); clonal B cells with the immunophenotype and genetic abnormalities associated with CLL, found in 3% to 5% of normal adults and >10% of those referred for evaluation of lymphocytosis (monoclonal B lymphocytosis) (91); clonal populations of CD10+ B cells found in lymph nodes with reactive lymphoid hyperplasia in children; and evidence of clonal B cells with the immunophenotype of follicular lymphoma (92) or mantle cell lymphoma (93), restricted to intrafollicular or mantle zone regions of otherwise reactive lymph nodes. Guidelines for dealing with these clinical situations are provided in the classification.

FUTURE DIRECTIONS IN LYMPHOMA CLASSIFICATION

Any classification of diseases must be considered a work in progress. The diseases recognized in the WHO classification

and their definitions represent our current best approximation; the list will need to be updated periodically as long as there continues to be progress in our understanding of the biology of the immune system and of cancer in general. Important new technologies such as deoxyribonucleic acid microarrays for assessing gene expression in hematologic and other malignancies should improve our understanding of these neoplasms, and provide additional markers for classification and diagnosis (94–96). The European Haematopathology Association and the Society for Hematopathology now have a >10-year record of collaboration on the development of classifications, with involvement of a broad range of hematologists and oncologists. This established mechanism will ensure periodic review and updates to the classification as new information warrants.

References

1. Callendar GR. Tumors and tumor-like conditions of the lymphocyte, the myelocyte, the erythrocyte, and the reticulum cell. *Am J Pathol* 1934;10:443–465.
2. Robb-Smith AHT. Reticulosis and reticulosarcoma. A histological classification. *J Pathol Bacteriol* 1938;47:457–480.
3. Gall EA, Mallory TB. Malignant lymphoma. A clinicopathologic survey of 618 cases. *Am J Pathol* 1942;18:381–395.
4. Rappaport H, Winter W, Hicks E. Follicular lymphoma. A re-evaluation of its position in the scheme of malignant lymphoma, based on a survey of 253 cases. *Cancer* 1956;9:792–821.
5. Rappaport H. Tumors of the hematopoietic system. In: *Atlas of tumor pathology. Series I.* Washington, DC: Armed Forces Institute of Pathology, 1966.
6. Dorfman RF. Letter: classification of non-Hodgkin's lymphomas. *Lancet* 1974;2:961–962.
7. Bennett M, Farrar-Brown G, Henry K, et al. Classification of non-Hodgkin's lymphomas. *Lancet* 1974;2:405–406.
8. Lukes R, Collins R. Immunologic characterization of human malignant lymphomas. *Cancer* 1974;34:1488–1503.
9. Gerard-Marchant R, Hamlin I, Lennert K, et al. Classification of non-Hodgkin's lymphomas. *Lancet* 1974;ii:406–408.
10. Kay HE. Letter: classification of non-Hodgkin's lymphomas. *Lancet* 1974;2:586.
11. Mathe G, Rappaport H, O'Conor GT, et al. Histological and cytological typing of neoplastic disease of hematopoietic and lymphoid tissue. In WHO International Histological Classification of Tumours, No. 14. Geneva: World Health Organization, 1976.
12. Lennert K, Mohri N, Stein H, et al. The histopathology of malignant lymphoma. *Br J Haematol* 1975;31(suppl):193–203.
13. Lennert K. *Malignant lymphomas other than Hodgkin's disease.* New York, NY: Springer-Verlag, 1978.
14. National Cancer Institute sponsored study of classifications of non-Hodgkin's lymphomas: summary and description of a working formulation for clinical usage. The Non-Hodgkin's Lymphoma Pathologic Classification Project. *Cancer* 1982;49:2112–2135.
15. Lennert K, Feller A. *Histopathology of non-Hodgkin's lymphomas*, 2nd ed. New York, NY: Springer-Verlag, 1992.
16. Dorfman RF. Hematopathology: a crescendo of scholarly activity. *Mod Pathol* 1994;7:226–241.
17. Jaffe ES, Harris NL, Stein H, et al. Classification of lymphoid neoplasms: the microscope as a tool for disease discovery. *Blood* 2008;112:4384–4399.
18. Alibert J. *Description des maladies de la peau observées à l'Hôpital St. Louis.* Paris, France: Barrois L'aîné et Fils, 1806.
19. Hodgkin T. On some morbid appearances of the absorbent glands. *Med-Chir Trans* 1832;17:69–97.
20. Symmers WS. Museum piece. *Pathol Annu* 1984;19:375.
21. Wilks S. Cases of enlargement of the lymphatic glands and spleen (or, Hodgkin's disease), with remarks. *Guy's Hosp Rep* 1865;11:56–67.
22. Kundrat H. Uber lymphosarkomatosis. *Wien klin Wochnschr* 1893;6:211–3 and 24–39.
23. Jackson H Jr, Parker F Jr. *Hodgkin's disease and allied disorders.* New York, NY: Oxford University Press, 1947.
24. Sternberg C. Uber ene eigenartige unter dem bilde der pseudoleukamie verlaufend tuberkulose des lymphatischen apparates. *Ztschr Heilk* 1898;19:21–90.
25. Reed D. On the pathological changes in Hodgkin's disease, with especial reference to its relation to tuberculosis. *Johns Hopkins Hosp Rep* 1902;10:133–196.

26. Sternberg C. Uber leukosarcomatose. *Wien Klin Wschr* 1908;21:475–480.
27. Barcos M, Lukes RJ. Malignant lymphoma of convoluted lymphocytes: a new entity of possible T-cell type. In: Sinks L, Godden J, eds. *Conflicts in childhood cancer an evaluation of current management.* New York, NY: Liss, 1975:147–178.
28. Gohn A, Roman D. Uber das lymphosarkom. *Franf Z Path* 1916;19:138.
29. Roulet F. Das primare retothelsarkom der lymphknoten. *Virchows Arch f Path Anat* 1930;277:15–47.
30. Parker F, Jackson H. Primary reticulum cell sarcoma of bone. *Surg Gynecol Obstet* 1939;68:45–53.
31. Bence Jones H. On a new substance occurring in the urine of a patient with millities and fragilitas ossium. *Phil Trans R Soc Lond* 1848;55:673.
32. Von Rustizky J. Multiples myelom. *Deutsche Zeitschrift für Chirurgie* 1873;3:162–172.
33. Wright JH. A case of multiple myeloma. *Bull Johns Hopkins Hosp* 1933;52:156.
34. Brill N, Baehr G, Rosenthal N. Generalized giant lymph follicle hyperplasia of the lymph nodes and spleen. A hitherto undescribed type. *JAMA* 1925;84:668–671.
35. Symmers D. Follicular lymphadenopathy with splenomegaly. a newly recognized disease of the lymphatic system. *Arch Pathol* 1927;3:816–820.
36. Symmers D. Giant follicular lymphadenopathy with or without splenomegaly. *Arch Pathol* 1938;26:603–647.
37. Gall EA, Morrison HR, Scott AT. The follicular type of malignant lymphoma: a survey of 63 cases. *Ann Int Med* 1941;14:2073–2090.
38. Sézary A, Bouvrain Y. Erythrodermie avec présence de cellules monstrueuses dans le derme et le sang circulant. *Bull Soc Franç Derm Syph* 1938;45:254–260.
39. Waldenström J. Incipient myelomatosis or "essential" hyperglobulinemia with fibrinogenopenia—a new syndrome? *Acta Med Scand* 1944;117:216–247.
40. Burkitt DP. A sarcoma involving the jaws in African children. *Br J Surg* 1958;59:46:218–223.
41. Burkitt D, O'Conor GT. Malignant lymphoma in African children. I. A clinical syndrome. *Cancer* 1961;14:258–69.
42. Burkitt DP, O'Conor GT. Malignant lymphoma in African children. I. A clinical syndrome. *Cancer* 1961;14:258–269.
43. O'Conor GT. Malignant lymphoma in African children. II. A pathological entity. *Cancer* 1961;14:270–283.
44. O'Conor GT, Rappaport H, Smith EB. Childhood lymphoma resembling "Burkitt tumor" in the United States. *Cancer* 1965;18:411–417.
45. Epstein M, Achong B, Barr Y. Virus particles in cultured lymphoblasts from Burkitt's lymphoma. *Lancet* 1964;1:702–703.
46. Willis R. The tumours of lymphoid tissue. In: *Pathology of tumours.* London, UK: Butterworth, 1948:760–783.
47. Jackson H Jr, Parker F Jr. Hodgkin's disease and allied disorders. *N Engl J Med* 1939;220:26–30.
48. Jackson H Jr, Parker F Jr. Hodgkin's disease I: general considerations. *N Engl J Med* 1944;230:1–8.
49. Jackson H Jr, Parker F Jr. Hodgkin's disease II: pathology. *N Engl J Med* 1944;231:35–44.
50. Gall EA, Rappaport H. *Proceedings of seminar on diseases of lymph node and spleen.* Chicago, IL: ASCP Press, 1958.
51. Nowell PC. Phytohemagglutinin: an initiator of mitosis in cultures of normal human leukocytes. *Cancer Res* 1960;20:462–426.
52. Jones S, Fuks Z, Bull M, et al. Non-Hodgkin's lymphomas IV. Clinicopathologic correlation in 405 cases. *Cancer* 1973;31:806–823.
53. Ezdinli E, Costello W, Wasser L, et al. Eastern Cooperative Oncology Group experience with the Rappaport classification of non-Hodgkin's lymphomas. *Cancer* 1979;43:544–550.
54. Murphy S. Management of childhood non-Hodgkin's lymphoma. *Cancer Treat Rep* 1977;61:1161–1173.
55. Cooper MD, Peterson RDA, Good RA. Delineation of the thymic and bursal lymphoid systems in the chicken. *Nature* 1965;205:143–146.
56. Cooper MD, Perey DY, McKneally MF, et al. A mammalian equivalent of the avian bursa of Fabricius. *Lancet* 1966;1:1388–1391.
57. Wilson JD, Nossal GJV. Identification of human T and B lymphocytes in normal peripheral blood and in chronic lymphocytic leukemia. *Lancet* 1971;II:788–791.
58. DeVita VT Jr, Canellos GP, Chabner B, et al. Advanced diffuse histiocytic lymphoma, a potentially curable disease. *Lancet* 1975;1:248–250.
59. Lennert K. Germinal centers and germinal center neoplasia. *Nippon Ketsueki Gakkai Zasshi* 1969;32:495–500.
60. Stein H, Lennert K, Parwaresch M. Malignant lymphomas of B-cell type. *Lancet* 1972;2:855–857.
61. Stansfeld A, Diebold J, Kapanci Y, et al. Updated Kiel classification for lymphomas. *Lancet* 1988;i:292–293.
62. Brittinger G, Bartels H, Common H, et al. Clinical and prognostic relevance of the Kiel classification of non-Hodgkin lymphomas: results of a prospective multicenter study by the Kiel lymphoma study group. *Hematol Oncol* 1984;2:269–306.
63. Schein PS, Chabner BA, Canellos GP, et al. Potential for prolonged disease-free survival following combination chemotherapy of non-Hodgkin's lymphoma. *Blood* 1974;43:181–189.
64. Strauchen J, Young R, De Vita V, et al. Clinical relevance of the histopathological subclassification of diffuse "histiocytic" lymphoma. *N Engl J Med* 1978;299:1382–1387.
65. Classification of non-Hodgkin's lymphomas. Reproducibility of major classification systems. *Cancer* 1985;55:91–95.
66. Fisher RI, Dahlberg S, Nathwani BN, et al. A clinical analysis of two indolent lymphoma entities: mantle cell lymphoma and marginal zone lymphoma (including the mucosa-associated lymphoid tissue and monocytoid B-cell subcategories): a Southwest Oncology Group study. *Blood* 1995;85:1075–1082.
67. Fisher R, Gaynor E, Dahlberg S, et al. Comparison of a standard regimen (CHOP) with three intensive chemotherapy regimens for advanced non-Hodgkin's lymphoma. *N Engl J Med* 1993;328:1002–1006.
68. Longo DL, DeVita VT, Jaffe ES, et al. Lymphocytic lymphomas. In: De Vita VT, Hellman S, Rosenberg S, eds. *Principles and practice of oncology,* 4th ed. Philadelphia, PA: J. B. Lippincott, 1993:1859–1927.
69. Hastrup N, Hamilton-Dutoit S, Ralfkiaer E, et al. Peripheral T-cell lymphomas: an evaluation of reproducibility of the updated Kiel classification. *Histopathology* 1991;18:99–105.
70. Chott A, Augustin I, Wra F, et al. Peripheral T-cell lymphomas—a clinicopathologic study of 75 cases. *Hum Pathol* 1990;21:1117–1125.
71. Banks P, Chan J, Cleary M, et al. Mantle cell lymphoma: a proposal for unification of morphologic, immunologic, and molecular data. *Am J Surg Pathol* 1992;16:637–640.
72. Mason D, Banks P, Chan J, et al. Nodular lymphocyte predominance Hodgkin's disease: a distinct clinico-pathological entity. *Am J Surg Pathol* 1994;18:528–530.
73. Harris NL, Jaffe ES, Stein H, et al. A revised European-American classification of lymphoid neoplasms: a proposal from the International Lymphoma Study Group. *Blood* 1994;84:1361–1392.
74. Weisenburger D. The International Lymphoma Study Group (ILSG) Classification of non-Hodgkin's lymphoma (NHL): pathology findings from a large multi-center study. *Mod Pathol* 1997;10:136A.
75. Weisenburger D. The International Lymphoma Study Group (ILSG) Classification of non-Hodgkin's lymphoma (NHL): clinical findings from a large multi-center study. *Mod Pathol* 1997;10:136A.
76. A clinical evaluation of the International Lymphoma Study Group classification of non-Hodgkin's lymphoma. The Non-Hodgkin's Lymphoma Classification Project. *Blood* 1997;89:3909–3918.
77. Armitage JO, Weisenburger DD. New Approach to classifying non-Hodgkin's lymphomas: clinical features of the major histologic subtypes. *J Clin Oncol* 1998;16:2780–2795.
78. Rosenberg SA. Classification of lymphoid neoplasms. *Blood* 1994;84:1359–1360.
79. Harris NL, Jaffe ES, Stein H, et al. Lymphoma classification proposal: clarification. *Blood* 1995;85:857–860.
80. Anderson JR, Armitage JO, Weisenburger DD. Epidemiology of the non-Hodgkin's lymphomas: distributions of the major subtypes differ by geographic locations. Non-Hodgkin's Lymphoma Classification Project. *Ann Oncol* 1998;9:717–720.
81. A predictive model for aggressive non-Hodgkin's lymphoma. The International non-Hodgkin's Lymphoma Project. *N Engl J Med* 1993;329:987–994.
82. Jaffe ES, Harris NL, Chan JKC, et al. Proposed World Health Organization classification of neoplastic diseases of hematopoietic and lymphoid tissues. *Am J Surg Pathol* 1997;21:114–121.
83. Jaffe ES, Harris NL, Diebold J, et al. World Health Organization classification of lymphomas: a work in progress. *Ann Oncol* 1998;(suppl 5):S25–S30.
84. Harris NL, Jaffe ES, Diebold J, et al. World Health Organization classification of neoplastic diseases of the hematopoietic and lymphoid tissues: report of the Clinical Advisory Committee meeting-Airlie House, Virginia, November 1997. *J Clin Oncol* 1999;17:3835–3849.
85. Harris NL, Jaffe ES, Diebold J, et al. The World Health Organization Classification of Hematological Malignancies. Report of the Clinical Advisory Committee Meeting - Airlie House, Virginia, November, 1997. *Ann Oncol* 1999;10:1419–1432.
86. Jaffe ES, Harris NL, Stein H, et al. *Pathology and genetics of tumours of haematopoietic and lymphoid tissues.* Lyon, France: IARC Press, 2001.
87. Swerdlow SH, Campo E, Harris NL, et al. *WHO classification of tumours of haematopoietic and lymphoid tissues,* 4th ed. Lyon, France: International Agency for Research on Cancer, 2008.
88. Feldman AL, Berthold F, Arceci RJ, et al. Clonal relationship between precursor T-lymphoblastic leukaemia/lymphoma and Langerhans-cell histiocytosis. *Lancet Oncol* 2005;6:435–437.
89. Feldman AL, Arber DA, Pittaluga S, et al. Clonally related follicular lymphomas and histiocytic/dendritic cell sarcomas: evidence for transdifferentiation of the follicular lymphoma clone. *Blood* 2008;111:5433–5439.
90. Roulland S, Navarro JM, Grenot P, et al. Follicular lymphoma-like B cells in healthy individuals: a novel intermediate step in early lymphomagenesis. *J Exp Med* 2006;203:2425–2431.
91. Rawstron AC, Green MJ, Kuzmicki A, et al. Monoclonal B lymphocytes with the characteristics of "indolent" chronic lymphocytic leukemia are present in 3.5% of adults with normal blood counts. *Blood* 2002;100:635–639.

92. Cong P, Raffeld M, Teruya-Feldstein J, et al. In situ localization of follicular lymphoma: description and analysis by laser capture microdissection. *Blood* 2002;99:3376–3382.

93. Aqel N, Barker F, Patel K, et al. In-situ mantle cell lymphoma—a report of two cases. *Histopathology* 2008;52:256–260.

94. Alizadeh AA, Eisen MB, Davis RE, et al. Distinct types of diffuse large B-cell lymphoma identified by gene expression profiling. *Nature* 2000;403:503–511.

95. Shipp MA, Ross KN, Tamayo P, et al. Diffuse large B-cell lymphoma outcome prediction by gene-expression profiling and supervised machine learning. *Nat Med* 2002;8:68–74.

96. Rosenwald A, Wright G, Chan WC, et al. The use of molecular profiling to predict survival after chemotherapy for diffuse large-B-cell lymphoma. *N Engl J Med* 2002;346:1937–1947.

NON-HODGKIN LYMPHOMAS

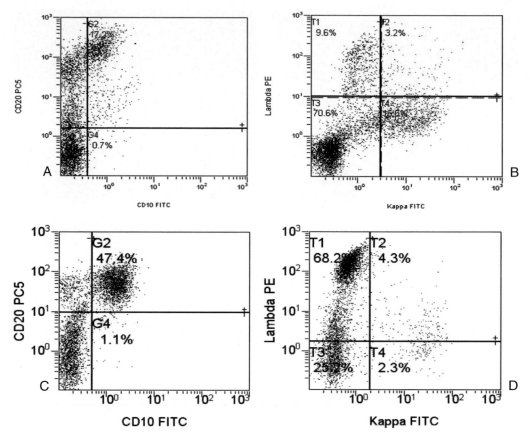

COLOR PLATE 1–4 A and B: Flow cytometry histograms for a lymph node with florid follicular hyperplasia. Note the presence of a CD20/CD10-positive population in (**A**). However, (**B**) clearly demonstrates polytypic expression (PE) of κ- and λ-light chains (See also Figure 9.2A and 9.2B). **C and D:** The same two histograms for flow cytometry of a lymph node with follicular lymphoma. Note again the presence of a CD20/CD10 positive population in (**C**). **D:** Clear λ-light chain restriction is demonstrated. FITC, fluorescein isothiocyanate (See also Figure 9.2C and 9.2D).

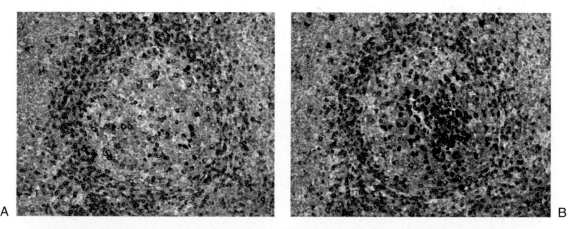

COLOR PLATE 5–6 A: IHC staining for κ-light chain (See also Figure 9.3A). **B:** λ-Light chain staining. These are both from the same lymph node with reactive follicular hyperplasia. These figures demonstrate optimized light chain IHC. Not only are the plasma cells staining but also the small B cells in the mantle zone, confirming polytypic light chain expression in both types of cells (See also Figure 9.3B).

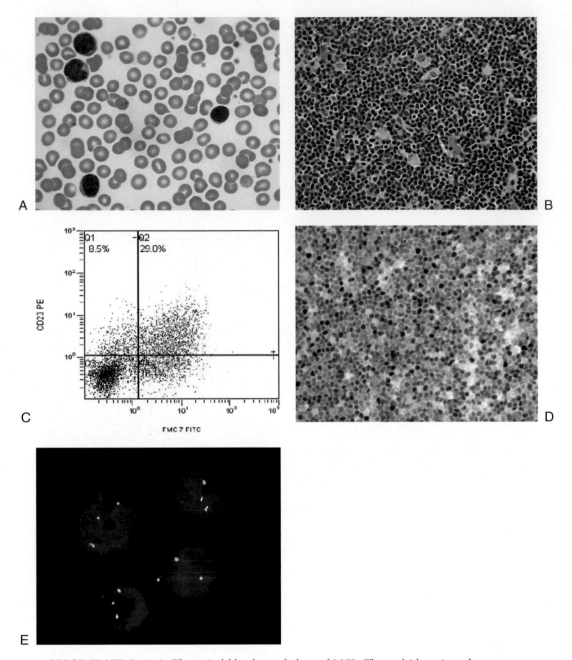

COLOR PLATE 7–11 A: The typical blood morphology of MCL. The nuclei have irregular contours, and there is a range of cell size, including larger lymphoid cells with more immature appearing chromatin (See also Figure 9.4A). **B:** The classic histologic appearance of MCL in a lymph node section. The cells are small and monomorphic with irregular nuclear contours. There are admixed epithelioid histiocytes, and the small blood vessels show fine sclerosis. Scattered mitotic figures are also present (See also Figure 9.4B). **C:** A flow cytometry histogram of CD23 and FMC-7 expression on a lymph node with MCL. This demonstrates the point that every case does not show a classic flow cytometry phenotype because there is clear coexpression of CD23 and FMC-7 in this instance. This diagnostic dilemma can be resolved either by cyclin D1 staining on the tissue section or by FISH analysis for t(11;14) on tissue, bone marrow, or peripheral blood specimens (See also Figure 9.4C). **D:** The same tissue section in (**B**), showing a positive result for an IHC stain for cyclin D1 (CCND1) (See also Figure 9.4D). **E:** FISH analysis for t(11;14) using a colocalization assay. A normal signal would show two red probes, localizing to the two alleles of the *CCND1* gene on chromosome 11 and two green probes localizing to the *IGH* gene on chromosome 14. In this case of a t(11;14) translocation, the red and green probes are brought in close proximity. FITC, fluorescein isothiocyanate (See also Figure 9.4E).

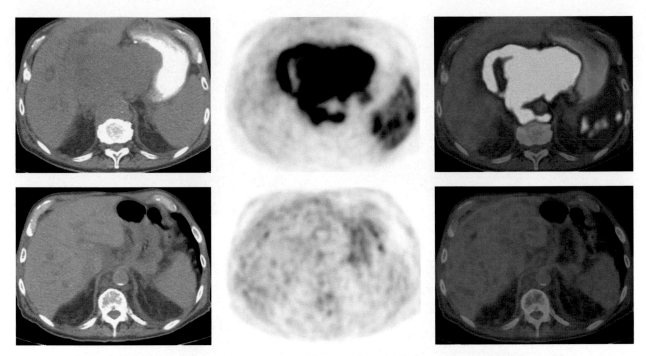

COLOR PLATE 12 This patient is a 52-year-old man with DLBCL who was started on therapy with rituximab plus CHOP. A PET/CT scan performed after two cycles demonstrated persistence of the mass on the CT, but no FDG avidity on the PET or fusion scan. The patient remains in CR. (Courtesy of Lale Kostakoglu.) (See also Figure 11.1).

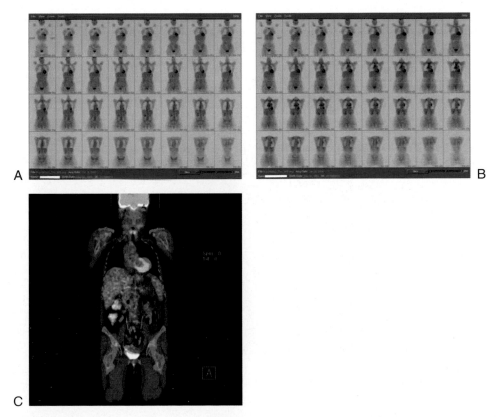

COLOR PLATE 13–15 A: This patient is a 56-year-old woman with stage IIIA DLBCL (See also Figure 11.2A). **B:** A normal CT-PET after completion of six cycles of rituximab plus CHOP. However, several months later, there was an FDG-avid mediastinal mass. Biopsy revealed sarcoidosis. At routine follow-up 4.5 years later, cervical and axillary lymphadenopathy were palpated (See also Figure 11.2B). **C:** CT/PET scan failed to identify either the previous sarcoid or any FDG-avid lymph nodes. The patient remains in a clinical remission (See also Figure 11.2C).

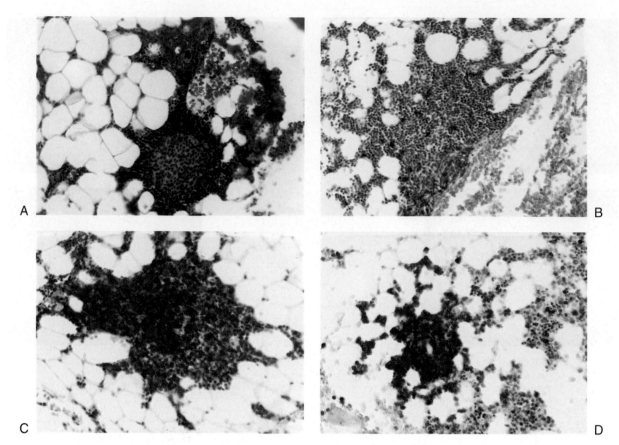

COLOR PLATE 16–19 Bone marrow biopsy of a patient with CLL/SLL following therapy. The residual lymphoid nodule (**A**) (See also Figure 11.3A) is demonstrated to represent residual disease because it is negative for CD3 (**B**) (See also Figure 11.3B), yet positive for CD20 (**C**) (See also Figure 11.3C) and CD 5 (**D**) (See also Figure 11.3D).

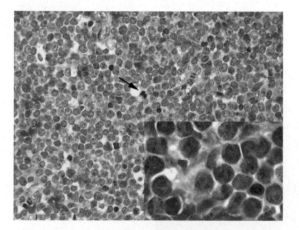

COLOR PLATE 20 Histologic section of lymphoblastic lymphoma, showing the characteristic uniform population of medium-sized cells, with mitotic figures *(arrow)*. At high power *(inset)*, the chromatin is finely dispersed, and nucleoli are inconspicuous (See also Chapter 12).

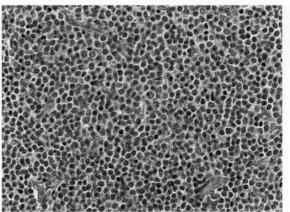

COLOR PLATE 21–22 Lymph node biopsy from a patient with CLL. **A:** At low magnification, there is a vaguely nodular (pseudofollicular) pattern (See also Figure 13.1A). **B:** Higher magnification shows a predominance of small lymphocytes with scattered larger cells known as prolymphocytes and paraimmunoblasts (See also Figure 13.1B).

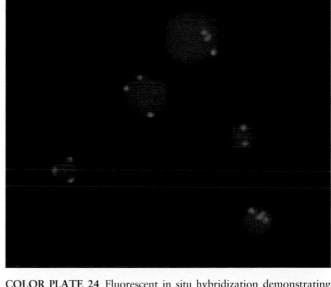

COLOR PLATE 24 Fluorescent in situ hybridization demonstrating trisomy 12 in chronic lymphocytic leukemia (See also Figure 13.4). (Courtesy of Dr. Randy Gascoyne, British Columbia Cancer Agency, Vancouver, British Columbia, Canada.)

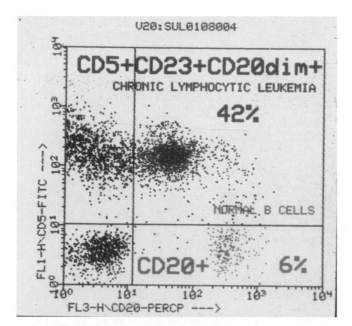

COLOR PLATE 23 Flow cytometry of chronic lymphocytic leukemia. The cells express dim CD20, dim CD5, and CD23 (See also Figure 13.2). (Courtesy of Dr. Frederick I. Preffer, Department of Pathology, Massachusetts General Hospital, Boston, MA.)

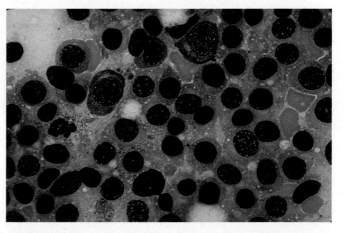

COLOR PLATE 25 Aspirate from a patient with WM demonstrating excess mature lymphocytes, lymphoplasmacytic cells, and plasma cells (See also Figure 14.1). (Courtesy of Marvin Stone, M.D.)

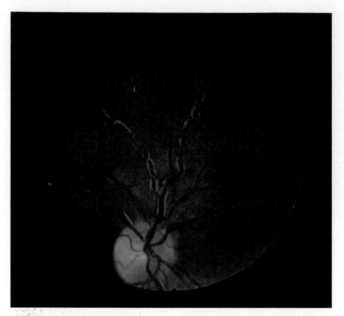

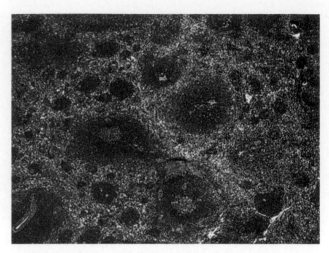

COLOR PLATE 27 Microscopic view of SMZL. Micronodular infiltration of the white pulp, with marginal zone differentiation, and involvement of red pulp (See also Figure 16.1).

COLOR PLATE 26 Funduscopic examination of a patient with WM demonstrating hyperviscosity related changes, including dilated retinal vessels, peripheral hemorrhages, and "venous sausaging" (See also Figure 14.2). (Courtesy of Marvin Stone, M.D.)

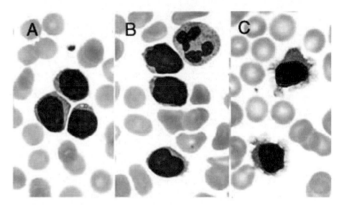

COLOR PLATE 28 Different cytologic aspects of blood involvement in SMZL. A: Aggregation of three cells with clumped chromatin and small round nucleus. B: Cells with notched nucleus. C: Typical villous lymphocytes with short cytoplasmic villi (See also Figure 16.2).

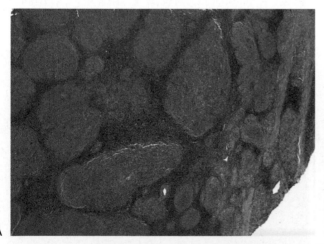

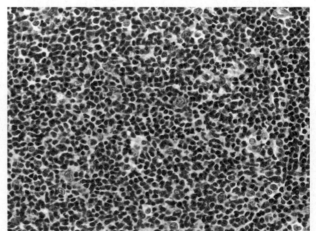

COLOR PLATE 29 A: Follicular lymphoma, low magnification. There are closely packed follicles of varying sizes, extending beyond the lymph node capsule into the fat, associated with sclerosis. B: Follicular lymphoma, grade 1/3, high magnification. The majority of the cells are small centrocytes with cleaved nuclei; there are rare large non-cleaved centroblasts with small nucleoli (See also Chapter 18).

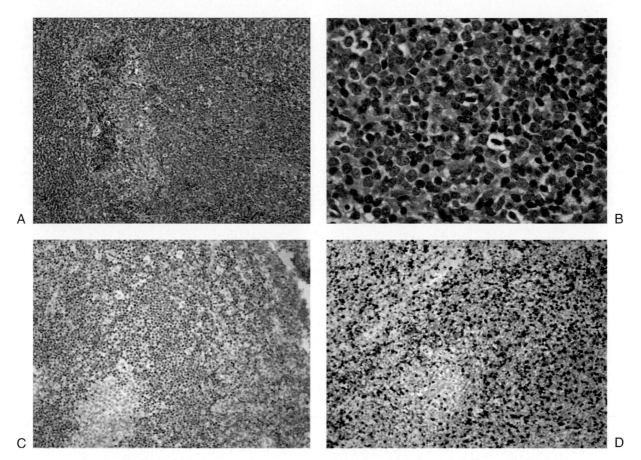

COLOR PLATE 30–33 Mantle zone lymphoma, nodular ("Mantle zone") pattern; a small reactive germinal center is seen surrounded by a markedly expanded mantle zone (Panel A, Hematoxylin & Eosin stain, original magnification 100X). The neoplastic lymphocytes have predominantly ovoid or irregular nuclear contours, fine chromatin, indistinct or small nucleoli, and scant cytoplasm (Panel B, Hematoxylin & Eosin stain, original magnification 400X). Cyclin D1 expressing lymphocytes are largely confined to the mantle zone (Panel C, original magnification 100X) and these cells show a moderately elevated proliferation index (approximately 30%), as assessed with a stain for Ki-67 (Panel D, original magnification 100X) (See also Figure 19.1A-D).

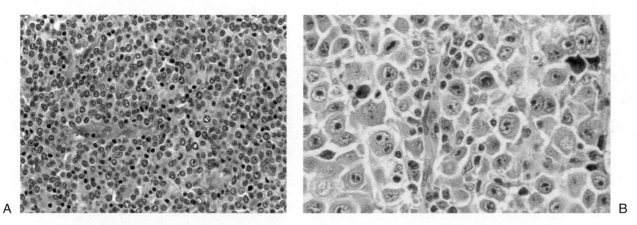

COLOR PLATE 34 Diffuse large B-cell lymphoma. **A:** The majority of cases contain a mixture of large cells that resemble centroblasts with peripheral nucleoli and a minority of large cells that resemble immunoblasts with central nucleoli. **B:** Occasional cases have a predominance of large cells with prominent central nucleoli and abundant cytoplasm, resembling immunoblasts (See also Chapter 20).

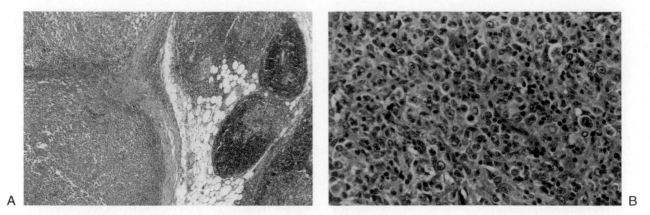

COLOR PLATE 35–36 Histopathology of PMBL. **A:** At low magnification, there is a focus of normal thymus (**right**) and a large mass of tumor cells (**left**) (See also Figure 21.A). **B:** At high magnification, the cells are large and range from round to oval to multiolobated, with moderately abundant, pale cytoplasm (hematoxylin and eosin stain) (See also Figure 21.B).

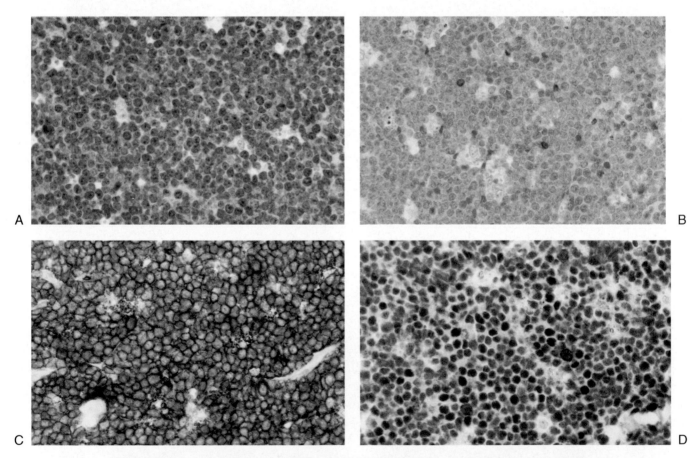

COLOR PLATE 37 Immunostains of MIB-1 (**A**), Bcl-2 (**B**), CD10 (**C**), and Bcl-6 (**D**) in a case of classic Burkitt's lymphoma. Note that all cells are proliferating as defined by positive MIB-1 staining, except the phagocytic histiocytes in the section. CD10 is strongly expressed by the malignant cells, and Bcl-2 is negative. Note several small, reactive lymphocytes in the section staining positively for Bcl-2 that serve as an internal control. Bcl-6 staining (**D**) shows strong nuclear expression (See also Figure 22.5A–D).

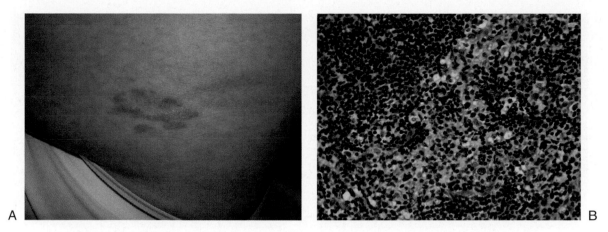

COLOR PLATE 38–39 A: A patient diagnosed with primary cutaneous MZL presenting with an irregularly shaped, erythematous plaque on the left flank (See also Figure 24.1A). **B:** Biopsy reveals a dense, pleomorphic infiltrate with atypical lymphocytes, plasma cells, and lymphoplasmacytoid cells (hematoxylin and eosin; original magnification ×200) (See also Figure 24.1B).

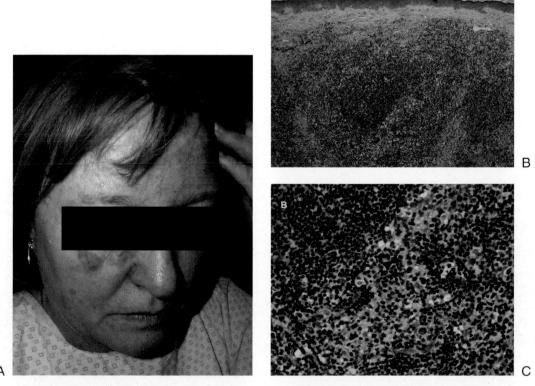

COLOR PLATE 40–42 A: This patient presented with erythematous papules and nodules on the face (See also Figure 24.2A). **B:** A skin biopsy shows a dense dermal infiltrate with a follicular growth pattern (hematoxylin and eosin; original magnification ×100). There is a grenz zone with uninvolved epidermis (See also Figure 24.2B). **C:** Follicles are composed of centrocytes and centroblasts surrounded by small lymphocytes (hematoxylin and eosin; original magnification ×200) (See also Figure 24.2C).

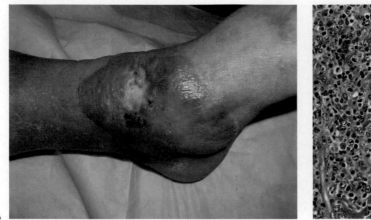
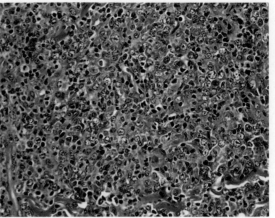

COLOR PLATE 43–44 A: DLBCL, leg type presenting as a thick, indurated, erythematous, and ulcerated plaque on the lower leg (See also Figure 24.3A). **B:** Histologic evaluation demonstrates a diffuse dermal infiltrate with predominately large lymphocytes with multilobulated nuclei, comprised of centroblasts and immunoblasts (hematoxylin and eosin; original magnification ×100) (See also Figure 24.3B).

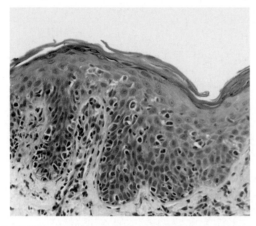

COLOR PLATE 45 Atypical cerebriform lymphocytes are arranged in a linear pattern along the dermoepidermal junction. Similar atypical lymphocytes are scattered within the upper epidermal layers, without accompanying spongiosis (See also Chapter 25).

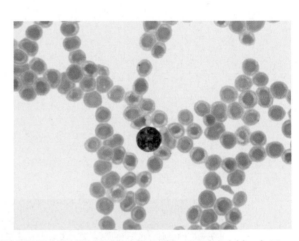

COLOR PLATE 47 Sézary cells within peripheral blood. Note the cerebriform nuclear convolution (See also Chapter 25).

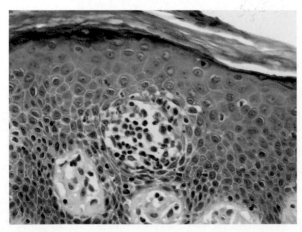

COLOR PLATE 46 Pautrier collections of atypical lymphocytes are characteristic of mycosis fungoides but are seen in only a minority of early-stage lesions (See also Chapter 25).

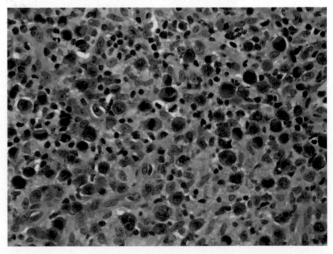

COLOR PLATE 48 In cases of large-cell transformation, the dermis demonstrates many large, cytologically atypical lymphocytes with prominent nucleoli and easily appreciated mitotic activity (See also Chapter 25).

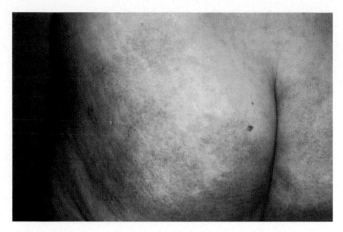

COLOR PLATE 49 Typical erythematosus patch disease in the bathing trunk distribution (See also Chapter 25).

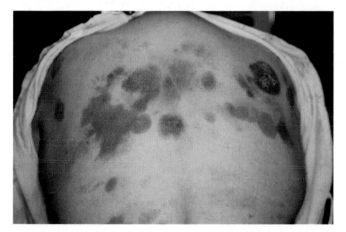

COLOR PLATE 50 Typical patch/plaque disease (See also Chapter 25).

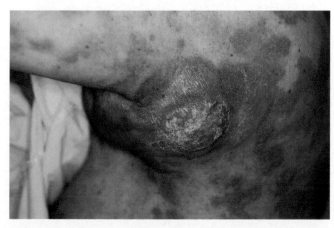

COLOR PLATE 51 A large cutaneous tumor of mycosis fungoides in a background of patch/plaque disease (See also Chapter 25).

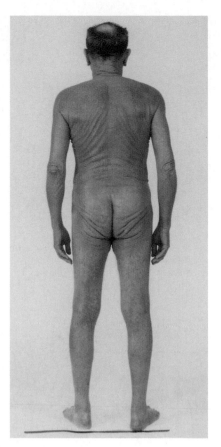

COLOR PLATE 52 Generalized erythroderma in the context of Sézary syndrome (See also Chapter 25).

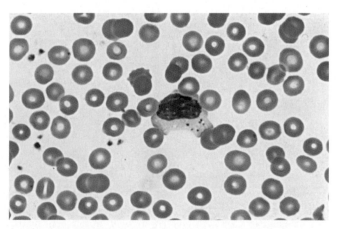

COLOR PLATE 53 A typical large granular lymphocyte is illustrated in this peripheral blood film. Note sparse, yet prominent, cytoplasmic granules in this mature-appearing lymphoid cell (Wright's stain.) (See also Chapter 26).

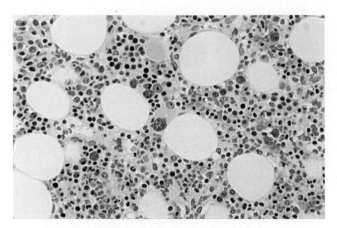

COLOR PLATE 54 Although inconspicuous on hematoxylin and eosin sections of this hypocellular bone marrow specimen, significant infiltration by T-cell large granular lymphocytic leukemia was documented by specialized techniques (See also Chapter 26).

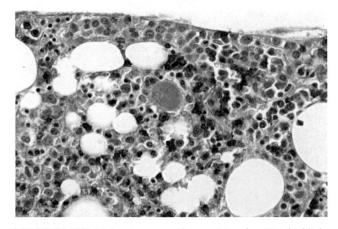

COLOR PLATE 55 Immunoperoxidase staining for CD3 highlights significant numbers of both clustered and individually dispersed T cells, in this case with subtle bone marrow involvement by T-cell large granular lymphocytic leukemia (Immunoperixodase staining for CD3.) (See also Chapter 26).

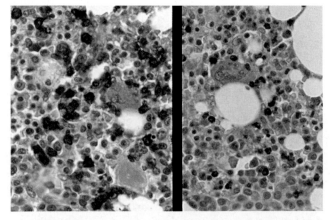

COLOR PLATE 56 This composite highlights the immunoperoxidase staining for CD8 *(left)* and TIA-1 *(right)* in this bone marrow biopsy section exhibiting subtle involvement by T –cell granular lymphocytic leukemia. Note sinusoidal involvement on CD8 stain (Immunoperoxidase staining for CD8 and TIA-1.) (See also Chapter 26).

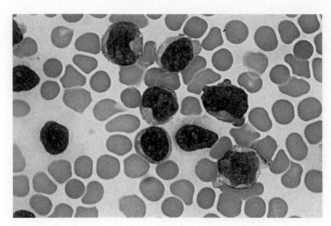

COLOR PLATE 57 Peripheral blood film from a 65-year-old man who presented with a white blood cell count of 280×10^9/L showing lymphocytes with distinct nucleoli and cytoplasmic blebbing. (Wright's stain.) (See also Chapter 26).

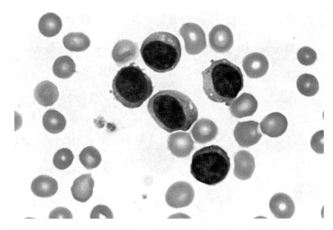

COLOR PLATE 58 Peripheral blood film from a 69-year-old man with a white blood cell count of 112×10^9/L, hemoglobin of 8 g/dL, and a platelet count of 50×10^9/L showing mature lymphocytes with condensed chromatin and inconspicuous nucleoli mimicking chronic lymphocytic leukemia (Wright's stain). This case represents an example of the small-cell variant of T-cell prolymphocytic leukemia (See also Chapter 26).

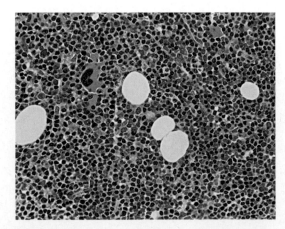

COLOR PLATE 59 A bone marrow clot section showing a hypercellular bone marrow in a 65-year-old man with T-cell prolymphocytic leukemia. Note extensive diffuse interstitial infiltration (Hematoxylin and eosin stain.) (See also Chapter 26).

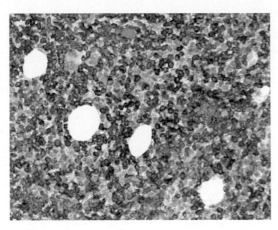

COLOR PLATE 60 Same bone marrow section as Color Plate 58 showing extensive CD3 positivity by the immunoperoxidase technique (See also Chapter 26).

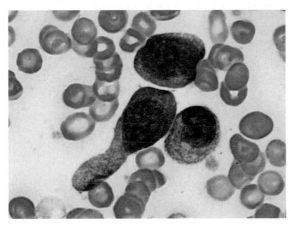

COLOR PLATE 61 Bone marrow aspirate smear showing several large immature NK leukemia cells with retained cytoplasmic granulation. Note more mature-appearing large granular lymphocyte (See also Chapter 26).

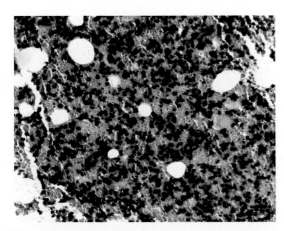

COLOR PLATE 62 *In situ hybridization* for EBER (Epstein-Barr virus RNA) in a case of aggressive natural killer-cell leukemia/lymphoma (See also Chapter 26).

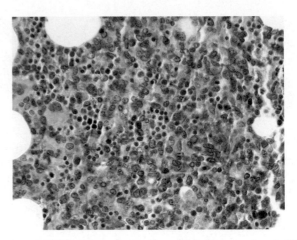

COLOR PLATE 63 Immunoperoxidase staining for cytoplasmic CD3ε in a case of aggressive natural killer-cell leukemia/lymphoma (See also Chapter 26).

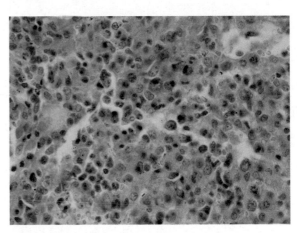

COLOR PLATE 64 Immunoperoxidase staining for TIA-1 cytoplasmic staining in a case of aggressive natural killer cell leukemia/lymphoma (See also Chapter 26).

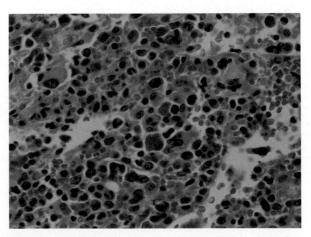

COLOR PLATE 65 Florid hemophagocytosis by benign histiocytes in conjunction with extensive subtle bone marrow infiltration by aggressive natural killer cell-leukemia/lymphoma in bone marrow core biopsy specimen (See also Chapter 26).

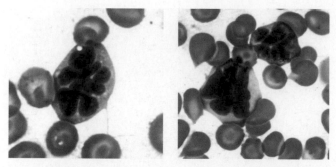

COLOR PLATE 66 The markedly polylobated neoplastic cells of adult T-cell leukemia-lymphoma in the peripheral blood. They have been termed *flower cells* based on the petal-like appearance of the nuclear lobes (See also Chapter 27).

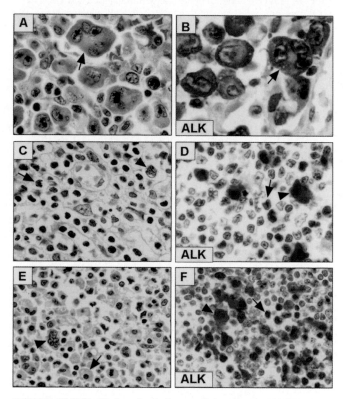

COLOR PLATE 67 Anaplastic large-cell lymphoma (ALCL): morphologic variants and anaplastic lymphoma kinase (ALK) expression. **A,B:** ALCL, common type (lymph node paraffin sections). **A:** The arrow points to a "hallmark cell" (hematoxylin and eosin; ×800). **B:** Tumor cells from the same case show cytoplasmic-restricted labeling for the ALK protein *(arrow)* (monoclonal antibody ALKc; APAAP technique; ×800). **C,D:** ALCL, small-cell variant (lymph node paraffin sections). **C:** Small *(arrow)* to medium-sized *(arrowhead)* tumor cells showing a clear cytoplasm and irregular nuclei (hematoxylin and eosin; ×800). **D:** Large anaplastic tumor cells show ALK expression both in the cytoplasm and the nucleus *(arrowhead)*. In the smaller cells with irregular nuclei, ALK labeling is restricted to the nucleus *(arrow)* (monoclonal antibody ALKc; APAAP technique; ×800). **E,F:** ALCL, lymphohistiocytic variant (lymph node paraffin sections). **E:** Small- and large-sized *(arrowhead)* tumor cells are admixed with a high number of reactive histiocytes *(arrow)* (hematoxylin and eosin; ×800). **F:** The small tumor cells show a nucleus-restricted positivity for the ALK protein *(arrow)*, whereas the large neoplastic elements are ALK+ both in the cytoplasm and the nucleus *(arrowhead)* (monoclonal antibody ALKc; APAAP technique; ×800) (See also Chapter 28). (C,D,E, and F from Falini B. Anaplastic large cell lymphoma: pathological, molecular and clinical features. *Br J Haematol* 2001; 114:741-760, with permission.)

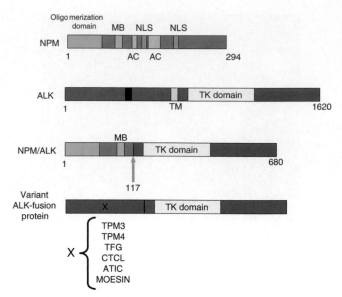

COLOR PLATE 68 Molecular structure of nucleophosmin (NPM), anaplastic lymphoma kinase (ALk), and ALK chimeric proteins. The NPM molecule consists of an oligomerization domain (residues 1-83), a metal binding domain (MB; residues 104-115), two acidic aminoacid clusters (AC; residues 120-132 and 161-188) functioning as acceptor regions for nucleolar targeting signals, and two nuclear localization signals (NLS). The ALK protein is a transmembrane tyrosine kinase (TK) receptor that contains an extracellular portion, a transmembrane domain (TM), and a TK domain in the N-terminal part of the intracytoplasmic tail. Approximately 85% of ALK+ ALCL bear ALK-variant fusion proteins in which the extracellular and TM domains of ALK are replaced by the oligomerization domains of proteins (X) other than NPM. In all ALK fusion proteins, with the exception of moesin-ALK (see Chapter 28), the fusion point is at codon 117 (See also Chapter 28).

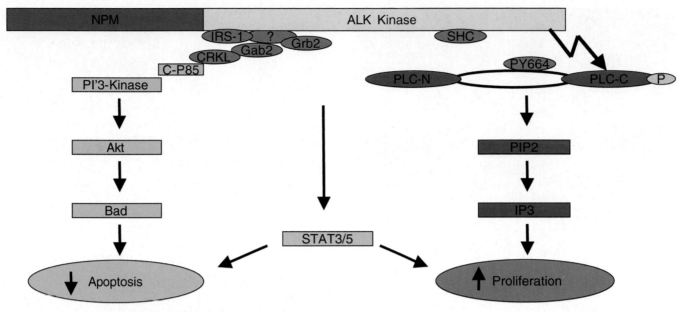

COLOR PLATE 69 Alterations of signaling pathways in anaplastic lymphoma kinase-positive (ALK+) anaplastic large-cell lymphoma. NPM, nucleophosmin (See also Chapter 28). [Modified from Duyster J, Bai Ry, Morris SW. Translocations involving anaplastic lymphoma kinase (ALK). *Oncogene* 2001;20:5623-5634, with permission.]

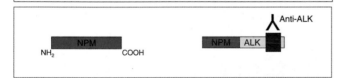

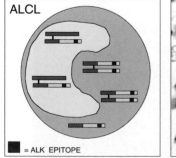

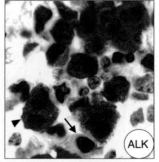

COLOR PLATE 70 Patterns of oligomerization and subcellular distribution of the nucleophosmin-anaplastic lymphoma kinase (NPM-ALK) fusion protein in ALK⁺ anaplastic large-cell lymphoma (ALCL) with t(2;5). ALK expression is localized only in the nucleus *(arrow)* or nucleus and cytoplasm *(arrowhead)* of tumor cells. Normal residual lymphoid cells are ALK⁻ (lymph node paraffin section; monoclonal antibody ALKc; APAAP technique; ×800) (See also Chapter 28).

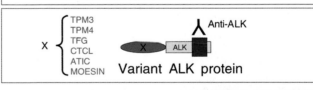

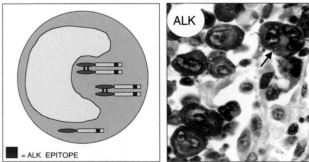

COLOR PLATE 71 Patterns of oligomerization and subcellular distribution of the anaplastic lymphoma kinase (ALK)-variant fusion proteins in ALK⁺ anaplastic large-cell lymphoma without t(2;5). ALK expression is localized only in the cytoplasm of tumor cells *(arrow)*. Normal residual lymphoid cells are ALK⁻ (lymph node paraffin section; monoclonal antibody ALKc; APAAP technique; ×800) (See also Chapter 28).

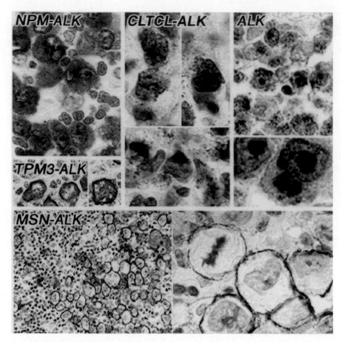

COLOR PLATE 72 Different patterns of anaplastic lymphoma kinase (ALK) immunostaining in lymphomas. All tumors contain a hybrid ALK protein, except for that marked ALK, an example of the rare subtype of large B-cell lymphoma in which full-length, wild-type ALK protein is expressed. Notice the typical granular cytoplasmic positivity for ALK in tumor cells bearing the chlatrin (CLTCL)-ALK and the surface expression for ALK in anaplastic large-cell lymphoma cells containing moesin (MSN)-ALK (immunoperoxidase technique in paraffin sections; ×800 to 1,000) (See also Chapter 28). (From Falini B, Mason DY. Proteins encoded by genes involved in chromosomal alterations in lymphoma and leukemia: clinical value of their detection by immunocytochemistry. *Blood* 2002;99:409-426, with permission.)

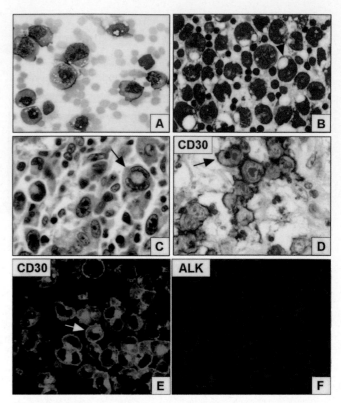

COLOR PLATE 73 Anaplastic large-cell lymphoma (ALCL): morphology and phenotype. **A:** ALCL, common type. Large tumor cells showing vacuolized cytopolasm (ascitic fluid; May-Grunwald Giemsa, ×800). **B:** ALCL with "signet-ring" appearance *(arrowhead)* (lymph node paraffin section). **C:** ALCL, common type (lymph node paraffin section). The arrow points to a large tumor cell with a bizarre nucleus (hematoxylin and eosin; ×800). **D:** ALCL cells show strong CD30 positivity at the surface and in the Golgi area (arrow) (APAAP technique; ×800). **E,F:** Double immunofluorescence labeling (rhodamin/fluorescein) of tumor cells for CD30 (E) and anaplastic lymphoma kinase (F) in lymph node paraffin sections from ALCL, common type. The arrow in (E) points to a neoplastic cell showing positivity on the cell surface and Golgi area (See also Chapter 28). (E and F from Falini B, Mason DY. Proteins encoded by genes involved in chromosomal alterations in lymphoma and leukemia: clinical value of their detection by immunocytochemistry. *Blood* 2002;99:409-426, with permission.)

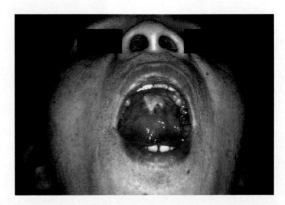

COLOR PLATE 74 Clinical photograph of a patient with nasal natural killer-cell lymphoma involving the hard palate (See also Chapter 29).

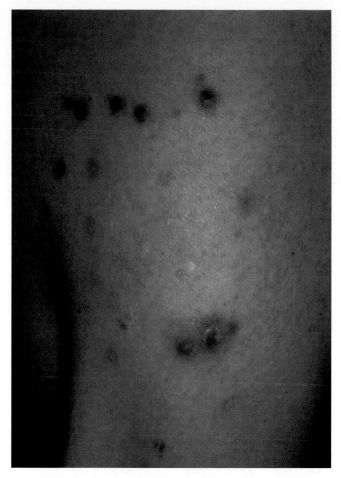

COLOR PLATE 75 Patient diagnosed with LyP presenting with multiple erythematous papules on the upper arm (See also Figure 30.1).

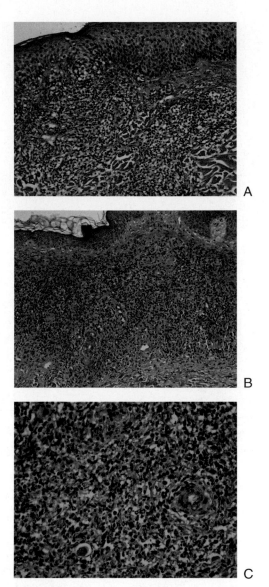

COLOR PLATE 76–78 LyP type A with large atypical cells intermingled with histiocytes, eosinophils, and small lymphocytes (See also Figure 30.2A) **(A)**, and type B with band-like infiltrate of small to medium-sized lymphocytes and epidermotropism resembling histologic features of MF (hematoxylin and eosin; original magnification ×200) **(B)** (See also Figure 30.2B). **C:** Type C reveals cohesive sheets of atypical lymphoid cells (hematoxylin and eosin; original magnification ×400) (See also Figure 30.2C).

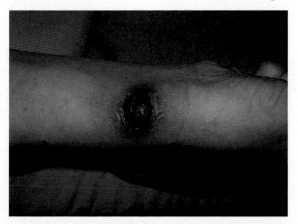

COLOR PLATE 79 Patient diagnosed with CD30+ CALCL revealing a solitary violaceous tumor with central necrosis on the forearm (See also Figure 30.3).

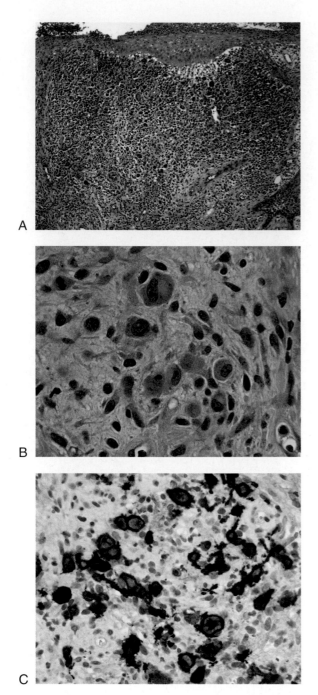

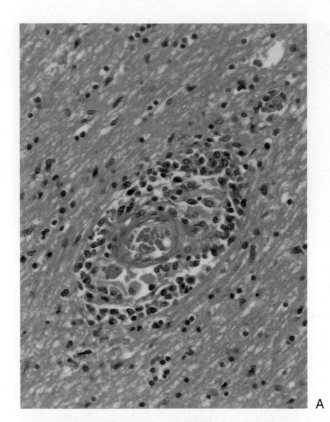

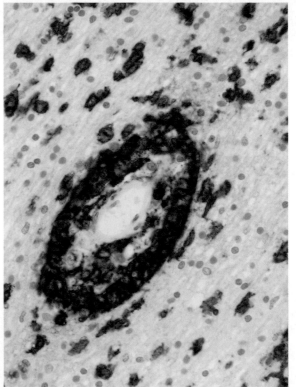

COLOR PLATE 80–82 Histologic features of CD30⁺ CALCL with a diffuse nonepidermotropic infiltrate with cohesive sheets of large atypical lymphocytes. **A:** Numerous inflammatory cells (T cells, eosinophils, and neutrophils) are present (hematoxylin and eosin; original magnification ×200) (See also Figure 30.4A). **B:** The tumor cells have the characteristic morphology of anaplastic cells, showing round, oval, or irregularly shaped nuclei with prominent (eosinophilic) nucleoli and abundant cytoplasm (hematoxylin and eosin; original magnification ×400) (See also Figure 30.4B). **C:** Immunostaining for CD30 antigen produced a strong cytoplasmic membrane staining of the tumor cells (hematoxylin and eosin; original magnification ×400) (See also Figure 30.4C).

COLOR PLATE 83 This blood vessel in the cerebral white matter is cuffed by large, atypical lymphoid cells—a growth pattern characteristic of primary cerebral non-Hodgkin lymphoma (×100). **B:** The same vessel is shown with an immunohistochemical preparation for CD20. Note labeling of nearly all perivascular cells for this B-lymphocyte antigen and the presence of lymphoma cells infiltrating the neural parenchyma (×100) (See also Chapter 36). (Photomicrographs from Dr. Marc Rosenblum, Department of Pathology, Memorial Sloan-Kettering Cancer Center, New York, NY).

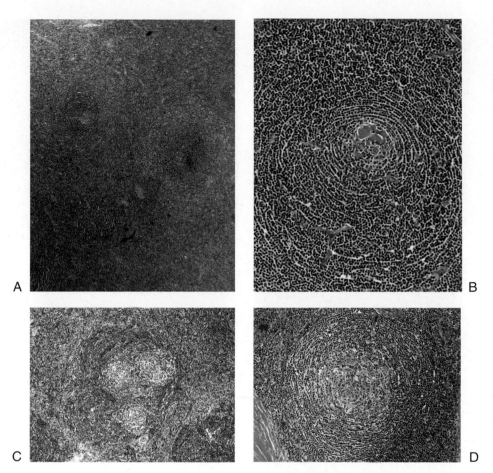

COLOR PLATE 84–87 CD, hyaline vascular variant. **A:** Hyaline vascular variant low-power view with reactive follicles and an interfollicular infiltrate of small lymphoid cells and fibrosis, as well as increased vascularization of the interfollicular region (Figures courtesy of Dr. Ahmet Dogan; reprinted with permission from Dispenzieri A. Castleman disease. Cancer Treat Res. 2008;142:293-330.) (See also Figure 38.1A). **B:** High-power view showing the B-cell follicle with typical expanded mantle zone showing "onion skin" pattern and depleted germinal center with increased vascularity and deposition of hyaline material (Figures courtesy of Dr. Ahmet Dogan.) (See also Figure 38.1B). **C:** Some mantle zones contain two germinal centers ("twinning") (See also Figure 38.1C). **D:** High magnification showing a regressed follicle with increased numbers of follicular dendritic cells and decreased germinal center cells. Note the penetrating blood vessel **(top)**, the so-called "lollipop" follicle (See also Figure 38.1D).

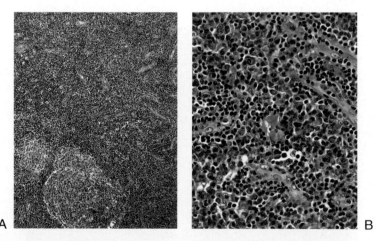

COLOR PLATE 88–89 CD, plasma cell variant. **A:** Plasma cell variant low-power view with small reactive follicles and an interfollicular infiltrate of plasma cells; vascular proliferation is present in the interfollicular region (See also Figure 38.2A). **B:** High-power view showing numerous plasma cells among HEVs. **Lower left corner:** A small part of a reactive follicle (Figures courtesy of Dr. Ahmet Dogan.) (See also Figure 38.2B).

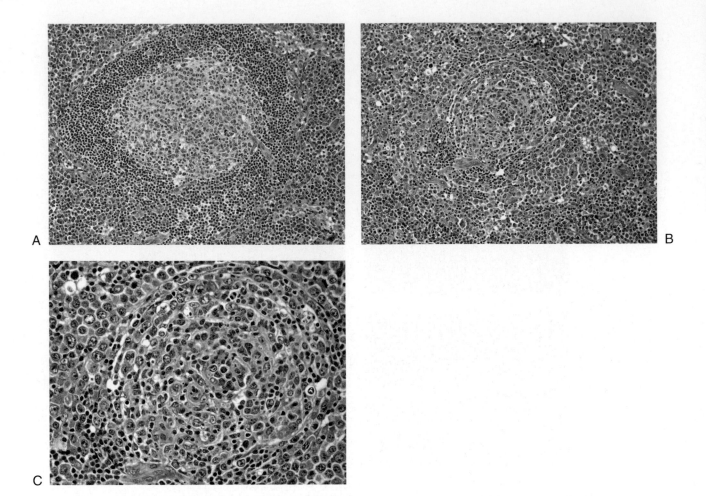

COLOR PLATE 90–92 CD, HHV-8+ multicentric. Reactive follicle surrounded by numerous plasma cells. **A:** Regressed follicle surrounded by plasmablasts (microlymphoma) (See also Figure 38.3A). **B:** Higher magnification of regressed follicle surrounded by plasmablasts (microlymphoma) (See also Figure 38.3B). **C:** Plasmablasts in these cases express λ light chain and contain nuclear HHV-8 LANA (See also Figure 38.3C).

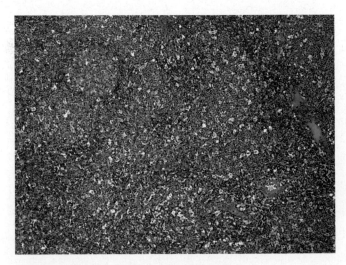

COLOR PLATE 93 ALPS (See also Figure 38.4).

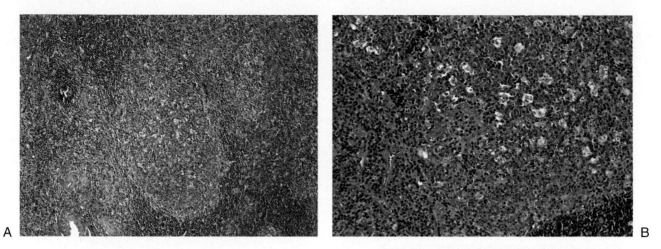

COLOR PLATE 94–95 Kimura disease. **A:** Low magnification showing florid follicular hyperplasia (See also Figure 38.5A). **B:** High magnification showing a follicle with numerous eosinophils (See also Figure 38.5B).

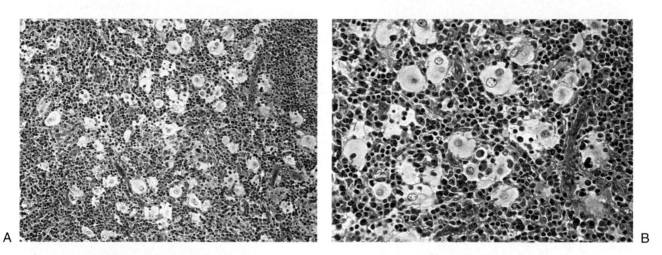

COLOR PLATE 96–97 SHML. **A:** Low magnification (See also Figure 38.6A). **B:** High magnification (See also Figure 38.6B).

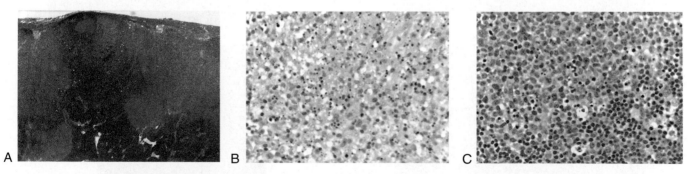

COLOR PLATE 98–100 Kikuchi disease. **A:** Low magnification of a lymph node shows a small reactive follicle and marked paracortical expansion with extensive necrosis (*pink areas*) (hematoxylin and eosin, 2.5×) (See also Figure 38.7A). **B:** Higher magnification of an area of necrosis shows amorphous eosinophilic material with nuclear debris but no neutrophils. Numerous histiocytes are present, many of which have eccentric, crescent-shaped nuclei (hematoxylin and eosin, 40×) (See also Figure 38.7B). **C:** A collection of PDCs is present adjacent to an area of necrosis (hematoxylin and eosin, 40×) (See also Figure 38.7C).

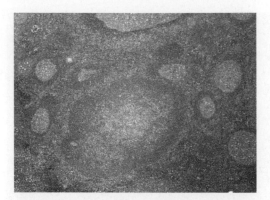

COLOR PLATE 101 PTGC (See also Figure 38.8).

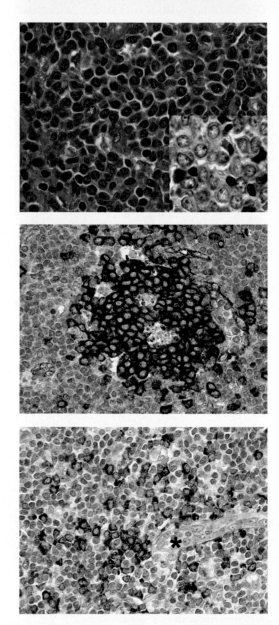

COLOR PLATE 102 PDCs in a large aggregate stained with hematoxylin and eosin (**top**): the cells are slightly larger than lymphocytes, the nucleus is round-oval or indented, chromatin is finely dispersed; note the cytoplasm that stains basophilic on Giemsa (**inset**). PDC may occur as distinct clusters (**middle**) or as scattered cells (**bottom**), and are readily identified using appropriate immunostains, such as anti-CD123 (**middle**) or anti-CD2AP (**bottom**). The *asterisk* (**bottom**) indicates an HEV, typically found in the vicinity of PDC. All images are taken from a reactive lymph node (See also Figure 38.9).

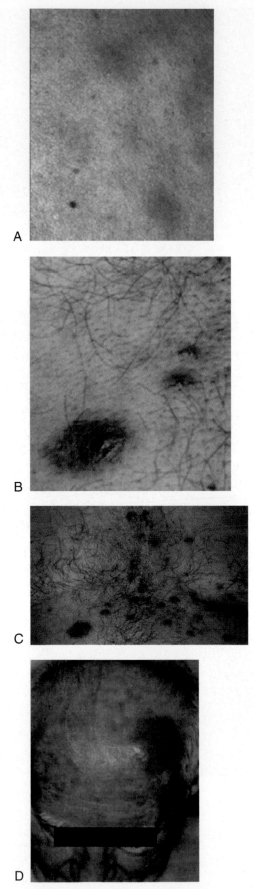

COLOR PLATE 103–106 A–D: Clinical aspects of blastic PDC skin lesions (See also Figure 38.10A–D).

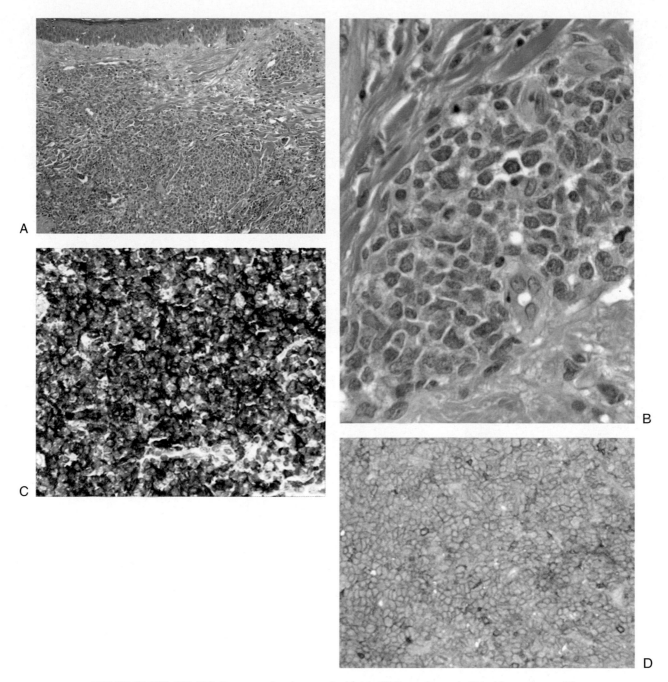

COLOR PLATE 107–110 Cutaneous involvement by blastic PDC neoplasm. **A:** Skin biopsy shows diffuse dermal infiltration and sparing of epidermis with a grenz zone. Cells have finely stippled chromatin (**B**), and are positive for CD56 (**C**), and CD4 (**D**) (See also Figure 38.11A–D).

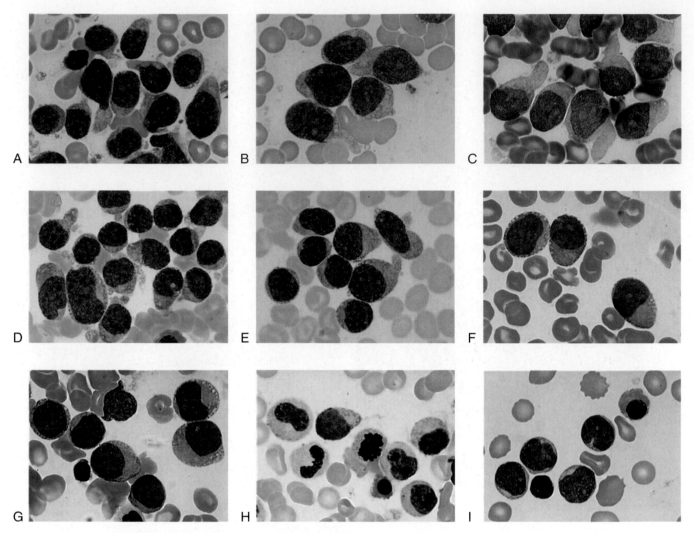

COLOR PLATE 111–119 Cytologic aspects of bone marrow infiltration (189,218). **A–E:** Typical cytologic aspects with pseudopodia-shaped cytoplasmic expansions, vacuoles along the cytoplasmic outline like a pearl necklace, and a blastic appearance of the chromatin (See also Figure 38.12A–E). **F and G:** Correspond to cytologic aspects resembling monoblastic acute leukemia (See also Figure 38.12F,G). **H:** A partial infiltration with features of myelodysplasia (See also Figure 38.12H). **I:** A cytologic aspect resembling those found in high-grade lymphoma (See also Figure 38.12I).

SECTION I ■ HISTORICAL ASPECTS

CHAPTER 1 ■ THE HISTORY OF CHEMOTHERAPY OF LYMPHOMAS

PAUL A. JIMENEZ AND JOSEPH R. BERTINO

ROOTS OF CHEMOTHERAPY

The first attempts to find drugs that are effective against neoplastic diseases are attributed to Paul Ehrlich, "the father of chemotherapy." His major efforts were directed at finding drugs to treat infectious diseases, and he was successful in finding drugs to treat trypanosome infections (Salvarsan) and syphilis (arsphenamine) in 1910. Although effective anticancer drugs were not found, his use of rodent models to screen compounds to treat infectious diseases provided the basis for the pioneering work of Clowes in the early 1900s, who developed inbred rodent lines to bear transplanted tumors. These models were used by Clowes and, subsequently, others to screen for potential anticancer agents.

Although arsenicals, Fowler's solution in particular, were used to treat leukemias and lymphomas in the late 19th century and early 1900s, the usefulness of this treatment was uncertain. It is somewhat ironic that the first effective agent to treat lymphoma was derived from the development of poisonous gases that were designed to kill and injure soldiers in World War I. Mustard gas, di-(2-chloroethyl) sulfide, not only had local tissue-damaging effects but also was found to have systemic effects on the marrow and gastrointestinal tract. The realization that this compound had effects on cell division led investigators in the 1930s to study its effects on experimental tumors and in man (1,2). This sulfur mustard was soon abandoned for clinical use because of its poor therapeutic index and the difficulties that were experienced in handling it.

World War II (1939 to 1945) again stimulated the search for compounds for chemical warfare, and attention was focused on a nitrogen mustard, tri-(2-chlorethyl)amine hydrochloride, which was synthesized by Ward (3) in 1935. During the war, this compound and other nitrogen mustards were actively investigated at Yale Medical School, the Army Chemical Center in Edgewood, Maryland, and in Oxford, England, and at the Sloan-Kettering Institute(4).

The beginnings of modern chemotherapy may be attributed to the remarkable tumor response of the first patient who was treated with a nitrogen mustard at Yale, New Haven Hospital, in 1942, although this treatment was not reported until 1946 (5) because of wartime security. This clinical trial was based on experiments in transplanted lymphosarcoma in mice by Dougherty and Gardner at Yale, which showed that the nitrogen mustards caused rapid disappearance of these tumors, albeit transiently. The following is a description of the first patient who was treated with nitrogen mustard (6).

At New Haven, when favorable results in animals with tumors of lymphoid tissue were reported, Dr. Alfred Gilman, in charge of the work there on the nitrogen mustards, decided to attempt control of similar tumors in man. A suitable case was made available by Dr. Gustaf Lindskog. This unfortunate patient had an extensive lymphosarcoma infiltrating widely the tissue of the neck and the mediastinum as well as the other lymphoid organs of the body. The tumor was said to have become wholly resistant to the therapeutic effects of x-rays. Because of its rapid growth, the trachea was rapidly being compressed below a point where a tracheostomy could be done, to an extent which bade fair to strangle the patient. With the permission and complete understanding on the part of the subject, an amount of nitrogen mustard was administered by vein, which if given on a similar weight basis to an animal, would have resulted in dissolution of a similar cellular structure. The mass in the neck melted away. Breathing became easier once more. Lymph nodes and spleen became smaller in size, but the effect on the bone marrow was extreme. Lymphopenia, leucopenia, granulocytopenia ensued, with severe and intractable purpura, and eventual aplastic anemia requiring repeated transfusions. The bone marrow depression was transient, however, and disappeared within a few weeks. No further treatment was given: the tumor grew again and eventually terminated the life of the patient. A new fact had been established, however. A chemical compound was at hand which would affect adversely and cause dissolution of a lymphoid neoplasm reputedly resistant to x-rays.

Several other patients were treated, but the trials were put on hold when Gilman and his associates entered military service, and continued their research on nitrogen mustards at the Edgewood Arsenal Laboratories. In a prescient statement in his review in 1947, Rhoads commented: "It is wholly possible that chemotherapeutic substances specifically destructive to one of the other forms of cancer tissue might be developed. There is at least ample precedent for this possibility. Time only will tell whether the public wished to have this sort of work done."

Following this lead, a Committee on Atypical Growth was established during wartime by the National Research Council, and work to establish these chemicals as therapeutic agents in civilian medicine was assigned to three institutions: the Memorial Hospital in New York, the Billings Hospital of the University of Chicago, and the Medical School of the University of Utah at Salt Lake. These investigators studied more than 150 patients and confirmed the antitumor activity of the nitrogen mustards in patients with Hodgkin disease and in patients with other lymphomas (7,8).

These observations were soon confirmed by others (9) and, after the end of the war, stimulated extensive research on alkylating agents as anticancer agents. For example, Burchenal et al. (10,11) tested more than 50 different nitrogen mustards against mouse leukemias; Haddow (12), at the Chester Beaty Institute, synthesized aromatic nitrogen mustards and sulphonic acid esters against the Walker 256 carcinosarcoma in the rat and discovered busulfan, which was used to treat chronic myelocytic leukemia for many years and is still in clinical use as part of transplant regimens for leukemia. At approximately the same time that nitrogen mustards were being tested, Dougherty and White (13) reported that adrenocorticotropic hormone caused lymphoid tissue to atrophy. This observation was followed by the report of Heilman and Kendall (14), in 1944, who showed that compound E (cortisone) treatment regressed lymphosarcoma in mice. When adrenocorticotropic hormone and cortisone became available for clinical use in 1949–1950, these drugs also proved to cause regressions in patients with lymphomas (15,16); however, similar to nitrogen mustard treatment, in most patients, these regressions were short lived. Other derivatives of cortisone were tested over the next 2 decades, thus leading to the discovery of other more potent corticosteroids, including prednisone and dexamethasone, which are now widely used in the clinic.

By the end of the 1940s, the demonstration that regressions could be obtained with nitrogen mustard and cortisone, together with the development of folate antagonists for the treatment of childhood leukemia (17), accelerated the search for additional anticancer drugs. The National Cancer Institute's (NCI's) Drug Development program was initiated and included large-scaling screening for anticancer drugs by using transplanted mouse tumors.

PRINCIPLES OF CHEMOTHERAPY

An important concept regarding human tumors is that growth is not exponential by nature, rather it follows a gompertzian model, a sigmoidal curve, in which the growth fraction reaches a maximum at approximately 30% of its tumor volume, then decreases with time. The slowing of the growth of tumor is due in part to hypoxia, decreased availability of nutrients, accumulation of toxic metabolites, and inhibitory cell-to-cell communication (18). In the growth curve, 1×10^9 cells represent the smallest number of cells required to be clinically detectable. This measurement is also equivalent to a mass of 1 cm in diameter on a chest x-ray film or by breast examination. Tumors with 10^{12} or 10^{13} cells usually result in damage to vital organs and death of the patient. The Gompertzian model suggests that the tumor's response to chemotherapy depends on the location of its growth curve with greater sensitivity along the mid portion of the curve—the best place to initiate drug therapy.

A major problem in cancer therapeutics is the development of drug resistance. Luria and Delbrück (19) pioneered the first experiments on drug resistance with their studies on bacteriophages during the 1940s. They discovered that some bacterial strains harbored mutants before exposure to the virus, which were selected after bacteriophage infection leading to resistance. A decade later, Law (20) also discovered the same pattern in the resistance of leukemia cells to methotrexate, i.e., the drug selected for preexistent mutants. In 1979, Goldie and Coldman (21) applied this principle to develop a mathematical model that predicted the mutation rate of a tumor. Its mutation properties were intrinsic to its genetic instability, which occurred in 1 to 1,000 and 1 million cells. These discoveries set forth the principles of modern medical oncology to treat most malignancies during the early stages with synergistic combinations of chemotherapy to prevent drug resistance. However, combination chemotherapy used simultaneously posed the problem of overlapping toxicities or competitive interference. Coldman and Goldie (22) thus proposed the administration of these drugs in an alternating sequence based on several assumptions of symmetry, i.e., two different cell populations would have similar characteristics of drug sensitivities, mutation rates, and growth rates or patterns. As an example, if a practitioner were to use two different drugs A and B, their administration could follow the pattern of ABABAB distributed in several weeks. Day (23) and Norton and Day (24), on the other hand, suggested a sequential approach in which the full course of one drug is completed before commencement of another drug as in AAABBB. They predicted that the sequential approach would outperform alternating cycles because the earlier hypotheses proposed by Coldman and Goldie (22) were unrealistic for the practical application of chemotherapy—no two combinations were likely to be strictly noncross-resistant or have equal cell-killing capacity. These two approaches were compared in a prospective randomized trial of intravenous cyclophosphamide, methotrexate, fluorouracil and doxorubicin in patients with high-risk breast cancer in Milan during the early 1980s. At a median follow-up of 59 months, the 5-year relapsefree survival was significantly superior for the sequential method at 61% compared with its alternating counterpart at 38% ($p = 0.001$) (25).

Another important principle is that chemotherapeutic agents could be classified as cycle active or noncycle active. The latter were the alkylating agents, nitrosoureas and radiation therapy, whereas cycle-active drugs were drugs such as methotrexate, which did not affect resting or G_0 cells. In a series of experiments in lymphoma cells, Bruce et al. (26) demonstrated that the noncycle-active agents were less schedule dependent than the cycle-active drugs, thus total dose rather than schedule was important. The increased sensitivity of spleen lymphoma colonies to cycle-active drugs compared with normal hematopoietic splenic colonies was explained by the idea that all of the lymphoma cells were in *cycle*, whereas an appreciable number of normal colony forming cells were temporarily out of cycle (G_0) and not affected by cell cycle-active agents. These experiments provided a rationale for the use of high doses of cycle-active drugs delivered in an intermittent fashion. One of the first combinations that was explored for the treatment of Hodgkin disease was the combination of vinblastine and chlorambucil. Lacher and Durant (27) treated patients with weekly vinblastine and daily chlorambucil. In this small series, ten of 16 patients had excellent responses, and three others had partial responses, lasting 1 to 2 years, but no long-term remissions were noted.

HODGKIN DISEASE

Radiation Therapy: Evidence that a Cure was Possible

After the description of Hodgkin disease in 1832 by Thomas Hodgkin, various systemic remedies were tried in the ensuing decades, including arsenicals and iodides. When radiation therapy became available in the early 1900s, the treatment of all stages of Hodgkin disease was radiation therapy because the arsenicals were considered to have minimal effectiveness. Until the 1950s, it was believed that Hodgkin disease was not curable despite the sensitivity of this tumor to irradiation. The early studies of Gilbert (28) elaborated the principles of radiation treatment of Hodgkin disease, namely to treat all involved areas with the highest dose possible, and to treat adjacent areas as well. Using these guidelines, Peters and Middlemiss (29) reported that a small percentage of patients with limited disease could be cured, if the involved nodes with contiguous areas were treated. Reports from Easson and Russell (30) also indicated that early stage disease was curable, thus setting the stage for the definitive work of Kaplan (31) at Stanford. Kaplan (31) used supervoltage irradiation to show that it was possible to irradiate involved lymph nodes to tumoricidal levels as well as to treat contiguous lymph node areas with large fields, such as "mantle" and "inverted Y," as well as "total nodal" irradiation. The result was the cure of early stage (stage I and II) Hodgkin disease in the majority of patients (31).

Single-Agent Chemotherapy

Cyclophosphamide

The synthesis of cyclophosphamide, a cyclic nitrogen mustard phosphamide ester, was described first by Arnold et al. (32a) in 1958. The attachment of a phosphoryl group to nitrogen mustard reduced the chemical activity of the parent compound. This process rendered the overall compound chemically inert until activated by cells containing enzymes found to be in increased amounts in cancerous cells such as phosphoamidases and phosphatases (32). A larger study on 66 patients with generalized "reticulum cell sarcoma" suggested an objective regression of disease in 42% of patients, with a median remission of more than 4 months (33).

Steroids

The use of steroids in the treatment of malignant tumors was inspired by the interpretation of Albright (34) regarding the pathophysiology of Cushing syndrome. The loss of body protoplasm due to adrenal cortical hyperfunction was interpreted as a failure in tissue production rather than destruction. In 1943, Dougherty and White (13) demonstrated that the increased adrenal cortical function in mice caused atrophy in normal lymphoid tissues, and in the following year, Heilman and Kendall (14) reported that administration of compound E caused regression of transplanted lymphoid tumor in mice. In addition, studies by Dobriner et al. (35) suggested an association between steroid metabolism and neoplastic diseases through the excretion of urinary steroids in patients with cancer. Corticosteroids were first tested in human subjects with lymphoma by Pearson et al. (36) in 1949. Adrenocorticotropic hormone and cortisone acetate were administered in seven patients with different malignancies, including chronic lymphocytic leukemia, Hodgkin disease, follicular lymphosarcoma, and prostate and breast cancer. Among those patients with lymphomatous tumors, there was a dramatic and progressive decrease in the size of enlarged lymph nodes and spleen (36).

Vinca Alkaloids

The discovery of vinca alkaloids, extracted from the periwinkle plant (*Catharanthus roseus*, formerly *Vinca rosea*), in the early 1960s proved to be an important advancement in the use of chemotherapy for Hodgkin disease. Before experimental studies, the periwinkle plant was used as indigenous medicine in various parts of the world, including the treatment of diabetes in the Philippines (37). This folklore led to the investigation of its hypoglycemic properties. Although the treatment for diabetes could not be substantiated, the laboratories at the University of Western Ontario observed granulocytopenia and bone marrow depression in experimental mice (38). Further investigations led to the discovery of various alkaloids, including vinblastine and vincristine. Both of these compounds were found to prolong life or cure experimental mice transplanted with a specific strain of acute lymphocytic leukemia (P-1534) (39). These vinca alkaloids were found to act as antimicrotubule agents, arresting cells in metaphase.

Early Trials in Hodgkin Disease

The first study that showed the successful use of sequential chemotherapy in the management of Hodgkin disease was published in 1963 by Scott (40). Induction chemotherapy with nitrogen mustard was used in 89 patients with advanced Hodgkin disease. Thereafter, randomization with no treatment versus maintenance therapy with the alkylating agent, chlorambucil, was administered in 40 patients shown to have a relatively successful induction response. The time to relapse was significantly different in patients who received chlorambucil with an average of 35 weeks compared with 12 weeks for the placebo group (40).

In 1968, a randomized trial of two combined clinical cooperative groups (Acute Leukemia B and the Eastern Solid Tumor Group) reported that vinblastine was superior to cyclophosphamide for remission induction in patients with Hodgkin disease, whereas cyclophosphamide was more effective than vincristine for remission induction for patients with non-Hodgkin lymphoma (41). Another conclusion from this study was that patients who had a complete remission had longer response durations than patients with partial responses. In the 1950s and early 1960s, a large number of other drugs were tested for anticancer activity in the clinic and were found to cause regression in patients with Hodgkin disease, but the corticosteroids, nitrogen mustards, the vincas, and procarbazine emerged as the most promising of these drugs. Table 1.1 lists the drugs that were found effective as single agents in the 1950s and early 1960s for the treatment of Hodgkin disease (42).

Combination Chemotherapy

Although the single chemotherapeutic agents produced significant tumor shrinkage, they rarely caused complete remissions. In addition, although patients with early stage Hodgkin disease responded well to radiation therapy, patients with higher stages had lower survival rates. As previously described in the comparative study with cyclophosphamide and vinca alkaloids, the achievement of a complete remission became an important goal for future studies. The

TABLE 1.1

SINGLE AGENTS THAT WERE FOUND TO BE EFFECTIVE IN THE TREATMENT OF HODGKIN'S DISEASE IN THE 1950s AND EARLY 1960s.

Alkylating agents
Nitrogen mustard
Trenimon
Degranol
Mannitol mustard
N-Formyl sarcolysine

Antimetabolites
6-Mercaptopurine
Cytosine arabinoside
5-Fluorouridine
Methotrexate

Antibiotics
Actinomycin C and D
Streptonigrin
Aurantin
Vinca alkaloids
Vinblastine
Vincristine

Miscellaneous agents
Methylglyoxal-bisguanylhydrazone
Desacetyl methylcolchine
Procarbazine

Adapted from Hall TC. New chemotherapeutic agents in Hodgkin's disease. *Cancer Res* 1966;26:1297–1302.

concepts derived from the experimental studies of Skipper (12a) were used by Freireich et al. (43) to develop combination chemotherapy programs to treat childhood leukemia, which led to increased complete remissions and duration of remissions and initial evidence that a cure could be obtained in this disease. Thus, the next logical step was to use combination chemotherapy in Hodgkin lymphoma.

A pilot study in 1963 by the researchers at the NCI tested the feasibility of combination chemotherapy in Hodgkin lymphoma. Moxley et al. (44) used the combination of mechlorethamine, vincristine, methotrexate, and prednisone in full doses followed by radiation therapy to investigate its use in Hodgkin disease. Vincristine was selected as the vinca alkaloid of choice because it showed less marrow toxicity than vinblastine. The study enrolled 14 patients ages 21 to 50 with predominantly stage II and III disease with a mean duration therapy of 2.3 months. Twelve of the 14 patients had rapid remission of the disease defined as absence of all detectable disease, including systemic signs and symptoms. The complete remission induction rate was 86%. Nine of the 12 patients remained in diseasefree remission at 3 years' follow-up (44).

Clinical studies of conventional doses of methotrexate by Frei et al. (45) showed that the drug had only marginal activity in the treatment of lymphomas. When it was shown that a new methylhydrazine derivative, procarbazine, was an active drug for the treatment of Hodgkin disease, Devita et al. (46) substituted this drug for methotrexate, thus formulating a new drug combination consisting of mechlorethamine, vincristine, procarbazine, and prednisone, otherwise known as MOPP.

This benchmark study, published in the *Ann Intern Med*, followed 43 patients with advanced Hodgkin disease stage III and IV from 1964 to 1967 treated with MOPP for 6 months. The response rate was highly encouraging with 35 of 43, or 81% of the patients achieving a complete remission, and 55% of these patients remained disease free at 5 years, thus raising, for the first time, the possibility of a cure of advanced Hodgkin disease (46). Studies from other institutions duplicated these results and confirmed that many patients with advanced Hodgkin disease could be cured with MOPP chemotherapy (47,48). During the next decade, many variations of MOPP were tried, including the substitution of cyclophosphamide for nitrogen mustard (cyclophosphamide, vincristine, procarbazine, and prednisone), the substitution of vinblastine for vincristine (mechlorethamine, vinblastine, procarbazine, and prednisone), or the addition of bleomycin (bleomycin, MOPP). None of these combinations produced superior complete remission rates or improved survival (49). Intensive chemotherapy with nitrogen mustard as a single agent was compared with MOPP chemotherapy by Hugeley et al. (50); nitrogen mustard produced complete remissions in only three of 23 patients.

Combined Modality Therapy: Chemotherapy and Radiation

The Yale program used three cycles of a combination of drugs that included nitrogen mustard, prednisone, and vincristine, followed by vinblastine and procarbazine, thus predating the concept of the use of sequential combinations. The rationale was to use an alkylating drug first to decrease the tumor mass, to convert the tumor-to-log phase growth, and, thus, to increase the sensitivity to antimetabolites. In addition, low-dose radiation was added to all known sites of disease after completion of chemotherapy. Like MOPP, the complete remission rate with this program was approximately 80%, however, this study was important in that it showed that the addition of low-dose radiation therapy after 6 months of chemotherapy resulted in an improvement in the percentage of patients who remained in a relapsefree remission (51). Other studies that compared MOPP alone with MOPP plus full-dose radiotherapy in patients with stage IV disease did not show any survival advantage with the addition of x-rays (52).

Development of an Effective, Less Toxic Combination: Doxorubicin (Adriamycin), Bleomycin, Vinblastine, and Dacarbazine (ABVD)

In the early 1970s, several other drugs were shown to have significant activity in Hodgkin disease, namely, bleomycin, dacarbazine, and doxorubicin. Bleomycin, which was isolated from the fungus *Streptomyces verticillus* by Umezawa et al. (53) in Japan, is a mixture of small molecular weight peptides that allows binding to deoxyribonucleic acid and subsequent strand breaks. This drug was of interest in that it caused regressions in patients with lymphoma with minimal marrow toxicity (54). The anthracyclines, doxorubicin (adriamycin), and daunomycin were antibiotics that were also produced by the *Streptomyces* species, and doxorubicin was shown to have a broad spectrum of activity against solid tumors as well as lymphomas (55,56).

Although MOPP therapy became the standard regimen for Hodgkin disease, there was still room for improvement. About 20% of patients treated with MOPP did not have complete remissions, and about 40% of those patients that initially responded relapsed within the first 5 years from the end of the treatment cycle (57). Thus, a search for a better drug combination was instigated by researchers at the Instituto Nationale Tumori in Milan, Italy. This four-drug regimen used new drugs that were not present in MOPP. These drugs included doxorubicin (adriamycin), bleomycin, vinblastine, and dacarbazine (ABVD). A randomized trial compared the efficacy of ABVD with MOPP chemotherapy in terms of complete induction remission. A total of 60 patients, 30 in each treatment group, with advanced Hodgkin disease stage III–IV were entered into the study in 1973 to 1974. Assessment of the results for complete remission utilized the skeletal survey, liver scan, and a bone marrow biopsy. Complete remissions occurred in 76% of patients treated with MOPP and 75% of patients treated with ABVD. In addition, crossover data for remission induction in five patients showed absence of cross-resistance between MOPP and ABVD. The conclusion from this study indicated that in terms of complete remission, ABVD could be used as an alternative to MOPP or in sequential combination with MOPP (57).

Over the next several years, clinicians investigated the use of alternating cyclical noncross-resistant chemotherapy such as MOPP and ABVD or MOPP and Cyclophosphamide, Adriamycin, bleomycin, and streptozocin (CABS), but the definitive study was published in 1992 by the Cancer and Acute Leukemia Group (58). In a randomized multicenter trial, 361 patients with advanced Hodgkin disease stages III and IV were divided into three groups: (a) MOPP alone, (b) MOPP alternating with ABVD, and (c) ABVD alone. Overall survival (OS) at 5 years was 66% for MOPP, 73% for ABVD, and 75% for MOPP-ABVD. The conclusion from the trial was that ABVD was just as effective as the alternating cycle of MOPP and ABVD, and that both were superior to MOPP alone. In addition, ABVD proved to be less carcinogenic and to have less antifertility effects than MOPP (59). In the 1990s, it replaced MOPP as first-line treatment for advanced Hodgkin disease. At a median follow-up of 14 years, Canellos et al. (58) reported the results of long-term follow-up of the patients enrolled in the trial. Although there was a significant difference in the failurefree survival distributions ($p = 0.03$), a difference was not seen in the OS distributions ($p = 0.35$). The patients treated with MOPP had 60 events, those treated with ABVD had 47 events, and those treated with MOPP alternating with ABVD had 47 events.

A New Regimen: Bleomycin, Etoposide, Adriamycin, Cyclophosphamide, Vincristine, Procarbazine, Prednisone

In 1992, the German Hodgkin Study Group developed the bleomycin, etoposide, adriamycin, cyclophosphamide, vincristine, procarbazine, prednisone (BEACOPP) regimen to attempt to further improve the rate of failurefree and OS for patients with advanced Hodgkin disease. Three different prospective randomized clinical trials (HD 9, HD 12, HD 15) were implemented to develop a regimen with maximal efficacy and least toxicity. In the three-armed HD 9 trial, dose-escalated and baseline BEACOPP regimens were compared with adriamycin, vincristine, procarbazine, prednisone /ABVD in 1,186 patients with advanced-stage Hodgkin lymphoma. At a median observation time of 7 years, escalated BEACOPP showed superior results in the rate for freedom from treatment failure (FFTF) and OS. Although the death rate due to treatment-induced toxicity was lower in the escalated BEACOPP arm compared with the adriamycin, vincristine, procarbazine, prednisone /ABVD arm, there was a higher number of secondary AML/MDS in the escalated BEACOPP arm. Thus, in an effort to reduce the risk of other hematologic disorders, subsequent trials were designed to compare escalated BEACOPP to de-escalated variations in terms of efficacy and toxicity. In the HD 12 trial, eight cycles of escalated BEACOPP was compared with four escalated and four baseline cycles. The results for FFTF and OS were similar: for the group getting eight cycles of escalated BEACOPP, FFTF: 90% and OS: 96%, whereas the group getting the combined escalated/baseline cycles, FFTF: 88% and OS: 94%. The rate of secondary AML/MDS was, at the same time point of observation, only half of that in the HD 9 study. In the current HD 15 trial, eight courses of escalated BEACOPP are compared with six courses of escalated BEACOPP or eight courses of the baseline BEACOPP given in 14-day intervals (BEACOPP-14) instead of the usual 21 days. Consolidative radiation therapy was given based on positron emission tomography scan positivity (60).

NON-HODGKIN LYMPHOMA

The response to treatment of lymphomas other than Hodgkin disease is related to the type of the lymphoma, and, as the recognition of the many types of non-Hodgkin lymphomas has evolved, the role of chemotherapy to treat these lymphomas has been more delineated. Fortunately, like Hodgkin disease, non-Hodgkin lymphoma proved to be a chemosensitive tumor.

As in Hodgkin disease, until the introduction of chemotherapy in the clinic in the late 1940s, the only treatment available for patients with non-Hodgkin lymphomas was palliative radiation therapy (31,61). When effective agents became available (alkylating agents, corticosteroids, and vincristine), single-agent chemotherapy was used only after radiation failure, except for patients with stage IV disease(62). Until the mid 1960s, the most widely used histologic classification of non-Hodgkin lymphomas included three major groups: reticulum cell sarcoma, lymphosarcoma, and giant follicular lymphomas (63). The classification of Rappaport et al. (64), which was described first in 1956 and later formalized in 1966 (65), considered pattern (nodular or diffuse) and differentiation (poorly or well-differentiated lymphocyte, histiocytic, or a mixture of the two) in defining categories of lymphoma. This classification was used to ascertain the relationship between the histopathologic category of lymphoma and the results of single agent chemotherapy by Jones et al. (66) in 1972. In this seminal study, it was found that patient with nodular lymphomas (now known as follicular lymphoma) had a higher response rate and longer survival after chemotherapy (alkylating agents or vincristine) than patients with diffuse histiocytic lymphoma (now known as *diffuse large B-cell lymphoma*). Furthermore, patients with follicular lymphomas that were composed of large cells (nodular histiocytic in the Rappaport classification, now known as grade-4 follicular lymphoma) had a shorter survival than patients with follicular lymphomas that were composed of small cells (poorly differentiated lymphocytic, now known as *grade-1 or -2 follicular lymphoma*).

Chemotherapy in Follicular Lymphomas

With the availability of three effective agents, cyclophosphamide, prednisone, and vincristine, to treat non-Hodgkin lymphoma, trials of this combination were initiated in the 1960s. These phase II trials demonstrated the effectiveness of this combination for follicular lymphomas, but they were less effective for diffuse large cell lymphoma (66,67). Surprisingly, when tested in a randomized trial against single-agent alkylating therapy (chlorambucil) in patients with follicular lymphomas, this combination did not prove to be better than single-agent treatment in regards to the response rate or to survival (68,69). Although the complete remission rate was higher in the combined chemotherapy group than in chlorambucil alone (83% vs. 74%), the overall response rate was the same for both groups, and there was no survival advantage. Neither groups resulted in a high proportion of complete remissions. Complete remissions were short and no longer than good partial remissions.

What was also clear from these studies was that were was no plateau in the survival curve, and patients with follicular lymphomas that were composed of predominantly small cells continued to relapse with time. Clinical and pathologic staging of these patients, including the use of staging laparotomies (70,71), showed that the follicular lymphomas were almost always disseminated at presentation, and chemotherapy was not curative. In the 5% to 10% of patients that had stage I disease, radiation therapy could be curative (72).

Another unique feature of follicular lymphomas was revealed by reports that indicated that many patients with this disease had indolent courses, and delay of therapy did not impact on survival. The concept of observation without treatment or expectant management for follicular lymphoma is supported by randomized trials. The first trial designed by the NCI randomized patients to receive either combined chemotherapy or observation alone. Eventually, however, the observed group was administered prednisone, methotrexate, doxorubicin, cyclophosphamide, and epipodophyllotoxin VP-16 (ProMACE)-MOPP as indicated. The analysis showed that early introduction of chemotherapy did not have a survival advantage over observation alone. At 5 years' follow-up, 75% of patients in each group were alive (73). The second trial from the Groupe d'Etude des Lymphomes de l'Adulte in France and Belgium randomized 193 patients with newly diagnosed follicular lymphomas into three arms: arm 1, no initial treatment; arm 2, prednimustine; or arm 3, interferon alpha. Overall response rates with prednimustine and interferon alpha were 78% and 70%, respectively. OS at 5 years was similar in the three arms: 78% in arm 1, 70% in arm 2, and 84% in arm 3 (74). A recent study supporting this concept was from the British National Lymphoma Investigation, which randomized patients to observation alone versus immediate treatment with chlorambucil. At a median follow-up of 16 years, there was no significant difference in OS between the two patient groups (75).

Development of Curative Combination Regimens for Diffuse Histiocytic Lymphoma

Although single chemotherapeutic agents were shown to produce tumor regression in 50% to 70% of patients with malignant lymphoma, only 10% to 20% of patients achieved a complete remission (62). In 1971, the Southwest Cancer Chemotherapy Study Group published an article in *Cancer* that investigated the use of combination chemotherapy in the treatment of lymphomas (76). James et al (76) used a combination of cyclophosphamide, vincristine, and prednisone (COP) on 262 patients with disseminated Hodgkin disease, lymphosarcoma, reticulum cell sarcoma, and follicular lymphomas. The results showed a complete remission in 36% of patients with Hodgkin disease, 50% of patients with lymphosarcoma, and 39% of patients with reticulum cell sarcoma. A comparison made between patients who received COP versus single agents showed a significantly superior survival advantage among patients who received the combination therapy (76).

Two important studies that used new combinations of drugs provided the first indication that diffuse large cell lymphomas could be cured with combination chemotherapy. The Yale group used a five-drug program sequencing cyclophosphamide-vincristine followed by weekly methotrexate-cytosine arabinoside and leucovorin rescue. The regimen was administered in 15 patients with advanced reticulum cell sarcoma. Nine patients achieved complete remission, whereas six had a partial response. When the results were reexamined using the Rappaport Classification, it was found that six of the eight patients who were classified as having diffuse histiocytic lymphoma had complete remissions and that five of these patients were still in remission 5 to 6 years after treatment, thus raising the possibility that diffuse large cell lymphoma could be cured by combination chemotherapy (77). Other studies confirmed the activity of this combination for diffuse large cell lymphoma (78). The NCI investigators used regimens that were shown to be effective for the treatment of Hodgkin disease (MOPP and C-MOPP), and of the 45% of patients who achieved a complete remission, 70% had an extended survival (79).

Then in the early 1970s, doxorubicin, an antitumor antibiotic of the anthracycline group, was found to be highly active in the treatment of non-Hodgkin lymphoma. When used as a single agent, doxorubicin was capable of producing responses in 30% of patients with refractory lymphocytic and histiocytic disease. Following these results, the Southwest Oncology Group (SWOG) incorporated doxorubicin in combination with COP (CHOP) in the treatment of stage III and stage IV non-Hodgkin lymphoma. Among 204 patients treated, there were 71% complete remissions with 92% overall responses (80).

Miller and Jones (81) were among the earliest investigators to use the CHOP regimen in the treatment of early stage lymphomas. In the study, 45 patients with stage I or II non-Hodgkin lymphoma, 41 of whom were diagnosed with the diffuse histiocytic type, were divided into two groups: CHOP alone or CHOP followed by radiotherapy. Forty-two patients (93%) remained alive, and 38 patients (84%) remained continuously free of disease with a median follow-up time of 41 months. There was no statistically significant difference found in survival and relapsefree survival between the two groups (81).

Following the initial success of the trials for the first-generation regimen, CHOP, the SWOG conducted other trials with CHOP based regimens: CHOP-bleomycin and CHOP-BCG in patients with aggressive lymphomas between 1974 and 1981. The complete remission rates for aggressive non-Hodgkin lymphoma varied from 44% to 61%, and that of diffuse large cell lymphoma from 58% to 62% (82–84). Coltman et al. (85), however, extended the follow-up to 12 years among 418 patients. The rate of complete remission was 53%, and the survival rate was only 30%—a value lower than the previous studies. Obviously, there was a need to improve on the results achieved with the CHOP regimen. Thus, during the 1970s and 1980s, several large lymphoma-referral centers developed second-generation and third-generation regimens by incorporating additional chemotherapeutic drugs not part of the original CHOP, e.g., methotrexate with leucovorin rescue, bleomycin, and etoposide. Initially, each of these centers reported complete remission rates of 70% to 85% and predicted long-term survival of 55% to 65% (86).

However, there were several criticisms raised regarding the validity of these studies. First, there was unequal comparison between the results of the new generation drugs with the historical data of the standard CHOP. The study populations were diverse with multiple important prognostic factors that could contribute to different responses to chemotherapy and, thus, different survival. Second, the duration of the follow-up periods made a substantial difference in the results for remission and survival. For example, long-term survival after treatment with ProMACE-MOPP (87) fell from 65% to 50% after 9 years of follow-up (88). Survival among patients treated with MACOP-B (94) fell from 76% to 65% (94). Third, succeeding phase II trials conducted by other single institutions and cooperative groups have reported lower rates of complete remission and survival (89–93).

In the mid 1980s to early 1990s, the SWOG and the Eastern Cooperative Oncology Group initiated a prospective, randomized phase III trial to compare CHOP against m-BACOD, ProMACE-CytaBOM, and MACOP-B. The study consisted of 899 eligible patients with intermediate-grade or high-grade non-Hodgkin lymphoma with at least 218 patients in each of the four treatment groups. The median ages of the groups ranged from 54 to 57 years. Most importantly, there were no differences in prognostic factors of bone marrow involvement, bulky disease, and high concentrations of lactate dehydrogenase. The results showed no significant differences in the rates of objective, partial, or complete responses, the curves for the time to treatment failure, or the estimated OS (50% at 3 years in the ProMACE-CytaBOM and MACOP-B groups, 52% in the m-BACOD group, and 54% in the CHOP group). However, the incidence of serious toxicity in relation to granulocytopenia and subsequent infections did differ significantly among the groups. Fatal toxic reactions occurred in 1% of the CHOP group, 3% of the ProMACE-CytaBOM group, 5% of the m-BACOD group, and 6% of the MACOP-B group. However, when the fatal and life-threatening reactions were combined, significant differences were found, with CHOP and ProMACE-CytaBOM being less toxic than m-BACOD and MACOP-B ($p = 0.001$). In addition, the cost of CHOP was the least expensive among the four treatment groups. To this date, CHOP remains the best available treatment for patients with advanced-stage, intermediate-grade, or high-grade non-Hodgkin lymphoma (94).

Rituximab

In 1997, rituximab (marketed as Rituxan) became the first monoclonal antibody approved for the treatment of cancer in the United States when approval was obtained for the treatment of relapsed or refractory low-grade or follicular, CD20+, B-cell non-Hodgkin lymphoma. Rituximab is a chimeric human-mouse anti-CD20 monoclonal antibody against cell-surface antigen CD20 expressed on more than 90% of B-cell lymphomas and chronic lymphocytic leukemias, and on 50% of pre-B-cell acute lymphoblastic leukemia (95–97). The success for its targeted therapy is that unlike other transmembrane proteins, the CD20 antigen does not shed, modulate, or internalize (98). In addition, it is specific to B-cells and not expressed on stem cells, plasma cells, or other cell lineages (97).

The pivotal trial that led to its Food and Drug Administration approval in November 1997 was based on a single-arm, multicenter trial of 166 patients with relapsed low-grade or follicular lymphoma. The overall response rate for the intent to treat group of all 166 patients was 48%, of which 6% were complete responders and the remainder partial responders. All patients were treated in an outpatient setting (99).

An earlier phase II trial of rituximab in combination with CHOP enrolled 33 patients with previously untreated advanced aggressive B-cell non-Hodgkin lymphoma. The overall response rate was 94%, which consisted of 61% complete responders and 33% partial responders. The most frequent adverse events attributed to rituximab were fever and chills, primarily during the first infusion (100). One of the definitive studies was published in the *N Engl J Med* in 2002, whereby the Groupe d'Etude des Lymphomes de l'Adulte group undertook a trial of 398 previously untreated patients with diffuse large B-cell lymphoma, ages 60 to 80 years old (101). The study was conducted at 86 centers in France, Belgium, and Switzerland between July 1998 and March 2000. The enrolled patients were randomized to receive either eight cycles of CHOP every 3 weeks (197 patients) or eight cycles of CHOP plus rituximab given on day 1 of each cycle (202 patients). The results showed an improvement in the complete response rate in the R-CHOP group than in the group that received CHOP alone (76% vs. 64%, $p = 0.005$). Moreover, with a median follow-up of 2 years, the R-CHOP group showed significantly better results in the eventfree and OS times, and the reduction in the risk of treatment failure and death without a clinically significant increase in toxicity (101).

Burkitt Lymphoma

In 1959, Burkitt (102) described an unusual tumor that involved the jaw in African children. Histopathologic examination revealed it to be a malignant lymphoma that was composed of uniformly undifferentiated lymphoid cells and that was diffuse in its pattern with other distinguishing features (103). What was remarkable about this tumor was that a single large dose of cyclophosphamide caused complete regression in 80% of these children and long-term survival in one-fourth of these patients (104,105). Methotrexate was also found to be effective in the treatment of this disease, and combination with both drugs increased the percentage of long-tem survivors, depending on the clinical stage of the patient (106). Photos of large, disfiguring jaw tumors that regressed completely with even one dose of cyclophosphamide attested to the unique sensitivity of this tumor to certain chemotherapy drugs and stimulated the search for other tumors that could be effectively treated with chemotherapy. This entity was subsequently recognized in other countries, including the United States, and although patients in this country were more likely to have Epstein-Barr virus negative and to present with large abdominal tumors rather than jaw tumors, the response to chemotherapy was also dramatic (107). Like African Burkitt lymphoma, early stage disease was more curable than disseminated disease. Rapid tumor lysis after chemotherapy was found to cause uric acid nephropathy and electrolyte disturbances, thus requiring close monitoring and even temporary dialysis in some patients (108,109). Interestingly, this tumor, perhaps unlike any other, has a high-growth fraction that is similar to the L1210 leukemia, and in part explains its sensitivity to chemotherapy agents.

High-Dose Chemotherapy and Bone Marrow Transplantation

Studies on the effects of whole body irradiation, particularly in patients who were exposed to radiation from nuclear explosions or accidents, showed that marrow failure, as well as gastrointestinal toxicity, were the major causes of death (110). The pioneering work of Thomas et al. (111,112), which began in Cooperstown, New York, using dogs as a model system, and then continued in Seattle, Washington, was first directed toward the reversal of bone marrow failure due to irradiation. The identification of various histocompatibility antigens in humans and the successful cryopreservation of bone marrow cells allowed clinical trials to be imitated in the late 1960s. When it became feasible to prevent marrow toxicity to not only x-rays, but also high doses of chemotherapy, this approach was used to treat patients who failed treatment with conventional doses of chemotherapy (113). Allogeneic transplants, initially in histocompatibility leukocyte antigen-identical twins, were followed by allogeneic transplants in histocompatibility leukocyte antigen-matched siblings. Marrow toxicity, as a limitation to the dose of many of the drugs that are used to treat lymphomas, and the information that response was a function of dose then led to autologous bone marrow transplants in patients with large cell diffuse lymphoma that relapsed from conventional doses of chemotherapy in the late 1970s (114). Allogeneic and autologous transplantation after high doses of chemotherapy or irradiation, or both, has saved many lives, and many centers now carry out these procedures in patients with relapsed or even high-risk lymphoma (115).

CONCLUSIONS

Perhaps not apparent to the current generation was the sometimes agonizingly slow, step-by-step progress in our ability to treat lymphoma. It is hoped that this review illustrates how each advance builds on a previous observation. Those of my generation realize that these gains have been made without a large amount of input from basic science discoveries, and, in a large measure, reflect the creativeness of the clinical scientist, and the bedside as the laboratory. Clearly, further advances (personal or more selective chemotherapy) will require chemists, molecular biologists, pharmacologists, immunologists, pathologists, and toxicologists, as well as clinicians. There is great anticipation that progress in the future toward the even more successful and minimally toxic treatment of all lymphomas will be accelerated and aided by the increased molecular understanding of these diseases.

References

1. Adair FE, Bogg HJ. Experimental and clinical studies on the treatment of cancer by dichloroethysulphide (mustard gas). *Ann Surg* 1931;93:190–199.
2. Berenblum I. Experimental inhibition of tumor induction by mustard gas and other compounds. *J Pathol Bacteriol* 1935;40:549–588.
3. Ward K. The chlorinated ethlamines—a new type of vesicant. *J Am Chem Soc* 1935;57:914–916.
4. Brookes P. The early history of the biological alkylating agents. *Mutat Res* 1990;233:3–14.
5. Goodman LS, Wintrobe MM, Dameshek W, et al. Nitrogen mustard therapy: use of methybis(b-chloroethyl) amino hydrochloride for Hodgkin's disease, lymphosarcoma, leukemia and certain allied disorders. *JAMA* 1946;132:126–132.
6. Rhoads CP. The sword and the plowshare. *J Mount Sinai Sch of Med.* 1947;13:299–309.
7. Jacobson LO, Spurr CL, Guzman Baron ES, et al. Nitrogen mustard therapy: studies on neoplastic disorders and allied disease of the hematopoietic system. *JAMA* 1946;132:263–271.
8. Karnofsky DA, Carver LF, Rhoads CP, et al. An evaluation of methyl-bis-(b-chloroethyl) amine hydrochloride and tris-(b-chloroethyl)amine hydrochloride (nitrogen mustards) in the treatment of lymphomas, leukemia and allied diseases. In: Moulton FR, ed. *Approaches to tumor chemotherapy.* Washington, DC: American Association for the Advancement of Science, 1952:319–337.
9. Dameshek W, Weifuse L, Stein T. Nitrogen mustard therapy in Hodgkin's disease. Analysis of 50 consecutive cases. *Blood* 1949;4:338–379.
10. Burchenal JH, Lester RA, Riley JB, et al. Studies on the chemotherapy of leukemia. Effect of certain nitrogen mustards and carbamates on transmitted mouse leukemia. *Cancer* 1949;1:399–412.
11. Burchenal JH, Curchenal JR, Johnston SF. Chemotherapy of leukemia, III. Further studies on the effect of nitrogen mustards and related compounds on transmitted mouse leukemia. *Cancer* 1951;4:353–356.
12. Haddow A. On the biological alkylating agents. *Perspect Biol Med* 1973;16:503–524.
13. Dougherty TF, White A. Effect of pituitary adrenotropic hormone on lymphoid tissue. *Proc Soc Exp Biol Med* 1943;53:132–133.
14. Heilman FR, Kendall ED. The influence of 11-dehydro-17-hydroxy-corticosterone (compound E) on the growth of a malignant tumor in the mouse. *Endocrinology* 1944;34:416–420.
15. Pearson OH, Eliel LP. Use of pituitary adrenocorticotropic hormone (ACTH) and cortisone in lymphomas and leukemias. *JAMA* 1950;144:1349–1350.
16. Kyle RA, McParland CE, Dameshek W. Large doses of prednisone and prednisolone in the treatment of malignant lymphoproliferative disorders. *Ann Intern Med* 1962;57:717–731.
17. Farber S, Diamond LK, Mercer RD, et al. Temporary remissions in acute leukemia in children produced by the folic acid antagonist, 4-aminopteroylglutamic acid (aminopterin). *N Engl J Med* 1948;238:787–793.
18. DeVita VT, Hellman S, Rosenberg SA. *Cancer: principles and practice of oncology,* 7th ed. Philadelphia: Lippincott Williams & Wilkins, 2005.
19. Luria SE, Delbrück M. Mutations of bacteria from virus sensitivity to virus resistance. *Genetics* 1943;28:491–511.
20. Law LW. Origin of resistance of leukaemic cells to folic acid antagonists. *Nature* 1952;169:628–629.
21. Goldie JH, Coldman AJ. A mathematical model for relating the drug sensitivity of tumors to the spontaneous mutation rate. *Cancer Treat Rep* 1979;63:1727–1733.
22. Coldman AJ, Goldie JH. A mathematical model of drug resistance in neoplasms. In: Bruchovsky N, Goldie JH, eds. *Drug and hormone resistance in neoplasia,* vol 1. Boca Raton, FL: CRC Press, 1982;1:55–78.
23. Day RS. Treatment sequencing, asymmetry, and uncertainty: protocol strategies for combination chemotherapy. *Cancer Res* 1986;46:3876–3885.

24. Norton L, Day RS. Potential innovations in scheduling in cancer chemotherapy. In: DeVita VT, Hellman S, Rosenberg SA, eds. *Important advances in oncology*. Philadelphia, PA: J.B. Lippincott, 1985:57.

25. Buzzoni R, Bonadoona G, Valagussa P, et al. Adjuvant chemotherapy with doxorubicin plus cyclophosphamide, methotrexate, and fluorouracil in the treatment of resectable breast cancer with more than three positive axillary nodes. *J Clin Oncol* 1991;9:2134–2140.

26. Bruce WR, Meeker BE, Valeriote FA. Comparison of the sensitivity of normal hematopoietic and transplanted lymphoma colony-forming cells to chemotherapeutic agents administered in vivo. *J Natl Cancer Inst* 1966;37:233–245.

27. Lacher MJ, Durant JR. Combined vinblastine and chlorambucil therapy of Hodgkin's disease. *Ann Intern Med* 1965;62:468–476.

28. Gilbert R. Radiotherapy in Hodgkin's disease (malignant granulomatosis): anatomic and clinical foundations: governing principles, results. *Am J Roentgenol* 1939;41:198–241.

29. Peters MV, Middlemiss KC. A study of Hodgkin's disease treated by irradiation. *Am J Roentgenol Radium Ther Nucl Med* 1958;79:114.

30. Easson EC, Russell MH. The cure of Hodgkin's disease. *Br Med J* 1963;1:1704–1707.

31. Kaplan HS. *Hodgkin's disease*, 2nd ed. Cambridge, MA: Harvard University Press, 1980.

32. Friedman OM, Seligman AM. Preparation of N-phosphorylated derivatives of bis-β-chloroethylamine. *J Am Chem Soc* 1954;76:655–658.

32a. Arnold H, Bourseaux F, Brock N. Neuartige Krebs-Chemotherapeutika aus der Gruppe der zyklicschen N-Lost-Phosphamidester. *Naturwissenschaften* 1958;45:64–66.

33. Hyman G, Cassileth P. Efficacy of cyclophosphamide in the management of reticulum cell sarcoma. *Cancer* 1966;19:1386–1392.

34. Albright F. Cushing's Syndrome; its pathological physiology, its relationship to the adrenogenital syndrome, and its connection with the problem of the reaction of the body to injurious agents ("alarm reaction of Selye"). *Harvey Lect* 1942;38:123–185.

35. Dobriner K, Lieberman S, Rhoads CP. The excretion in the urine of metabolites of adrenal cortical hormones in health and disease, including neoplastic growth. *Cancer Res* 1947;7:711.

36. Pearson OH, Eliel LP, Rawson RW, et al. Adrenocorticotropic hormone- and cortisone-induced regression of lymphoid tumors in man; a preliminary report. *Cancer* 1949;2:943–945.

37. Garcia F. *A botany symposium on medicinal plants: Proceedings of the Eighth Pacific Science Congress of the National Research Council of the Philippines, IVA*. 1954:182–194.

38. Cutts JH. Biological effects of extracts of *Vinca rosea*. *Proc Am Assoc Cancer Res* 1958;2:289.

39. Johnson IS, Armstrong JG, Gorman M, et al. The vinca alkaloids: a new class of oncolytic agents. *Cancer Res* 1963;23:1390–1427.

40. Scott JL. The effect of nitrogen mustard and maintenance chlorambucil in the treatment of advanced Hodgkin's disease. *Cancer Chemother Rep* 1963;27:27–32.

41. Carbone PP, Spurr C, Schneiderman M, et al. Management of patients with lymphoma, a comparative study with cyclophosphamide and vinca alkaloids. *Cancer Res* 1968;28:811–822.

42. Hall TC. New chemotherapeutic agents in Hodgkin's disease. *Cancer Res* 1966;26:1297–1302.

42a. Skipper HE, Schabel FM, Wilcox WS. Experimental evaluation of potential anticancer agents XIII. On the criteria and kinetics associated with "Curability" of experimental leukemia. *Cancer chemotherapy reports* 1964;35:1–111.

43. Freireich EJ, Karon M, Frie E III. Quadruple combination therapy (VAMP) or acute lymphocytic leukemia of childhood. *Proc Am Assoc Cancer Res* 1964;5:20.

44. Moxley JH 3rd, De Vita VT, Brace K, et al. Intensive combination chemotherapy and x-irradiation of Hodgkin's disease. *Cancer Res* 1967;27:1258–1263.

45. Frei E III, Spurr CI, Brindley CO, et al. Clinical studies of dichloromethotrexate. *Clin Pharmacol Ther* 1965;6:160–171.

46. Devita VT Jr, Serpick AA, Carbone PP. Combination chemotherapy in the treatment of advanced Hodgkin's disease. *Ann Intern Med* 1970;73:881–895.

47. Frei E III, Luce JK, Gamble GE, et al. Combination chemotherapy in advanced Hodgkin's disease: induction and maintenance of remission. *Ann Intern Med* 1973;79:376–382.

48. Moore MR, Jones SE, Bull JM, et al. MOPP chemotherapy for advanced Hodgkin's disease. Prognostic factors in 81 patients. *Cancer* 1973;32: 52–60.

49. DeVita VT, Lewis BT, Rozencweig M, et al. The chemotherapy of Hodgkin's disease. Past experiences and future directions. *Cancer* 1978;42:979–990.

50. Hugeley CM Jr, Durant JR, Moores RR, et al. Comparison of nitrogen mustard, vincristine, procarbazine and prednisone (MOPP) to nitrogen mustard in advanced Hodgkin's disease. *Cancer* 1975;36:1227–1240.

51. Prosnitz LR, Farber LR, Fischer JJ, et al. Low dose radiation therapy and combination chemotherapy in the treatment of advanced Hodgkin's disease. *Radiology* 1973;107:187–193.

52. Rosenberg SA, Kaplan HS, Portlock CS, et al. Combined modality therapy of Hodgkin's disease, a report on the Stanford trials. *Cancer* 1978;42:991–1000.

53. Umezawa H. Bleomycin and other tumor antibiotics of high molecular weight. *Antimicrob Agents Chemother (Bethesda)* 1965;17:1079–1085.

54. Kimura I, Onoshi T, Kunimasa I, et al. Treatment of malignant lymphomas with bleomycin. *Cancer* 1972;29:58–60.

55. Bonadonna G, Monfardini S, De Lena M, et al. Phase I and preliminary phase II evaluation of adriamycin (NSC 123127). *Cancer Res* 1970;30:2572–2582.

56. Gottlieb J, Gutterman J, McCredie K, et al. Chemotherapy of malignant lymphoma with adriamycin. *Cancer Res* 1973;33:3024–3028.

57. Bonadonna G, Zucali R, Monfardini S, et al. Combination chemotherapy of Hodgkin's disease with adriamycin, bleomycin, vinblastine and imidazole carboxamide versus MOPP. *Cancer* 1975;36:252–259.

58. Canellos GP, Anderson JR, Propert KJ, et al. Chemotherapy of advanced Hodgkin's disease with MOPP, ABVD or MOPP alternating with ABVD. *N Engl J Med* 1992;327:1478–1484.

59. Valagussa P, Santoro A, Fassati Bellani F, et al. Absence of treatment induced second neoplasms after ABVD in Hodgkin's disease. *Blood* 1982;59:4388–4982.

60. Diehl V, Behringer K. Could BEACOPP be the new standard for the treatment of advanced Hodgkin's lymphoma? *Cancer Invest* 2006;24:461–465.

61. Peckham MJ. Radiation therapy of the non-Hodgkin's lymphomas. *Semin Hematol* 1974;11:41–45.

62. Jones SE, Rosenberg SA, Kaplan HS, et al. Non-Hodgkin's lymphomas. II. Single agent chemotherapy. *Cancer* 1972;30:31–38.

63. Gall EA, Mallory TB. Malignant lymphoma: a clinicopathologic survey of 618 cases. *Am J Pathol* 1942;18:381–395.

64. Rappaport H, Winter WJ, Hicks EB. Follicular lymphoma: re-evaluation of its position in the scheme of malignant lymphomas based on survey of 253 cases. *Cancer* 1956;9:792–821.

65. Rappaport H. Tumors of the hematopoietic system. In: *Atlas of tumor pathology*. *Third Series*, fasc 8. Section III. Washington, DC: Armed Forces Institute of Pathology, 1966.

66. Bagley CM, DeVita VT, Berard CW, et al. Advanced lymphosarcoma: intensive cyclic combination chemotherapy with cyclophosphamide, vincristine and prednisone. *Ann Intern Med* 1972;76:227–234.

67. Canellos GP, Lester E, Skarin AT. Chemotherapy of the non-Hodgkin's lymphomas. *Cancer* 1978;42:932–940.

68. Portlock CS, Rosenberg SA, Glatstein E, et al. Treatment of advanced non-Hodgkin's lymphomas with favorable histologies. Preliminary results of a prospective trial. *Blood* 1976;47:747–756.

69. Lister TA, Cullen MH, Beard ME, et al. Comparison of combined and single-agent chemotherapy in non-Hodgkin's lymphoma of favourable histological type. *Br Med J* 1978;1:533–537.

70. Goffinet DR, Castellino RA, Kim H, et al. Staging laparotomies in unselected previously untreated patients with non-Hodgkin's lymphoma. *Cancer* 1973;32:672–681.

71. Lotz MJ, Chabner B, DeVita VT. Pathologic staging of 100 consecutive untreated patients with non-Hodgkin's lymphoma. *Cancer* 1976;37:266–270.

72. Fuks Z, Kaplan HS. Recurrence rates following radiation therapy of nodular and diffuse malignant lymphomas. *Radiology* 1973;108:675–684.

73. Young R, Longo D, Glatstein E, et al. The treatment of indolent lymphomas: watchful waiting vs aggressive combined modality treatment. *Semin Hematol* 1988;2(suppl 2):11–16.

74. Brice P, Bastion Y, Lepage E, et al. Comparison in low-tumor-burden follicular lymphomas between an initial no-treatment policy, prednimustine, or interferon alfa: a randomized study from the Groupe d'Etude des Lymphomes Folliculaires. Groupe d'Etude des Lymphomes de l'Adulte. *J Clin Oncol* 1997;15:1110–1117.

75. Ardeshna K, Smith P, Norton A, et al. Long-term effect of a watch and wait policy vs. immediate systemic treatment for asymptomatic advanced stage non-Hodgkin's lymphoma: a randomized controlled trial. *Lancet* 2003;362:516–522.

76. Luce JK, Gamble JFE, Wilson HE, et al. Combined cyclophosphamide, vincristine, and prednisone therapy of malignant lymphoma. *Cancer* 1971;28:306–317.

77. Berd D, Cornog J, DeConti RC, et al. Long term remission in diffuse histiocytic lymphoma treated with combination sequential therapy. *Cancer* 1975;35:1050–1054.

78. Sweet DL, Golomb HM, Ultmann JE, et al. Cyclophosphamide, vincristine, methotrexate with leucovorin rescue, and cytarabine (COMLA) combination sequential chemotherapy for advanced diffuse histiocytic lymphoma. *Ann Intern Med* 1980;92:785–790.

79. Shein PS, Chabner BA, Canellos GP, et al. Potential for prolonged disease-free survival following combination chemotherapy of non-Hodgkin's lymphoma. *Blood* 1974;43:181–189.

80. McKelvey E, Gottlieb J, Wilson H, et al. Hydroxyldaunomycin (Adriamycin) combination chemotherapy in malignant lymphoma. *Cancer* 1976;38:1484–1493.

81. Miller TP, Jones SE. Initial chemotherapy for clinically localized lymphomas of unfavorable histology. *Blood* 1983;62:413–418.

82. Jones SE, Grozea PN, Metz EN, et al. Superiority of Adriamycin-containing combination chemotherapy in the treatment of diffuse lymphoma: a Southwest Oncology Group Study. *Cancer* 1979;43:417–425.

83. Jones SE, Grozea PN, Metz EN, et al. Improved complete remission rates and survival I for patients with large cell lymphoma treated with

chemoimmunotherapy: a Southwest Oncology Group Study. *Cancer* 1983;51:1083–1090.

84. Jones SE, Grozea PN, Miller TP, et al. Chemotherapy with cyclophosphamide, doxorubicin, vincristine, and prednisone alone or with levamisole or with levamisole plus BCG for malignant lymphoma: a Southwest Oncology Group Study. *J Clin Oncol* 1985;3:1318–1324.

85. Coltman CA, Dahlberg S, Jones SE, et al. Southwest Oncology Group studies in diffuse large cell lymphoma: a subset analysis. In: Kimura K, ed. *Cancer chemotherapy: challenges for the future.* Tokyo, Japan: Excerpta Medica, 1988:194–202.

86. Fisher RI, DeVita VT Jr, Hubbard SM, et al. Diffuse aggressive lymphomas: increased survival after alternating flexible sequences of ProMACE and MOPP chemotherapy. *Ann Intern Med* 1983;98:304–309.

87. Longo DL, DeVita VT Jr, Duffey PL, et al. Superiority of ProMACE-CytaBOM over ProMACE-MOPP in the treatment of advanced diffuse aggressive lymphoma: results of a prospective randomized trial [published correction appears in *J Clin Oncol* 1991;9:710]. *J Clin Oncol* 1991;9:25–38.

88. Klimo P, Connors JM. MACOP-B chemotherapy for the treatment of diffuse large-cell lymphoma. *Ann Intern Med* 1985;102:596–602.

89. Connors JM, Klimo P. MACOP-B chemotherapy for malignant lymphomas and related conditions: 1987 update and additional observations. *Semin Hematol* 1988;25(suppl 2):41–46.

90. Dana BW, Dahlberg S, Miller TP, et al. m-BACOD treatment for intermediate- and high-grade malignant lymphomas: a Southwest Oncology Group phase II trial. *J Clin Oncol* 1990;8:1155–1162.

91. Miller TP, Dahlberg S, Weick JK, et al. Unfavorable histologies of non-Hodgkin's lymphoma treated with ProMACE-CytaBOM: a groupwide Southwest Oncology Group study. *J Clin Oncol* 1990;8:1951–1958.

92. Weick JK, Dahlberg S, Fisher RI, et al. Combination chemotherapy of intermediate-grade and high-grade non-Hodgkin's lymphoma with MACOP-B: a Southwest Oncology Group study. *J Clin Oncol* 1991;9:748–753.

93. Schneider AM, Straus DJ, Schluger AE, et al. Treatment results with an aggressive chemotherapeutic regimen (MACOP-B) for intermediate-and some high-grade non-Hodgkin's lymphomas. *J Clin Oncol* 1990;8:94–102.

94. Fisher RI, Gaynor ER, Dalberg S, et al. Comparison of a standard regimen (CHOP) with three intensive chemotherapy regimens for advanced on-Hodgkin's lymphoma. *N Engl J Med* 1993;328:1002–1006.

95. Stashenko P, Nadler LM, Hardy R, et al. Characterization of a human B lymphocyte-specific antigen. *J Immunol* 1980;125:1678–1685.

96. Anderson KC, Bates MP, Slaughenhoupt BL, et al. Expression of human B cell-associated antigens on leukemias and lymphomas: a model of human B cell differentiation. *Blood* 1984;63:1424–1433.

97. Zhou LJ, Tedder T.: CD20 Workshop Panel Report. In: Schlossman SF, Boumsell L, Gilks W, et al. *Leucocyte typing V: white cell differentiation antigens: proceedings of the fifth international workshop and conference held in Boston, USA, 3-7 November, 1993.* Oxford, UK: Oxford University, 1995:511–514.

98. Einfeld DA, Brown JP, Valentine MA, et al. Molecular cloning of the human B cell CD20 receptor predicts a hydrophobic protein with multiple transmembrane domains. *EMBO J* 1988;7:711–717.

99. McLaughlin P, Grillo-Lopez AJ, Link BK, et al. Rituximab chimeric anti-CD20 monoclonal antibody therapy for relapsed indolent lymphoma: half of patients respond to a four-dose treatment program. *J Clin Oncol* 1998;16:2825–2833.

100. Vose JM, Link BK, Grossbard ML, et al. Phase II study of rituximab in combination with CHOP chemotherapy in patients with previously untreated, aggressive non-Hodgkin's lymphoma. *J Clin Oncol* 2001;19:389–397.

101. Coiffer B, Lepage E, Briere J, et al. CHOP chemotherapy plus rituximab compared with CHOP alone in elderly patients with diffuse large B-cell lymphoma. *N Engl J Med* 2002;346:235–2424.

102. Burkitt DP. Sarcomas involving jaws in African children. *Br J Surg* 1969;46:218–223.

103. Histopathological definition of Burkitt's lymphoma. *Bull World Health Organ* 1969;40:601–607.

104. Burkitt D. Long-term remissions following one and two dose chemotherapy for African lymphoma. *Cancer* 1967;20:756–759.

105. Burkitt D, Hutt MS, Wrigt DH. The African lymphoma: preliminary observations on response to therapy. *Cancer* 1965;18:399–410.

106. Ramirez I, Sullivan M, Wang Y, et al. Effective therapy for Burkitt's lymphoma: high-dose cyclophosphamide + high-dose methotrexate with coordinated intrathecal therapy. *Cancer Chemother Pharmacol* 1979;3:103–109.

107. Ziegler JL. Treatment results of 54 American patients with Burkitt's lymphoma are similar to the African experience. *N Engl J Med* 1977;3:75–80.

108. Arsenau JC, Bagley CM, Anderson T, et al. Hyperkalemia, a sequel to chemotherapy of Burkitt's lymphoma. *Lancet* 1973;1:10–14.

109. Cadman EC, Lunberg WB, Bertino JR. Hyperphosphatemia and hypocalcemia accompanying rapid lysis in a patient with Burkitt's lymphoma and Burkitt cell leukemia. *Am J Med* 1977;62:283–290.

110. Cronkite EP, Bond VP. *Radiation injury in man; its chemical and biological basis, pathogenesis and therapy.* Springfield, IL.: Thomas, 1960:138–139.

111. Thomas ED, Lochte HL Jr, Lu WC, et al. Intravenous infusion of bone marrow in patients receiving radiation and chemotherapy. *N Engl J Med* 1957;257:491–496.

112. Thomas ED, Lochte HL Jr, Cannon JH, et al. Supra-lethal whole body irradiation and isologous marrow transplantation in man. *J Clin Invest* 1959;38:1709–1716.

113. Thomas ED, Storb R, Clift RA, et al. Bone-marrow transplantation. *N Engl J Med* 1975;292:895–902.

114. Appelbaum FR, Herzig GP, Ziegler JL, et al. Successful engraftment of cryopreserved autologous bone marrow in patients with malignant lym phoma. *Blood* 1978;52:85–95.

115. Armitage JO, Vose JM. Bone marrow transplantation for malignant lymphoma. In: Canellos GP, Lister TA, Sklar JL, eds. *The lymphomas.* Philadelphia, PA: Lippincott Williams & Wilkins, 1998:247–226.

CHAPTER 2 ■ THE HISTORY OF RADIATION THERAPY OF LYMPHOMAS

LENA SPECHT

FIRST 50 YEARS—THE KILOVOLT ERA

In December 1895, Wilhelm Conrad Röntgen first published his discovery of x-rays in a short communication to the Medical Physics Society of Würzburg, Germany, entitled "Über eine neue Art von Strahlen" ("On a New Type of Rays") (1–3). The news spread rapidly within the medical and scientific community on both sides of the Atlantic, the paper was translated into several languages, and, during the year 1896, more than 1,000 oral and written communications on x-rays were presented. It was soon discovered that the x-rays had biologic effects, and many started using them in dermatology and for superficial cancers. The first radiotherapy for cancer was probably given to a patient with pharyngeal cancer by Voight in Germany in January 1896 (4,5), possibly followed closely by Grubbé in Chicago (2,6–8). The first documented cure of cancer was a case of skin cancer on the nose that was treated by Stenbeck in Stockholm, Sweden, in 1899 (9). Shortly afterwards, cases of mycosis fungoides were treated with x-rays, which resulted in the healing of tumors, as well as patches and plaques in the irradiated area (10–12).

In Chicago, in 1902, Pusey (13) published what appear to be the first documented cases of radiotherapy of extracutaneous lymphomas; he reported excellent local effect, at least in the short term. Figure 2.1 shows a 24-year-old man, who was treated by Pusey, with a "small round cell sarcoma" (undoubtedly a lymphoma, judging from the description of the clinical signs and response to radiation). The patient was treated in September 1901 with "21 x-ray exposures, with a hard tube and a weak light. The distance of the tube from the surface was maintained at 5 cm. And the length of the exposures varied from 10 to 15 minutes." The effect on the tumor was described as "almost magical." Two weeks after the end of treatment, "there was no trace of the disease left except a small, freely movable, painless gland not larger than an almond kernel." Equally impressive results were published by Senn (14), Williams (15), and others in the following couple of years (16,17). In 1904, Krause (18), from Breslau (now Wroclaw, Poland), gave an overview of the published cases of radiotherapy of lymphomas (and other hematologic diseases). In 1903 and 1905, in Leipzig, Germany, Heineke (19,20) published experimental and clinical data that showed the radiosensivity of lymphoid cells, and he described some cases of lymphomas that were treated with x-rays, although with only transient responses. The optimism that was fostered by these early reports of what were regularly described as almost miraculous responses to x-ray therapy was soon to be tempered by reports of almost inevitable recurrences (21–24). In the words of Foster (25) (in 1906): "As has happened frequently before in the history of medicine, the world was doomed to a bitter disappointment."

The equipment for radiotherapy was, at first, rather primitive and difficult to control. The maximum energy that was available ranged from 50 to 100 kV, the x-ray tube was placed at a short distance from or in contact with the skin, and no filter was used (2,26). Gradually, better equipment was developed that could operate at 250 to 400 kV, filters were introduced, and the treatment distance increased, typically to 50 cm, thus allowing much larger volumes to be treated with better control of dosage. Still, for several decades, the treatment of lymphomas was considered palliative in all but a few exceptional cases, and radiation doses were limited to doses that did not cause too much discomfort for the patients (27–33). It was realized that most cases had advanced disease that could not be cured by radiotherapy, but these patients could often be effectively palliated with relatively small doses (32,34–39). In these circumstances, wide regional irradiation (the so-called x-ray bath) or total-body irradiation was regularly used with good palliative effect that lasted up to several years (33,36,40–43). It was noted that, with generalized body irradiation, a considerably smaller dose was required to cause tumor regression than was necessary for equal regression of tumors that were treated locally. A certain technique that was called the Heublein method, after its inventor, was developed at the Memorial Hospital in New York for continuously irradiating several patients at a time in a specially designed room with treatment times over 10 days (44). Patient safety was ostensibly ensured by monitoring the effect of the irradiation on a canary that was placed in the same room halfway between the x-ray tube and the patients. A series of 30 patients with widely disseminated lymphosarcoma who were treated with the Heublein method at the Memorial Hospital was published in 1942; it indicated some prolongation of survival in these patients (45). Total-body irradiation with radioactive isotopes, particularly radiophosphorus, was also tried but generally proved unsatisfactory (33).

The bewildering diversity within the lymphomas was recognized early, and attempts were made to determine the radiosensivity of different lymphoma types (30,39,46,47). The striking radiosensivity of the lymphoid tissue and lymphomatous lesions was acknowledged (20,32,39,47–50). Of the lymphomas, the follicular type and mycosis fungoides were found to be the most sensitive of all; complete regression was often seen after total doses of only 400 to 800 R (30,46,51–55). It was noticed that the tumor cells died soon after irradiation, often within the first 2 weeks (50), and

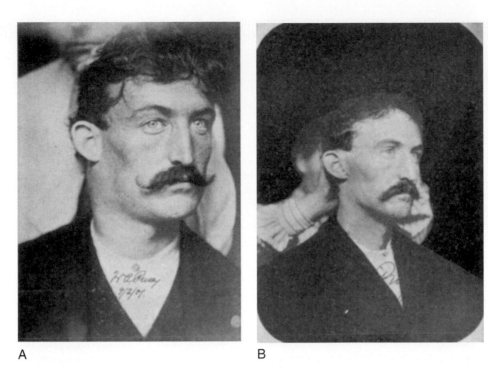

A   B

FIGURE 2.1 A case of lymphoma that was treated in September 1901 by W. A. Pusey, Professor of Dermatology in the Medical Department of the University of Illinois. **A:** The patient on September 2, before the start of radiotherapy. **B:** The patient on October 11, 2 weeks after the end of treatment. This seems to be the first documented case of radiotherapy for lymphoma. (Reprinted with permission from Pusey WA. Cases of sarcoma and of Hodgkin's disease treated by exposures to x-rays—a preliminary report. *JAMA* 1902;38:166–169.)

Coutard (48), in Paris, observed that the daily repetition of irradiation in small doses and an increase in the number of days of treatment of these tumors "enable us mainly to achieve the preservation of the general tissues and to avoid early or late accidents." Radiotherapy in this era was the only effective treatment for patients with malignant lymphomas. However, treatment was regarded throughout as merely palliative in nearly all cases, and recommended radiation doses varied greatly: from 600 to 4,000 R (30,32,39,46,47,50). The techniques also varied, but it was recognized early on that even localized cases needed fairly large treatment volumes to encompass not only the overt lymphoma, but also occult disease in the adjacent areas. It, thus, became apparent that moderate- to high-voltage x-ray treatment was clearly superior to radium treatment, which has only rarely been used for lymphomas (29,32,47,49,50).

Despite the prevailing skepticism regarding the curative potential of radiotherapy, in 1931, Berven (56), in Stockholm, Sweden, had already reported 35 cases of lymphosarcoma of the tonsil that were treated with x-rays and local application of radium during the period 1916 to 1927, with a 5-year relapse-free survival of 37%. In his thesis for the Karolinska Institute in Stockholm, Sweden, he meticulously described his cases with illustrations in watercolor showing patients before treatment and at later follow-up; see Figure 2.2. In the following years, other reports began to appear that documented the possibility of a cure for localized cases by repeated treatments and radical radiotherapy techniques with large fields. Some of these studies advised the inclusion of neighboring noninvolved regions (41,47,57,58), whereas others did not

(50,59–61). Long-term survivors were seen in series that were treated with minimum doses of 2,000 to 3,500 R (skin dose) to all manifest lesions, in lymphosarcomas and reticulosarcomas, although more frequently in the former (48,50,54, 61–69). Exceptional cases, even of reticulosarcoma, were reported to be cured with lower doses (70). The great prognostic impact of the size of the tumor on the outcome after radiotherapy was demonstrated (67). Combined treatment with operation followed by radiotherapy for localized cases was advocated by some (35,71), but this strategy did not ultimately seem to produce better results than radiotherapy alone in comparable cases (50,67). Still, most authorities questioned whether x-ray therapy alone appreciably prolonged life in patients with malignant lymphomas (27,29,35,72). A large series that was published by Rosenberg et al. (73) from the Memorial Center in New York, with more than 1,200 patients who were treated from the late 1920s to the early 1950s, showed a 5-year survival of 54% for giant follicle lymphosarcoma, 27% for lymphosarcoma, and 23% for reticulum cell sarcoma, with no indication of an improvement of results during the period that was covered. Rosenberg et al. (73) cautiously stated that "the comparative radiosensitivity of these tumors generally permits some degree of symptomatic improvement, but it is not known whether this treatment has significantly prolonged survival." They rightly deplored the lack of randomized, well-controlled comparisons of different therapeutic regimens. Other studies were not quite so guarded. Easson and Russell (74) reported long-term follow-up (15 years) of 202 patients who were treated with large-field regional x-ray therapy in the Christie Hospital,

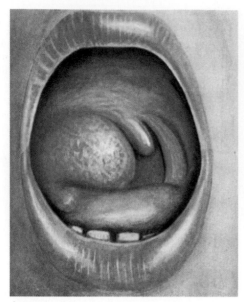 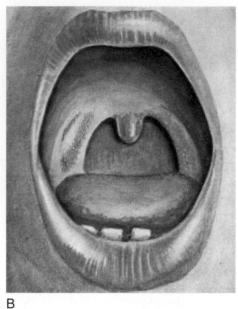

A   B

FIGURE 2.2 A case of lymphosarcoma of the right tonsil. **A:** Before treatment November 1916. **B:** Local condition April 1930. The patient was still alive, free from signs and symptoms 13 years after treatment. (Reprinted with permission from Berven E. Malignant tumours of the tonsil. A clinical study with special reference to radiological treatment. *Acta Radiologica* 1931;11[Suppl]:1–285.)

Manchester, United Kingdom, during the period from 1933 to 1949. They concluded that, for patients with localized disease (over one-half of their patients), the definitive cure rate was 49% (74). Peters (75) reported that 414 patients from Toronto were treated during the period from 1934 to 1952 with fairly aggressive irradiation to tumor in doses of 2,000 to 6,500 rad, with prophylactic irradiation of uninvolved lymphatic regions in approximately one half the patients. For patients with localized disease, Peters (75) reported crude 5-, 10-, and 15-year survivals of 51%, 43%, and 36%, respectively, with no indication that prophylactic irradiation of uninvolved regions improved results. Fuller and Fletcher (76), from Houston, reported 278 patients who were treated from 1947 to 1959; the majority were treated with 250 kV, but some were treated with cobalt 60. Patients with localized dis-

ease had a 5-year survival of 47%. Van der Werf-Messing (77), from Rotterdam, The Netherlands, reported a series of 113 cases with localized disease; between 1953 and 1963, the patients were treated with orthovoltage x-rays to the clinically involved area with a fairly large margin. She reported a 5-year survival of greater than 50% in these patients (77). Hansen (78), from Copenhagen, Denmark, reported a series of patients who were treated during the period from 1940 to 1966; this series included 66 patients with localized disease who were treated with 180 or 250 kV, with a 5-year survival of 45%. Results from these and other series (79) of patients with localized disease who were treated with kilovolt irradiation are shown in Table 2.1. Results were best for giant follicular lymphomas and poorest for reticulum cell sarcoma, with results for lymphosarcoma in the middle of the result

TABLE 2.1

STUDIES OF PRIMARY RADIOTHERAPY FOR LOCALIZED NON-HODGKIN LYMPHOMA THAT WAS TREATED IN THE KILOVOLT ERA

Reference	Number of patients	Histology	5-year survival (%)	10-year survival (%)	15-year survival (%)
Rosenberg et al. (73)	245	Lymphosarcoma	41	—	—
Easson and Russell (74)	107	Lymphoreticular sarcoma	52	49	49
Peters (75)	102	Lymphoma	51	43	36
Fuller and Fletcher (76)	131	Lymphoma	47	—	—
Van der Werf-Messing (77)	113	Reticulum cell sarcoma and lymphosarcoma	66 (1 region) 50 (2 contiguous regions)	—	—
Hansen (78)	66	Reticulum cell sarcoma	45	30	—
Cook et al. (79)	211	Lymphosarcoma and reticulum cell sarcoma	30	—	—

spectrum, but few of the studies split localized cases into the different histologic groups. Results for patients with widespread disease were, not unexpectedly, much poorer, with few long-term survivors.

NEXT 50 YEARS: THE MEGAVOLT ERA

Scientific and technologic developments before and during World War II created new opportunities for improvements in radiotherapy. Thus, the production of radionuclides in nuclear reactors made possible the construction of telegamma devices with cobalt 60 that produced x-rays of approximately 1.2 MV of high intensity, which represented a great technical improvement over conventional kilovolt x-ray tubes and teleradium cannons. Eventually, the construction of electron accelerators enabled the production of high-energy x-rays (4 to 50 MV) with high intensity from a small focus, thus allowing the treatment distance to be increased to 100 cm, with treatment times of a duration of typically less than 1 minute. The x-ray beam from these devices is characterized by high tissue penetration and dose homogeneity in the irradiated field, and by sharp field boundaries. Electron accelerators have the added advantage of being able to deliver high-energy electron irradiation, as well. Because of the limited penetration of electron irradiation (depth depending on the energy of the electrons), it is particularly suitable for treating superficial lesions. Linear accelerators, which were based on microwave technology that was developed during World War II, became available in the early 1950s, and this device now dominates the market.

These huge advances in technology allowed for the treatment of all lymphoid tissues in the body with acceptable normal tissue toxicity. Many of the techniques that were used for nodal lymphomas are copied to a great extent from the techniques that were developed for the treatment of Hodgkin disease. Treatment volumes may roughly be divided into involved-field radiotherapy, extended-field radiotherapy, or total lymphoid irradiation. Problems with the classification of non-Hodgkin lymphomas, however, made analyses and trials more difficult than in Hodgkin disease. In the following discussion, lymphomas have been roughly divided into the categories of favorable and unfavorable. In studies in which cases are subdivided according to follicular or diffuse histology, the former are considered favorable, the latter unfavorable.

The new technology was implemented in most large centers during the 1950s and 1960s. Some of the first linear accelerators were installed at Stanford University, and series of patients who were treated from the early 1960s were published by Fuks and Kaplan (80), Fuks (81), Glatstein (82), Goffinet (83), Hoppe (84) et al., Jacobs and Hoppe (85), Jones et al. (86,87), Mac-Manus and Hoppe (88,89), Murtha (90), Paryani (91–93), and Rosenberg (94) et al. Patients with localized lymphomas were treated with involved-field radiotherapy, extended-field radiotherapy, or total lymphoid irradiation. In patients with favorable histology, total lymphoid irradiation resulted in superior relapse-free survival compared with extended-field radiotherapy and involved-field radiotherapy, but there was no difference in overall survival (88,89,91). In patients with unfavorable histology and extra-nodal involvement, neither the extent of irradiation nor the addition of chemotherapy had a significant influence on outcome (92). Table 2.2 shows results of radiotherapy for localized lymphomas from Stanford and other centers. At Stanford, total lymphoid irradiation for patients with favorable stage III disease, a group that was often considered incurable, was also tested, demonstrating that this treatment may be a potentially curative modality in these patients (89,90,93). Table 2.3 shows the results from Stanford and other centers of total lymphoid irradiation for stage III disease with favorable histology. Based on the data from Stanford, for patients with all stages, Fuks and Kaplan (80) made retrospective calculations on the dose-response relationship for the different types of lymphomas (Table 2.4), although they were aware of the pitfall that patients with relatively advanced disease (and, hence, an inherently poorer prognosis) tend to receive lower doses. These data were for a long time highly influential on the choice of dose levels.

Hellman (95,96) and Mauch (97) et al., at Harvard, reported on patients who were treated at the Joint Center for Radiation Therapy in the late 1960s and 1970s. Their results for patients with localized disease who were treated with radiotherapy alone are shown in Table 2.2. From the Princess Margaret Hospital in Toronto, Bush et al. (98), Bush and Gospodarowicz (99), and Gospodarowicz (100) and Sutcliffe (101) et al. published large series of patients with localized lymphomas who were treated with irradiation in the late 1960s and 1970s (Table 2.2). They defined subgroups with high cure rates based on tumor bulk, age, and histology. Their large database allowed important analyses of the dose-response relationship (Table 2.4). At the M.D. Anderson Hospital, Fuller et al. (103,104) and others (102,105–108), made several publications on their patients who were treated in the 1960s and 1970s (Table 2.2). Cox continued his interest in total lymphoid irradiation for patients with favorable stage III disease (109–112), having previously combined data from his own institution with data from other centers (Table 2.3) (113–116). This innovative treatment for an otherwise incurable group of patients is now receiving renewed interest (117). Cox (118) and Kun (119) et al. also contributed data on the dose-response relationship in lymphomas (Table 2.4). In Florida, Kamath (120), Nathu (121), and De Los Santos (122) et al., and Mendenhall and Million (123) have reported series of patients who were treated from the mid-1960s with irradiation for localized disease (Table 2.2) (120,121) and with total lymphoid irradiation for stage III disease (Table 2.3) (122,123). They too contributed to our knowledge of the dose-response relationship (Table 2.4). Other American centers also contributed series of patients who were treated with irradiation in the 1960s and 1970s. Among them are: Chen et al. (124), at Yale; Bitran (125), Hallahan (126), and Vokes (127) et al., in Chicago; and Levitt et al. (128–131) and Lee and Levitt (132), in Minnesota. Data from some of these studies are summarized in Table 2.2.

In Europe, Musshoff and Schmidt-Vollmer (133), in Freiburg, Germany, published series of patients who were treated during the 1950s and 1960s, thus encompassing patients who were treated with kilovolt and megavolt equipment. They reported survival data on patients with localized disease, dividing them into patients with primary extranodal involvement and patients with primary nodal involvement.

TABLE 2.2

STUDIES OF PRIMARY RADIOTHERAPY FOR LOCALIZED NON-HODGKIN LYMPHOMA THAT WAS TREATED IN THE MEGAVOLT ERA

Location of study (reference)	Number of patients	Histology	5-year RFS (%)	5-year OS (%)	10-year RFS (%)	10-year OS (%)	15-year RFS (%)	15-year OS (%)
Stanford (88)	177	F	55	82	44	64	40	44
Stanford (92)	111	U (extranodal)	49	46	49	36	—	—
Stanford (84)	35	U (Waldeyer)	50 (CS I)	50 (CS I)	—	—	—	—
			25 (CS II)	20 (CS II)	—	—	—	—
Harvard (97)	28	U	35	45	—	—	—	—
	26	F	47	91	—	—	—	—
Princess Margaret Hospital (101)	496	332 U, 143 F	54	62	49	49	—	—
M.D. Anderson (105)	113	U + F (Waldeyer)	37	47	26	32	—	—
M.D. Anderson (102)	45	F	48	—	45	—	35	53
Florida (120)	159	92 U	60	—	50	—	50	—
		67 F	80	—	80	—	—	—
Yale (124)	78	53 U	37	59	—	—	—	—
		25 F	83	100	—	—	—	—
Chicago (127)	31	U	78	80	54	58	—	—
Minnesota (131)	19	U	83	88	64	88	—	—
Freiburg (133)	39 CS I	U + F	75	75	65	65	65	60
	42 CS II		36	27	36	18	36	18
	35 CS IE, IIE		52	60	52	60	52	52
Institut Gustave Roussy (136)	134	123 U	—	40	—	—	—	—
		11 F	—	60	—	—	—	—
European Organization for Research and Treatment of Cancer (139)	43 CS I	U + F	60	87	50	75	—	—
	21 CS II	F	62	75	—	—	—	—
	15 CS II	U	10	10	—	—	—	—
British National Lymphoma Investigation (141,144,146)	243 CS I	U	—	—	45	61	—	—
	208 CS I	F	—	—	47	64	—	—
	46 CS II	U	—	40	—	—	—	—
	43 CS II	F	—	75	—	60	—	—
The Royal Marsden Hospital (148,151)	12	U	—	83	—	—	—	—
	58	F	59	93	43	79	36	58
St. Bartholomew's Hospital (152)	57 CS I	U + F	68	78	58	64	—	—
	43 CS II	—	38	48	32	43	—	—
Sweden (154)	99 CS I	U + F	64	78	—	—	—	—
	48 CS II	U + F	8	30	—	—	—	—

CS, clinical stage; F, favorable; OS, overall survival; RFS, relapse-free survival; U, unfavorable.

For patients with stage I disease, survival was roughly the same for these two groups; for patients with stage II disease, survival was actually better for patients with primary extranodal involvement. Altogether, prognosis for patients with localized extranodal involvement was much better than for patients with disseminated extranodal involvement, thus confirming the importance of the E stages that Musshoff and Schmidt-Vollmer (133) had previously introduced in the staging classification for Hodgkin disease. Data regarding localized disease are summarized in Table 2.2. Musshoff and Leopold (134) also contributed analyses of the dose-response relationship (Table 2.4). At the Institut Gustave Roussy in Paris, Brugere (135) and Tubiana (136) et al. published large series of patients with localized disease treated in the late 1950s and the 1960s with involved-field radiotherapy to doses of 3,000 to 5,000 rad (Tables 2.2 and 2.4). Tubiana was instrumental in creating the Lymphoma Group of the European Organization for Research and Treatment of Cancer, which has carried out important randomized trials in non-Hodgkin lymphomas (137–139) (Table 2.2). The British National Lymphoma Investigation, a large multi-institutional collaboration that was based at the Middlesex Hospital in London and coordinated by Jelliffe and G. and B. Vaughan Hudson for many years, managed to gather together large

TABLE 2.3

STUDIES OF PRIMARY RADIOTHERAPY FOR PATIENTS WITH STAGE III DISEASE WITH FAVORABLE HISTOLOGY

Location of study (reference)	Number of patients	5-year RFS (%)	5-year OS (%)	10-year RFS (%)	10-year OS (%)	15-year RFS (%)	15-year OS (%)
Stanford (90)	66	57	76	42	48	37	38
M.D. Anderson (112)	23	50	91	—	—	—	—
Wisconsin (116)	34	58	70	40	50	40	28
Florida (122)	11	—	—	—	—	45	34

OS, overall survival; RFS, relapse-free survival.

numbers of patients in its many trials (140–146). Data from some of its series of patients with localized disease who were treated with irradiation are summarized in Table 2.2. At the Royal Marsden Hospital, London, Horwich and Peckham (147), Horwich et al. (148), Peckham (149), and Peckham (150) and Pendlebury (151) et al. have published series of patients with localized disease who were treated with irradiation alone in the 1970s and 1980s (Tables 2.2 and 2.4). At St. Bartholomew's Hospital, London, Timothy (152) and Richards (153) et al. also published data on patients with localized disease who were treated in the 1960s and 1970s with irradiation, which, in a few cases, was supplemented with adjuvant chemotherapy. Most of their cases had unfavorable histology (Table 2.2). In Sweden, Hagberg et al. (154) published a series of patients who were treated in the 1970s, two-thirds of whom had stage I disease (Table 2.2). A later series of 129 patients with stage I high-grade disease who were treated with radiotherapy showed a relapse rate of 29% (155).

The overall conclusion from these and other studies is that a significant number of patients with truly localized disease are cured with radiotherapy. This is true for indolent as well as aggressive subtypes of lymphoma, although it is true more frequently in the former.

Addition of Chemotherapy

With the advent of single-drug chemotherapy in the 1940s and 1950s and the development of combinations of drugs in the 1960s, the idea arose to combine radiotherapy and chemotherapy with the aim of further improving outcome. Early nonrandomized studies showed promising results for combined modality treatment in localized disease (97,156–158); however, the assessment of the true value of this novel approach had to await the results of randomized trials. A number of randomized trials of radiotherapy alone versus combined modality treatment in localized disease have since been carried out. Early trials that tested the addition of single-drug therapy, or combinations without anthracycline, to radiotherapy are summarized in Table 2.5 (143,145,159–165). Some of the trials that included patients with unfavorable histology showed a significant improvement in relapse-free survival, but only one trial showed an improvement in survival. Two randomized trials of adjuvant chemotherapy with the combination of cyclophosphamide, adriamycin, vincristine, and prednisone in addition to radiotherapy for localized disease have been published (166,167); see Table 2.6.

TABLE 2.4

RADIATION DOSES RECOMMENDED FOR LOCAL CONTROL IN DIFFERENT STUDIES

Location of study (reference)	Histology	Minimum total dose (cGy)
Stanford (80)	U	— (No correlation found between 1,500 and 6,500)
	F	4,400
Princess Margaret Hospital (101)	U	3,000
	F	2,000
M.D. Anderson (105)	U + F	3,500
Wisconsin (119)	U	4,000
Walter Reed General Hospital (118)	U	4,200
	F	2,200
Florida (120)	U	4,000
	F	3,000
Freiburg (134)	F	2,500
Institut Gustave Roussy (136)	U + F	3,500 to 4,000
The Royal Marsden Hospital (150)	U	— (No correlation found between 3,500 and 5,500)
	F	3,000

F, favorable histology; U, unfavorable histology.

TABLE 2.5

EARLY RANDOMIZED STUDIES OF RADIOTHERAPY ALONE VERSUS COMBINED MODALITY TREATMENT IN LOCALIZED DISEASE

Reference	Number of patients	Histology	Chemotherapy	RT alone		RT + CT		p value
				5-year RFS (%)	5-year OS (%)	5-year RFS (%)	5-year OS (%)	RFS/OS
Landberg et al. (161)	55	U + F	CVP	41[a]	92[a]	86[a]	91[a]	0.02/NS
Monfardini et al. (162)	96	U + F	CVP	46	56	72	83	0.005/0.03
Kelsey et al. (143)	148	F	Chlorambucil	33[b]	52[b]	42[b]	42[b]	NS/NS
Phillips (145)	80	U	CVP	—	68	—	48	NS
Nissen et al. (163)	73	U + F	CVPS	49	58	90	71	0.001/NS
Kaminski et al. (160)	46	U	CVP	68	62	54	60	NS/NS
Gomez et al. (159)	21	F	BMCVP	—	—	—	—	NS/NS
Somers et al. (165)	124	U + F	CVP	55	86	75	84	0.002/NS
Panahon et al. (164)	63 (some stage III)	U + F	BMCVP	80[c] (CS I) / 75[c] (CS II)	90[c] (CS I) / 100[c] (CS II)	66[c] (CS I) / 75[c] (CS II)	100[c] (CS I) / 75[c] (CS II)	NS/NS
		—	—					—

B, bischloroethylnitrosourea; C, cyclophosphamide; CS, clinical stage; CT, chemotherapy; F, favorable; M, mechlorethamine; NS, not significant; OS, overall survival; P, prednisone; RFS, relapse-free survival; RT, radiotherapy; S, streptonigrin; U, unfavorable; V, vincristine.
[a] 30-month figures only.
[b] 10-year figures only.
[c] 3-year figures only.

TABLE 2.6

RANDOMIZED STUDIES OF RADIOTHERAPY ALONE VERSUS COMBINED MODALITY TREATMENT WITH CYCLOPHOSPHAMIDE, ADRIAMYCIN, VINCRISTINE, AND PREDNISONE IN LOCALIZED DISEASE

| Reference | Number of patients | Histology | RT alone | | RT + CT | | p value |
			5-year RFS (%)	5-year OS (%)	5-year RFS (%)	5-year OS (%)	RFS/OS
Yahalom et al. (167)	44	U + F	47[a]	66[a]	83[a]	88[a]	0.03/NS
Avilés et al. (166)	224	U	48	56	83	90	0.001/0.001

CT, chemotherapy; F, favorable; NS, not significant; OS, overall survival; RFS, relapse-free survival; RT, radiotherapy; U, unfavorable.
[a] 7-year figures.

With effective modern chemotherapy, relapse-free and overall survival is improved with combined modality treatment for patients with aggressive localized lymphomas, but not for patients with indolent localized lymphomas.

When chemotherapy was first introduced in the treatment of lymphomas, radiotherapy was the standard treatment. Consequently, chemotherapy was introduced as an adjuvant and was given after what was considered the standard treatment. In all except one of the previously mentioned randomized trials, radiotherapy was given initially, followed by chemotherapy after 4 to 8 weeks. However, in some series, relapses occurred in approximately 10% of patients in the interval between radiotherapy and chemotherapy (161,162). Consequently, Nissen et al. (163) introduced in their trial concurrent chemoradiotherapy, which improved the early relapse rate, but at the expense of more toxicity. Furthermore, in some trials, radiotherapy was given to extended fields, which sometimes precluded full doses of chemotherapy afterwards (159). With the introduction in the 1980s of the more effective anthracycline-containing chemotherapy regimens, the sequence of combined modality in aggressive localized lymphomas has changed, with chemotherapy assuming a primary role for induction of response and with radiotherapy being used for consolidation (167). This approach has the added advantage of reducing disease bulk before radiotherapy, thus allowing the use of lower doses of irradiation.

Total-Body Irradiation

In the kilovolt era, irradiation of the whole body with low doses in patients with advanced disease had been used already with good palliative effect (see First 50 Years—The Kilovolt Era). In the 1960s, interest in low-dose total-body irradiation was renewed. The treatment was given with total doses of 100 to 300 cGy in 10 to 30 cGy fractions in various protocol schedules over several weeks. In America, Johnson et al. (168–170) at the National Cancer Institute, Carabell (171) and Chaffey (172–174) et al. at the Joint Center for Radiation Therapy (171–174), Hoppe et al. (175) at Stanford, and Mendenhall et al. (176) and Thar and Million (177) in Florida published series of patients, some with aggressive and some with indolent lymphomas, who were treated in this way. In Europe, series were published by the British National Lymphoma Investigation (178), Pettingale (179) and Dobbs et al. (180) at the Royal Marsden Hospital,

and De Neve (181) and Lybeert (182) et al., and Qasim (183) in Rotterdam. Results are summarized in Table 2.7. In aggressive lymphomas, the results of total-body irradiation were poor. In indolent lymphomas, approximately 30% of patients were recurrence free at 5 years. This result was similar to that that could be obtained with chemotherapy, which was substantiated by the results of the two randomized studies, from Stanford and National Cancer Institute, which compared total-body irradiation with the chemotherapy combination of cyclophosphamide, vincristine, and prednisone (170,175). The notion that a radiation dose as low as 2 Gy should be able to induce long-lasting remission remains something of a puzzle. This effect may possibly be mediated through mechanisms of immune modulation and induction of apoptosis (184).

Total Skin Electron-Beam Therapy

Mycosis fungoides, or cutaneous T-cell lymphoma, was probably the first type of lymphoma ever to be treated with x-rays (11), and, as mentioned above, it was found to be an extremely radiosensitive disease. Local x-ray therapy remained the most effective palliative therapy for mycosis fungoides until the 1950s. The problem with conventional x-ray therapy is that, if it is administered over large areas, the dose to the underlying internal organs exceeds their tolerance. Electrons, by contrast, have a limited range of penetration and deposit their total energy within that range. The effect of electrons is, therefore, limited to superficial tissues, the depth depending on the energy of the electrons. The possibility of using artificially accelerated high-energy electrons (cathode rays) in radiotherapy was envisaged as far back as the 1920s and 1930s (185,186), but energies at the time were not high enough. In the 1940s, Trump et al. (187), at the Massachusetts Institute of Technology, constructed a Van de Graaff generator that was able to produce a 1,500 keV electron beam; experiments were conducted, but this technique still only yielded a maximum range of electrons in tissue of approximately 7 mm. Trump et al. gradually improved their technology, and, by 1950, they were able to produce electron beams for therapy with energies of up to 2.5 MeV. They published the first two cases of mycosis fungoides that were treated with total skin electron-beam therapy by using a four-field technique, with the patient lying on a couch and moving under the machine (188). With the introduction of linear accelerators, it became possible to generate electrons for therapy with energies from 4

TABLE 2.7

STUDIES OF TOTAL-BODY IRRADIATION IN ADVANCED DISEASE

Location of study (reference)	Number of patients	Histology	5-year RFS (%)	5-year OS (%)	10-year RFS (%)	10-year OS (%)
National Cancer Institute (170)	13	U	8	27	—	—
	22	F	14	84	—	—
Harvard (171)	15	U	10	42	0[a]	42[a]
	43	F	23	65	15[a]	57[a]
Stanford (175)	17	F	34	95	—	—
Florida (176)	17	U	0	17	0	0
	27	F	28	56	12	32
British National Lymphoma Investigation (178)	48	U	0	0	—	—
The Royal Marsden Hospital[b] (180)	15	U	—	0	—	0
	22	F	—	30	—	30[a]
Rotterdam Radiotherapeutic Institute (182)	20	U	0	15	0	0
	25	F	32	48	27	35

CT, chemotherapy; F, favorable; OS, overall survival; RFS, relapse-free survival; RT, radiotherapy; U, unfavorable.
[a] 7.5-year figures.
[b] 13 patients previously treated.

to more than 20 MeV, and techniques were enhanced to yield a more uniform dose to the entire skin surface. At Stanford, Cox (189) and Karzmark (190) et al. refined the physical aspects of the technique, and Fuks (191–193) and Hoppe (194–197) et al. refined the clinical aspects of total skin electron-beam therapy, by using a six-field standing technique (191–197). The Stanford technique has gained wide acceptance, but other techniques have also been used with largely similar results. Published series from different centers are summarized in Table 2.8 (197–202). Complete remission is attained in 70% to 100% of patients with plaque disease and less often in patients with tumors. Most patients relapse within 5 years, but often with quite limited disease, which may be managed with limited irradiation or other topical therapies. When relapse is widespread in the skin, total skin electron-beam therapy may be repeated (203). Although total skin electron-beam therapy is rarely curative, it offers significant palliation in most patients.

TABLE 2.8

STUDIES OF TOTAL SKIN ELECTRON-BEAM THERAPY FOR MYCOSIS FUNGOIDES

Location of study (reference)	Number of patients	Subset	Complete remission (%)	5-year relapse-free survival (%)	5-year overall survival (%)
Stanford (196)	43	Limited plaques	98	50	80
	104	Generalized plaques	71	25	45
	47	Tumors	36	—	25
Lahey Clinic and Massachusetts Institute of Technology (200)	89	Generalized plaques	—	19	48
	54	Tumors	—	17	32
Ontario Cancer Foundation (198)	68	Limited plaques	88	38	93
	59	Generalized plaques	80	25	81
	13	Tumors	62	—	53
Montreal (197)	11	Generalized plaques	91	—	64
	21	Tumors	71	—	20
Henri Mondor University Hospital, France (199)	46	Plaques <50% of surface	100	62	93
	20	Plaques >50% of surface	44	19	79
		Tumors or Sézary syndrome	39	0	44
University Hospital Leiden, The Netherlands (201)	30	Mixed	90	—	70

FUTURE

Radiotherapy is a highly effective treatment modality for lymphomas that, as demonstrated by the previous discussion, has been used to the benefit of vast numbers of patients with lymphoma for more than a century. The benefit has depended on scientific and technologic ingenuity, and the intelligent employment of specific innovations by oncologists with a profound knowledge of lymphomas and an understanding of the strengths and weaknesses of all available treatment modalities. The coming years hold great promise for further significant advances in the use of radiotherapy for lymphomas. The new lymphoma classification defines far more disease entities with distinctive clinical features than before (204), thus enabling us to tailor treatment, including radiation fields and doses, more specifically to each recognized disease entity. The technical side of radiotherapy is also changing dramatically. Advances in computer hardware and software have led to the development of sophisticated three-dimensional treatment planning and computer-controlled radiation therapy delivery systems. This three-dimensional conformal radiation therapy and the even more sophisticated intensity-modulated radiation therapy allow us to shape the high-dose volume precisely to the tumor volume while minimizing the dose to the surrounding normal structures. Even further reductions in the dose to normal structures may be achievable with particle therapy, primarily protons. The implementation of these techniques to the treatment of lymphomas is still in its early phase. However, these technical innovations already show significant potential for improving and expanding the use of radiotherapy, alone or in combination with chemotherapy or biologic therapies, with the aim of further optimizing the treatment that can be offered to patients with lymphoma in the future.

References

1. Röntgen WC. Über eine neue Art von Strahlen. *Sitzungsberichte Physikalisch-Medicinischen Gesellschaft zu Würzburg* 1895;30:132–141.
2. Lederman M. The early history of radiotherapy: 1895–1939. *Int J Radiat Oncol Biol Phys* 1981;7:639–648.
3. Dubois JB, Ash D. The discovery of x-rays and radioactivity. In: Bernier J, ed. *Radiation oncology: a century of progress and achievement.* Brussels, Belgium: The European Society for Therapeutic Radiology and Oncology, 1995:77–98.
4. Case JT. History of radiation oncology. *Prog Radiat Ther* 1958;1:13–41.
5. McCarty PJ, Million R. History of radiation oncology. *J Fla Med Assoc* 1995;82:745–748.
6. Grubbé EH. Priority in the therapeutic use of x-rays. *Radiology* 1933;21:156–162.
7. Walstam R. A historical review on radiotherapeutic applications. In: Bernier J, ed. *Radiation oncology: a century of progress and achievement.* Brussels, Belgium: The European Society for Therapeutic Radiology and Oncology, 1995:17–46.
8. Mould RF. Invited review: the early years of radiotherapy with emphasis on x-ray and radium apparatus. *Br J Radiol* 1995;68:567–582.
9. Berven E. The development and organization of therapeutic radiology in Sweden. *Radiology* 1962;79:829–841.
10. Riehl. Vereine, Kongresse. Gesellschaft der Ärzte in Wien. 1903. 15. Mai. *Fortschr Geb Rontgenstr* 1903:7:41.
11. Scholz W. Ueber den Einfluss der Röntgenstrahlen auf die Haut in gesundem und krankem Zustande. III. Klinischer Theil. *Archiv F Dermatol Syphilis* 1902;59:421–445.
12. Kienböck R. Der gegenwärtige Stand der Radiotherapie. *Fortschr Geb Rontgenstr* 1903;7:343–346.
13. Pusey WA. Cases of sarcoma and of Hodgkin's disease treated by exposures to x-rays—a preliminary report. *JAMA* 1902;38:166–169.
14. Senn N. The therapeutical value of the Röntgen ray in the treatment of pseudoleukemia. *N Y Med J* 1903;77:665–668.
15. Williams FH. The use of the x-rays in the treatment of diseases of the skin, of new-growths, of the glandular system, and of other diseases, and as a means of relieving pain. *Trans Assoc Am Physicians* 1903;18:89–96.
16. Chrysospathes JG. Erfolgreiche Behandlung eines inoperablen Sarkoms mittels Röntgenstrahlen. *Munch Med Wochenschr* 1903;50:2182–2185.
17. Cohn M. Die Bedeutung der Röntgenstrahlen für die Behandlung der lymphatischen Sarkome. *Berliner Klin Wochenschr* 1906;43:14–17.
18. Krause P. Zur Röntgenbehandlung von Bluterkrankungen (Leukaemie, Pseudoleukaemie, Lymphomatosis, perniciöse Anaemie, Anaemia splenica, Polycythaemia mi Milztumor). *Fortschr Geb Rontgenstr* 1904;8:209–235.
19. Heineke H. Experimentelle Untersuchungen über die Einwirkung der Röntgenstrahlen auf innere Organe. *Mitteilungen aus den Grenzgebieten der Medizin und Chirurgie* 1903;14.
20. Heineke H. Experimentelle Untersuchungen über die Einwirkung der Röntgenstrahlen auf das Knochenmark, nebst einigen Bemerkungen über die Röntgentherapie der Leukämie und Pseudoleukämie und des Sarcoms. *Dtsch Zeitschrift Chirurgie* 1905;78:196–230.
21. Ewald CA. Ein Fall von geheiltem Lymphosarkom, mit Röntgen und Arsen behandelt. *Berliner Klin Wochenschr* 1906;43:910–911.
22. Forssell G. Kort öfversikt öfver nyare rön inom Röntgenterapien. *Almänna Svenska Läkartidningen* 1904;1:481–509.
23. Coley WB. The present status of the x-ray treatment of malignant tumors. *Med Rec N Y* 1903;63:441–451.
24. Coley WB. Primary neoplasms of the lymphatic glands including Hodgkin's disease. In: Binnie JF, ed. *Transactions of the American Surgical Association.* Philadelphia, PA: William J. Dornan, 1915:499–644.
25. Foster B. The present state of our knowledge concerning the therapeutic value of the x-ray. *J Minn State Med Assoc Northwest Lancet* 1906;26:23–26.
26. Ewing J. Early experiences in radiation therapy. Janeway memorial lecture. *AJR Am J Roentgenol* 1934;31:153–163.
27. Desjardins AU, Ford F. Hodgkin's disease and lymphosarcoma: clinical and statistical study. *JAMA* 1923;81:925–927.
28. Minot GR. Lymphoblastoma. *Radiology* 1926;7:119–120.
29. Desjardins AU. Radiotherapy for Hodgkin's disease and lymphosarcoma. *JAMA* 1932;99:1231–1236.
30. Craver LF. The treatment of the more important lymphadenopathies, with special reference to irradiation. *Med Clin North Am* 1934;18:703–726.
31. Desjardins AU, Habein HC, Watkins CH. Unusual complications of lymphoblastoma and their radiation treatment. *AJR Am J Roentgenol* 1936;36:169–179.
32. Arons I. Further studies on radiotherapy of lymphoblastoma. *Radiology* 1941;37:164–173.
33. Craver LF. Lymphomas and leukemias. *Bull N Y Acad Med* 1947;23:79–100.
34. Fabian E. Ueber die Behandlung des Lymphosarkoms. *Munch Med Wochenschr* 1913;43:1876–1878.
35. Minot GR, Isaacs R. Lymphoblastoma (malignant lymphoma). *JAMA* 1926;86:1185–1189.
36. Cutler M. Lymphosarcoma: a clinical, pathologic and radiotherapeutic study, with a report of thirty cases. *Arch Surg* 1935;30:405–441.
37. Scott RB. Some clinical aspects of the reticuloses. *Br J Radiol* 1951;24:475–478.
38. Elkins HB. Treatment of malignant lymphoma and blood dyscrasias by conventional roentgen therapy. *AJR Am J Roentgenol* 1956;76:960–964.
39. Gall EA, Mallory TB. Malignant lymphoma: a clinico-pathologic survey of 618 cases. *Am J Pathol* 1942;18:381–429.
40. Cottenot P, Sluys F. La Téléroentgenthérapie totale. *J Radiol Électrol* 1935;19:347–359.
41. Finzi NS. The Roentgen treatment of lymphadenoma. *AJR Am J Roentgenol* 1938;39:261–262.
42. Levitt WM. Regional x-ray baths in the treatment of lymphadenoma. *Br J Radiol* 1938;11:183–188.
43. Teschendorf W. Über Bestrahlung des ganzen menschlichen Körpers bei Blutkrankheiten. *Strahlentherapie* 1927;26:720–728.
44. Heublein AC. A preliminary report on continuous irradiation of the entire body. *Radiology* 1932;18:1051–1062.
45. Medinger FG, Craver LF. Total body irradiation with review of cases. *AJR Am J Roentgenol* 1942;48:651–671.
46. Gall EA, Morrison HR, Scott AT. The follicular type of malignant lymphoma: a survey of 63 cases. *Ann Intern Med* 1941;14:2073–2090.
47. Paterson R, Tod M. The reticuloendothelial system. In: Paterson R, ed. *The treatment of malignant disease by radium and X-rays, being a practice of radiotherapy.* Baltimore, MD: J.B. Lippincott, 1948:414–437.
48. Coutard H. Principles of x-ray therapy of malignant diseases. *Lancet* 1934;2:1–8.
49. Ewing J. Radiosensitivity. *Radiology* 1929;13:313–318.
50. Sugarbaker ED, Craver LF. Lymphosarcoma. *JAMA* 1940;115:112–117.
51. Meyer OO. Follicular lymphoblastoma. *Blood* 1948;3:921–933.
52. Craver LF. Treatment of chronic forms of malignant lymphomas and leukemias. *Med Clin North Am* 1949;33:527–540.
53. Cocchi U. Die Therapie des grossfollikulären Lymphoblastoms (Brill-Symmersche Erkrankung). *Schweiz Med Wochenschr* 1950;17:440–442.

54. Gilbert RJ. Lymphogranulome, lymphosarcome, réticulosarcome; radiothérapie. *Radiol Clin (Basel)* 1951;20:313–336.

55. Bauer R. Die Strahlentherapie der Retikulosen unter besonderer Berücksichtigung der Lymphogranulomatose. *Strahlentherapie* 1953;91:65–80.

56. Berven E. Malignant tumours of the tonsil. A clinical study with special reference to radiological treatment. *Acta Radiol* 1931;11(suppl):1–285.

57. Decker FH, Leddy ET, Desjardins AU. Leukopenia and leukocytosis in lymphoblastoma: their reaction to Roentgen therapy. *AJR Am J Roentgenol* 1938;39:747–766.

58. Hynes JF, Frelick RW. Roentgen therapy of malignant lymphoma with special reference to segmental radiation therapy. Results 1935–1945. *AJR Am J Roentgenol* 1953;70:247–257.

59. Catlin D. Lymphosarcoma of head and neck. *AJR Am J Roentgenol* 1948;59:354–358.

60. Oeser H. *Strahlenbehandlung der Geschwülste. Technik, Ergebnisse und Probleme.* München, Germany: Urban & Schwarzenberg, 1954.

61. Hilton G, Sutton PM. Malignant lymphomas: classification, prognosis, and treatment. *Lancet* 1962:283–287.

62. Baumann-Schenker R. Über das Rundzellensarkom. Lymphosarkom, Retothelsarkom, Rundzellensarkom im engeren Sinne. Zürcher Erfahrungen aus den Jahren 1919–1934. *Strahlentherapie* 1934;51:201–236.

63. Stout AP. Is lymphosarcoma curable? *JAMA* 1942;118:968–970.

64. Stout AP. The results of treatment of lymphosarcoma. *N Y J Med* 1947;47:158–164.

65. Gardini GF. La radioterapia dei reticulo-sarcomi. *Radiol Clin (Basel)* 1952;21:219–222.

66. Scheel A, Myhre E. Malignant lymphomata: a review of the pathology, clinic features and therapy. *Acta Radiol* 1953;40:63–80.

67. Goes M. Zur Klinik der Lympho- und Retothelsarkome. *Strahlentherapie* 1953;89:554–566.

68. Hancock PE. Malignant tumours of the reticulo-endothelial system. In: Raven RW, ed. *Cancer* vol 4, part VIII. London, UK: Butterworth, 1958:412–441.

69. Levitt WM. Cancer of the reticulo-endothelial system. In: Raven RW, ed. *Cancer,* vol 5. London, UK: Butterworth, 1959:363–374.

70. Lawrence KB, Lenson N. Reticulum cell sarcoma. Report of a thirteen-year survival following one thousand roentgens of x-ray therapy. *JAMA* 1952;149:361–362.

71. Verhagen A. Strahlenbehandlung bei Rerothelsarkomen. *Strahlentherapie* 1948;77:605–612.

72. Ross JF, Ebaugh FG. Current trends in the management of the leukemias and the malignant lymphomas. *Med Clin North Am* 1951;35:1381–1401.

73. Rosenberg SA, Diamond HD, Jaslowitz B, et al. Lymphosarcoma: a review of 1269 cases. *Medicine (Baltimore)* 1961;40:31–84.

74. Easson EC, Russell MH. *The curability of cancer in various sites; 4th statistical report.* London, UK: Pitman, 1968.

75. Peters MV. The contribution of radiation therapy in the control of early lymphomas. *AJR Am J Roentgenol* 1963;90:956–967.

76. Fuller LM, Fletcher GH. The radiotherapeutic management of the lymphomatous diseases. *Am J Roentgenol Radium Ther Nucl Med* 1962;88:909–923.

77. Van der Werf-Messing B. Reticulum cell sarcoma and lymphosarcoma. A retrospective study of potential survival in loco-regional disease. *Eur J Cancer* 1968;4:549–557.

78. Hansen HS. Reticulum cell sarcoma treated by radiotherapy. Significance of clinical features upon the prognosis. *Acta Radiol Ther Phys Biol* 1969;8:439–458.

79. Cook JC, Krabbenhoft KL, Leucutia T. Lymphosarcoma, reticulum cell sarcoma and giant follicular lymphoma; long term results following radiation therapy. *Am J Roentgenol Radium Ther Nucl Med* 1960;84:656–665.

80. Fuks Z, Kaplan HS. Recurrence rates following radiation therapy of nodular and diffuse malignant lymphomas. *Radiology* 1973;108:675–684.

81. Fuks Z, Glatstein E, Kaplan HS. Patterns of presentation and relapse in the non-Hodgkin's lymphomata. *Br J Cancer* 1975;31:286–297.

82. Glatstein E, Fuks Z, Goffinet DR, et al. Non-Hodgkin's lymphomas of stage III extent. Is total lymphoid irradiation appropriate treatment? *Cancer* 1976;37:2806–2812.

83. Goffinet DR, Glatstein E, Fuks Z, et al. Abdominal irradiation in non-Hodgkin's lymphomas. *Cancer* 1976;37:2797–2805.

84. Hoppe RT, Burke JS, Glatstein E, et al. Non-Hodgkin's lymphoma: involvement of Waldeyer's ring. *Cancer* 1978;42:1096–1104.

85. Jacobs C, Hoppe RT. Non-Hodgkin's lymphoma of head and neck extranodal sites. *Int J Radiat Oncol Biol Phys* 1985;11:357–364.

86. Jones SE, Kaplan HS, Rosenberg SA. Non-Hodgkin's lymphomas. III. Preliminary results of radiotherapy and a proposal for new clinical trials. *Radiology* 1972;103:657–662.

87. Jones SE, Fuks Z, Kaplan HS, et al. Non-Hodgkin's lymphomas. V. Results of radiotherapy. *Cancer* 1973;32:682–691.

88. Mac-Manus MP, Hoppe RT. Is radiotherapy curative for stage I and II low-grade follicular lymphoma? Results of a long-term follow-up study of patients treated at Stanford University. *J Clin Oncol* 1996;14:1282–1290.

89. Mac-Manus MP, Hoppe RT. Overview of treatment of localized low-grade lymphomas. *Hematol Oncol Clin North Am* 1997;11:901–918.

90. Murtha AD, Knox SJ, Hoppe RT, et al. Long-term follow-up of patients with stage III follicular lymphoma treated with primary radiotherapy at Stanford University. *Int J Radiat Oncol Biol Phys* 2001;49:3–15.

91. Paryani SB, Hoppe RT, Cox RS, et al. Analysis of non-Hodgkin's lymphomas with nodular and favorable histologies, stages I and II. *Cancer* 1983;52:2300–2307.

92. Paryani S, Hoppe RT, Burke JS, et al. Extralymphatic involvement in diffuse non-Hodgkin's lymphoma. *J Clin Oncol* 1983;1:682–688.

93. Paryani SB, Hoppe RT, Cox RS, et al. The role of radiation therapy in the management of stage III follicular lymphomas. *J Clin Oncol* 1984;2:841–848.

94. Rosenberg SA, Dorfman RF, Kaplan HS. A summary of the results of a review of 405 patients with non-Hodgkin's lymphoma at Stanford University. *Br J Cancer* 1975;31:168–173.

95. Hellman S, Rosenthal DS, Moloney WC, et al. The treatment of non-Hodgkin's lymphoma. *Cancer* 1975;36:804–808.

96. Hellman S, Chaffey JT, Rosenthal DS, et al. The place of radiation therapy in the treatment of non-Hodgkin's lymphomas. *Cancer* 1977;39:843–851.

97. Mauch P, Leonard R, Skarin A, et al. Improved survival following combined radiation therapy and chemotherapy for unfavorable prognosis stage I–II non-Hodgkin's lymphoma. *J Clin Oncol* 1985;3:1301–1308.

98. Bush RS, Gospodarowicz M, Sturgeon J, et al. Radiation therapy of localized non-Hodgkin's lymphoma. *Cancer Treat Rep* 1977;61:1129–1136.

99. Bush RS, Gospodarowicz M. The place of radiation therapy in the management of patients with localized non-Hodgkin's lymphoma. In: Rosenberg SA, Kaplan HS, eds. *Malignant lymphomas. Etiology, immunology, pathology, treatment.* Orlando, FL: Academic Press, 1982:485–502.

100. Gospodarowicz MK, Bush RS, Brown TC, et al. Prognostic factors in nodular lymphomas: a multivariate analysis based on the Princess Margaret Hospital experience. *Int J Radiat Oncol Biol Phys* 1984;10:489–497.

101. Sutcliffe SB, Gospodarowicz MK, Bush RS, et al. Role of radiation therapy in localized non-Hodgkin's lymphoma. *Radiother Oncol* 1985;4:211–223.

102. Besa PC, McLaughlin PW, Cox JD, et al. Long term assessment of patterns of treatment failure and survival in patients with stage I or II follicular lymphoma. *Cancer* 1995;75:2361–2367.

103. Fuller LM, Banker FL, Butler JJ, et al. The natural history of non-Hodgkin's lymphomata stages I and II. *Br J Cancer* 1975;31:270–285.

104. Fuller LM, Gamble JF, Butler JJ, et al. Team approach to management of non-Hodgkin's lymphomas: past and present. *Cancer Treat Rep* 1977;61:1137–1148.

105. Kong JS, Fuller LM, Butler JJ, et al. Stages I and II non–Hodgkin's lymphomas of Waldeyer's ring and the neck. *Am J Clin Oncol* 1984;7:629–639.

106. McLaughlin P, Fuller LM, Velasquez WS, et al. Stage I-II follicular lymphoma. Treatment results for 76 patients. *Cancer* 1986;58:1596–1602.

107. Seymour JF, McLaughlin P, Fuller LM, et al. High rate of prolonged remissions following combined modality therapy for patients with localized low-grade lymphoma. *Ann Oncol* 1996;7:157–163.

108. Wong DS, Fuller LM, Butler JJ, et al. Extranodal non-Hodgkin's lymphomas of the head and neck. *Am J Roentgenol Radium Ther Nucl Med* 1975;123:471–481.

109. Ha CS, Cabanillas F, Lee MS, et al. Serial determination of the bcl-2 gene in the bone marrow and peripheral blood after central lymphatic irradiation for stages I-III follicular lymphoma: a preliminary report. *Clin Cancer Res* 1997;3:215–219.

110. Ha CS, Tucker SL, Blanco AI, et al. Salvage central lymphatic irradiation in follicular lymphomas following failure of chemotherapy: a feasibility study. *Int J Radiat Oncol Biol Phys* 1999;45:1207–1212.

111. Ha CS, Tucker SL, Lee MS, et al. The significance of molecular response of follicular lymphoma to central lymphatic irradiation as measured by polymerase chain reaction for t(14;18)(q32;q21). *Int J Radiat Oncol Biol Phys* 2001;49:727–732.

112. Ha CS, Kong JS, Tucker SL, et al. Central lymphatic irradiation for stage I-III follicular lymphoma: report from a single-institutional prospective study. *Int J Radiat Oncol Biol Phys* 2003;57:316–320.

113. Cox JD. Total central lymphatic irradiation for stage III nodular malignant lymphoreticular tumors. *Int J Radiat Oncol Biol Phys* 1976;1:491–496.

114. Cox JD. Central lymphatic irradiation to low dose for advanced nodular lymphoreticular tumors (non-Hodgkin's lymphoma). *Radiology* 1978;126:767–772.

115. Cox JD, Komaki R, Kun LE, et al. Stage III nodular lymphoreticular tumors (non-Hodgkin's lymphoma): results of central lymphatic irradiation. *Cancer* 1981;47:2247–2252.

116. Jacobs JP, Murray KJ, Schultz CJ, et al. Central lymphatic irradiation for stage III nodular malignant lymphoma: long-term results. *J Clin Oncol* 1993;11:233–238.

117. Yahalom J. Radiation therapy for stage III follicular lymphoma—often ignored, but still effective. *Int J Radiat Oncol Biol Phys* 2001;49:1–2.

118. Cox JD, Koehl RH, Turner WM, et al. Irradiation in the local control of malignant lymphoreticular tumors (non-Hodgkin's malignant lymphoma). *Radiology* 1974;112:179–185.

119. Kun LE, Cox JD, Komaki R. Patterns of failure in treatment of stage I and II diffuse malignant lymphoid tumors. *Radiology* 1981;141:791–794.
120. Kamath SS, Marcus RB, Lynch JW, et al. The impact of radiotherapy dose and other treatment-related and clinical factors on in-field control in stage I and II non-Hodgkin's lymphoma. *Int J Radiat Oncol Biol Phys* 1999;44:563–568.
121. Nathu RM, Mendenhall NP, Almasri NM, et al. Non-Hodgkin's lymphoma of the head and neck: a 30-year experience at the University of Florida. *Head Neck* 1999;21:247–254.
122. De Los Santos JF, Mendenhall NP, Lynch JW. Is comprehensive lymphatic irradiation for low-grade non-Hodgkin's lymphoma curative therapy? Long-term experience at a single institution. *Int J Radiat Oncol Biol Phys* 1997;38:3–8.
123. Mendenhall NP, Million RR. Comprehensive lymphatic irradiation for stage II-III non-Hodgkin's lymphoma. *Am J Clin Oncol* 1989;12:190–194.
124. Chen MG, Prosnitz LR, Gonzalez-Serva A, et al. Results of radiotherapy in control of stage I and II non-Hodgkin's lymphoma. *Cancer* 1979;43:1245–1254.
125. Bitran JD, Kinzie J, Sweet DL, et al. Survival of patients with localized histiocytic lymphoma. *Cancer* 1977;39:342–346.
126. Hallahan DE, Farah R, Vokes EE, et al. The patterns of failure in patients with pathological stage I and II diffuse histiocytic lymphoma treated with radiation therapy alone. *Int J Radiat Oncol Biol Phys* 1989;17:767–771.
127. Vokes EE, Ultmann JE, Golomb HM, et al. Long-term survival of patients with localized diffuse histiocytic lymphoma. *J Clin Oncol* 1985;3:1309–1317.
128. Levitt SH, Bloomfield CD, Lee CK, et al. Extended field radiotherapy in non-Hodgkin's lymphoma. *Radiology* 1976;118:457–459.
129. Levitt SH. The treatment of non-Hodgkin's lymphoma with radiation therapy. *Prog Clin Biol Res* 1978;25:27–31.
130. Levitt SH, Bloomfield CD, Frizzera G, et al. Curative radiotherapy for localized diffuse histiocytic lymphoma. *Cancer Treat Rep* 1980;64:175–177.
131. Levitt SH, Lee CK, Bloomfield CD, et al. The role of radiation therapy in the treatment of early stage large cell lymphoma. *Hematol Oncol* 1985;3:33–37.
132. Lee CK, Levitt SH. Long-term follow-up of pathologic stage I large cell non-Hodgkin's lymphoma patients after primary radiotherapy. *Am J Clin Oncol* 1996;19:93–98.
133. Musshoff K, Schmidt-Vollmer H. Prognostic significance of primary site after radiotherapy in non-Hodgkin's lymphomata. *Br J Cancer* 1975;31:425–434.
134. Musshoff K, Leopold H. On the question of the tumoricidal dose in non-Hodgkin's lymphomas. In: Mathé G, Seligmann M, Tubiana M, eds. *Lymphoid neoplasias.* Berlin, Germany: Springer-Verlag, 1978:203–206.
135. Brugere J, Schlienger M, Gerard-Marchant R, et al. Non-Hodgkin's malignant lymphomata of upper digestive and respiratory tract: natural history and results of radiotherapy. *Br J Cancer Suppl* 1975;2:435–440.
136. Tubiana M, Pouillart P, Hayat M, et al. Results of radiotherapy in stage I and II lymphosarcomas and reticulosarcomas [in French]. *Bull Cancer* 1974;61:93–110.
137. Carde P, Burgers JM, van Glabbeke M, et al. Combined radiotherapy-chemotherapy for early stages non-Hodgkin's lymphoma: the 1975–1980 EORTC controlled lymphoma trial. *Radiother Oncol* 1984;2:301–312.
138. Tubiana M, Carde P, Burgers JM, et al. Non-Hodgkin's lymphoma. *Cancer Surv* 1985;4:377–398.
139. Tubiana M, Carde P, Burgers JM, et al. Prognostic factors in non-Hodgkin's lymphoma. *Int J Radiat Oncol Biol Phys* 1986;12:503–514.
140. Denham JW, Denham E, Dear KB, et al. The follicular non-Hodgkin's lymphomas—I. The possibility of cure. *Eur J Cancer* 1996;32A:470–479.
141. Vaughn Hudson B, Vaughn Hudson G, Maclennan KA, et al. Clinical stage 1 non-Hodgkin's lymphoma: long-term follow-up of patients treated by the British National Lymphoma Investigation with radiotherapy alone as initial therapy. *Br J Cancer* 1994;69:1088–1093.
142. Vaughn Hudson B. The BNLI: past and present. British National Lymphoma Investigation. *Clin Oncol (R Coll Radiol)* 1998;10:212–218.
143. Kelsey SM, Newland AC, Vaughn Hudson G, et al. A British National Lymphoma Investigation randomised trial of single agent chlorambucil plus radiotherapy versus radiotherapy alone in low grade, localised non-Hodgkins lymphoma. *Med Oncol* 1994;11:19–25.
144. Lamb DS, Vaughn Hudson G, Easterling MJ, et al. Localised grade 2 non-Hodgkin's lymphoma: results of treatment with radiotherapy (BNLI Report No. 24). *Clin Radiol* 1984;35:253–260.
145. Phillips DL. Radiotherapy in the treatment of localised non-Hodgkin's lymphoma (Report no 16). *Clin Radiol* 1981;32:543–546.
146. Spry NA, Lamb DS, Vaughn Hudson G, et al. Localized grade I non-Hodgkin's lymphoma: results of treatment with radiotherapy alone in 88 patients. *Clin Oncol (R Coll Radiol)* 1989;1:33–38.
147. Horwich A, Peckham M. "Bad risk" non-Hodgkin's lymphomas. *Semin Hematol* 1983;20:35–56.
148. Horwich A, Catton CN, Quigley M, et al. The management of early-stage aggressive non-Hodgkin's lymphoma. *Hematol Oncol* 1988;6:291–298.
149. Peckham MJ. Radiation therapy of the non-Hodgkin's lymphomas. *Semin Hematol* 1974;11:41–58.
150. Peckham MJ, Guay JP, Hamlin IM, et al. Survival in localized nodal and extranodal non-Hodgkin's lymphomata. *Br J Cancer* 1975;31:413–424.
151. Pendlebury S, el Awadi M, Ashley S, et al. Radiotherapy results in early stage low grade nodal non-Hodgkin's lymphoma. *Radiother Oncol* 1995;36:167–171.
152. Timothy AR, Lister TA, Katz D, et al. Localized non-Hodgkin's lymphoma. *Eur J Cancer* 1980;16:799–807.
153. Richards MA, Gregory WM, Hall PA, et al. Management of localized non-Hodgkin's lymphoma: the experience at St. Bartholomew's Hospital 1972–1985. *Hematol Oncol* 1989;7:1–18.
154. Hagberg H, Glimelius B, Sundstrom C. Radiation therapy of non-Hodgkin's lymphoma stages I and II. *Acta Radiol Oncol* 1982;21:145–150.
155. Osterman B, Cavallin-Stahl E, Hagberg H, et al. High-grade non-Hodgkin's lymphoma stage I. A retrospective study of treatment, outcome and prognostic factors in 213 patients. *Acta Oncol* 1996;35:171–177.
156. Ossenkoppele GJ, Mol JJ, Snow GB, et al. Radiotherapy versus radiotherapy plus chemotherapy in stages I and II non-Hodgkin's lymphoma of the upper digestive and respiratory tract. *Cancer* 1987;60:1505–1509.
157. Taylor RE, Allan SG, McIntyre MA, et al. Influence of therapy on local control and survival in stage I and II intermediate and high grade non-Hodgkin's lymphoma. *Eur J Cancer Clin Oncol* 1988;24:1771–1777.
158. Toonkel LM, Fuller LM, Gamble JF, et al. Laparotomy staged I and II non-Hodgkin's lymphomas: preliminary results of radiotherapy and adjunctive chemotherapy. *Cancer* 1980;45:249–260.
159. Gomez GA, Barcos M, Krishnamsetty RM, et al. Treatment of early—stages I and II—nodular, poorly differentiated lymphocytic lymphoma. *Am J Clin Oncol* 1986;9:40–44.
160. Kaminski MS, Coleman CN, Colby TV, et al. Factors predicting survival in adults with stage I and II large-cell lymphoma treated with primary radiation therapy. *Ann Intern Med* 1986;104:747–756.
161. Landberg TG, Hakansson LG, Moller TR, et al. CVP-remission-maintenance in stage I or II non-Hodgkin's lymphomas: preliminary results of a randomized study. *Cancer* 1979;44:831–838.
162. Monfardini S, Banfi A, Bonadonna G, et al. Improved five year survival after combined radiotherapy-chemotherapy for stage I–II non-Hodgkin's lymphoma. *Int J Radiat Oncol Biol Phys* 1980;6:125–134.
163. Nissen NI, Ersboll J, Hansen HS, et al. A randomized study of radiotherapy versus radiotherapy plus chemotherapy in stage I–II non-Hodgkin's lymphomas. *Cancer* 1983;52:1–7.
164. Panahon A, Kaufman JA, Grasso JA, et al. A randomized study of radiation therapy (RT) vs. RT and chemotherapy (CT) in stage IA–IIIB non-Hodgkin's lymphoma. *Proc Am Assoc Cancer Res Am Soc Clin Oncol* 1977;18:321.
165. Somers R, Burgers JM, Qasim M, et al. EORTC trial non-Hodgkin lymphomas. *Eur J Cancer Clin Oncol* 1987;23:283–293.
166. Avilés A, Delgado S, Ruiz H, et al. Treatment of non-Hodgkin's lymphoma of Waldeyer's ring: radiotherapy versus chemotherapy versus combined therapy. *Eur J Cancer B Oral Oncol* 1996;32B:19–23.
167. Yahalom J, Varsos G, Fuks Z, et al. Adjuvant cyclophosphamide, doxorubicin, vincristine, and prednisone chemotherapy after radiation therapy in stage I low-grade and intermediate-grade non-Hodgkin's lymphoma. Results of a prospective randomized study. *Cancer* 1993;71:2342–2350.
168. Johnson RE. Total body irradiation (TBI) as primary therapy for advanced lymphosarcoma. *Cancer* 1975;35:242–246.
169. Johnson RE. Management of generalized malignant lymphomata with "systemic" radiotherapy. *Br J Cancer* 1975;31:450–456.
170. Johnson RE, Canellos GP, Young RC, et al. Chemotherapy (cyclophosphamide, vincristine, and prednisone) versus radiotherapy (total body irradiation) for stage III–IV poorly differentiated lymphocytic lymphoma. *Cancer Treat Rep* 1978;62:321–325.
171. Carabell SC, Chaffey JT, Rosenthal DS. Results of total body irradiation in the treatment of advanced non-Hodgkin's lymphomas. *Cancer* 1979;43:994–1000.
172. Chaffey JT, Rosenthal DS, Pinkus G, et al. Advanced lymphosarcoma treated by total body irradiation. *Br J Cancer Suppl* 1975;2:441–449.
173. Chaffey JT, Rosenthal DS, Moloney WC, et al. Total body irradiation as treatment for lymphosarcoma. *Int J Radiat Oncol Biol Phys* 1976;1:399–405.
174. Chaffey JT, Hellman S, Rosenthal DS, et al. Total-body irradiation in the treatment of lymphocytic lymphoma. *Cancer Treat Rep* 1977;61:1149–1152.
175. Hoppe RT, Kushlan P, Kaplan HS, et al. The treatment of advanced stage favorable histology non-Hodgkin's lymphoma: a preliminary report of a randomized trial comparing single agent chemotherapy, combination chemotherapy, and whole body irradiation. *Blood* 1981;58:592–598.
176. Mendenhall NP, Noyes WD, Million RR. Total body irradiation for stage II–IV non-Hodgkin's lymphoma: ten-year follow-up. *J Clin Oncol* 1989;7:67–74.
177. Thar TL, Million RR. Total body irradiation in non-Hodgkin's lymphoma. *Cancer* 1978;42:926–931.
178. A prospective comparison of combination chemotherapy with total body irradiation in the treatment of advanced non-Hodgkin's lymphoma. British National Lymphoma Investigation Report. *Clin Oncol* 1981;7:193–200.

179. Pettingale KW. The management of generalised Grade 2 non-Hodgkin's lymphomas (Report No 18). *Clin Radiol* 1981;32:553–556.
180. Dobbs HJ, Barrett A, Rostom AY, et al. Total-body irradiation in advanced non-Hodgkin's lymphoma. *Br J Radiol* 1981;54:878–881.
181. De Neve WJ, Lybeert ML, Meerwaldt JH. Low-dose total body irradiation in non-Hodgkin lymphoma: short- and long-term toxicity and prognostic factors. *Am J Clin Oncol* 1990;13:280–284.
182. Lybeert ML, Meerwaldt JH, Deneve W. Long-term results of low dose total body irradiation for advanced non-Hodgkin lymphoma. *Int J Radiat Oncol Biol Phys* 1987;13:1167–1172.
183. Qasim MM. Total body irradiation as a primary therapy in non-Hodgkin lymphoma. *Clin Radiol* 1979;30:287–289.
184. Safwat A. The role of low-dose total body irradiation in treatment of non-Hodgkin's lymphoma: a new look at an old method. *Radiother Oncol* 2000;56:1–8.
185. Brasch A, Lange F. Aussichten und Möglichkeiten einer Therapie mit schnellen Kathodenstrahlen. *Strahlentherapie* 1934;51:119–128.
186. Coolidge WD, Moore CN. Some experiments with high voltage cathode rays outside of the generating tube. *J Franklin Inst* 1926;202: 722–735.
187. Trump JG, van de Graaff RJ, Cloud RW. Cathode rays for radiation therapy. *Am J Roentgenol Radium Ther Nucl Med* 1940;43:728–734.
188. Trump JG, Wright KA, Evans WW, et al. High energy electrons for the treatment of extensive superficial malignant lesions. *AJR Am J Roentgenol* 1953;69:623–629.
189. Cox RS, Heck RJ, Fessenden P, et al. Development of total-skin electron therapy at two energies. *Int J Radiat Oncol Biol Phys* 1990;18:659–669.
190. Karzmark CJ, Loevinger R, Steele RE, et al. A technique for large-field, superficial electron therapy. *Radiology* 1960;74:633–644.
191. Fuks Z, Bagshaw MA. Total-skin electron treatment of mycosis fungoides. *Radiology* 1971;100:145–150.
192. Fuks Z, Bagshaw MA, Farber EM. New concepts in the management of mycosis fungoides. *Br J Dermatol* 1974;90:355–356.
193. Fuks Z, Hoppe T, Bagshaw MA. The role of total skin irradiation with electrons in the management of mycosis fungoides. *Bull Cancer* 1977;64: 291–304.
194. Hoppe RT, Fuks Z, Bagshaw MA. The rationale for curative radiotherapy in mycosis fungoides. *Int J Radiat Oncol Biol Phys* 1977;2:843–851.
195. Hoppe RT, Cox RS, Fuks Z, et al. Electron-beam therapy for mycosis fungoides: the Stanford University experience. *Cancer Treat Rep* 1979;63:691–700.
196. Hoppe RT, Fuks Z, Bagshaw MA. Radiation therapy in the management of cutaneous T-cell lymphomas. *Cancer Treat Rep* 1979;63:625–632.
197. Hoppe RT, Wood GS, Abel EA. Mycosis fungoides and the Sézary syndrome: pathology, staging, and treatment. *Curr Probl Cancer* 1990;14: 295–361.
198. Freeman CR, Suissa S, Shenouda G, et al. Clinical experience with a single field rotational total skin electron irradiation technique for cutaneous T-cell lymphoma. *Radiother Oncol* 1992;24:155–162.
199. Jones GW, Tadros A, Hodson DI, et al. Prognosis with newly diagnosed mycosis fungoides after total skin electron radiation of 30 or 35 GY. *Int J Radiat Oncol Biol Phys* 1994;28:839–845.
200. Kirova YM, Piedbois Y, Haddad E, et al. Radiotherapy in the management of mycosis fungoides: indications, results, prognosis. Twenty years experience. *Radiother Oncol* 1999;51:147–151.
201. Lo TC, Salzman FA, Moschella SL, et al. Whole body surface electron irradiation in the treatment of mycosis fungoides. An evaluation of 200 patients. *Radiology* 1979;130:453–457.
202. van Vloten WA, de Vroome H, Noordijk EM. Total skin electron beam irradiation for cutaneous T-cell lymphoma (mycosis fungoides). *Br J Dermatol* 1985;112:697–702.
203. Becker M, Hoppe RT, Knox SJ. Multiple courses of high-dose total skin electron beam therapy in the management of mycosis fungoides. *Int J Radiat Oncol Biol Phys* 1995;32:1445–1449.
204. Jaffe ES, Harris NL, Stein H, et al. *Pathology and genetics of tumours of haematopoietic and lymphoid tissues.* Lyon, France: IARC Press, 2001.

SECTION II ■ ETIOLOGY, EPIDEMIOLOGY, AND BIOLOGY

CHAPTER 3 ■ DEVELOPMENTAL AND FUNCTIONAL BIOLOGY OF B LYMPHOCYTES

RALF KÜPPERS

B lymphocytes are central components of the adaptive immune response. Their important role in the control of infections becomes evident from the fact that humans with deficiencies in the generation of functional B cells suffer from severe diseases (1). The main task of B cells is to search for foreign antigens, such as infectious agents, and to produce large amounts of specific antibody once activated by such antigens to mediate their elimination from the body. To be able to combat an extremely diverse variety of foreign antigens, each newly generated B cell in the body is equipped with a distinct antigen receptor. This formidable task is accomplished by the structure of the gene segments coding for the variable part of the antibody molecule. Antibodies are composed of heavy and light chains, and the variable regions of both are encoded by distinct gene segments (called V, D, and J for the heavy chain, and V and J for the two types of light chain genes, κ and λ) that need to be somatically rearranged to give rise to functional V region genes (Fig. 3.1). This modal structure of the immunoglobulin (Ig) loci allows an essentially limitless diversity of antibodies to be generated. Even further diversity is accomplished in later stages of B-cell development, when antigen-activated B lymphocytes undergo the process of somatic hypermutation. As the production of antigen-specific antibodies is the main role of B cells in the immune response, it is perhaps not surprising that the life of these cells is dominated from the beginning to the end by selection of the appropriate cell surface receptor in the various stages of development (2).

THE GENERATION OF B LYMPHOCYTES

Development of B-Cell Precursors

B lymphocytes are generated in the bone marrow from hematopoietic stem cells. The development of B cells is regulated by an ordered rearrangement of the antigen receptor genes and selection of the cells at successive stages of development for appropriate receptor molecules (2). The first B-lineage cells are called *pro-B cells*. In these cells, D_H to J_H gene rearrangements occur, often, but not always on both IgH alleles, which are located on chromosome 14 in humans. There are 27 D_H and six J_H gene segments available for this process (3,4). In the next step, one of approximately 50 functional V_H gene segments is rearranged to a D_HJ_H joint (Fig. 3.1) (5). As the joining sites of the V_H, D_H, and J_H gene segments are variable and often modified by the addition of nongerm-

line encoded nucleotides, the V_H to D_HJ_H rearrangement can be either productive or nonproductive (discussed in more detail in section 'V Gene Recombination and Antibody Diversity'). Only productive IgH gene rearrangements can give rise to a heavy chain protein. If the first $V_HD_HJ_H$ rearrangement is nonproductive, the B-cell precursor has a second chance to generate a productive IgH gene rearrangement by using the second IgH allele. Productively rearranged IgH genes are expressed together with a surrogate light chain that

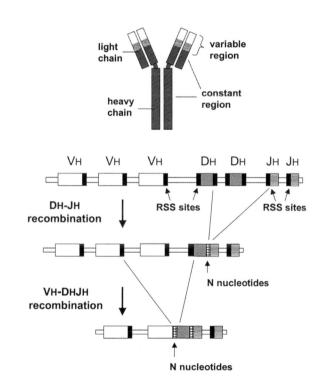

FIGURE 3.1 Structure of the antibody and outline of V(D)J recombination. The upper part depicts the structure of the antibody molecule, which is composed of two identical heavy and two identical light chains. Heavy, as well as light, chains consist of a variable and a constant part. The variable regions mediate antigen binding, whereas the constant region of the heavy chain determines the effector functions of the antibody. The lower part depicts the principle of V(D)J recombination at the heavy chain locus. During heavy chain gene rearrangements, first one of 27 D_H gene segments is joined to one of six J_H gene segments. The intervening DNA is deleted from the chromosome as a circle and later lost from the cell. The recombination is mediated by cutting the DNA at the recombination signal sequence (RSS) sites. In the second step, one of approximately 50 functional V_H genes is recombined to a D_HJ_H joint. At the V-D and D-J joining sites, additional diversity is generated by the removal of nucleotides from the ends of the gene segments and the addition of nongermline encoded N nucleotides.

is composed of two proteins, λ5 and VpreB, and the signal transducing molecules Igα and Igβ (CD79a and CD79b); this structure is called the *pre-B-cell receptor*. Cells are then selected for expression of the pre-B-cell receptor. It is, however, not yet clarified whether expression on the cell surface is needed or whether assembly of this complex in the endoplasmatic reticulum is sufficient; it is also not known whether the receptor needs to bind to some ligand for signaling. Expression of this receptor has several consequences. The cells, which are now called *pre-B cells*, discontinue further IgH gene rearrangements, divide several times, and then initiate light chain gene rearrangements (2). As further IgH gene rearrangements are prevented once a pre-B cell carries a productive V_H gene rearrangement, B cells usually express only one IgH allele, a phenomenon called *allelic exclusion*.

There are two light chain loci in the human, the Igκ locus on chromosome 2 and the Igλ locus on chromosome 22. In the κ locus, there are, depending on the haplotype, 30 to 35 functional Vκ gene segments and five Jκ segments, whereas in the λ locus, there are 30 to 37 functional Vλ gene segments and four functional Jλ gene segments available for recombination (6–10). Pre-B cells usually first perform light chain gene rearrangements on κ loci, and only if these fail to give rise to a productive light chain gene, the Igλ locus is rearranged. This is suggested by the fact that the normal and malignant human κ-expressing B cells in most cases have the λ locus in germline configuration, whereas λ-expressing B cells carry rearranged κ loci (11–13). A productive light chain gene rearrangement is then expressed. If the corresponding light chain cannot pair with the heavy chain of the cell, further light chain gene rearrangements can be performed. In case the light chain can pair with the heavy chain and be expressed on the cell surface, the cells are now called *immature B cells*. These cells undergo a further selection process before they can become mature B cells. The immature B cells are tested for binding of the B-cell receptor to autoantigens. Cells that show strong binding to such antigens are either removed by apoptosis, or they reinitiate light chain gene rearrangements to replace the originally expressed light chain by a novel one (receptor editing), so that the cells may now express a B-cell receptor without autoreactivity (14). If the immature B cells pass also this last selection process, they become mature B cells and are allowed to leave the bone marrow microenvironment to enter the peripheral immune system. Mature B cells express, with rare exceptions, only one light chain gene, either of the κ or λ isotype (allelic and isotype exclusion). Whereas immature B cells carry only IgM on their surface, mature B cells coexpress IgM and IgD. About 60% of mature human B cells express κ light chains; 40% express λ light chains.

V Gene Recombination and Antibody Diversity

V gene recombination is guided by specific sequences flanking the V, D, and J gene segments, the recombination signal sequences. These sites are composed of a conserved heptamer, a spacer of either 12 or 23 base pairs' length and a conserved nonamer (15). The sites are present at the 3′ end of V gene segments, at the 5′ ends of J gene segments, and at both ends of D_H gene segments (Fig. 3.1). Rearrangement takes place only between gene segments with different spacer lengths (12/23 base pair rule). For example, in the human IgH locus, V and J gene segments have recombination signal sequences with 23 base pair spacers, whereas the recombination signal sequences of D_H gene segments contain 12 base pair spacers. This ensures that rearrangement cannot happen between two V gene segments, and that a V_H gene is not directly joined to a J_H gene.

The enzymatic machinery that controls V gene recombination is largely known [reviewed in (15)]. Only two of the enzymes involved in the process are lymphocyte specific, namely the recombination activating genes RAG-1 and RAG-2. These enzymes recognize the recombination signal sequences and introduce deoxyribonucleic acid (DNA) double-strand breaks precisely between the heptamer of the recombination signal sequences and the respective gene segment (16). This happens in a complex in which the ends of the two rearranging gene segments are brought close to each other. The ends of the gene segments (coding ends) are closed by the generation of hairpin loops, whereas the ends of the recombination signal sequences (signal ends) have a blunt end structure. In the next step, the coding ends are opened at a variable position along the hairpin. This may create short palindromic sequences (P nucleotides) that contribute to the diversity of the joining sites. The coding ends are usually further modified, either by the exonucleolytic loss of some base pairs or by the introduction of additional, nongermline-encoded bases (N nucleotides). The latter is mediated by the enzyme terminal desoxynucleotidyltransferase. After these modifications, the coding ends are joined. These modifications of the joining sites vastly increase the diversity of the antigen-binding sites, thereby significantly contributing to the essentially limitless diversity of antibody molecules. The signal ends of the intervening DNA are usually closed to a circle, which is released from the complex and later lost from the cell. However, when the rearranging gene segments are not in the same transcriptional orientation, as it is the case for approximately one half of the human Vκ gene segments in relation to the Jκ genes, V gene recombination does not result in the deletion of the intervening DNA but in an inversion, without loss of DNA from the chromosome (8).

Besides the lymphocyte-specific RAG proteins (and optionally terminal deoxynucleotidyl transferase), the enzymatic recombination machinery is composed of ubiquitously expressed enzymes involved in double-stranded DNA repair, i.e., DNA-PKcs, the Ku70 and Ku80 proteins, XRCC4, DNA ligase IV, and the Artemis protein (15). Artemis in a complex with DNA-PKcs mediates opening of the hairpin and trimming of the overhangs (17). If any of the components of the V gene recombination machinery is lacking, V gene recombination is blocked, and no or only few mature lymphocytes develop.

Due to the modifications introduced at the ends of the rearranging gene segments, the correct reading frame of the Ig gene, defined by the start codon in the leader peptide of the V gene segment, can be either retained or lost in the V(D)J joining reaction. In in-frame rearrangements, the J gene segment and the following C gene to which the V region gene is precisely spliced are read in the correct reading frame and can thus be translated into protein (note that many D_H elements can be read in all three possible reading frames). However, if the reading frame is lost, the C gene is not read in the correct reading frame, and the rearrangement

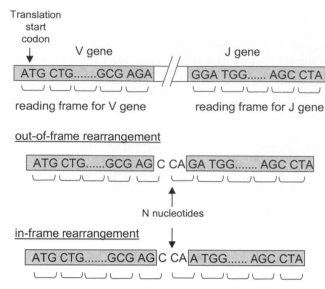

FIGURE 3.2 V gene rearrangements can be in frame or out-of-frame. Shown are two possible outcomes of a V_L to J_L joining. The reading frame of the V gene segment is defined by the start codon of the leader exon (leader exon and V segment are not distinguished here). There is also only one functional reading frame for the J gene segment, as this is directly spliced to the constant region gene, which codes for an Ig light chain protein only in one reading frame. If the removal of nucleotides from the ends of the V and J segments and the addition of N nucleotides result in a reading frame in which the J gene segment (and consequently the C gene) is read in the correct frame, the rearrangement is in frame (note that in-frame rearrangements can be nonfunctional if a stop codon is generated at the V-J joint). In out-of-frame rearrangements, the number of nucleotides between the last complete V codon and the first complete J codon is not a multiple of three, so that the J segment and, consequently, the C segment are not translated in the correct reading frame. Such rearrangements are nonfunctional, as they do not code for an Ig light chain protein. Note that out-of-frame rearrangements do not necessarily generate stop codons at the joining site or in the J gene. Usually, stop codons are encountered in the C-gene segments if they are translated in the wrong reading frame, resulting in premature translation stop. The correct codons defined in the germline and the codons used after rearrangement are indicated below the sequences.

is out-of-frame (Fig. 3.2). Often, premature stop codons are encountered in the incorrectly translated C genes. As the codons are nucleotide triplets, only one-third of the rearrangements will be in frame.

The high frequency of nonproductive V gene rearrangements potentially results in a massive wastage of B-cell precursors that did not succeed in generating productive heavy and light chain gene rearrangements. However, the loss of cells is reduced, as on the heavy chain locus, a second recombination attempt can be made on the second IgH allele. For the light chains, there are even four loci available (two κ and two λ). Moreover, the structure of the light chain loci allows for repeated V-J rearrangements on a given allele. If a first rearrangement is nonproductive, a second attempt can be made if upstream unrearranged V and downstream germline J segments are still present. For the heavy chain locus, this kind of additional rearrangement is not possible, as all germline D_H gene segments are deleted in the first $V_H D_H J_H$ recombination, and a direct V_H to J_H joining is not allowed, as discussed previously. However, most human V_H gene segments contain an internal heptamer sequence close to the 3' end of the coding sequence, and the analysis of pre-B-cell leukemias indicates

that this internal heptamer can be used to perform a V_H gene replacement, in which an upstream V_H germline gene replaces a V_H gene segment in a $V_H D_H J_H$ joint (18). However, it is not known whether V_H gene replacement is used at a significant frequency in the development of normal B cells.

B CELLS IN T-CELL-DEPENDENT IMMUNE RESPONSES

Initiating T-Cell-Dependent Immune Responses

If foreign antigens cross the epithelial layers of the body and enter human tissues, they are taken up by resident dendritic cells. These dendritic cells then migrate to the T-cell zone of local lymph nodes where they present antigenic peptides on major histocompatibility complex class II molecules. This results in the specific recruitment and activation of antigen-specific T-helper cells. B cells that enter lymph nodes through high endothelial venules also migrate through the T-cell zones on their way to the B-cell follicles. If a B cell encounters cognate antigen in the T-cell zone, it is retained in this area and becomes activated (19). Antigen-specific T and B cells can now interact and stimulate each other. As a consequence, B cells start to proliferate, and clusters of proliferating B cells, called *primary foci*, become visible a few days after initiation of the immune response (19). A fraction of these B cells differentiates into short-lived plasma cells and produces a first wave of antibody (20). Other antigen-specific B cells of the foci migrate into primary B-cell follicles where they then initiate the germinal center reaction (Fig. 3.3). Experiments in the mouse indicate that the primary foci usually involute after a few days (21).

Germinal Center Reaction

Antigen-activated B cells that migrate from the T-cell zone into primary B-cell follicles start to vigorously proliferate and differentiate into centroblasts (22). The resident resting B cells of the primary follicle are moved away from the follicle center and build a corona of resting cells around the germinal center, the mantle zone. After some days, two distinct compartments of the germinal center can be histologically recognized, the dark zone and the light zone (Fig. 3.4). The dark zone is dominated by proliferating centroblasts and harbors a loose network of follicular dendritic cells, whereas the light zone is mainly composed of noncycling centrocytes, a dense network of follicular dendritic cells and T-helper cells (22). In the course of their clonal expansion, centroblasts activate the process of somatic hypermutation, which introduces mutations at a high rate into the V region genes of the antigen receptor (23–25) (see section 'Somatic Hypermutation'). Thereby, antibody variants are generated. The centroblasts then move to the light zone where they are selected based on the affinity of their B-cell receptor to the respective antigen (Fig. 3.4). Germinal center B cells expressing a B-cell receptor with increased affinity will be able to appropriately interact with germinal center T cells and follicular dendritic cells, and be positively selected (26,27). Likely, the vast majority of germinal center B cells acquire disadvantageous mutations and

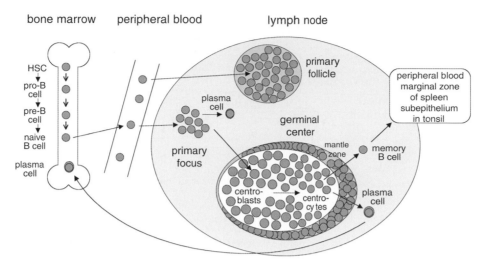

FIGURE 3.3 B-cell developmental pathways. B cells are generated in the bone marrow (or during fetal development in the liver) from hematopoietic stem cells. B-cell precursors that performed D_H-J_H rearrangements at their Ig H loci are called *pro-B cells*. D_H-J_H rearrangements are usually followed by V_H to $D_H J_H$ rearrangements, and the cells expressing a functional heavy chain rearrangement are termed *pre-B cells*. The cells then perform rearrangements at their light chain loci. Cells expressing a functional (and nonautoreactive) B-cell receptor are allowed to mature and leave the bone marrow as naive B cells. Naive B cells are found in the peripheral blood; in secondary lymphoid organs, they constitute primary B-cell follicles and the mantle zone of secondary B-cell follicles. Early steps in adaptive immune responses usually take place in the T-cell area of lymphoid organs, where antigen-activated B cells are in contact with T cells and dendritic cells. The interaction of these cells stimulates B-cell proliferation, leading to the generation of primary B-cell foci in the T-cell area. Some of the B cells differentiate into (presumably short-lived) plasma cells. Other activated B cells migrate into B-cell follicles, where they undergo massive clonal expansion and establish germinal centers (see Fig. 3.4 for details of the germinal center reaction). Positively selected germinal center B cells differentiate to memory B cells or plasmablasts and leave the germinal center. Many plasma cell precursors migrate to the bone marrow, where these long-lived cells can secrete large amounts of antibody. Memory B cells are found in the peripheral blood and also in lymphoid organs. In tonsils, they are mainly located in the subepithelial region; in the spleen, they are a major constituent of the marginal zone.

undergo apoptosis. These cells are taken up by macrophages, which are also present in the germinal center (28). Recent in vivo imaging studies revealed that germinal center B cells are highly motile, and likely undergo repeated rounds of proliferation, mutation, and selection, resulting in a very efficient selection of germinal center B cells with high-affinity B-cell receptors (29–31).

In many germinal center B cells, the Ig genes are not only modified at the level of the V region genes by somatic hypermutation, but also by altering the isotype of the IgH constant region genes. This change from IgM and IgD expression to IgG, IgA, or IgE is performed by a somatic recombination process, termed *class-switch recombination* (see section 'Class-Switch Recombination').

Based on the detection of RAG transcripts or protein in germinal center B cells and V gene recombination intermediates in both human and mouse, it has been suggested that V gene recombination may be reinitiated in germinal center B cells (32–34). This would enable these cells to revise their antigen receptors, e.g., by replacing the originally expressed light chain gene by a novel one, and would represent a further means of antibody diversification in germinal center B cells. However, other studies question the original reports (35). In the human, RAG- and terminal deoxynucleotidyl transferase-expressing tonsillar B cells are mostly found outside germinal centers, perhaps representing immature B cells (36). Hence, the contribution of receptor revision to shaping the memory B-cell compartment in the human seems to be modest at most (37).

Finally, the selected germinal center B cells differentiate either into memory B cells or plasma cell precursors and leave the germinal center microenvironment. The signals that regulate these different developmental pathways are not yet fully understood. However, in vitro experiments suggest that incubation of germinal center B cells with interleukin (IL)-2 and IL-10 and cross-linking of CD40, or cross-linking of the B-cell receptor together with IL-4 stimulation induces differentiation of the cells to a resting B-cell population resembling memory B cells (38,39). Treatment of germinal center B cells with recombinant CD23 and IL-1α results in the development of cells sharing features with plasma cells (40). Intriguingly, the CD40 ligand is expressed by germinal center T cells (41), and CD23 is highly expressed by follicular dendritic cells (42). Studies in the mouse indicate that plasma cells generated in the germinal center are very long lived, so that they are able to sustain high serum antibody levels (43,44).

Somatic Hypermutation

Somatic hypermutation is a process by which point mutations are introduced into productively or nonproductively rearranged V region genes at a high rate (10^{-3} to 10^{-4}/bp/cell division) (45). The mutations are introduced into the DNA over a distance of 1.5 to 2 kilobases, beginning downstream of the V gene promoter and extending into the intron between variable and constant region genes. The constant region genes

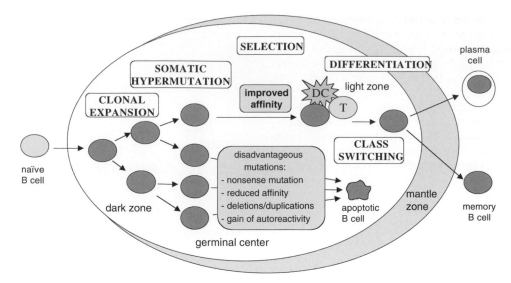

FIGURE 3.4 The germinal center reaction. Antigen-activated B cells that receive appropriate T-cell help are driven into primary B-cell follicles where they establish germinal centers. In the germinal center, a dark zone and a light zone can be distinguished. The dark zone mainly consists of proliferating germinal center B cells, the centroblasts, whereas the germinal center B cells in the light zone, the centrocytes, are mostly resting B cells. The germinal center is surrounded by a mantle of resting, naive B cells, which constitute the primary follicle. In proliferating germinal center B cells, the process of somatic hypermutation is activated, which leads to the introduction of mutations at a high rate specifically into the Ig V region genes of the proliferating B cells. Most mutations are disadvantageous for the cells such as when they result in reduced affinity of the B-cell receptor to the respective antigen. B cells acquiring such mutations undergo apoptosis. Only a few germinal center B cells acquire affinity increasing mutations, and these cells are positively selected. The selection process presumably takes place mainly in the light zone, where the centrocytes are in close contact with CD4 T cells and follicular dendritic cells. A fraction of the centrocytes undergoes class-switch recombination. Finally, antigen-selected germinal center B cells will differentiate to memory B cells or plasma cells and leave the germinal center microenvironment.

themselves are not targeted by somatic hypermutation. Most of the mutations are single nucleotide exchanges, but deletions and duplications of various length can also be found, accounting for approximately 4% to 5% of the mutation events in human B cells (46). The generation of such deletions and duplications is likely related to the fact that somatic hypermutation is accompanied by DNA strand breaks in the V region genes (46–48). The pattern of somatic mutations is not random. There is an intrinsic preference for transitions (replacement of a purine by a purine base or a pyrimidine by a pyrimidine base) over transversions (replacement of a purine by a pyrimidine base or vice versa), and several hot-spot motifs of somatic hypermutation have been identified (49). The most prominent hot spot is the RGYW motif (with R representing A or G, Y representing C or T, and W defining A or T) (49,50).

Somatic hypermutation depends on transcription of the target sequence, although the V gene promoter can be replaced by other promoters (51,52). Likewise, the target sequence does not have to be a rearranged V gene but can be any sequence downstream of the promoter (53). In contrast, the Ig enhancers represent indispensable elements for somatic hypermutation, as their deletion severely impairs somatic hypermutation (51). Hence, the target for hypermutation of Ig V genes is defined by an active promoter in close association with the Ig-specific enhancers.

Somatic hypermutation appears to be not absolutely specific for rearranged Ig genes. So far, three genes have been identified in humans that acquire mutations in germinal center B cells at a significant frequency and with a mutation pattern consistent with somatic hypermutation. The bcl-6 gene

is found mutated in its 5′ region in about one-third of human germinal center and memory B cells (54,55). Also, the CD95 and the CD79b genes carry mutations in their 5′ regions in a small fraction of germinal center B cells (56,57). The molecular features of these genes causing them to be targeted by the hypermutation machinery are still unclear.

Several years ago, the enzyme activation-induced cytidine deaminase (AID) was identified as an essential component of both somatic hypermutation and class-switch recombination (58,59). The role of AID as a master regulator of these processes is suggested by the fact that AID deficiency in humans results in the autosomal recessive form of the hyper-IgM syndrome, which is characterized by the absence of class-switch recombination and a lack of somatic hypermutation (59), and that ectopic AID expression is sufficient to cause somatic hypermutation and class switching of transgenic constructs in non-B cells (60,61). AID initiates somatic hypermutation by deaminating cytosine bases in the DNA, resulting in the generation of uracil, which is not a normal base in DNA. This lesion can be resolved in several ways, by error-prone DNA repair (62). DNA repair enzymes involved in hypermutation include uracil-DNA glycosylase and the mismatch binding factor MSH2. Several error-prone DNA polymerases are presumably also involved in somatic hypermutation, including the polymerases η, ζ, and Rev1 (63–65).

Although it is clear that somatic hypermutation is a hallmark of germinal center B cells and that at least the vast majority of B cells with mutated Ig genes are derived from germinal center B cells, it is an intriguing question whether hypermutation may occur in human B cells also outside of the germinal center microenvironment. Two mouse models have been described in which somatic mutations occur in the absence of or outside of germinal centers (66,67). Importantly, patients with hyper-IgM syndrome who appear to lack germinal centers due to a deficiency in the CD40-ligand gene, lack classic memory B cells, but have an IgM+IgD+CD27+ B-cell population with somatically mutated Ig genes (68). This raises the interesting possibility that the mutated IgD+ B cells are generated in a germinal center-independent way. However, it may well be that CD40L-independent germinal center (-like) structures supporting somatic hypermutation but not class switching exist in some lymphoid organs of patients with hyper-IgM syndrome. This would be reminiscent of the situation in CD19-deficient mice, which do not develop germinal centers in spleen and lymph nodes upon immunization, but that have these structures in Peyer patches (69). It is also noteworthy that patients with hyper-IgM with a deficiency in the CD40 gene apparently lack a population of somatically mutated IgD+CD27+ B cells (70). In conclusion, some human B cells may acquire somatic mutations in a germinal center-independent manner, but direct evidence for this is still weak.

Class-Switch Recombination

Class-switch recombination is, besides V gene recombination and somatic hypermutation, the third B-cell-specific process that modifies the Ig genes. By class switching, the Ig heavy chain constant region gene expressed by a B cell is changed. Naive B cells express IgM and IgD on their surface as a result of differential splicing of the corresponding messenger ribonucleic acid (mRNA) transcripts, but after antigen activation, the IgH class of the B-cell receptor is often changed to IgG, IgA, or IgE. This alters the effector functions of the antibody molecule. For example, IgA dimers can cross epithelial layers and can be secreted into the gut lumen, and IgG can bind to specific receptors on phagocytic cells (Fcγ receptors), thereby improving pathogen recognition and binding by those cells.

In the human, there are nine IgH constant (C_H) region genes, one Cμ, one Cδ, four Cγ, two Cα, and one Cε gene (71). These gene segments are located downstream of the V, D, and J gene segments on chromosome 14. Class switching is mediated by a somatic recombination process that results in deletion of the originally expressed IgH genes (usually IgM and IgD) and their replacement by one of the further downstream-located IgH genes.

The class-switch recombination process is initiated by transcription from promoters upstream of the C_H genes (72). These transcripts contain a first exon (I exon) located upstream of repetitive elements, the switch regions, that is spliced to the C_H exons. The generation of these germline transcripts and their splicing is mandatory for the class-switch recombination process, but it is not yet clarified whether the role of this transcription is mainly in regulating the accessibility of the IgH locus for the recombination machinery, or whether the germline transcripts are directly involved in the recombination process (73,74).

In the next step, DNA breaks (either double-strand breaks or staggered single-strand breaks) are introduced into the repetitive switch regions of the two C_H genes involved in the class-switching process (Fig. 3.5). The intervening DNA is excised as a circle (switch circle) that is later lost from the cell, and the two switch regions are joined. Class switching usually

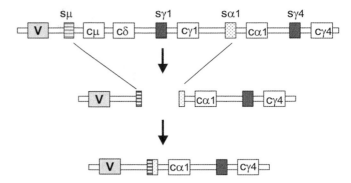

FIGURE 3.5 Class-switch recombination. Class switching is initiated by transcription through the repetitive switch regions and the C_H genes involved in the recombination process, followed by splicing of the transcripts (not shown). In the next step, DNA strand breaks are introduced in the switch regions. The DNA between the two switch sites is deleted as a circle (not shown) and later lost from the cell. As a result of the class-switch recombination process, a downstream C_H gene is now juxtaposed to the V region gene, so that this C_H gene is now expressed instead of the original one.

results in replacement of the originally expressed Cμ (and Cδ) gene by a downstream C_H gene, but there is also indication that sequential class-switching processes can take place (75).

The enzymes involved in the regulation of class-switch recombination are only partly known. The later steps of the process appear to be mediated by the components of nonhomologous end-joining DNA repair. A master regulator and perhaps the only B-cell–specific component of class switching is the AID protein, as its ectopic expression is sufficient to induce class switching of an extrachromosomal construct even in fibroblasts (60).

Most class switching takes place in the germinal center microenvironment, which is evident from the fact that nearly all class-switched B cells and plasma cells in the human carry somatically mutated V region genes and, hence, the hallmark of a germinal center passage. However, class-switch recombination, mostly to Cγ2, can also take place in T-cell-independent immune responses (76,77).

B CELLS IN T-INDEPENDENT IMMUNE RESPONSES

Although humoral immune responses against most protein antigens are dependent on T-helper cells, antibodies against many bacterial antigens can also be produced in humans or mice lacking a thymus or with other T-cell deficiencies. Such thymus independent (TI) antigens fall into two classes: TI-1 and TI-2 antigens. TI-1 antigens result in a polyclonal B-cell activation, and can thus also be considered as B-cell mitogens. TI-2 antigens are characterized by highly repetitive structures (78). This allows for a strong cross-linking of the B-cell receptor on the surface of the B cells. TI-2 antigens are typically bacterial capsular polysaccharides. Immune responses of the TI-II-type are, however, not completely T cell independent, because mouse strains lacking all T cells are impaired in immune responses against TI-2 antigens (78). The exact role of T cells in these responses is not yet understood. There are indications that specific subsets of B cells are mainly involved in T-independent immune responses, namely CD5+ B cells and a fraction of marginal zone B cells.

REGULATION OF B-CELL DEVELOPMENT AND DIFFERENTIATION BY TRANSCRIPTION FACTORS AND MICRO-RIBONUCLEIC ACIDS

The appropriate expression of genes needed for the generation of B cells and the execution of specific functions at distinct stages of differentiation is regulated by the coordinated activity of a series of transcription factors (Fig. 3.6). One of the factors needed for the earliest stages of B-cell development is PU.1, which is expressed exclusively in hematopoietic cells (79). PU.1 plays a role not only for the development of B cells but also of macrophages. Although very high expression of this ets-type transcription factor favors the development of macrophages, moderate expression results in a preferential generation of B cells (80).

The E12 and E47 gene products of the E2A gene are members of the basic helix-loop-helix family of transcription factors. They are widely expressed, but homodimeric complexes appear to be restricted to B-lineage cells (81). The E2A proteins are involved in the expression and rearrangement of Ig genes. Hence, E2A is essential for the development of pro-B cells from common lymphoid precursors. Another transcription factor needed for the development of pro-B cells is the early B-cell factor (EBF), which is expressed at all stages of B-cell differentiation, excluding plasma cells (82). Genes activated by EBF include: the transcription factor Pax-5; the B-cell receptor-associated signal-transducing mole-

cule CD79b; $\lambda 5$, a component of the pre-B-cell receptor; and κ light chains. EBF also contributes to B-cell fate commitment by repressing the expression of alternative lineage genes (83).

The key molecule for the commitment of cells to the B lineage is the transcription factor B-cell-specific activating protein, the product of the Pax-5 gene. Mouse models revealed that in the absence of Pax-5, B-cell development is arrested at the pro-B-cell stage, and that these cells that carry $D_H J_H$ joints have retained the capacity to give rise to other lineages, such as T cells and monocytes (84,85). Thus, one of the main functions of Pax-5 appears to be the suppression of alternative developmental pathways in B-lineage precursors and the commitment of these cells to the B-lymphoid lineage. Critical B-cell-specific genes are positively controlled by B-cell-specific activating protein, including CD19 and CD79a. The Pax-5 gene is also expressed in mature B cells and appears to play a role in these cells to maintain their B-cell identity (86).

For the differentiation of activated B cells to germinal center B cells, the transcriptional repressor Bcl-6 is critical, as Bcl-6-deficient mice are unable to generate germinal centers (87,88). Bcl-6 is highly up-regulated and expressed in germinal center B cells and down-regulated before the cells differentiate to memory or plasma cells (89,90). Bcl-6 regulates a large number of genes in germinal center B cells (91). Rapid proliferation of germinal center B cells is mediated by Bcl-6 through repression of the cell cycle inhibitors p21 and p27kip1 (91,92). Bcl-6 may also allow germinal center B cells to sustain the physiologic genotoxic stress caused by the vigorous proliferation of these cells, and the DNA strand breaks associated with somatic hypermutation and class-switch

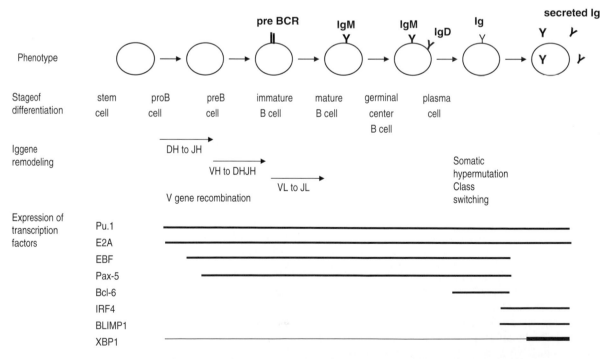

FIGURE 3.6 Stages of B-cell development. Given are the main stages of B-cell development in the human. It is indicated at which stages Ig genes are remodeled by V gene recombination, somatic hypermutation, or class-switch recombination. The expression pattern of several key transcription factors for B-cell development is shown. Note that this list does not include all known transcription factors involved in B-cell development. IRF4 and Blimp1 are starting to be expressed in a small subset of germinal center B cells in the light zone with plasmacytoid features. These cells are already Bcl-6$^-$.

recombination by suppressing p53 and ATR, two main components of the DNA damage response (93,94). Moreover, Bcl-6 represses transcription factors important for plasma cell differentiation (see next paragraph), thereby arresting cells at the germinal center B-cell stage of development as long as Bcl-6 is expressed.

When germinal center B cells differentiate into plasma cells, major changes in gene expression happen. This is accompanied by down-regulation of several transcription factors that are expressed during early B-cell development and in mature B cells, such as EBF and Pax-5. Moreover, as already discussed, down-regulation of Bcl-6 is needed to allow germinal center B cells to terminally differentiate. However, several transcription factors are up-regulated in plasma cells, namely the B-lymphocyte-induced maturation protein-1 (Blimp-1), interferon regulatory factor-4 (IRF-4, also called *MUM-1*), and X-box-binding protein-1 (XBP-1). Expression of Blimp-1 and IRF-4 is already detectable in a small subset of germinal center B cells that are located in the light zone and resemble early plasma cells, suggesting that the differentiation of germinal center B cells toward plasma cells is initiated in the germinal center microenvironment (95,96).

Blimp-1 is a transcriptional repressor that is involved in the repression of many genes, including Bcl-6, Pax-5, c-Myc, CD19, CD20, and major histocompatibility complex class II [summarized in (97)]. Thus, Blimp-1 down-regulates many germinal center B-cell functions and activates plasma cell functions. Blimp-1 is repressed by Bcl-6 (91); hence, the balance between Bcl-6 and Blimp-1 is a key determinant for the switch from a germinal center B cell to a plasma cell fate. IRF-4 can associate with several other transcription factors, such as PU.1 and SpiB, and the lack of plasma cells in IRF-4 deficient mice suggests an important role in plasma cell development (98). So far, little is known about the genes regulated by this factor besides a potential involvement in the regulation of Ig transcription and class-switch recombination (99). XBP-1 is an activating ubiquitously expressed transcription factor that it is highly up-regulated in plasma cells (100). The critical target genes of XBP-1 are still unknown, but like in the case of IRF-4, no plasma cells develop in mice in the absence of XBP-1. This transcription factor is repressed by the Pax-5 gene product (101), which is likely one of the reasons why down-regulation of Pax-5 is a prerequisite for the development of plasma cells.

It has recently become clear that B-cell differentiation processes are not only regulated at the transcriptional level by transcription factors, but also at the posttranscriptional level by small, noncoding ribonucleic acids (RNAs), the *micro-RNAs* (miRNAs). These approximately 22-nucleotide long molecules bind to complementary sequences in the $3'$ ends of mRNAs and regulate gene expression either by inducing degradation of the target mRNAs or by inhibiting their translation. For several miRNAs, important roles in B-cell development and differentiation have been revealed. miR-181 promotes differentiation of hematopoietic precursors into B-lineage cells (102), miR-155 is a regulator of the germinal center reaction and involved in the generation of class-switched plasma cells (103,104), and miR-150 controls B-cell differentiation by targeting the transcription factor c-Myb (105). That deregulated activity of miRNAs can also contribute to B-lymphoid malignancies is evident from a recent study showing that enforced expression of miR-17-92

causes lymphoproliferative disease in mice (106). Notably, in humans, the miR-17-92 cluster is located in a genomic region frequently amplified in lymphomas and other cancers. It is likely that additional miRNAs controlling particular B-cell differentiation processes will be revealed in the near future.

THE PERIPHERAL B-CELL COMPARTMENT

B Cells in the Peripheral Blood

The largest distinct population of B cells in the peripheral blood is conventional (i.e., CD5$^-$) naive B cells (Table 3.1). These cells usually account for 45% of the B-cell pool in adults (108). Naive B cells coexpress IgM and IgD on their surface, and are characterized by unmutated V region genes, lack of expression of the CD27 surface molecule, a member of the tumor necrosis factor receptor family, and expression of the adenosine 5'-triphosphate-binding cassette (ABC)B1 transporter (108,109).

In the fetus and in the first years after birth, most B cells in the peripheral blood express the CD5 antigen (110). Studies in the mouse suggested that CD5 B cells are mainly involved in T-cell-independent immune responses (type II) and are responsible for production of a large fraction of "natural" serum antibodies (111). It has been speculated that they represent a separate, perhaps evolutionary old, B-cell lineage important as a first line of defense against common infectious agents. There is indeed indication for separate progenitors of CD5$^+$ and conventional, CD5$^-$ B cells in mice (112). However, other experiments suggest that B-cell receptor engagement is critical for the development of CD5 B cells, leading to the "induced differentiation" model for the generation of these cells (111). Whether human CD5 B cells are equivalent to murine CD5 B cells is debatable. Human CD5 B cells share with murine CD5 B cells that they are the predominant B-cell population early in life, and that they only very rarely have participated in germinal center reactions as they mostly carry unmutated V region genes (113–115). In adult humans, CD5 B cell account for approximately 15% of the peripheral blood B-cell pool.

Class-switched B cells, expressing IgG, IgA, or IgE, were classically considered to represent the population of memory B cells that were generated in germinal center reactions. Most if not all of these cells, which represent about 10% to 15% of B cells in the peripheral blood (Table 3.1), indeed carry somatically mutated V region genes. Most class-switched cells express CD27, which plays a role in promoting plasma cell differentiation upon stimulation (116). A fraction of IgG$^+$ B cells, however, lacks CD27 expression (109,117). These cells have a lower level of somatic mutations in their rearranged V genes and show an IgG subclass distribution distinct from CD27$^+$IgG$^+$ memory B cells (109,117,118).

Class-switched cells appear to be not the only memory B cells in the human. Somatically mutated Ig genes are also a hallmark of cells expressing IgM without significant levels of IgD (IgM-only B cells) (119). These cells share several other features with class-switched cells, supporting their close relationship. Both B-cell subsets can under similar stimulation conditions differentiate into plasma cells, whereas naive B

TABLE 3.1

CELLULAR COMPOSITION OF THE PERIPHERAL BLOOD B-CELL COMPARTMENT[a]

B-cell subset	sIg	Phenotype				Average frequency (%)	Average mutation frequency of V_H genes (%)
		CD20	CD27	CD5	CD10		
Pregerminal center							
Naive conventional	IgM⁺IgD⁺	+	−	−	−	45	0
CD5⁺	IgM⁺IgD⁺	+	−	+	−	15	0[b]
V-preB⁺L⁺	IgM⁺IgD⁺	+	+/−	−	−	0.5–1	0[b]
Transitional	IgM⁺IgD⁺	+	−	+	+	2–4	0
Postgerminal center							
IgM⁺IgD⁺ memory	IgM⁺IgD⁺	+	+	−	−	15	5
IgM only	IgM⁺IgD^low/−	+	+	−	−	5	5
Class switched CD27⁺	IgG⁺or IgA⁺	+	+	−	−	15	6
IgG⁺CD27⁻	IgG⁺	+	−	−	−	1–4	3
IgD only	IgM⁻IgD⁺	+	+	−	−	<1	12
Plasmablasts	sIg^low/−	−	+	−	−	<2	7[c]

L, light chain; sIg, surface immunoglobulin.

[a] The average frequency of the various B-cell subsets in the peripheral blood of healthy adults and their Ig gene mutation loads can vary between individuals. Whether IgM⁺IgD⁺CD27⁺ B cells are a postgerminal center B-cell subset is debated (68).

[b] A small fraction carries mutated V genes.

[c] So far, mutation frequency only determined for plasmablasts from a patient affected by systemic lupus erythematosus (107).

cells are resistant to these stimuli (120). Both subsets are lacking in patients with hyper-IgM who apparently lack germinal centers due to a defect in the CD40 ligand gene (68). Moreover, IgM-only B cells are CD27⁺, as most class-switched memory B cells.

Interestingly, a subset of IgM⁺IgD⁺ B cells also expresses CD27 (120). These B cells, which represent up to 20% of IgD⁺ B cells and about 10% to 15% of all B cells in the peripheral blood, also carry somatically mutated V region genes, suggesting that they also represent a subset of memory B cells and that CD27 thus likely represents a marker for memory B cells in the human (108). That IgM⁺IgD⁺CD27⁺ B cells belong to the memory B-cell compartment is also supported by phenotypic and functional similarities to IgM-only and class-switched memory B cells (108,120). However, the presence of IgM⁺IgD⁺CD27⁺ B cells with mutated Ig genes in patients with CD40-ligand deficient hyper-IgM may indicate that these cells derive from a separate developmental pathway independent of germinal centers, as discussed previously (68).

Besides these main peripheral blood B-cell subsets, there are a few additional distinct populations of B-lineage cells in the peripheral blood. One of these is transitional B cells, which represent an intermediate differentiation stage between bone marrow immature B cells and mature, naive B cells. Transitional B cells are characterized by the phenotype IgM⁺IgD⁺ CD5⁺CD10⁺CD24⁺CD38^high (Table 3.1) (121,122). They harbor unmutated Ig V genes and usually represent 2% to 4% of peripheral B cells in adults.

A peculiar and rare peripheral blood B-cell subset is the population of B cells expressing IgD without IgM (IgD-only B cells), which are also found in tonsillar tissues (108,123). These cells performed an unusual class-switch recombination resulting in the deletion of the Cμ gene, although retaining the Cδ

gene, so that they express IgD in the complete absence of IgM. These cells carry the highest Ig V gene mutation load of all human B-cell subsets (average of 12% to 14%). The frequency of IgD-only B cells among all B cells in the peripheral blood is usually less than 1% (108). A further peculiarity of these cells is their predominant expression of λ light chains. The role of these cells in humoral immunity is presently unclear.

Another peculiar peripheral blood B-cell subset is defined by coexpression of κ or λ light chains and surrogate light chains (124). These cells account for 0.5% to 1% of the B cells in peripheral blood. A fraction of the cells express CD27, but nearly all cells carry unmutated V region genes, indicating that they represent pregerminal center B cells (124,125). As the light chain and surrogate light chain coexpressing B cells express low levels of RAG mRNA and show a significantly biased antibody repertoire, it has been suggested that they may represent cells expressing autoreactive and edited B-cell receptors. Indeed, these cells are enriched in the joints of patients with rheumatoid arthritis (124).

Plasma cells are mainly found in lymphoid tissues (see next section), and they are rare in the peripheral blood. The frequency of CD38^high CD20^low cells, which include plasma cells and their immediate precursors, plasmablasts, usually is in the range of 1% to 2% among all B-lineage cells (107,126).

B-Cell Subsets in Tissues

In secondary lymphoid tissues (i.e., lymph nodes, spleen, and Peyer patches of the mucosa-associated lymphatic tissue [MALT]), mature B cells of distinct differentiation stages can be found in distinct histologic structures (Fig. 3.7). Naive B

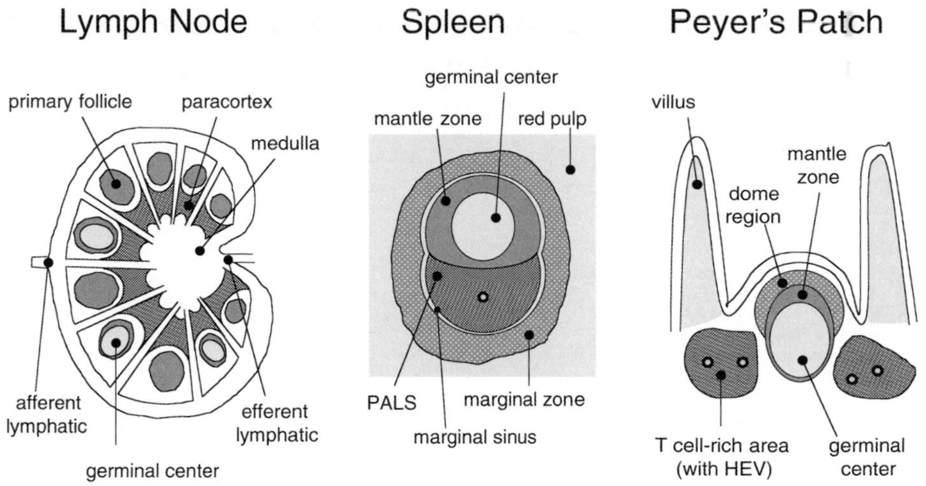

Lymph Node

Spleen

Peyer's Patch

FIGURE 3.7 Schematic structures of secondary lymphoid organs. Lymph node: the cortex of lymph nodes consists mainly of primary B-cell follicles or germinal centers. The paracortex is an area rich in T lymphocytes. In the medulla, macrophages and plasma cells are found. The lymph enters the lymph node through afferent lymphatics and leaves the lymph node through efferent lymphatics. The structure of blood vessels is not shown. Spleen: a detailed view of a white pulp area surrounded by red pulp is shown. The white pulp is composed of a germinal center surrounded by a mantle zone, and the T-cell-rich periarteriolar lymphoid sheath (PALS). A high endothelial venule (HEV) is shown in the center of the T-cell zone. The white pulp is surrounded by the marginal zone. The space between the marginal zone and the central parts of the white pulp is called the marginal sinus. The mantle zone is mainly composed of IgD$^+$ naive B cells, whereas many marginal zone B cells show features of IgD$^-$ memory B cells. Many plasma cells migrate to the red pulp. Peyer patch: a Peyer patch lymph node and two villi are shown. In the villi, many plasma cells are found. In the lymph node area, one can distinguish a T-cell-rich area with high endothelial venules and a B-cell area. In the B-cell area, a germinal center, surrounded by a mantle zone, is shown. Adjacent to the mantle zone, a dome region is found. Whereas the mantle zone is populated mainly by naive B cells, the dome region consists mainly of memory B cells.

cells populate primary follicles in lymph nodes and spleen. As already discussed earlier, when a germinal center develops in a primary follicle, these cells are pushed aside and constitute the mantle zone of the germinal center in the secondary follicle.

In the white pulp of the spleen, a distinct B-cell compartment is located around the mantle zone of germinal centers, the marginal zone. Many of the B cells in this area are IgM$^+$IgD$^{/low}$, and most of the cells carry somatically mutated V region genes (127–129). Hence, the marginal zone is a reservoir of (IgM-only) memory B cells. However, a subset of marginal zone B cells is responsive to T-cell-independent type II antigens, suggesting that naive B cells, albeit at a low frequency, are also present in the marginal zone (130). In Peyer patches, a structure corresponding to the marginal zone of the spleen is seen around the mantle zones of germinal centers. Like in the spleen, these cells mostly represent memory B cells as they harbor mutated Ig genes and lack IgD expression (131). In human tonsils, which are also components of the MALT, a distinct marginal zone is missing. Here, memory B cells are located mainly in the subepithelial region (132). A clear marginal zone is also lacking in lymph nodes. However, in several types of infections, a population of B cells can be discerned near sinus structures of the lymph node. These B cells have a more pronounced cytoplasm than naive B cells, similar to memory B cells in the spleen and tonsil. Because of morphologic similarities to monocytes, these cells are designated *monocytoid B cells*. The monocytoid B-cell population appears to be a mixture of pregerminal center and memory B cells (129,133).

Plasma cells show a typical distribution in lymphoid tissues, too. In the spleen, plasma cells are mainly found in the red pulp, whereas their numbers are relatively low in lymph nodes. Many plasma cells generated in germinal centers migrate to the bone marrow, which is, therefore, an important microenvironment for serum antibody production. However, approximately 80% of human plasma cells are found in extrafollicular areas of Peyer patches along the intestine (134). Most of these plasma cells carry mutated Ig V genes, suggesting that they developed in germinal centers (135,136).

RELATIONSHIP OF NORMAL B CELLS TO B-CELL NEOPLASMS

Typing B-Cell Tumors to Their Normal Counterparts

As outlined in more detail in other chapters of this book, considerable efforts have been made to identify the cellular origin of the various types of lymphomas. Often, the immunophenotype of the tumor cells and/or the histology was suggestive for the normal counterpart of the lymphoma cells. For example, the derivation of follicular lymphoma cells from transformed germinal center B cells is suggested by the observations that the tumor cells share several surface markers with normal germinal center B cells (e.g., bcl-6, CD10) and morphologically resemble these cells, by the follicular growth pattern of the lymphoma and the association of the tumor B cells with follicular dendritic cells and CD4 T cells. However, for other B-cell lymphomas, the origin of the lymphoma cells was less evident. When V gene mutation patterns turned out to identify distinct stages of B-cell development, Ig gene sequence analyses were performed by many groups to gain insight into the cellular origin of B-cell lymphomas [reviewed in (137-139)]. These studies revealed that a surprisingly large number of mature B-cell lymphomas are derived from germinal center or postgerminal center B cells, as they carry somatically mutated Ig genes (Fig. 3.8). Among B-cell non-Hodgkin lymphomas, somatically mutated Ig V genes were found in diffuse large cell lymphomas, follicular lymphomas, Burkitt lymphomas, MALT lymphomas, hairy cell leukemia, prolymphocytic leukemia, lymphoplasmacytoid lymphomas, and monocytoid B-cell lymphoma (138,139). Also, the Hodgkin and Reed/Sternberg cells of classic and lymphocyte-predominant Hodgkin lymphoma, and multiple myelomas are characterized by somatically mutated Ig genes (141-145). Unmutated V region genes are typical for mantle cell lymphomas, although a small fraction of cases carries

mutated V region genes (146,147). The situation is also diverse in B-cell chronic lymphocytic leukemia. Here, about half of the cases harbor unmutated Ig genes, whereas the other half is characterized by mutated Ig genes (148,149). It is interesting that the lack of somatic mutations in B-cell chronic lymphocytic leukemia is associated with a poorer prognosis for the patients.

As the somatic hypermutation process is active in germinal center B cells but silenced when the cells further differentiate into memory B or plasma cells, the detection of intraclonal sequence diversity in the rearranged V genes of a lymphoma B-cell clone indicates that somatic hypermutation is still active (at least during the early phase of tumor clone expansion) in the lymphoma and, hence, that the tumor derives from malignant transformation of germinal center B cells. Such intraclonal V gene diversity is typical for follicular lymphoma, Burkitt lymphoma, many MALT lymphomas, a subset of diffuse large cell lymphomas, and lymphocyte-predominant Hodgkin lymphoma (138,139). The Reed-Sternberg cells in classic Hodgkin lymphoma carry mutated Ig genes but lack ongoing

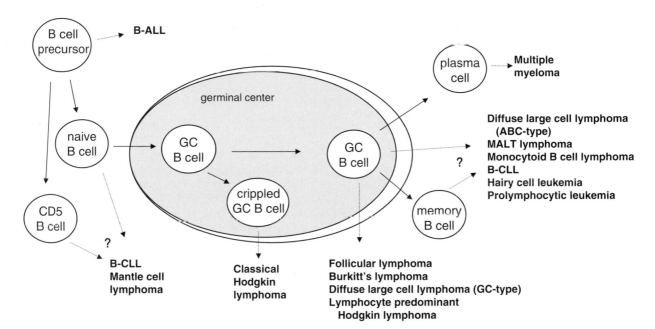

FIGURE 3.8 Cellular origin of human B-cell lymphomas. Human B-cell lymphomas are assigned to their putative normal counterparts. Mantle cell lymphomas are assigned to naive or CD5 B cells, as they carry unmutated Ig genes in most cases. However, a few cases with mutated Ig genes have been described. In B-cell chronic lymphocytic leukemia (B-CLL), about half of the cases carry unmutated Ig genes, whereas the other half is characterized by mutated Ig genes. In mantle cell lymphoma and B-cell chronic lymphocytic leukemia, the expression of CD5 by the leukemic cells indicates a derivation from CD5 B cells. However, a derivation from conventional naive B cells that up-regulated CD5 expression after transformation cannot be excluded. As somatic hypermutation is considered a germinal center (GC) B cell-specific process, the detection of ongoing mutation (at least during early phases of tumor clone expansion) is an indication for a germinal center B-cell origin of the tumor clone. Intraclonal V gene diversity is typical for follicular lymphoma and lymphocyte-predominant Hodgkin lymphoma. Moreover, a fraction of Burkitt lymphomas and MALT lymphomas and approximately one half of diffuse large cell lymphomas show ongoing V gene mutation. A derivation of these diffuse large cell lymphomas from germinal center B cells is also supported by their gene expression profile that closely resembles normal germinal center B cells (germinal center-type diffuse large cell lymphomas). For a number of lymphomas, it is not clear whether the tumor precursors are germinal center or post germinal center B cells, including diffuse large cell lymphomas with a gene expression profile resembling in vitro-activated B cells (ABC-type diffuse large cell lymphomas) (140). However, it is also likely that in most of these instances, important steps in the transformation process take place in the germinal center. ABC, activated B cell; B-ALL, B-cell acute lymphoblastic leukemia.

mutation (143,150). Nevertheless, there is strong indication that these cells also represent transformed germinal center B cells. In approximately one fourth of cases, somatic mutations were detected in originally productive V gene rearrangements that rendered these rearrangements nonfunctional (143,145). As such mutations usually result in a very efficient elimination of the cells in the germinal center, the Reed-Sternberg cells likely derive from preapoptotic germinal center B cells that were rescued by some transforming event(s).

Role of the Germinal Center Reaction and Immunoglobulin Gene Remodeling Processes in Lymphomagenesis

The cellular origin of most human B-cell lymphomas from germinal center or postgerminal center B cells suggests that the development of these lymphomas occurs or is at least initiated in the germinal center microenvironment. One important feature of germinal center B cells in this regard is likely the vigorous proliferation of these cells, which may by itself represent a risk for malignant transformation. Moreover, reciprocal chromosomal translocations involving Ig loci and resulting in the dysregulated expression of oncogenes are a hallmark of many B-cell lymphomas (151,152). The molecular structure of the translocations suggests that many of them are generated as by-products of class-switch recombination or somatic hypermutation (153). Hence, occasional failures in the control of these molecular processes likely plays a decisive role in the generation of chromosomal translocations and consequently the pathogenesis of B-cell lymphomas. Somatic hypermutation may be involved in lymphomagenesis not only by causing chromosomal translocations, but also by targeting non Ig genes. The bcl-6 gene is mutated in many B-cell lymphomas, and some of these mutations may well cause deregulated expression of the protein. The CD95 gene is mutated in a small fraction of germinal center B cells, and a considerable fraction of germinal center B-cell-derived lymphomas, in particular those associated with autoimmune phenomena (56,154,155). Destructive CD95 gene mutations may rescue germinal center B cells from apoptosis mediated via the CD95 pathway, and may enable lymphoma cells to avoid elimination by CD95 ligand-expressing T cells.

Somatic hypermutation may play a particularly important role in the pathogenesis of diffuse large cell lymphomas. In these lymphomas, targeting of multiple protooncogenes (c-myc, Pax-5, Rho/TTF, Pim-1) by somatic hypermutation was observed (156). These genes were found mutated only in diffuse large cell lymphomas, but not at significant frequency in other B-cell lymphomas or normal germinal center B cells, pointing to a diffuse large cell lymphoma-specific process. The aberrant hypermutation activity in these lymphoma cells (or their precursors) may cause lymphomagenesis not only by changing gene regulation and/or the coding sequence, but also by mediating chromosomal translocations involving these protooncogenes. Indeed, each of these genes is involved in chromosomal translocations, and the translocation breakpoints in these genes overlap with the regions that are targeted by hypermutation (156).

Besides somatic hypermutation and class switching, V gene recombination is also likely involved in the generation of chromosomal translocations, such as bcl-1/IgH translocations in mantle cell lymphoma and bcl-2/IgH translocations in follicular lymphomas (153). As V gene recombination predominantly, if not exclusively, takes place in the bone marrow and likely only rarely if at all in the germinal center, V gene recombination-associated chromosomal translocations presumably happen in the bone marrow during early B-cell development. Notably, in the case of follicular lymphoma, the bcl-2 translocation, although likely acquired already during development of the respective cell in the bone marrow, may become effective only when a cell with such a translocation becomes a germinal center B cell. These cells normally downregulate bcl-2 expression and become sensitive to apoptosis (157), which is prevented in cells with bcl-2 translocation.

Taking these aspects together, it becomes evident that the germinal center plays a decisive role not only for normal B-cell differentiation and effective immune responses, but also for the development of most mature B-cell lymphomas in the human.

ACKNOWLEDGMENTS

I thank Klaus Rajewsky for many stimulating discussions.

REFERENCES

1. Buckley RH. Primary immunodeficiency diseases due to defects in lymphocytes. *N Engl J Med* 2000;343:1313–1324.
2. Rajewsky K. Clonal selection and learning in the antibody system. *Nature* 1996;381:751–758.
3. Corbett SJ, Tomlinson IM, Sonnhammer EL, et al. Sequence of the human immunoglobulin diversity (D) segment locus: a systematic analysis provides no evidence for the use of DIR segments, inverted D segments, "minor" D segments or D-D recombination. *J Mol Biol* 1997;270:587–597.
4. Ravetch JV, Siebenlist U, Korsmeyer S, et al. Structure of the human immunoglobulin mu locus: characterization of embryonic and rearranged J and D genes. *Cell* 1981;27:583–591.
5. Cook GP, Tomlinson IM. The human immunoglobulin VH repertoire. *Immunol Today* 1995;16:237–242.
6. Hieter PA, Maizel JV, Leder P. Evolution of human immunoglobulin kappa J region genes. *J Biol Chem* 1982;257:1516–1522.
7. Kawasaki K, Minoshima S, Nakato E, et al. One-megabase sequence analysis of the human immunoglobulin lambda gene locus. *Genome Res* 1997;7:250–261.
8. Schäble KF, Zachau HG. The variable genes of the human immunoglobulin kappa locus. *Biol Chem Hoppe Seyler* 1993;374:1001–1022.
9. Vasicek TJ, Leder P. Structure and expression of the human immunoglobulin lambda genes. *J Exp Med* 1990;172:609–620.
10. Williams SC, Frippiat JP, Tomlinson IM, et al. Sequence and evolution of the human germline V lambda repertoire. *J Mol Biol* 1996;264:220–232.
11. Bräuninger A, Goossens T, Rajewsky K, et al. Regulation of immunoglobulin light chain gene rearrangements during early B cell development in the human. *Eur J Immunol* 2001;31:3631–3637.
12. Hieter PA, Korsmeyer SJ, Waldmann TA, et al. Human immunoglobulin kappa light-chain genes are deleted or rearranged in lambda-producing B cells. *Nature* 1981;290:368–372.
13. Korsmeyer SJ, Hieter PA, Sharrow SO, et al. Normal human B cells display ordered light chain gene rearrangements and deletions. *J Exp Med* 1982;156:975–985.
14. Nemazee D. Receptor editing in B cells. *Adv Immunol* 2000;74:89–126.
15. Fugmann SD, Lee AI, Shockett PE, et al. The RAG proteins and V(D)J recombination: complexes, ends, and transposition. *Annu Rev Immunol* 2000;18:495–527.
16. McBlane JF, van Gent DC, Ramsden DA, et al. Cleavage at a V(D)J recombination signal requires only RAG1 and RAG2 proteins and occurs in two steps. *Cell* 1995;83:387–395.
17. Ma Y, Pannicke U, Schwarz K, et al. Hairpin opening and overhang processing by an Artemis/DNA-dependent protein kinase complex in nonhomologous end joining and V(D)J recombination. *Cell* 2002;108:781–794.
18. Wasserman R, Yamada M, Ito Y, et al. VH gene rearrangement events can modify the immunoglobulin heavy chain during progression of B-lineage acute lymphoblastic leukemia. *Blood* 1992;79:223–228.

19. MacLennan IC, Gulbranson-Judge A, Toellner KM, et al. The changing preference of T and B cells for partners as T-dependent antibody responses develop. *Immunol Rev* 1997;156:53–66.
20. Jacob J, Kelsoe G. In situ studies of the primary immune response to (4-hydroxy-3- nitrophenyl)acetyl. II. A common clonal origin for periarteriolar lymphoid sheath-associated foci and germinal centers. *J Exp Med* 1992;176:679–687.
21. Jacob J, Kassir R, Kelsoe G. In situ studies of the primary immune response to (4-hydroxy-3- nitrophenyl)acetyl. I. The architecture and dynamics of responding cell populations. *J Exp Med* 1991;173:1165–1175.
22. MacLennan IC. Germinal centers. *Annu Rev Immunol* 1994;12:117–139.
23. Berek C, Berger A, Apel M. Maturation of the immune response in germinal centers. *Cell* 1991;67:1121–1129.
24. Jacob J, Kelsoe G, Rajewsky K, et al. Intraclonal generation of antibody mutants in germinal centres. *Nature* 1991;354:389–392.
25. Küppers R, Zhao M, Hansmann ML, et al. Tracing B cell development in human germinal centres by molecular analysis of single cells picked from histological sections. *EMBO J* 1993;12:4955–4967.
26. Jacob J, Przylepa J, Miller C, et al. In situ studies of the primary immune response to (4-hydroxy-3- nitrophenyl)acetyl. III. The kinetics of V region mutation and selection in germinal center B cells. *J Exp Med* 1993;178:1293–1307.
27. Weiss U, Zoebelein R, Rajewsky K. Accumulation of somatic mutants in the B cell compartment after primary immunization with a T cell-dependent antigen. *Eur J Immunol* 1992;22:511–517.
28. Nakamura M, Yagi H, Kayaba S, et al. Death of germinal center B cells without DNA fragmentation. *Eur J Immunol* 1996;26:1211–1216.
29. Allen CD, Okada T, Tang HL, et al. Imaging of germinal center selection events during affinity maturation. *Science* 2007;315:528–531.
30. Hauser AE, Junt T, Mempel TR, et al. Definition of germinal-center B cell migration in vivo reveals predominant intrazonal circulation patterns. *Immunity* 2007;26:655–667.
31. Schwickert TA, Lindquist RL, Shakhar G, et al. In vivo imaging of germinal centres reveals a dynamic open structure. *Nature* 2007;446:83–87.
32. Han S, Dillon SR, Zheng B, et al. V(D)J recombinase activity in a subset of germinal center B lymphocytes. *Science* 1997;278:301–305.
33. Meffre E, Papavasiliou F, Cohen P, et al. Antigen receptor engagement turns off the V(D)J recombination machinery in human tonsil B cells. *J Exp Med* 1998;188:765–772.
34. Papavasiliou F, Casellas R, Suh H, et al. V(D)J recombination in mature B cells: a mechanism for altering antibody responses. *Science* 1997;278:298–301.
35. Monroe RJ, Seidl KJ, Gaertner F, et al. RAG2:GFP knockin mice reveal novel aspects of RAG2 expression in primary and peripheral lymphoid tissues. *Immunity* 1999;11:201–212.
36. Meru N, Jung A, Baumann I, et al. Expression of the recombination-activating genes in extrafollicular lymphocytes but no apparent reinduction in germinal center reactions in human tonsils. *Blood* 2002;99:531–537.
37. Goossens T, Bräuninger A, Klein U, et al. Receptor revision plays no major role in shaping the receptor repertoire of human memory B cells after the onset of somatic hypermutation. *Eur J Immunol* 2001;31:3638–3648.
38. Arpin C, Dechanet J, Van Kooten C, et al. Generation of memory B cells and plasma cells in vitro. *Science* 1995;268:720–722.
39. Choe J, Kim HS, Armitage RJ, et al. The functional role of B cell antigen receptor stimulation and IL-4 in the generation of human memory B cells from germinal center B cells. *J Immunol* 1997;159:3757–3766.
40. Liu YJ, Cairns JA, Holder MJ, et al. Recombinant 25-kDa CD23 and interleukin 1 alpha promote the survival of germinal center B cells: evidence for bifurcation in the development of centrocytes rescued from apoptosis. *Eur J Immunol* 1991;21:1107–1114.
41. Vyth-Dreese FA, Dellemijn TA, Majoor D, et al. Localization in situ of the co-stimulatory molecules B7.1, B7.2, CD40 and their ligands in normal human lymphoid tissue. *Eur J Immunol* 1995;25:3023–3029.
42. Johnson GD, Hardie DL, Ling NR, et al. Human follicular dendritic cells (FDC): a study with monoclonal antibodies (MoAb). *Clin Exp Immunol* 1986;64:205–213.
43. Manz RA, Thiel A, Radbruch A. Lifetime of plasma cells in the bone marrow. *Nature* 1997;388:133–134.
44. Slifka MK, Antia R, Whitmire JK, et al. Humoral immunity due to long-lived plasma cells. *Immunity* 1998;8:363–372.
45. Kocks C, Rajewsky K. Stable expression and somatic hypermutation of antibody V regions in B-cell developmental pathways. *Annu Rev Immunol* 1989;7:537–559.
46. Goossens T, Klein U, Küppers R. Frequent occurrence of deletions and duplications during somatic hypermutation: Implications for oncogene translocations and heavy chain disease. *Proc Natl Acad Sci U S A* 1998;95:2463–2468.
47. Bross L, Fukita Y, McBlane F, et al. DNA double-strand breaks in immunoglobulin genes undergoing somatic hypermutation. *Immunity* 2000;13:589–597.
48. Sale JE, Neuberger MS. TdT-accessible breaks are scattered over the immunoglobulin V domain in a constitutively hypermutating B cell line. *Immunity* 1998;9:859–869.
49. Wagner SD, Neuberger MS. Somatic hypermutation of immunoglobulin genes. *Annu Rev Immunol* 1996;14:441–457.
50. Rogozin IB, Kolchanov NA. Somatic hypermutagenesis in immunoglobulin genes. II. Influence of neighbouring base sequence on mutagenesis. *Biochim Biophys Acta* 1992;1171:11–18.
51. Betz AG, Milstein C, Gonzalez-Fernandez A, et al. Elements regulating somatic hypermutation of an immunoglobulin kappa gene: critical role for the intron enhancer/matrix attachment region. *Cell* 1994;77:239–248.
52. Fukita Y, Jacobs H, Rajewsky K. Somatic hypermutation in the heavy chain locus correlates with transcription. *Immunity* 1998;9:105–114.
53. Yelamos J, Klix N, Goyenechea B, et al. Targeting of non-Ig sequences in place of the V segment by somatic hypermutation. *Nature* 1995;376:225–229.
54. Pasqualucci L, Migliazza A, Fracchiolla N, et al. BCL-6 mutations in normal germinal center B cells: evidence of somatic hypermutation acting outside Ig loci. *Proc Natl Acad Sci U S A* 1998;95:11816–11821.
55. Shen HM, Peters A, Baron B, et al. Mutation of BCL-6 gene in normal B cells by the process of somatic hypermutation of Ig genes. *Science* 1998;280:1750–1752.
56. Müschen M, Re D, Jungnickel B, et al. Somatic mutation of the CD95 gene in human B cells as a side-effect of the germinal center reaction. *J Exp Med* 2000;192:1833–1840.
57. Gordon MS, Kanegai CM, Doerr JR, et al. Somatic hypermutation of the B cell receptor genes B29 (Igbeta, CD79b) and mb1 (Igalpha, CD79a). *Proc Natl Acad Sci U S A* 2003;100:4126–4131.
58. Muramatsu M, Kinoshita K, Fagarasan S, et al. Class switch recombination and hypermutation require activation-induced cytidine deaminase (AID), a potential RNA editing enzyme. *Cell* 2000;102:553–563.
59. Revy P, Muto T, Levy Y, et al. Activation-induced cytidine deaminase (AID) deficiency causes the autosomal recessive form of the Hyper-IgM syndrome (HIGM2). *Cell* 2000;102:565–575.
60. Okazaki IM, Kinoshita K, Muramatsu M, et al. The AID enzyme induces class switch recombination in fibroblasts. *Nature* 2002;416:340–345.
61. Yoshikawa K, Okazaki IM, Eto T, et al. AID enzyme-induced hypermutation in an actively transcribed gene in fibroblasts. *Science* 2002;296:2033–2036.
62. Di Noia JM, Neuberger MS. Molecular mechanisms of antibody somatic hypermutation. *Annu Rev Biochem* 2007;76:1–22.
63. Faili A, Aoufouchi S, Flatter E, et al. Induction of somatic hypermutation in immunoglobulin genes is dependent on DNA polymerase iota. *Nature* 2002;419:944–947.
64. Zan H, Komori A, Li Z, et al. The translesion DNA polymerase zeta plays a major role in Ig and bcl-6 somatic hypermutation. *Immunity* 2001;14:643–653.
65. Weill JC, Reynaud CA. DNA polymerases in adaptive immunity. *Nat Rev Immunol* 2008;8:302–312.
66. Matsumoto M, Lo SF, Carruthers CJ, et al. Affinity maturation without germinal centres in lymphotoxin-alpha- deficient mice. *Nature* 1996;382:462–466.
67. William J, Euler C, Christensen S, et al. Evolution of autoantibody responses via somatic hypermutation outside of germinal centers. *Science* 2002;297:2066–2070.
68. Weller S, Faili A, Garcia C, et al. CD40-CD40L independent Ig gene hypermutation suggests a second B cell diversification pathway in humans. *Proc Natl Acad Sci U S A* 2001;98:1166–1170.
69. Gardby E, Lycke NY. CD19-deficient mice exhibit poor responsiveness to oral immunization despite evidence of unaltered total IgA levels, germinal centers and IgA-isotype switching in Peyer's patches. *Eur J Immunol* 2000;30:1861–1871.
70. Ferrari S, Giliani S, Insalaco A, et al. Mutations of CD40 gene cause an autosomal recessive form of immunodeficiency with hyper IgM. *Proc Natl Acad Sci U S A* 2001;98:12614–12619.
71. Hofker MH, Walter MA, Cox DW. Complete physical map of the human immunoglobulin heavy chain constant region gene complex. *Proc Natl Acad Sci U S A* 1989;86:5567–5571.
72. Honjo T, Kinoshita K, Muramatsu M. Molecular mechanism of class switch recombination: linkage with somatic hypermutation. *Annu Rev Immunol* 2002;20:165–196.
73. Hein K, Lorenz MG, Siebenkotten G, et al. Processing of switch transcripts is required for targeting of antibody class switch recombination. *J Exp Med* 1998;188:2369–2374.
74. Lorenz M, Jung S, Radbruch A. Switch transcripts in immunoglobulin class switching. *Science* 1995;267:1825–1828.
75. Zhang K, Mills FC, Saxon A. Switch circles from IL-4-directed epsilon class switching from human B lymphocytes. Evidence for direct, sequential, and multiple step sequential switch from mu to epsilon Ig heavy chain gene. *J Immunol* 1994;152:3427–3435.
76. Barrett DJ, Ayoub EM. IgG2 subclass restriction of antibody to pneumococcal polysaccharides. *Clin Exp Immunol* 1986;63:127–134.
77. Shackelford PG, Granoff DM. IgG subclass composition of the antibody response of healthy adults, and normal or IgG2-deficient children to immunization withH. influenzae type b polysaccharide vaccine or Hib PS-protein conjugate vaccines. *Monogr Allergy* 1988;23:269–281.
78. Mond JJ, Lees A, Snapper CM. T cell-independent antigens type 2. *Annu Rev Immunol* 1995;13:655–692.

79. Scott EW, Simon MC, Anastasi J, et al. Requirement of transcription factor PU.1 in the development of multiple hematopoietic lineages. *Science* 1994;265:1573–1577.

80. DeKoter RP, Singh H. Regulation of B lymphocyte and macrophage development by graded expression of PU.1. *Science* 2000;288:1439–1441.

81. Kee BL, Quong MW, Murre C. E2A proteins: essential regulators at multiple stages of B-cell development. *Immunol Rev* 2000;175:138–149.

82. Reya T, Grosschedl R. Transcriptional regulation of B-cell differentiation. *Curr Opin Immunol* 1998;10:158–165.

83. Pongubala JM, Northrup DL, Lancki DW, et al. Transcription factor EBF restricts alternative lineage options and promotes B cell fate commitment independently of Pax5. *Nat Immunol* 2008;9:203–215.

84. Nutt SL, Heavey B, Rolink A, et al. Commitment to the B-lymphoid lineage depends on the transcription factor Pax5. *Nature* 1999;401:556–562.

85. Rolink AG, Nutt SL, Melchers F, et al. Long-term in vivo reconstitution of T-cell development by Pax5-deficient B-cell progenitors. *Nature* 1999;401:603–606.

86. Horcher M, Souabni A, Busslinger M. Pax5/BSAP maintains the identity of B cells in late B lymphopoiesis. *Immunity* 2001;14:779–790.

87. Dent AL, Shaffer AL, Yu X, et al. Control of inflammation, cytokine expression, and germinal center formation by BCL-6. *Science* 1997;276:589–592.

88. Ye BH, Cattoretti G, Shen Q, et al. The BCL-6 proto-oncogene controls germinal-centre formation and T<h2>-type inflammation. *Nat Genet* 1997;16:161–170.

89. Cattoretti G, Chang CC, Cechova K, et al. BCL-6 protein is expressed in germinal-center B cells. *Blood* 1995;86:45–53.

90. Onizuka T, Moriyama M, Yamochi T, et al. BCL-6 gene product, a 92- to 98-kD nuclear phosphoprotein, is highly expressed in germinal center B cells and their neoplastic counterparts. *Blood* 1995;86:28–37.

91. Shaffer AL, Yu X, He Y, et al. BCL-6 represses genes that function in lymphocyte differentiation, inflammation, and cell cycle control. *Immunity* 2000;13:199–212.

92. Phan RT, Saito M, Basso K, et al. BCL6 interacts with the transcription factor Miz-1 to suppress the cyclin-dependent kinase inhibitor p21 and cell cycle arrest in germinal center B cells. *Nat Immunol* 2005;6:1054–1060.

93. Phan RT, Dalla-Favera R. The BCL6 proto-oncogene suppresses p53 expression in germinal-centre B cells. *Nature* 2004;432:635–639.

94. Ranuncolo SM, Polo JM, Dierov J, et al. Bcl-6 mediates the germinal center B cell phenotype and lymphomagenesis through transcriptional repression of the DNA-damage sensor ATR. *Nat Immunol* 2007;8:705–714.

95. Angelin-Duclos C, Cattoretti G, Lin KI, et al. Commitment of B lymphocytes to a plasma cell fate is associated with Blimp-1 expression in vivo. *J Immunol* 2000;165:5462–5471.

96. Falini B, Fizzotti M, Pucciarini A, et al. A monoclonal antibody (MUM1p) detects expression of the MUM1/IRF4 protein in a subset of germinal center B cells, plasma cells, and activated T cells. *Blood* 2000;95:2084–2092.

97. Calame KL. Plasma cells: finding new light at the end of B cell development. *Nat Immunol* 2001;2:1103–1108.

98. Mittrucker HW, Matsuyama T, Grossman A, et al. Requirement for the transcription factor LSIRF/IRF4 for mature B and T lymphocyte function. *Science* 1997;275:540–543.

99. Klein U, Casola S, Cattoretti G, et al. Transcription factor IRF4 controls plasma cell differentiation and class switch recombination. *Nat Immunol* 2006;7:773–782.

100. Reimold AM, Iwakoshi NN, Manis J, et al. Plasma cell differentiation requires the transcription factor XBP-1. *Nature* 2001;412:300–307.

101. Reimold AM, Ponath PD, Li YS, et al. Transcription factor B cell lineage-specific activator protein regulates the gene for human X-box binding protein 1. *J Exp Med* 1996;183:393–401.

102. Chen CZ, Li L, Lodish HF, et al. MicroRNAs modulate hematopoietic lineage differentiation. *Science* 2004;303:83–86.

103. Thai TH, Calado DP, Casola S, et al. Regulation of the germinal center response by microRNA-155. *Science* 2007;316:604–608.

104. Vigorito E, Perks KL, Abreu-Goodger C, et al. microRNA-155 regulates the generation of immunoglobulin class-switched plasma cells. *Immunity* 2007;27:847–859.

105. Xiao C, Calado DP, Galler G, et al. MiR-150 controls B cell differentiation by targeting the transcription factor c-Myb. *Cell* 2007;131:146–159.

106. Xiao C, Srinivasan L, Calado DP, et al. Lymphoproliferative disease and autoimmunity in mice with increased miR-17-92 expression in lymphocytes. *Nat Immunol* 2008;9:405–414.

107. Odendahl M, Jacobi A, Hansen A, et al. Disturbed peripheral B lymphocyte homeostasis in systemic lupus erythematosus. *J Immunol* 2000;165:5970–5979.

108. Klein U, Rajewsky K, Küppers R. Human immunoglobulin (Ig)M+IgD+ peripheral blood B cells expressing the CD27 cell surface antigen carry somatically mutated variable region genes: CD27 as a general marker for somatically mutated (memory) B cells. *J Exp Med* 1998;188:1679–1689.

109. Wirths S, Lanzavecchia A. ABCB1 transporter discriminates human resting naive B cells from cycling transitional and memory B cells. *Eur J Immunol* 2005;35:3433–3441.

110. Bhat NM, Kantor AB, Bieber MM, et al. The ontogeny and functional characteristics of human B-1 (CD5+ B) cells. *Int Immunol* 1992;4: 243–252.

111. Berland R, Wortis HH. Origins and functions of B-1 cells with notes on the role of CD5. *Annu Rev Immunol* 2002;20:253–300.

112. Montecino-Rodriguez E, Leathers H, Dorshkind K. Identification of a B-1 B cell-specified progenitor. *Nat Immunol* 2006;7:293–301.

113. Brezinschek HP, Foster SJ, Brezinschek RI, et al. Analysis of the human VH gene repertoire. Differential effects of selection and somatic hypermutation on human peripheral CD5(+)/IgM+ and CD5(-)/IgM+ B cells. *J Clin Invest* 1997;99:2488–2501.

114. Fischer M, Klein U, Küppers R. Molecular single-cell analysis reveals that CD5-positive peripheral blood B cells in healthy humans are characterized by rearranged Vkappa genes lacking somatic mutation. *J Clin Invest* 1997;100:1667–1676.

115. Geiger KD, Klein U, Bräuninger A, et al. CD5-positive B cells in healthy elderly humans are a polyclonal B cell population. *Eur J Immunol* 2000;30:2918–2923.

116. Agematsu K, Nagumo H, Oguchi Y, et al. Generation of plasma cells from peripheral blood memory B cells: synergistic effect of interleukin-10 and CD27/CD70 interaction. *Blood* 1998;91:173–180.

117. Fecteau JF, Cote G, Neron S. A new memory CD27-IgG+ B cell population in peripheral blood expressing VH genes with low frequency of somatic mutation. *J Immunol* 2006;177:3728–3736.

118. Wei C, Anolik J, Cappione A, et al. A new population of cells lacking expression of CD27 represents a notable component of the B cell memory compartment in systemic lupus erythematosus. *J Immunol* 2007;178:6624–6633.

119. Klein U, Küppers R, Rajewsky K. Evidence for a large compartment of IgM-expressing memory B cells in humans. *Blood* 1997;89:1288–1298.

120. Agematsu K, Nagumo H, Yang FC, et al. B cell subpopulations separated by CD27 and crucial collaboration of CD27+ B cells and helper T cells in immunoglobulin production. *Eur J Immunol* 1997;27:2073–2079.

121. Marie-Cardine A, Divay F, Dutot I, et al. Transitional B cells in humans: characterization and insight from B lymphocyte reconstitution after hematopoietic stem cell transplantation. *Clin Immunol* 2008;127:14–25.

122. Sims GP, Ettinger R, Shirota Y, et al. Identification and characterization of circulating human transitional B cells. *Blood* 2005;105:4390–4398.

123. Liu YJ, de Bouteiller O, Arpin C, et al. Normal human IgD+IgM- germinal center B cells can express up to 80 mutations in the variable region of their IgD transcripts. *Immunity* 1996;4:603–613.

124. Meffre E, Davis E, Schiff C, et al. Circulating human B cells that express surrogate light chains and edited receptors. *Nat Immunol* 2000;1:207–213.

125. Meffre E, Schaefer A, Wardemann H, et al. Surrogate light chain expressing human peripheral B cells produce self-reactive antibodies. *J Exp Med* 2004;199:145–150.

126. Arce E, Jackson DG, Gill MA, et al. Increased frequency of pre-germinal center B cells and plasma cell precursors in the blood of children with systemic lupus erythematosus. *J Immunol* 2001;167:2361–2369.

127. Dunn-Walters DK, Isaacson PG, Spencer J. Analysis of mutations in immunoglobulin heavy chain variable region genes of microdissected marginal zone (MGZ) B cells suggests that the MGZ of human spleen is a reservoir of memory B cells. *J Exp Med* 1995;182:559–566.

128. Tangye SG, Liu YJ, Aversa G, et al. Identification of functional human splenic memory B cells by expression of CD148 and CD27. *J Exp Med* 1998;188:1691–1703.

129. Tierens A, Delabie J, Michiels L, et al. Marginal-zone B cells in the human lymph node and spleen show somatic hypermutations and display clonal expansion. *Blood* 1999;93:226–234.

130. Martin F, Kearney JF. Marginal-zone B cells. *Nat Rev Immunol* 2002;2:323–335.

131. Dunn-Walters DK, Isaacson PG, Spencer J. Sequence analysis of rearranged IgVH genes from microdissected human Peyer's patch marginal zone B cells. *Immunology* 1996;88:618–624.

132. Liu YJ, Barthelemy C, de Bouteiller O, et al. Memory B cells from human tonsils colonize mucosal epithelium and directly present antigen to T cells by rapid up-regulation of B7-1 and B7-2. *Immunity* 1995;2:239–248.

133. Stein K, Hummel M, Korbjuhn P, et al. Monocytoid B cells are distinct from splenic marginal zone cells and commonly derive from unmutated naive B cells and less frequently from postgerminal center B cells by polyclonal transformation. *Blood* 1999;94:2800–2808.

134. Brandtzaeg P, Halstensen TS, Kett K, et al. Immunobiology and immunopathology of human gut mucosa: humoral immunity and intraepithelial lymphocytes. *Gastroenterology* 1989;97:1562–1584.

135. Dunn-Walters DK, Isaacson PG, Spencer J. Sequence analysis of human IgVH genes indicates that ileal lamina propria plasma cells are derived from Peyer's patches. *Eur J Immunol* 1997;27:463–467.

136. Fischer M, Küppers R. Human IgA- and IgM-secreting intestinal plasma cells carry heavily mutated VH region genes. *Eur J Immunol* 1998;28: 2971–2977.

137. Klein U, Goossens T, Fischer M, et al. Somatic hypermutation in normal and transformed human B cells. *Immunol Rev* 1998;162:261–280.

138. Küppers R, Klein U, Hansmann ML, et al. Cellular origin of human B-cell lymphomas. *N Engl J Med* 1999;341:1520–1529.

139. Stevenson FK, Sahota SS, Ottensmeier CH, et al. The occurrence and significance of V gene mutations in B cell-derived human malignancy. *Adv Cancer Res* 2001;83:81–116.

140. Alizadeh AA, Eisen MB, Davis RE, et al. Distinct types of diffuse large B-cell lymphoma identified by gene expression profiling. *Nature* 2000;403:503–511.

141. Bakkus MH, Heirman C, Van Riet I, et al. Evidence that multiple myeloma Ig heavy chain VDJ genes contain somatic mutations but show no intraclonal variation. *Blood* 1992;80:2326–2335.

142. Braeuninger A, Küppers R, Strickler JG, et al. Hodgkin and Reed-Sternberg cells in lymphocyte predominant Hodgkin disease represent clonal populations of germinal center-derived tumor B cells. *Proc Natl Acad Sci U S A* 1997;94:9337–9342.

143. Kanzler H, Küppers R, Hansmann ML, et al. Hodgkin and Reed-Sternberg cells in Hodgkin's disease represent the outgrowth of a dominant tumor clone derived from (crippled) germinal center B cells. *J Exp Med* 1996;184:1495–1505.

144. Marafioti T, Hummel M, Anagnostopoulos I, et al. Origin of nodular lymphocyte-predominant Hodgkin's disease from a clonal expansion of highly mutated germinal-center B cells. *N Engl J Med* 1997;337:453–458.

145. Küppers R. Molecular biology of Hodgkin's lymphoma. *Adv Cancer Res* 2002;44:277–312.

146. Hummel M, Tamaru J, Kalvelage B, et al. Mantle cell (previously centrocytic) lymphomas express VH genes with no or very little somatic mutations like the physiologic cells of the follicle mantle. *Blood* 1994;84:403–407.

147. Thorselius M, Walsh S, Eriksson I, et al. Somatic hypermutation and V(H) gene usage in mantle cell lymphoma. *Eur J Haematol* 2002;68:217–224.

148. Damle RN, Wasil T, Fais F, et al. Ig V gene mutation status and CD38 expression as novel prognostic indicators in chronic lymphocytic leukemia. *Blood* 1999;94:1840–1847.

149. Hamblin TJ, Davis Z, Gardiner A, et al. Unmutated Ig V(H) genes are associated with a more aggressive form of chronic lymphocytic leukemia. *Blood* 1999;94:1848–1854.

150. Bräuninger A, Hansmann ML, Strickler JG, et al. Identification of common germinal-center B-cell precursors in two patients with both Hodgkin's disease and non-Hodgkin's lymphoma. *N Engl J Med* 1999;340:1239–1247.

151. Siebert R, Rosenwald A, Staudt LM, et al. Molecular features of B-cell lymphoma. *Curr Opin Oncol* 2001;13:316–324.

152. Willis TG, Dyer MJ. The role of immunoglobulin translocations in the pathogenesis of B-cell malignancies. *Blood* 2000;96:808–822.

153. Küppers R, Dalla-Favera R. Mechanisms of chromosomal translocations in B cell lymphomas. *Oncogene* 2001;20:5580–5594.

154. Gronbaek K, Straten PT, Ralfkiaer E, et al. Somatic Fas mutations in non-Hodgkin's lymphoma: association with extranodal disease and autoimmunity. *Blood* 1998;92:3018–3024.

155. Müschen M, Rajewsky K, Krönke M, et al. The origin of CD95 gene mutations in B cell lymphoma. *Trends Immunol* 2002;23:75–80.

156. Pasqualucci L, Neumeister P, Goossens T, et al. Hypermutation of multiple proto-oncogenes in B-cell diffuse large-cell lymphomas. *Nature* 2001;412:341–346.

157. Liu YJ, Mason DY, Johnson GD, et al. Germinal center cells express bcl-2 protein after activation by signals which prevent their entry into apoptosis. *Eur J Immunol* 1991;21:1905–1910.

CHAPTER 4 ■ DEVELOPMENTAL AND FUNCTIONAL BIOLOGY OF T LYMPHOCYTES

JACQUES J. M. VAN DONGEN, FRANK J. T. STAAL, AND ANTON W. LANGERAK

The development of T lymphocytes in the thymus and their regulatory and cytotoxic cellular functions in peripheral lymphoid organs play a central role in the antigen-specific immune response. The tightly regulated process of T-cell differentiation with the stepwise rearrangements in the T-cell receptor (TCR) genes and selection processes are essential to mediate T-cell responses with well-suited antigen-specific receptors.

Multistep deregulation and malignant transformation can occur at multiple stages of T-cell differentiation and T-cell-mediated immune responses, resulting in immature (thymocytic) or mature (post-thymic) T-cell malignancies. This chapter summarizes the molecular background of the TCR repertoire, the stepwise T-cell differentiation processes, the T-cell effector functions, and the immunophenotypic and genotypic characteristics of normal, as compared with malignant, T cells.

T-CELL RECEPTOR MOLECULES AND T-CELL RECEPTOR REPERTOIRE

T-Cell Receptor Molecules and Their Encoding Genes

The ability of human T lymphocytes to specifically recognize millions of different antigens and antigenic epitopes is based on the enormous diversity (at least 10^{10}) of their antigen-specific receptors, better known as *TCR molecules* (1–3). Being distinct per T lymphocyte, each single T lymphocyte expresses approximately 10^5 TCR molecules with identical antigen specificity. TCR molecules consist of two generally disulfide-linked chains. Two different types of TCR are known: the "classical" TCRαβ receptor, consisting of a TCRα and a TCRβ chain; and the "alternative" TCRγδ receptor, comprised of a TCRγ and a TCRδ chain (2,4). The majority of mature T lymphocytes (85% to 98%) in peripheral blood and in most lymphoid tissues are TCRαβ$^+$, whereas only a minority (2% to 15%) express TCRγδ (4). Both types of TCR molecules are closely associated with CD3 protein chains, required for transmembrane signal transduction of the TCR-CD3 complex (Fig. 4.1) (3).

Each TCR chain consists of two domains: one variable domain involved in actual recognition of antigens and one constant domain that mediates the effector function resulting in signaling through CD3. To recognize all antigenic epitopes, an extensive repertoire of variable domains of TCR molecules is needed. If this entire repertoire is encoded by separate genes, these would occupy a major part of the human genome. However, because the variable domains are encoded by a single exon that is formed through distinct combinations of gene segments, only a limited set of gene segments is able to encode the required diversity of TCR molecules (2,5). In the case of the *TCRB* and *TCRD* loci, this concerns the combination of variable (V), diversity (D), and joining (J) gene segments, whereas the *TCRA* and *TCRG* gene complexes only contain V and J gene segments (Fig. 4.2) (2,4).

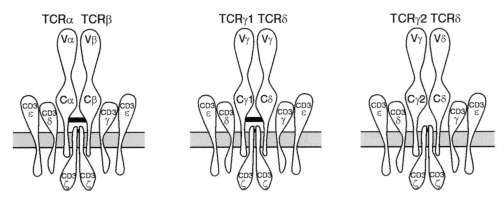

FIGURE 4.1 Schematic diagram of human TCRαβ and TCRγδ molecules. Both types of TCR molecules are associated with CD3 protein chains, which are involved in signal transduction. The proteins of TCRγδ receptor that are derived from Cγ1 sequences are disulfide linked, whereas this interchain disulfide bond is lacking if the TCRγ chain is derived from Cγ2 sequences. Most TCRγδ$^+$ T lymphocytes in peripheral blood use disulfide-linked TCR chains because of selection for Vδ2-Jδ1/Vγ9-Jγ1.2 receptors. Vα, Vβ, Vγ, and Vδ are variable domains of TCR chains; Cα, Cβ, Cγ, and Cδ are constant domains of TCR chains.

TCRA and TCRD gene complex (# 14q11)

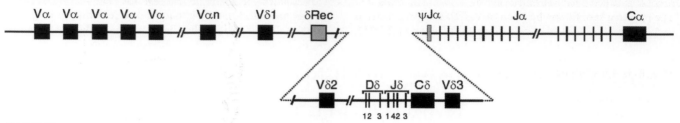

TCRB gene complex (# 7q35)

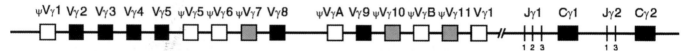

TCRG gene complex (# 7p14-15)

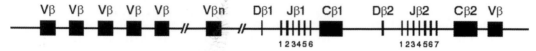

FIGURE 4.2 Schematic diagram of the human TCR gene complexes. The *TCRA* gene complex consists of approximately 60 V gene segments, a stretch of 61 J gene segments, and one C gene segment. The *TCRB* gene complex contains approximately 65 V gene segments and two C gene segments, both of which are preceded by a D gene segment and six or seven J gene segments. The *TCRG* gene complex consists of a restricted number of V gene segments (six functional segments and nine pseudosegments) and two C gene segments, each preceded by two to three J gene segments. The *TCRD* gene complex comprises several V (three true Vδ segments and several Vα/Vδ segments), three D, four J, and one C gene segment. The major part of the *TCRD* gene complex is located between the Vα and Jα gene segments, and is flanked by the δREC and ΨJα gene segments, which are involved in *TCRD* gene deletions that occur before *TCRA* gene rearrangements. Pseudogenes (Ψ) are indicated as *open symbols*.

TABLE 4.1

ESTIMATED NUMBER OF HUMAN V, D, AND J GENE SEGMENTS THAT CAN POTENTIALLY BE INVOLVED IN TCR GENE REARRANGEMENTS[a]

Gene segment	*TCRA*	*TCRB*	*TCRG*	*TCRD*
V (family)	~60 (32)	~65 (30)	9 (4)	7[b]
D	—	2	—	3
J (family)	61[b]	13	5 (3)	4

[a] Numbers are based on the international ImMunoGeneTics database (161). Numbers in parentheses reflect families.
[b] These numbers include the nonfunctional ΨJα gene segment (*TCRA* locus) and the δREC gene segment (*TCRD* locus).

The human *TCRA* and *TCRB* loci contain large sets of Vα and Vβ gene segments (60–65), which can be further subdivided into families based on homology at the deoxyribonucleic acid (DNA) level (Table 4.1). The nine V gene segments of the human *TCRG* gene complex are generally subdivided into four families, three of which are single-member families; the human *TCRD* locus consists of six V segments. Human J gene segments are generally sparser than V gene segments, ranging from four for *TCRD*, five for *TCRG*, to 13 for *TCRB*; the 61 different J segments of the *TCRA* locus are exceptional. Finally, two Dβ and three Dδ gene segments

exist (Table 4.1). The constant domains of the TCR chains are encoded by C gene segments; *TCRA* and *TCRD* loci each contain a single C-gene segment, whereas *TCRB* and *TCRG* loci comprise two C-gene segments (Fig. 4.2) (6–14).

Gene Rearrangement or V(D)J Recombination

During early T-cell differentiation, V, (D), and J gene segments from the germline repertoire of the various TCR gene complexes are coupled via a tightly regulated process; this process is called *gene rearrangement* or *V(D)J recombination*. The resulting specific combination of V, (D), and J segments in each T lymphocyte is also known as *V(D)J exon* (1,2,5,15). V(D)J recombination is a complex process involving several proteins, which together form the recombinase enzyme system. Next to regulatory DNA binding proteins, the products of the lymphoid-specific recombinase-activating genes 1 and 2 (RAG1 and RAG2 proteins) are the main constituents of the recombinase complex (16–18). RAG 1 and RAG 2 specifically bind to the recombination signal sequences (RSSs), which flank the 3′ side of V gene segments, both sides of D gene segments, and the 5′ side of J gene segments (19–21). These RSS elements consist of conserved palindromic heptamer (CACAGTG) and nonamer (ACAAAAACC) sequences, separated by either 12 or 23 base pair spacer regions (19–21). After the introduction of double-strand breaks between the RSS and the rearranging gene segment, a hairpin structure is formed at the coding end of the break (Fig. 4.3). This hairpin has to be opened before relegation to another gene segment via several enzymes known to be involved in double-strand break repair; this results in the so-called coding joint. During the coding joint formation, deletion and random insertion of nucleotides can occur, leading to imprecise coupling of gene segments. The RSS ends of the breaks fuse head to tail to form the so-called signal joint, which is generally removed from the genomic DNA in the form of an excision circle (Fig. 4.3) (2,19,20). Such TCR excision circles (TRECs) are relatively stable molecules, which do not replicate on cell division; consequently, they are diluted out on proliferation of the developing T cells. This characteristic has prompted the development of quantitative assays for analysis of TREC levels as measure for thymic output of recent thymic emigrants (22,23). TREC analysis has been used to study thymic output in different age groups and different pathophysiologic conditions (e.g., during human immunodeficiency virus type 1 infection) (22,24).

In Figure 4.4, an example of a *TCRB* gene rearrangement is illustrated. Initially, a coding joint is formed between a Jβ gene segment and one of the Dβ gene segments, whereas the 3′ Dβ RSS and the Jβ RSS form a signal joint in the excision circle or TREC. In a second-step rearrangement, coupling of one of many Vβ gene segments results in a complete V(D)J exon, as well as another TREC with the signal joint of the Vβ RSS and the 5′ Dβ RSS. The rearranged gene is subsequently transcribed into a precursor messenger ribonucleic acid (mRNA), which is further processed into mature mRNA by splicing out all intronic, noncoding sequences and coupling of the V(D)J exon and the C exons (Fig. 4.4) (2). Similar rearrangement and transcription processes occur in all other TCR loci as well. Although the signal joints that are formed during TCR gene recombination are generally present on TRECs, this is not the case for one exceptional type of rearrangement. On inversional rearrangement, which occurs in the case of V gene segments in inverted orientation (e.g., the Vβ20 or Vδ3 gene segments) (13), the signal joint and other intervening sequences between the two coding elements are not removed as TREC but are preserved on the genome.

As TCR recombinations are complex processes with imprecise joining of gene segments, approximately two out

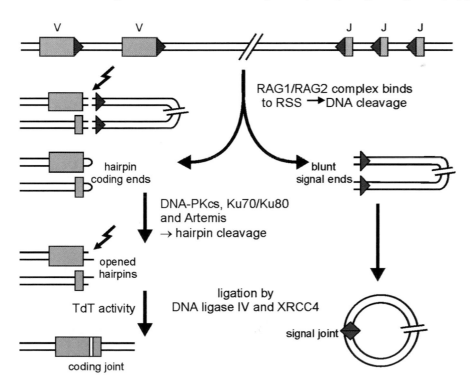

FIGURE 4.3 Scheme of the V(D)J recombination mechanism. RAG1 and RAG2 bind to RSSs, resulting in double-strand breaks. After cleavage, hairpin structures are formed at the coding ends, whereas the RSS blunt ends fuse to form a signal joint. Further processing results in opening of the hairpins via several enzymes known to be involved in double-strand break repair (DNA-PK_CS, Ku70/Ku80, and Artemis). Finally, opened hairpins are relegated (involving DNA ligase IV and XRCC4) to a coding joint and are further diversified by the action of TdT, which introduces nucleotides in a template-independent way.

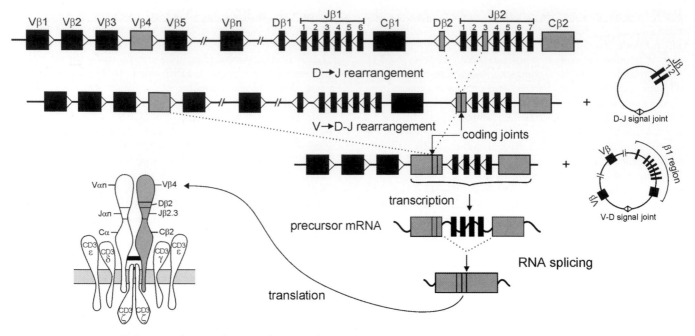

FIGURE 4.4 Schematic diagram of sequential rearrangement steps, transcription, and translation of the *TCRB* gene during T-cell differentiation. In this example, first a Dβ2 to Jβ2.3 rearrangement occurs, followed by Vβ4 to Dβ2-Jβ2.3 rearrangement, resulting in the formation of a Vβ4Dβ2Jβ2.3 coding joint. The rearranged *TCRB* gene is transcribed into precursor mRNA, spliced into mature mRNA, and finally translated into a TCRβ protein. The two extrachromosomal TRECs that are formed during this recombination process are indicated as well; they contain the D-J signal joint and V-D signal joint, respectively.

of three joinings are out-of frame (1). This high frequency of out-of-frame rearrangements may explain why most T cells have biallelic *TCRB* and *TCRG* gene rearrangements (5,25). In addition, replacement gene rearrangements appear to occur that are assumed to rescue precursor T cells with non-productive TCR genes. In *TCRB* and *TCRD* loci, this concerns D-J replacements, whereas V-J replacements replace preexisting V-J joinings in *TCRA* and *TCRG* loci (26–28). Both types of replacements can occur repeatedly in the same TCR gene complex as long as germline V, (D), and J gene segments are available. Another type of secondary rearrangement concerns V gene segment replacement in a complete V(D)J exon by an upstream V gene segment. This process is mediated via an internal heptamer RSS in the 3′ part of the V gene segments (29,30).

T-Cell Receptor Repertoire

The complete repertoire of TCR molecules of T lymphocytes is shaped by V(D)J recombination mechanisms in the TCR gene loci. The extent of this potential primary repertoire is determined by two levels of diversity: combinatorial diversity [different V(D)J combinations] and junctional diversity (due to imprecise joining of V, D, and J gene segments) (1).

Combinatorial diversity results from all possible combinations of available functional V, D, and J gene segments per TCR locus and the pairing of two different functional protein chains per TCR molecule (TCRα with TCRβ and TCRγ with TCRδ) (1). As the *TCRB* gene complex probably contains at least approximately 45 functional Vβ gene segments, two Dβ

gene segments, and 13 functional Jβ gene segments, coupling results in many possible Vβ-Dβ-Jβ combinations (more than 1,000). Together with the many combinations of the approximately 45 functional Vα and 50 functional Jα gene segments, a potential combinatorial diversity of more than 2×10^6 can be obtained (Table 4.2).

The combinatorial diversity of TCRγδ molecules is less extensive due to the limited number of functional V, D, and J gene segments in the encoding gene complexes. Still, because of multiple Dδ gene segment usage, a potential combinatorial repertoire of more than 5,000 TCRγδ molecules can be produced. The numbers of different TCRαβ and TCRγδ molecules are based on the assumption of random usage of available functional V, D, and J gene segments. However, there are indications for preferential gene segment usage. TCRαβ+ cells tend to use Jβ2 gene segments more frequently than Jβ1 gene segments (31), whereas peripheral TCRγδ+ T lymphocytes exhibit preferential usage of Vγ9-Jγ1.2 and Vδ2-Jδ1 gene segments (32,33). Alternatively, gene segment usage might be random, but overrepresentation of certain receptor types would be explained by clonal selection and expansion of particular receptor specificities in peripheral tissues (34).

The other type of diversity, *junctional diversity*, is based on deletion of nucleotides at the ends of the rearranging gene segments as well as random insertion of nucleotides (N region nucleotides) between the coupled gene segments (junctional region). Insertion of N-region nucleotides at the 3′ ends of DNA breakpoints is mediated by terminal deoxynucleotidyl transferase (TdT) and occurs in a template-independent way (35). Absence or decreased TdT activity, as in

TABLE 4.2

ESTIMATION OF POTENTIAL PRIMARY REPERTOIRE OF HUMAN TCR MOLECULES

Repertoire	TCRαβ molecules		TCRγδ molecules	
	TCRα	TCRβ	TCRγ	TCRδ
Number of functional gene segments[a]				
V gene segments	45	44–47	6	6
D gene segments	—	2[b]	—	3[b]
J gene segments	50	13	5	4
Combinatorial diversity	$>2 \infty 10^6$		>5000	
Junctional diversity	+	++	+	+++
Estimation of total repertoire	$>10^{12}$		$>10^{12}$	

+, limited (range 0–20 nt); ++, extensive (range 0–35 nt); +++, very extensive (range 7–55 nt).
[a] Numbers are based on the international ImMunoGeneTics database (161).
[b] In *TCRD* gene rearrangements, multiple D segments might be used; this implies that the number of junctions can vary from one to four. In *TCRB* gene rearrangements, generally only one D gene segment is used.

early fetal thymocytes, leads to the virtual absence of N-region insertion in TCR gene rearrangement, but the junctional regions of rearranged TCR genes in late fetal and postnatal thymocytes do contain N regions (36,37). The junctional regions of TCR genes encode the so-called complementarity determining regions 3, which are involved in antigen recognition and which function as unique lymphocyte-specific ("fingerprint-like") sequences. N-region insertion thus drastically increases diversity of antigen recognition by TCR chains and TCR molecules. This especially holds true for *TCRB* and *TCRD* gene rearrangements in which multiple couplings (V-D, D-J, and even D-D) can be present within a junctional region. The enormous junctional diversity of TCRδ chains thereby compensates for the relatively low number of different V, D, and J combinations (Table 4.2).

STAGES OF T-CELL DIFFERENTIATION

Immunophenotype of Thymocyte Subsets

T cells develop from common lymphoid progenitor cells that seed the thymus from the fetal liver or bone marrow (38). In most differentiation schemes, thymocyte subsets are phenotypically distinguished by the expression of CD4 and CD8 coreceptors. Thymocytes are either double negative (DN), double positive (DP), or single positive (SP) for these two cell surface antigens (Fig. 4.5). During the DN stage, thymocytes can be subdivided into subpopulations based on the expression of the CD34 stem cell marker and CD1a [for a recent review, see (39)]. The earliest cells in the human thymus phenotypically resemble hematopoietic stem cells and are CD34$^+$CD38$^-$CD1a$^-$ (40). CD38 expression is rapidly acquired, and the CD34$^+$CD38$^+$CD1a$^-$ cells represent cells that behave as multipotent progenitor cells having the capacity to develop not only into the T-cell lineage but also into natural

killer (NK) cells, dendritic cells, and B cells. The thymus is an important site for the development of NK cells and probably dendritic cells but a very minor site for B-cell development (41). After acquisition of CD1a expression on the progenitor cells (CD34$^+$CD1a$^+$), T-cell commitment is established (Fig. 4.5). This is because the first TCR gene rearrangements occur at this transition, concomitant with increased expression of the pre-Tα gene.

During transition to the next stage of T-cell maturation, the pre-T-cell stage (DN3 in the mouse), the cells shut down proliferation (42), and *TCRB* genes start to rearrange. During the immature SP stage, the TCRβ protein chain is expressed at the cell surface, complexed to pre-Tα as the pre-TCR complex. In the mouse, these immature SP cells express CD8, whereas in humans, they express CD4 (Fig. 4.5). In both species, the immature SP cells represent a stage of rapid proliferation, driven by signals via the pre-TCR complex (TCRβ selection). This process generates DP cells, which comprise 85% to 90% of thymocytes. As soon as the DP thymocytes express CD3/TCRαβ, they undergo positive selection (for self-major histocompatibility complex [MHC]) and negative selection (against autoreactivity) (43). The selected cells develop into CD4 or CD8 SP cells with high CD3/TCRαβ expression, which exit the thymus and become circulating T cells that reside in blood and peripheral lymphoid organs (Fig. 4.5).

Rearrangement Processes during T-Cell Differentiation

Antigen recognition by T lymphocytes is dependent on successful rearrangement of TCR genes through the process of V(D)J recombination. During early T-cell differentiation, *TCRD* genes rearrange first, followed by *TCRG* gene rearrangements (44). This might result in TCRγδ$^+$ T lymphocytes, provided that these rearrangements are functional. TCRαβ$^+$ T lymphocytes most probably develop via a separate differentiation lineage, with *TCRB* gene rearrangements

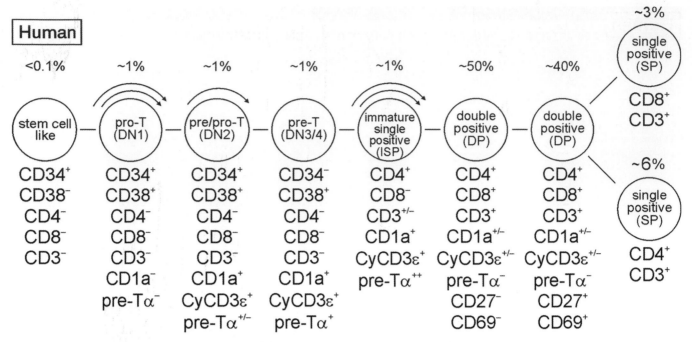

FIGURE 4.5 Stages of human T-cell development in the thymus. This scheme is designed to highlight similarities with mouse T-cell development. Cells that are not yet T-cell committed seed the thymus. These first two stages represent a minute fraction (less than 1%) of all thymocytes. The most common cell type in the thymus is the DP thymocyte (85% to 90%), which gives rise to both CD4 (4% to 9%) and CD8 (2% to 5%) single-positive (SP) cells. ISP, immature single positive.

taking place before *TCRA* gene rearrangements (Fig. 4.6). *TCRA* gene rearrangements are preceded by deletion of the *TCRD* gene, which is for the major part located between the Vα and Jα gene segments (Fig. 4.2). This *TCRD* gene deletion process is primarily mediated via rearrangement of the flanking δREC and ?Jα gene segments. These rearrangement and deletion processes in the *TCRA/TCRD* locus probably play a crucial role in the divergence of the TCRγδ and TCRαβ differentiation pathways, although it is still unclear in which differentiation stage this divergence occurs. The fact that virtually all TCRαβ⁺ T lymphocytes have rearranged *TCRG* genes and that a large part of the TCRγδ⁺ T lymphocytes have rearranged *TCRB* genes is remarkable and suggests that both differentiation lineages might share a common origin (Fig. 4.6).

In the earliest human thymocyte subset (CD34⁺CD1a⁻), recombination is initiated in the *TCRD* locus, with incomplete Dδ2-Dδ3 and Vδ2-Dδ3 couplings as the earliest rearrangements. *TCRG* recombinations start in the next stage (CD34⁺CD1a⁺), in which *TCRD* rearrangements are further completed, and incomplete *TCRB* (Dβ-Jβ) rearrangements start (45). During transition to the next stage (pre-T-cell stage), the thymocytes stop proliferating, and the *TCRB* genes further rearrange into complete Vβ-Jβ joints. During the immature SP stage in humans, the protein product of the *TCRB* gene is expressed at the cell surface together with the pre-Tα chain, forming the pre-TCR complex, leading to expansion of cells expressing a functional TCRβ chain (45). Finally, after rearranging their *TCRA* gene, the DP cells express TCRαβ and undergo (positive and negative) selection, followed by maturation into CD4⁺ or CD8⁺ SP cells with high TCRαβ expression (Fig. 4.6).

Positive and Negative Selection during T-Cell Differentiation

The rescue of DP thymocytes from programmed cell death via interaction of their TCR with peptide/self-MHC complexes is called *positive selection*. When a DP thymocyte recognizes no MHC molecules with appreciable affinity, neither a positive nor a negative signal is given, and the thymocyte dies "by neglect." Positive selection ensures that mature T cells can recognize foreign antigens preferentially in the context of self-MHC molecules (46,47) (Fig. 4.7). DP thymocytes also undergo *negative selection*, which refers to the process of eliminating potentially self-reactive cells via apoptosis. In general, these cells bear TCR molecules with high affinity for self-peptide/self-MHC complexes and are likely to be autoreactive (Fig. 4.7). Selection for low-affinity interaction with peptide/MHC determines that CD4⁺ T cells become helper T cells, and CD8⁺ T cells become cytotoxic T cells. That is, almost all CD4⁺ T cells have TCR molecules that recognize peptides bound to self-MHC class II and are programmed to become cytokine-secreting helper T cells, whereas most of the CD8⁺ T cells have receptors recognizing self-MHC class I molecules and are determined to become cytotoxic effector cells (48).

Specialized cells in the thymic cortex mediate positive and negative selection. Positive selection involves interaction of DP thymocytes with cortical epithelial cells, whereas negative selection is driven by a variety of antigen-presenting cells in the thymic stroma that are bone marrow derived such as dendritic cells and macrophages (Fig. 4.7) (49).

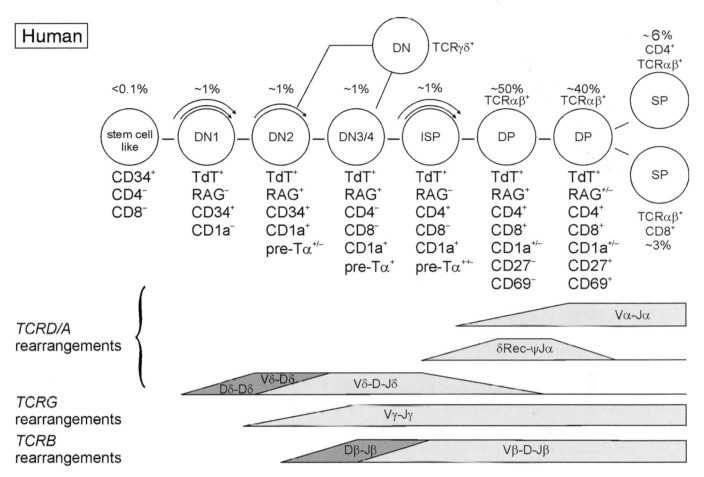

FIGURE 4.6 TCR rearrangements during thymocyte differentiation. The major stages of T-cell development are depicted with the corresponding start of rearrangements of the TCR loci. The δREC-ΨJα elements are involved in deletion of the *TCRD* locus, which is necessary for efficient rearrangement of the *TCRA* locus (Fig. 48.2). ISP, immature single positive.

Signal Transduction via the Pre-T-Cell Receptor and T-Cell Receptor Molecules

Signaling via the pre-TCR complex and mature TCR molecules provides important signals during T-cell differentiation (proliferation, positive selection, apoptosis). The events from triggering of a receptor and transmission of this signal inside the cell via signaling molecules to activation of transcription factors leading to specific changes in gene expression are referred to as *signal transduction*. Because of its relevance to both thymocyte differentiation and activation of mature T lymphocytes, we briefly discuss signaling via TCR molecules (50,51).

The complete TCR complex consists of a highly diverse TCR chain, complexed to nonvariant CD3 molecules (one CD3γ, one CD3δ, two CD3ε, and two CD3ζ molecules), which are responsible for transduction of the signals via the TCR complex. The TCR molecules themselves have very short intracellular domains incapable of signaling. Signaling from the TCR complex is dependent on the presence of so-called immunoreceptor tyrosine-based activation motif in the CD3 chains. Immunoreceptor tyrosine-based activation motifs are composed of two tyrosine residues separated by 13 amino acids. The pre-TCR complex has a similar makeup, except

that the TCRβ chain is not associated with a TCRα chain but with the invariant pre-Tα protein.

When antigen binds the TCR molecule, the tyrosines of the immunoreceptor tyrosine-based activation motifs become phosphorylated by the protein tyrosine kinases Lck and Fyn. Lck is constitutively associated with CD4 and CD8; Fyn associates with CD3ζ and ε on receptor clustering. Lck is activated when CD4 or CD8 is clustered with the TCR when it binds its peptide/MHC ligand. Both Lck and Fyn phosphorylate the immunoreceptor tyrosine-based activation motifs in the CD3 complex (Fig. 4.8). This then recruits another tyrosine kinase, ZAP-70, to bind to the immunoreceptor tyrosine-based activation motifs of the CD3ζ chains. Lck subsequently activates ZAP-70, which then phosphorylates the linker proteins LAT (linker of activation in T cells) and SLP-76. Several signaling routes are subsequently activated, one of which involves the small G protein Ras, which via the Raf kinase activates the so-called mitogen-activated protein (MAP) kinase pathway, which consists of several serine/threonine protein kinases that are activated by subsequent phosphorylation steps (Ras, Raf, extracellular signal-regulated kinase kinase, and extracellular signal-regulated kinase). Ultimately, the MAP kinase pathway activates transcription factors important for cell proliferation (Fig. 4.8), such as nuclear factor-κB (NF-κB), nuclear factor of activated T-cell (NFAT), and Elk.

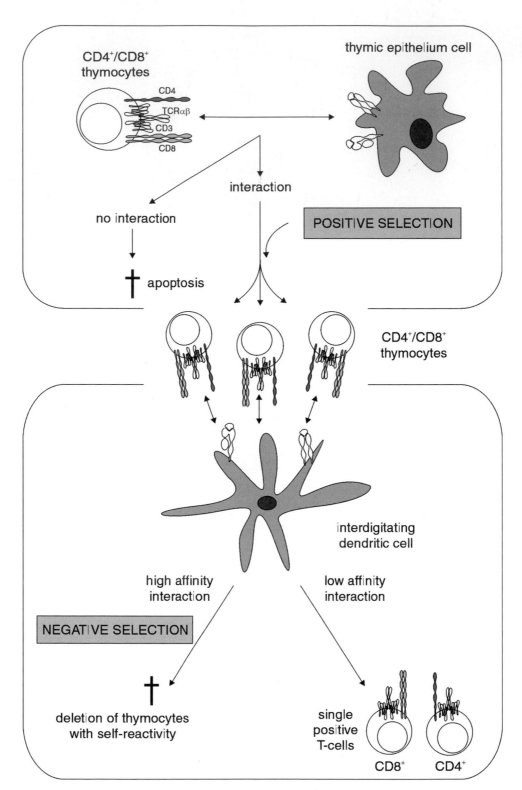

FIGURE 4.7 Positive and negative selection in the thymus. The thymic stroma selects for those TCR $\alpha\beta^+$ T cells that have useful TCRs by contact of the TCR and its coreceptor with self-MHC on thymic cortical epithelial cells (positive selection). Also within the thymus, professional antigen-presenting cells of bone marrow origin delete potentially harmful cells that recognize self-antigens (negative selection).

ZAP-70 also activates PLC-γ1, which cleaves phosphatidyl-inositol bisphosphate (PIP$_2$) into diacylglycerol (DAG) and inositol trisphosphate (IP$_3$). IP$_3$ is responsible for increasing intracellular levels of free calcium, which is an important signal for various calcium-binding proteins and kinases involved in cell proliferation and apoptosis. DAG together with calcium can activate protein kinase C (PKC). PKC activates the important NF-κB transcription factor by phosphorylation and activation of a series of kinases that phosphorylate an inhibitor molecule, IκB, that traps the NF-κB transcription factor in the

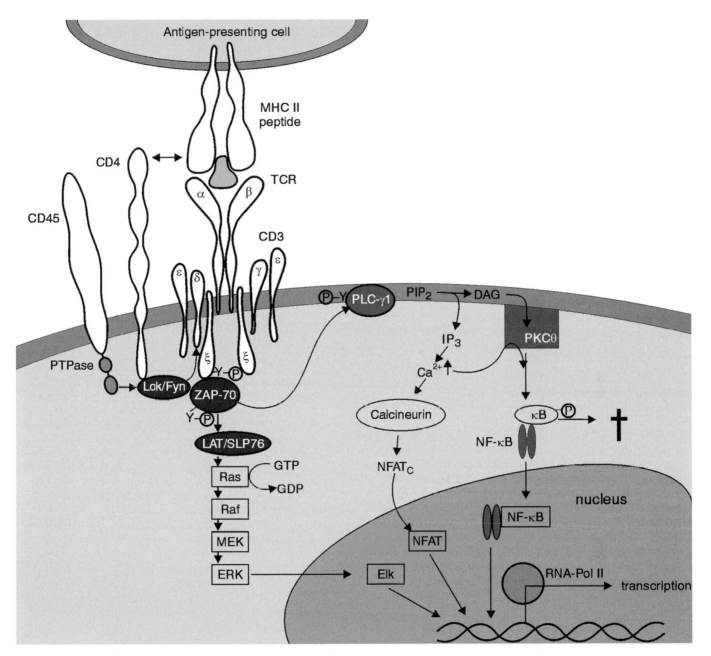

FIGURE 4.8 Signal transduction pathways emanating from the TCR. Stimulation of the TCR via antigen/MHC and the CD4 or CD8 coreceptor leads to activation of the Lck and Fyn tyrosine kinases (PTK). These kinases phosphorylate the immunoreceptor tyrosine-based activation motif in the CD3 chains. CD3ζ now recruits the ZAP-70 PTK, which then activates SOS adapter molecule and the phospholipase PLCγ1. The latter cleaves phosphatidylinositol bisphosphate (PIP$_2$) into IP$_3$ and DAG, leading to increases in intracellular-free calcium and activation of PKC θ. PKC and other kinases can phosphorylate IκB, which is subsequently degraded, releasing the NF-κB transcription factor from cytoplasmic retention to activate target genes in the nucleus. The NFAT transcription factor is activated via the phosphatase calcineurin. The Ras/Raf/MAP kinase pathway activates the Elk transcription factor. Ultimately, target genes involved in proliferation, apoptosis, and differentiation are activated. GDP, guanosine diphosphate; GTP, guanosine triphosphate; PTPase, protein tyrosine phosphatase.

cytoplasm. Phosphorylation of IκB leads to its breakdown and release of NF-κB from its inhibition in the cytoplasm. NF-κB then migrates to the nucleus to activate its target genes (Fig. 4.8). The calcium signal also is important to activate the calcineurin phosphatase. This phosphatase dephosphorylates NFAT, thereby activating nuclear import of this transcription factor.

Transcriptional Regulation of T-Cell Differentiation

Regulation of gene expression, resulting in cell-specific or differentiation stage-specific gene expression profiles, can occur

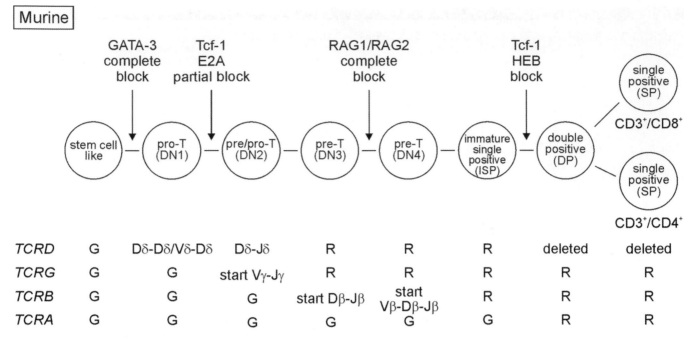

Murine								
TCRD	G	Dδ-Dδ/Vδ-Dδ	Dδ-Jδ	R	R	R	deleted	deleted
TCRG	G	G	start Vγ-Jγ	R	R	R	R	R
TCRB	G	G	G	start Dβ-Jβ	start Vβ-Dβ-Jβ	R	R	R
TCRA	G	G	G	G	G	G	R	R

FIGURE 4.9 Transcription factors in T-cell development. Shown is a scheme of murine T-cell development and those stages of differentiation in which development is blocked in mice with specific targeted mutations in the transcription factor indicated. The basic mechanisms governing murine and human T-cell development are conserved, as evidenced from blocks at similar stages in in vitro experiments with human thymocytes. ISP, immature single position.

at multiple levels, such as induction of locus accessibility, transcription initiation, RNA splicing, mRNA stability, translation, and posttranslational modification (52). Transcription initiation is probably the most critical regulatory step in control of gene expression. Several different (types of) transcription factors have been shown to be essential for T-cell differentiation. Evidence for this has, for a large part, come from studies on mice with targeted disruptions in the genes encoding these transcription factors, leading to characteristic blocks in thymocyte differentiation. The most important transcription factors known to date to be involved in T-cell differentiation are summarized here: ikaros, GATA-3, E2A, and Tcf-1 (Fig. 4.9). These factors may become important markers for staging of malignant counterparts of immature thymocytes in the future. For instance, the transcription factor Tcf-1 is already in use to distinguish immature myeloid leukemias from immature T-cell leukemias (53). *Ikaros* is a lymphoid-restricted, zinc-finger transcription factor (54,55) related to Helios and Aiolos. Mice expressing a stable dominant-negative form of Ikaros lacked all T, B, and NK cells and their precursors.

GATA-3 expression is confined to stem cells, common lymphoid precursors, and pro-T and pre-T cells but not to precursors of other hematopoietic lineages. Data from several different experimental approaches demonstrate an essential role for GATA-3 in T-cell commitment, probably already at the stage of development of T-lineage precursors in fetal liver and bone marrow.

Basic helix-loop-helix (bHLH) transcription factors consist of a basic (DNA binding) domain and a helix-loop-helix (dimerization) region, and have been implicated in gene regulation and differentiation of many cell types, including lymphoid cells. Class I bHLH proteins comprise E2A, HEB, and E2-2, which are also known as *E proteins* for their capacity to bind

to E-box sequences (CANNTG) within regulatory elements. During lymphoid differentiation, E-protein dimers are the major players. In addition to their B-cell deficiency, E2A$^{-/-}$ mice exhibit a defect in T-cell differentiation (56). HEB$^{-/-}$ mice display a partial block in T-cell differentiation at the transition from DN to DP cells, which is later than in E2A$^{-/-}$ mice. E-box binding sites have been recognized in enhancers of the *TCRD/TCRA* locus as well as the *TCRB* locus, suggesting a role for E proteins in regulation of TCR recombination (57).

Tcf-1 is a highly T-cell-specific transcription factor in mice and humans. Complete disruption of Tcf-1 results in a partial block of T-cell differentiation at the DN 1 to DN 2 and immature SP to DP transitions. Tcf-1 is not an active transcription factor by itself but requires the interaction with the Wnt effector β-catenin (58).

Interaction between membrane-bound *Notch* and one of its ligands results in proteolytic cleavage of Notch (59). On cleavage, the intracellular Notch domain is released and translocates to the nucleus to interact with *CBF-1/RBP-Jκ*, thereby converting it from a repressor to an activator of gene transcription. Recent data from reconstitution experiments suggest that Notch signaling may play a critical role in promoting progression through several major checkpoints during T-cell differentiation, including: the choice of T-lineage or B-lineage commitment; the choice between TCRαβ and TCRγδ lineages; and, in the case of TCRαβ T cells, between CD4$^+$ and CD8$^+$ lineages (60).

Post-Thymic T-Cell Maturation and Effector Function

Once T cells have completed their development in the thymus, they enter the bloodstream. The relative frequency and

TABLE 4.3

ABSOLUTE COUNTS OF BLOOD T LYMPHOCYTES AND THEIR SUBSETS[a]

Age group	TCRαβ+	CD4+CD3+	CD8+CD3	TCRγδ+	Natural killer cells
Neonatal cord blood ($n = 35$)	1.5–3.5	1.0–2.5	0.4–1.5	0.05–0.20	0.5–1.5
Children <9 mo ($n = 164$)	2.5–6.0	1.7–4.0	0.7–1.8	0.05–0.30	0.3–0.8
Children 9–24 mo ($n = 103$)	2.0–5.0	1.2–3.8	0.5–1.5	0.10–0.40	0.2–0.8
Children 2–15 yr ($n = 91$)	1.0–3.0	0.5–1.8	0.4–1.2	0.10–0.40	0.1–0.6
Adults ($n = 51$)	0.8–1.7	0.4–1.2	0.2–0.7	0.05–0.20	0.1–0.4

[a] The indicated values concern the 25–75 percentiles in 10^9 /L.

the absolute numbers of T lymphocytes and their subsets in peripheral blood are age dependent, with high numbers in younger age groups (particularly younger than 2 years of age) (Table 4.3). These higher numbers are probably directly related to the encountering of many new antigens and the subsequent immune responses during the first 2 years of life.

The blood T lymphocytes migrate to peripheral lymphoid organs (Peyer patches, tonsil, lymph nodes) where they encounter antigen and where immune responses are initiated. The naive T lymphocytes mature into effector T lymphocytes after interaction with antigen/MHC complexes on antigen-presenting cells. The initial activation of naive T lymphocytes requires a costimulatory signal in addition to the signal via the TCR. Costimulatory signals are given via CD28, but other molecules, including adhesion molecules (LFA-1, ICAM-3), can serve this function as well (61,62).

Naive CD8+ T lymphocytes emerging from the thymus are already predestined to become cytotoxic cells, even though they do not yet express high levels of cytotoxic molecules. Virus-infected cells present viral antigens via their MHC class I molecules to the CD8+ T lymphocytes, which subsequently are activated. The activated CD8+ T lymphocytes can kill the target cells that display the viral antigens (Fig. 4.10A). This killing is done via specialized molecules such as perforin, which makes holes in the cell membrane of the target cell, proteases called *granzymes*, and cytokines, such as tumor necrosis factor-α (TNFα). Also, cell-cell mediated apoptotic signals are given via interaction of Fas ligand on the cytotoxic T cells, with Fas on the virus-infected target cell (Fig. 4.10A).

Uncommitted (naive) CD4+ T-helper precursor (Thp) cells can be induced to differentiate toward T helper 1 (T<h1>), T<h2>, T regulatory (Treg), or T<h1>7 phenotypes according to the local cytokine milieu and their first encounter with antigen (63,64). This has been demonstrated both in vitro and in vivo for murine CD4+ Thp cells, and convincing data are available for human Thp cells as well. The division between the four types of T-helper cells mostly relates to the type of cytokines they produce and the type of immune responses they are involved in (Fig. 4.10B).

T<H1> cells activate macrophages and induce B lymphocytes to produce opsonizing antibodies. They are mostly involved in cell-mediated immunity (e.g., for the response against intracellular pathogens) and produce large amounts of interferon-γ (IFNγ), interleukin (IL)-12, and tumor TNFα and TNPβ.

T<H2> cells activate B cells to make neutralizing antibodies; they help induce class switching in B cells and have variable effects on macrophages. Typical T<H2> cytokines are IL-4, IL-5, IL-6, and IL-13 (Fig. 4.10B).

The CD4+ CD25+ Treg cells have the ability to inhibit proliferation and production of cytokines by bystander CD4+ T cells, as well as to down-modulate the responses of CD8+ T cells, NK cells, and CD4+ cells to specific antigens. In vivo the range of functions is far broader and includes maintenance of tolerance to self-components (i.e., prevention of autoimmune disease), as well as the ability to prevent transplant rejection and to maintain gastrointestinal tolerance (65). Tregs are also involved in maternal tolerance to semiallogeneic fetal antigens during pregnancy (66).

T<h1>7 T cells have been linked with the proinflammatory cytokine IL-23 and induction of autoimmunity because IL-23-deficient mice contain very few T<h1>7 cells and are protected from autoimmune diseases such as experimental autoimmune encephalomyelitis, and collagen-induced arthritis (67). However, although IL-23 seems to be involved in T<h1>7-mediated immune pathology, it is not required for the differentiation of T<h1>7 from naive CD4 Thp cells, as transforming growth factor (TGF)β and IL-6 are responsible for this process (68).

The differential development of the CD4+ Th subsets is regulated via cytokine-induced transcription factor activities. IL-12 signaling and IFNγ through "signal transduction and activator of transcription" (STAT)-4 skew toward T<h1>, IL-4 (signaling through STAT-6) toward T<h2>, TGFβ toward Treg, and IL-6 and TGFβ toward T<h1>7. The committed cells are characterized by expression of specific transcription factors, T-bet for T<h1>, GATA-3 for T<h2>, forkhead box P3 for Tregs, and RORγT for T<h1>7 cells. Recently, it has been demonstrated that the skewing of murine Thp toward T<h1>7 and Treg is mutually exclusive. Although human Thp can also be skewed toward T<h1>, T<h2>, and Treg phenotypes, there is as yet no direct evidence for the existence of discrete T<h1>7 cells in humans or of mutually antagonistic development of T<h1>7 cells and Tregs. There is considerable evidence, however, both in man and in mice for the importance of IFNγ and IL-17 in the development and progression of inflammatory and autoimmune diseases (Fig. 4.10B) (69).

In recent years yet another type of T cell has been identified that shares characteristics with NK cells. These NKT

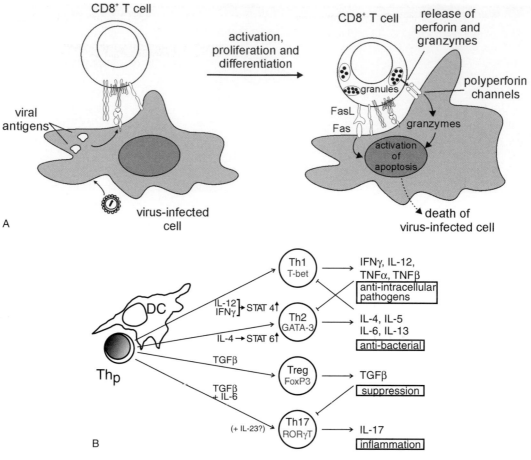

FIGURE 4.10 Effector cell functions of mature CD4+ and CD8+ T cells. **A:** After encounter of viral antigens on infected cells, antigens are presented via MHC class I to CD8+ cytotoxic T cells. The activated CD8+ T cells kill then target cells that display fragments of cytosolic pathogens (mostly viruses). Via release of perforin and granzymes and interaction of Fas-FasL, the virally infected cell is killed. **B:** CD4+ T helper cell commitment toward specific lineages

Thps cells can be skewed toward T<h1>, T<h2>, Treg, or T<h1>7 phenotypes on the basis of the cytokine environment and antigens contacted. Presence of IL-12 promotes skewing toward T<h1> commitment that are characterized by expression of T-bet and produce IFNγ and TNFα and β. T<h2> cell commitment is promoted by IL-4 via STAT-6 signaling. T<h2> committed cells are characterized by expression of GATA-3. Development of Treg and T<h1>7 phenotypes both require the presence of TGFβ, but the presence of IL-6 preferentially skews the response toward a T<h1>7 phenotype. Tregs are characterized in mice and man by expression of forkhead box P3 transcription factor, whereas RORγT is an important factor in the development of proinflammatory T<h1>7 cells.

cells differentiate from mainstream thymocytes through instructive signals through TCR engagement by CD1d-expressing cortical thymocytes, rather than via MHCI or MHCII. Their semi-invariant TCR molecules (Vα10/Vβ11) recognize mammalian glycosphingolipids, as well as ceramides found in the cell wall of Gram-negative, lipopolysaccharide-negative bacteria (70). This dual recognition of self and microbial ligands underlies innate-like antimicrobial functions mediated by CD40L induction and massive T<h1> and T<h2> cytokine and chemokine release. It is now apparent that CD1d-dependent NKT cells are a unique T-cell subset with the ability to regulate the immune system in response to a broad range of diseases. Details of their involvement in various types of disease are the subject of intense research in many laboratories worldwide (71).

The term *NK cells* was originally assigned on a merely functional basis to lymphoid cells capable of lysing certain

tumor cells in the absence of prior stimulation [for review, see (72)]. Regarding their origin, clear evidence has now been provided both in mice and humans that NK cells and T lymphocytes may derive from a common precursor. That is, mature NK cells can be obtained in vitro from CD34+ cells isolated from umbilical cord blood, bone marrow, and even human thymus when cultured in the presence of appropriate feeder cells or IL-15.

The molecular mechanism allowing NK cells to discriminate between normal cells and tumor cells, predicted by the "missing self hypothesis," has been clarified only in recent years. Thus, NK cells recognize MHC class I molecules through surface receptors delivering signals that inhibit, rather than activate, NK cells. As a consequence, NK cells lyse target cells that have lost expression of MHC class I molecules, as frequently occurs in tumors and in cells infected by certain viruses.

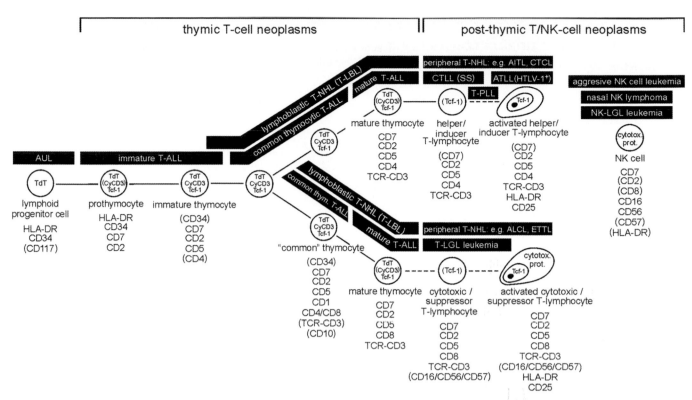

FIGURE 4.11 Hypothetic scheme of T/NK-lymphoid differentiation. The expression of relevant immunologic markers is indicated for each differentiation stage; markers in *parentheses* are not always expressed. The *bars* represent the various types of leukemias and non-Hodgkin lymphomas (NHL) as presumed malignant counterparts of lymphoid T cells on maturational arrest. AITL, angioimmunoblastic T-cell lymphoma; ALCL, anaplastic large-cell lymphoma; ATLL, adult T-cell leukemia lymphoma; AUL, acute undifferentiated leukemia; CTCL, cutaneous T-cell lymphoma; CTLL (SS), cutaneous T-cell leukemia lymphoma (mycosis fungoides/Sézary syndrome); ETTL, enteropathy-type T-cell lymphoma; HTLV-1, human T-cell leukemia virus type I; LBL, lymphoblastic lymphoma; LGL, large granular lymphocyte; PLL, prolymphocytic leukemia.

Several mechanisms control discrimination between self and non-self, including the thymic deletion of autoreactive T cells and the induction of anergy in the periphery. In addition to these passive mechanisms, evidence has accumulated for the active suppression of autoreactivity by a population of regulatory or suppressor T cells that coexpress CD4 and CD25 (the IL-2 receptor α-chain) (73). CD4+ CD25+ Treg cells are powerful inhibitors of T-cell activation both in vivo and in vitro. These cells have received a lot of interest lately from basic researchers as well as clinicians. Obviously, they could play a critical regulatory role in many pathologic conditions.

NORMAL T LYMPHOCYTES AND THEIR RELATIONSHIP TO T-CELL NEOPLASIA

Immunophenotype

The various types of acute and chronic T-cell leukemias and T-cell lymphomas can be regarded as the malignant counterparts of immature (thymic) or more mature (post-thymic) T-lymphoid cells (Fig. 4.11). Apart from morphologic and cytochemical features, the normal (precursor) T cells and their malignant counterparts can be characterized by immunophenotyping, using antibodies directed against (membrane bound or intracellular) leukocyte antigens.

Immunophenotype of Thymic-Derived T-Cell Neoplasms

Approximately 15% to 20% of childhood acute lymphoblastic leukemias (ALLs) and 20% to 25% of adult ALLs belong to the T lineage. Virtually all T-cell ALLs (T-ALLs) are positive for TdT, CD2, CD7, and CyCD3; further discrimination of subtypes is possible on the basis of CD1, CD3, CD4, CD5, and CD8 reactivity (Table 4.4) (74–79). T-ALLs are often classified in three main subtypes using CD1 and CD3: immature T-ALL (CD1−/CD3−), common (cortical) thymocytic T-ALL (CD1+/CD3+ or −), and mature T-ALL (CD1−/CD3+). Immature T-ALL can be further subdivided into the rare CD5− prothymocytic T-ALL and the CD5+ immature thymocytic T-ALL. These immature T-ALLs have a poor prognosis, whereas the CD1+ common thymocytic T-ALL is characterized by a much better outcome under intensive treatment. This difference in outcome probably reflects the apoptosis sensitivity of the normal thymocytic counterparts of these T-ALLs (76,77,80,81). Membrane CD3+ T-ALLs,

TABLE 4.4

IMMUNOPHENOTYPIC CHARACTERISTICS OF T-ALL

| Marker | Immature T-ALL | | Common thymocytic T-ALL | | Mature T-ALL |
	Prothymocytic (pro T-ALL)	Immature thymocytic (pre- T-ALL)	SmCD3$^-$	SmCD3$^+$	
TdT	++	++	++	++	++
CD1	−	−	++	++	−
CD2	+	++	++	++	++
CyCD3	++	++	++	++	++
CD3	−	−	−	++	++
CD4$^-$/CD8$^-$	++	+	−	−	−
CD4$^+$/CD8$^-$	−	±	±	±	+
CD4$^-$/CD8$^+$	−	±	±	±	±
CD4$^+$/CD8$^+$	−	−	+	+	±
CD5	−	++	++	++	++
CD7	++	++	++	++	++
TCR$\alpha\beta$	−	−	−	60% to 70%	60% to 70%
TCR$\gamma\delta$	−	−	−	30% to 40%	30% to 40%

−, <10% of T-ALL positive; ±, 10–25% of T-ALL positive; +, 25–75% of T-ALL positive; ++, >75% of T-ALL positive.

which constitute approximately 35% of all T-ALLs, are further subdivided in TCR$\alpha\beta^+$ (20% of T-ALLs) and TCR$\gamma\delta^+$ (15% of T-ALLs) subgroups (4); event-free survival is better in TCR$\gamma\delta^+$ T-ALL. The various types of T-ALLs and the T-cell lymphoblastic lymphomas (T-LBLs) form a continuous spectrum of lymphoblastic T-cell malignancies. CD3$^+$ T-ALL and T-LBL seem to be highly comparable in many features, despite a single report claiming a difference in the type of TCR molecule (TCR$\alpha\beta$ vs. TCR$\gamma\delta$) that is expressed (82).

Immunophenotype of Post-Thymic T-Cell Neoplasms

Mature T/NK-cell neoplasms are also called *post-thymic T-cell neoplasms* because they do not express TdT or CD1 antigen. This group consists of several types of chronic T/NK-cell leukemias and mature T/NK-cell lymphomas (83–86). They comprise approximately 5% to 10% of all mature lymphoid neoplasms. Immunophenotypic analysis helps to identify these subtypes as separate entities that show their characteristic disease course, prognosis, and treatment possibilities. Consequently, in the recent World Health Organization classification of hematopoietic tumors, immunologic marker analysis plays a major role next to morphology [reviewed in (87,88)]. One of the most important antibodies is CD3, which enables discrimination between CD3$^+$ T-cell neoplasms and CD3$^-$ NK cell neoplasms, such as the aggressive NK cell leukemia and the mostly NK-type extranodal/nasal lymphoma (Table 4.5). Most post-thymic CD3$^+$ T-cell neoplasms express TCR$\alpha\beta$, with only a minority expressing TCR$\gamma\delta$. Nevertheless, in some entities, such as T-cell large granular lymphocytic leukemia or hepatosplenic T-cell lymphoma, TCR$\gamma\delta$ cases are more abundant than in others

(89–91). However, generally TCR$\gamma\delta^+$ mature T-cell neoplasms are more rare than TCR$\gamma\delta^+$ T-ALLs. A major subdivision within the group of post-thymic TCR$\alpha\beta^+$ T-cell neoplasms concerns CD4 or CD8 positivity, largely reflecting the helper or cytotoxic origin of their normal counterparts, respectively. Most chronic T-cell leukemias, including T-cell prolymphocytic leukemia and adult T-cell leukemia/lymphoma, are largely of CD4 phenotype, except for T-cell large granular lymphocytic leukemia, which generally shows a CD8$^+$/CD57$^+$ cytotoxic origin (Table 4.5). T-cell prolymphocytic leukemia and adult T-cell leukemia/lymphoma typically express CD7 and CD25 antigens, respectively. Also, the various T-cell lymphomas are generally characterized as CD4$^+$ or CD8$^+$. Angioimmunoblastic lymphoma, peripheral T-cell lymphoma unspecified, and various types of cutaneous T-cell lymphoma (including mycosis fungoides and its leukemic variant Sézary syndrome) are mostly CD4$^+$, whereas others are CD8$^+$, such as the enteropathy type and subcutaneous panniculitis-like T-cell lymphoma (Table 4.5). In many of the CD8$^+$ post-thymic neoplasms as well as in TCR$\gamma\delta^+$ and NK cell types, cytotoxic granule proteins can be detected; this also holds for anaplastic large cell lymphomas and their cutaneous variants, which are both often CD4$^+$ (Table 4.5).

Immunogenotype

Given the observation that the various types of T-cell lymphomas and leukemias strongly resemble normal lymphoid (precursor) cells (75), the vast majority also contain rearranged TCR genes. However, neoplasms might exhibit curious types of rearrangements, which are rare or absent in normal T lymphocytes. One example concerns the so-called cross-lineage *IGH* gene rearrangements, which are found in

TABLE 4.5

MAJOR IMMUNOPHENOTYPIC CHARACTERISTICS OF POST-THYMIC T/NK-CELL NEOPLASMS

Post-thymic T/NK-cell neoplasms[a]	TCRαβ phenotype		TCRγδ phenotype	NK phenotype	Cytotoxic granule proteins
	CD4	CD8			
T-cell prolymphocytic leukemia	+	±	−	−	−
T-cell large granular lymphocytic leukemia	Rare	~70%	~10%	~15%	+
Aggressive NK cell leukemia	−	−	−	+	+
Adult T-cell leukemia/lymphoma	+	Rare	−	−	−
Extranodal/nasal T/NK lymphoma	−	−	−	+	+
Enteropathy type T-cell lymphoma	−	±	−	−	−
Hepatosplenic T-cell lymphoma	−	−	+	−	+
Subcutaneous panniculitis-like T-cell lymphoma	−	75%	25%	−	+
Mycosis fungoides/Sézary syndrome	+	Rare	Rare	−	−
Primary cutaneous anaplastic large-cell lymphoma	+	−	−	−	+
Peripheral T-cell lymphoma, unspecified	+	−	−	−	Rare
Angioimmunoblastic T-cell lymphoma	+	±	−	−	−
Anaplastic large cell lymphoma	±	Rare	−	−	+

−, negative; ±, occasionally positive; +, positive.
[a] Post-thymic T/NK-cell neoplasms as defined according to the World Health Organization Classification of tumors of hematopoietic and lymphoid tissues.

10% to 15% of T-ALLs (25,92–95) and which are probably due to the continuous activity of the recombinase enzyme system after malignant transformation in these precursor T-cell leukemias.

T-Cell Receptor Gene Recombination Patterns in Thymic-Derived T-Cell Neoplasms

CD3⁻, TCRαβ⁺, and TCRγδ⁺ T-ALLs/T-LBLs show major differences in TCR gene rearrangement patterns (Table 4.6) (4,25). Although the frequency of TCR gene rearrangements in T-ALL in general is very high, approximately 10% of CD3⁻ T-ALLs still have all TCR genes in germline configuration (4,25); this mainly concerns immature CD1⁻/CD3⁻ T-ALL of the prothymocytic T-ALL type. The TCRD genes in CD3⁻ T-ALL are rearranged in most cases (approximately 80%) and contain biallelic deletions in approximately 10% of cases (4,13). As expected, all TCRγδ⁺ T-ALLs have TCRG and TCRD gene rearrangements, and the vast majority (approximately 95%) also contain TCRB gene rearrangements (Table 4.6) (13,96). All TCRαβ⁺ T-ALLs contain TCRB and TCRG genes, and have at least one deleted TCRD allele (equals TCRA rearrangement); the second TCRD allele is also deleted in two thirds of cases(13,25). Despite persistent V(D)J recombinase activity in the T-ALL blasts, a comparative diagnosis-relapse study in 26 patients with T-cell lymphoblastic leukemia revealed a high stability of clonal TCR rearrangements; continuing and

secondary rearrangements were apparent in 0%, 14%, and 20% of TCRD, TCRG, and TCRB gene rearrangements, respectively (97). Oligoclonality at diagnosis is rarely seen in T-ALL (25,97), except for a few CD3⁻ T-ALLs showing polyclonal δREC-ΨJα rearrangements that can be interpreted as continuing rearrangements aiming at TCRαβ expression (98). TCRA rearrangements have not been studied in detail so far.

T-Cell Receptor Gene Recombination Patterns in Post-Thymic T-Cell Neoplasms

As the vast majority of chronic T-cell leukemias (T-cell prolymphocytic leukemia, adult T-cell leukemia/lymphoma, T-cell large granular lymphocytic leukemia) concern TCRαβ⁺ T-cell malignancies, TCRB rearrangements are found in virtually all samples (95% to 100%) (Table 4.6). Only the small subgroup of TCRγδ⁺ T-cell large granular lymphocytic leukemia lacks TCRB recombinations in approximately 50% of cases. TCRG rearrangements are very frequent in both TCRγδ⁺ and TCRαβ⁺ chronic leukemias. In contrast, most TCRαβ⁺ T-cell leukemias show monoallelic or biallelic deletions of their TCRD loci, which correlates with their expression of TCRα chains. Only a minority of cases, including all TCRγδ⁺ T-cell large granular lymphocytic leukemias, have rearranged TCRD genes (Table 4.6). NK large granular lymphocytic leukemias completely lack TCR rearrangements.

The membrane TCR expression of post-thymic T-cell non-Hodgkin lymphoma also largely reflects its TCR gene recombination patterns. Because most T-cell non-Hodgkin

TABLE 4.6

FREQUENCIES OF TCR GENE REARRANGEMENTS AND DELETIONS IN HUMAN T/NK-CELL NEOPLASMS

T/NK-cell neoplasm	*TCRB* R (%)	*TCRG* R (%)	*TCRD* R (%)	*TCRD* D (%)
Thymic derived				
CD3⁻ T-ALL (T-LBL)	85	90	80	10
TCRγδ⁺ T-ALL (T-LBL)	95	100	100	0
TCRαβ⁺ T-ALL (T-LBL)	100	100	35	65
Post-thymic				
ATLL, CTLL, T-PLL[a]	100	100	10–25	75–90
TCRαβ⁺ T-LGL[b]	100	100	<25	>75
TCRγδ⁺ T-LGL[b]	~50	100	100	0
NK-LGL[b]	0	0	0	0
T-NHL[c]	80	60–100	<35?	>60?

ATLL, adult T-cell leukemia/lymphoma; CTLL, cutaneous T-cell leukemia/lymphoma; D, both alleles deleted; R, at least one allele rearranged; T-LGL, T-cell large granular lymphocytic leukemia; T-NHL, T-cell non-Hodgkin lymphoma; T-PLL, T-cell prolymphocytic leukemia.
[a] The majority of adult T-cell leukemia/lymphoma, cutaneous T-cell leukemia/lymphoma, and T-cell prolymphocytic leukemia are of TCRαβ⁺ type.
[b] Most T-cell large granular lymphocytic leukemiaproliferations are TCRαβ⁺ (70% to 80%), and minorities are TCRγδ⁺ (10% to +15%) or belong to the NK lineage (10% to 15%).
[c] Except for γδ hepatosplenic lymphoma and some cases of TCR⁻ anaplastic large cell lymphoma, many post-thymic T-cell non-Hodgkin lymphomas are TCRαβ⁺.

lymphoma types are TCRαβ⁺, except for (TCRγδ⁺) hepatosplenic T-cell lymphomas and some TCR⁻ anaplastic large cell lymphomas, *TCRB* and *TCRG* rearrangements are very frequent but (slightly) less than those found in chronic T-cell leukemias (Table 4.6). The frequency of *TCRD* rearrangements is not exactly known but is estimated to be less than 35%, whereas *TCRD* deletions are probably found in more than 60% of cases.

TCR Clonality Detection in T-Cell Neoplasms

Because T-cell leukemias are clonal cell proliferations, the TCR gene rearrangements are assumed to be identical in all cells of the leukemic clone (25,99–102). This is the basis of clonality assessment in lymphoproliferations (25). Detection of clonal TCR gene rearrangements is possible via polymerase chain reaction methods. As *TCRG* and *TCRD* loci contain a limited number of V and J gene segments (Table 4.1 and Fig. 4.2) (10,13), only a restricted number of polymerase chain reaction primers is sufficient to analyze the various *TCRG* and *TCRD* gene rearrangements. In contrast, polymerase chain reaction analysis of *TCRA* and *TCRB* gene rearrangements requires many more (family) primers, especially for the many different V and J gene segments in *TCRA* and *TCRB* genes (7,8,103–106). Reverse-transcriptase polymerase chain reaction analysis of *TCRA* and *TCRB* V(D)J-C transcripts still requires many different V (family) primers but in combination with only a single C primer (103–105,107). False-negative results, due to primer sets that do not recognize all involved TCR gene segments, might be overcome by using specific primers for every individual V and J gene segment in multiplex polymerase chain reactions.

Polymerase chain reaction-based detection of clonal TCR gene rearrangements is relatively easy if the percentage of

leukemic cells is high (e.g., greater than 90%). In such cell samples, the background of TCR gene rearrangements of normal, polyclonal cells generally does not hamper proper interpretation. However, if a sample contains substantial numbers of polyclonal T cells, many polyclonal TCR polymerase chain reaction products are present as well, stressing the need to discriminate between clonal (leukemia derived) and polyclonal (reactive) polymerase chain reaction products. Methods exploiting the junctional diversity of rearranged TCR genes to discriminate between identical (clonal) and heterogeneous (polyclonal) polymerase chain reaction products include a.o. heteroduplex analysis (108,109) and GeneScan/fragment analysis (Fig. 4.12) (110,111).

T-Cell Receptor Vβ Detection via Monoclonal Antibodies

Molecular methods for clonality detection and repertoire analysis of (aberrant) T-cell populations can be time consuming and labor intensive, and, most important, do not allow precise quantitative evaluation. However, the recent availability of a set of well-defined Vβ antibodies enables flow cytometric analysis of the TCR Vβ repertoire. Using normal values in healthy controls of different age groups as a reference (Fig. 4.13), clonal T-cell populations can be identified in a quantitative manner (112,113). In a comparative study using 28 thymic-derived T-cell neoplasms and 47 post-thymic mature T-cell neoplasms, Vβ flow cytometric results appeared to correlate completely with *TCRB* polymerase chain reaction results. As the complete set of antibodies covers 65% to 70% of all TCR Vβ domains, flow cytometric assays served to identify restricted Vβ usage in two thirds of the monoclonal T-cell neoplasms (Fig. 4.14); in the other cases, a major T-cell population did not stain with any of the antibodies, which is indirect evidence

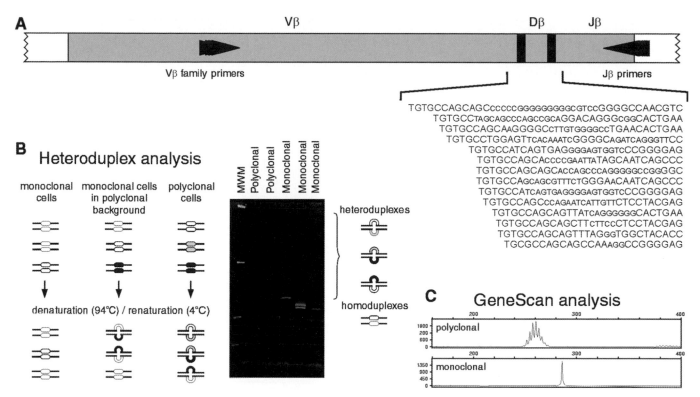

FIGURE 4.12 Schematic diagram of the heteroduplex analysis and GeneScan analysis techniques. Rearranged TCR genes (*TCRB* in the example) show heterogeneity (in size and nucleotide composition) in their junctional regions. This heterogeneity of rearranged TCR polymerase chain reaction (PCR) products is used in heteroduplex analysis (size and composition) and GeneScan analysis (size) to discern between products derived from monoclonal and polyclonal lymphoid cell populations. In heteroduplex analysis, PCR products are heat denatured (5 minutes, 94°C) and subsequently rapidly cooled (1 hour, 4°C) to induce duplex (homo- or heteroduplex) formation. In cell samples consisting of clonal lymphoid cells, the polymerase chain reaction products of rearranged TCR genes give rise to homoduplexes after denaturation and renaturation, whereas in samples that contain polyclonal lymphoid cell populations, the single-strand polymerase chain reaction fragments mainly form heteroduplexes, which result in a background smear of slowly migrating fragments on electrophoresis. In GeneScan analysis, fluorochrome-labeled rearranged TCR products are first denatured before high-resolution fragment analysis of the resulting single-strand fragments. Monoclonal cell samples give rise to polymerase chain reaction products of identical size, whereas in polyclonal samples, many different TCR polymerase chain reaction products are formed, which show a characteristic gaussian size distribution.

for the homogenous character of these samples in line with the molecular data (107,114). In the future, quantitative flow cytometric Vβ analyses might, thus, (partly) replace the more expensive and cumbersome molecular TCR repertoire studies. Likewise, Vγ and Vδ analysis in the case of TCR$\gamma\delta$ T-cell proliferations might also (partly) be performed by flow cytometry using Vγ and Vδ antibodies, although the small Vγ/Vδ repertoire makes this more difficult than Vβ analysis (91,96).

DEREGULATED DIFFERENTIATION LEADING TO T-CELL NEOPLASIA

Illegitimate V(D)J Recombination Leading to Chromosome Aberrations in Thymocytes

T-cell neoplasms harbor characteristic TCR gene recombination patterns (13,96,102,115–117), and also nonphysiologic

rearrangements between TCR loci and protooncogenes can occur (118). This is particularly the case in T-cell lymphoblastic leukemias, in which several types of chromosome aberrations involving the *TCRD* (chromosome region 14q11) and *TCRB* (7q34-35) loci have been described (Table 4.7). Such translocations are most likely mediated via mechanisms closely resembling physiologic V(D)J gene rearrangements (type I aberrations) (119,120). This is supported by the presence of RSS-like or cryptic RSS elements in the breakpoint regions of several of these genes. However, in the majority of cases, no such cryptic RSSs are observed, suggesting that breaks occur through distinct, as yet unknown, molecular mechanisms (type II aberrations) (119,120). As a result of these illegitimate V(D)J recombinations, protooncogenes on the partner chromosomes are either activated through regulatory elements of the translocated TCR gene or through removal of negative regulatory elements that normally inhibit expression of the protooncogene (120). One of the best-known examples concerns ectopic expression of the transcription factor TAL1 upon t(1;14)(p32;q11) and t(1;7)(p32;q35) (Table 4.7). Together with microdeletions of chromosome region 1p32

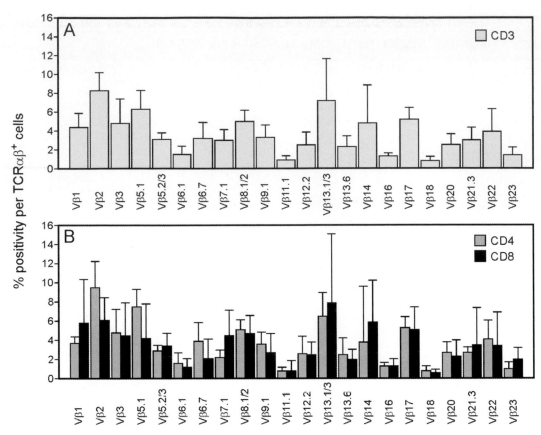

FIGURE 4.13 Flow cytometric Vβ analysis in healthy individuals. Schematic overview of mean values and standard deviations for Vβ positivity within TCR αβ⁺/CD3⁺ T lymphocytes (**A**) and within TCRαβ⁺/CD4⁺ and TCRαβ⁺/CD8⁺ T lymphocytes (**B**).

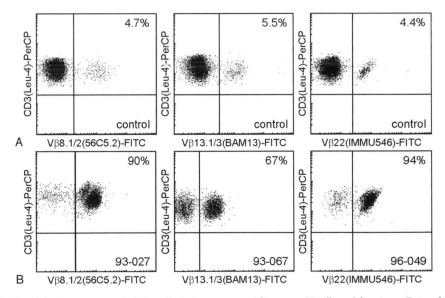

FIGURE 4.14 Flow cytometric Vβ analysis in patients with mature T-cell proliferations. Examples of Vβ8.1/2, Vβ13.1/3, and Vβ22 reactivity within CD3⁺ T lymphocytes of healthy controls (**A**) and three different monoclonal T-cell neoplasms (**B**).

that also give rise to TAL1 overexpression, these aberrations are found in a considerable subgroup of 20% to 25% of all T-ALLs (121–123). In addition to TAL1, other transcription factors can be activated inappropriately by translocation of

TCR genes. This concerns other bHLH transcription factors, such as MYC, TAL2, and LYL1, the LIM domain factors LMO1 and LMO2, and homeobox factors HOX11, HOX11L2, HOXA, and NKX2-5 (Table 4.7) (124–134).

TABLE 4.7

MOST FREQUENT NONRANDOM CHROMOSOME ABERRATIONS IN T-ALL

Chromosome aberration	Relative frequency of T-ALL (%)	Involved gene	Involved T-cell receptor gene
1p32 aberrations	20–25	TAL1	TCRD/TCRB
t(1;7)(p32;q34)	1	LCK	TCRB
t(5;14) (q35;q11)/t(5;14)(q35;q32)	15–20	HOX11L2 / NKX2-5	TCRD/(BCL11B)
t(6;7) (q23;q32-36)	1–2	MYB	TCRB
t(7;7) (q34;p14)/inv(7) (q35p14)	5	HOXA	TCRB
t(7;9)(q34;q32)	2	TAL2	TCRB
t(7;9)(q34;q34)	2	TAN1 Notch1	TCRB
t(7;12) (q34;p13)	1–2	CCND2	TCRB
t(7;19)(q34;p13)	1	LYL1	TCRB
t(8;14)(q24;q11)	2	MYC	TCRD
t(10;14)(q24;q11)/t(7;10)(q35;q24)	4	HOX11	TCRD/TCRB
t(11;14)(p13;q11)/t(7;11)(q35;p13)	7	LMO2	TCRD/TCRB
t(11;14)(p15;q11)	1	LMO1	TCRD

So far, illegitimate V(D)J recombination involving TCR loci has not been described in more mature T-cell neoplasms. One exceptional type of TCR rearrangement is found in lymphocytes of patients with ataxia-telangiectasia and Nijmegen breakage syndrome, as well as in T-cell neoplasms that develop in patients with ataxia-telangiectasia and Nijmegen breakage syndrome. This concerns the so-called transrearrangements between the *TCRB* and *TCRG* loci through t(7;7) or inversion seven (135–138). However, though described in isolated T-ALL cases (139), these transrearrangements are not believed to play a direct role in oncogenesis; they are rather considered to be a general indicator of genomic instability and the risk of lymphoma development in such patients. Many of the molecular genetic events involved in lymphomagenesis and leukemogenesis of post-thymic T lymphocytes, therefore, still remain to be identified.

Inappropriate Transcriptional Activation in Thymocytes

As a general result of translocations in human T-ALL, transcription factors are inappropriately activated, leading to ectopic expression and deregulated thymocyte differentiation. In the case of tissue-specific bHLH factors, it has been hypothesized that their ectopic expression in T-lymphocyte precursors causes heterodimerization with class I bHLH factors (e.g., E2A and HEB). As a result, key regulator functions of these E proteins in thymocyte differentiation are blocked, which contributes to malignant transformation and subsequently T-ALL development (140,141). Consistent with the E-protein inactivation hypothesis is the rapid development of immature T-cell lymphomas in E2A$^{-/-}$ mice (56).

Another family of regulatory factors known to be involved in human T-ALL is the Notch receptor family, which normally controls cell fate decisions (142,143). Notc<h1>, truncated by a chromosomal translocation leading to a constitutively active intracellular domain (TAN-1), plays a role in T-ALL leukemogenesis (144). However, Notc<h1>-activating mutations, resulting in increased intracellular Notc<h1> levels, are far more important, given their occurrence in >50% of T-ALL cases (145,146).

Even though only 30-40% of human T-ALLs have chromosomal TCR translocations, gene-profiling studies have revealed that T-ALLs cluster into groups with common gene expression signatures (147). This is due to the fact that the *LYL1*, *HOX11*, *HOX11L2*, and *TAL1* oncogenes that define these groups can also be overexpressed via other mechanisms than translocations. These groups represent distinct clinical subtypes with different prognosis. HOX11+ T-ALLs are associated with a relatively favorable prognosis, whereas LYL1+, TAL1+, and probably also HOX11L2+ cases show a less favorable outcome.

Interestingly, the gene expression-based groups appeared to correspond to different thymic subsets, showing a maturational arrest through ectopic expression of the involved transcription factor (147). Thus, high *LMO2* expression was especially associated with the immature and $\alpha\beta$-lineage T-ALL cases, whereas high *LYL1* expression mainly occurred in immature and TCR$\gamma\beta$+ T-ALL, *HOX11* was exclusively expressed in $\alpha\beta$-lineage preselected T-ALL and *HOX11L2* predominantly in TCR$\gamma\delta$+ T-ALL, and finally, high *TAL1* expression was especially associated with the $\alpha\beta$-lineage T-ALL (122,148–150).

These data suggest specific associations between the stage of maturational arrest of T-ALL and the expressed oncogenes. However, gene expression profiling studies on all major human T-cell developmental stages revealed that several well-known T-ALL oncogenes are also expressed during certain stages of normal human T-cell development (151). This implies that knowledge on the expression of T-ALL oncogenes during normal T-cell development is a prerequisite for correct biologic interpretation of oncogene expression in T-ALL. Such comparison showed that expression of *TAL1*, *HOX11*, or *HOX11L2* in T-ALL at any maturational stage is ectopic and, hence, oncogenic. Importantly, however, *LMO2* and *LYL1* expression in immature and TCR$\gamma\delta$ T-ALL mostly reflects a T-cell developmental program rather than oncogenic activation, whereas expression in $\alpha\beta$-lineage restricted T-ALL is truly oncogenic (150,151).

Although inappropriate transcriptional activation, either due to translocation or other mechanisms responsible for increased expression of several classes of transcription factors, seems to be a general principle contributing to aberrant thymocyte development and subsequent malignant transformation, much less is known yet about similar mechanisms in more mature T-cell neoplasias. Many of the molecular genetic events involved in lymphomagenesis and leukemogenesis of post-thymic T lymphocytes, therefore, still remain to be identified.

LMO2 Oncogene Activation by Retroviral Insertion in Gene Therapy

An interesting, albeit, tragic type of T-ALL has been documented in five children as a side effect in an otherwise successful gene therapy trial for the most common form of human severe combined immunodeficiency, termed severe combined immunodeficiency-X1 (152–154). In this X-linked immunodeficiency, the IL2Rγ chain is nonfunctional due to inactivating mutations. IL2Rγ is also called "common γ chain" because it functions as the signal-transducing component for a number of cytokine receptors [reviewed in (155,156)]. Together with specific α and/or β chains, the common γ-chain forms receptors for IL2, IL4, IL7, IL9, IL15, and IL21. These side effects of gene therapy have emphasized insertional mutagenesis and its oncogenic consequence as an unexpectedly common adverse effect of the γ-retroviral gene transfer technology used. As it turns out, integration of retroviruses is by no means at random as previously assumed, but favors transcriptionally active loci in hematopoietic stem cells, thereby marking "stemness" genes (157–159). If such an integration event occurs nearby an oncogene, its expression may be deregulated, leading to arrest in differentiation and a preleukemic condition. In four out of five children, integration occurred near the *LMO2* oncogene, leading to very high expression of this gene. During normal human T-cell development, expression of LMO2 is rapidly down-regulated during the early thymocyte stages (160). Using human CD34+ cells, we recently demonstrated that retrovirus-mediated expression of LMO2 only hampers T-cell development, whereas differentiation into other blood lineages was not affected. We showed that overexpression of LMO2 in human cells leads to a block in early T-cell development, consistent with earlier findings in *Lmo2*-transgenic mice. The activation of LMO2 by insertional mutagenesis is clearly an important oncogenic factor but is by itself probably insufficient to cause full-blown leukemia. Additional genetic abnormalities are likely required (152–154).

CONCLUSION

Insight into normal T-cell differentiation and T-cell function is essential to understand the origin and characteristics of T-cell malignancies. Although malignantly transformed cells differ in some aspects from their normal counterparts, most phenotypic and genotypic characteristics are identical.

Transformation of T-cells might be mediated via several different events, such as aberrant TCR gene rearrangements leading to oncogene activation, inappropriate apoptosis leading to proliferation instead of cell death, or unwanted activation and subsequent proliferation. This implies that malignant transformation might be caused by seemingly minor defects in

several molecular steps during normal T-cell differentiation, TCR gene rearrangement processes, positive and negative selection processes, activation and TCR molecule signaling processes, and T-helper and cytotoxic functions. Understanding the regulation of these processes supports the understanding of malignant transformation.

Over the last decade, progress in the immunodiagnosis of T-cell malignancies was based on:

1. Advances in immunophenotyping of normal and malignant T cells, particularly by use of multiparameter flow cytometry with quadruple labelings. This progress allowed more detailed characterization and classification of T-cell malignancies (Fig. 4.11 and Table 4.5).
2. Novel developments in clonality diagnostics, particularly based on the polymerase chain reaction-mediated detection of clonal TCR gene rearrangements (Fig. 4.12 and Table 4.6) and TCR gene-related chromosome aberrations (Table 4.7). Clonality assessment appeared to be highly valuable in the diagnosis of mature T-cell malignancies, particularly in patients who have many reactive T lymphocytes in suspect lesions.
3. New possibilities for evaluation of treatment effectiveness by detection of minimal residual disease in blood and bone marrow during and after treatment. Minimal residual disease detection in T-cell malignancies is possible by use of Vβ antibodies in part of the patients. However, in virtually all patients, polymerase chain reaction-based techniques can be applied for minimal residual disease detection, using the junctional regions of rearranged TCR genes as leukemia-specific polymerase chain reaction targets.

It can be foreseen that current developments in genomics and proteomics (including gene expression profiling and antibody or tissue arrays) will further contribute to the insight in normal and malignant T-cell development. Subsequent multidisciplinary translational research will play a key role in the further improvement of diagnostics and treatment of patients with T-cell malignancies.

REFERENCES

1. Davis MM, Bjorkman PJ. T-cell antigen receptor genes and T-cell recognition. *Nature* 1988;334:395–402.
2. Owen MJ, Lamb JR. *Immune recognition*. Oxford, UK: IRL Press, 1988.
3. Borst J, Brouns GS, de Vries E, et al. Antigen receptors on T and B lymphocytes: parallels in organization and function. *Immunol Rev* 1993;132:49–84.
4. van Dongen JJ, Comans-Bitter WM, Wolvers-Tettero IL, et al. Development of human T lymphocytes and their thymus-dependency. *Thymus* 1990;16:207–234.
5. van Dongen JJ, Wolvers-Tettero IL. Analysis of immunoglobulin and T cell receptor genes. Part I: basic and technical aspects. *Clin Chim Acta* 1991;198:1–91.
6. Yoshikai Y, Clark SP, Taylor S, et al. Organization and sequences of the variable, joining and constant region genes of the human T-cell receptor alpha-chain. *Nature* 1985;316:837–840.
7. Griesser H, Champagne E, Tkachuk D, et al. The human T cell receptor alpha-delta locus: a physical map of the variable, joining and constant region genes. *Eur J Immunol* 1988;8:641–644.
8. Toyonaga B, Yoshikai Y, Vadasz V, et al. Organization and sequences of the diversity, joining, and constant region genes of the human T-cell receptor beta chain. *Proc Natl Acad Sci U S A* 1985;82:8624–8628.
9. Quertermous T, Strauss WM, Van Dongen JJ, et al. Human T cell gamma chain joining regions and T cell development. *J Immunol* 1987;138:2687–2690.
10. Lefranc MP, Rabbitts TH. The human T-cell receptor gamma (TRG) genes. *Trends Biochem Sci* 1989;14:214–218.
11. Zhang XM, Tonnelle C, Lefranc MP, et al. T cell receptor gamma cDNA in human fetal liver and thymus: variable regions of gamma chains are

restricted to V gamma I or V9, due to the absence of splicing of the V10 and V11 leader intron. *Eur J Immunol* 1994;24:571–578.

12. Takihara Y, Tkachuk D, Michalopoulos E, et al. Sequence and organization of the diversity, joining, and constant region genes of the human T-cell delta-chain locus. *Proc Natl Acad Sci U S A* 1988;85:6097–6101.

13. Breit TM, Wolvers-Tettero IL, Beishuizen A, et al. Southern blot patterns, frequencies, and junctional diversity of T-cell receptor-delta gene rearrangements in acute lymphoblastic leukemia. *Blood* 1993;82:3063–3074.

14. Davodeau F, Peyrat MA, Hallet MM, et al. Characterization of a new functional TCR J delta segment in humans. Evidence for a marked conservation of J delta sequences between humans, mice, and sheep. *J Immunol* 1994;153:137–142.

15. Tonegawa S. Somatic generation of antibody diversity. *Nature* 1983;302:575–581.

16. Schatz DG, Oettinger MA, Baltimore D. The V(D)J recombination activating gene, RAG-1. *Cell* 1989;59:1035–1048.

17. Oettinger MA, Schatz DG, Gorka C, Baltimore D. RAG-1 and RAG-2, adjacent genes that synergistically activate V(D)J recombination. *Science* 1990;248:1517–1523.

18. McBlane JF, van Gent DC, Ramsden DA, et al. Cleavage at a V(D)J recombination signal requires only RAG1 and RAG2 proteins and occurs in two steps. *Cell* 1995;83:387–395.

19. Lieber MR. The mechanism of V(D)J recombination: a balance of diversity, specificity, and stability. *Cell* 1992;70:873–876.

20. Lieber MR. The role of site-directed recombinases in physiologic and pathologic chromosomal rearrangements. In: Kirsch IR, ed. *The causes and consequences of chromosomal aberrations.* Boca Raton, FL: CRC Press, 1993;239–275.

21. van Gent DC, Ramsden DA, Gellert M. The RAG1 and RAG2 proteins establish the 12/23 rule in V(D)J recombination. *Cell* 1996;85:107–113.

22. Hazenberg MD, Verschuren MC, Hamann D, et al. T cell receptor excision circles as markers for recent thymic emigrants: basic aspects, technical approach, and guidelines for interpretation. *J Mol Med* 2001;79:631–640.

23. Ye P, Kirschner DE. Reevaluation of T cell receptor excision circles as a measure of human recent thymic emigrants. *J Immunol* 2002;168:4968–4979.

24. Hazenberg MD, Otto SA, Cohen Stuart JW, et al. Increased cell division but not thymic dysfunction rapidly affects the T-cell receptor excision circle content of the naive T cell population in HIV-1 infection. *Nat Med* 2000;6:1036–1042.

25. van Dongen JJ, Wolvers-Tettero IL. Analysis of immunoglobulin and T cell receptor genes. Part II: possibilities and limitations in the diagnosis and management of lymphoproliferative diseases and related disorders. *Clin Chim Acta* 1991;198:93–174.

26. Marolleau JP, Fondell JD, Malissen M, et al. The joining of germ-line V alpha to J alpha genes replaces the preexisting V alpha-J alpha complexes in a T cell receptor alpha, beta positive T cell line. *Cell* 1988;55:291–300.

27. McCormack WT, Liu M, Postema C, et al. Excision products of TCR V alpha recombination contain in-frame rearrangements: evidence for continued V(D)J recombination in TCR+ thymocytes. *Int Immunol* 1993;5:801–804.

28. Huang C, Kanagawa O. Ordered and coordinated rearrangement of the TCR alpha locus: role of secondary rearrangement in thymic selection. *J Immunol* 2001;166:2597–2601.

29. Golub R, Huang CY, Kanagawa O, Wu GE. Valpha gene replacement in a TCRalpha knock-in mouse. *Eur J Immunol* 2001;31:2919–2925.

30. Golub R. V gene replacement in T and B lymphocytes: illicit or regimented rearrangement? *Arch Immunol Ther Exp (Warsz)* 2002;50:255–262.

31. Leiden JM, Dialynas DP, Duby AD, et al. Rearrangement and expression of T-cell antigen receptor genes in human T-lymphocyte tumor lines and normal human T-cell clones: evidence for allelic exclusion of Ti beta gene expression and preferential use of a J beta 2 gene segment. *Mol Cell Biol* 1986;6:3207–3214.

32. Triebel F, Hercend T. Subpopulations of human peripheral T gamma delta lymphocytes. *Immunol Today* 1989;10:186–188.

33. Borst J, Wicherink A, Van Dongen JJ, et al. Non-random expression of T cell receptor gamma and data variable gene segments in functional T lymphocyte clones from human peripheral blood. *Eur J Immunol* 1989;19:1559–1568.

34. Breit TM, Wolvers-Tettero IL, van Dongen JJ. Unique selection determinant in polyclonal V delta 2-J delta 1 junctional regions of human peripheral gamma delta T lymphocytes. *J Immunol* 1994;152:2860–2864.

35. Desiderio SV, Yancopoulos GD, Paskind M, et al. Insertion of N regions into heavy-chain genes is correlated with expression of terminal deoxytransferase in B cells. *Nature* 1984;311:752–755.

36. Elliott JF, Rock EP, Patten PA, et al. The adult T-cell receptor delta-chain is diverse and distinct from that of fetal thymocytes. *Nature* 1988;331:627–631.

37. Breit TM, Wolvers-Tettero IL, Bogers AJ, et al. Rearrangements of the human TCRD-deleting elements. *Immunogenetics* 1994;40:70–75.

38. Kondo M, Weissman IL, Akashi K. Identification of clonogenic common lymphoid progenitors in mouse bone marrow. *Cell* 1997;91:661–672.

39. Spits H. Development of alphabeta t cells in the human thymus. *Nat Rev Immunol* 2002;2:760–772.

40. Peault B. Human T-cell lineage development in foetal thymus-engrafted SCID mice. *Res Immunol* 1994;145:124–128.

41. Spits H, Blom B, Jaleco AC, et al. Early stages in the development of human T, natural killer and thymic dendritic cells. *Immunol Rev* 1998;165:75–86.

42. Shortman K, Wu L. Early T lymphocyte progenitors. *Annu Rev Immunol* 1996;14:29–47.

43. Hogquist KA, Jameson SC, Bevan MJ. The ligand for positive selection of T lymphocytes in the thymus. *Curr Opin Immunol* 1994;6:273–278.

44. McVay LD, Carding SR. Generation of human gammadelta T-cell repertoires. *Crit Rev Immunol* 1999;19:431–460.

45. Blom B, Verschuren MC, Heemskerk MH, et al. TCR gene rearrangements and expression of the pre-T cell receptor complex during human T-cell differentiation. *Blood* 1999;93:3033–3043.

46. Pawlowski TJ, Staerz UD. How are alpha beta T cells positively selected in the thymus? *Behring Inst Mitt* 1994;94–103.

47. Hogquist KA. Signal strength in thymic selection and lineage commitment. *Curr Opin Immunol* 2001;13:225–231.

48. Germain RN. T-cell development and the CD4-CD8 lineage decision. *Nat Rev Immunol* 2002;2:309–322.

49. Anderson G, Harman BC, Hare KJ, Jenkinson EJ. Microenvironmental regulation of T cell development in the thymus. *Semin Immunol* 2000;12:457–464.

50. Sen J. Signal transduction in thymus development. *Cell Mol Biol (Noisy-le-grand)* 2001;47:197–215.

51. Rothenberg EV. Signaling mechanisms in thymocyte selection. *Curr Opin Immunol* 1994;6:257–265.

52. Ernst P, Smale ST. Combinatorial regulation of transcription. I: general aspects of transcriptional control. *Immunity* 1995;2:311–319.

53. Castrop J, van Wichen D, Koomans-Bitter M, et al. The human TCF-1 gene encodes a nuclear DNA-binding protein uniquely expressed in normal and neoplastic T-lineage lymphocytes. *Blood* 1995;86:3050–3059.

54. Georgopoulos K, Moore DD, Derfler B. Ikaros, an early lymphoid-specific transcription factor and a putative mediator for T cell commitment. *Science* 1992;258:808–812.

55. Georgopoulos K, Bigby M, Wang JH, et al. The Ikaros gene is required for the development of all lymphoid lineages. *Cell* 1994;79:143–156.

56. Bain G, Engel I, Robanus Maandag EC, et al. E2A deficiency leads to abnormalities in alphabeta T-cell development and to rapid development of T-cell lymphomas. *Mol Cell Biol* 1997;17:4782–4791.

57. Bain G, Murre C. The role of E-proteins in B- and T-lymphocyte development. *Semin Immunol* 1998;10:143–153.

58. van de Wetering M, Cavallo R, Dooijes D, et al. Armadillo coactivates transcription driven by the product of the *Drosophila* segment polarity gene dTCF. *Cell* 1997;88:789–799.

59. Struhl G, Adachi A. Nuclear access and action of notch in vivo. *Cell* 1998;93:649–660.

60. Pui JC, Allman D, Xu L, et al. Notc<h1> expression in early lymphopoiesis influences B versus T lineage determination. *Immunity* 1999;11:299–308.

61. Schwartz JC, Zhang X, Nathenson SG, et al. Structural mechanisms of costimulation. *Nat Immunol* 2002;3:427–434.

62. Bour-Jordan H, Blueston JA. CD28 function: a balance of costimulatory and regulatory signals. *J Clin Immunol* 2002;22:1–7.

63. Reiner SL. Helper T cell differentiation, inside and out. *Curr Opin Immunol* 2001;13:351–355.

64. Rautajoki KJ, Kylaniemi MK, Raghav SK, et al. An insight into molecular mechanisms of human T helper cell differentiation. *Ann Med* 2008;40:322–335.

65. Baecher-Allan C, Hafler DA. Human regulatory T cells and their role in autoimmune disease. *Immunol Rev* 2006;212:203–216.

66. Aluvihare VR, Kallikourdis M, Betz AG. Regulatory T cells mediate maternal tolerance to the fetus. *Nat Immunol* 2004;5:266–271.

67. Langrish CL, Chen Y, Blumenschein WM, et al. IL-23 drives a pathogenic T cell population that induces autoimmune inflammation. *J Exp Med* 2005;201:233–240.

68. Veldhoen M, Hocking RJ, Atkins CJ, et al. TGFβ in the context of an inflammatory cytokine milieu supports de novo differentiation of IL-17-producing T cells. *Immunity* 2006;24:179–189.

69. Ouyang W, Kolls JK, Zheng Y. The biological functions of T helper 17 cell effector cytokines in inflammation. *Immunity* 2008;28:454–467.

70. Kronenberg M. Toward an understanding of NKT cell biology: progress and paradoxes. *Annu Rev Immunol* 2005;26:877–900.

71. Sidobre S, Hammond KJ, Bénazet-Sidobre L, et al. The T cell antigen receptor expressed by Valpha14i NKT cells has a unique mode of glycosphingolipid antigen recognition. *Proc Natl Acad Sci U S A* 2004;101:12254–12259.

72. Colucci F, Di Santo JP, Leibson PJ. Natural killer cell activation in mice and men: different triggers for similar weapons? *Nat Immunol* 2002;3:807–813.

73. Shevach EM. CD4+ CD25+ suppressor T cells: more questions than answers. *Nat Rev Immunol* 2002;2:389–400.

74. Foon KA, Todd RF 3rd. Immunologic classification of leukemia and lymphoma. *Blood* 1986;68:1–31.

75. van Dongen JJ, Adriaansen HJ, Hooijkaas H. Immunophenotyping of leukaemias and non-Hodgkin's lymphomas. Immunological markers and their CD codes. *Neth J Med* 1988;33:298–314.

76. Pui CH, Behm FG, Crist WM. Clinical and biologic relevance of immunologic marker studies in childhood acute lymphoblastic leukemia. *Blood* 1993;82:343–362.

77. Ludwig WD, Raghavachar A, Thiel E. Immunophenotypic classification of acute lymphoblastic leukaemia. *Baillieres Clin Haematol* 1994;7:235–262.

78. Bene MC, Castoldi G, Knapp W, et al. Proposals for the immunological classification of acute leukemias. European Group for the Immunological Characterization of Leukemias. *Leukemia* 1995;9:1783–1786.

79. Craig FE, Foon KA. Flow cytometric immunophenotyping for hematologic neoplasms. *Blood* 2008;111:3941–3967.

80. Niehues T, Kapaun P, Harms DO, et al. A classification based on T cell selection-related phenotypes identifies a subgroup of childhood T-ALL with favorable outcome in the COALL studies. *Leukemia* 1999;13:614–617.

81. Pullen J, Shuster JJ, Link M, et al. Significance of commonly used prognostic factors differs for children with T cell acute lymphocytic leukemia (ALL), as compared to those with B-precursor ALL. A Pediatric Oncology Group (POG) study. *Leukemia* 1999;13:1696–1707.

82. Gouttefangeas C, Bensussan A, Boumsell L. Study of the CD3-associated T-cell receptors reveals further differences between T-cell acute lymphoblastic lymphoma and leukemia. *Blood* 1990;75:931–934.

83. Bain BJ. *Leukemia diagnosis: a guide to the FAB classification.* Philadelphia, Pa: J.B. Lippincott, 1990.

84. Bennett JM, Catovsky D, Daniel MT, et al. Proposals for the classification of chronic (mature) B and T lymphoid leukaemias. French-American-British (FAB) Cooperative Group. *J Clin Pathol* 1989;42:567–584.

85. Catovsky D, Matutes E. Leukemias of mature T cells. In: Knowles DM, ed. *Neoplastic hematopathology.* Baltimore, MD: J.B. Lippincott, 1992:1267.

86. Matutes E, Brito-Babapulle V, Swansbury J, et al. Clinical and laboratory features of 78 cases of T-prolymphocytic leukemia. *Blood* 1991;78:3269–3274.

87. Harris NL, Jaffe ES, Diebold J, et al. World Health Organization classification of neoplastic diseases of the hematopoietic and lymphoid tissues: report of the Clinical Advisory Committee meeting-Airlie House, Virginia, November 1997. *J Clin Oncol* 1999;17:3835–3849.

88. Jaffe ES, Harris NL, Stein H, World Health Organization, et al. *Pathology and genetics of tumours of the haematopoietic and lymphoid tissues.* Lyon, France: IARC Press, 2001.

89. Loughran TP Jr. Clonal diseases of large granular lymphocytes. *Blood* 1993;82:1–14.

90. Semenzato G, Zambello R, Starkebaum G, et al. The lymphoproliferative disease of granular lymphocytes: updated criteria for diagnosis. *Blood* 1997;89:256–260.

91. Sandberg Y, Almeida J, Gonzalez M, et al. TCRgammadelta+ large granular lymphocyte leukemias reflect the spectrum of normal antigen-selected TCRgammadelta+ T-cells. *Leukemia* 2006;20:505–513.

92. Greaves MF, Chan LC, Furley AJ, et al. Lineage promiscuity in hemopoietic differentiation and leukemia. *Blood* 1986;67:1–11.

93. Adriaansen HJ, Soeting PW, Wolvers-Tettero IL, et al. Immunoglobulin and T-cell receptor gene rearrangements in acute non-lymphocytic leukemias. Analysis of 54 cases and a review of the literature. *Leukemia* 1991;5:744–751.

94. Beishuizen A, Verhoeven MA, van Wering ER, et al. Analysis of Ig and T-cell receptor genes in 40 childhood acute lymphoblastic leukemias at diagnosis and subsequent relapse: implications for the detection of minimal residual disease by polymerase chain reaction analysis. *Blood* 1994;83:2238–2247.

95. Szczepanski T, Pongers-Willemse MJ, Langerak AW, et al. Ig heavy chain gene rearrangements in T-cell acute lymphoblastic leukemia exhibit predominant DH6-19 and DH7-27 gene usage, can result in complete V-D-J rearrangements, and are rare in T-cell receptor alpha beta. *Blood* 1999;93:4079–4085.

96. Langerak AW, Wolvers-Tettero IL, van den Beemd MW, et al. Immunophenotypic and immunogenotypic characteristics of TCRgammadelta+ T cell acute lymphoblastic leukemia. *Leukemia* 1999;13:206–214.

97. Sczepanski T, Van der Velden VHJ, Ratt T, et al. Comparative analysis of T-cell receptor gene rearrangements at diagnosis and relapse of T-cell acute lymphoblastic leukemia (T-ALL) shows high stability of clinical markers for monitoring of minimal residual disease and reveals the occurrence of second T-ALL. *Leukemia* In press.

98. Breit TM, Verschuren MC, Wolvers-Tettero IL, et al. Human T cell leukemias with continuous V(D)J recombinase activity for TCR-delta gene deletion. *J Immunol* 1997;159:4341–4349.

99. Furley AJ, Mizutani S, Weilbaecher K, et al. Developmentally regulated rearrangement and expression of genes encoding the T cell receptor-T3 complex. *Cell* 1986;46:75–87.

100. Felix CA, Wright JJ, Poplack DG, et al. T cell receptor alpha-, beta-, and gamma-genes in T cell and pre-B cell acute lymphoblastic leukemia. *J Clin Invest* 1987;80:545–556.

101. Williams ME, Innes DJ Jr, Borowitz MJ, et al. Immunoglobulin and T cell receptor gene rearrangements in human lymphoma and leukemia. *Blood* 1987;69:79–86.

102. van Dongen JJ, Quertermous T, Bartram CR, et al. T cell receptor-CD3 complex during early T cell differentiation. Analysis of immature T cell acute lymphoblastic leukemias (T-ALL) at DNA, RNA, and cell membrane level. *J Immunol* 1987;138:1260–1269.

103. Oksenberg JR, Stuart S, Begovich AB, et al. Limited heterogeneity of rearranged T-cell receptor V alpha transcripts in brains of multiple sclerosis patients. *Nature* 1991;353:94.

104. Broeren CP, Verjans GM, Van Eden W, et al. Conserved nucleotide sequences at the 5′ end of T cell receptor variable genes facilitate polymerase chain reaction amplification. *Eur J Immunol* 1991;21:569–575.

105. Doherty PJ, Roifman CM, Pan SH, et al. Expression of the human T cell receptor V beta repertoire. *Mol Immunol* 1991;28:607–612.

106. Wei S, Charmley P, Robinson MA, et al. The extent of the human germline T-cell receptor V beta gene segment repertoire. *Immunogenetics* 1994;40:27–36.

107. Langerak AW, van Den Beemd R, Wolvers-Tettero IL, et al. Molecular and flow cytometric analysis of the Vbeta repertoire for clonality assessment in mature TCRalphabeta T-cell proliferations. *Blood* 2001;98:165–173.

108. Bottaro M, Berti E, Biondi A, et al. Heteroduplex analysis of T-cell receptor gamma gene rearrangements for diagnosis and monitoring of cutaneous T-cell lymphomas. *Blood* 1994;83:3271–3278.

109. Langerak AW, Szczepanski T, van der Burg M, et al. Heteroduplex PCR analysis of rearranged T cell receptor genes for clonality assessment in suspect T cell proliferations. *Leukemia* 1997;11:2192–2199.

110. Kneba M, Bolz I, Linke B, et al. Analysis of rearranged T-cell receptor beta-chain genes by polymerase chain reaction (PCR) DNA sequencing and automated high resolution PCR fragment analysis. *Blood* 1995;86:3930–3937.

111. Linke B, Bolz I, Pott C, et al. Use of UITma DNA polymerase improves the PCR detection of rearranged immunoglobulin heavy chain CDR3 junctions. *Leukemia* 1995;9:2133–2137.

112. McCoy JP Jr, Overton WR, Schroeder K, et al. Immunophenotypic analysis of the T cell receptor V beta repertoire in CD4+ and CD8+ lymphocytes from normal peripheral blood. *Cytometry* 1996;26:148–153.

113. van den Beemd R, Boor PP, van Lochem EG, et al. Flow cytometric analysis of the Vbeta repertoire in healthy controls. *Cytometry* 2000;40:336–345.

114. Lima M, Almeida J, Santos AH, et al. Immunophenotypic analysis of the TCR-Vbeta repertoire in 98 persistent expansions of CD3(+)/TCR-alpha-beta(+) large granular lymphocytes: utility in assessing clonality and insights into the pathogenesis of the disease. *Am J Pathol* 2001;159:1861–1868.

115. Langerak AW, Wolvers-Tettero IL, van Dongen JJ. Detection of T cell receptor beta (TCRB) gene rearrangement patterns in T cell malignancies by Southern blot analysis. *Leukemia* 1999;13:965–974.

116. Moreau EJ, Langerak AW, van Gastel-Mol EJ, et al. Easy detection of all T cell receptor gamma (TCRG) gene rearrangements by Southern blot analysis: recommendations for optimal results. *Leukemia* 1999;13:1620–1626.

117. Szczepanski T, Langerak AW, Willemse MJ, et al. T cell receptor gamma (TCRG) gene rearrangements in T cell acute lymphoblastic leukemia reflect "end-stage" recombinations: implications for minimal residual disease monitoring. *Leukemia* 2000;14:1208–1214.

118. Hwang LY, Baer RJ. The role of chromosome translocations in T cell acute leukemia. *Curr Opin Immunol* 1995;7:659–664.

119. Marculescu R, Vanura K, Montpellier B, et al. Recombinase, chromosomal translocations and lymphoid neoplasia: targeting mistakes and repair failures. *DNA Repair (Amst)* 2006;8:1246–1258.

120. Dik WA, Nadel B, Przybylski GK, et al. Different chromosomal breakpoints impact the level of LMO2 expression in T-ALL. *Blood* 2007;110:388–392.

121. Begley CG, Aplan PD, Denning SM, et al. The gene SCL is expressed during early hematopoiesis and encodes a differentiation-related DNA-binding motif. *Proc Natl Acad Sci U S A* 1989;86:10128–10132.

122. Breit TM, Mol EJ, Wolvers-Tettero IL, et al. Site-specific deletions involving the tal-1 and sil genes are restricted to cells of the T cell receptor alpha/beta lineage: T cell receptor delta gene deletion mechanism affects multiple genes. *J Exp Med* 1993;177:965–977.

123. Fitzgerald TJ, Neale GA, Raimondi SC, et al. c-tal, a helix-loop-helix protein, is juxtaposed to the T-cell receptor-beta chain gene by a reciprocal chromosomal translocation: t(1;7)(p32;q35). *Blood* 1991;78:2686–2695.

124. Mellentin JD, Smith SD, Cleary ML. lyl-1, a novel gene altered by chromosomal translocation in T cell leukemia, codes for a protein with a helix-loop-helix DNA binding motif. *Cell* 1989;58:77–83.

125. Xia Y, Brown L, Yang CY, et al. TAL2, a helix-loop-helix gene activated by the t(7;9)(q34;q32) translocation in human T-cell leukemia. *Proc Natl Acad Sci U S A* 1991;88:11416–11420.

126. Kennedy MA, Gonzalez-Sarmiento R, Kees UR, et al. HOX11, a homeobox-containing T-cell oncogene on human chromosome 10q24. *Proc Natl Acad Sci U S A* 1991;88:8900–8904.
127. Hatano M, Roberts CW, Minden M, et al. Deregulation of a homeobox gene, HOX11, by the t(10;14) in T cell leukemia. *Science* 1991;253:79–82.
128. Royer-Pokora B, Rogers M, Zhu TH, et al. The TTG-2/RBTN2 T cell oncogene encodes two alternative transcripts from two promoters: the distal promoter is removed by most 11p13 translocations in acute T cell leukaemia's (T-ALL). *Oncogene* 1995;10:1353–1360.
129. Valge-Archer V, Forster A, Rabbitts TH. The LMO1 and LDB1 proteins interact in human T cell acute leukaemia with the chromosomal translocation t(11;14)(p15;q11). *Oncogene* 1998;17:3199–3202.
130. Bernard OA, Busson-LeConiat M, Ballerini P, et al. A new recurrent and specific cryptic translocation, t(5;14)(q35;q32), is associated with expression of the Hox11L2 gene in T acute lymphoblastic leukemia. *Leukemia* 2001;15:1495–1504.
131. Mauvieux L, Leymarie V, Helias C, et al. High incidence of Hox11L2 expression in children with T-ALL. *Leukemia* 2002;16:2417–2422.
132. Soulier J, Clapppier E, Cayuela JM, et al. HOXA genes are included in genetic and biologic networks defining human acute T-cell leukemia (T-ALL). *Blood* 2005;106:274–286.
133. Przybylski GK, Dik WA, Wanzeck J, et al. The effect of a novel recombination between the homeobox gene NKX2-5 and the TRD locus in T-cell acute lymphoblastic leukemia on activation of the NKX2-5 gene. *Haematologica* 2006;91:317–321.
134. Cauwelier B, Cavé H, Gervais C, et al. Clinical, cytogenetic and molecular characteristics of 14 T-ALL patients carrying the TCRbeta-HOXA rearrangement: a study of the Groupe Francophone de Cytogénétique Hématologique. *Leukemia* 2007;21:121–128.
135. Stern MH, Lipkowitz S, Aurias A, et al. Inversion of chromosome 7 in ataxia telangiectasia is generated by a rearrangement between T-cell receptor beta and T-cell receptor gamma genes. *Blood* 1989;74:2076–2080.
136. Kobayashi Y, Tycko B, Soreng AL, et al. Transrearrangements between antigen receptor genes in normal human lymphoid tissues and in ataxia telangiectasia. *J Immunol* 1991;147:3201–3209.
137. Retiere C, Halary F, Peyrat MA, et al. The mechanism of chromosome 7 inversion in human lymphocytes expressing chimeric gamma beta TCR. *J Immunol* 1999;162:903–910.
138. Hinz T, Allam A, Wesch D, et al. Cell-surface expression of transrearranged Vgamma-cbeta T-cell receptor chains in healthy donors and in ataxia telangiectasia patients. *Br J Haematol* 2000;109:201–210.
139. Bernard O, Groettrup M, Mugneret F, et al. Molecular analysis of T-cell receptor transcripts in a human T-cell leukemia bearing a t(1;14) and an inv(7); cell surface expression of a TCR-beta chain in the absence of alpha chain. *Leukemia* 1993;7:1645–1653.
140. Murre C. Intertwining proteins in thymocyte development and cancer. *Nat Immunol* 2000;1:97–98.
141. Herblot S, Steff AM, Hugo P, et al. SCL and LMO1 alter thymocyte differentiation: inhibition of E2A-HEB function and pre-T alpha chain expression. *Nat Immunol* 2000;1:138–144.
142. Osborne B, Miele L. Notch and the immune system. *Immunity* 1999;11:653–663.
143. Screpanti I, Bellavia D, Campese AF, et al. Notch, a unifying target in T-cell acute lymphoblastic leukemia? *Trends Mol Med* 2003;9:30–35.
144. Ellisen LW, Bird J, West DC, et al. TAN-1, the human homolog of the *Drosophila* notch gene, is broken by chromosomal translocations in T lymphoblastic neoplasms. *Cell* 1991;66:649–661.
145. Weng AP, Ferrando AA, Lee W, et al. Activating mutations of NOTC<H1> in human T cell acute lymphoblastic leukemia. *Science* 2004;306:269–271.
146. Pear WS, Aster JC. T cell acute lymphoblastic leukemia/lymphoma: a human cancer commonly associated with aberrant NOTC<H1> signaling. *Curr Opin Hematol* 2004;11:426–433.
147. Ferrando AA, Neuberg DS, Staunton J, et al. Gene expression signatures define novel oncogenic pathways in T cell acute lymphoblastic leukemia. *Cancer Cell* 2002;1:75–87.
148. Asnafi V, Beldjord K, Libura M, et al. Age-related phenotypic and oncogenic differences in T-cell acute lymphoblastic leukemias may reflect thymic atrophy. *Blood* 2004;104:4173–4180.
149. Van Grotel M, Meijerink JP, van Wering ER, et al. Prognostic significance of molecular-cytogenetic abnormalities in pediatric T-ALL is not explained by immunophenotypic differences. *Leukemia* 2008;22:124–131.
150. Dik WA, Van der Velden VHJ, Hoogeveen PG, et al. Biological relevance of oncogene expression in T-ALL is determined by the normal thymic counterpart. Submitted.
151. Dik WA, Pike-Overzet K, Weerkamp F, et al. New insights on human T cell development by quantitative T cell receptor gene rearrangement studies and gene expression profiling. *J Exp Med* 2005;201:1715–1723.
152. Hacein-Bey-Abina S, von Kalle C, Schmidt M, et al. A serious adverse event after successful gene therapy for X-linked severe combined immunodeficiency. *N Engl J Med* 2003;348:255–256.
153. Hacein-Bey-Abina S, Von Kalle C, Schmidt M, et al. LMO2-associated clonal T cell proliferation in two patients after gene therapy for SCID-X1. *Science* 2003;302:415–419.
154. Howe S, Mansour M, Schwarzwaelder K, et al. Insertional mutagenesis combined with acquired somatic mutations causes leukemogenesis following gene therapy of SCID-X1 patients. *J Clin Invest* 2008;118:3143–3150.
155. Baum C, von Kalle C, Staal FJ, et al. Chance or necessity? Insertional mutagenesis in gene therapy and its consequences. *Mol Ther* 2004;9:5–13.
156. Pike-Overzet K, van der Burg M, Wagemaker G, et al. New insights and unresolved issues regarding insertional mutagenesis in X-linked SCID gene therapy. *Mol Ther* 2007;15:1910–1916.
157. Deichmann A, Hacein-Bey-Abina S, Schmidt M, et al. Vector integration is nonrandom and clustered and influences the fate of lymphopoiesis in SCID-X1 gene therapy. *J Clin Invest* 2007;117:2225–2232.
158. Schwarzwaelder K, Howe SJ, Schmidt M, et al. Gammaretrovirus-mediated correction of SCID-X1 is associated with skewed vector integration site distribution in vivo. *J Clin Invest* 2007;117:2241–2249.
159. Aiuti A, Cassani B, Andolfi G, et al. Multilineage hematopoietic reconstitution without clonal selection in ADA-SCID patients treated with stem cell gene therapy. *J Clin Invest* 2007;117:2233–2240.
160. Pike-Overzet K, de Ridder D, Weerkamp F, et al. Ectopic retroviral expression of LMO2, but not IL2gamma, blocks human T-cell development from CD34+ cells: implications for leukemogenesis in gene therapy. *Leukemia* 2007;21:754–763.
161. Lefranc MP. IMGT, the international ImMunoGeneTics database. *Nucleic Acids Res* 2001;29:207–209.

CHAPTER 5 ■ EPIDEMIOLOGY

SOPHIA S. WANG AND PATRICIA HARTGE

The epidemiology of non-Hodgkin lymphoma (NHL) has undergone a remarkable transformation in the last decade. A number of large epidemiologic studies of NHL have been completed, leading to many consortial efforts and pooled analyses. These have clarified the etiologic risk estimates for several factors for NHL. With large sample sizes, there also has been adequate power for evaluating NHL subtypes. Both environmental and genetic susceptibility factors have been investigated intensively, revealing new clues to our understanding of NHL etiology. Continued efforts in this direction will prove essential for uncovering the epidemiologic causes of NHL.

Cancer registries around the world reported a steady unexplainable increase in the occurrence of NHL during the second half of the 20th century that has now, just as mysteriously, plateaued. It is well recognized that the human immunodeficiency virus (HIV) epidemic produced a second NHL epidemic superimposed on this unexplained long-term rise of NHL. The subsequent use of highly active antiretroviral therapy (HAART) among populations infected with HIV has led to a decline of NHL among individuals infected with HIV but does not account for the current leveling of rates reported in the general population. As of this writing, most cases of NHL that occur still remain unexplained.

Several features of NHL make the tumor particularly challenging to investigate epidemiologically. Most notably, NHL constitutes not one but many diseases, and these subtypes have different incidence rates and patterns. It is well established that some rare lymphoma subtypes, e.g., Burkitt lymphoma (BL), mycosis fungoides, mucosa-associated lymphoid tissue (MALT) lymphomas, primary effusion lymphoma (PEL), and adult T-cell leukemia/lymphomas (ATLs), have distinctive etiologies. In addition, there is now evidence for distinct etiologies between more common lymphoma subtypes.

In general, the cause of all lymphomas is immune dysregulation. Epidemiologic studies have targeted their evaluations on specific immune defects at work, and the influence of viruses, genes, chemicals, radiation, diet, and aging on the complex natural history of the immune system. In particular, severe immune suppression, whether inborn, medication induced, or viral, dramatically increases NHL risk. Lymphomas arise quite soon after HIV infection or after organ transplantation. Common immune gene polymorphisms also have been demonstrated to influence NHL risk. Exposures to pesticides, organic solvents, and other chemicals on the job and in the general environment, and dietary and other factors also may act via immune dysregulation. The evidence for a small set of underlying immune mechanisms is mounting, but the fundamental explanation remains to be found.

The recognition that NHL subtypes may have distinct etiologies and the recent efforts to evaluate subtypes by pooling data from multiple studies will continue to contribute to our understanding of NHL etiology. Except for the small proportion of NHL cases that are strikingly caused by inherited or acquired immune dysregulation, most NHL likely is caused by a convergence of risk factors that, although individually have modest effects on the immune system, together achieve a threshold of immune dysregulation that creates a microenvironment conducive for lymphomagenesis.

PATTERNS OF OCCURRENCE

More than 2% of white non-Hispanic men in the United States (US) will develop NHL at some point in their lives if current age-specific rates hold constant. By comparison, 17% will develop prostate cancer and 7% lung cancer, with NHL as the fifth-ranked cancer diagnosis. At current rates of incidence and survival, about 1% of white men will die of NHL, as compared with 6% for lung cancer and 3% for prostate cancer (1). During the period 2001 to 2005, 24.3 NHL diagnoses were recorded among white, non-Hispanic men per 100,000 person-years, as shown in Figure 5.1. At the same time, 9.7 deaths from NHL were recorded per 100,000 person-years.

Rates of NHL diagnosis and death are about one-third lower among women than men. Among both men and women, rates are about one-third lower in the African-American and Hispanic populations than in the non-Hispanic white population. Among American Indians and Alaskan natives, women showed 11.1 cases and 3.8 deaths per 100,000 person-years.

A geographic gradient in risk persists in the US, with highest rates in the north-central region, but the gap in rates between the highest and the lowest region has narrowed in recent years. During the period 1990 to 2004, 10% of state economic areas had mortality rates exceeding 9.3 deaths per 100,000 person-years, whereas 10% had rates below 7.1 (2). Incidence and mortality vary appreciably more among nations (3). As shown in Figure 5.2, NHL rates generally were higher in wealthier nations.

Although NHL risk varies markedly according to place and person, the most dramatic feature of the patterns of risk is the remarkable trend of increase over time. For the entire 50-year period ending in 1999, the rate of death due to NHL rose steadily in the US and elsewhere. Among men in the US, for example, mortality rates for NHL rose from 4.4 to 10.8 deaths per 100,000 person-years between the early 1950s and the late 1990s. Among women, the rates rose from 3.0 to 7.1 over the same period. NHL deaths due to HIV infection contributed to the rising rates beginning in the 1980s. With the success of HAART, and improved survival, mortality rates have started to fall for men and women (Fig. 5.3).

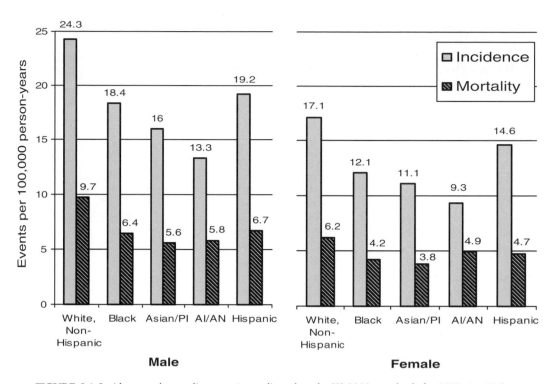

FIGURE 5.1 Incidence and mortality rates (age adjusted to the US 2000 standard) for NHL, in 17 Surveillance, Epidemiology, and End Results (SEER) registries, 2001–2005. (From SEER*Stat, http://seer.cancer.gov/statfacts/ with permission. Accessed March 17, 2008.) AI, American Indian; AN, Alaska Native; PI, Pacific Islander.

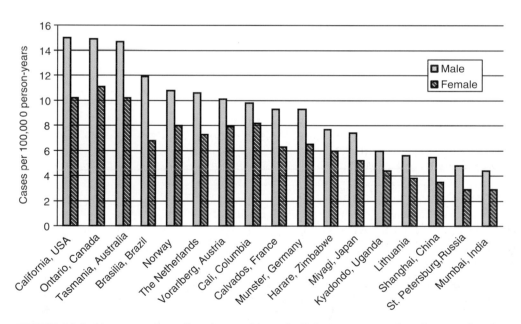

FIGURE 5.2 Incidence rates (age adjusted to world standard) for NHL. (From Curado MP, Edwards B, Shin HR, et al. *Cancer incidence in five continents*, vol IX, no 160. Lyon, France: IARC Scientific Publications, 2007, with permission. From: http://www-dep.iarc.fr. Accessed March 18, 2008.)

The complete explanation for the long-term NHL epidemic remains obscure, but several features warrant attention. Declines in the rates of Hodgkin lymphoma (HL) were far smaller than the increases in NHL. Many investigations have concluded that diagnostic improvements and classification changes cannot account for the level of increase. The increase occurred in men and women and in most populations. Finally, the rates rose most dramatically at older ages at diagnosis (Fig. 5.4). Indeed, among people older than 60 years, rates have not yet fallen.

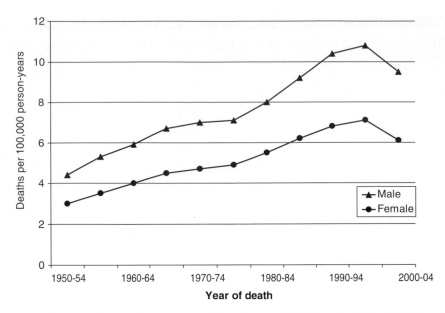

FIGURE 5.3 Trends in US mortality rates (age adjusted to the 2000 US standard) for NHL. [From Surveillance, Epidemiology, and End Results (SEER) Program (www.seer.cancer.gov) SEER*Stat Database: Mortality–Cancer, Total US (1950–2004), National Cancer Institute, DCCPS, Surveillance Research Program, Cancer Statistics Branch, released March 2007, with permission. Underlying mortality data provided by NCHS (www.cdc.gov/nchs).]

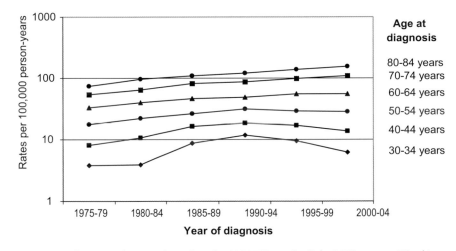

FIGURE 5.4 Incidence trends (age adjusted to the 2000 US standard) for NHL among US white males. [From: Surveillance, Epidemiology, and End Results (SEER) Program (www.seer.cancer.gov) SEER*Stat Database: Incidence–SEER 9 Regs Limited-Use, Nov 2006 Sub (1973–2004)–Linked to County Attributes–Total US, 1969–2004 Counties, National Cancer Institute, DCCPS, Surveillance Research Program, Cancer Statistics Branch, released April 2007, based on the November 2006 submission, with permission.]

These overall patterns of occurrence reflect an average of the many distinct lymphoid neoplasms that NHL comprises (Table 5.1). Indeed, several specific lymphomas exhibit unusual patterns of risk among demographic groups. For example, diffuse large B-cell lymphoma (DLBCL) shows predominance in men, but marginal zone does not (4). Follicular lymphoma (FL) shows only a slight male excess, whereas small lymphocytic lymphoma/chronic lymphocytic leukemia (SLL/CLL) shows nearly a two-fold male excess. Rates of most B-

cell neoplasms in the white population generally exceed those in the Black or Hispanic population, but T-cell neoplasms occur equally often in Black and White populations.

Geographic patterns also differ among subtypes, sometimes for evident reasons. In Japan and the Caribbean, human T-cell lymphotropic virus I (HTLV-1) is endemic, and peripheral T-cell lymphomas are correspondingly common. Where HIV rates are highest, DLBCL rates are notably higher. DLBCL rates are elevated in some agricultural areas,

TABLE 5.1

INCIDENCE OF LYMPHOID NEOPLASM SUBTYPES AS DEFINED BY THE INTERLYMPH PROPOSED NESTED CLASSIFICATION, 17 SEER REGISTRIES, 2001–2004

Lymphoid neoplasms	Number of cases	Rate[a]	% of NHL
NHL	89,777	31.22	
NHL, B-cell[b]	79,007	27.53	88.0
Mature NHL, B-cell	71,625	25.02	79.8
CLL/SLL/PLL/MCL	16,975	5.98	18.9
CLL/SLL	14,949	5.27	16.7
Prolymphocytic leukemia, B-cell	76	0.03	0.1
Mantle cell lymphoma	1,950	0.68	2.2
LPL/Waldenstrom	1,801	0.64	2.0
Lymphoplasmacytic lymphoma	786	0.28	0.9
Waldenstrom macroglobulinemia	1015	0.36	1.1
DLBCL	19,713	6.85	22.0
DLBCL, NOS	19,154	6.66	21.3
Intravascular large B-cell lymphoma	15	0.01	0.0
PEL	71	0.02	0.1
Mediastinal large B-cell lymphoma	473	0.16	0.5
BL/leukemia	1,151	0.39	1.3
Marginal zone lymphoma	4,932	1.72	5.5
Splenic marginal zone lymphoma	324	0.11	0.4
Extranodal marginal zone lymphoma, MALT type	3,244	1.13	3.6
Nodal marginal zone lymphoma	1,364	0.48	1.5
FL	10,376	3.58	11.6
Hairy cell leukemia	879	0.30	1.0
Plasma cell neoplasms	15,786	5.55	17.6
Plasmacytoma	1,047	0.36	1.2
MM/plasma cell leukemia	14,739	5.19	16.4
Heavy chain disease	12	0.00	0.0
NHL, NOS, B-cell	4,090	1.43	4.6
NHL, T-cell[b]	5,972	2.03	6.7
Mature NHL, T-cell	4,973	1.70	5.5
Mycosis fungoides/Sézary syndrome	1,281	0.44	1.4
Mycosis fungoides	1,252	0.43	1.4
Sézary syndrome	29	0.01	0.0
Peripheral T-cell lymphoma	3,273	1.12	3.6
Peripheral T-cell lymphoma, NOS	1,187	0.41	1.3
Angioimmunoblastic T-cell lymphoma	280	0.10	0.3
Subcutaneous panniculitis-like T-cell lymphoma	31	0.01	0.0
Anaplastic large cell lymphoma, T-cell or null-cell type	829	0.28	0.9
Hepatosplenic T-cell lymphoma	19	0.01	0.0
Enteropathy-type T-cell lymphoma	31	0.01	0.0
Cutaneous T-cell lymphoma, NOS	638	0.22	0.7
Primary cutaneous anaplastic large cell lymphoma	258	0.09	0.3
ATL	109	0.04	0.1
NK/T-cell lymphoma, nasal-type/aggressive NK-cell leukemia	185	0.06	0.2
T-cell large granular lymphocytic leukemia	48	0.02	0.1
Prolymphocytic leukemia, T-cell	77	0.03	0.1
NHL, NOS, T-cell	195	0.07	0.2
Precursor NHL	5,202	1.72	5.8
Precursor lymphoblastic leukemia/lymphoma, B-cell	3,292	1.09	3.7
Precursor lymphoblastic leukemia/lymphoma, T-cell	804	0.26	0.9
Precursor lymphoblastic leukemia/lymphoma, unknown lineage	1,106	0.37	1.2
NHL, unknown lineage[b]	3,692	1.29	4.1
Prolymphocytic leukemia, unknown lineage	3645	1.27	4.1
NHL, NOS, unknown lineage	47	0.02	0.1

LPL, lymphoplasmacytic lymphoma; MALT, mucosa associated lymphoid tissue; MCL, mantle cell lymphoma; NK, natural killer cell; NOS, not otherwise specified; PLL, prolymphocytic leukemia; SEER, Surveillance, Epidemiology, and End Results.
[a] Incidence rates are age adjusted to the 2000 US population and are expressed per 100,000 person-years.
[b] Includes both mature and precursor neoplasms.
(Adapted from Morton LM, Turner JJ, Cerhan JR, et al. Proposed classification of lymphoid neoplasms for epidemiologic research from the Pathology Working Group of the International Lymphoma Epidemiology Consortium (InterLymph). *Blood* 2007;110:695–708.)

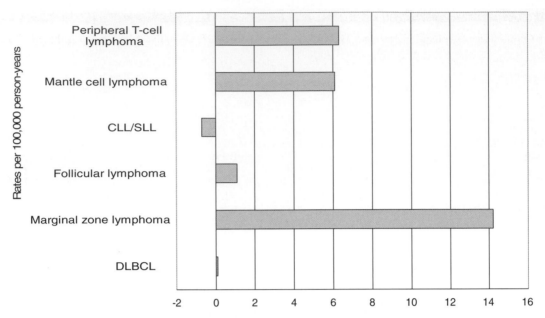

FIGURE 5.5 Annual percent change in NHL incidencerates, selected subtypes, 1992–2004. (From: Surveillance, Epidemiology, and End Results (SEER) Program (www.seer.cancer.gov) SEER*Stat Database: Incidence–SEER 9 Regs Limited-Use, Nov 2006 Sub (1973–2004)–Linked to County Attributes–Total US 1969–2004 Counties, National Cancer Institute, DCCPS, Surveillance Research Program, Cancer Statistics Branch, released April 2007, based on the November 2006 submission, with permission.)

suggesting a role for pesticides, fertilizers, or other agricultural chemicals. For both FL and DLBCL, rates are higher in the northern US, possibly because of a protective effect of sunlight in the southern US.

Differences in time trends also suggest that the clinically and histologically distinct subtypes often have distinct sets of causes (Fig. 5.5). Incidence of DLBCL changed little from 1992 to 2004, whereas incidence of FL rose 1.1% per annum. Marginal zone, mantle cell, peripheral T-cell, and BL all increased more than 5% per annum, partly due to changes in recognition of these entities.

Most lymphomas arise in lymph nodes (Table 5.2). The numbers diagnosed elsewhere have risen over time, in part because of improved diagnosis. For some extranodal tumors, the site of origin points to likely etiology. For example, MALT lymphomas can be caused by infection with *Helicobacter pylori*, and probably also by hepatitis C (5–7). Many such lymphomas regress after the infection is eradicated. Salivary gland lymphomas also have been linked to hepatitis C virus (HCV) (8).

Migrant studies have given less information on NHL than on more common malignancies, but one study of Asian migrants (9) suggested a change in FL rates toward the levels in the new country. Similarly, a few clusters have been noted, but few have been confirmed or explained (10–12).

RISK FACTORS FOR NON-HODGKIN LYMPHOMA

Epidemiologists have examined a wide range of potential risk factors as they relate to the broad spectrum of lymphomas, with particular emphasis on risk factors that affect the immune system (summarized in Table 5.3). Family and personal history of cancer and of immune-related conditions

have been studied extensively. Medical conditions and viral infections characterized by marked or moderate immune suppression also have been explored in detail. There have been dozens of studies of occupational and environmental exposures, including evaluation of exposure to radiation (ionizing, ultraviolet, and electric and magnetic fields). Numerous chemical exposures have been evaluated, with most consistent evidence found for pesticides and various organic solvents. Behavioral factors such as dietary and reproductive patterns also have been explored, along with personal exposures such as hair coloring.

Personal and Family History of Cancers

The absolute lifetime risk for developing NHL among those with a first-degree relative with NHL is approximately 3.6% in the most accurate studies, which are based upon registries that capture all confirmed cancers in a population over several generations such as those from Sweden and Denmark. Equivalently, people with one or more first-degree relatives who had NHL face about twice the average risk of developing NHL, as reported from registry based studies in Utah (13), Denmark (14), and Sweden (15,16). Additional information comes from the numerous case-control studies of NHL, including a pooled analysis of 10,211 NHL cases and 11,905 controls from US and European case-control studies that reported the same magnitude of risk (17). Results from the pooled analysis demonstrated that NHL conferred a consistently stronger familial association among men than women, and that siblings were a more powerful marker of personal risk for NHL than history of NHL in a parent, consistent with previous reports (15,16,18). Several other cancers consistently appear in excess in families of patients with NHL: leukemia, HL, and multiple myeloma (MM). Higher

TABLE 5.2

NUMBERS OF CASES AND INCIDENCE RATES FOR NHL BY SITE OF ORIGIN, AMONG MALES AND FEMALES, 2000–2004

Site of origin	Total		Male		Female	
	Rate	Count	Rate	Count	Rate	Count
All sites	19.9	26,315	24.2	14,157	16.6	12,158
Nodal	13.2	17,452	16.1	9,447	10.9	8,005
Extranodal - total	6.7	8,863	8	4,710	5.7	4,153
Skin	1.4	1,919	1.9	1,145	1.1	774
Stomach	0.9	1,152	1.1	589	0.8	563
Brain	0.4	471	0.4	274	0.3	197
Small intestine	0.4	561	0.6	347	0.3	214
Lung	0.3	339	0.3	156	0.3	183
Soft tissue	0.3	432	0.4	211	0.3	221
Colon	0.3	337	0.4	206	0.2	131
Eye	0.3	411	0.3	166	0.3	245
Thyroid	0.2	224	0.1	72	0.2	152

Rates are per 100,000 and age adjusted to the 2000 US population standard.
[From Surveillance, Epidemiology, and End Results (SEER) Program (www.seer.cancer.gov) SEER*Stat Database: Incidence–SEER 9 Regs Limited-Use, Nov 2006 Sub (1973–2004)–Linked to County Attributes–Total US 1969–2004 Counties, National Cancer Institute, DCCPS, Surveillance Research Program, Cancer Statistics Branch, released April 2007, based on the November 2006 submission, with permission.]

NHL risk has been reported for individuals with a parent with either HL or MM (16,17). There is also evidence that familial risk varies according to histologic subtypes; e.g., higher risk for SLL/CLL has been observed among those with family history of leukemia. Further follow-up of these reports in twin registries may prove fruitful for confirming the mode of inheritance. Interaction of familial risk with other factors and determining whether environmental risks vary according to family history also require further investigation. Although a US case-control study previously reported differential risk factors by those with family history of NHL and other lymphoid neoplasms (19), a registry based Swedish study did not (16).

People who have survived certain other cancers are also at increased risk for developing NHL. Some of these second cancers result from therapy for the first cancer, but some reflect common etiology, including the other lymphoproliferative and the hematopoietic malignancies (Hodgkin, lymphoid leukemia, myeloid leukemia, MM) that tend to cluster in many studies of second primary cancers. Overall, those with a history of a previous primary NHL have a relative risk (RR) of 2.4 for developing another primary NHL, a risk that persists for 10 years after their first primary diagnosis (20). In a recent review, risk of secondary lymphomas increased after the first 5 years of completion of chemotherapy or radiotherapy and persisted for more than 3 decades (21). Survivors of childhood HL appear to have seven times the ordinary risk of NHL (22). In a large Swedish series, survivors of Hodgkin lymphoma diagnosed in middle and late adulthood also had greatly increased NHL risk. Survivors of lymphoid leukemias had four times the usual NHL risk, and survivors of MM had two times the usual NHL risk (20). Similarly, people who survive NHL are also at increased risk for other lymphoproliferative and the hematopoietic malignancies. In an analysis of survivors of NHL, risks were at least doubled for HL, leukemias, melanoma, and brain can-

cers (23). Similar risks were reported in a US childhood cancer survivor study (24). Risks for lymphoma were also found elevated in a study that followed patients with mycosis fungoides and Sézary syndrome (25).

The development of skin cancers following NHL has received special attention because of the associations reported between sunlight and NHL. People diagnosed with either basal cell or squamous cell skin cancers had twice the risk of NHL in a Swiss registry study (26). In US registry data on 55,000 survivors of melanoma, NHL risk was increased 40% following skin melanoma, especially in the first few years after melanoma (23). In a recent cancer registry study of 62,000 US survivors of NHL, skin melanoma risk was also increased 75% (23). In a pooled analysis of 137,612 patients with NHL and 109,532 patients with primary cutaneous melanoma, a standard incidence ratio (SIR) of 2.01 was reported for increased NHL risk among survivors of cutaneous melanoma, and a SIR of 1.41 for cutaneous melanoma among survivors of NHL (27). It may be relevant that skin cancers and lymphomas are the most common cancers to arise from post-transplant immunosuppression, fueling speculation that chronic immunosuppression is a risk factor for both cutaneous melanoma and NHL (27,28). Few other cancers have been reported consistently to be in excess either as additional primaries in patients with NHL or in their families.

Primary Immunosuppression

Children and adults with primary or acquired immune deficiencies face enormous and well-documented increases in risk for lymphoproliferative diseases, including NHL. Immune deficiencies associated with NHL risk include congenital immune deficiency diseases, immunosuppression following organ transplant, autoimmune disorders, and immunosuppression by

TABLE 5.3

OVERVIEW OF RISK FACTORS FOR DEVELOPING NHLS

Risk	Subtype-specificity	Factor
↑ ↑ ↑		Age
↑		Male gender
↑ ↑		NHLs in family
↑		Hodgkin disease or MM in family
↑		History of Hodgkin disease
↑ ↑ ↑		Inherited immunodeficiency
↑ ↑ ↑	B-cell lymphomas	Ataxia telangiectasia
↑ ↑ ↑		WAS
↑ ↑ ↑		CVID
↑ ↑ ↑		XLP
↑ ↑ ↑		Severe combined immunodeficiency
↑ ↑ ↑	DLBCL, MZ	SS
↑ ↑ ↑	T cell lymphomas	Celiac disease
↑ ↑ ↑	B-cell lymphomas (DLBCL, MZ, MALT)	SLE
↑ ↑		HIV infection
↑ ↑ ↑		AIDS
↑ ↑ ↑	ATL	HTLV1
↑ ↑	MALT	*H. pylori*
↑ ↑ ↑	BL	EBV
↑ ↑ ↑	PEL	HHV-8
↑	DLBCL	Common genetic variations
↑		HCV
—		SV40
↑		Severe arthritis
? ↑		Infectious mononucleosis
? ↑		Blood transfusions
? ↓		Asthma
? ↓		Allergies
? ↓		Birth order (early)
↑		Occupational pesticides (farmers, grain handlers, applicators)
↑		Occupational solvent exposures (benzene, TCE)
? ↑		Serum dioxin level
↑		Serum polychlorinated biphenyl level
—		Ionizing radiation
↓	B-cell lymphomas	Nonionizing radiation - sunlight
? ↑	Follicular	Smoking
↓		Alcohol
? ↑ ↓	Follicular, CLL/SLL	Hair dyes
? ↑		Nitrates, nitrosamines
? ↑		Diet: meat, protein
? ↓		Diet: vegetables and fruits

↑ ↑ ↑, RR 5+; ↑ ↑, RR 3–4; ↑, RR 2; ↓, decreased risk; ?, uncertain; —, no association; ↑ ↓, conflicting data.; H. pylori = Heliobacter pylori, MALT = mucosa associated lymphoid tissue, EBV = Epstein Barr virus, HHV-8 = human herpesvirus-8, PEL = primary effusion lymphoma, TCE = trichloroethylene, XLP = X-linked proliferative disease

infectious agents such as HIV. In general, the strength of association between immune deficiencies and NHL risk mirrors the degree of immune deficiency.

Rare congenital or primary immune deficiencies carry high absolute risks for lymphoma that are independent of other risk factors. These conditions include ataxia telangiectasia, Wiskott-Aldrich syndrome (WAS), common variable immunodeficiency (CVID), X-linked lymphoproliferative disease (XLP), and severe combined immunodeficiency (29). As many as one-quarter of all patients with congenital immune deficiencies develop cancers during their lifetime (half of them lymphomas) (30). As resulting lymphomas correlate to the degree of immune dysregulation, congenital or primary immune defi-

ciencies, which produce a large degree of immune deficiency, result in high-grade lymphomas that are clinically aggressive.

Specifically, approximately 10% of children with ataxia telangiectasia develop lymphomas that are largely B-cell in type (31). WAS is an X-linked recessive disorder, and 14% of boys with WAS will develop Epstein-Barr virus (EBV) related lymphomas. CVID is a heterogeneous collection of rare genetic immunodeficiency disorders, and approximately 1.4% to 7% of persons with CVID will develop lymphoproliferative disease and lymphoma (32). XLP causes EBV-related lymphoma in 20% to 35% of affected boys (31). Other congenital immunodeficiencies associated with higher frequency of NHL include hyperimmunoglobulin (Ig)M syndrome, Chédiak-Higashi syndrome, B-cell proliferative syndrome, and Bruton agammaglobulinemia.

Autoimmune Disorders

NHL occurs in higher frequencies in several autoimmune disorders, notably Sjögren syndrome (SS), systemic lupus erythematosus (SLE), celiac disease, and rheumatoid arthritis (RA) (33). SS largely affects women, and is characterized by progressive destruction of salivary and lachrymal glands and an increased risk for developing lymphoproliferative diseases, mainly NHL. Very high risk estimates have been reported; data from the Finnish Cancer Registry, where 676 patients with primary SS and 709 with secondary SS were followed for malignancies, shows that NHL risk rises four-fold with secondary SS and nine-fold with primary SS (34). A meta-analysis of five studies on SS demonstrated high NHL risks (SIR = 18.8) (35). A recent pooled analyses of 12 case-control studies including over 29,000 participants further confirmed the association between SS and NHL, particularly for marginal zone and DLBCL (36). Strikingly, the pooled analyses reported a 250-fold increase in risk of parotid gland NHL and a 1000-fold increase in risk of parotid gland MALT lymphoma.

Patients with SLE also have a well-documented increased risk for B-cell lymphomas, and initial studies reported high magnitudes of risk (four- to eight-fold). Animal models also provide convincing evidence for causality (37). A meta-analyses of six studies reported a consistent SIR of 7.4 for SLE and NHL risk (35). However, recent large-scale efforts now consistently show three- to four-fold risk increases in both the largest cohort study to date and in the pooled InterLymph analyses of 12 case-control studies (36). Subtypes most affected are marginal zone lymphoma, predominantly MALT, and DLBCL.

Patients with celiac disease exhibit elevated rates of NHL with a predominance for T-cell lymphomas. High risk for NHL mortality (standard mortality ratio = 69) has been reported from an Italian cohort study (38), and a six- to 11-fold risk increase reported in both US (39) and Swedish cohort studies (40). Elevated NHL incidence has also been reported in a Swedish registry based study (41). Results from the pooled analysis of case-control studies provided further evidence of an association between celiac disease and extranodal T-cell lymphoma (36).

RA, a common inflammatory connective tissue disease, has been linked to lymphoma in several cohort studies. Finnish investigators have demonstrated a two-fold increase in risk for lymphoma in a registry based study (42); Swedish and Danish investigators also have reported similar excess risks (43,44). A recent meta-analysis of nine studies reported SIRs of NHL above two (35). Among patients with Felty syndrome, a rare complication affecting 1% of RA patients, a higher eight-fold increase in risk for NHL has been reported based on a retrospective cohort study of US men (45).

Determining whether an independent association between RA and NHL exists is complicated by use of medication among those with RA. A Finnish study using registry data demonstrated excess risk of NHL for patients with RA receiving cyclophosphamide (42), but a 3-year prospective French study reported no risk increase among patients with RA treated with methotrexate (46). In a review of autoimmune rheumatic diseases (47), patients with RA who were on immunosuppressive therapies (e.g., azathioprine, cyclophosphamide, and chlorambucil) had 10 times the risk for NHL, with longer use and higher doses correlating with level of risk. In the recent pooled analysis of case-control studies, increased NHL risk was observed among patients with self-reported RA treated with corticosteroids or immunosuppressants (36). Analyses of an 18,572 US RA cohort, however, found little differences between therapies (e.g., methotrexate vs. anti tumor necrosis factor [TNF] therapy), and concluded that there was insufficient evidence to establish a causal relationship between RA treatments and NHL (48).

Although there is clinical evidence supporting a specific biologic role for RA and EBV-related NHL, the epidemiologic evidence remains inconclusive at the time of this writing. Increased NHL risk has also been reported for patients with hemolytic anemia (49) and Crohn disease (50) but requires further confirmation. Reports on the association between psoriases and NHL remain inconsistent (33). Data also remain inconsistent but largely null for other syndromes that affect immune function and NHL risk, including inflammatory bowel disorders, type 1 diabetes, sarcoidosis, pernicious anemia, and multiple sclerosis.

Organ Transplant

EBV-related lymphomas arising in organ transplant recipients on immunosuppressive therapy has long been recognized (51,52). This association is correlated with the type of transplantation, the size of the organ transplanted, and the degree of immunosuppression needed to forestall rejection. Data from a large, multicenter study in Europe and North America show NHL occurring in 0.2% of kidney transplant recipients and in 1.2% of heart transplant recipients during the first year, rates that are 20 and 120 times higher than those seen in the general population (53,54). Among a large cohort of Swedish patients with kidney transplant, risks for NHL were 9.9 in the first year (55). Among a large series of patients with renal transplant in the United Kingdom, post-transplant lymphoma occurred in 2% of the population in the first and subsequent years (56). Interestingly, there is some evidence suggesting that lymphomas occurring over 1 year after transplantation may be more likely to be EBV negative and less likely to respond to reductions in immunosuppressive therapies when compared with the lymphomas occurring within 1 year after transplantation (57).

Among organ transplant recipients, the medications used (e.g., cyclosporin A, monoclonal antibodies for T-cell depletion, prednisone, azathioprine, and cyclosporin), which vary in their degree of immunosuppression, correlate with the risk of developing post-transplant lymphoma. In the Collaborative Transplant Study, higher doses of cyclosporin and azathioprine were used in heart transplant recipients compared with kidney transplant recipients (58). This corresponded to NHL incidence in patients with heart transplant that was three-fold higher than in patients with kidney transplant; individuals administered cyclosporin A, azathioprine, and steroids simultaneously showed the highest NHL incidence (54). Notably, cessation of immunosuppressive therapies appears to lead to regression of lymphomas (59).

Common Medical Conditions, Medications, and Procedures

Two-fold risk increases for NHL have been reported in several cohort studies among recipients of allogeneic blood transfusions (60–62) but not confirmed in subsequent case-control studies (63,64). Other common diseases and medications associated with NHL but not established as risk factors include asthma, allergies and eczema (33), vaccinations (65), steroid use (66), nonsteroidal anti-inflammatory drug use (66), injection drug use (67), and amphetamine use (65). Much research effort has been focused on understanding whether atopic conditions that exhibit mild, subclinical immune deficiencies, such as that reflected in those with asthma, allergies, and eczema, and are characterized by a T<h2>-driven immune response, are associated with decreased NHL risk. Early birth order, hypothesized to reflect a T<h2>-dominated immune response, has also garnered much recent attention with a growing number of reports showing an association with reduced NHL risk (68,69). Cohort studies, which avoid disease bias whereby NHL itself leads to altered immunity, likely will be important for clarifying this hypothesis.

Viruses and Other Infectious Agents

A growing number of viruses and other infectious agents are associated with NHL. Infections operate by depressing immune function such as the case for HIV, or by contributing to chronic inflammation or by other mechanisms. The associations between specific infectious agents and NHL risk vary by preexisting immunosuppressive conditions, by the nature of the infectious agents and by NHL subtype. The evidence for epidemiologic associations relies on the identification of viral or bacterial deoxyribonucleic acid in the tumors and/or by the host serologic response to infections. Based on such measurements, well-established associations now include those between specific retroviruses (e.g., HTLV-I and ATL, HIV, and NHL) and herpesviruses (e.g., human herpesvirus [HHV] 8 /Kaposi sarcoma herpesvirus, and PEL; EBV and BL). There is now also strong epidemiologic evidence supporting the association between *H. pylori* infection and the development of MALT lymphomas in the gastrointestinal tract, and between HCV and NHL. Associations with NHL also have been suggested but largely null for simian virus 40 (SV40).

Retroviruses

HTLV-I was the first retrovirus established as a cause of lymphoma, specifically of ATL. HTLV-I infection is endemic in southern Japan and the Caribbean, where 56% and 78% of ATL cases, respectively, are attributable to HTLV-I infection (70). Coinfection with strongyloides stercoralis, a gastrointestinal parasite endemic in the same geographic regions as HTLV-I, may further increase the risk for ATL (71). HTLV-I is also found in isolated parts of Africa, the Middle East, South America, and Papua New Guinea but is rare elsewhere (<1% seroprevalence) (72). Mode of HTLV-I transmission includes mother to infant, sexual activity, injection drug use, and whole blood transfusion. NHL risk is most pronounced among those with early HTLV-I infection (70), and the 20 to 40-year incubation period required for ATL development means that fewer than 5% of individuals infected with HTLV-I will develop ATL (73).

HIV is a well-established cause of NHL. NHL and specific subtypes are considered acquired immunodeficiency syndrome (AIDS) defining illnesses by the US Centers for Disease Control (74,75) and account for 3% to 5% of all initial AIDS diagnoses (76). NHL is the second most frequent cancer occurring in patients with HIV (77), and among specific populations with AIDS, such as intravenous drug abusers and hemophiliacs, NHL is the most frequent cancer (29). HIV is thought to cause lymphoma via disruption of immune surveillance and resulting immunosuppression, rather than through HIV infection itself (78).

Individuals infected with HIV face very high risks for NHL, with RR estimates generally ranging 50 to 100. Although risks for all NHL subtypes are elevated among individuals infected with HIV, there is a preponderance of high-grade and extranodal B-cell lymphomas. Risks appear highest (>100) for Burkitt and Burkitt-like lymphoma and DLBCL (79), and lower for low-grade lymphomas (approximately 15) (80). NHL risk also varies with the duration and degree of immunosuppression. The widespread use of HAART beginning in 1996 has resulted in a reported decline of NHL incidence and improved survival among individuals infected with HIV in some populations but not all. These discrepancies likely reflect methodological differences between different studies. A meta-analysis of 23 prospective studies on AIDS-related lymphomas examining the effect of widespread HAART usage demonstrated a decline in AIDS-related NHL incidence, particularly for central nervous system and immunoblastic lymphomas (81) that, before HAART, accounted for much of the extranodal NHL. A recent review showed that not only has survival of AIDS-related lymphomas improved with HAART but that it is now comparable to that of patients with aggressive lymphomas in the general population (82). Verifying the continued effects of HAART on NHL incidence worldwide will require on-going surveillance of populations infected with HIV.

Herpesviruses

HHV-8 is endemic in the Mediterranean basin and sub-Saharan Africa but rare elsewhere (83). First identified as the cause of Kaposi sarcoma and termed Kaposi sarcoma herpesvirus, HHV-8 was linked to NHL in 1995 (84). Specifically, HHV-8 is associated with multicentric Castleman disease-plasmablastic lymphoma and body cavity based lymphoma or PEL (85), where HHV-8 has been identified in all tumors (84). Notably, NHL arises in those infected with HHV-8 in settings of profound immunosuppression (86), including HIV infection. Among male homosexuals, HHV-8 seroprevalence is high and ranges from 20% to 40% (83). Coinfection with HHV-8 and EBV is also common (87). Although the numbers of NHL resulting from HHV-8 infection account for only a small fraction of NHL, a clear understanding of this association may further clarify mechanisms of NHL pathogenesis.

EBV infection is ubiquitous; greater than 90% of the world's population is thought to be infected with EBV. The International Agency for Research on Cancer (IARC) has determined that there is sufficient evidence to classify EBV as a proven human carcinogen (87). EBV was first identified among children with BL in equatorial Africa, where EBV infection is endemic and occurs early in life. EBV infection occurs later in life in developed countries (88). Nearly all BL arising in endemic regions is associated with EBV infection, whereas most BL (20% to 34%) arising in Western countries harbors EBV (89).

EBV occurs in lymphomas other than Burkitt but presumably as a passenger rather than a cause in many of them. The strength of association between EBV and NHL differs among subtype and correlates closely with degree of immunosuppression. EBV has been detected in 33% to 67% of AIDS-related lymphomas, depending on the detection method (90), but in few high-grade lymphomas of patients with HIV-1 negative. Notably, EBV appears in virtually all post-transplant lymphomas and in lymphomas of the central nervous system among immunocompromised patients. In two hereditary diseases characterized by severe immunosuppression (WAS and XLP), the resulting lymphomas also contain EBV (31). Among the general population, cohort studies such as a 240,000-person cohort in Norway and the US reported two-fold to three-fold increases in risk for NHL associated with EBV antibody titers (91). Similarly, a Finnish cohort followed for 12 years reported a three-fold increase in risk for NHL in people with elevated EBV antibodies (92). The modest serology effects, the variation in viral detection in tumors, and the studies of immunocompromised cohorts implicate EBV as a cofactor but not the major agent in many forms of NHL. Although the association between EBV and lymphoma is established, immunosuppression appears to be a prerequisite (87).

There is little evidence that other members of the herpesviruses family, including human T-cell lymphotrophic virus type II, HHV-6, and cytomegalovirus, are associated with NHL (29,93).

Other Viruses

Clinical and laboratory studies have provided some biologic evidence linking HCV infection with NHL, which is hypothesized to cause NHL via chronic immune stimulation (94). In a small series of patients with splenic marginal zone lymphoma, complete tumor remission was attained in patients infected with HCV whose infection was successfully treated with antiviral medications, whereas tumors did not regress in patients with HCV negative who received the same antiviral regimen (95). In laboratory studies, antigens to the HCV envelope protein have been shown to bind to some HCV lymphoma Igs but not non-HCV lymphoma Igs (96).

Although epidemiologic studies previously have provided conflicting reports for an association between HCV and NHL risk, a more consistent picture has recently emerged. A recent meta-analysis, despite demonstrating high heterogeneity across HCV prevalence, reported elevated NHL risks in both case-control studies (RR = 2.5) and cohort studies (RR = 2.0); risks were elevated for all major B-cell NHL subtypes, and T-cell NHL with no evident risk difference by subtype (97). Similarly, a pooled analyses of seven case-control studies comprising 4,784 NHL cases and 6,269 controls and using third-generation enzyme-linked immunosorbent assays to detect antibodies against HCV in serum samples reported a nearly two-fold risk elevation (seroprevalence among cases,

3.6%; controls, 2.7%) with risks of 1.8 for all NHL and over two-fold risk elevation for marginal zone lymphoma, DLBCL, and lymphoplasmacytic lymphoma (98). In addition, a large retrospective cohort study of US veterans reported modest but statistically significant increased NHL risk (hazard ratio =1.28) (99). These findings are supported further by data from a large Danish-Swedish population-based case-control study of 2,819 cases and 1,856 controls using enzyme-linked immunosorbent assay and confirming recombinant immunoblot assay where a stringent definition of HCV positivity that required HCV RNA detection revealed an NHL risk of 1.7 (100). Further clarification of NHL risk in relation to coinfections such as from hepatitis B virus and further demonstration of temporality in cohort studies will be essential.

Early experimental studies in laboratory animals demonstrated SV40 to be oncogenic, and first suggested the link between the polyomavirus SV40 and lymphoma (101). Poliovirus vaccines were found to be contaminated with SV40 in 1960, largely affecting those immunized in the US, Canada, Europe, Japan, Mexico, and Central and South America between 1955 and 1963. The true exposure, though, varies due to the varying extent in which the different batches were contaminated.

In case series, SV40 deoxyribonucleic acid sequences have been reported in a large proportion of lymphomas in some but not all studies (102,103). Epidemiologic studies evaluating the risks among those likely to have been vaccinated with contaminated polio vaccine have reported no association with NHL. Epidemiologic studies measuring seroprevalence of SV40 also have reported no associations, and consistently find SV40 seroprevalence to be low. Age-period-cohort analyses comparing those in exposed cohorts versus those in unexposed cohorts also have not supported an association in Norway (104), Denmark (105), or among US veterans (106). The Institute of Medicine of the National Academies recently reviewed the scientific evidence, and concluded that there is moderate evidence that SV40 can lead to human cancers, including lymphomas, in natural conditions (107). However, recent reviews of the laboratory, clinical, and epidemiologic data have concluded that the contribution of SV40 to NHL remains uncertain (102) and likely does not contribute to human cancers in general (103).

Initial reports of an association between hepatitis B virus infection and NHL have been reported in Singapore (108), Italy (109), China (110), Japan (111), and the US (112), but hepatitis B virus reactivation has been reported to occur in patients with NHL after therapy, such as rituximab (113). Further studies are needed to clarify whether an independent association exists.

Nonviral and Other Infections

A growing number of epidemiologic studies implicate infection with *H. pylori* and resulting chronic gastritis with increased risk of gastric B-cell lymphoma. *H. pylori*-associated gastritis is found in up to 98% of gastric low-grade MALT lymphomas (114). In a prospective study of populations in the US and Norway, individuals with detectible *H. pylori* IgG antibodies possessed a six-fold increase in risk for gastric NHL, largely DLBCL (115). Investigators examining a series of Japanese patients with gastric lymphoma (116) also pinpointed MALT lymphoma as most strongly linked. This observation is consistent with the epidemiologic studies of peptic ulcer and gastric lymphoma, which demonstrate a stronger association for MALT (117). Furthermore, low-grade gastric B-cell MALT lymphoma regresses after antibiotic treatment eradicates *H. pylori* infection (118–120). Because lymphocytes are not present normally at sites in which MALT develops, investigators infer that *H. pylori* attracts and activates the lymphocytes that develop into lymphoma at those sites (121).

Small case series also have reported highly specific associations with MALT lymphomas, including *Campylobacter jejuni* with small intestine NHL, *Chlamydia psittaci* and ocular adnexa NHL, and *Borrelia burgdorferi* and cutaneous NHL (94), but require additional confirmation.

Finally, there is some evidence, largely indirect, that there may be other infectious causes of NHL. For example, increased hospitalization in the first year of life due to infection has been associated with increased NHL risk in one population-based cohort study in Jerusalem (122). Delayed exposure to common infectious agents such as population mixing among isolated (and presumably unexposed) populations has also been proposed as a risk factor for NHL (11). Results from a large United Kingdom cohort of childhood cancer and population mixing showed that low population diversity was associated with risk of childhood leukemia and lymphoma (123). A review of 17 published studies of childhood cancer and population mixing also concluded that patterns of childhood exposure to infectious diseases were likely to play a role in the etiology of childhood hematopoietic cancers. Future investigations determining patterns of childhood exposure to infectious diseases are warranted to understand the potential biologic basis and to identify specific organisms accounting for these associations.

Ionizing Radiation

Ionizing radiation causes most forms of malignancy, but it plays a relatively minor role in lymphomagenesis (124). This lack of radiosensitivity of lymphoid tissue stands out in comparison to bone marrow with leukemia risk rising rapidly after exposure. For example, atomic bomb survivors had a slightly increased risk of death (RR = 1.3) from lymphomas, compared with 4.9 for leukemia (125). Similarly, among men who participated in the United Kingdom atmospheric nuclear weapons test, risk of leukemia, but not lymphoma, was seen in excess (126).

Most studies of workers who are exposed routinely to low levels of ionizing radiation have found no excess risk of lymphomas. For example, Japanese nuclear industry workers had no elevated risk of lymphoma (127). Similarly, large case-control studies of lymphoma comparing job histories typically found no association with ionizing radiation (128). Among radiation technologists in the US, there was no excess NHL risk in women, who comprise the majority of workers, but there was an increase among men (129). Canadian dental workers showed elevated risks of leukemia but not NHL (130). Diagnostic x-rays do not appear to increase risk. For example, twins exposed in utero had increased risk of leukemia but not lymphoma (131).

Ionizing radiation does increase lymphoma risk in one setting, namely when medical treatments involve high-dose radi-

ation as for infertility or ankylosing spondylitis (132,133). Among patients exposed to Thorotrast, an excess of NHL was found, but with a very small number of cases (134).

Nonionizing Radiation

Populations in geographic areas with stronger exposure to sunlight and individuals with higher personal exposures because of recreational activities, sun behaviors, or residential history have decreased risk of developing NHL. At present, it is not clear whether one subtype of lymphoma is disproportionately affected. A pooled case-control analysis of more than 8,000 cases in 10 studies at widely varying latitudes yielded an overall RR of 0.76 for people in the highest versus the lowest quartile of exposure (135). Solar radiation indicators were associated with all forms of B-cell, but not T-cell, lymphomas.

Few cohort studies have addressed the role of recreational sunlight in NHL. Various ecologic studies have compared NHL rates with ambient ultraviolet levels. In the US, the correlation is consistent and inverse (136), but patterns elsewhere are less clear, possibly because of confounding by skin coloring, sun sensitivity, or sun behaviors. Vitamin D, a possible mediator of the protective effect of sunlight, varies markedly with latitude in Europe (137). Occupational exposure to ultraviolet radiation has not been consistently associated with NHL risk (138–140). Lighter pigmentation has not shown consistent association with risk in the US, Australia, and Scandinavia (141–143).

Electromagnetic fields (EMFs) and radiofrequency radiation have been studied extensively in relation to leukemia, brain cancer, and breast cancer (144). EMFs around power lines have been investigated as a potential cause of lymphomas in childhood or adulthood. Early case-control studies of childhood cancer and EMFs reported some evidence of an association with lymphomas, often with very few lymphoma cases combined with more leukemias, but subsequent studies have had widely varying results. In adults, various occupational studies have been conducted. For example, investigators studying lymphoma within a cohort of Canadian electric utility workers interpreted their results as favoring an association, but the risk estimates were very imprecise because of the small sample size and did not show dose response (145). A larger study in a cohort of US electric workers showed a weakly positive association (146). A US NHL case-control study investigated the hypothesis in depth and found no association (147).

Occupational Exposures

Farmers, livestock workers, printers, teachers, woodworkers, dry cleaners, barbers, and hairdressers have elevated risks of developing NHL (148,149). For most of these high-risk occupations, the responsible agent has not been established. For several agents that have been suggested to account for the excess lymphoma risk, especially those with major economic impact or widespread use, there is an extensive body of meta-analysis, critical review, and commentary. IARC expert review panels have judged nonarsenical insecticides, tetrachloroethylene and trichloroethylene (TCE), 2,3,7,8-tetrachlorodibenzo-*para*-dioxin, and 1,3-butadiene to be "probable human carcinogens" with NHL as one of the sites of malignancy (150–153). They also have found hairdressers and barbers to have probable increased risk of NHL (154).

Farmers appear to have increased risk in the range of 10% to 15%, for the major subtypes (149). A large prospective study of US farmers (155) is focusing on specific chemical exposures such as alachlor, atrazine, carbofuran, chlorpyrifos, diazinon, glyphosate, metachlor, and pendimethalin, with NHL RR to date ranging from 1.0 to 2.4, but the number of lymphomas is too small for firm conclusions yet.

For TCE, as for other organic solvents, associations with NHL have been seen in many studies, but the interpretation remains controversial. A summary estimate was derived in 2006 showing a RR of 1.29 for NHL among workers in cohorts potentially exposed and 1.39 for workers known to be exposed (156). The authors judged that limitations in exposure measurement, inconsistent dose response, supporting toxicology results, and heterogeneity in findings produced insufficient evidence to suggest a causal link between trichloroethylene exposure and NHL. A recent cohort study collected data from 347 Danish companies with fewer than 200 employees each in which TCE was used in the course of the metal, electronic, painting, printing, chemical, dry cleaning, or other work. Using a national identification number, investigators linked each person to cancer registry data and found elevated NHL incidence with a RR of 1.2 overall and 1.5 in the subcohort that was more highly exposed (157). A few cohort studies in Nordic countries used urinary trichloroacetic acid as an exposure measure and found elevated NHL risk but had small study sizes (158). A US Environmental Protection Agency review of the literature in 2006 found further support for the lymphatic system as a target of trichloroethylene toxicity but noted various methodological challenges to estimating the risk with confidence (159).

Exposure to benzene, a major industrial chemical and a component of gasoline, occurs at very low levels in the general environment and at higher levels in petroleum refineries, natural gas production, and fuel and solvent distribution. Leukemia clearly occurs in excess following benzene exposure, but whether lymphoma also does remains controversial (160,161). One recent review noted that 40 of 43 NHL case-control studies found increased risk, with 23 of those statistically significant. In addition, 23 of 26 cohort studies of petroleum refinery workers also showed excess risk. They concluded that an association probably exists, possibly via immunotoxicity or chromosomal damage (160).

By contrast, another review of the literature, after eliminating studies in which workers had exposures to solvents other than benzene, found no association (161). It concluded that it was critical to document benzene exposure and separate non-benzene exposure. Epidemiology and laboratory work underway may resolve the controversy; in the meantime, benzene might best be characterized as a probable cause of lymphoma but with much lower excess risk than for leukemia.

Organochlorines that persist in the environment and accumulate in fat and blood include polychlorinated biphenyls (PCBs), dioxins, and furans. Each has been associated with NHL in one or more studies, but the imputation of exposure from self-report is difficult (162). Recent studies have used biologic and environmental sampling to clarify exposure. Plasma levels of PCBs and furans were linked to risk in a case-control study in the US (163). Body burden of PCBs

was related to risk in a Swedish case-control study (164). Organochlorine pesticide levels in fat tissues from cadavers were linked to NHL risk (165). A 2005 record linkage study in a farm workers labor union showed increased risks for 2,4-dichlorophenoxyacetic acid (2,4-D) as did earlier studies in Sweden and the US (166). Occupational cohort studies with record or questionnaire data have not consistently supported an association between PCBs and risk of NHL, but the emerging evidence from studies with biospecimen tends to support an association (162).

Pursuing the occupational exposures that may cause lymphomas requires accurate and detailed exposure data, information on factors that could confound, and adequate expected numbers of lymphomas (particularly subtypes) in specific jobs. In many cohort studies, details of occupational exposures are measured, but other possible lymphoma risk factors are unknown, leading to possible confounding. Many recent case-control interview studies have industrial hygienists review the occupational histories and assess likely exposures. In these studies, confounders usually are measured, but the number of subjects in any particular job is small, leading to imprecise results and chance associations. Studies created by linking population registries gain statistical power but generally lack confounder data and detailed exposure data, which tends to obscure any real risks. Occupational epidemiologists use a mixture of these approaches to balance strengths and weaknesses of the evidence.

Environmental Exposures

Air, water, and soil can be a source of exposure to many organic compounds. Samples taken from the home or personal environment are expensive and, therefore, have had limited use in lymphoma epidemiology to date, but they may be more widely used in the future.

Pesticides in the home environment are of interest because of the risk for farmers. A US population-based study showed increased risk with dichlorodiphenyldichloroethylene (167) and α-chlordane (168) as measured in the carpet dust of cases and controls. On the other hand, no increased risk was seen either for self-reported herbicide use, or carpet dust levels of 2,4-D or dicamba (169). Studies of possible effects of such environmental exposures vary greatly in design. Some are ecologic studies, which use counties, towns, or other administrative units to compare rates of disease with local exposure levels. Some use records, for example, from water utilities, and many use questionnaires. Nitrate in water supplies was linked to NHL in early case-control data (170), but subsequent studies have found no excess risks below the level of 3 mg/L (171).

Childhood lymphoma, often HL or BL, has been included with leukemias in some studies of environmental factors (172). Generally, the studies include small numbers of childhood lymphomas, and differences in etiology between leukemia and lymphoma appear likely.

In summary, a few specific chemicals in the general environment, many of them present in higher concentrations in work environment, have been linked to NHL risk. It is likely that this area of research will expand greatly, and increasingly use environmental monitoring to refine exposure assessment. Furthermore, the expansion of research using geographic information systems likely will produce more hypotheses regarding NHL risk and environmental contaminants.

Smoking

Current and former cigarette smokers have approximately the same overall risk of NHL as do nonsmokers. It is not yet clear whether smoking, especially current smoking, increases the risk of FL. Although a substantial body of evidence suggests they do, a few other strong studies fail to confirm. It may be important to distinguish case-control from cohort data even though most respondents can recall and report cigarette smoking fairly accurately. In pooled data from 6,594 cases in nine case-control studies, risk of FL, but not other types, was elevated in smokers (173). A similar pattern appeared in a study of 1,742 cases in six European case-control studies (174). A Scandinavian case-control study found increased risk of FL for female but not male smokers (175). Cohort studies, which avoid the possibility of bias in recall or reporting but often lack detail on timing of exposure, also show that overall risk is similar in smokers and nonsmokers. The risk of FL, but not other types, was elevated in a cohort of Iowa women and a cohort of Kaiser Permanente health maintenance organization enrollees (9,176), but it was not in a US cohort of retirees (177) or in a large multicenter European cohort (178). The absence of an effect on most forms of NHL seems clear, and further investigations should resolve whether FL risk is elevated.

Alcohol

A reduced risk of NHL has been consistently associated with alcohol consumption, but it is not yet clear whether the association reflects a casual mechanism or an unidentified aspect of lifestyle that is correlated with alcohol consumption. In a large pooled analysis of nine case-control studies, the RR was estimated as 0.73 for current drinkers and 0.95 for former drinkers, with no apparent variation by type of beverage (179). Reports from other case-control data also have shown an inverse association between NHL and consumption of alcohol, regardless of whether in the form of beer, wine, or spirits (174,180). Cohort studies have tended to support the association, including cohorts of physicians, Iowa women, and US retirees (177,181,182). Moderate alcohol intake might plausibly affect immunity or inflammation, but the explanation for the decreased risk is speculative at present.

Weight, Height, and Physical Activity

It appears that risk of NHL is moderately elevated with excess weight and higher among taller individuals. Risk is somewhat decreased with greater physical activity, but the literature shows considerable difference in findings depending on the study design and the timing of the measurement of weight or activity in relation to the occurrence of lymphoma (183).

A pooled analysis of more than 10,000 cases from 18 case-control studies found a positive association between NHL risk and height, which is often a surrogate for social class (184). The same pooled analysis showed no consistent effect of overweight or obesity, except for an increase in DLBCL with severe obesity. Cohort studies, which avoid possible bias in retrospective reporting, have yielded rather different results. Increased risk with higher body mass index was seen in the US Multi-Ethnic Cohort (185), a cohort of Swedish hospital patients (186), Korean men (187), US retirees (177), the Whitehall study (188), and the America Cancer Society cohort (189). In the Swedish Construction Workers Cohort, obesity increased risk in women but not men (190), whereas no effect was seen in Iowa women (191).

Physical activity has not been studied as extensively in association with lymphoma risk. To date, workers with physically active jobs have shown typical NHL risks (192,193). Among Iowa women, self-reported physical activity did influence subsequent NHL risk (191). Activity in college did not predict NHL risk (194,195). On the other hand, a Canadian and a US case-control study reported a protective effect (196,197). It is likely that pooled data from cohorts will reveal whether a protective effect exists.

Diet

Diet has been suggested to influence lymphoma risk apart from its effect on weight and apart from the effects of food supply contaminants like PCBs. Dozens of studies have been reported in recent years. Lymphoma is not one of the malignancies most strongly associated with diet, but the reported associations follow the general pattern reported for many cancers (183). High-fat intake may increase risk slightly, whereas high-vegetable intake may decrease it. Less consistent are effects reported for dairy, fruits, antioxidants, and one-carbon nutrients. For lymphomas arising in the gastrointestinal tract, diet may play a different and highly specific role. For instance, celiac disease is associated with a rare T-cell lymphoma, and dietary control reduces risk. Diet will continue to be studied in relation to these more common lymphomas because so few means of prevention exist. Future studies may include genetic polymorphisms that either affect or mimic diet.

Hair Dyes

Overall, users of hair coloring products have approximately the same risk of NHL as nonusers. The topic has been extensively studied after early reports of elevated risk, possibly only among users of darker colors. A pooled analysis of more than 4,400 cases from studies in 13 regions in Europe and the US showed that women who used any hair dye (a large majority of women) had no increased risk (198). Those who had used hair dyes before many manufacturers switched formulations in 1980 had increased risk (RR = 1.3), more for FL and CLL/SLL than for other types. Use of darker colors after 1980 was associated with risk, with sparser data. One cohort study reported no overall risk (199), and another reported an effect, especially for longer use of darker colors (200). A recent case-control study found the effect of hair dyes dependent on genetic variation in N-acetyltransferases 1 and 2, which encode enzymes metabolizing aromatic amines found in dyes, but replication is needed (201).

Reproductive and Hormonal

Pregnancy produces transient changes in immunity, and several studies have assessed whether the number or timing of pregnancies or births affects NHL risk. Despite initial reports of an association, a number of subsequent cohort and case-control studies have yielded inconsistent but largely no associations (202–204). Other reproductive factors, including menarche and menopause, similarly show little or no association with NHL (205), but a recent study did report an association between preeclampsia in the mother and increased NHL risk (206). Initial reports of increased NHL risk among those with a history of endometriosis (207,208) and of increased childhood NHL risk among children delivered by cesarean section (209) also require further confirmation.

Estrogen and estrogen-like compounds influence B-cell development. Oral contraceptive use and postmenopausal hormones, thus, have been evaluated in case-control and cohort studies for associations with NHL. Among the modest number of reports, the association is not presently convincing (210). Two studies reported decreased NHL risk associated with use of oral contraceptives (203,211) and lactation suppressants (203). Despite a report from a cohort study of increased NHL risk among those using postmenopausal hormones (210), this association has not been consistently observed (203,210).

Genetic Susceptibility

Numerous studies now implicate common host genetic variation in NHL etiology, as recently reviewed (212). Most of these reports comprise evaluation of *a priori* candidate genes with a large emphasis on immune genes but also include evaluation of deoxyribonucleic acid repair, oxidative stress, cell cycle/apoptosis, innate immunity, one-carbon metabolism, environmental and chemical metabolism, and genes involved in hormone production and metabolism. To date, the most convincing evidence of a role for common genetic polymorphisms in NHL risk comes from a large pooled analysis of eight European, Canadian, and US case-control studies comprising 3,586 NHL cases and 4,018 controls (213). The analysis showed that a polymorphism in the promoter region of the *TNF* gene ($-308G->A$) was associated with increased NHL risk (p for trend = 0.005 for each additional G allele), particularly for DLBCL (odds ratio = 1.3 for GA and 1.6 for AA, p for trend <0.0001), but not for FL. Similarly, the interleukin 10 (*IL10*) $-3575T->A$ polymorphism was also associated with increased NHL risk (p for trend = 0.02) and DLBCL (p for trend = 0.006), but not FL. Joint effects between the two polymorphisms further increased DLBCL risk. The pooled analysis convincingly implicates common polymorphisms in *TNF* and *IL10*, key cytokines for the inflammatory response and T<h1>/T<h2> balance, as susceptibility loci for NHL. Notably, TNF-$\alpha\alpha$, the protein product of *TNF*, activates the nuclear factor-$\kappa\kappa$B pathway, a hallmark of inflammation. Further investigation of the role that nuclear factor-$\kappa\kappa$B plays in lymphoma may, thus, provide additional mechanistic clues in our understanding of lymphomagenesis. Further evaluation of the major histocompatibility region where *TNF* resides may also be of interest (214).

Replication of other reported associations will be required, but the search for genetic polymorphisms related to NHL risk has proved a promising one thus far. Further gene-gene and gene-environment interactions may also prove fruitful, as suggested by some preliminary reports. In one such US report, the effects of established and hypothesized NHL risk factors were evaluated in relation to the *TNF* G308A or *IL10* T3575A genotypes (215). The study reported increased DLBCL risk among those with variant *TNF* or *IL10* alleles and those with an autoimmune condition, or who were last-born status or obese. These results support the hypothesis that autoimmune conditions, late birth order, and obesity act partly through a common inflammatory pathway, posing a greater risk to individuals with variant *TNF* and *IL10* genotypes than those with wild-type alleles. Similar gene-environment evaluations have been reported for one-carbon metabolism genes and folate intake (216), sunlight exposure and vitamin D gene polymorphisms (217), and N-acetyltransferase enzymes and cigarette smoking and hair dye use (218). All results require replication in larger populations such as in the context of consortia to identify true positive associations.

Large-scale genotyping efforts in targeted pathways (219) and genome-wide association studies are emerging now, and likely will implicate new pathways and genes of interest. These recent approaches largely employ tagging algorithms to identify gene variations for investigation. Subsequent efforts to identify causal variants with functional evidence certainly will add to our knowledge of NHL etiology (220,221) and are underway also.

Molecular Subtyping

Gene expression profiling with microarrays has provided important new insights in lymphomagenesis in recent years. Although much of this research has focused on delineating differences in response to therapy and survival outcomes, the relevance of new molecular subtypes within NHL may also contribute to our understanding of NHL etiology. Notably, gene-expression profiles have been reported for DLBCL, FL, and BL. For DLBCL, two distinct signatures, i.e., the germinal enter (GC) B-cell signature and activated B-cell-like subgroup, indicate that DLBCL arises at different stages of normal B-cell development and has differential prognosis. The GC subtype has a higher rate of overall survival 5 years after chemotherapy (222). Genetic characteristics of DLBCL subgroups also are distinct; GCB-DLBCL has frequent gains of 21q12, and activated B-cell-DLBCL has frequent trisomy 3, gains of 3q, and losses of 6q21-q22 (223). Gene signatures delineating differential survival in FL also have been reported, and implicate the immunologic microenvironment and, specifically, nonmalignant tumor-infiltrating immune cells (224). Gene expression signature for BL has also been reported (225). The technology is rapidly evolving, and efforts are being made to translate this knowledge to clinical and population-based efforts (226) that may potentially be useful for etiologic studies. For example, a recent study of patients with RA suggested that severe RA is particularly associated with the non-GC subtype of DLBCL (227).

Finally, other molecular characteristics such as higher ataxia telangiectasia mutated mutations in mantle cell lymphomas (228) and t(14;18) translocations in NHL may be markers of interest for pinpointing epidemiologic risk factors as reported in one Nebraska case-control study where insecticides and herbicides were associated specifically with t(14;18)-related NHL (229). These results are intriguing but require confirmation.

FUTURE EPIDEMIOLOGIC RESEARCH ON NON-HODGKIN LYMPHOMA

Although much of NHL and the epidemic of the last half of the 20th century still remain unexplained, we have steadily increased our understanding of NHL etiology. In general, epidemiologists have been methodically pursuing hypotheses raised earlier, considering one homogeneous subset of lymphoma at a time. We now know that a growing number of infectious agents often produce lymphomas that are clinically or immunohistochemically distinctive. We now know also that proinflammatory immune gene variations increase risk for DLBCL. Investigative teams of geneticists and epidemiologists currently are scanning the human genome for genetic variations related to NHL risk in the pursuit of uncovering the biologic and causal mechanisms of lymphomagenesis. Environmental and behavioral exposures also are being evaluated in the context of immune or inflammatory response along with previously hypothesized genotoxic mechanisms. As refined biologic measurements of these exposures in the environment or as absorbed in the body have yielded important clues, their accurate measurements applied before diagnosis in cohort studies, such as the case for persistent organochlorine exposure and increased NHL risk, will be important for further illuminating the causal mechanisms for lymphoma.

The recent identification and confirmation of NHL risk factors coincides with a paradigm shift in epidemiologic studies of NHL that now also evaluate NHL by subtypes rather than considering NHL only as a whole, as done previously. Classification of NHL according to their molecular or genetic characteristics may further reveal etiologically distinctive subsets. It is fortuitous that this research direction has been met with another paradigm shift in epidemiology where meta-analyses, cooperative parallel studies, and consortia are regarded as a way forward for identifying true epidemiologic associations with adequate sample size and power. This latter effort is critical and already yielding important clues to understanding the etiology of NHL and its subtypes.

Striking clinical case reports also will continue to yield new clues. Epidemiologists will continue to examine unique populations with distinct exposures, including the development of lymphoma in patients with AIDS and transplants, to understand co-factors and late natural history of lymphoma development. They also will study agricultural workers, populations exposed to particular viruses, and other especially informative groups to measure their risks of developing lymphoma. Advances in MM, chronic lymphocytic, and other leukemias and nonmalignant immune conditions also will be examined for possible relevance to NHL.

Research advances of the last decade, including improved biologic measures of infection or environmental exposures, genome-wide interrogation of genetic variations, identifica-

tion of molecular subtypes, to name a few, surely will merge in the years to come. When they do, sophisticated analyses of these data should provide a detailed model of the biologic processes critical for NHL and its various subtypes and the controlling genetic pathways involved. Confirming associations from case-control studies in cohort studies where NHL is rare but prediagnostic biospecimens are precious also will prove essential for establishing temporality and identifying characteristics that may predict NHL risk. With major research efforts and advancing technology, a clearer understanding of the causal mechanisms undoubtedly will emerge, brightening our prospects for the intervention and prevention of NHL.

ACKNOWLDGMENTS

We thank Dr. Susan Devesa for expert guidance on descriptive statistics. We thank Sarah Del Castillo for editorial assistance, graphical presentation, and careful review of the chapter. We also thank J. Daniel Carreon for editorial assistance.

ABBREVIATIONS

AIDS, acquired immunodeficiency syndrome
ATL, adult T-cell leukemia/lymphoma
BL, Burkitt lymphoma
CVID, common variable immunodeficiency
DLBCL, diffuse large B-cell lymphoma
EBV, Epstein-Barr virus
FL, follicular lymphoma
GC, germinal center
HAART, highly active antiretroviral therapy
HCV, hepatitis C virus
HHV, human herpesvirus
HIV, human immunodeficiency virus
HL, Hodgkin lymphoma
HTLV-1, human T-cell lymphotropic virus I
IARC, International Agency for Research on Cancer
IL10, interleukin 10
MALT, mucosa associated lymphoid tissue
MM, multiple myeloma
NHL, non-Hodgkin lymphoma
PCB, polychlorinated biphenyl
PEL, primary effusion lymphoma
RA, rheumatoid arthritis
RR, relative risk
SIR, standard incidence ratio
SLE, systemic lupus erythematosus
SLL/CLL, small lymphocytic lymphoma/chronic lymphocytic leukemia
SS, Sjogren syndrome
SV40, simian virus 40
TCE, tetrachloroethylene and trichloroethylene
TNF, tumor necrosis factor
US, United States
WAS, Wiskott-Aldrich syndrome
XLP, X-linked lymphoproliferative disease

References

1. Surveillance Research Program. National Cancer Institute SEER*Stat software, version 5.3.1. Available at: www.seer.cancer.gov/seerstat. Accessed March 7, 2003.

2. National Cancer Institute. Cancer Mortality Maps and Graphs. Atlas of Cancer Mortality in the United States: 1950–94 2008. Available at: http://ratecalc.nci.nih.gov/ratecalc/.

3. Curado MP, Edwards B, Shin HR, et al. *Cancer incidence in five continents*, vol IX, no 160. Lyon, France: IARC Scientific Publications, 2007.

4. Morton LM, Wang SS, Devesa SS, et al. Lymphoma incidence patterns by WHO subtype in the United States, 1992–2001. *Blood* 2006;107:265–276.

5. Dohden K, Kaizaki Y, Hosokawa O, et al M. Regression of rectal mucosa-associated lymphoid tissue lymphoma but persistence of Helicobacter pylori infection of gastric mucosa after administration of levofloxacin: report of a case. *Dis Colon Rectum* 2004;47:1544–1546.

6. Tursi A, Brandimarte G, Torello M. Disappearance of gastric mucosa-associated lymphoid tissue in hepatitis C virus-positive patients after antihepatitis C virus therapy. *J Clin Gastroenterol* 2004;38:360–363.

7. Alpen B, Robbecke J, Wundisch T, e al. Helicobacter pylori eradication therapy in gastric high grade non Hodgkin's lymphoma (NHL). *Ann Hematol* 2001;80(suppl 3):B106–B107.

8. Engels EA, Chatterjee N, Cerhan JR, Davis S, Cozen W, Severson RK et al. Hepatitis C virus infection and non-Hodgkin lymphoma: results of the NCI-SEER multi-center case-control study. *Int J Cancer* 2004;111:76–80.

9. Herrinton LJ, Friedman GD. Cigarette smoking and risk of non-Hodgkin's lymphoma subtypes. *Cancer Epidemiol Biomarkers Prev* 1998;7:25–28.

10. Masala G, Di Lollo S, Picoco C, et al. Incidence rates of leukemias, lymphomas and myelomas in Italy: geographic distribution and NHL histotypes. *Int J Cancer* 1996;68:156–159.

11. Kinlen LJ, Dickson M, Stiller CA. Childhood leukaemia and non-Hodgkin's lymphoma near large rural construction sites, with a comparison with Sellafield nuclear site. *BMJ* 1995;310:763–768.

12. Alexander FE, McKinney PA, Moncrieff KC, et al. Residential proximity of children with leukaemia and non-Hodgkin's lymphoma in three areas of northern England. *Br J Cancer* 1992;65:583–588.

13. Goldgar DE, Easton DF, Cannon-Albright LA, et al. Systematic population-based assessment of cancer risk in first-degree relatives of cancer probands. *J Natl Cancer Inst* 1994;86:1600–1608.

14. Goldin LR, Landgren O, McMaster ML, et al. Familial aggregation and heterogeneity of non-Hodgkin lymphoma in population-based samples. *Cancer Epidemiol Biomarkers Prev* 2005;14:2402–2406.

15. Dong C, Hemminki K. Modification of cancer risks in offspring by sibling and parental cancers from 2,112,616 nuclear families. *Int J Cancer* 2001;92:144–150.

16. Chang ET, Smedby KE, Hjalgrim H, et al. Family history of hematopoietic malignancy and risk of lymphoma. *J Natl Cancer Inst* 2005;97:1466–1474.

17. Wang SS, Slager SL, Brennan P, et al. Family history of hematopoietic malignancies and risk of non-Hodgkin lymphoma (NHL): a pooled analysis of 10 211 cases and 11 905 controls from the International Lymphoma Epidemiology Consortium (InterLymph). *Blood* 2007;109:3479–3488.

18. Altieri A, Bermejo JL, Hemminki K. Familial risk for non-Hodgkin lymphoma and other lymphoproliferative malignancies by histopathologic subtype: the Swedish Family-Cancer Database. *Blood* 2005;106:668–672.

19. Zhu K, Levine RS, Brann EA, et al. Risk factors for non-Hodgkin's lymphoma according to family history of haematolymphoproliferative malignancies. *Int J Epidemiol* 2001;30:818–824.

20. Dong C, Hemminki K. Second primary neoplasms among 53 159 haematolymphoproliferative malignancy patients in Sweden, 1958–1996: a search for common mechanisms. *Br J Cancer* 2001;85:997–1005.

21. Krishnan B, Morgan GJ. Non-Hodgkin lymphoma secondary to cancer chemotherapy. *Cancer Epidemiol Biomarkers Prev* 2007;16:377–380.

22. Metayer C, Lynch CF, Clarke EA, et al. Second cancers among long-term survivors of Hodgkin's disease diagnosed in childhood and adolescence. *J Clin Oncol* 2000;18:2435–2443.

23. Goggins WB, Finkelstein DM, Tsao H. Evidence for an association between cutaneous melanoma and non-Hodgkin lymphoma. *Cancer* 2001;91:874–880.

24. Friedman DL, Kadan-Lottick NS, Whitton J, et al. Increased risk of cancer among siblings of long-term childhood cancer survivors: a report from the childhood cancer survivor study. *Cancer Epidemiol Biomarkers Prev* 2005;14:1922–1927.

25. Huang KP, Weinstock MA, Clarke CA, et al. Second lymphomas and other malignant neoplasms in patients with mycosis fungoides and Sezary syndrome: evidence from population-based and clinical cohorts. *Arch Dermatol* 2007;143:45–50.

26. Levi F, Randimbison L, Te VC, et al C. Non-Hodgkin's lymphomas, chronic lymphocytic leukaemias and skin cancers. *Br J Cancer* 1996;74:1847–1850.

27. Lens MB, Newton-Bishop JA. An association between cutaneous melanoma and non-Hodgkin's lymphoma: pooled analysis of published data with a review. *Ann Oncol* 2005;16:460–465.

28. McKenna DB, Doherty VR, McLaren KM, et al. Malignant melanoma and lymphoproliferative malignancy: is there a shared aetiology? *Br J Dermatol* 2000;143:171–173.

29. Knowles DM. Immunodeficiency-associated lymphoproliferative disorders. *Mod Pathol* 1999;12:200–217.

30. Filipovich AH, Mathur A, Kamat D, et al. Lymphoproliferative disorders and other tumors complicating immunodeficiencies. *Immunodeficiency* 1994;5:91–112.

31. Levine AM. Lymphoma complicating immunodeficiency disorders. *Ann Oncol* 1994;5(suppl 2):29–35.

32. Elenitoba-Johnson KS, Jaffe ES. Lymphoproliferative disorders associated with congenital immunodeficiencies. *Semin Diagn Pathol* 1997;14:35–47.

33. Grulich AE, Vajdic CM, Cozen W. Altered immunity as a risk factor for non-Hodgkin lymphoma. *Cancer Epidemiol Biomarkers Prev* 2007;16:405–408.

34. Kauppi M, Pukkala E, Isomaki H. Elevated incidence of hematologic malignancies in patients with Sjogren's syndrome compared with patients with rheumatoid arthritis (Finland). *Cancer Causes Control* 1997;8:201–204.

35. Zintzaras E, Voulgarelis M, Moutsopoulos HM. The risk of lymphoma development in autoimmune diseases: a meta-analysis. *Arch Intern Med* 2005;165:2337–2344.

36. Ekstrom SK, Vajdic CM, Falster M, et al. Autoimmune disorders and risk of non-Hodgkin lymphoma subtypes: a pooled analysis within the InterLymph Consortium. *Blood* 2008;111:4029–4038.

37. Mellors RC. Autoimmune and immunoproliferative diseases of NZB/Bl mice and hybrids. *Int Rev Exp Pathol* 1966;5:217–252.

38. Corrao G, Corazza GR, Bagnardi V, et al. Mortality in patients with coeliac disease and their relatives: a cohort study. *Lancet* 2001;358:356–361.

39. Green PH, Fleischauer AT, Bhagat G, et al. Risk of malignancy in patients with celiac disease. *Am J Med* 2003;115:191–195.

40. Peters U, Askling J, Gridley G, et al. Causes of death in patients with celiac disease in a population-based Swedish cohort. *Arch Intern Med* 2003;163:1566–1572.

41. Askling J, Linet M, Gridley G, et al. Cancer incidence in a population-based cohort of individuals hospitalized with celiac disease or dermatitis herpetiformis. *Gastroenterology* 2002;123:1428–1435.

42. Hakulinen T, Isomaki H, Knekt P. Rheumatoid arthritis and cancer studies based on linking nationwide registries in Finland. *Am J Med* 1985;78:29–32.

43. Gridley G, McLaughlin JK, Ekbom A, et al. Incidence of cancer among patients with rheumatoid arthritis. *J Natl Cancer Inst* 1993;85:307–311.

44. Mellemkjaer L, Linet MS, Gridley G, et al. Rheumatoid arthritis and cancer risk. *Eur J Cancer* 1996;32A:1753–1757.

45. Gridley G, Klippel JH, Hoover RN, et al. Incidence of cancer among men with the Felty syndrome. *Ann Intern Med* 1994;120:35–39.

46. Mariette X, Cazals-Hatem D, Warszawki J, et al. Lymphomas in rheumatoid arthritis patients treated with methotrexate: a 3-year prospective study in France. *Blood* 2002;99:3909–3915.

47. Leandro MJ, Isenberg DA. Rheumatic diseases and malignancy—is there an association? *Scand J Rheumatol* 2001;30:185–188.

48. Wolfe F, Michaud K. Lymphoma in rheumatoid arthritis: the effect of methotrexate and anti-tumor necrosis factor therapy in 18,572 patients. *Arthritis Rheum* 2004;50:1740–1751.

49. Soderberg KC, Jonsson F, Winqvist O, et al. Autoimmune diseases, asthma and risk of haematological malignancies: a nationwide case-control study in Sweden. *Eur J Cancer* 2006;42:3028–3033.

50. von Roon AC, Reese G, Teare J, et al. The risk of cancer in patients with Crohn's disease. *Dis Colon Rectum* 2007;50:839–855.

51. Penn I, Hammond W, Brettschneider L, et al. Malignant lymphomas in transplantation patients. *Transplant Proc* 1969;1:106–112.

52. Hoover R, Fraumeni JFJ. Risk of cancer in renal-transplant recipients. *Lancet* 1973;2:55–57.

53. Opelz G, Henderson R. Incidence of non-Hodgkin lymphoma in kidney and heart transplant recipients. *Lancet* 1993;342:1514–1516.

54. Opelz G, Schwarz V, Henderson R, et al. Non-Hodgkin's lymphoma after kidney or heart transplantation: frequency of occurrence during the first post-transplant year. *Transpl Int* 1994;7(suppl 1):S353–S356.

55. Adami J, Gabel H, Lindelof B, et al. Cancer risk following organ transplantation: a nationwide cohort study in Sweden. *Br J Cancer* 2003;89:1221–1227.

56. Bates WD, Gray DW, Dada MA, et al. Lymphoproliferative disorders in Oxford renal transplant recipients. *J Clin Pathol* 2003;56:439–446.

57. Penn I. Some new problems with post-transplant lymphoproliferative disease. *Transplantation* 2000;69:705–706.

58. Swinnen LJ, Costanzo-Nordin MR, Fisher SG, et al. Increased incidence of lymphoproliferative disorder after immunosuppression with the monoclonal antibody OKT3 in cardiac- transplant recipients. *N Engl J Med* 1990;323:1723–1728.

59. Bayerdorffer E, Neubauer A, Rudolph B, et al. Regression of primary gastric lymphoma of mucosa-associated lymphoid tissue type after cure of Helicobacter pylori infection. MALT Lymphoma Study Group. *Lancet* 1995;345:1591–1594.

60. Cerhan JR, Wallace RB, Folsom AR, et al. Transfusion history and cancer risk in older women. *Ann Intern Med* 1993;119:8–15.

61. Cerhan JR, Wallace RB, Dick F, et al. Blood transfusions and risk of non-Hodgkin's lymphoma subtypes and chronic lymphocytic leukemia. *Cancer Epidemiol Biomarkers Prev* 2001;10:361–368.
62. Blomberg J, Moller T, Olsson H, et al. Cancer morbidity in blood recipients–results of a cohort study. *Eur J Cancer* 1993;29A:2101–2105.
63. Chow EJ, Holly EA. Blood transfusions as a risk factor for non-Hodgkin's lymphoma in the San Francisco Bay Area: a population-based study. *Am J Epidemiol* 2002;155:725–731.
64. Zhang Y, Holford TR, Leaderer B, et al. Blood transfusion and risk of non-Hodgkin's lymphoma in Connecticut women. *Am J Epidemiol* 2004;160:325–330.
65. Holly EA, Lele C. Non-Hodgkin's lymphoma in HIV-positive and HIV-negative homosexual men in the San Francisco Bay Area: allergies, prior medication use, and sexual practices. *J Acquir Immune Defic Syndr Hum Retrovirol* 1997;15:211–222.
66. Bernatsky S, Lee JL, Rahme E. Non-Hodgkin's lymphoma—meta-analyses of the effects of corticosteroids and non-steroidal anti-inflammatories. *Rheumatology Oxford* 2007;46:690–694.
67. Bernstein L, Ross RK. Prior medication use and health history as risk factors for non- Hodgkin's lymphoma: preliminary results from a case-control study in Los Angeles County. *Cancer Res* 1992;5219 suppl): 5510s–5515s.
68. Grulich AE, Vajdic CM, Kaldor JM, et al. Birth order, atopy, and risk of non-Hodgkin lymphoma. *J Natl Cancer Inst* 2005;97:587–594.
69. Bracci PM, Dalvi TB, Holly EA. Residential history, family characteristics and non-Hodgkin lymphoma, a population-based case-control study in the San Francisco Bay Area. *Cancer Epidemiol Biomarkers Prev* 2006; 15:1287–1294.
70. Manns A, Cleghorn FR, Falk RT, et al. Role of HTLV-I in development of non-Hodgkin lymphoma in Jamaica and Trinidad and Tobago. The HTLV Lymphoma Study Group. *Lancet* 1993;342:1447–1450.
71. Mortreux F, Gabet AS, Wattel E. Molecular and cellular aspects of HTLV-1 associated leukemogenesis in vivo. *Leukemia* 2003;17:26–38.
72. Mueller NE, Blattner WA. Retroviruses-human T-cell lymphotropic virus. In: Evans AS, Kaslow RA, eds. *Viral Infections of humans: epidemiology and control*, 4th ed. New York, NY: Plenum Publishing Co., 1997:785–813.
73. Siegel R, Gartenhaus R, Kuzel T. HTLV-I associated leukemia/lymphoma: epidemiology, biology, and treatment. *Cancer Treat Res* 2001;104:75–88.
74. Council of State and Territorial Epidemiologists. Revision of the CDC surveillance case definition for acquired immunodeficiency syndrome. Council of State and Territorial Epidemiologists; AIDS Program, Center for Infectious Diseases. *MMWR Morb Mortal Wkly Rep* 1987;36(suppl 1):1S–15S.
75. Centers for Disease Control. Revision of the CDC surveillance case definition for acquired immunodeficiency syndrome. 1987. Report No.: 36suppl).
76. Dal Maso L, Franceschi S. Epidemiology of non-Hodgkin lymphomas and other haemolymphopoietic neoplasms in people with AIDS. *Lancet Oncol* 2003;4:110–119.
77. Bower M. Acquired immunodeficiency syndrome-related systemic non-Hodgkin's lymphoma. *Br J Haematol* 2001;112:863–873.
78. Grulich AE, Wan X, Law MG, et al. B-cell stimulation and prolonged immune deficiency are risk factors for non-Hodgkin's lymphoma in people with AIDS. *AIDS* 2000;14:133–140.
79. Beral V, Peterman T, Berkelman R, et al. AIDS-associated non-Hodgkin lymphoma. *Lancet* 1991;337:805–809.
80. Cote TR, Biggar RJ, Rosenberg PS, et al. Non-Hodgkin's lymphoma among people with AIDS: incidence, presentation and public health burden. AIDS/Cancer Study Group. *Int J Cancer* 1997;73:645–650.
81. International Collaboration on HIV and Cancer. Highly active antiretroviral therapy and incidence of cancer in human immunodeficiency virus-infected adults. *J Natl Cancer Inst* 2000;92:1823–1830.
82. Lim ST, Levine AM. Recent advances in acquired immunodeficiency syndrome (AIDS)-related lymphoma. *CA Cancer J Clin* 2005;55:229–241.
83. Schulz TF. Kaposi's sarcoma-associated herpesvirus (human herpesvirus 8): epidemiology and pathogenesis. *J Antimicrob Chemother* 2000;45(suppl T3):15–27.
84. Cesarman E, Chang Y, Moore PS, et al. Kaposi's sarcoma-associated herpesvirus-like DNA sequences in AIDS- related body-cavity-based lymphomas. *N Engl J Med* 1995;332:1186–1191.
85. Hengge UR, Ruzicka T, Tyring SK, et al. Update on Kaposi's sarcoma and other HHV8 associated diseases. Part 2: pathogenesis, Castleman's disease, and pleural effusion lymphoma. *Lancet Infect Dis* 2002;2:344–352.
86. Cesarman E, Knowles DM. Kaposi's sarcoma-associated herpesvirus: a lymphotropic human herpesvirus associated with Kaposi's sarcoma, primary effusion lymphoma, and multicentric Castleman's disease. *Semin Diagn Pathol* 1997;14:54–66.
87. International Agency for Research on Cancer. *IARC monographs. Epstein-Barr virus and Kaposi's sarcoma herpes virus/human herpes virus 8*. Lyon, France: International Agency for Research on Cancer, 1997.
88. Hsu JL, Glaser SL. Epstein-Barr virus-associated malignancies: epidemiologic patterns and etiologic implications. *Crit Rev Oncol Hematol* 2000;34:27–53.
89. Hummel M, Anagnostopoulos I, Korbjuhn P, et al. Epstein-Barr virus in B-cell non-Hodgkin's lymphomas: unexpected infection patterns and different infection incidence in low- and high-grade types. *J Pathol* 1995;175:263–271.
90. Cohen K, Scadden DT. Non-Hodgkin's lymphoma: pathogenesis, clinical presentation, and treatment. *Cancer Treat Res* 2001;104:201–230.
91. Mueller N, Mohar A, Evans A, et al. Epstein-Barr virus antibody patterns preceding the diagnosis of non- Hodgkin's lymphoma. *Int J Cancer* 1991;49:387–393.
92. Lehtinen T, Lumio J, Dillner J, et al. Increased risk of malignant lymphoma indicated by elevated Epstein-Barr virus antibodies—a prospective study. *Cancer Causes Control* 1993;4:187–193.
93. Rezk SA, Weiss LM. Epstein-Barr virus-associated lymphoproliferative disorders. *Hum Pathol* 2007;38:1293–1304.
94. Engels EA. Infectious agents as causes of non-Hodgkin lymphoma. *Cancer Epidemiol Biomarkers Prev* 2007;16:401–404.
95. Hermine O, Lefrere F, Bronowicki JP, et al. Regression of splenic lymphoma with villous lymphocytes after treatment of hepatitis C virus infection. *N Engl J Med* 2002;347:89–94.
96. Quinn ER, Chan CH, Hadlock KG, et al. The B-cell receptor of a hepatitis C virus (HCV)-associated non-Hodgkin lymphoma binds the viral E2 envelope protein, implicating HCV in lymphomagenesis. *Blood* 2001;98:3745–3749.
97. Dal ML, Franceschi S. Hepatitis C virus and risk of lymphoma and other lymphoid neoplasms: a meta-analysis of epidemiologic studies. *Cancer Epidemiol Biomarkers Prev* 2006-;15:2078–2085.
98. De SS, Benavente Y, Vajdic CM, et al. Hepatitis C and non-Hodgkin lymphoma among 4784 cases and 6269 controls from the International Lymphoma Epidemiology Consortium. *Clin Gastroenterol Hepatol* 2008;6:451–458.
99. Giordano TP, Henderson L, Landgren O, et al. Risk of non-Hodgkin lymphoma and lymphoproliferative precursor diseases in US veterans with hepatitis C virus. *JAMA* 2007;297:2010–2017.
100. Schollkopf C, Smedby KE, Hjalgrim H, et al. Hepatitis C infection and risk of malignant lymphoma. *Int J Cancer* 2008;122:1885–1890.
101. Diamandopoulos GT. Leukemia, lymphoma, and osteosarcoma induced in the Syrian golden hamster by simian virus 40. *Science* 1972;176:173–175.
102. Engels EA. Does simian virus 40 cause non-Hodgkin lymphoma? A review of the laboratory and epidemiological evidence. *Cancer Invest* 2005;23:529–536.
103. Shah KV. SV40 and human cancer: a review of recent data. *Int J Cancer* 2007;120:215–223.
104. Thu GO, Hem LY, Hansen S, et al. Is there an association between SV40 contaminated polio vaccine and lymphoproliferative disorders? An age-period-cohort analysis on Norwegian data from 1953 to 1997. *Int J Cancer* 2006;118:2035–2039.
105. Engels EA, Katki HA, Nielsen NM, et al. Cancer incidence in Denmark following exposure to poliovirus vaccine contaminated with simian virus 40. *J Natl Cancer Inst* 2003;95:532–539.
106. Rollison DE, Page WF, Crawford H, et al. Case-control study of cancer among US Army veterans exposed to simian virus 40-contaminated adenovirus vaccine. *Am J Epidemiol* 2004;160:317–324.
107. Stratton K, Amario DA, McCormick MC. *SV40 contamination of polio vaccine and cancer*. Washington, DC: The National Academies Press, 2002.
108. Lim ST, Fei G, Quek R, et al. The relationship of hepatitis B virus infection and non-Hodgkin's lymphoma and its impact on clinical characteristics and prognosis. *Eur J Haematol* 2007;79:132–137.
109. Marcucci F, Mele A, Spada E, et al. High prevalence of hepatitis B virus infection in B-cell non-Hodgkin's lymphoma. *Haematologica* 2006;91:554–557.
110. Wang F, Xu RH, Han B, et al. High incidence of hepatitis B virus infection in B-cell subtype non-Hodgkin lymphoma compared with other cancers. *Cancer* 2007;109:1360–1364.
111. Kuniyoshi M, Nakamuta M, Sakai H, et al. Prevalence of hepatitis B or C virus infections in patients with non-Hodgkin's lymphoma. *J Gastroenterol Hepatol* 2001;16:215–219.
112. Ulcickas YM, Quesenberry CP Jr, Guo D, et al. Incidence of non-Hodgkin's lymphoma among individuals with chronic hepatitis B virus infection. *Hepatology* 2007;46:107–112.
113. Tsutsumi Y, Kanamori H, Mori A, et al. Reactivation of hepatitis B virus with rituximab. *Expert Opin Drug Saf* 2005;4:599–608.
114. Eidt S, Stolte M, Fischer R. Helicobacter pylori gastritis and primary gastric non-Hodgkin's lymphomas. *J Clin Pathol* 1994;47:436–439.
115. Parsonnet J, Friedman GD, Vandersteen DP, et al. Helicobacter pylori infection and the risk of gastric carcinoma. *N Engl J Med* 1991;325:1127–1131.
116. Nakamura S, Yao T, Aoyagi K, et al. Helicobacter pylori and primary gastric lymphoma. A histopathologic and immunohistochemical analysis of 237 patients. *Cancer* 1997;79:3–11.
117. Vineis P, Crosignani P, Sacerdote C, et al. Hematopoietic cancer and peptic ulcer: a multicenter case-control study. *Carcinogenesis* 1999;20:1459–1463.
118. Ruskone-Fourmestraux A, Lavergne A, Aegerter PH, et al. Predictive factors for regression of gastric MALT lymphoma after anti-Helicobacter pylori treatment. *Gut* 2001;48:297–303.

119. Wotherspoon AC, Doglioni C, Diss TC, et al. Regression of primary low-grade B-cell gastric lymphoma of mucosa- associated lymphoid tissue type after eradication of Helicobacter pylori. *Lancet* 1993;342:575–577.

120. Neubauer A, Thiede C, Morgner A, et al. Cure of Helicobacter pylori infection and duration of remission of low-grade gastric mucosa-associated lymphoid tissue lymphoma. *J Natl Cancer Inst* 1997;89:1350–1355.

121. Beales IL, Calam J. Pathogenic mechanisms in Helicobacter pylori infection. *Hosp Med* 1998;59:186–190.

122. Paltiel O, Laniado DE, Yanetz R, et al. The risk of cancer following hospitalization for infection in infancy: a population-based cohort study. *Cancer Epidemiol Biomarkers Prev* 2006;15:1964–1968.

123. Law GR, Parslow RC, Roman E. Childhood cancer and population mixing. *Am J Epidemiol* 2003;158:328–336.

124. Boice JD Jr. Ionizing radiation. In: Schottenfeld D, Fraumeni JF Jr, eds. *Cancer epidemiology and prevention*, 3rd ed. New York, NY: Oxford University Press, Inc., 2006:259–293.

125. Preston DL, Kusumi S, Tomonaga M, et al. Cancer incidence in atomic bomb survivors. Part III. Leukemia, lymphoma and multiple myeloma, 1950–1987. *Radiat Res* 1994;1372 (suppl):S68–S97.

126. Muirhead CR, Bingham D, Haylock RG, et al. Follow up of mortality and incidence of cancer 1952–98 in men from the UK who participated in the UK's atmospheric nuclear weapon tests and experimental programmes. *Occup Environ Med* 2003;60:165–172.

127. Iwasaki T, Murata M, Ohshima S, et al. Second analysis of mortality of nuclear industry workers in Japan, 1986–1997. *Radiat Res* 2003;159:228–238.

128. Eheman CR, Tolbert PE, Coates RJ, et al. Case-control assessment of the association between non-Hodgkin's lymphoma and occupational radiation with doses assessed using a job exposure matrix. *Am J Ind Med* 2000;38:19–27.

129. Linet MS, Freedman DM, Mohan AK, et al. Incidence of haematopoietic malignancies in US radiologic technologists. *Occup Environ Med* 2005;62:861–867.

130. Zielinski JM, Garner MJ, Krewski D, et al. Decreases in occupational exposure to ionizing radiation among Canadian dental workers. *J Can Dent Assoc* 2005;71:29–33.

131. Inskip PD, Harvey EB, Boice JD Jr, et al. Incidence of childhood cancer in twins. *Cancer Causes Control* 1991;2:315–324.

132. Ron E, Boice JD Jr, Hamburger S, et al. Mortality following radiation treatment for infertility of hormonal origin or amenorrhoea. *Int J Epidemiol* 1994;23:1165–1173.

133. Weiss HA, Darby SC, Doll R. Cancer mortality following X-ray treatment for ankylosing spondylitis. *Int J Cancer* 1994;59:327–338.

134. dos Santos Silva I, Malveiro F, Jones ME, et al. Mortality after radiological investigation with radioactive Thorotrast: a follow-up study of up to fifty years in Portugal. *Radiat Res* 2003;159:521–534.

135. Kricker A, Armstrong BK, Hughes AM, et al. Personal sun exposure and risk of non Hodgkin lymphoma: a pooled analysis from the InterLymph Consortium. *Int J Cancer* 2008;122:144–154.

136. Hartge P, Devesa SS, Grauman D, et al. Non-Hodgkin's lymphoma and sunlight. *J Natl Cancer Inst* 1996;88:298–300.

137. Ovesen L, Andersen R, Jakobsen J. Geographical differences in vitamin D status, with particular reference to European countries. *Proc Nutr Soc* 2003;62:813–821.

138. Freedman DM, Zahm SH, Dosemeci M. Residential and occupational exposure to sunlight and mortality from non-Hodgkin's lymphoma: composite threefold) case-control study. *BMJ* 1997;314:1451–1455.

139. Adami J, Gridley G, Nyren O, et al. Sunlight and non-Hodgkin's lymphoma: a population-based cohort study in Sweden. *Int J Cancer* 1999;80:641–645.

140. Hakansson N, Floderus B, Gustavsson P, et al. Occupational sunlight exposure and cancer incidence among Swedish construction workers. *Epidemiology* 2001;12:552–557.

141. Hartge P, Lim U, Freedman DM, et al. Ultraviolet radiation, dietary vitamin D, and risk of non-Hodgkin lymphoma United States). *Cancer Causes Control* 2006;17:1045–1052.

142. Hughes AM, Armstrong BK, Vajdic CM, et al. Pigmentary characteristics, sun sensitivity and non-Hodgkin lymphoma. *Int J Cancer* 2004;110:429–434.

143. Smedby KE, Hjalgrim H, Melbye M, et al. Ultraviolet radiation exposure and risk of malignant lymphomas. *J Natl Cancer Inst* 2005;97:199–209.

144. Savitz DA, Ahlbom A. Electromagnetic fields and radiofrequency radiation. In: Schottenfeld D, Fraumeni JF, eds. *Cancer epidemiology and prevention*, 3rd ed. New York, NY: Oxford University Press, 2006:306–321.

145. Villeneuve PJ, Agnew DA, Miller AB, et al. Non-Hodgkin's lymphoma among electric utility workers in Ontario: the evaluation of alternate indices of exposure to 60 Hz electric and magnetic fields. *Occup Environ Med* 2000;57:249–257.

146. Schroeder JC, Savitz DA. Lymphoma and multiple myeloma mortality in relation to magnetic field exposure among electric utility workers. *Am J Ind Med* 1997;32:392–402.

147. Linet MS, Taggart T, Severson RK, et al. Cellular telephones and non-Hodgkin lymphoma. *Int J Cancer* 2006;119:2382–2388.

148. Siemiatycki J, Richardson L, Boffetta P. Occupation. In: Schottenfeld D, Fraumeni JF, eds. *Cancer epidemiology and prevention*, 3rd ed. New York, NY: Oxford University Press, 2006:322–354.

149. Boffetta P, de Vocht F. Occupation and the risk of non-Hodgkin lymphoma. *Cancer Epidemiol Biomarkers Prev* 2007;16:369–372.

150. Occupational exposures in insecticide application, and some pesticides. IARC Working Group on the Evaluation of Carcinogenic Risks to Humans. Lyon, 16–23 October 1990. *IARC Monogr Eval Carcinog Risks Hum* 1991;53:5–586.

151. International Agency for Research on Cancer. *IARC monographs on the evaluation of carcinogenic risks to humans: dry cleaning, some chlorinated solvents and other industrial chemicals*. Lyon, France: International Agency for Research on Cancer, 1995.

152. IARC Working Group on the Evaluation of Carcinogenic Risks to Humans: Polychlorinated Dibenzo-Para-Dioxins and Polychlorinated Dibenzofurans. Lyon, France, 4–11 February 1997. *IARC Monogr Eval Carcinog Risks Hum* 1997;69:1–631.

153. Re-evaluation of some organic chemicals, hydrazine and hydrogen peroxide. Proceedings of the IARC Working Group on the Evaluation of Carcinogenic Risks to Humans. Lyon, France, 17–24 February 1998. *IARC Monogr Eval Carcinog Risks Hum* 1999;71(pt 1):1–315.

154. IARC working group on the evaluation of carcinogenic risks to humans: occupational exposures of hairdressers and barbers and personal use of hair colourants; some hair dyes, cosmetic colourants, industrial dyestuffs and aromatic amines. Proceedings. Lyon, France, 6–13 October 1992. *IARC Monogr Eval Carcinog Risks Hum* 1993;57:7–398.

155. Blair A, Sandler DP, Tarone R, et al. Mortality among participants in the agricultural health study. *Ann Epidemiol* 2005;15:279–285.

156. Mandel JH, Kelsh MA, Mink PJ, et al. Occupational trichloroethylene exposure and non-Hodgkin's lymphoma: a meta-analysis and review. *Occup Environ Med* 2006;63:597–607.

157. Raaschou-Nielsen O, Hansen J, McLaughlin JK, et al. Cancer risk among workers at Danish companies using trichloroethylene: a cohort study. *Am J Epidemiol* 2003;158):1182–1192.

158. Hansen J, Raaschou-Nielsen O, Christensen JM, et al. Cancer incidence among Danish workers exposed to trichloroethylene. *J Occup Environ Med* 2001;43:133–139.

159. Scott CS, Chiu WA. Trichloroethylene cancer epidemiology: a consideration of select issues. *Environ Health Perspect* 2006;114:1471–1478.

160. Smith MT, Jones RM, Smith AH. Benzene exposure and risk of non-Hodgkin lymphoma. *Cancer Epidemiol Biomarkers Prev* 2007;16:385–391.

161. Lamm SH, Engel A, Byrd DM. Non-Hodgkin lymphoma and benzene exposure: a systematic literature review. *Chem Biol Interact* 2005;153–154:231–237.

162. Engel LS, Lan Q, Rothman N. Polychlorinated biphenyls and non-Hodgkin lymphoma. *Cancer Epidemiol Biomarkers Prev* 2007;16:373–376.

163. De Roos AJ, Hartge P, Lubin JH, et al. Persistent organochlorine chemicals in plasma and risk of non-Hodgkin's lymphoma. *Cancer Res* 2005;65:11214–11226.

164. Hardell L, Eriksson M, Lindstrom G, et al. Case-control study on concentrations of organohalogen compounds and titers of antibodies to Epstein-Barr virus antigens in the etiology of non-Hodgkin's lymphoma. *Leuk Lymphoma* 2001;42:619–629.

165. Quintana PJ, Delfino RJ, Korrick S, et al. Adipose tissue levels of organochlorine pesticides and polychlorinated biphenyls and risk of non-Hodgkin's lymphoma. *Environ Health Perspect* 2004;112:854–861.

166. Mills PK, Yang R, Riordan D. Lymphohematopoietic cancers in the United Farm Workers of America (UFW), 1988–2001. *Cancer Causes Control* 2005;16:823–830.

167. Colt JS, Severson RK, Lubin J, et al. Organochlorines in carpet dust and non-Hodgkin lymphoma. *Epidemiology* 2005;16:516–525.

168. Colt JS, Davis S, Severson RK, et al. Residential insecticide use and risk of non-Hodgkin's lymphoma. *Cancer Epidemiol Biomarkers Prev* 2006;15:251–257.

169. Hartge P, Colt JS, Severson RK, et al. Residential herbicide use and risk of non-Hodgkin's lymphoma. *Cancer Epidemiol Biomarkers Prev* 2005;14:934–937.

170. Ward MH, Mark SD, Cantor KP, et al. Drinking water nitrate and the risk of non-Hodgkin's lymphoma. *Epidemiology* 1996;7:465–471.

171. Ward MH, Cerhan JR, Colt JS, et al. Risk of non-Hodgkin lymphoma and nitrate and nitrite from drinking water and Diet. *Epidemiology* 2006;17:375–382.

172. McNally RJ, Parker L. Environmental factors and childhood acute leukemias and lymphomas. *Leuk Lymphoma* 2006;47:583–598.

173. Morton LM, Hartge P, Holford TR, et al. Cigarette smoking and risk of non-Hodgkin lymphoma: a pooled analysis from the International Lymphoma Epidemiology Consortium (interLymph). *Cancer Epidemiol Biomarkers Prev* 2005;14:925–933.

174. Besson H, Brennan P, Becker N, et al. Tobacco smoking, alcohol drinking and non-Hodgkin's lymphoma: a European multicenter case-control study (Epilymph). *Int J Cancer* 2006;119:901–908.

175. Schollkopf C, Smedby KE, Hjalgrim H, et al. Cigarette smoking and risk of non-Hodgkin's lymphoma—a population-based case-control study. *Cancer Epidemiol Biomarkers Prev* 2005;14:1791–1796.

176. Parker AS, Cerhan JR, Dick F, et al. Smoking and risk of non-Hodgkin lymphoma subtypes in a cohort of older women. *Leuk Lymphoma* 2000;37:341–349.

177. Lim U, Morton LM, Subar AF, et al. Alcohol, smoking, and body size in relation to incident Hodgkin's and non-Hodgkin's lymphoma risk. *Am J Epidemiol* 2007;166:697–708.

178. Nieters A, Kallinowski B, Brennan P, et al. Hepatitis C and risk of lymphoma: results of the European multicenter case-control study EPI-LYMPH. *Gastroenterology* 2006;131:1879–1886.

179. Morton LM, Zheng T, Holford TR, et al. Alcohol consumption and risk of non-Hodgkin lymphoma: a pooled analysis. *Lancet Oncol* 2005;6:469–476.

180. Nieters A, Deeg E, Becker N. Tobacco and alcohol consumption and risk of lymphoma: results of a population-based case-control study in Germany. *Int J Cancer* 2006;118:422–430.

181. Gaziano JM, Gaziano TA, Glynn RJ, et al. Light-to-moderate alcohol consumption and mortality in the Physicians' Health Study enrollment cohort. *J Am Coll Cardiol* 2000;35:96–105.

182. Chiu BC, Cerhan JR, Gapstur SM, et al. Alcohol consumption and non-Hodgkin lymphoma in a cohort of older women. *Br J Cancer* 1999;80:1476–1482.

183. Skibola CF. Obesity, diet and risk of non-Hodgkin lymphoma. *Cancer Epidemiol Biomarkers Prev* 2007;16:392–395.

184. Willett EV, Morton LM, Hartge P, et al. Non-Hodgkin lymphoma and obesity: a pooled analysis from the InterLymph Consortium. *Int J Cancer* 2008;122:2062–2070.

185. Maskarinec G, Erber E, Gill J, et al. Overweight and obesity at different times in life as risk factors for non-Hodgkin's lymphoma: the multiethnic cohort. *Cancer Epidemiol Biomarkers Prev* 2008;17:196–203.

186. Wolk A, Gridley G, Svensson M, et al. A prospective study of obesity and cancer risk (Sweden). *Cancer Causes Control* 2001;12:13–21.

187. Oh SW, Yoon YS, Shin SA. Effects of excess weight on cancer incidences depending on cancer sites and histologic findings among men: Korea National Health Insurance Corporation Study. *J Clin Oncol* 2005;23:4742–4754.

188. Batty GD, Shipley MJ, Jarrett RJ, et al. Obesity and overweight in relation to organ-specific cancer mortality in London (UK): findings from the original Whitehall study. *Int J Obes (Lond)* 2005;29:1267–1274.

189. Calle EE, Rodriguez C, Walker-Thurmond K, et al. Overweight, obesity, and mortality from cancer in a prospectively studied cohort of U.S. adults. *N Engl J Med* 2003;348:1625–1638.

190. Fernberg P, Odenbro A, Bellocco R, et al. Tobacco use, body mass index and the risk of malignant lymphomas—a nationwide cohort study in Sweden. *Int J Cancer* 2006;118:2298–2302.

191. Cerhan JR, Janney CA, Vachon CM, et al. Anthropometric characteristics, physical activity, and risk of non-Hodgkin's lymphoma subtypes and B-cell chronic lymphocytic leukemia: a prospective study. *Am J Epidemiol* 2002;156:527–535.

192. Brownson RC, Chang JC, Davis JR, et al. Physical activity on the job and cancer in Missouri. *Am J Public Health* 1991;81:639–642.

193. Zahm SH, Hoffman-Goetz L, Dosemeci M, et al. Occupational physical activity and non-Hodgkin's lymphoma. *Med Sci Sports Exerc* 1999;31:566–571.

194. Polednak AP. College athletics, body size, and cancer mortality. *Cancer* 1976;38:382–387.

195. Paffenbarger RS Jr, Lee IM, Wing AL. The influence of physical activity on the incidence of site-specific cancers in college alumni. *Adv Exp Med Biol* 1992;322:7–15.

196. Pan SY, Mao Y, Ugnat AM. Physical activity, obesity, energy intake, and the risk of non-Hodgkin's lymphoma: a population-based case-control study. *Am J Epidemiol* 2005;162:1162–1173.

197. Cerhan JR, Bernstein L, Severson RK, et al. Anthropometrics, physical activity, related medical conditions, and the risk of non-Hodgkin lymphoma. *Cancer Causes Control* 2005;16:1203–1214.

198. Zhang Y, Sanjose SD, Bracci PM, et al. Personal use of hair dye and the risk of certain subtypes of non-Hodgkin lymphoma. *Am J Epidemiol* 2008;167:1321–1331.

199. Grodstein F, Hennekens CH, Colditz GA, et al. A prospective study of permanent hair dye use and hematopoietic cancer. *J Natl Cancer Inst* 1994;86:1466–1470.

200. Altekruse SF, Henley SJ, Thun MJ. Deaths from hematopoietic and other cancers in relation to permanent hair dye use in a large prospective study (United States). *Cancer Causes Control* 1999;10:617–625.

201. Morton LM, Bernstein L, Wang SS, et al. Hair dye use, genetic variation in N-acetyltransferase 1 (NAT1) and 2 (NAT2), and risk of non-Hodgkin lymphoma. *Carcinogenesis* 2007;28:1759–1764.

202. Adami HO, Tsaih S, Lambe M, et al. Pregnancy and risk of non-Hodgkin's lymphoma: a prospective study. *Int J Cancer* 1997;70:155–158.

203. Nelson RA, Levine AM, Bernstein L. Reproductive factors and risk of intermediate- or high-grade B-Cell non-Hodgkin's lymphoma in women. *J Clin Oncol* 2001;19:1381–1387.

204. Cerhan JR, Habermann TM, Vachon CM, et al. Menstrual and reproductive factors and risk of non-Hodgkin lymphoma: the Iowa women's health study (United States). *Cancer Causes Control* 2002;13:131–136.

205. Zhang Y, Holford TR, Leaderer B, et al. Menstrual and reproductive factors and risk of non-Hodgkin's lymphoma among Connecticut women. *Am J Epidemiol* 2004;160:766–773.

206. Roman E, Simpson J, Ansell P, et al. Perinatal and reproductive factors: a report on haematological malignancies from the UKCCS. *Eur J Cancer* 2005;41:749–759.

207. Brinton LA, Gridley G, Persson I, et al. Cancer risk after a hospital discharge diagnosis of endometriosis. *Am J Obstet Gynecol* 1997;176:572–579.

208. Olson JE, Cerhan JR, Janney CA, et al. Postmenopausal cancer risk after self-reported endometriosis diagnosis in the Iowa Women's Health Study. *Cancer* 2002;94:1612–1618.

209. Adami J, Glimelius B, Cnattingius S, et al. Maternal and perinatal factors associated with non-Hodgkin's lymphoma among children. *Int J Cancer* 1996;65:774–777.

210. Cerhan JR, Vachon CM, Habermann TM, et al. Hormone replacement therapy and risk of non-Hodgkin lymphoma and chronic lymphocytic leukemia. *Cancer Epidemiol Biomarkers Prev* 2002;11:1466–1471.

211. Schiff D, Suman VJ, Yang P, et al. Risk factors for primary central nervous system lymphoma: a case-control study. *Cancer* 1998;82:975–982.

212. Skibola CF, Curry JD, Nieters A. Genetic susceptibility to lymphoma. *Haematologica* 2007;92:960–969.

213. Rothman N, Skibola CF, Wang SS, et al. Genetic variation in TNF and IL10 and risk of non-Hodgkin lymphoma: a report from the InterLymph Consortium. *Lancet Oncol* 2006;7:27–38.

214. Wang SS, Cerhan JR, Hartge P, et al. Common genetic variants in proinflammatory and other immunoregulatory genes and risk for non-Hodgkin lymphoma. *Cancer Res* 2006;66:9771–9780.

215. Wang SS, Cozen W, Cerhan JR, et al. Immune mechanisms in non-Hodgkin lymphoma: joint effects of the TNF G308A and IL10 T3575A polymorphisms with non-Hodgkin lymphoma risk factors. *Cancer Res* 2007;67:5042–5054.

216. Lim U, Wang SS, Hartge P, et al. Gene-nutrient interactions among determinants of folate and one-carbon metabolism on the risk of non-Hodgkin lymphoma: NCI-SEER case-control study. *Blood* 2007;109:3050–3059.

217. Purdue MP, Hartge P, Davis S, et al. Sun exposure, vitamin D receptor gene polymorphisms and risk of non-Hodgkin lymphoma. *Cancer Causes Control* 2007;18:989–999.

218. Morton LM, Schenk M, Hein DW, et al. Genetic variation in N-acetyltransferase 1 (NAT1) and 2 (NAT2) and risk of non-Hodgkin lymphoma. *Pharmacogenet Genomics* 2006;16:537–545.

219. Cerhan JR, Ansell SM, Fredericksen ZS, et al. Genetic variation in 1253 immune and inflammation genes and risk of non-Hodgkin lymphoma. *Blood* 2007;110:4455–4463.

220. Novik KL, Spinelli JJ, Macarthur AC, et al. Genetic variation in <H2>AFX contributes to risk of non-Hodgkin lymphoma. *Cancer Epidemiol Biomarkers Prev* 2007;16:1098–1106.

221. Skibola CF, Nieters A, Bracci PM, et al. A functional TNFRSF5 gene variant is associated with risk of lymphoma. *Blood* 2008;111:4348–4354.

222. Alizadeh AA, Eisen MB, Davis RE, et al. Distinct types of diffuse large B-cell lymphoma identified by gene expression profiling. *Nature* 2000;403:503–511.

223. Bea S, Zettl A, Wright G, et al. Diffuse large B-cell lymphoma subgroups have distinct genetic profiles that influence tumor biology and improve gene-expression-based survival prediction. *Blood* 2005;106:3183–3190.

224. Dave SS, Wright G, Tan B, et al. Prediction of survival in follicular lymphoma based on molecular features of tumor-infiltrating immune cells. *N Engl J Med* 2004;351:2159–2169.

225. Dave SS, Fu K, Wright GW, et al. Molecular diagnosis of Burkitt's lymphoma. *N Engl J Med* 2006;354:2431–2442.

226. Hans CP, Weisenburger DD, Greiner TC, et al. Confirmation of the molecular classification of diffuse large B-cell lymphoma by immunohistochemistry using a tissue microarray. *Blood* 2004;103:275–282.

227. Baecklund E, Backlin C, Iliadou A, et al. Characteristics of diffuse large B cell lymphomas in rheumatoid arthritis. *Arthritis Rheum* 2006;54:3774–3781.

228. Fang NY, Greiner TC, Weisenburger DD, et al. Oligonucleotide microarrays demonstrate the highest frequency of ATM mutations in the mantle cell subtype of lymphoma. *Proc Natl Acad Sci U S A* 2003;100:5372–5377.

229. Chiu BC, Dave BJ, Blair A, et al. Agricultural pesticide use and risk of t(14;18)-defined subtypes of non-Hodgkin lymphoma. *Blood* 2006;108:1363–1369.

CHAPTER 6 ■ INFECTIOUS ETIOLOGY OF LYMPHOMA

RICHARD F. AMBINDER

Among the infectious agents associated with lymphoma, there is great diversity. Viral, bacterial, and parasitic infections have all been implicated. Several very different mechanisms of lymphomagenesis seem to be operative. Viruses may immortalize or transform lymphocytes yielding tumor cells that harbor viral genomes as episomes or integrated viral or proviral genomes; whereas other viruses, bacteria, and parasites may stimulate proliferation and activation of uninfected lymphocytes through antigen-specific or other receptors and signaling pathways. Infectious agents may also lead to immune dysfunction that is permissive for the emergence of lymphoma. This chapter is organized by classes of agents (gammaherpesviruses, retroviruses, hepatitis C virus [HCV], *Helicobacter* and other bacterial agents, and malaria). Each section begins with a discussion of the pathogen and proceeds to a discussion of associated lymphomas. Table 6.1 provides a compilation organized by lymphoma types. The chapter concludes with a discussion of common features and themes in pathogenesis among diverse infectious agents.

THE GAMMAHERPESVIRUSES AND ASSOCIATED LYMPHOMAS

Recognition of endemic Burkitt lymphoma (BL) led to the discovery of Epstein-Barr virus (EBV) and provided the first evidence that some human tumors might be viral in origin (1,2) (Fig. 6.1 and Table 6.1). Although initially greeted with skepticism, the notion that a herpesvirus might be a cancer virus was made biologically plausible by the discovery that EBV immortalized B cells in vitro. Appreciation that viral infection was not confined to equatorial Africa, but was nearly universal and was associated with acute infectious mononucleosis dashed any hopes that the relationship between virus and tumor might be simple (3). The observation that the EBV produced lymphomas following experimental infection in cotton-top marmosets and owl monkeys, and that viral deoxyribonucleic acid (DNA) was present in several different types of lymphomas as well as other malignancies indicated that the presence of viral DNA in tumor tissue was more than an epiphenomenon. Decades later the link between human gammaherpesvirus Kaposi sarcoma-associated herpesvirus (KSHV), also referred to as human herpesvirus 8, and lymphoma was much more rapidly accepted (4).

EBV and KSHV have a life cycle that involves two alternative states of infection (5,6) (Table 6.2). Viral gene expression associated with the production of virions is referred to as lytic (Fig. 6.2A). In virions, viral genomes are packaged as double-stranded linear DNA molecules in enveloped icosahedral capsids. Viral gene expression not associated with the production of new virions is referred to as latent (Fig. 6.2B). In latently infected cells, viral genomes are maintained as multicopy circular DNA episomes. These episomes replicate once per cell cycle using cellular replication machinery. During latent infection, viral gene expression may profoundly affect cellular function. Thus, expression of EBV latency viral proteins drives proliferation of infected lymphocytes, increasing the numbers of cells harboring viral genomes. It is predominantly in states of latency that EBV and KSHV are found in lymphoma cells.

Aspects of Epstein-Barr Virus Infection

EBV is a ubiquitous virus found in all adult populations throughout the world (2,5,7). The virus is transmitted in saliva (Fig. 6.3). Primary infection is usually asymptomatic and occurs in childhood. However, when delayed until adolescence or adulthood, infection is commonly associated with the syndrome of infectious mononucleosis characterized by cervical lymphadenopathy, pharyngitis, hepatosplenomegaly, atypical lymphocytosis, and the appearance of heterophile antibodies. The determinants of symptomatology are poorly understood. Symptomatic infection leaves an "immune scar" (8). Expression of interleukin (IL)-15Rα is lost in acute infectious mononucleosis, and remains undetectable in peripheral T and natural killer (NK) cells. This correlates with defective IL-15 responsiveness in vitro and appears to persist for years.

EBV has a tropism for B lymphocytes, although other cell types, including T cells, monocytes, and epithelial cells, are infected in vitro and in vivo. Virion attachment and virion entry are distinct processes (9). B-cell attachment involves an interaction between CD21, a component of the complement receptor, and the viral envelope glycoprotein gp350/220; entry requires a complex of three additional viral glycoproteins: gH, gL, and gp42, and an interaction with human leukocyte antigen class II acting as a coreceptor. Infection of resting B cells leads to cell proliferation. This proliferation leads to the spread of virus-infected cells throughout the B-cell compartment. In acute infectious mononucleosis, as many as several percentages of B cells may be EBV infected (10). Viral antigen expression in proliferating cells leads to a massive T-cell response characterized in part by expansion of activated CD45RO$^+$CD8$^+$ T cells (11). Tetramer staining shows that epitopes from immediate early and early lytic

TABLE 6.1

LYMPHOMA AND ASSOCIATED INFECTIOUS AGENTS

Cell type	Lymphoma	Associated infectious agent	Comments about mechanisms
B cell	Bl	EBV	Viral genes may drive proliferation early in pathogenesis; later more restricted expression of viral genes may protect against apoptosis.
		P. falciparum	Chronic activation of signaling pathways leads to polyclonal B-cell lymphoproliferation, T-cell immunosuppression.
		HIV	HIV activation of polyclonal B-cell proliferation and AID expression.
	PEL	KSHV	Viral genes may protect against apoptosis, drive proliferation.
		EBV	Viral genes may protect against apoptosis and suppress KSHV lytic reactivation.
		HIV	Immunosuppression and/or chronic B-cell activation may be important.
	Primary central nervous system lymphoma	EBV	Viral genes likely drive tumor proliferation and protect against apoptosis.
		HIV	Immunosuppression.
	Plasmablastic lymphoma	KSHV	Viral genes may protect against apoptosis and suppress KSHV lytic reactivation.
		EBV	Viral genes likely drive tumor proliferation and protect against apoptosis.
		HIV	Immunosuppression and/or chronic B-cell activation may be important.
	Polymorphic posttransplant lymphoproliferative disease	EBV	Viral genes likely drive tumor proliferation and protect against apoptosis.
	Monomorphic posttransplant lymphoproliferative disease	EBV	Viral genes likely drive tumor proliferation and protect against apoptosis.
	Splenic lymphoma with villous lymphocytes	HCV	Chronic B-cell activation.
	Marginal zone lymphoma	HCV	Chronic B-cell activation.
	Gastric MALT lymphoma	H. pylori	Chronic B-cell activation.
	Extranodal marginal zone lymphoma (immunoproliferative small intestinal disease)	C. jejuni	Chronic antigen stimulation.
	Primary cutaneous B-cell lymphoma	B. burgdorferi	Chronic B-cell activation.
	Ocular adenexal lymphoma	C. psittaci	Chronic B-cell activation.
	Age-related EBV lymphoproliferative disease	EBV	Viral genes may protect against apoptosis and drive proliferation.
T or NK cell	ATL	HTLV-1	Viral genes likely drive tumor proliferation early in pathogenesis, engender genetic instability, and protect against apoptosis.
		Strongyloides	May activate cognate T-cell clones harboring HTLV-1.
	Nasal and nasal type NK/T lymphoma	EBV	Viral genes may protect against apoptosis and drive lymphoproliferation.

proteins and the Epstein-Barr nuclear antigen (EBNA) 3 family of latency nuclear antigens (EBNA3A, 3B, and 3C) are immunodominant. As the cellular immune response is established, expression of viral antigens serves to target latently infected proliferating B cells for immune destruction. Ultimately, EBV persists in resting B lymphocytes with very limited viral gene expression (12–14).

Virus is periodically shed in the saliva of individuals who are seropositive. Acyclovir treatment eliminates lytic viral replication as evidenced by the inability to detect EBV in throat washings (15). However, the number of latently infected B cells in the blood is unaffected. Treatment with the monoclonal antibody rituximab that targets the pan B-cell antigen CD20, depletes B lymphocytes from peripheral blood, and leads to a fall in viral DNA in lymphocytes (13). However, such treatment does not abolish salivary shedding of virus (16). Thus, although there may be interactions between the two compartments, in the short term, the levels of viral DNA are independent of each other. Patients with the congenital absence of B cells (X-linked agammaglobulinemia) appear not to maintain EBV infection in either the oropharynx or lymphocytes (17).

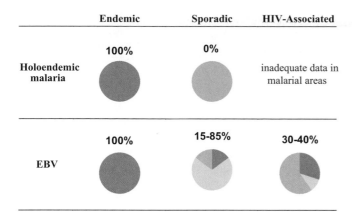

	Endemic	Sporadic	HIV-Associated
Holoendemic malaria	100%	0%	inadequate data in malarial areas
EBV	100%	15-85%	30-40%

FIGURE 6.1 Three distinct forms of BL. Endemic BL is associated with holoendemic malaria and with EBV. Sporadic BL is not associated with malaria and is variably (15% to 85%) associated with EBV. HIV-associated BL in Western Europe and North America is associated with EBV in only 30% to 40% of cases.

Epstein-Barr Virus Genes and B-Lymphocyte Immortalization

Viral infection of primary B cells yields lymphoblastoid cell lines that proliferate indefinitely (5). This functional property is variously referred to as immortalization or as lymphocyte transformation. The resultant lymphoblastoid cell lines are tumorigenic in immunodeficient mice (18). Recombinant genetic analysis has identified the viral genes required for immortalization (Fig. 6.4). These include EBNA1, EBNA2, EBNA3A, EBNA3C, and latency membrane protein (LMP) 1.

EBNA1 is necessary for episomal maintenance. It binds to the viral origin of replication used in latency and interacts with chromatin. Thus, it serves to tether viral episomes to chromatin. It also acts as a transcriptional transactivator (19). Studies of EBNA1 expression in transgenic mice have yielded conflicting results with regards to possible roles in tumorigenesis (20,21). EBNA2 is a transcriptional transactivator that regulates viral and cellular gene expression stimulating G0 to G1 cell cycle progression (22). In these effects,

TABLE 6.2

HUMAN GAMMAHERPESVIRUSES AND LYMPHOMA

		Virion	Lytic	Latent
EBV				
	Viral genome	ds DNA	Linear	Episome
	Sensitivity to antivirals such as ganciclovir		Yes	No
	Associated disease		Oral hairy leukoplakia	Lymphoma, carcinoma
KSHV				
	Viral genome	ds DNA	Linear	Episome
	Sensitivity to antivirals such as ganciclovir		Yes	No
	Associated disease		Castleman disease	Lymphoma, KS

ds, double-strand; KS, Karposi sarcoma.

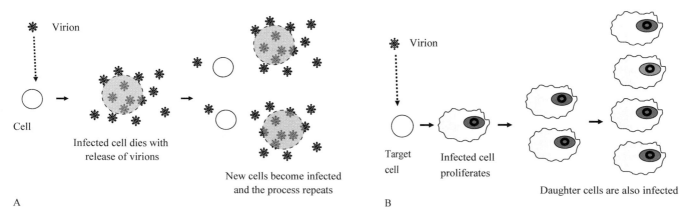

FIGURE 6.2 A: Lytic infection. A virion infects a cell. The viral DNA replicates, is packaged into virions, the cell is killed, and virions are released. New cells are infected, and the process repeats. **B:** Latent infection. A virion infects a cell. The cell expresses latency viral proteins that drive proliferation. No new virions are produced, but viral episomes that replicate in tandem with cellular DNA are passed on to daughter cells.

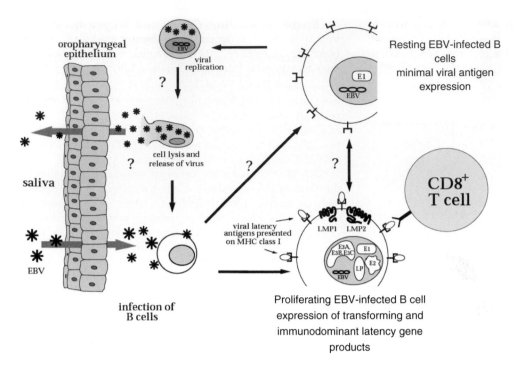

FIGURE 6.3 The EBV life cycle. Virus (*) is transmitted in saliva. B cells become infected. Viral protein expression leads to proliferation with expansion of the infected B-cell pool. Viral DNA is in episomal form (¥). Proliferating cells express EBNA1, 2, 3A, 3B, 3C, LP(leader protein), and LMP1 and LMP2. Expression of these antigens, particularly the immundominant EBNA3A, 3B, and 3C, renders infected cells susceptible to killing by CD8⁺ cytotoxic T cells. Some infected cells with limited antigen expression elude this surveillance. The viral proteins that drive proliferation are not expressed in these cells, and the cells are not cycling. These infected cells constitute the major latency reservoir of infection. Intermittently lytic cycle yields new virions that are released into saliva. Question marks (?) indicate transitions that are poorly understood. LP, leader protein; MHC, major histocompatibility complex. (Artwork courtesy of M. Victor Lemas.)

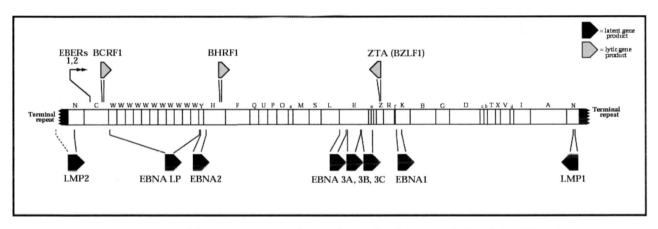

FIGURE 6.4 Map of the EBV genome. Viral genes discussed in the text are indicated. BamHI restriction fragments are designated by letters and associated vertical bars. A variable number of terminal repeats are present at the ends of the genome. LP, leader protein. (Artwork courtesy of M. Victor Lemas.)

EBNA2 mimics activated Notch, an evolutionarily conserved, surface receptor that mediates cell-cell signaling and influences cell fate. Both activated Notch and EBNA2 target promoters through the cellular DNA binding protein CSL (CBF1/SuH/Lag-1). CSL is highly conserved from worms to mammals, and influences cell fate decisions and proliferation versus differentiation. Bound to DNA, CSL acts as a transcriptional repressor, bringing to target promoters a histone deacetylase complex (23). EBNA2 and Notch compete away the corepressor complex and interact with coactivator proteins, including pCAF, CBP, and p300. Target viral promoters include the C promoter driving EBNA2 and the other EBNAs, as well as the LMP1 promoter and the promoters of a variety of cellular genes, including CD23. Members of the EBNA3 family (EBNA3A, 3B, 3C) have a common structure. They also share aspects of function insofar

as they each modulate the Notch signaling pathway. EBNA3A and 3C are required for immortalization, whereas EBNA3B is dispensable.

LMP1 is a member of the tumor necrosis factor (TNF) receptor (TNFR) superfamily (2,24). LMP1 is an integral membrane protein with cytoplasmic aminoterminus, cytoplasmic carboxyterminus, and six hydrophobic transmembrane domains that spontaneously oligomerize, leading to constitutive aggregation and signaling in the absence of ligand. In vitro expression is associated with transformation of immortalized rodent fibroblast cell lines, as marked by loss of contact inhibition, anchorage independent growth, and tumorigenesis in nude mice. In transgenic mice, expression under the control of an immunoglobulin (Ig) heavy chain regulatory locus leads to B-cell lymphomagenesis (25).

LMP1 expression leads to: activation of stress-activated protein kinases, nuclear factor-κB (NF-κB), c-Jun N-terminal kinase, mitogen-activated protein kinase, and p38 kinases; induction of activation markers (CD23, CD30, CD40); induction of cell adhesion molecules (intercellular adhesion molecule-1, lymphocyte function-associated antigen-3); antiapoptotic genes, including bcl2; and induction of IL-6. LMP1 also recruits signaling adapter molecules, including TNFR-associated factors 1, 2, and 3 to lipid rafts (26). In all of these regards, LMP1 resembles activated CD40. However, whereas activated CD40 also mediates TNFR-associated factor degradation, LMP1 does not (24). Activating protein 1 and signal transduction and activator of transcriptions 1 and 3 are also activated. Strain variation, particularly in the carboxyl terminus, is well recognized with some variants activating NF-κB more efficiently, whereas others activate protein 1 more efficiently.

Epstein-Barr Virus Latency Genes Relevant to Lymphomagenesis

Other EBV genes are not required for lymphocyte immortalization but are expressed in immortalized lymphocytes, and may play important roles in the viral life cycle and in tumorigenesis. LMP2A contains immunoreceptor tyrosine activation motifs, and LMP2A modulates the signaling pathways associated with the B-cell receptor (BCR) complex such that neither BCR engagement by antigen nor the absence of such engagement is fatal to the virus-harboring B cell (27,28). BCR engagement normally leads to Ca2$^+$ flux, and would precipitate lytic replication (Ca2$^+$ flux being a potent lytic cycle activator) and B-cell death. However, LMP2A recruitment of Lyn and Syk prevents the Ca2$^+$ flux. Conversely, LMP2A also substitutes for a BCR-mediated survival signal such that, in a transgenic mouse model, expression of LMP2A prevents death of B cells lacking membrane Ig (24,27). Both properties may contribute to the survival of EBV-infected B cells in vivo and to the survival of tumor cells expressing the protein. The Epstein-Barr-encoded ribonucleic acids (EBERs) 1 and 2 are the most abundant viral transcripts in EBV-infected lymphocytes (29). These ribonucleic acid (RNA) polymerase III transcripts do not code for protein, and their function remains uncertain. Other RNAs collectively referred to as the BamHI A rightward transcripts give rise to multiple micro-RNAs (30,31). Their functions remain poorly understood, but their tissue-specific differential expression may account for differences in viral antigen expression in epithelial and lymphoid tissues.

EBV lytic cycle is initiated by expression of the viral ZTA protein (32–35). This is a DNA-binding bZIP transcription factor whose expression initiates a cascade of events that leads to expression of delayed early genes, late genes, and ultimately packaging and release of infectious virus. ZTA mediates viral DNA replication at the lytic origin of replication and induces cell cycle arrest. Among the lytic genes encoded by the virus are two with homology to cellular genes implicated in tumorigenesis and another with homology to a cellular gene that regulates immune function. These are viral BCL2 family members, BHRF1 and BALF1, and a viral IL (vIL)-10 homologue vIL-10. BHRF1 shares functional properties with BCL2, whereas BALF1 appears to serve as an inhibitor of BHRF1 antiapoptotic activity (36). Insofar as the expression of the BCL2 family members is lim-

ited to lytically infected cells, any contributions to immortalization or maintenance of the malignant phenotype remain poorly understood. vIL-10 is presumed to modulate immune responses to viral infection. This is a function that presumably might impact on the ability of tumors to escape immune surveillance. However, there is very little evidence to date of expression by tumor cells (37).

Antiviral agents such as acyclovir and ganciclovir inhibit lytic cycle viral DNA replication (Table 6.2). These agents are phosphorylated by one of two viral kinases (viral thymidine kinase or viral protein kinase), and their phosphorylated products inhibit the viral DNA polymerase (38,39). The growth of the latently infected cells and replication of the episomal genome is not inhibited by these agents.

Epstein-Barr Virus Strain

Two viral strains have been recognized. In vitro and in murine studies suggest that A strain or type 1 virus is more efficient in immortalization and transformation than the less common B strain (5). The A strain predominates in most studies of tumors. However, B-strain virus is detected in some African BL and in tumors arising in homosexual patients with acquired immunodeficiency syndrome (AIDS). Whether A-strain predominance in tumors reflects increased pathogenicity or just prevalence is not clear. Many variations in viral genes have been described, including variants in EBNA1, LMP1, and ZTA (40). However, the role of strain variation in tumorigenesis remains uncertain.

Animal Models of Epstein-Barr Virus Lymphomagenesis

Several animal models have provided insights into EBV-associated tumorigenesis (41). Most Old World nonhuman primates harbor EBV-like herpesviruses. Cross-reactive immunity protects against EBV infection. However, in the setting of pharmacologic or viral immunosupression and perhaps other factors, lymphoproliferative disease with EBV-like viruses may emerge (42,43). New World primates are naturally infected by more distant gammaherpesviruses (44). Inoculation of some of these primates with EBV, notably tamarins, leads to B-cell lymphoproliferative disease, and vaccine studies have often focused on these animals (45–47). Mice with severe combined immunodeficiency develop EBV-associated B-cell tumors following transfer of peripheral blood mononuclear cells (PBMCs) from EBV-seropositive donors or transfer of PBMCs from EBV-seronegative donors followed by inoculation with EBV, or simply transfer of EBV-immortalized B-cell lines (18,48). In all of these models, whether primate or human engrafted into mouse, the lymphoproliferative disease is B cell, and patterns of viral gene expression resemble that seen in posttransplant lymphoproliferative disease.

Specific Tumors

Burkitt Lymphoma

BL occurs in three epidemiologically distinct forms (Fig. 6.1) (49). Endemic BL is among the most common cancers of childhood in equatorial areas of Africa and New Guinea (49–51). Elsewhere, sporadic BL occurs in children at a low to intermediate incidence depending on the geographic area.

A third form of BL occurs in individuals infected with human immunodeficiency virus (HIV), with incidence rates far above even that of the endemic tumor (51,52). The tumor is characterized by chromosome translocations involving the c-myc locus on chromosome 8 and an Ig locus, most commonly the heavy chain locus on chromosome 14. Although chromosomal translocations are similar in endemic and sporadic BL, characteristic breakpoints differ (53,54).

Endemic BL (in areas holoendemic for malaria) is uniformly associated with EBV. EBNA1 is the only viral protein consistently expressed in these tumors, although rare cells expressing other latency antigens or lytic antigens have been described (55). As noted previously, expression of EBNA1 does not drive the proliferation of cells in vitro. In transgenic mouse models, the association with lymphomagenesis is either weak or nonexistent (20,21). Thus, the contribution of the viral episome to tumor maintenance is poorly understood. The viral genes that drive lymphocyte immortalization (EBNA2, LMP1, EBNA3A, EBNA3C) are not expressed in BL (Fig. 6.5). The growth effects of these genes have often been invoked with regard to the biologic plausibility of EBV as a causative agent in BL, and it is possible that expression of these genes is important in early stages of the pathogenesis of the tumor. However, present evidence suggests that they do not contribute to tumor maintenance.

BL cells are shielded from CD8$^+$ T-cell immune surveillance because immunodominant viral proteins are not expressed and because they lack antigen-processing machinery (49,56). High-level c-myc expression characteristic of BL may account for both. High-level c-myc and EBNA2 expression are antagonistic in cell lines, and high-level c-myc expression leads to down-regulation of antigen-processing machinery (57–59).

The origin of BL, with respect to the cell type initially infected by EBV (naive or mature B cell), the timing of the c-myc translocation, passage through the germinal center, and possible evolution of patterns of viral gene expression during pathogenesis have generated considerable controversy (2,60). Expression of phenotypic markers characteristic of the germinal center and somatic hypermutation the V region of Ig genes suggests a germinal center origin for the lymphoma to some investigators. Study of chromosomal breakpoints that suggest errors in V-D-J joining (something that would occur before lymphocytes enter the germinal center) and the very restricted pattern of viral gene expression in BL (which parallels that in memory B cells) suggest a more complex pathogenesis. A review of the controversy and a detailed proposal for the evolution of the pattern of viral gene expression and the chromosomal translocations in BL have been presented (2).

Other B-Lineage Lymphoma

Hodgkin lymphoma (HL) requires mention in this context. EBV is detected in the tumor cells of approximately one-third of cases in Western Europe and North America, with a much higher percentage in areas of Africa and Latin America (61–63). Infectious mononucleosis is associated with an increased incidence of EBV-associated HL but not other HL or non-HL in Denmark (64). The interval between symptomatic primary infection and HL is typically several months to several years. Tumor cells express EBNA-1, LMP1, and LMP2 (Fig. 6.5). Virtually all cases of HL show Ig rearrangement as characterized by microdissection. Sequencing studies identify stop codons in a fraction of cases, and these may be consistently associated with EBV infection (65).

Lymphomatoid granulomatosis is a rare angiocentric and angiodestructive B-cell lymphoproliferative disease that often involves skin, lungs, brain, kidney, and other organs (66,67). Lesions consist of reactive T cells and neoplastic EBV-infected B cells. Only a few cases have been studied by immunohistochemistry to identify the pattern of EBV gene expression, but those reports indicate that EBNA2, LMP1, and the EBERs are expressed (68). It is associated with systemic symptoms and areas of necrosis within the tumor. The disease generally arises in older patients and may be associated with diminished immune surveillance (69).

Pyothorax-associated lymphoma arises in the setting of long-standing pyothorax and pulmonary tuberculosis, and is EBV associated (70,71). This is a solid lymphoma arising in

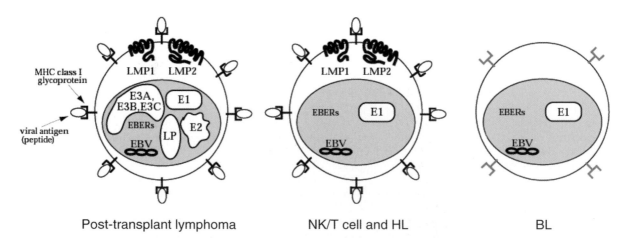

FIGURE 6.5 Viral gene expression in three types of lymphoma. Posttransplant lymphoproliferative disease is often associated with expression of the full range of viral latency antigens expressed in immortalized B cells. HL is associated with a more restricted pattern. BL is associated with the most restricted pattern. In BL, major histocompatibility complex (MHC) class I molecules are often down-regulated, and antigens are not processed for presentation. (Artwork courtesy of M. Victor Lemas.)

the pleural space (vs. primary effusion lymphoma [PEL] that may present in the pleural space as a malignant effusion). Patients had previously been treated for tuberculosis in the preantibiotic era with therapeutic pneumothorax maintained by placement of Ping-Pong balls in the pleural space. Typically, chronic suppurative infection and pyothorax developed. Tumors are diagnosed with a latency of >20 years from the time of the pneumothorax.

Senile or Age-Associated Lymphoproliferative Disease

EBV-associated lymphoproliferative disorders arising in older patients without history of immunodeficiency have recently received attention (67,72,73). Tumors have a predilection for extranodal sites. Tumors have been subdivided into polymorphous type (broad range of differentiation in an inflammatory background) and large cell type (monomorphic large cells). EBV expression includes LMP1 and often EBNA2. Attention has been drawn to the entity by reports from Japan, but it may be more widespread. Immunodeficiency associated with aging may be an important aspect of the pathogenesis.

Lymphoma Arising in the Setting of Immunodeficiency

Congenital immunodeficiencies associated with lymphoproliferative diseases include severe combined immunodeficiency, ataxia telangiectasia, Wiskott-Aldrich syndrome, hyper-IgM syndrome, and X-linked lymphoproliferative disease (74–77). EBV infection in such patients may manifest as fatal infectious mononucleosis, dysgammaglobulinemia, and lymphoma. Diffuse large B-cell lymphoma, including primary central nervous system lymphoma, BL, and polymorphic lymphoproliferations, resembles those seen in the posttransplant setting and EBV-associated HL. Some lymphomas in congenital immunodeficiency syndromes, notably ataxia telangiectasia, but even in X-linked lymphoproliferative disease, are not EBV associated.

Following solid organ or bone marrow transplantation, lymphoproliferative diseases arise in approximately 0.5% to 10% of recipients (78). Allogeneic immune responses, whether those associated with organ rejection in solid organ transplant recipients or those associated with graft versus host disease in bone marrow and stem cell recipients, are associated with an increased incidence of lymphoproliferative disorder. Similarly, many immunosuppressive therapies used to prevent or reduce these responses are also associated with increased risk, such as the use of OKT3 antibodies in either setting. However, not all such therapies are associated with increased risk. In particular, in the bone marrow or hematopoietic stem cell setting, the selective removal of T cells from the graft product (such as is accomplished with OKT3 antibody that targets CD3 on T cells) dramatically increases risk, whereas balanced removal of T cells and B cells (such as is accomplished with either the Campath antibody that targets CD52 on T cells and B cells) is not associated with any increased risk (79–82). Whether B-cell depletion protects against the development of EBV tumors because it reduces the pool of virus-infected cells or because it reduces the pool of cells that might potentially be infected by virus is unknown.

Another difference in risk factors between organ and bone marrow or hematopoietic transplantation is that EBV seronegativity in the recipient is only important as a risk factor in organ transplantation (79). This is presumably because

in that setting the organ transplant recipient has no immunologic experience with EBV. In contrast, in the bone marrow/hematopoietic transplant setting, the recipient's immune system is generally replaced by the donor's, and, thus, the recipient's immunologic experience is largely irrelevant.

EBV is usually associated with B-cell lymphoproliferative disease arising soon after transplantation. Lesions arising several years after transplantation are often but not always EBV associated. Some of these tumors express the full spectrum of antigens expressed by EBV-immortalized lymphoblastoid cell lines, whereas others much more restricted patterns of viral gene expression (Fig. 6.5). Lack of immune surveillance is thought to play a critical role in the pathogenesis of posttransplant lymphoma (83,84). This idea was strengthened when it was demonstrated that adoptive cellular immunotherapy was useful, particularly in the bone marrow transplant setting (85,86). In some instances, tumors regressed with administration of EBV-specific T cells. In other instances, patients at high risk received EBV-specific T-cell prophylaxis.

An antibody targeting CD20, a B-cell surface antigen, has proven very useful in the management of posttransplant lymphoproliferative disease (13,87). Approximately half of patients will respond to this therapy. However, following its administration, there is virtually always a fall in EBV copy number in PBMCs that accompanies the depletion of B cells. This B-cell depletion and fall in EBV copy number occur independently of tumor response, and, thus, rituximab therapy may render viral copy number measurement in PBMC irrelevant.

Immunosuppressive drugs used in nontransplant settings may also be associated with EBV lymphoma. Attention has particularly focused on lymphoma arising in the context of methotrexate or anti-TNF therapy for rheumatoid arthritis (88) and fludarabine for the treatment of lymphoid malignancies or as part of a conditioning regimen for allogeneic transplant (89–92). However, the risk associated with treatments for rheumatoid arthritis has been called into question (93).

Approximately half of AIDS lymphomas are EBV associated (94). Primary central nervous system lymphomas in patients with AIDS are virtually always EBV associated (95,96). Other large B-cell lymphomas, particularly those with immunoblastic features, are also usually EBV associated, as are plasmablastic oral lymphomas (94,97–99). Low CD4+ T-cell counts identify patients with AIDS at especially high risk for EBV non-HL. Patients with brain lymphoma generally have CD4+ counts that are <20 per μL (100). Higher but not normal CD4+ counts (>200 per μL) that are often seen in patients receiving antiretroviral therapy are associated with an increased risk of HL (99).

Natural Killer/T-Cell Lymphoma and Leukemia and Peripheral T-Cell Tumors

EBV has been associated with a variety of peripheral T-cell tumors 67 (Table 6.1). Nasal and nasal type NK/T-cell lymphomas are very closely linked with EBV (101,102). The pattern of viral gene expression is similar to that in EBV-associated HL, i.e., EBNA1, LMP1, and LMP2 are expressed, but not EBNA2, 3A, 3B, or 3C (Fig. 6.5) (103). EBV is also present in most cases of NK-cell leukemia, and the presence of virus is one of the features that distinguishes it from a more indolent NK-cell lymphoproliferative disorder (101,104,105).

Aspects of Kaposi Sarcoma-Associated Herpesvirus Infection and Associated Lymphoproliferative Disease

KSHV was discovered in association with Kaposi sarcoma. Subsequently, viral DNA was identified in lymphoma (106). Serologic evidence of viral infection is most common in men who have sex with men, and in certain Southern European, Mediterranean, African, and indigenous South American populations. The mode of transmission is poorly understood, but in men who have sex with men, seroprevalence is increased in men with many sexual partners. Increasing evidence suggests salivary transmission in areas where viral infection is endemic (107,108). In vivo the virus is found in B cells, endothelial cells, epithelial cells, and macrophages (109,110).

KSHV infects but does not immortalize primary lymphocytes in vitro. Viral genes expressed in lymphoma tumor cell lines are shown in Table 6.3 (94,111–113). Latent-associated nuclear antigen tethers the viral episome to chromatin, and interacts with cellular transcriptional regulatory proteins, including p53, Rb, and components of the SAP30 corepressor complex, to bring about alterations in increased cell survival and proliferation. Latent-associated nuclear antigen also sequesters glycogen synthase kinase 3 in the nucleus, resulting in elevated levels of β catenin, which promotes cell proliferation (114). Viral FLICE inhibitory protein protects against apoptosis and is a potent activator of the NF-κB pathway. Viral cyclin associates with cycle-dependent kinase proteins, and promotes phosphorylation of retinoblastoma protein and other cellular targets modulating cell cycle checkpoints and DNA damage responses. The kaposin transcript encodes three different proteins corresponding to different protein start sites and reading frames (115,116) and 11 micro-RNAs. Kaposin A leads to focus formation, anchorage-independent growth, and tumorigenicity in immortalized murine cell lines (117). Some of its effects are mediated through its association with cytohesin-1, a guanine nucleotide exchange factor, which regulates integrin activity. Kaposin B modulates the mitogen-activated protein kinase pathways prolonging the half-life of various labile cytoplasmic messenger RNAs (mRNAs), including many cytokine and growth factor transcripts (116). miR-K12-11 targets cellular mRNAs regulating the germinal center reaction during B-cell maturation. In this regard it parallels the cellular micro-RNA miR-155.

Several other proteins expressed in lytic cycle may contribute to transformation. Some may be expressed in both latent and lytic infection, whereas others may act as cytokines or chemokines, leading to growth changes in nearby cells. K15 is a 12-transmembrane spanning constitutive signaling receptor. Interactions between K15 and TNFR-associated factors lead to activation of mitogen-activated protein kinases extracellular signal-regulated kinase, c-Jun N-terminal kinase, and NF-κB and activating protein 1. Similar to LMP2 of EBV, K15 interrupts BCR signal transduction. K15 is expressed in lytic infection but may also be expressed in latency and is sometimes referred to as latency associated membrane protein. There are four viral interferon regulatory factors (vIRFs) encoded by KSHV. vIRF3 differs from the others in that it appears only to be expressed in B cells (both in PELs and in Castleman disease). vIRF3 binds to and inhibits the apoptotic activity of p53, and interferes with cellular interferon regulatory factors (118–120). An IL-6 homologue, vIL-6, is encoded by the virus (121,122). It induces proliferation and angiogenesis in IL-6-dependent cell lineages, induces vascular endothelial growth factor, and serves as an autocrine growth factor for PEL cell lines. Immunohistochemistry shows high-level expression in some PEL primary tissues (123). The viral cytokine promoter is similar in its actions to IL-6 but differs in the details. For example, cells that express only gp130 (one of two subunits that bind human IL-6) respond to vIL-6, vascular endothelial growth factor production, and B-cell growth in vitro. Expression is increased following lytic cycle induction. Yet other proteins encoded by the virus and expressed in lytic infection with properties that suggest a possible role in transformation are K1, vIRF1, and viral glucorticoid receptor (94,113).

TABLE 6.3

VIRAL GENES EXPRESSED IN EBV AND KSHV ASSOCIATED LYMPHOMA

Virus	Viral gene	BL	Nasal NK and HL	Polymorphous posttransplant lymphoproliferative disease	PEL
EBV	EBNA1	x	x	x	x
	EBNA2			x	
	EBNA3A,B,C			x	
	LMP1		x	x	
	LMP2		x	x	
	EBERs	x	x	x	x
	LANA				x
	vFLIP				x
	vCYC				x
KSHV	Kaposin A, B				x
	vIRF3				x
	vIL6				x

LANA, latent-associated nuclear antigen; vCYC, viral cyclin; vFLIP, viral FLICE inhibitory protein.

Whereas Kaposi sarcoma is always associated with KSHV, most B-cell lymphomas are not associated with KSHV. PEL usually arises in body cavities, and the tumor cells are often present as malignant effusions (106,124). These tumor cells harbor KSHV and often EBV. The cells are monoclonal with Ig gene rearrangement but express few of the usual markers of B-cell differentiation. In contrast with BL, there is no consistent cytogenetic abnormality identified, but cells are consistently aneuploid.

The virus is also often associated with a benign nonclonal lymphoproliferative disease, multicentric Castleman disease. The association is particularly strong in patients with HIV infection and in organ transplant recipients (125). Immunohistochemistry and in situ hybridization show the presence of virus in the B cells of the follicular mantle. Phenotypic analysis consistently shows cytoplasmic λ light chain expression (126). However, Ig gene analysis shows that multicentric Castleman disease is not a clonal disease.

THE RETROVIRUSES

The discovery of the human retroviruses implicated in human malignancy, human T-cell lymphotropic virus I (HTLV-1) and HIV, followed the clinical characterization of associated diseases. Thus, the description of the syndrome of adult T-cell leukemia/lymphoma (ATL) and its peculiar geographic clustering in 1977 led to the study of T-cell lymphoblastoid cell lines and peripheral T cells harboring HTLV-1 (127–129) (Fig. 6.6). Similarly, recognition of the AIDS led to culture and characterization of HIV-1 (130).

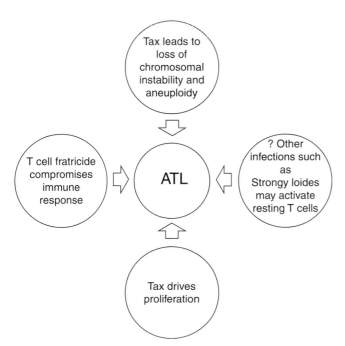

FIGURE 6.6 Pathogenesis of ATL. HTLV-1 and perhaps another infectious cofactor or factors are important in pathogenesis. The Tax protein is known to drive the proliferation of infected lymphocytes, to lead to chromosomal instability and aneuploidy. Activation of T cells may render them especially susceptible to infection and, thus, lead to fratricidal killing. Antigen-receptor interaction may also directly stimulate proliferation of the malignant clone.

Since the early 1900s, retroviruses had been known to be associated with malignancies in animals. Acutely transforming retroviruses induce tumors within days of infection. These viruses carry viral homologues of cellular protooncogenes. Expression of the viral onc genes led to transformation of infected cells, whereas the loss of required viral genes rendered them replication defective, except in the presence of a helper virus that supplies required functions. Although integration of proviral DNA is part of the viral life cycle, the locus of the integration site is not important to their ability to transform. Chronically transforming retroviruses produce tumors slowly. They lack a viral onc gene. Transformation is the result of integration of the viral genome adjacent to cellular genes that regulate proliferation or signaling pathways (insertional mutagenesis). Thus, the site of integration is central to their role in transformation. The study of acute and chronic transforming retroviruses has led to many insights into the molecular biology of tumorigenesis, but neither of these general mechanisms of transformation appears to be involved with human retroviruses and their associated tumors. In contrast to these acutely or chronically transforming retroviruses, HTLV-1 leads to the development of malignancy only after decades and in <5% of individuals who are infected (129). There is no targeted integration site or sites that are crucial to tumorigenesis, although a preference for A/T-rich sequences has been suggested (131). HIV-1 infection also leads to malignancy, but the pathogenesis of AIDS-related lymphoma is entirely distinct from the retroviruses discussed previously, and HIV is not present in the tumors it engenders.

The acute and chronic transforming retroviruses and the human retroviruses have in common two identical, plus-sense single-stranded RNA molecules that are noncovalently linked. Viral proteins include coat proteins encoded by the env gene, nonglycosylated core proteins encoded by the gag gene, and nonstructural proteins encoded by the pol gene. The latter include the reverse transcriptase and ribonuclease H, which together generate double-stranded circular proviral DNA from single-stranded viral RNA, the viral integrase that mediates integration of the proviral DNA into the host genome, and the protease that processes large precursor polyproteins. Following cell entry, reverse transcriptase within the viral capsid initiates synthesis of DNA from plus-sense RNA. The RNA is displaced, and the DNA is used as a template to generate a complementary DNA strand. The double-stranded proviral DNA is ultimately transported into the nucleus. Then the viral integrase (also carried within the virion) mediates integration into the host genome.

The human genome carries endogenous and exogenous retroviruses. The endogenous retroviruses are inherited as genetic elements in chromosomal DNA. Most, but not all, are defective or incomplete. None of the endogenous human retroviruses has yet been shown to be associated with malignancy. The exogenous human retroviruses, in contrast, are horizontally transmitted, and at least two are associated with lymphoma. These are HTLV-1 associated with ATL and HIV-1 associated with a variety of B-lineage lymphomas. In addition to the gag, pol, and env proteins encoded by all replication competent retroviruses, the human retroviruses use alternative splicing and internal initiation codons to produce several additional regulatory and accessory proteins, some of which are essential for efficient viral replication.

Aspects of Human T-Cell Lymphotropic Virus-1 Infection

HTLV-1 is endemic in parts of southwestern Japan, the Caribbean basin, sub-Saharan Africa, South America, and the Southeastern United States (129). Worldwide, an estimated 10 to 20 million people are infected (51). In the highest prevalence, endemic areas up to 15% of normal blood donors are infected, whereas in nonendemic areas, <1% are positive. Transmission is believed to require infected cells because little if any cell-free virus is found in plasma (132). Virus-infected cells may be transmitted in breast milk or semen. Sexual transmission occurs rarely (133). The virus is associated with HTLV-1-associated myelopathy and tropical spastic paraparesis, uveitis, infectious dermatitis, and arthropathy in addition to ATL (134).

Infected $CD4^+$ T cells typically contain a single integrated provirus (135). Cellular replication of integrated proviral DNA involves proofreading, whereas the viral reverse transcriptase lacks proofreading and is highly error prone. The genetic stability of the viral genome (in contrast to HIV-1 or HCV) provides evidence that expansion of proviral DNA is mainly mediated by cellular proliferation rather than lytic viral replication. These infected cells engender a very active cytotoxic T-cell response targeting the tax protein. Up to 10% of $CD8^+$ T cells may target a single tax epitope (136,137). Tax-expressing cells are efficiently killed (138). Ultimately, this includes $CD8^+$ T cells specific for HTLV-1 targets. Activation of $CD8^+$ T cells specific for HTLV-1 by HTLV-1-infected $CD4^+$ T cells or dendritic cells enhances their susceptibility to HTLV-1 infection. HTLV-1-specific $CD8^+$ T cells thus become infected, making them targets for a fratricidal immune response (139). Resulting specific immune impairment may contribute to viral persistence. Viral mRNA is detectable only at low levels in PBMCs, probably reflecting the powerful cytotoxic T-cell response and resultant short half-life of tax-expressing cells (140,141).

Tax and other regulatory proteins are encoded in the Px region at the 3' end of the genome. Tax drives transcription from the viral long terminal repeat, and modulates the expression or function of many cellular genes involved in proliferation, apoptosis, differentiation, cell cycle control, and DNA repair (135,142,143). These include the NF-κB pathway, serum response factor and activating transcription factor/cyclic adenosine monophosphate responsive element binding protein (artificial transcription factor/adenosine 3c,5c-cyclic monophosphate response element binding)-responsive genes, cycle-dependent kinase 4, and cellular DNA repair pathways (144–146). Tax alone can immortalize primary human T cells, morphologically transform rodent fibroblasts, and induce tumors in transgenic mice (142,147–149).

Human T-Cell Lymphotropic Virus-1 and Lymphoma

HTLV-1 infection acquired at birth or in infancy is associated with ATL (150). Acquisition in adulthood by blood transfusion, injection drug use, or sexual contact is not associated with ATL, suggesting that HTLV-1 tumorigenesis is a multistep process requiring decades. Oligoclonal expansions of virus-infected cells as reflected by unique proviral integration sites in PBMCs of individuals infected with disease are well documented (135). The frequency of abundant circulating clones varies among patient populations with the highest frequency in patients with ATL, an intermediate frequency in patients with tropical spastic paraparesis and HTLV-1-associated myelopathy, and the lowest frequency in asymptomatic carriers.

Geographic factors seem to be important in the natural history of HTLV-1 infection (151). The risk of ATL is higher in Japan, and the risk of tropical spastic paraparesis and HTLV-1-associated myelopathy is higher in the Caribbean. Comparison of immune marker patterns in HTLV-1-endemic populations shows evidence of diminished T-cell immunity in Japanese seropositives but activated T-cell immunity in Jamaican seropositives.

Chromosomal instability is a key feature of ATL that may be the result of Tax expression (129). Centrosomes serve as the microtubule-organizing centers that form bipolar mitotic spindle poles. Tax interacts with one centrosome protein so as to yield hyperamplification of centrosomes and interacts with a protein at the spindle poles, leading to centrosome fragmentation. Both interactions contribute to the disruption of the correct segregation of replicated chromosomes. Missegregation of chromosomes in mitosis is guarded against by the spindle assembly checkpoint. Tax also interacts with proteins involved in the spindle assembly checkpoint effectively weakening the checkpoint. The micronuclei and aneuploid genomes that are common findings in HTLV-1-transformed lymphocytes are believed to be the result of these effects of Tax on the centrosomes, spindle proteins, and the spindle assembly checkpoint. DNA repair is also affected by Tax. Damage to DNA bases caused by a variety of mutagenic agents is repaired by nucleotide excision. Tax activates proliferating cell nuclear antigen, which inhibits such repair. In the presence of a functional p53, DNA damage leads to growth arrest until the damage is repaired or apoptosis, eliminating the damaged cell. Tax inactivates p53 as well as the retinoblastoma protein. These effects of the Tax protein likely explain the progression to malignancy, the aneuploid multilobulated nuclei "flower cells" characteristic of ATL, and perhaps the poor responses to chemotherapy (145,152,153).

Escape from immune surveillance may be important for the pathogenesis of tumor. Down-regulation of viral gene expression, major histocompatibility complex class I expression, mutation or deletion of T-cell epitopes in the tax protein, and T-cell deficiency possibly reflecting T-cell fratricide may all contribute to such immune evasion (139,154–156). Evidence in favor of the role of immune surveillance comes from the observation that organ transplantation and associated immunosupression in patients with HTLV-1 may increase the incidence of ATL (157).

Immune stimulation may contribute to pathogenesis. The possibility has also been raised that strongyloidiasis is a cofactor in the development of ATL (135). Both Strongyloides stercoralis and HTLV-1 are endemic in the same regions. Proviral load is higher in PBMCs from patients with dual infection than in those with HTLV-1 alone. The incidence of strongyloidiasis in Martinique in the French West Indies is higher in patients with ATL than in asymptomatic HTLV-1 carriers, and the incubation period for ATL may be shortened in patients with S. stercoralis infection. In a patient who presented with HTLV-1-associated chronic ATL and Strongyloides infection, viral RNA levels demonstrated stimulation of HTLV-1 replication by Strongyloides and resolution with antihelminthic therapy (158).

Aspects of Human Immunodeficiency Virus-1 Infection

HIV-1 infection is worldwide but is endemic in central Africa. HIV-2 is a related virus that is most closely related to simian immunodeficiency virus and is found in West Africa. Both cause AIDS. In nonendemic regions, HIV is found mainly in homosexual and bisexual men, injection drug users, transfusion recipients, sexual partners of infected persons, and infants born to infected mothers. Sexual contact, blood exposure, and perinatal exposure are all modes of transmission. Following infection there is a slow progressive depletion of CD4+ T cells. HIV infection is associated with opportunistic infections and specific malignancies.

The HIV genome is similar to the HTLV in that it encodes regulatory tat and rev proteins analogous to tax and rex. In addition, it encodes at least four regulatory proteins: nef, vif, vpu, and vpr. HIV infects CD4+ T cells, monocytes, macrophages, follicular dendritic cells, and a variety of neural, glial, and intestinal cells. CD4 and a chemokine receptor (CCR), CCR5 or CXCR4, are required for cellular entry. CCR5 mutations are rare, but when homozygous, are protective from HIV infection. In contrast to HTLV-1, viral infection typically results in cell lysis with budding of numbers of virions from the cell surface, releasing free virus. Infected CD4+ T cells die rather than proliferate. There is considerable genomic variation and antigenic heterogeneity, even in isolates obtained from individuals over the course of their infection. HIV infection is associated with polyclonal B-cell activation and hypergammaglobulinemia (159,160). However, B-cell stimulatory activity has been attributed to the Nef protein, to gp41, and most recently to CD40 ligand carried on the viral envelope (161,162).

Human Immunodeficiency Virus and Lymphoma

HIV-associated lymphoma is seen in all populations of people infected with HIV worldwide (163–165). The lymphomas that are seen in association with HIV infection include BL, diffuse large B-cell lymphoma, PEL, plasmablastic lymphoma, and HL. The aforementioned non-HLs are all formally recognized as AIDS-defining diseases.

In the era before highly active antiretroviral therapy, primary central nervous system lymphoma occurred with a 3,600-fold greater incidence among people with a diagnosis of AIDS than in the general population (166). With the advent of highly active antiretroviral therapy, the incidence of primary central nervous system lymphoma and perhaps some other lymphomas in patients with AIDS appears to have declined (167–169).

Lymphomagenesis in the setting of HIV infection is often associated with EBV, and is sometimes complex and multifactorial. Approximately 40% to 0% of lymphomas arising in patients with HIV are EBV associated (94). PELs are associated with both EBV and KSHV, or KSHV alone (170). BL in patients with HIV is not generally EBV associated (171). Immunocom-

promise is almost certainly an important contributing factor in many instances, but it is likely that other factors contribute as well. Marked CD4+ T-cell lymphopenia (often <20 per μL) is associated with primary central nervous system lymphoma (172), whereas BL and HL are generally associated with CD4+ T-cell counts >100 per μL (173,174).

Little evidence suggests that HIV directly infects malignant clones of B cells, and HIV proviral DNA is rarely found in tumors. The precise role that HIV-1 plays, particularly in the lymphomas that do not carry EBV, is not well characterized. Chronic antigenic stimulation is often presumed to be a contributing factor. Evidence in support of the idea comes from the observation that B-cell activation, hypergammaglobulinemia, and generalized lymphadenopathy commonly precede lymphoma development (175). In patients with paraproteins monoclonal IgG κ paraproteins that specifically recognized the HIV-1 p24 gag antigen have been identified. However, when lymphoma-derived Ig genes from HIV-related lymphomas were assayed for HIV reactivity, none of the tumor-related Igs bound to HIV proteins (176). The observation that activation-induced deaminase (AID) is upregulated in PBMC from patients with HIV destined to develop B-cell lymphoma suggested the possibility that as in large B-cell lymphoma arising in other settings, AID might contribute to the tumorigenesis (177–179).

HEPATITIS C VIRUS

Appreciation of the relationship between HCV infection and essential mixed cryoglobulinemia, a disorder characterized by oligoclonal proliferation of B cells, led to investigation of HCV and lymphoma (Fig. 6.7) (180). The relationship between the virus and lymphomagenesis remains poorly understood, but the idea that a robust immune response was likely to be important in the pathogenesis of the disease was widely accepted after reports of regression of B-cell lymphoma following successful treatment of HCV infection with antivirals (181).

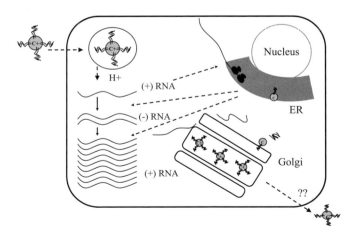

FIGURE 6.7 Hepatitis C life cycle. Hepatitis C binds to receptors and is endocytosed. The viral RNA is translated to synthesize a viral polyprotein that is cleaved to yield the nucleocapsid protein, glycoproteins, and nonstructural replication proteins, including an RNA-dependent RNA polymerase. Many copies of the original positive-strand RNA are made. mRNA is transported into the proteins of the viral envelope. The capsid assembles around the viral RNA, and the virus buds from the host membrane. ER (endoplasmic reticulum).

Aspects of Hepatitis C Virus Infection

HCV infection is usually acquired through blood-borne exposures, particularly injection drug use or unsafe uses of medical equipment. Before 1990, transfusion was also a major source of infection. HCV infection is usually asymptomatic but may lead to chronic hepatitis, cirrhosis, and hepatocellular carcinoma. HCV is a single-stranded, positive-sense RNA virus of 9.6 kb (182). The viral genome never enters the nucleus of infected cells. Viral RNA functions directly as an mRNA in the cytoplasm of the host cell. It encodes a polyprotein of approximately 3,000 amino acids that is processed to yield a nucleocapsid core protein and two N-glycosylated envelope glycoproteins (E1 and E2), and nonstructural proteins. Nonstructural proteins and viral RNA form replication complexes that catalyze the transcription of negative-strand RNA intermediates from which progeny positive-strand RNA molecules are generated. Genomic RNA and capsid proteins assemble into nucleocapsids and bud through intracellular membranes into cytoplasmic vesicles. CD81 serves as a cellular receptor for viral infection (183–185).

Humoral immune responses in patients infected with HIV predominantly target the E2 protein. The protein includes a hypervariable region with rapid mutations suggesting immune selection. One manifestation of the humoral response in some individuals is type II mixed cryoglobulinemia, a systemic vasculitis characterized by deposition of immune complexes in blood vessel walls (186). The complexes consist of a monoclonal IgM (typically κ) with specificity for IgG, polyclonal IgG with specificity for HCV antigens, and HCV antigens themselves.

Hepatitis C Virus and Lymphoma

Splenic and nodal marginal zone lymphomas have been most commonly linked to HCV (187–191). Epidemiologic evidence in favor of the association comes from Italy, Southern California, and Japan, where the prevalence of HCV infection among patients with B-cell non-HL is 9% to 32%. Although the epidemiologic evidence is clearest for low-grade lymphomas, higher-grade lymphomas may also be HCV associated (Fig. 6.8).

One explanation for the association of HCV with lymphoma relates to chronic antigenic stimulation. Evidence in support of this idea comes from the observations suggesting that lymphoma cell proliferation is antigen driven. A restricted V-gene repertoire (VH1-69 and Vκ3-A27) is common to human monoclonal antibodies established from HCV carriers, mixed cryoglobulinemia, and HCV-associated lymphoma (192,193). The restricted Ig gene usage is all the more striking given that it differentiates HCV-associated marginal zone lymphomas from other marginal zone lymphomas (194). In HCV-associated lymphomas, there is homology in the CDR3 regions consistent with response to a common epitope, and in at least one case, Ig rescued from HCV-associated lymphoma was shown to bind a conserved epitope of the E2 glycoprotein (195). Further evidence comes from studies of patients with HCV treated with antiviral therapy. Patients without clinically evident lymphoma, but with clonally expanded B cells as detected by polymerase chain reaction (PCR), were treated with α interferon alone or in combination with ribavirin. In 77% of patients with monoclonal IgH rearrangement and 86% of patients with

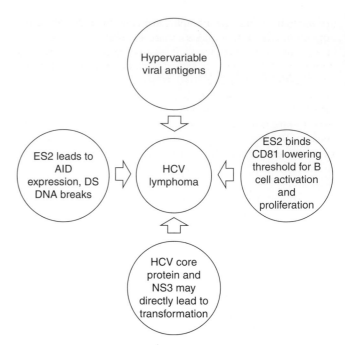

FIGURE 6.8 Pathogenesis of HCV-associated lymphoma. HCV antigens drive an intense polyclonal immune response. ES2 is an envelope protein that binds to the B-cell coreceptor (CD81) and lowers the threshold for B-cell activation, and drives proliferation. The interaction also leads to expression of AID and double-strand (DS) DNA breaks and hypermutation. The core and NS3 may directly contribute to transformation of infected cells.

t(14;18), these PCR markers of clonality disappeared, an effect that was closely associated with HCV clearance (196). In a series of nine patients with a splenic lymphoma with villous lymphocytes, tumor regression followed the disappearance of viral RNA in ten of 11 patients treated with interferon or interferon and ribavirin (181,197). However, PCR assays showed persistence of clonal B cells.

Whether antigen and antigen variation are sufficient for lymphomagenesis or whether there must be another sort of interaction between virus and B cells is not clear. As noted previously, the HCV envelope proteins engage the CD19/CD21/CD81 complex as well as the BCR (198). Dual engagement is believed to reduce the threshold for B-cell activation and proliferation (195,199). In addition, the interaction induces expression of AID and double-strand DNA breaks in B cells (200). A lymphotropic HCV strain has been isolated from a lymphoma cell line (198). The HCV core protein and the nonstructural protein NS3 have been reported to transform cells in tissue culture, cooperate with other genes in transforming cells, or to lead to malignancy when expressed as transgenes in mice (201–203). Thus, HCV infection leads to chronic antigenic stimulation, activates B-cell signaling coreceptor pathways, and leads to expression of AID that may lead to mutagenesis and chromosomal translocation.

SIMIAN VIRUS 40 AND POLYMOMA VIRUSES

Other DNA viruses have well-documented transforming properties and may play a role in lymphomagenesis. Possible links with polyomaviruses and particularly simian virus 40

(SV40) with human lymphoma have recently attracted attention (204,205). Polyomaviruses are commonly transforming in animals, which are not their natural hosts. Viral proteins (tumor or "T" antigens) lead to an alteration in cell cycle. Cells from species that are not permissive for viral replication progeny virus are not produced, and the cells that harbor these cell cycle perturbing viral genes are not killed by viral lysis, resulting in transformation. Possible mass cross-species infection might have been a consequence of the poliovirus vaccination program. Before 1963, SV40 contaminated tissue cultures used to grow the poliovirus used in vaccines. Two PCR-based studies identified SV40 T-antigen sequences in 43% and 42% of non-HLs (204,206). However, a study of lymphoma specimens from Italy and Spain utilizing PCR with the sensitivity to detect ten copies of the viral genome in 200,000 genome equivalents detected SV40 sequences much less commonly, and never detected both right and left ends of the genome in lymphoma (205). The discrepancies are not readily attributed to geographic differences because contaminated poliovaccines were distributed in the United States and Southern Europe over similar periods. The recent discovery of a novel polyomavirus integrated into the genome of most Merkel cell tumors (207) suggests that there are polyomaviruses and associations with human malignancy yet to be characterized, but at present any polyomavirus human lymphoma association remains yet to be clearly established.

HELICOBACTER AND OTHER BACTERIAL INFECTIONS

Helicobacter pylori colonizes gastric mucosa, leading to chronic inflammation and the appearance of mucosa-associated lymphoid tissue (MALT) in some individuals. The organism is present in most gastric lymphomas, with the association being strongest in early lesions. Antibiotic treatment to eradicate the infection results in regression of a substantial fraction of such tumors (180,208).

Aspects of *Helicobacter* Infection

Transmission is thought to be person to person (fecal-oral, oral-oral), and the major reservoir is human, but waterborne transmission may also be important in some regions (209). The prevalence of infection varies widely between populations, but approximately one-half of the world's population is infected. The lifetime risk of infection is greatest in developing countries, where more than half the population is infected by the age of 10 years. Infection rates increase with age. In adults in developed countries, the annual incidence of infection is approximately 1%. Both environmental and host genetic factors have been implicated in explaining infection rates among different groups. High titers of serum IgA and IgG antibodies develop in people who are infected.

Helicobacters are microaerophilic, nonsporulating, gram-negative curved, or spiral rods distinguished by multiple, sheathed flagellae (210). *H. pylori* may adhere to gastric epithelium or reside in the mucus layer of the stomach, but the organism does not invade tissues. Adherence to gastric epithelium is facilitated by the appearance of adherence pedestals on epithelial cells (211,212). The process is orchestrated

by the bacteria through secretion of the CagA protein, CagA insertion into mucosal cells, CagA phosphorylation by a tyrosine kinase, and resultant actin polymerization. Urease production from ammonia neutralizes gastric acid, making these organisms uniquely adapted to colonization of the stomach. *H. pylori* resides in the mucus layer of the stomach and adheres to the epithelium. Urease production allows these microorganisms to degrade host urea into ammonia and, thus, neutralize gastric acid, thus making them uniquely adapted to colonize the human stomach. The organism does not invade tissues. *H. pylori* is linked to gastritis, peptic ulcer disease, and gastric malignancy. Infection is usually associated with a superficial gastritis characterized by a mononuclear infiltrate, disruption of the epithelial gland structure, and decrease in overlying mucus (210). Inflammation has been attributed to production of urease, a vaculolating cytotoxin, and the CagA protein. Duodenal ulcer disease seems to follow antral gastritis and to be associated with excessive acid production. Progressive gastric atrophy and, less commonly, gastric cancer follow gastritis involving the acid-secreting corpus region, and are associated with hypochlorhydria. Duodenal ulceration and gastric cancer appear to be mutually exclusive consequences of infection. Host genetic polymorphisms may play an important role in determining the outcome of infection (213,214). *Helicobacter* infection has been shown to trigger aberrant expression of AID in gastric epithelial cells (215).

Helicobacter and Lymphoma

In vitro low-grade gastric lymphoma cells proliferate only in the presence of *H. pylori* and autologous T lymphocytes (180,216). The specificity of the malignant B cells has been the subject of conflicting reports. There is agreement that the malignant B cells are not specific for *H. pylori* antigens. Some have suggested specificity for autoantigens expressed in the gastric mucosa, whereas others have not confirmed this specificity (217). With antibiotic treatment, gastric MALT regresses, and a substantial fraction of gastric MALT lymphomas regress. Gastric marginal zone lymphoma-MALTs with t(11;18)(q21;q21) are generally resistant to *H. pylori* eradication (218).

Animal models (ferrets, mice, cats, and dogs among others) have provided some insight (219). None mimic the full spectrum of human *Helicobacter*-associated disease, particularly ulceration or gastric carcinoma. However, lymphocytic infiltrates are common consequences of accompanying infection in several. *Helicobacter felis*, *Helicobacter. heilmannii*, and *H. pylori* will all colonize in the mouse stomach indefinitely. Each will produce MALT-like lesions that, in some instances, evolve into low-grade and even high-grade lymphomas in murine and other animal models (219,220). Antibiotic treatment results in regression of the lymphomas in some instances.

Other Bacterial Infections and Lymphoma

Other bacterial infections have also been implicated in lymphomagenesis. Borrelia burgdorferi, the spirochete that causes Lyme disease, has been associated with cutaneous B-cell lymphoma (221). Evidence of the association comes from PCR-detection studies, culture, or serology. In some cases, tumors have regressed following antibiotic treatment.

Others have failed to confirm the association (222,223). Similarly, Campylobacter jejuni has been associated with immunoproliferative small intestinal disease, also called α heavy chain disease, which often responds to antibacterials (224). Chlamydia psittaci has been linked with ocular adenexal and other indolent lymphomas by some investigators, although others have failed to replicate the findings (225–227).

MALARIA AND BURKITT LYMPHOMA

Evidence for a link between malaria and lymphoma is mainly geographic. The distribution of endemic BL parallels holoendemic *Plasmodium falciparum*. In addition, there is some evidence that malarial prophylaxis with choloroquine may impact on the frequency of BL, but alternative explanations for the observations have been presented (228,229).

P. falciparum is the malarial parasite associated with the most severe forms of disease, causing in excess of 1 million deaths annually, most of them in young children in Africa (230,231). Climate is a key determinant of its geographic distribution. In equatorial Africa, there is sustained and intense exposure to *P. falciparum*, with the prevalence of the parasite in children <5 years of age as high as 90% (232).

The pathogenesis of BL in association with malaria has not been extensively investigated. However, *P. falciparum* leads to polyclonal B-cell activation, and this may provide clues to pathogenesis. The cysteine-rich interdomain region 1α of the erythrocyte membrane protein 1 is a T-cell-independent polyclonal B-cell activator and Ig binding protein that activates B lymphocytes, rescues B cells from apoptosis, and increases the proportion of cycling cells (233). *P. falciparum*-infected erythrocytes also have Toll-like receptor 9 ligand activity that may also drive the proliferation and differentiation of memory B lymphocytes (234). These effects on B-cell populations might drive lymphomagenesis directly. Alternatively, because endemic BL is consistently associated with EBV, malarial effects on B-cell populations may have downstream effects on the viral infection. Several groups of investigators have noted that malarial infection is associated with increased EBV copy number in blood (49,232). Whether this reflects chronic B-cell activation or suppression of EBV-

specific T-cell surveillance is not clear. Evidence has been presented that malaria leads to exhaustion of EBV-specific T-cell responses after repeated malaria infections, and that malaria inhibits of dendritic cell maturation by engagement of CD36 and suppression of CD4$^+$ T-cell responses (234).

SPECTRUM OF INFECTION-ASSOCIATED LYMPHOMA

Some infection-associated lymphomas (primary central nervous system lymphoma associated with EBV in patients with HIV, PEL associated with EBV and KSHV in patients with HIV) occur in the setting of immunodeficiency; others occur in hosts with apparently normal immune function (gastric MALT lymphoma associated with *Helicobacter* infection, nasal NK/T-cell lymphoma associated with EBV) (Table 6.4). Some develop rapidly after primary infection (EBV-associated posttransplant lymphoma); others, decades after primary infection (ATL associated with HTLV-1). Some show striking geographics (BL, ATL) in their degree of association with the virus; others show a very consistent association with the virus (nasal NK/T cell). Some have well-characterized genetic underpinnings in their hosts, such as X-linked lymphoproliferative disease.

The association of agents with regard to specific lymphoma types is poorly understood. Several agents are associated only with a specific B-cell disease: malaria with BL, and *Helicobacter* with gastric MALT lymphoma. Other agents are associated with a spectrum of B-cell malignancies (HIV with aggressive NHL and HL, HCV with typically low-grade B-cell malignancies). HTLV-1 is associated with a specific T-cell malignancy, although a multitude of presentations are recognized. EBV is associated with B and T and NK malignancies.

Even for a given infectious agent, the tissue distribution is not well understood. CD21, a complement receptor, is well characterized as important for the infection of B cells by EBV (235,236). However, CD21 expression is not an absolute requirement for EBV infection in vitro, and the cell types of EBV-associated tumors could not be predicted from patterns of CD21 expression. Thus, CD21 is not expressed on BL or HL. But CD21 is expressed on follicular lymphoma, and follicular lymphoma is never associated with EBV.

TABLE 6.4

NK/T AND PERIPHERAL T-CELL LYMPHOMA

Tumor	EBV association	Comment	Reference
Nasal NK/T lymphoma	100%	More common in Asia and central America	(101,244)
Peripheral T-cell lymphoma, NOS	<20%		
Angioimmunoblastic	NA	EBV is commonly found in infiltrating B lymphocytes in this T-cell tumor. When a B cell tumor arises in this setting, it is usually EBV-associated.	
Hepatosplenic γδ T-cell lymphoma	Rare or not associated	Sinusoidal infiltration by lymphoma cells in liver and spleen	(245)
Nonhepatosplenic γδ T-cell lymphoma	Common	Sinusoidal infiltration by lymphoma cells in skin, gut, lymph nodes, and other sites	(246)
Subcutaneous panniculitis-like	Rare		(247)

NA, not appliable; NOS, not otherwise specified.

Time from infection to the clinical appearance of tumor varies among tumor types (64,237,238). Posttransplant lymphoma may develop in weeks after primary infection in the setting of immunosuppression. HL may develop in 6 months to 10 years after primary symptomatic EBV infection in the normal host. In patients who have undergone organ transplantation, non-Hodgkin B-cell lymphomas typically arise in the 1st year after transplantation, whereas HL arises several years after transplantation. In patients with HIV, non-HLs also appear to arise earlier in the course of HIV disease than HL. Indeed, several years of moderate immunodeficiency (with CD4 T cell counts >200 per mm^2) may be required for the development of HL. Pyothorax lymphoma (see above) typically arises at least 2 decades after tuberculosis.

Tumor genetics are very different among infection-associated tumors. Thus, gastric MALT lymphoma shows a characteristic family of karyotypic abnormalities. Particular translocations may identify tumors that will no longer respond to antibiotic therapy. HTLV-1 and KSHV-associated lymphoma show complex cytogenetics, but little has been made of specific abnormalities. Well-defined families of translocations help to define BL with or without EBV.

Clinical Importance of the Associations

A better understanding of the pathogenesis of these infection-related lymphomas may ultimately lead to successful prevention strategies. The association of hepatitis B virus with hepatoma and the widespread use of hepatitis B vaccine in Taiwan has led to a documented decline in the incidence of this tumor. Although there has been interest in vaccines, there has yet to be evidence that any vaccines have been effective at preventing lymphoma. Agents associated with lymphoma appear to have a common feature in that humeral responses provide modest protection at best.

For established tumors, understanding the association may facilitate diagnosis. Detection of HTLV-1 in tumor is sometimes useful in helping to establish a diagnosis of ATL, and detecting EBV DNA in cerebrospinal fluid may obviate the need for a brain biopsy in a patient with AIDS with appropriate radiologic findings. There are few clinical settings in which the detection of infection alters the prognosis or therapy. For gastric MALT lymphoma associated with *H. pylori* and for marginal zone lymphoma associated with HCV, there is a general consensus that therapy aimed at the infection is an appropriate consideration for first-line therapy. There is less consensus with regard to other marginal zone or MALT lymphoma entities. An aggressive diagnostic and antibiotic-based therapeutic strategy has been explored for patients with nonbulky indolent lymphoma with some encouraging results (239).

The presence of viral nucleic acids and proteins has suggested other strategies for killing tumors associated with infection where the therapy is focused on the tumor, but the infectious agent provides a mechanism for targeting therapy. The greatest successes have been achieved with adoptive cellular immunotherapy for EBV-associated posttransplant lymphoma, particularly in the hematopoietic stem cell transplant setting (240,241). Approaches are evolving for targeted pharmacologic approaches as well. Patients with EBV-associated lymphomas have been treated with arginine butyrate and ganciclovir. Ganciclovir is selectively phosphorylated by the EBV thymidine kinase, and after further phosphorylations, the ganciclovir triphosphate will inhibit the cellular DNA polymerase and kill such cells. Insofar as the EBV thymidine kinase is not expressed in lymphomas, the hope was that arginine butyrate would up-regulate the viral thymidine kinase and allow selective killing. Encouraging results were reported in a pilot trial (242). An alternative approach that involves the use of bortezomib to up-regulate viral kinases and a ^{131}I-labeled nucleoside analog to target 2'-fluoro-2'-deoxy-beta-D-5-iodouracil-arabinofuranoside to EBV tumor cells so as to deliver targeted radiation has also been described but not yet studied in patients (243).

References

1. Epstein MA. Historical background. *Philos Trans R Soc Lond B Biol Sci* 2001;356:413–420.
2. Thorley-Lawson DA, Allday MJ. The curious case of the tumour virus: 50 years of Burkitt's lymphoma. *Nat Rev Microbiol* 2008;6;913–924.
3. Diehl V, Henle G, Henle W, et al. Demonstration of a herpes group virus in cultures of peripheral leukocytes from patients with infectious mononucleosis. *J Virol* 1968;2:663–669.
4. Cesarman E, Nador RG, Aozasa K, et al. Kaposi's sarcoma-associated herpesvirus in non-AIDS related lymphomas occurring in body cavities. *Am J Pathol* 1996;149:53–57.
5. Cohen JI, Bollard CM, Khanna R, et al. Current understanding of the role of Epstein-Barr virus in lymphomagenesis and therapeutic approaches to EBV-associated lymphomas. *Leuk Lymphoma* 2008; 49(suppl 1):27–34.
6. Moore PS, Chang Y. Molecular virology of Kaposi's sarcoma-associated herpesvirus. *Philos Trans R Soc Lond B Biol Sci* 2001;356:499–516.
7. Williams H, Crawford DH. Epstein-Barr virus: the impact of scientific advances on clinical practice. *Blood* 2006;107:862–869.
8. Sauce D, Larsen M, Curnow SJ, et al. EBV-associated mononucleosis leads to long-term global deficit in T-cell responsiveness to IL-15. *Blood* 2006;108:11–18.
9. Hutt-Fletcher LM. Epstein Barr virus entry. *J Virol* 2007;81:7825–7832.
10. Ryon JJ, Hayward SD, MacMahon EM, et al. In situ detection of lytic Epstein-Barr virus infection: expression of the NotI early gene and viral interleukin-10 late gene in clinical specimens. *J Infect Dis* 1993;168:345–351.
11. Hislop AD, Annels NE, Gudgeon NH, et al. Epitope-specific evolution of human CD8(+) T cell responses from primary to persistent phases of Epstein-Barr virus infection. *J Exp Med* 2002;195:893–905.
12. Miyashita EM, Yang B, Babcock GJ, et al. Identification of the site of Epstein-Barr virus persistence in vivo as a resting B cell. *J Virol* 1997;71:4882–4891.
13. Yang J, Tao Q, Flinn IW, et al. Characterization of Epstein-Barr virus-infected B cells in patients with posttransplantation lymphoproliferative disease: disappearance after rituximab therapy does not predict clinical response. *Blood* 2000;96:4055–4063.
14. Thorley-Lawson DA. Epstein-Barr virus: exploiting the immune system. *Nat Rev Immunol* 2001;1:75–82.
15. Yao QY, Ogan P, Rowe M, et al. Epstein-Barr virus-infected B cells persist in the circulation of acyclovir-treated virus carriers. *Int J Cancer* 1989;43:67–71.
16. Hoover SE, Kawada J, Wilson W, et al. Oropharyngeal shedding of Epstein-Barr virus in the absence of circulating B cells. *J Infect Dis* 2008;198:318–323.
17. Faulkner GC, Burrows SR, Khanna R, et al. X-Linked agammaglobulinemia patients are not infected with Epstein-Barr virus: implications for the biology of the virus. *J Virol* 1999;73:1555–1564.
18. Mosier DE. Viral pathogenesis in hu-PBL-SCID mice. *Semin Immunol* 1996;8:255–262.
19. Wu H, Kapoor P, Frappier L. Separation of the DNA replication, segregation, and transcriptional activation functions of Epstein-Barr nuclear antigen 1. *J Virol* 2002;76:2480–2490.
20. Tsimbouri P, Drotar ME, Coy JL, et al. bcl-xL and RAG genes are induced and the response to IL-2 enhanced in EmuEBNA-1 transgenic mouse lymphocytes. *Oncogene* 2002;21:5182–5187.
21. Kang MS, Soni V, Bronson R, et al. Epstein-Barr virus nuclear antigen 1 does not cause lymphoma in C57BL/6J mice. *J Virol* 2008;82:4180–4183.
22. Lee JM, Lee KH, Weidner M, et al. Epstein-Barr virus EBNA2 blocks Nur77- mediated apoptosis. *Proc Natl Acad Sci U S A* 2002;99:11878–11883.

23. Hsieh JJ, Zhou S, Chen L, et al. CIR, a corepressor linking the DNA binding factor CBF1 to the histone deacetylase complex. *Proc Natl Acad Sci U S A* 1999;96:23–28.
24. Bishop GA, Busch LK. Molecular mechanisms of B-lymphocyte transformation by Epstein-Barr virus. *Microbes Infect* 2002;4:853–857.
25. Kulwichit W, Edwards RH, Davenport EM, et al. Expression of the Epstein-Barr virus latent membrane protein 1 induces B cell lymphoma in transgenic mice. *Proc Natl Acad Sci U S A* 1998;95:11963–11968.
26. Lam N, Sugden B. CD40 and its viral mimic, LMP1: similar means to different ends. *Cell Signal* 2003;15:9–16.
27. Caldwell RG, Wilson JB, Anderson SJ, et al. Epstein-Barr virus LMP2A drives B cell development and survival in the absence of normal B cell receptor signals. *Immunity* 1998;9:405–411.
28. Rovedo M, Longnecker R. Epstein-barr virus latent membrane protein 2B (LMP2B) modulates LMP2A activity. *J Virol* 2007;81:84–94.
29. Nanbo A, Takada K. The role of Epstein-Barr virus-encoded small RNAs (EBERs) in oncogenesis. *Rev Med Virol* 2002;12:321–326.
30. Pfeffer S, Zavolan M, Grasser FA, et al. Identification of virus-encoded microRNAs. *Science* 2004;304:734–736.
31. Lo AK, To KF, Lo KW, et al. Modulation of LMP1 protein expression by EBV-encoded microRNAs. *Proc Natl Acad Sci U S A* 2007;104:16164–16169.
32. Wu FY, Chen H, Wang SE, et al. CCAAT/enhancer binding protein alpha interacts with ZTA and mediates ZTA-induced p21(CIP-1) accumulation and G(1) cell cycle arrest during the Epstein-Barr virus lytic cycle. *J Virol* 2003;77:1481–1500.
33. Deng Z, Chen CJ, Zerby D, et al. Identification of acidic and aromatic residues in the Zta activation domain essential for Epstein-Barr virus reactivation. *J Virol* 2001;75:10334–10347.
34. Wiedmer A, Wang P, Zhou J, et al. Epstein-Barr virus immediate-early protein Zta co-opts mitochondrial single-stranded DNA binding protein to promote viral and inhibit mitochondrial DNA replication. *J Virol* 2008;82:4647–4655.
35. Countryman JK, Gradoville L, Miller G. Histone hyperacetylation occurs on promoters of lytic cycle regulatory genes in Epstein-Barr virus-infected cell lines which are refractory to disruption of latency by histone deacetylase inhibitors. *J Virol* 2008;82:4706–4719.
36. Bellows DS, Howell M, Pearson C, et al. Epstein-Barr virus BALF1 is a BCL-2-like antagonist of the herpesvirus antiapoptotic BCL-2 proteins. *J Virol* 2002;76:2469–2479.
37. Boulland ML, Meignin V, Leroy-Viard K, et al. Human interleukin-10 expression in T/natural killer-cell lymphomas: association with anaplastic large cell lymphomas and nasal natural killer-cell lymphomas. *Am J Pathol* 1998;153:1229–1237.
38. Moore SM, Cannon JS, Tanhehco YC, et al. Induction of Epstein-Barr virus kinases to sensitize tumor cells to nucleoside analogues. *Antimicrob Agents Chemother* 2001;45:2082–2091.
39. Feng WH, Israel D, Raab-Traub N, et al. Chemotherapy induces lytic EBV replication and confers ganciclovir susceptibility to EBV-positive epithelial cell tumors. *Cancer Res* 2002;62:1920–1926.
40. Gutierrez MI, Kingma DW, Sorbara L, et al. Association of EBV strains, defined by multiple loci analyses, in non-Hodgkin lymphomas and reactive tissues from HIV positive and HIV negative patients. *Leuk Lymphoma* 2000;37:425–429.
41. Johannessen I, Crawford DH. In vivo models for Epstein-Barr virus (EBV)-associated B cell lymphoproliferative disease (BLPD). *Rev Med Virol* 1999;9:263–277.
42. Castanos-Velez E, Heiden T, Ekman M, et al. Proliferation and apoptosis-related gene expression in experimental acquired immunodeficiency syndrome-related simian lymphoma. *Blood* 1999;93:1364–1371.
43. Schmidtko J, Wang R, Wu CL, et al. Posttransplant lymphoproliferative disorder associated with an Epstein-Barr-related virus in cynomolgus monkeys. *Transplantation* 2002;73:1431–1439.
44. Cho Y, Ramer J, Rivailler P, et al. An Epstein-Barr-related herpesvirus from marmoset lymphomas. *Proc Natl Acad Sci U S A* 2001;98:1224–1229.
45. Young LS, Finerty S, Brooks L, et al. Epstein-Barr virus gene expression in malignant lymphomas induced by experimental virus infection of cottontop tamarins. *J Virol* 1989;63:1967–1974.
46. Wilson AD, Lovgren-Bengtsson K, Villacres-Ericsson M, et al. The major Epstein-Barr virus (EBV) envelope glycoprotein gp340 when incorporated into Iscoms primes cytotoxic T-cell responses directed against EBV lymphoblastoid cell lines. *Vaccine* 1999;17:1282–1290.
47. Morgan AJ. Epstein-Barr virus vaccines. *Vaccine* 1992;10:563–571.
48. Rowe M, Young LS, Crocker J, et al. Epstein-Barr virus (EBV)-associated lymphoproliferative disease in the SCID mouse model: implications for the pathogenesis of EBV-positive lymphomas in man. *J Exp Med* 1991;173:147–158.
49. Njie R, Bell AI, Jia H, et al. The effects of acute malaria on Epstein-Barr virus (EBV) load and EBV-specific T cell immunity in Gambian children. *J Infect Dis* 2009;199:31–38.
50. Burkitt D. A sarcoma involving the jaws in African children. *Br J Surg* 1958;46:218–223.
51. Parkin DM. The global health burden of infection-associated cancers in the year 2002. *Int J Cancer* 2006;118:3030–3044.
52. Parkin DM, Bray F, Ferlay J, et al. Global cancer statistics, 2002. *CA Cancer J Clin* 2005;55:74–108.
53. Shiramizu B, Barriga F, Neequaye J, et al. Patterns of chromosomal breakpoint locations in Burkitt's lymphoma: relevance to geography and Epstein-Barr virus association. *Blood* 1991;77:1516–1526.
54. Gutierrez MI, Bhatia K, Barriga F, et al. Molecular epidemiology of Burkitt's lymphoma from South America: differences in breakpoint location and Epstein-Barr virus association from tumors in other world regions. *Blood* 1992;79:3261–3266.
55. Niedobitek G, Agathanggelou A, Rowe M, et al. Heterogeneous expression of Epstein-Barr virus latent proteins in endemic Burkitt's lymphoma. *Blood* 1995;86:659–665.
56. Khanna R, Burrows SR, Suhrbier A, et al. EBV peptide epitope sensitization restores human cytotoxic T cell recognition of Burkitt's lymphoma cells. Evidence for a critical role for ICAM-2. *J Immunol* 1993;150:5154–5162.
57. Kelly G, Bell A, Rickinson A. Epstein-Barr virus-associated Burkitt lymphomagenesis selects for downregulation of the nuclear antigen EBNA2. *Nat Med* 2002;8:1098–1104.
58. Pajic A, Staege MS, Dudziak D, et al. Antagonistic effects of c-myc and Epstein-Barr virus latent genes on the phenotype of human B cells. *Int J Cancer* 2001;93:810–816.
59. Staege MS, Lee SP, Frisan T, et al. MYC overexpression imposes a non-immunogenic phenotype on Epstein-Barr virus-infected B cells. *Proc Natl Acad Sci U S A* 2002;99:4550–4555.
60. Kuppers R. B cells under influence: transformation of B cells by Epstein-Barr virus. *Nat Rev Immunol* 2003;3:801–812.
61. Glaser SL, Lin RJ, Stewart SL, et al. Epstein-Barr virus-associated Hodgkin's disease: epidemiologic characteristics in international data. *Int J Cancer* 1997;70:375–382.
62. Ambinder RF, Browning PJ, Lorenzana I, et al. Epstein-Barr virus and childhood Hodgkin's disease in Honduras and the United States. *Blood* 1993;81:462–467.
63. Chang KL, Albujar PF, Chen YY, et al. High prevalence of Epstein-Barr virus in the Reed-Sternberg cells of Hodgkin's disease occurring in Peru. *Blood* 1993;81:496–501.
64. Hjalgrim H, Askling J, Rostgaard K, et al. Characteristics of Hodgkin's lymphoma after infectious mononucleosis. *N Engl J Med* 2003;349:1324–1332.
65. Brauninger A, Schmitz R, Bechtel D, et al. Molecular biology of Hodgkin's and Reed/Sternberg cells in Hodgkin's lymphoma. *Int J Cancer* 2006;118:1853–1861.
66. Katzenstein AL, Carrington CB, Liebow AA. Lymphomatoid granulomatosis: a clinicopathologic study of 152 cases. *Cancer* 1979;43:360–373.
67. Rezk SA, Weiss LM. Epstein-Barr virus-associated lymphoproliferative disorders. *Hum Pathol* 2007;38:1293–1304.
68. Taniere P, Thivolet-Bejui F, Vitrey D, et al. Lymphomatoid granulomatosis—a report on four cases: evidence for B phenotype of the tumoral cells. *Eur Respir J* 1998;12:102–106.
69. Wilson WH, Kingma DW, Raffeld M, et al. Association of lymphomatoid granulomatosis with Epstein-Barr viral infection of B lymphocytes and response to interferon-alpha 2b. *Blood* 1996;87:4531–4537.
70. Aozasa K, Takakuwa T, Nakatsuka S. Pyothorax-associated lymphoma: a lymphoma developing in chronic inflammation. *Adv Anat Pathol* 2005;12:324–331.
71. Copie-Bergman C, Niedobitek G, Mangham DC, et al. Epstein-Barr virus in B-cell lymphomas associated with chronic suppurative inflammation. *J Pathol* 1997;183:287–292.
72. Shimoyama Y, Oyama T, Asano N, et al. Senile Epstein-Barr virus-associated B-cell lymphoproliferative disorders: a mini review. *J Clin Exp Hematop* 2006;46:1–4.
73. Oyama T, Ichimura K, Suzuki R, et al. Senile EBV+ B-cell lymphoproliferative disorders: a clinicopathologic study of 22 patients. *Am J Surg Pathol* 2003;27:16–26.
74. Filipovich AH, Mertens A, Robison L, et al. Lymphoproliferative disorders associated with primary immunodeficiencies. In: Margath I, ed. *The non-Hodgkin's lymphomas*, 2nd ed. London, UK: Oxford University Press, 1995:459–471.
75. Morra M, Howie D, Grande MS, et al. X-linked lymphoproliferative disease: a progressive immunodeficiency. *Annu Rev Immunol* 2001;19:657–682.
76. Strahm B, Rittweiler K, Duffner U, et al. Recurrent B-cell non-Hodgkin's lymphoma in two brothers with X-linked lymphoproliferative disease without evidence for Epstein-Barr virus infection. *Br J Haematol* 2000;108:377–382.
77. Sharifi R, Sinclair JC, Gilmour KC, et al. SAP mediates specific cytotoxic T-cell functions in X-linked lymphoproliferative disease. *Blood* 2004;103:3821–3827.
78. Swinnen LJ. Organ transplant-related lymphoma. *Curr Treat Options Oncol* 2001;2:301–308.
79. Curtis RE, Travis LB, Rowlings PA, et al. Risk of lymphoproliferative disorders after bone marrow transplantation: a multi-institutional study. *Blood* 1999;94:2208–2216.
80. Meijer E, Slaper-Cortenbach IC, Thijsen SF, et al. Increased incidence of EBV-associated lymphoproliferative disorders after allogeneic stem cell

transplantation from matched unrelated donors due to a change of T cell depletion technique. *Bone Marrow Transplant* 2002;29:335–339.

81. Gross TG, Hinrichs SH, Davis JR, et al. Depletion of EBV-infected cells in donor marrow by counterflow elutriation. *Exp Hematol* 1998;26:395–399.

82. Lucas KG, Small TN, Heller G, et al. The development of cellular immunity to Epstein-Barr virus after allogeneic bone marrow transplantation. *Blood* 1996;87:2594–2603.

83. Starzl TE, Nalesnik MA, Porter KA, et al. Reversibility of lymphomas and lymphoproliferative lesions developing under cyclosporin-steroid therapy. *Lancet* 1984;1:583–587.

84. Porcu P, Eisenbeis CF, Pelletier RP, et al. Successful treatment of post-transplantation lymphoproliferative disorder (PTLD) following renal allografting is associated with sustained CD8(+) T-cell restoration. *Blood* 2002;100:2341–2348.

85. Papadopoulos EB, Ladanyi M, Emanuel D, et al. Infusions of donor leukocytes to treat Epstein-Barr virus-associated lymphoproliferative disorders after allogeneic bone marrow transplantation. *N Engl J Med* 1994;330:1185–1191.

86. Rooney CM, Smith CA, Ng CY, et al. Infusion of cytotoxic T cells for the prevention and treatment of Epstein-Barr virus-induced lymphoma in allogeneic transplant recipients. *Blood* 1998;92:1549–1555.

87. Gruhn B, Meerbach A, Hafer R, et al. Pre-emptive therapy with rituximab for prevention of Epstein-Barr virus-associated lymphoproliferative disease after hematopoietic stem cell transplantation. *Bone Marrow Transplant* 2003;31:1023–1025.

88. Mariette X, Cazals-Hatem D, Warszawki J, et al. Lymphomas in rheumatoid arthritis patients treated with methotrexate: a 3-year prospective study in France. *Blood* 2002;99:3909–3915.

89. Ho AY, Adams S, Shaikh H, et al. Fatal donor-derived Epstein-Barr virus-associated post-transplant lymphoproliferative disorder following reduced intensity volunteer-unrelated bone marrow transplant for myelodysplastic syndrome. *Bone Marrow Transplant* 2002;29:867–869.

90. Milpied N, Coste-Burel M, Accard F, et al. Epstein-Barr virus-associated B cell lymphoproliferative disease after non-myeloablative allogeneic stem cell transplantation. *Bone Marrow Transplant* 1999;23:629–630.

91. Shields DJ, Byrd JC, Abbondanzo SL, et al. Detection of Epstein-Barr virus in transformations of low-grade B-cell lymphomas after fludarabine treatment. *Mod Pathol* 1997;10:1151–1159.

92. Abruzzo LV, Rosales CM, Medeiros LJ, et al. Epstein-Barr virus-positive B-cell lymphoproliferative disorders arising in immunodeficient patients previously treated with fludarabine for low-grade B-cell neoplasms. *Am J Surg Pathol* 2002;26:630–636.

93. Balandraud N, Guis S, Meynard JB, et al. Long-term treatment with methotrexate or tumor necrosis factor alpha inhibitors does not increase epstein-barr virus load in patients with rheumatoid arthritis. *Arthritis Rheum* 2007;57:762–767.

94. Carbone A, Cesarman E, Spina M, et al. HIV-associated lymphomas and gamma-herpesviruses. *Blood* 2009;113:1213–1224.

95. MacMahon EM, Glass JD, Hayward SD, et al. Epstein-Barr virus in AIDS-related primary central nervous system lymphoma. *Lancet* 1991;338:969–973.

96. Camilleri-Broet S, Davi F, Feuillard J, et al. AIDS-related primary brain lymphomas: histopathologic and immunohistochemical study of 51 cases. The French Study Group for HIV-Associated Tumors. *Hum Pathol* 1997;28:367–374.

97. Knowles DM. Immunodeficiency-associated lymphoproliferative disorders. *Mod Pathol* 1999;12:200–217.

98. Horenstein MG, Nador RG, Chadburn A, et al. Epstein-Barr virus latent gene expression in primary effusion lymphomas containing Kaposi's sarcoma-associated herpesvirus/human herpesvirus-8. *Blood* 1997;90:1186–1191.

99. Glaser SL, Clarke CA, Gulley ML, et al. Population-based patterns of human immunodeficiency virus-related Hodgkin lymphoma in the Greater San Francisco Bay Area, 1988–1998. *Cancer* 2003;98:300–309.

100. Ambinder RF, Lee S, Curran WJ, et al. Phase II intergroup trial of sequential chemotherapy and radiotherapy for AIDS-related primary central nervous system lymphoma. *Cancer Ther* 2003;1:215–221.

101. Cheung MM, Chan JK, Wong KF. Natural killer cell neoplasms: a distinctive group of highly aggressive lymphomas/leukemias. *Semin Hematol* 2003;40:221–232.

102. Jaffe ES, Krenacs L, Raffeld M. Classification of cytotoxic T-cell and natural killer cell lymphomas. *Semin Hematol* 2003;40:175–184.

103. Chiang AK, Tao Q, Srivastava G, et al. Nasal NK- and T-cell lymphomas share the same type of Epstein-Barr virus latency as nasopharyngeal carcinoma and Hodgkin's disease. *Int J Cancer* 1996;68:285–290.

104. Kawa-Ha K, Ishihara S, Ninomiya T, et al. CD3-negative lymphoproliferative disease of granular lymphocytes containing Epstein-Barr viral DNA. *J Clin Invest* 1989;84:51–55.

105. Hart DN, Baker BW, Inglis MJ, et al. Epstein-Barr viral DNA in acute large granular lymphocyte (natural killer) leukemic cells. *Blood* 1992;79:2116–2123.

106. Cesarman E, Mesri EA. Kaposi sarcoma-associated herpesvirus and other viruses in human lymphomagenesis. *Curr Top Microbiol Immunol* 2007;312:263–287.

107. Mbulaiteye S, Marshall V, Bagni RK, et al. Molecular evidence for mother-to-child transmission of Kaposi sarcoma-associated herpesvirus in Uganda and K1 gene evolution within the host. *J Infect Dis* 2006;193:1250–1257.

108. Anderson LA, Lauria C, Romano N, et al. Risk factors for classical Kaposi sarcoma in a population-based case-control study in Sicily. *Cancer Epidemiol Biomarkers Prev* 2008;17:3435–3443.

109. Lin L, Lee JY, Kaplan LD, et al. Effects of chemotherapy in AIDS-associated non-Hodgkin's lymphoma on Kaposi's sarcoma herpesvirus DNA in blood. *J Clin Oncol* 2009;27:2496–2502.

110. Harrington WJ Jr, Bagasra O, Sosa CE, et al. Human herpesvirus type 8 DNA sequences in cell-free plasma and mononuclear cells of Kaposi's sarcoma patients. *J Infect Dis* 1996;174:1101–1105.

111. Dupin N, Fisher C, Kellam P, et al. Distribution of human herpesvirus-8 latently infected cells in Kaposi's sarcoma, multicentric Castleman's disease, and primary effusion lymphoma. *Proc Natl Acad Sci U S A* 1999;96:4546–4551.

112. Dittmer DP. Transcription profile of Kaposi's sarcoma-associated herpesvirus in primary Kaposi's sarcoma lesions as determined by real-time PCR arrays. *Cancer Res* 2003;63:2010–2015.

113. Schulz TF. The pleiotropic effects of Kaposi's sarcoma herpesvirus. *J Pathol* 2006;208:187–198.

114. Fujimuro M, Wu FY, ApRhys C, et al. A novel viral mechanism for dysregulation of beta-catenin in Kaposi's sarcoma-associated herpesvirus latency. *Nat Med* 2003;9:300–306.

115. McCormick C, Ganem D. The kaposin B protein of KSHV activates the p38/MK2 pathway and stabilizes cytokine mRNAs. *Science* 2005;307:739–741.

116. McCormick C, Ganem D. Phosphorylation and function of the kaposin B direct repeats of Kaposi's sarcoma-associated herpesvirus. *J Virol* 2006;80:6165–6170.

117. Li H, Komatsu T, Dezube BJ, et al. The Kaposi's sarcoma-associated herpesvirus K12 transcript from a primary effusion lymphoma contains complex repeat elements, is spliced, and initiates from a novel promoter. *J Virol* 2002;76:11880–11888.

118. Burysek L, Pitha PM. Latently expressed human herpesvirus 8 encoded interferon regulatory factor 2 inhibits double-stranded RNA-activated protein kinase. *J Virol* 2001;75:2345–2352.

119. Rivas C, Thlick AE, Parravicini C, et al. Kaposi's sarcoma-associated herpesvirus LANA2 is a B-cell-specific latent viral protein that inhibits p53. *J Virol* 2001;75:429–438.

120. Wies E, Mori Y, Hahn A, et al. The viral interferon-regulatory factor-3 is required for the survival of KSHV-infected primary effusion lymphoma cells. *Blood* 2008;111:320–327.

121. Nicholas J. Human herpesvirus 8 encoded proteins with potential roles in virus-associated neoplasia. *Front Biosci* 2007;12:265–281.

122. Chen D, Sandford G, Nicholas J. Intracellular signaling mechanisms and activities of human herpesvirus 8 interleukin-6. *J Virol* 2009;83:722–733.

123. Cannon JS, Nicholas J, Orenstein JM, et al. Heterogeneity of viral IL-6 expression in HHV-8-associated diseases. *J Infect Dis* 1999;180:824–828.

124. Carbone A, Gloghini A. KSHV/HHV8-associated lymphomas. *Br J Haematol* 2008;140:13–24.

125. Soulier J, Grollet L, Oksenhendler E, et al. Kaposi's sarcoma-associated herpesvirus-like DNA sequences in multicentric Castleman's disease. *Blood* 1995;86:1276–1280.

126. Chadburn A, Hyjek EM, Tam W, et al. Immunophenotypic analysis of the Kaposi sarcoma herpesvirus (KSHV; HHV-8)-infected B cells in HIV+ multicentric Castleman disease (MCD). *Histopathology* 2008;53:513–524.

127. Uchiyama T, Yodoi J, Sagawa K, et al. Adult T-cell leukemia: clinical and hematologic features of 16 cases. *Blood* 1977;50:481–492.

128. Morgan DA, Ruscetti FW, Gallo R. Selective in vitro growth of T lymphocytes from normal human bone marrows. *Science* 1976;193:1007–1008.

129. Jeang KT. Retrovirology highlights a quarter century of HTLV-I research. *Retrovirology* 2005;2:15.

130. Armitage AE, McMichael AJ, Drakesmith H. Reflecting on a quarter century of HIV research. *Nat Immunol* 2008;9:823–826.

131. Leclercq I, Mortreux F, Cavrois M, et al. Host sequences flanking the human T-cell leukemia virus type 1 provirus in vivo. *J Virol* 2000;74:2305–2312.

132. Wodarz D, Nowak MA, Bangham CR. The dynamics of HTLV-I and the CTL response. *Immunol Today* 1999;20:220–227.

133. Iga M, Okayama A, Stuver S, et al. Genetic evidence of transmission of human T cell lymphotropic virus type 1 between spouses. *J Infect Dis* 2002;185:691–695.

134. Yoshida M. Discovery of HTLV-1, the first human retrovirus, its unique regulatory mechanisms, and insights into pathogenesis. *Oncogene* 2005;24:5931–5937.

135. Mortreux F, Gabet AS, Wattel E. Molecular and cellular aspects of HTLV-1 associated leukemogenesis in vivo. *Leukemia* 2003;17:26–38.

136. Bieganowska K, Hollsberg P, Buckle GJ, et al. Direct analysis of viral-specific CD8+ T cells with soluble HLA-A2/Tax11-19 tetramer complexes in patients with human T cell lymphotropic virus-associated myelopathy. *J Immunol* 1999;162:1765–1771.

137. Jeffery KJ, Usuku K, Hall SE, et al. HLA alleles determine human T-lymphotropic virus-I (HTLV-I) proviral load and the risk of HTLV-I-associated myelopathy. *Proc Natl Acad Sci U S A* 1999;96:3848–3853.

138. Hanon E, Hall S, Taylor GP, et al. Abundant tax protein expression in CD4+ T cells infected with human T-cell lymphotropic virus type I (HTLV-I) is prevented by cytotoxic T lymphocytes. *Blood* 2000;95:1386–1392.

139. Hanon E, Stinchcombe JC, Saito M, et al. Fratricide among CD8(+) T lymphocytes naturally infected with human T cell lymphotropic virus type I. *Immunity* 2000;13:657–664.

140. Asquith B, Hanon E, Taylor GP, et al. Is human T-cell lymphotropic virus type I really silent? *Philos Trans R Soc Lond B Biol Sci* 2000;355:1013–1019.

141. Richardson JH, Hollsberg P, Windhagen A, et al. Variable immortalizing potential and frequent virus latency in blood-derived T-cell clones infected with human T-cell leukemia virus type I. *Blood* 1997;89:3303–3314.

142. Grassmann R, Aboud M, Jeang KT. Molecular mechanisms of cellular transformation by HTLV-1 Tax. *Oncogene* 2005;24:5976–5985.

143. Yoshida M. Multiple viral strategies of HTLV-1 for dysregulation of cell growth control. *Annu Rev Immunol* 2001;19:475–496.

144. Haller K, Wu Y, Derow E, et al. Physical interaction of human T-cell leukemia virus type 1 Tax with cyclin-dependent kinase 4 stimulates the phosphorylation of retinoblastoma protein. *Mol Cell Biol* 2002;22:3327–3338.

145. Jin DY, Spencer F, Jeang KT. Human T cell leukemia virus type 1 oncoprotein Tax targets the human mitotic checkpoint protein MAD1. *Cell* 1998;93:81–91.

146. Van PL, Yim KW, Jin DY, et al. Genetic evidence of a role for ATM in functional interaction between human T-cell leukemia virus type 1 Tax and p53. *J Virol* 2001;75:396–407.

147. Grassmann R, Berchtold S, Radant I, et al. Role of human T-cell leukemia virus type 1 X region proteins in immortalization of primary human lymphocytes in culture. *J Virol* 1992;66:4570–4575.

148. Portis T, Grossman WJ, Harding JC, et al. Analysis of p53 inactivation in a human T-cell leukemia virus type 1 Tax transgenic mouse model. *J Virol* 2001;75:2185–2193.

149. Portis T, Harding JC, Ratner L. The contribution of NF-kappa B activity to spontaneous proliferation and resistance to apoptosis in human T-cell leukemia virus type 1 Tax-induced tumors. *Blood* 2001;98:1200–1208.

150. Blattner WA. Human T-lymphotrophic viruses and diseases of long latency. *Ann Intern Med* 1989;111:4–6.

151. Birmann BM, Breen EC, Stuver S, et al. Population differences in immune marker profiles associated with human T-lymphotropic virus type I infection in Japan and Jamaica. *Int J Cancer* 2009;124:614–621.

152. Marriott SJ, Lemoine FJ, Jeang KT. Damaged DNA and miscounted chromosomes: human T cell leukemia virus type I tax oncoprotein and genetic lesions in transformed cells. *J Biomed Sci* 2002;9:292–298.

153. Kasai T, Iwanaga Y, Iha H, et al. Prevalent loss of mitotic spindle checkpoint in adult T-cell leukemia confers resistance to microtubule inhibitors. *J Biol Chem* 2002;277:5187–5193.

154. Kannagi M, Matsushita S, Harada S. Expression of the target antigen for cytotoxic T lymphocytes on adult T-cell-leukemia cells. *Int J Cancer* 1993;54:582–588.

155. Ohashi T, Hanabuchi S, Suzuki R, et al. Correlation of major histocompatibility complex class I downregulation with resistance of human T-cell leukemia virus type 1-infected T cells to cytotoxic T-lymphocyte killing in a rat model. *J Virol* 2002;76:7010–7019.

156. Furukawa Y, Kubota R, Tara M, et al. Existence of escape mutant in HTLV-I tax during the development of adult T-cell leukemia. *Blood* 2001;97:987–993.

157. Kawano N, Shimoda K, Ishikawa F, et al. Adult T-cell leukemia development from a human T-cell leukemia virus type I carrier after a living-donor liver transplantation. *Transplantation* 2006;82:840–843.

158. Ratner L, Grant C, Zimmerman B, et al. Effect of treatment of Strongyloides infection on HTLV-1 expression in a patient with adult T-cell leukemia. *Am J Hematol* 2007;82:929–931.

159. Rosenberg ZF, Fauci AS. Immunopathogenesis of HIV infection. *FASEB J* 1991;5:2382–2390.

160. De Silva FS, Venturini DS, Wagner E, et al. CD4-independent infection of human B cells with HIV type 1: detection of unintegrated viral DNA. *AIDS Res Hum Retroviruses* 2001;17:1585–1598.

161. Chirmule N, Kalyanaraman VS, Saxinger C, et al. Localization of B-cell stimulatory activity of HIV-1 to the carboxyl terminus of gp41. *AIDS Res Hum Retroviruses* 1990;6:299–305.

162. Chirmule N, Oyaizu N, Saxinger C, et al. Nef protein of HIV-1 has B-cell stimulatory activity. *AIDS* 1994;8:733–734.

163. Ziegler JL, Beckstead JA, Volberding PA, et al. Non-Hodgkin's lymphoma in 90 homosexual men. Relation to generalized lymphadenopathy and the acquired immunodeficiency syndrome. *N Engl J Med* 1984;311:565–570.

164. Franceschi S, Dal Maso L, La Vecchia C. Advances in the epidemiology of HIV-associated non-Hodgkin's lymphoma and other lymphoid neoplasms. *Int J Cancer* 1999;83:481–485.

165. Goedert JJ, Cote TR, Virgo P, et al. Spectrum of AIDS-associated malignant disorders. *Lancet* 1998;351:1833–1839.

166. Cote TR, Manns A, Hardy CR, et al. Epidemiology of brain lymphoma among people with or without acquired immunodeficiency syndrome. AIDS/Cancer Study Group. *J Natl Cancer Inst* 1996;88:675–679.

167. Jacobson LP, Yamashita TE, Detels R, et al. Impact of potent antiretroviral therapy on the incidence of Kaposi's sarcoma and non-Hodgkin's lymphomas among HIV-1-infected individuals. Multicenter AIDS Cohort Study. *J Acquir Immune Defic Syndr* 1999;21(suppl 1):S34–S41.

168. Rabkin CS. AIDS and cancer in the era of highly active antiretroviral therapy (HAART). *Eur J Cancer* 2001;37:1316–1319.

169. Grulich AE, Law MG. Long-term high-dose acyclovir and AIDS-related non-Hodgkins lymphoma. *Clin Infect Dis* 2001;32:989–990.

170. Cesarman E, Chadburn A, Liu YF, et al. BCL-6 gene mutations in post-transplantation lymphoproliferative disorders predict response to therapy and clinical outcome. *Blood* 1998;92:2294–2302.

171. Subar M, Neri A, Inghirami G, et al. Frequent c-myc oncogene activation and infrequent presence of Epstein-Barr virus genome in AIDS-associated lymphoma. *Blood* 1988;72:667–671.

172. Pedersen C, Gerstoft J, Lundgren JD, et al. HIV-associated lymphoma: histopathology and association with Epstein-Barr virus genome related to clinical, immunological and prognostic features. *Eur J Cancer* 1991;27:1416–1423.

173. Gabarre J, Raphael M, Lepage E, et al. Human immunodeficiency virus-related lymphoma: relation between clinical features and histologic subtypes. *Am J Med* 2001;111:704–711.

174. Davi F, Delecluse HJ, Guiet P, et al. Burkitt-like lymphomas in AIDS patients: characterization within a series of 103 human immunodeficiency virus-associated non-Hodgkin's lymphomas. Burkitt's Lymphoma Study Group. *J Clin Oncol* 1998;16:3788–3795.

175. Grulich AE, Wan X, Law MG, et al. B-cell stimulation and prolonged immune deficiency are risk factors for non-Hodgkin's lymphoma in people with AIDS. *AIDS* 2000;14:133–140.

176. Cunto-Amesty G, Przybylski G, Honczarenko M, et al. Evidence that immunoglobulin specificities of AIDS-related lymphoma are not directed to HIV-related antigens. *Blood* 2000;95:1393–1399.

177. Martinez-Maza O, Breen EC. B-cell activation and lymphoma in patients with HIV. *Curr Opin Oncol* 2002;14:528–532.

178. Epeldegui M, Breen EC, Hung YP, et al. Elevated expression of activation induced cytidine deaminase in peripheral blood mononuclear cells precedes AIDS-NHL diagnosis. *AIDS* 2007;21:2265–2270.

179. He B, Qiao X, Klasse PJ, et al. HIV-1 envelope triggers polyclonal Ig class switch recombination through a CD40-independent mechanism involving BAFF and C-type lectin receptors. *J Immunol* 2006;176:3931–3941.

180. Suarez F, Lortholary O, Hermine O, et al. Infection-associated lymphomas derived from marginal zone B cells: a model of antigen-driven lymphoproliferation. *Blood* 2006;107:3034–3044.

181. Hermine O, Lefrere F, Bronowicki JP, et al. Regression of splenic lymphoma with villous lymphocytes after treatment of hepatitis C virus infection. *N Engl J Med* 2002;347:89–94.

182. Rehermann B, Nascimbeni M. Immunology of hepatitis B virus and hepatitis C virus infection. *Nat Rev Immunol* 2005;5:215–229.

183. Cocquerel L, Kuo CC, Dubuisson J, et al. CD81-dependent binding of hepatitis C virus E1E2 heterodimers. *J Virol* 2003;77:10677–10683.

184. Machida K, Cheng KT, Pavio N, et al. Hepatitis C virus E2-CD81 interaction induces hypermutation of the immunoglobulin gene in B cells. *J Virol* 2005;79:8079–8089.

185. Rosa D, Saletti G, De Gregorio E, et al. Activation of naive B lymphocytes via CD81, a pathogenetic mechanism for hepatitis C virus-associated B lymphocyte disorders. *Proc Natl Acad Sci U S A* 2005;102:18544–18549.

186. De Vita S, De Re V, Gasparotto D, et al. Oligoclonal non-neoplastic B cell expansion is the key feature of type II mixed cryoglobulinemia: clinical and molecular findings do not support a bone marrow pathologic diagnosis of indolent B cell lymphoma. *Arthritis Rheum* 2000;43:94–102.

187. Silvestri F, Pipan C, Barillari G, et al. Prevalence of hepatitis C virus infection in patients with lymphoproliferative disorders. *Blood* 1996;87:4296–4301.

188. Izumi KM, Kaye KM, Kieff ED. The Epstein-Barr virus LMP1 amino acid sequence that engages tumor necrosis factor receptor associated factors is critical for primary B lymphocyte growth transformation. *Proc Natl Acad Sci U S A* 1997;94:1447–1452.

189. Izumi T, Sasaki R, Shimizu R, et al. Hepatitis C virus infection in Waldenstrom's macroglobulinemia. *Am J Hematol* 1996;52:238–239.

190. Zuckerman E, Zuckerman T, Levine AM, et al. Hepatitis C virus infection in patients with B-cell non-Hodgkin lymphoma. *Ann Intern Med* 1997;127:423–428.

191. Schollkopf C, Smedby KE, Hjalgrim H, et al. Hepatitis C infection and risk of malignant lymphoma. *Int J Cancer* 2008;122:1885–1890.

192. Arima N, Tei C. HTLV-I Tax related dysfunction of cell cycle regulators and oncogenesis of adult T cell leukemia. *Leuk Lymphoma* 2001;40:267–278.

193. Ivanovski M, Silvestri F, Pozzato G, et al. Somatic hypermutation, clonal diversity, and preferential expression of the VH 51p1/VL kv325

immunoglobulin gene combination in hepatitis C virus-associated immunocytomas. *Blood* 1998;91:2433–2442.

194. Marasca R, Vaccari P, Luppi M, et al. Immunoglobulin gene mutations and frequent use of VH1-69 and VH4-34 segments in hepatitis C virus-positive and hepatitis C virus-negative nodal marginal zone B-cell lymphoma. *Am J Pathol* 2001;159:253–261.

195. Quinn ER, Chan CH, Hadlock KG, et al. The B-cell receptor of a hepatitis C virus (HCV)-associated non-Hodgkin lymphoma binds the viral E2 envelope protein, implicating HCV in lymphomagenesis. *Blood* 2001;98:3745–3749.

196. Zuckerman E, Zuckerman T, Sahar D, et al. The effect of antiviral therapy on t(14;18) translocation and immunoglobulin gene rearrangement in patients with chronic hepatitis C virus infection. *Blood* 2001;97:1555–1559.

197. El-Sabban ME, Merhi RA, Haidar HA, et al. Human T-cell lymphotropic virus type 1-transformed cells induce angiogenesis and establish functional gap junctions with endothelial cells. *Blood* 2002;99:3383–3389.

198. Machida K, Kondo Y, Huang JY, et al. Hepatitis C virus (HCV)-induced immunoglobulin hypermutation reduces the affinity and neutralizing activities of antibodies against HCV envelope protein. *J Virol* 2008;82:6711–6720.

199. Fearon DT, Carroll MC. Regulation of B lymphocyte responses to foreign and self-antigens by the CD19/CD21 complex. *Annu Rev Immunol* 2000;18:393–422.

200. Lai CK, Jeng KS, Machida K, et al. Hepatitis C virus NS3/4A protein interacts with ATM, impairs DNA repair and enhances sensitivity to ionizing radiation. *Virology* 2008;370:295–309.

201. Sakamuro D, Furukawa T, Takegami T. Hepatitis C virus nonstructural protein NS3 transforms NIH 3T3 cells. *J Virol* 1995;69:3893–3896.

202. Ray RB, Meyer K, Ray R. Hepatitis C virus core protein promotes immortalization of primary human hepatocytes. *Virology* 2000;271:197–204.

203. Moriya K, Fujie H, Shintani Y, et al. The core protein of hepatitis C virus induces hepatocellular carcinoma in transgenic mice. *Nat Med* 1998;4:1065–1067.

204. Vilchez RA, Madden CR, Kozinetz CA, et al. Association between simian virus 40 and non-Hodgkin lymphoma. *Lancet* 2002;359:817–823.

205. Capello D, Rossi D, Gaudino G, et al. Simian virus 40 infection in lymphoproliferative disorders. *Lancet* 2003;361:88–89.

206. Shivapurkar N, Harada K, Reddy J, et al. Presence of simian virus 40 DNA sequences in human lymphomas. *Lancet* 2002;359:851–852.

207. Feng H, Shuda M, Chang Y, et al. Clonal integration of a polyomavirus in human Merkel cell carcinoma. *Science* 2008;319:1096–1100.

208. Nakamura S, Yao T, Aoyagi K, et al. Helicobacter pylori and primary gastric lymphoma. A histopathologic and immunohistochemical analysis of 237 patients. *Cancer* 1997;79:3–11.

209. Parsonnet J, Shmuely H, Haggerty T. Fecal and oral shedding of Helicobacter pylori from healthy infected adults. *JAMA* 1999;282:2240–2245.

210. Passaro DJ, Chosy EJ, Parsonnet J. Helicobacter pylori: consensus and controversy. *Clin Infect Dis* 2002;35:298–304.

211. Odenbreit S, Puls J, Sedlmaier B, et al. Translocation of Helicobacter pylori CagA into gastric epithelial cells by type IV secretion. *Science* 2000;287:1497–1500.

212. Segal ED, Cha J, Lo J, et al. Altered states: involvement of phosphorylated CagA in the induction of host cellular growth changes by Helicobacter pylori. *Proc Natl Acad Sci U S A* 1999;96:14559–14564.

213. El-Omar EM, Carrington M, Chow WH, et al. Interleukin-1 polymorphisms associated with increased risk of gastric cancer. *Nature* 2000;404:398–402.

214. El-Omar EM, Carrington M, Chow WH, et al. The role of interleukin-1 polymorphisms in the pathogenesis of gastric cancer. *Nature* 2001;412:99.

215. Matsumoto Y, Marusawa H, Kinoshita K, et al. Helicobacter pylori infection triggers aberrant expression of activation-induced cytidine deaminase in gastric epithelium. *Nat Med* 2007;13:470–476.

216. Hussell T, Isaacson PG, Crabtree JE, et al. The response of cells from low-grade B-cell gastric lymphomas of mucosa-associated lymphoid tissue to Helicobacter pylori. *Lancet* 1993;342:571–574.

217. Lenze D, Berg E, Volkmer-Engert R, et al. Influence of antigen on the development of MALT lymphoma. *Blood* 2006;107:1141–1148.

218. Wang G, Auerbach A, Wei M, et al. t(11;18)(q21;q21) in extranodal marginal zone B-cell lymphoma of mucosa-associated lymphoid tissue in stomach: a study of 48 cases. *Mod Pathol* 2009;22:79–86.

219. Chiang KY, Hazlett LJ, Godder KT, et al. Epstein-Barr virus-associated B cell lymphoproliferative disorder following mismatched related T cell-depleted bone marrow transplantation. *Bone Marrow Transplant* 2001;28:1117–1123.

220. Enno A, O'Rourke J, Braye S, et al. Antigen-dependent progression of mucosa-associated lymphoid tissue (MALT)-type lymphoma in the stomach. Effects of antimicrobial therapy on gastric MALT lymphoma in mice. *Am J Pathol* 1998;152:1625–1632.

221. Hofbauer GF, Kessler B, Kempf W, et al. Multilesional primary cutaneous diffuse large B-cell lymphoma responsive to antibiotic treatment. *Dermatology* 2001;203:168–170.

222. Munksgaard L, Frisch M, Melbye M, et al. Incidence patterns of lyme disease and cutaneous B-cell non-Hodgkin's lymphoma in the United States. *Dermatology* 2000;201:351–352.

223. van Maldegem F, van Dijk R, Wormhoudt TA, et al. The majority of cutaneous marginal zone B-cell lymphomas expresses class-switched immunoglobulins and develops in a T-helper type 2 inflammatory environment. *Blood* 2008;112:3355–3361.

224. Lecuit M, Abachin E, Martin A, et al. Immunoproliferative small intestinal disease associated with Campylobacter jejuni. *N Engl J Med* 2004;350:239–248.

225. Ferreri AJ, Ponzoni M, Guidoboni M, et al. Regression of ocular adnexal lymphoma after Chlamydia psittaci-eradicating antibiotic therapy. *J Clin Oncol* 2005;23:5067–5073.

226. Rosado MF, Byrne GE Jr, Ding F, et al. Ocular adnexal lymphoma: a clinicopathologic study of a large cohort of patients with no evidence for an association with Chlamydia psittaci. *Blood* 2006;107:467–472.

227. Ponzoni M, Ferreri AJ, Guidoboni M, et al. Chlamydia infection and lymphomas: association beyond ocular adnexal lymphomas highlighted by multiple detection methods. *Clin Cancer Res* 2008;14:5794–5800.

228. Geser A, Brubaker G, Draper CC. Effect of a malaria suppression program on the incidence of African Burkitt's lymphoma. *Am J Epidemiol* 1989;129:740–752.

229. Dang CV. Antimalarial therapy prevents Myc-induced lymphoma. *J Clin Invest* 2008;118:15–17.

230. Greenwood BM, Fidock DA, Kyle DE, et al. Malaria: progress, perils, and prospects for eradication. *J Clin Invest* 2008;118:1266–1276.

231. Rainey JJ, Mwanda WO, Wairiumu P, et al. Spatial distribution of Burkitt's lymphoma in Kenya and association with malaria risk. *Trop Med Int Health* 2007;12:936–943.

232. Rochford R, Cannon MJ, Moormann AM. Endemic Burkitt's lymphoma: a polymicrobial disease? *Nat Rev Microbiol* 2005;3:182–187.

233. Donati D, Mok B, Chene A, et al. Increased B cell survival and preferential activation of the memory compartment by a malaria polyclonal B cell activator. *J Immunol* 2006;177:3035–3044.

234. Pichyangkul S, Yongvanitchit K, Kum-arb U, et al. Malaria blood stage parasites activate human plasmacytoid dendritic cells and murine dendritic cells through a Toll-like receptor 9-dependent pathway. *J Immunol* 2004;172:4926–4933.

235. Kasprzak A, Spachacz R, Wachowiak J, et al. Epstein-Barr virus (EBV) infection in B-cell non-Hodgkin's lymphomas in children: virus latency and its correlation with CD21 and CD23 molecules. *Folia Histochem Cytobiol* 2007;45:169–179.

236. Young KA, Chen XS, Holers VM, et al. Isolating the Epstein-Barr virus gp350/220 binding site on complement receptor type 2 (CR2/CD21). *J Biol Chem* 2007;282:36614–36625.

237. Loren AW, Porter DL, Stadtmauer EA, et al. Post-transplant lymphoproliferative disorder: a review. *Bone Marrow Transplant* 2003;31:145–155.

238. Raab-Traub N. Epstein-Barr virus in the pathogenesis of NPC. *Semin Cancer Biol* 2002;12:431–441.

239. Portlock CS, Hamlin P, Noy A, et al. Infectious disease associations in advanced stage, indolent lymphoma (follicular and nonfollicular): developing a lymphoma prevention strategy. *Ann Oncol* 2008;19:254–258.

240. Gottschalk S, Heslop HE, Rooney CM. Adoptive immunotherapy for EBV-associated malignancies. *Leuk Lymphoma* 2005;46:1–10.

241. Savoldo B, Goss JA, Hammer MM, et al. Treatment of solid organ transplant recipients with autologous Epstein Barr virus-specific cytotoxic T lymphocytes (CTLs). *Blood* 2006;108:2942–2949.

242. Perrine SP, Hermine O, Small T, et al. A phase 1/2 trial of arginine butyrate and ganciclovir in patients with Epstein-Barr virus-associated lymphoid malignancies. *Blood* 2007;109:2571–2578.

243. Fu D, Tanhehco Y, Chen J, et al. Bortezomib-induced enzyme-targeted radiotherapy in herpesvirus-associated tumors. *Nat Med* 2008;14:1118–1122.

244. Chan JK, Yip TT, Tsang WY, et al. Detection of Epstein-Barr viral RNA in malignant lymphomas of the upper aerodigestive tract. *Am J Surg Pathol* 1994;18:938–946.

245. Belhadj K, Reyes F, Farcet JP, et al. Hepatosplenic gammadelta T-cell lymphoma is a rare clinicopathologic entity with poor outcome: report on a series of 21 patients. *Blood* 2003;102:4261–4269.

246. Kagami Y, Suzuki R, Taji H, et al. Nodal cytotoxic lymphoma spectrum: a clinicopathologic study of 66 patients. *Am J Surg Pathol* 1999;23:1184–1200.

247. Kong YY, Dai B, Kong JC, et al. Subcutaneous panniculitis-like T-cell lymphoma: a clinicopathologic, immunophenotypic, and molecular study of 22 Asian cases according to WHO-EORTC classification. *Am J Surg Pathol* 2008;32:1495–1502.

CHAPTER 7 ■ NON-HODGKIN LYMPHOMA IN IMMUNODEFICIENT HOSTS

THOMAS G. GROSS, PIERLUIGI PORCU, AND ROBERT A. BAIOCCHI

In 1959, Lewis Thomas (1) proposed that immune surveillance was an active process controlling the emergence of malignant clones from somatic cells that undergo precancerous mutations during the lifetime of a normal, immune competent individual. This hypothesis predicted that subjects that were immune deficient should experience much higher rates of all types of cancers compared with the general population. Since that time, it has been observed that individuals with compromised immunity indeed have an increased incidence of cancer; however, not all types of cancer, but predominantly lymphoproliferative disorders. In this chapter, etiology, diagnosis, and current therapeutic options will be reviewed for lymphoproliferative disorders that are associated with: (a) iatrogenic immunosuppression, such as transplantation; (b) acquired immunodeficiency following HIV infection; (c) certain primary immunodeficiencies; and finally, (d) lymphoproliferative disease that is associated with autoimmune disease (Table 7.1).

EPSTEIN-BARR VIRUS BIOLOGY AND PATHOGENESIS OF LYMPHOPROLIFERATIVE DISORDERS IN IMMUNODEFICIENT HOSTS

Not all lymphoproliferative disorders in the immune-deficient host are associated with Epstein-Barr virus (EBV), but the majority are. Therefore, a brief discussion of the biology and immunologic control of EBV-driven B-cell proliferation is warranted.

EBV is one of eight known human herpesviruses (HHVs) and is subgrouped into the gammaherpesvirus subfamily. The only natural host for EBV is humans. The natural route of transmission of EBV is via saliva. However, following transplantation, infection from donor lymphocytes is common. Following transmission of infective virions in saliva, EBV first infects epithelium of the oropharynx, though the mechanism of how this occurs is not well known because epithelium does not express CD21, the receptor for EBV (2). Epithelium is not permissive to viral infection, and viral replication occurs, resulting in cell lysis and the release of large quantities of viral particles, which leads to infection of B cells located in the lymphoid tissues of the Waldeyer ring, via the EBV receptor, CD21. These EBV-infected B cells may remain latently infected in the lymphoid tissue of the oropharynx or disseminate throughout the body, residing in secondary lymphatic organs, i.e., lymph nodes, spleen, or gut. Viral reactivation and replication can occur in latently infected B cells, also resulting in production of infectious virions and cell lysis. The conditions favoring viral replication are not well understood, though differentiation toward plasma cells does trigger viral replication (3). When latently infected B cells of the oropharynx undergo viral replications, the virus is shed into the saliva and can potentially be transmitted to another host. EBV has been found in other tissues, e.g., T cells, gastric mucosa, smooth muscle cells, etc. Again the mechanism of infection is unknown, though virion internalization is suspected.

Completion of viral replication results in the lysis and death of the host cell, which has implications for the use of therapies that inhibit viral replication in the treatment of EBV-associated lymphoproliferative disease. During viral replication, two key early immediate genes are first transcribed, BRLF1 and BZLF-1, which encodes Z EBV replication activator protein (4). These proteins then up-regulate the expression of early gene products essential for viral replication, including viral deoxyribonucleic acid (DNA) polymerase and viral thymidine kinase.

The reservoir for latent EBV infection is a small percentage of postgerminal center, antigen-selected resting memory B cells (3). Latent infection is characterized by the expression of nine virally encoded proteins, Epstein-Barr nuclear antigen (EBNA)-1, EBNA-2, EBNA-3A, EBNA-3B, EBNA-3C, and EBNA leader protein, latent membrane protein (LMP)-1, LMP-2A, and LMP-2B (2–4). Two EBV-encoded ribonucleic acids (Epstein-Barr-encoded RNA [EBER]-1 and EBER-2) are expressed abundantly in all EBV-infected cells and are valuable for making the diagnosis of EBV disease, but do not code for proteins, and their function remains to be determined. Additionally, the Bam HI-A rightward transcript is generally found in infected cells, but its function also remains to be fully delineated. Expression of EBV genes varies among the spectrum of EBV-associated diseases and often differs from in vitro immortalized B cells or normal human resting B cells infected by EBV (3,4). In type I latency, only EBNA-1, EBER-1, and EBER-2, and Bam HI-A rightward transcript are expressed. Type I latency is observed in Burkitt lymphoma (BL) and a portion of EBV-positive gastric carcinoma. Type II latency is characterized by the expression of EBNA-1, LMP-1, LMP-2A and B, EBER-1. and EBER-2. and is observed in nasopharyngeal carcinoma and other EBV-positive T-cell or natural killer (NK)-cell non-Hodgkin lymphoma (NHL), as well as Reed-Sternberg (R-S) cells of Hodgkin lymphoma (HL). In the lymphoproliferative disease that is observed in patients with immunodeficiency, EBV gene expression resembles in vitro immortalized B cells, e.g., generally expressing all nine of the EBV-related latent proteins (type III latency). The site of EBV latency in seropositive healthy individuals, the

TABLE 7.1

LYMPHOPROLIFERATIVE DISEASE IN IMMUNE COMPROMISED HOSTS

PTLD
- Early lesions
  - Plasmacytic hyperplasia
  - IM-like
- Polymorphic PTLD
- Monomorphic PTLD
  - DLBCL
  - Burkitt/Burkitt-like
  - Plasmacytoma/plasma cell myeloma
  - Peripheral T/NK cell lymphoma
- Hodgkin/Hodgkin-like PTLD

AIDS-related NHL
- Lymphomas frequently seen in immunocompetent hosts
  - DLBCL
  - BL
  - PCNSL
- Lymphomas occurring in patients with HIV
  - PEL
  - PBL
- Lymphomas in other immunodeficiency states
  - Polymorphic B cell lymphoma

NHL associated with primary immunodeficiency
- DLBCL
- BL
- PCNSL
- Lymphoblastic lymphoma (DNA repair defects)
- Peripheral T-cell lymphoma (XLP)

NHL associated with autoimmune disease
- ALPS
  - Aggressive B-cell lymphoma (diffuse large B cell and Burkitt)
  - Indolent B-cell lymphoma (follicular, marginal zone)
  - Peripheral T-cell lymphoma
- Sjögren syndrome
  - Marginal zone lymphoma (especially parotid gland)
  - DLBCL
  - Follicular lymphoma
- Systemic lupus erythematous
  - DLBCL
  - Marginal zone lymphoma
- Rheumatoid arthritis
  - Aggressive B-cell lymphoma (diffuse large B cell and Burkitt)
  - Indolent B-cell lymphoma (follicular and extranodal marginal zone)
- Inflammatory bowel disease
  - Enteropathy type T-cell lymphoma (celiac disease)
  - Hepatosplenic T-cell lymphoma (Crohn disease)

resting memory B cells do not appear to express EBNA-1 but do express LMP-2, EBER-1, and EBER-2 together with Bam HI-A rightward transcript (type IV latency).

Understanding the immune response to EBV infection is essential to comprehend the pathogenesis of EBV-related disease. EBV is a very potent immune stimulus. The immune system must control lymphoproliferation in the normal host and maintain a host/virus symbiosis. In a healthy individual, although only 10^{-5} to 10^{-6} B cells are latently infected with EBV (5), approximately 1% to 5% of all circulating CD8+ cytotoxic T cells (CTLs) are capable of reacting against EBV (6). Following primary infection the majority of EBV-specific CTLs (EBV-CTLs) are reactive against lytic viral antigens, but over time the number of EBV-CTLs against latent viral antigens predominates (7). The reservoir of viral latency is found among the resting memory B cells (3). These resting memory B cells do not express high levels of adhesion molecules or T-cell costimulatory molecules, making them poor antigen-presenting cells. However, activated EBV-infected B cells readily express major histocompatibility complex class I antigens and various adhesion molecules, making them good antigen-presenting cells. Proliferating, latently infected B cells express all latent proteins, including EBNA-2, EBNA-3A, EBNA-3C, LMP-1, and LMP-2 (type III latency). These activated, proliferating EBV-infected B cells are highly susceptible to cellular lysis by EBV-CTL and are eliminated (3,4,7). Therefore, any deficient EBV-CTL response, either quantitative or qualitative, may result in an EBV-driven B-cell proliferative process.

POSTTRANSPLANT LYMPHOPROLIFERATIVE DISORDERS

The term posttransplant lymphoproliferative disease (PTLD) does not refer to a single disease, but defines a spectrum of lymphoproliferative disorders linked to the iatrogenic immunosuppression required to prevent rejection of cell and organ allografts or graft versus host disease (GVHD) (8). The occurrence of lymphoma in solid organ transplantation (SOT) was first reported in 1968 (9). The association of PTLD with allogeneic bone marrow transplantation was first reported in 1982 (10). Studies over the next several decades described the heterogeneous clinical course and pathological spectrum of PTLD, as well as the strong association with EBV (11,12). Greater than 90% of PTLD observed with blood or marrow transplantation (BMT) and about 70% of PTLD following SOT are associated with EBV (13,14). However, the pathogenesis of PTLD that is not related to EBV is much less understood. EBV-negative PTLD typically occurs many years after transplantation (15), and a higher proportion of late-developing PTLD (>12 months after transplant) is of T cell, NK cell of Hodgkin-like disease.

Studies on the cell of origin have shown that at least 90% of PTLDs in SOT originate from host cells, whereas the converse is true for BMT, due to the myeloablative nature of the conditioning regimen. Whether the use on nonmyeloablative regimens will change the source of PTLD in BMT remains to be seen. The prognostic significance of donor versus host-derived PTLD is unclear, though the origin of the PTLD has implications when considering adoptive cellular therapy, as discussed below (see Treatment of Posttransplant Lymphoproliferative Disease).

Incidences and Risk Factors for Posttransplant Lymphoproliferative Disease

The incidence of PTLD varies from 1% to 15%, depending on the graft, the age of the recipient, and the immunosuppressive agents used (13,16–19). Data from the United Network for Organ Sharing (UNOS) in the United States show that the incidence of PTLD is highest in intestinal transplants (8% to 20%), followed by thoracic organs (2% to 10%), liver (2% to 8%), and kidney transplants (1%) (17). A potential reason for different rates of PTLD among different allografts may be the amount of lymphoid tissue that is transferred, which may serve as a reservoir for EBV. However, allografts with the highest incidence of PTLD also tend to require higher levels of immunosuppression to maintain the allograft. The incidence of PTLD after allogeneic BMT is low (0.5% to 2%), except in patients receiving T-cell–depleted allografts, where the incidence may be as high as 20% to 25% (13,19). The period of risk for PTLD is much shorter following BMT, due to the fact that immunosuppression can be discontinued often within the first year after transplant, as opposed to the lifetime immunosuppression required for the vast majority of recipients of SOT.

In SOT, a consistent finding is that the incidence of PTLD is highest in the pediatric age group. United Network for Organ Sharing data suggest that the relative risk for PTLD for pediatric patients is 2.81 compared with adult recipients (17). The risk may be even higher in patients younger than 5 years (20). Age may be a surrogate marker for EBV seronegativity at transplant (17,21). The single most important risk factor for PTLD is the EBV status of the recipient at transplant (17,22).

Over the past 30 years, the improvement in immunosuppressive drugs has contributed greatly to the success of both SOT and allogeneic BMT. At present, no single laboratory assay can reliably measure the global burden of immunosuppression in individual patients (23). Retrospective analyses of PTLD incidence in different transplant eras have shown that the overall intensity of the immunosuppression is a significant factor for the risk of developing PTLD (16–18,22,24). The specific PTLD-promoting effect of any individual immunosuppressive drug has been difficult to tease out. In general, the more T-cell specific the immunosuppression is, the greater the risk of PTLD. Another general finding is that there is a "learning curve" for immunosuppressive agents, with the highest risk of PTLD associated with the introduction of newer agents. With the advent of calcineurin inhibitors, i.e., cyclosporine A, a dramatic improvement in allograft and patient survival was observed, but also a dramatic increase in PTLD. Similar results were observed when tacrolimus was introduced with early studies suggesting increased risk of PTLD compared with cyclosporine A, but more current data suggest similar risks with either of these agents (25). Rapamycin (sirolimus), a mammalian target of rapamycin (mTOR) inhibitor, has antitumor effects and has been demonstrated to directly inhibit the proliferation of EBV-infected B cells, both in vitro and in vivo (26). A recent study by United Network for Organ Sharing revealed a decreased risk for malignancy with the use of mammalian target of rapamycin inhibitors compared with calcineurin inhibitors (27). Antimetabolites have been used as chronic immunosuppression for a long time, e.g., azathioprine. Although PTLD can occur with any immunosuppressive agent, recent studies suggest that mycophenolate mofetil, an inhibitor of purine synthesis, is less associated with PTLD (27,28). The use of T-cell-depleting serotherapies, e.g., OKT3 and antithymocyte globulin, is associated with the highest risk of PTLD (16,18). There are conflicting results about the risk of PTLD when using monoclonal anti-T-cell–nondeplet-

ing antibodies, such as the anti-interleukin (IL)-2R antibodies basiliximab and daclizumab (16,18,29). These differences may be related to different databases and follow-up time periods. In conclusion, the overall intensity of immunosuppression is likely to play a more significant role in PTLD development than each individual drug's effect on DNA repair, cell cycling, growth, and survival.

There are other factors that have been identified in various studies to possibly increase the risk of PTLD. The recipient's underlying disease may affect the risk of developing PTLD. For example, patients who receive BMT for primary immunodeficiencies may have a higher risk of PTLD (13). There are reports that suggest that recipients of liver transplant for autoimmune hepatitis, or primary biliary cirrhosis (30), hepatitis C virus infection (31), or cystic fibrosis (32) may have an increased risk for PTLD. However, due to very small numbers and a variety of confounding factors, the strength of these associations remains to be determined. Data from several North American registries have demonstrated a significant higher risk in white recipients compared with other races (17,33). The biologic reason for this difference remains to be explained. There have been reports suggesting that other viral infections, such as *Cytomegalovirus*, HHV-8, and simian virus 40, may play a role in some patients with PTLD. However, the data in the literature are conflicting, so the impact of these other viruses as risk factors and/or the mechanisms of interaction with EBV and other well-established cofactors remain to be determined. And finally, individual genetic polymorphisms that affect the innate immune responses of the host may play a role in the development of PTLD (34).

Diagnosis and Classification of Posttransplant Lymphoproliferative Disease

The diagnosis of PTLD requires a tissue biopsy. Other tests can support the diagnosis but lack specificity and sensitivity as diagnostic tests. Tests for detection of EBV infection, i.e., monospot or serology, can be difficult to interpret in a patient who is immunocompromised. The finding of EBV DNA by polymerase chain reaction (PCR) is very specific for EBV infection, but is not 100% sensitive. Although elevated levels of EBV DNA in the peripheral blood of patients with radiographic evidence of lymphoproliferation provides strong evidence of PTLD, this is insufficient to make the diagnosis. A determination of EBV-associated PTLD is best made by in situ hybridization with EBV-encoded ribonucleic acid (EBER) probes with the finding of EBV in tumor cells. Immunohistochemical staining for EBV proteins, e.g., LMP, does result in some false negatives (35). Perhaps the greatest difficulty in making the diagnosis of PTLD occurs when mass lesions are not evident. This form of PTLD rapidly disseminates and infiltrates organs, resulting in death within days to weeks, and diagnosis is often made at autopsy (13). When mass lesions are not present or accessible for biopsy, examination of the peripheral blood, bone marrow, cerebrospinal fluid, or other body fluids for the presence of plasmacytoid cells or large B cells can be helpful.

Currently, PTLD is classified according to the World Health Organization (WHO) schema for hematopoietic neoplasms, based on clinical, histologic, immunophenotypic, genetic, and virologic criteria (14). The WHO classification divides PTLD into four major categories: (a) early lesions, (b) polymorphic PTLD, (c) monomorphic PTLD, and (d) HL or HL-like PTLD. These categories represent a pathologic spectrum that can be observed synchronously or metachronously within a single specimen or within multiple specimens from a single patient.

Early lesions consist of two morphologic types, plasmacytic hyperplasia and infectious mononucleosis (IM)-like PTLD; both are characterized by preservation of the architecture of the involved tissue. Early lesions are more common in EBV-naive transplant recipients following primary infection, usually via the allograft. Plasmacytic hyperplasia is characterized by numerous plasma cells with rare immunoblasts. IM-like lesions demonstrate marked paracortical expansion with a mixed T-cell and plasma cell infiltrate, and a prominent immunoblastic proliferation. Immunophenotyping of early lesions usually shows polyclonal B cells, with variable mixtures of T cells, plasma cells, monocytes and NK cells. In situ hybridization for EBER often highlights the immunoblasts, but other EBV-associated antigens are not consistently expressed (14). These lesion may be polyclonal or oligoclonal.

In contrast to early lesions, polymorphic PTLD lesions are characterized by effacement of the lymph node or destruction of the normal architecture of the involved tissue (14). However, in contrast to monomorphic PTLD, a full, heterogeneous spectrum of B-cell differentiation can be seen, small to intermediate-size lymphocytes, to immunoblasts all the way to mature plasma cells. Atypia, necrosis, R-S-like cells, and numerous mitotic figures are often present. Variable mixtures of B cells and T cells can be found. Polymorphic PTLD can be either polyclonal or monoclonal, and though rare, cytogenetic abnormalities may be found.

Monomorphic PTLDs are destructive, infiltrating proliferations characterized by complete architectural effacement atypia with necrosis commonly observed. Morphologic features are sufficient to be classified as a lymphoma (14). In general, monomorphic PTLDs show large aggregates and/or confluent sheets of transformed cells with large nuclei with prominent nucleoli. The neoplastic cells can be markedly pleomorphic, or may have significant plasmacytoid or plasmablastic differentiation. It is not uncommon for a single biopsy to demonstrate histology that is consistent with both polymorphic and monomorphic PTLD. These cases are difficult to classify within a single category, and there is significant interpretation bias among pathologists. The presence of areas of monomorphic PTLD, however, should always be noted.

Monomorphic PTLDs are subclassified according to the WHO classification of lymphomas in patients with immunocompetence (14). The majority of monomorphic PTLDs will be monoclonal, though polyclonal disease can be observed. Monomorphic B-cell PTLD is the prototypic monomorphic PTLD. Diffuse large B-cell lymphoma (DLBCL) with variants, including immunoblastic, centroblastic, and less commonly, anaplastic morphology, predominates. The next most common histology observed is Burkitt or Burkitt-like; however, many of these cases are not associated with c-myc translocations. The majority of B-PTLDs show presence of EBV infection within the transformed cells, with variable latency patterns, though type III latency occurs in the majority of tumors (3,4). Currently, the evaluation of germinal center or postgerminal center phenotype is not required

because the clinical and prognostic implications remain to be determined. Rare cases of B-PTLD are morphologically and immunophenotypically identical to plasma cell neoplasms (14). Plasma cell myeloma and plasmacytoma-like PTLD are EBV associated in only about 50% of the cases. Clinically, these can present as extramedullary plasmacytic neoplasms similar to plasmacytomas or plasma cell myeloma. Plasma cell PTLDs need to be differentiated from plasmacytic hyperplasia, a nondestructive early lesion, and DLBCL with marked plasmacytic differentiation, a monomorphic PTLD. Due to the rarity of plasma cell PTLD, it is currently unclear if plasma cell directed, B-cell directed, or both, is the most effective therapy. The evaluation for urine and serum M components, serum immunoglobulin levels, and lytic bone lesions, although not always conclusive, can be helpful in the diagnosis of plasma cell myeloma PTLD. Most T-cell PTLDs lack EBV; however, a minor subset may be EBV positive (14). T-cell PTLDs resemble peripheral T-cell lymphoma (PTCL); though as opposed to immune competent hosts, anaplastic large cell histology is rarely observed. NK-cell PTLD is very rare but will frequently express CD56 and cytotoxic markers, and lack surface CD3. Unlike T-cell PTLDs, the vast majority of true NK-cell PTLDs show EBV infection.

HL and HL-like PTLD is a rare category of PTLD that is classified independently from other monomorphic PTLD (14). HL PTLDs show the morphologic features characteristic of classic HL in nontransplant patients. These include the proper background inflammatory infiltrate and R-S cells with the characteristic phenotype (CD45−, CD3−, CD20−/weak+, CD15+, CD30+). HL PTLD must be distinguished from polymorphic PTLD with R-S–like cells that are CD45+, CD20+, and CD15- (36). Although currently HL and HL-like PTLD are considered similar, there is evidence suggesting that HL-like PTLD may be more related clinically and pathologically to B-cell polymorphic PTLD (36). The HL-like PTLD frequently shows an atypical immunophenotype for HL, such as strong expression of CD20. HL and HL-like PTLD usually arise late in transplantation and frequently show evidence of EBV infection (14).

The current WHO classification does not recognize low-grade B-cell lymphoproliferative disorders as PTLD. Follicular lymphoma, extranodal marginal zone B-cell lymphomas of mucosa-associated lymphoid tissue (MALT), and hairy cell leukemia that are morphologically and immunophenotypically identical to counterparts in patients with immune competence have been reported in transplant recipients. These lymphomas do not show evidence of EBV, but the MALT lymphomas are frequently associated with *Helicobacter* infections, especially in gastric sites (37). These lesions are exceedingly rare and may represent coincidental events, as opposed to a consequence of immunosuppression.

Treatment of Posttransplant Lymphoproliferative Disease

Successful treatment of PTLD necessitates controlling the lymphocyte proliferation while awaiting or ideally facilitating the development of an appropriate memory cytotoxic T-cell (EBV-CTL) response to maintain a homeostasis. Additional factors that contribute to the difficulty of treating these patients include: increased toxicity from therapy and/or secondary infections; and potential enhancement of alloreactive T-cell immunity, which increases the patient's risk of developing life-threatening GVHD or allograft rejection/loss. Additionally, it is difficult to compare results in the literature because of differing definitions of disease, and interventions, e.g., how immunosuppression is reduced.

There are few proven methods to reduce the incidence of PTLD. Some retrospective analyses have suggested that the use of ganciclovir prophylaxis can reduce the incidence of PTLD (38,39). However, changes in immunosuppression over time might also explain the observed decrease in incidence. One review of a large database suggests that the use of anti-*Cytomegalovirus* intravenous immunoglobulin reduced the incidence of PTLD (40), but prospective randomized trials have not been able to demonstrate benefit (41,42). The use of pan-lymphocyte depletion, as opposed to T-cell-specific depletion, can reduce the incidence of PTLD (19).

Because the problem in most cases of PTLD is an inadequate number of EBV-CTLs (43,44), replacement of EBV-CTLs would be a logical therapeutic intervention. Infusion of donor lymphocytes has been demonstrated to be successful in the prevention and treatment of PTLD after BMT (45). To avoid the GVHD and other associated toxicities with infusion of donor lymphocytes, ex vivo–generated EBV-specific CTLs have been shown to be effective in treating and preventing PTLD after BMT (46). The ex vivo generation of EBV-specific CTLs takes several weeks (46–48), and requires a high level of technology and cost. Therefore, due to the cost and regulatory oversight necessary to generate and administer the ex vivo-generated EBV-CTLs, this approach is not feasible for most centers. The use of adoptive T-cell therapy in an organ transplant recipient is more complex. First, cadaver organs are most widely used; therefore, donor lymphocytes are often not available. Second, as opposed to BMT, after organ transplant, the PTLD cells are usually of recipient origin, so the immunologic recognition, specificity, and efficacy of donor lymphocytes are uncertain. Third, the use of closely matched relatives' lymphocytes runs the risk of both rejection and GVHD. It has been shown that in organ transplant patients, EBV-specific CTLs can be given safely, and when given prophylactically, no PTLD developed (46). However, despite detection of increased number of EBV-specific CTLs, EBV DNA levels in the peripheral blood decreased very little, and the infused EBV-specific CTLs persisted only several months (48). EBV-specific CTLs have been used to treat PTLD successfully following organ transplant, but multiple infusions are required (47,48). One strategy to overcome the time it takes to generate EBV-CTLs from patients with PTLD is to utilize human leukocyte antigens-matched EBV-CTLs that are banked (49). Although a logical and exciting therapeutic strategy, at present, adoptive cellular therapy is not available for the majority of patients with PTLD.

Preemptive therapy has been very successful for reducing the incidence of posttransplant *Cytomegalovirus* disease. For preemptive therapy to be successful, one must have a method of reliably identifying patients who are at high risk before they develop disease and an effective intervention. There are many reports that correlate increased EBV viral load with PTLD (43,50). Other than in the setting of T-cell-depleted BMT, the predictive value of EBV PCR monitoring is unclear (51). In both BMT and SOT, it has been shown that the predictive value of EBV viremia is vastly improved by including

measures of anti-EBV T-cell immunity, though these assays are not presently commercially available (44,52). Although there are no well-controlled trials to support the practice, it is common following BMT using T-cell depletion, either ex vivo or in vivo, to monitor for EBV for 3 to 6 months and to give anti-CD20 antibody (rituximab) as preemptive therapy (53). This approach appears to reduce the incidence of PTLD; however, disease that does occur tends to be very resistant to other therapies (54). In SOT, despite the lack of well-controlled trials, many centers monitor EBV regularly and reduce immunosuppression for elevated or persistent EBV positivity (39,55). It is unclear the efficacy of this strategy.

Reports of mortality due to PTLD vary from 50% to 90%. A reduction or complete withdrawal of immunosuppression remains the cornerstone of PTLD treatment. The response varies greatly, which probably reflects the differences in the practice of reduction of immunosuppression and the wide spectrum of PTLD, with localized or polymorphic disease more likely to respond (56). Even for patients who have disease that is responsive to a reduction of immunosuppression, rejection may threaten the viability of the allograft or produce GVHD (57). Reduction of immunosuppression is rarely successful following BMT because the defect is delayed EBV-CTL recovery, not suppression of EBV-CTL function (13). The efficacy of antiviral drugs in treating PTLD is controversial because they are seldom used without other interventions (e.g., reduction of immunosuppression) (57). In addition, if viral replication, which is lytic to the infected B cells, is suppressed, B-cell proliferation could theoretically be enhanced. A novel approach using arginine butyrate, which up-regulates expression of EBV thymidine kinase and stimulates viral replication, given with ganciclovir, which causes an abortive replicative cycle so no virions are produced but cell death occurs, has been shown to be effective in highly refractory PTLD (58). Strategies to target viral replication to treat PTLD is an interesting approach and warrants further investigation.

The first report using anti-B-cell therapy used anti CD21 and anti-CD23 antibodies demonstrated that they were well tolerated, but only 35% of patients achieved long-term survival, and only patients with monoclonal disease survived (59). More recently, anti-CD20, or rituximab, has been used. All reports to date have had small numbers, and results vary. But it appears that about 50% of patients will achieve complete remission with rituximab (60–62). However, relapse has been reported in up to 25% of patients (63). Additionally, one must keep in mind the significant effect of rituximab on normal B cells, and monitor patients' immunoglobulin levels closely (64).

Chemotherapy has been used to treat resistant PTLD following SOT. Chemotherapy is attractive because it kills proliferating B cells and is immunosuppressive enough to treat or prevent allograft rejection. However, at conventional doses used in the treatment of NHL, posttransplant patients have significantly more end-organ toxicity and susceptibility to infection, with as many as 35% of patients dying of toxicity of the therapy (62,65,66). One study demonstrated that outcome was the same when chemotherapy was reserved for patients who failed rituximab (67). Therefore, a common practice at present is to treat patients who have failed reduction of immunosuppression with rituximab and reserve chemotherapy for patients who fail rituximab (62,67). A low-dose chemotherapy approach has been shown to be very effective in treating PTLD in children following organ transplant with little toxicity; however, it remains to be determined if this approach will be successful in treating adult PTLD (68).

Non-EBV-associated PTLD, B cell, T cell, Hodgkin, or plasmacytic/myeloma tends to occur late and rarely resolves with reduction of immunosuppression (15,69). Despite the associated toxicity, standard dosed chemotherapy regimens are usually required to achieve remissions. Remissions are rare, and if achievable, recurrences are common. The possible exception is Hodgkin PTLD. Although more toxicity and outcomes are inferior compared with nontransplant HL patients, the use of standard HL regimens has produced a significant number of cures (70).

In summary, PTLD can range from a benign, self-limited polyclonal or oligoclonal lymphoproliferation to an aggressive, widely disseminated, monoclonal, and fatal malignant lymphoma. PTLD remains a challenge, and a significant cause of morbidity and mortality in transplant recipients. Due to low numbers of patients in any one center, pathologic and clinical heterogeneity, and wide variation in the use of immunosuppressive regimens, progress in improving the outcome of PTLD remains a challenge due to the lack of consensus in terminology in classification and difficulty of conducting large, controlled clinical trials.

ACQUIRED IMMUNODEFICIENCY SYNDROME-RELATED LYMPHOMA (SEE CHAPTER 35)

Human immunodeficiency virus (HIV)/acquired immunodeficiency syndrome (AIDS) remains the fourth leading cause of death in the world (71). In the early years of the HIV epidemic, the majority of complications were related to infectious diseases; lymphoma typically occurred in the later stages of HIV infection, with CD4 counts less than 200/mm^3 and a history of other AIDS-defining illnesses (72). In the pre–highly active antiretroviral therapy (HAART) era, the incidence of NHL was 60 to 200 times greater in patients infected with HIV than in the HIV seronegative population (73). Since the advent of HAART in 1996, primary central nervous system (CNS) lymphoma (PCNSL) and NHL have declined in areas where HAART is routinely available, but in the developing world, the incidence of NHL has increased. And though there has been a decrease in NHL, a higher prevalence of non-AIDS-defining lymphomas and other malignancies has been observed since the introduction of HAART (74).

Pathogenesis and Pathology of Acquired Immunodeficiency Syndrome–Related Non-Hodgkin Lymphoma

In individuals infected with HIV, the incidence of EBV-associated lymphomas is high (75% of all AIDS-NHL). EBV-associated NHL in this population is typically aggressive and includes both CNS and systemic lymphomas (75). It has been shown that patients with HIV have lower numbers of functioning EBV-specific CTLs. Studies have shown that EBV-specific CTLs are not physically lost, but rather cease to

function properly (76–78). This phenomenon has been shown to correlate with both lower CD4 counts and increasing EBV viral load (77).

Classification of Acquired Immunodeficiency Syndrome-Related Lymphoma

The WHO classifies HIV-associated lymphomas into three categories:

1. Lymphomas that also occur in patients with immunocompetence. The majority of these are high-grade B-cell lymphomas, including BL and DLBCL with plasmablastic or immunoblastic features. These are further classified as extranodal/nodal lymphomas or PCNSL. Nearly half of these cases are associated with EBV infection.
2. Lymphomas occurring more specifically in patients with HIV, including primary effusion lymphoma (PEL) and plasmablastic lymphoma (PBL) of the oral cavity.
3. Lymphomas also occurring in other immunodeficiency states, such as PTLD-like polymorphic B-cell lymphoma (79).

DBLCLs constitute about 60% to 70% of AIDS-related lymphoma (ARL), and include immunoblastic lymphomas and large noncleaved cell lymphomas. DLBCLs may present with nodal or extranodal disease. These lymphomas exhibit an association with EBV in approximately 75% of cases. Rearrangements of BCL-6 and MYC have been noted in some patients (80). Proliferation rates are typically high, but not at the level characteristically seen with BL. In the HAART era, patients with DBLCL have median survival times of 6 months to 4 years, which is comparable to patients without HIV with aggressive lymphoma (81).

BL comprises 30% of ARLs, and tends to occur at relatively higher CD4 counts (>200) (82). Patients are typically diagnosed with advanced-stage disease, B symptoms, and extranodal and bone marrow involvement (81). In the pre-HAART era, median survival was similar in patients with BL and DLBCL when treated with the same chemotherapy regimen. Since the advent of HAART, the median survival of BL lags significantly behind that of DLBCL (8 vs. 22 months) (81). This suggests the possibility that in the HAART era, patients with BL and DLBCL should be treated with different approaches.

PCNSL is a universally EBV-associated lymphoma that occurs in patients with severe immunodeficiency. The incidence of PCNSL is markedly increased in the HIV population, and these patients tend to have the poorest prognosis. Since the advent HAART, the incidence of PCNSL has significantly decreased, but it is seen more frequently as the AIDS-defining illness. Tissue biopsy is the definitive diagnostic test, but in some cases, biopsy is not possible. EBV-DNA by PCR on cerebrospinal fluid has been shown to have a sensitivity and specificity of 80% and 100%, respectively, for detection of PCNSL (83). Tumor expression of BCL-6 is a potentially important prognostic factor that has been correlated with improved survival (84).

PELs are HHV-8 and EBV-associated lymphomas characterized by malignant effusions as the predominant feature and lack of nodal involvement. PELs comprise 1% to 5% of ARLs, and tend to be associated with severe immunosuppression (85). PEL cells do not express surface immunoglobulin, but immunoglobulin gene rearrangements typically demonstrate clonal B-cell origin. Median survival for patients with PEL is 6 months. Extracavitary HHV-8-associated lymphomas, also referred to as "solid PEL," have been reported to be associated temporally with PEL, and are essentially extranodal counterparts of PEL, with identical morphology, immunophenotype, and immunoglobulin light-chain rearrangements (86). The spectrum of HHV-8 lymphomas has been expanded to include extracavitary solid lymphomas without serous effusions. These ARLs are typically composed of an immunoblastic-like cell population, but some reported cases have been noted to have anaplastic-like features, and greater pleomorphism than their noneffusion-associated counterparts.

Multicentric Castleman disease has also been reported in patients with HIV. Castleman disease is an HHV-8-associated process thought to be in part related to cytokine dysregulation, particularly IL-6 (85). The disorder is characterized by plasmacytosis, polyclonal hypergammaglobulinemia, hepatosplenomegaly, generalized lymphadenopathy, and may present with constitutional symptoms, including autoimmune cytopenias. The HHV-8-infected lymphocytes have a plasma-cell morphology and phenotype, and occasionally display light chain restriction (79). Aggregates of these plasmablasts form clusters, or microlymphomas, in the spleen, which can sometimes develop into mass lesions. The median survival of patients with multicentric Castleman disease is only 14 months. Potentially beneficial treatment options suggested by recent reports include HAART alone, splenectomy, antiherpesvirus drugs such as ganciclovir, and/or rituximab, but at present no therapy has been demonstrated to consistently be effective (85).

First described in 1997, PBL is a rare form of B-cell lymphoma that commonly presents extranodally, with an affinity for the oral cavity, though about a third have been noted to be extraoral, and marrow involvement occurs in less than one fourth of cases (73). PBL is a highly aggressive lymphoma, affecting predominantly young males. It is often mistaken for an oral abscess or infected tooth, leading to critical delays in appropriate diagnosis and treatment. PBL is strongly associated with severe immune suppression. Since its initial description, 151 cases have been reported, 120 (79%) of which have been HIV associated, and 135 (89%) of which involved some form of immune suppression. Despite this association, PBL is currently not classified as an AIDS-defining illness (73). Given the strong association of PBL with HIV, combined with evidence of improved prognosis when appropriate chemotherapy is combined with HAART, it is recommended that all patients diagnosed with PBL be tested for HIV. PBL is recognized by the WHO as a subtype of DLBCL. Histologically, large neoplastic cells with a squared-off appearance display a diffuse and cohesive growth pattern, featuring a single, prominent, centrally located nucleolus, or several peripheral ones, and abundant, deeply basophilic cytoplasm (73). Immunophenotypically, the cells display weak or absent expression of the most common B-cell antigens, particularly CD20 and CD79a, but stain strongly for plasma-cell markers CD138/B-B4, CD38, and VS38c (79). Cells invariably display λ-light chain restriction. Proliferation index typically exceeds 90%. The presence of EBV has frequently been described in biopsy specimens (73). The clinical course of PBL is typically rapidly progressive, with only 38% of patients surviving 1 year after diagnosis (87,88). Increased survival times have been observed with the combination of

HAART and lymphoma-specific chemotherapy (73). The role of rituximab is questionable because PBL is CD20 negative.

Salivary gland enlargement is relatively common in individuals infected with HIV, occurring in about 5% of the population with HIV. Patients may present with salivary gland enlargement as part of a generalized lymphadenopathy secondary to reactive lymphoid hyperplasia (89). This typically occurs in the form of multiple bilateral parotid lymphoepithelial cysts that develop along a spectrum of disease from initial lymphoid infiltration of salivary lobules to lymphoepithelial duct lesions. This is thought to be due to ductal obstruction as a result of basal cell and intraglandular lymphofollicular hyperplasia (90). The lymphoid proliferation is polyclonal and not associated with lymphoma. However, extranodal marginal zone lymphoma, MALT lymphoma, has been rarely reported in individuals with HIV. They have been described in the salivary glands, and also involving other sites, including the stomach and lung (91). The relationship between pulmonary MALT lymphoma and lymphocytic interstitial pneumonitis suggests a possible infectious etiology (92).

Polymorphic B-cell lymphomas are composed of small lymphocytes, plasma cells, and plasmacytoid immunoblasts that are typically monoclonal, and occur infrequently in patients with HIV (93). In high-grade lesions, tumor necrosis and prominent large cells may be seen. Their polymorphic appearance and EBV association are similar to PTLD.

Lymphomatoid granulomatosis is a rare angiocentric and angiodestructive lymphoproliferative disorder that is associated with immunosuppression. It is strongly linked to EBV, with nearly 100% of cases being EBV associated (94). It has been previously described in the oral cavity and gingival areas in individuals with HIV (95).

T-cell lymphomas have recently been noted to occur more frequently in the HIV-infected population (96). These lymphomas typically occur in the skin and subcutaneous tissues, presenting with tumor-like masses, vascular invasion, and tissue necrosis. They have been noted to be associated with skin and bone marrow involvement more commonly than B-cell ARLs, but median survival is similar (97). Morphologically, they tend to resemble peripheral T-cell lymphomas but lack the epidermotropism displayed by mycosis fungoides.

Clinical Presentation of Acquired Immunodeficiency Syndrome-Related Lymphoma

Most patients with ARL present with constitutional B symptoms, and lymphoma should be considered in the differential diagnosis of patients with HIV presenting with B symptoms (81). CNS involvement occurs in over 20% of ARLs and conveys a poor prognosis (98). Finding EBV DNA by PCR in cerebrospinal fluid has been shown to be nearly 100% predictive of CNS involvement and may aid in selecting appropriate patients for CNS prophylaxis (83). Current recommendations for CNS prophylaxis in ARL include all patients with BLs involving the head and neck, and those with stage IV disease. The best results for treatment of CNS disease have been obtained using methotrexate, steroids, and HAART, with or without craniospinal radiation (99). About 25% of patients will have marrow involvement at diagnosis for ARL, with over half of patients with BL having marrow involvement. Of note, thrombocytopenia and anemia can occur with or without macroscopic marrow involvement (100). Although marrow involvement itself is not an independent prognostic factor for survival in ARL, gross leukemic involvement, i.e., >50%, confers a poor prognosis. Due to the correlation of marrow and CNS involvement, CNS prophylaxis should be considered for any patient with marrow involvement. Gastrointestinal tract involvement is noted in about 25% of ARLs, and liver involvement occurs in 10% to 25% of cases (101,102). However, any anatomic site may be involved in patients with ARL (81).

LYMPHOPROLIFERATIVE DISEASE ASSOCIATED WITH PRIMARY IMMUNODEFICIENCY

Due to advances in prevention and treatment of opportunistic infections, patients with primary immunodeficiencies now enjoy longer lives than ever before. However, neoplastic disorders, particularly lymphoproliferative complications, remain the second most common cause of premature mortality, still preceded by infections. The incidence of lymphomas is estimated to be between 15% and 25%, and this risk increases with age (103). Table 7.2 is a summary of tumor types reported for the various primary immunodeficiency diseases, with NHL predominating. Although EBV has been identified as a common cofactor, not all NHLs are EBV associated, suggesting that the specific immune defect is not in recognition of viral-specific antigens, but perhaps a defect in immune surveillance necessary in the elimination of cells with abnormalities of proliferation, function, and/or apoptosis.

Historically, NHL treatment with conventional doses of chemotherapy and radiation has met with limited success in patients with primary immunodeficiency (104,105). This is primarily due to opportunistic infections and increase in treatment-related mortality due to end organ dysfunction. In the current era, improved antiviral and antifungal therapies have allowed many patients with immunodeficiencies who have cancer to be treated more aggressively. However, even for patients who achieve complete remission, relapses are common. It is unclear if relapse is always truly a recurrence of the same clonal process, or a "new" disease, because "recurrences" with a different clonal origin compared with the original lymphoma have been documented (106). Because the primary risk factor for cancer is the underlying immunodeficiency, immune system replacement with allogeneic hematopoietic stem cell transplantation is ideal, if a suitable donor is available.

Severe Combined Immunodeficiencies

Severe combined immunodeficiency (SCID) is not a disease, but a collection of more than a dozen genetically distinct disorders with severe impairment of both cellular and humoral immune function, leading to early mortality from opportunistic infections during infancy in the absence of aggressive medical intervention (107). Patients with SCID who develop lymphoma share the characteristics of severe quantitative or qualitative defects in T cells and presence of B cells. Examples of types of SCID with increased risk of NHL are X-linked SCID, the defect results from mutations in the X-linked common γ chain gene of multiple IL receptors, IL-7 receptor deficiency, and JAK3 deficiency. In these diseases, T cell development is inhibited, but B-cell numbers are generally plentiful.

Wiskott-Aldrich Syndrome

Wiskott-Aldrich syndrome (WAS), an X-linked disorder of broad-ranging and variable immunodeficiency and microthrombocytopenia, results from mutations in the WASP gene (108). The WASP gene encodes a large intracellular protein involved with cytoskeletal integrity and signal transduction. Several molecules reported to be associated with WASP are

---

TABLE 7.2

IMMUNODEFICIENCY CANCER REGISTRY CASES: DISTRIBUTION OF TUMORS AND IMMUNODEFICIENCIES

	Adenocarcinoma	Lymphoma	Hodgkin disease	Leukemia	Other immunodeficiency tumors	Total (%)
Severe combined immunodeficiency	1 (2.4%)	3 (73.8%)	4 (9.5%)	5 (11.9%)	1 (2.4%)	42 (8.4)
X-linked agammaglobulinemia	3 (14.3%)	7 (33.3%)	3 (14.3%)	7 (33.3%)	1 (4.8%)	21 (4.2)
Common variable immunodeficiency	20 (16.7%)	55 (45.8%)	8 (6.7%)	8 (6.7%)	29 (24.2%)	120 (24.0)
IgA deficiency	8 (21.1%)	6 (15.8%)	3 (7.9%)	0 (0%)	21 (55.3%)	38 (7.6)
Hyper-IgM syndrome	0 (0%)	9 (56.3%)	4 (25.0%)	0 (0%)	3 (18.8%)	16 (3.2)
WAS	0 (0%)	59 (75.6%)	3 (3.8%)	7 (9.0%)	9 (11.5%)	78 (15.6)
AT	13 (8.7%)	69 (46.0%)	16 (10.7%)	32 (21.3%)	20 (13.3%)	150 (30.0)
Other immunodeficiencies	1 (4.0%)	12 (48.0%)	1 (4%)	4 (16.0%)	7 (28.0%)	25 (5.0)
Total immunodeficiency	46 (9.2%)	252 (50.4%)	43 (8.6%)	63 (12.6%)	96 (19.2%)	500 (100)

Modified from Shiloh Y, Rotman G. Ataxia-telangiectasia and the ATM gene: linking neurodegeneration, immunodeficiency, and cancer to cell cycle checkpoints. *J Clin Immunol* 1996;16:254—260.

involved in normal progression through the cell cycle. Experimental evidence suggests that B cells from patients with WAS are relatively resistant to apoptosis, and there have been reports of EBV-negative B-cell lymphomas, especially among adult males with clinically milder forms of WAS that are sometimes termed X-linked thrombocytopenia (108).

X-Linked Lymphoproliferative Syndrome

Males affected with X-linked lymphoproliferative syndrome (XLP) were originally recognized for fatal complications of EBV infection and high risk of lymphoma (109). The defective gene has been identified as SH2D1A or SLAM-associated protein (110). SLAM-associated protein is a small adaptor protein of only a SH2 binding domain and short C and N terminus. Although the function of SLAM-associated protein is still being delineated, it has been shown to bind to at least four regulatory molecules known to alter T- and NK-cell functions by both activation and suppression, and it is thought to be involved in T-B-cell interactions through cytokine regulation (111).

Clinical features of XLP include an excessive immune reaction to EBV associated with hemophagocytosis and liver failure that is clinically indistinguishable from other forms of hemophagocytic syndromes, and has been called fulminant infectious mononucleosis (FIM) or EBV-associated hemophagocytic lymphohistiocytosis (112). Both FIM and EBV-associated hemophagocytic lymphohistiocytosis can be seen in patients without XLP. Patients with XLP may also present with lymphoproliferative disease, hypogammaglobulinemia, or hematologic cytopenias (109). Patients who develop FIM may initially present with the usual signs and symptoms of IM, but these symptoms are often more severe. The course and progression of the disease are variable, ranging from presentation in multiorgan failure developing over hours, to persistent or recurring symptoms of IM for months. FIM is characterized by extensive infiltration of parenchymal organs by lymphoid cells, primarily CD8 (+) cells in varying degrees of transformation and histiocytes with surprisingly few B cells. If this aggressive immune reaction goes unabated, ultimately all organs and even vessels will sustain extensive damage. This reaction culminates in the phagocytosis, tissue destruction, and cellular depletion, with death usually following shortly thereafter due to multisystem organ failure. The only successful treatment is early use of etoposide and immunosuppression with corticosteroids and cyclosporin A or tacrolimus (113). Even with remission of symptoms, recurrences are common, and recurrences tend to be more difficult to control, resulting in an extremely poor prognosis. When control of symptoms can be achieved, allogeneic BMT is recommended and is the felt to be the only curative therapy (114).

Lymphoma develops in approximately one-fourth of patients with XLP (109,115). Over 90% of lymphomas are of B-cell phenotype, but HL, T-cell NHL, lymphomatoid granulomatosis, or angiocentric immunoproliferative lesions can occur (109). Half of the boys with lymphoma have had no evidence of prior EBV infection, and EBV is detectable in only 25% of tumor specimens (115). Again, as in other immunodeficiency, allogeneic hematopoietic stem cell transplant should be considered if remission can be achieved (114).

X-Linked Hyperimmunoglobulin M Syndrome (X-Linked CD40 Ligand Deficiency)

X-linked hyperimmunoglobulin M syndrome results in a failure of immunoglobulin switching by B cells that requires signaling through CD40, and in decreased development and maintenance of type 1 cell-mediated responses (including NK-cell function) due to impaired responsiveness of CD40 expressing monocyte-derived antigen-presenting cells (115). Patients with X-linked hyperimmunoglobulin M syndrome appear to have an increased risk of lymphomas, and a higher incidence of HL compared with other primary immunodeficiencies (116).

Common Variable Immunodeficiency

Common variable immunodeficiency is not a single disease but a heterogenous group of patients who have varying degrees of antibody production defects, and many have subtle to more pronounced T-cell defects. Patients with common variable immunodeficiency are at increased risk for lymphomas similar to other primary immunodeficiencies, but also are at increased risk for MALT lymphomas in adulthood (117). It has been suggested that strict adherence to immuneoglobulin replacement and prophylactic antibiotics may reduce the risk of lymphoma.

Immunodeficiency and Cancer in Genetic Disorders of Deoxyribonucleic Acid Repair

There are several genetic diseases where the primary defect is in DNA repair, but they may also manifest with varying degrees of immunodeficiency. These diseases have a substantially increased risk of lymphoma, as well as other cancers, because generation of immunologic diversity among both B and T cells requires a well-orchestrated "creation" of DNA breaks followed by rearrangement of immunoglobulin and T-cell receptor gene sequences and repair to stabilize the final genetic product. The treatment of these patients with NHL is indeed challenging.

Ataxia Telangiectasia

Ataxia telangiectasia (AT) is an autosomal disorder with cancer predisposition that has variable and profound immunologic and other systemic manifestations, principally cerebellar degeneration (118). For some time it has been recognized that AT cells fail to normally activate cell-cycle checkpoints after exposure to γ-irradiation. The mutant gene (AT mutated) is a member of the phosphatidyl inositol kinase family of molecules involved in signal transduction, and has also been implicated in meiotic recombination (119). AT lymphocytes demonstrate a 25-fold increase in nonrandom rearrangements of immunoglobulin and T-cell receptor genes compared with lymphocytes from normal individuals (120). Although lymphomas and leukemias predominate, patients with AT also experience high rates of epithelial cancers involving the skin, gastrointestinal tract, genitourinary tract, and CNS. Outcome for NHL in patients with AT is dismal, with a median survival of 1 year and <20% at 5 years, with toxicity, primarily infection and pulmonary toxicities and secondary malignancies being significant causes of mortality (104).

Nijmegen Breakage Syndrome

Nijmegen Breakage syndrome (NBS) is another rare autosomal recessive syndrome, which like AT is associated with both humoral and T-cell defects, clinical radiosensitivity, chromosomal instability, and predisposition to lymphoid and epithelial cancers (121). Other characteristics of patients with NBS are growth retardation, microcephaly, and "birdlike" facies. The protein defective in NBS-NBS1, nibrin, or p95, appears to function together with AT mutated to "sense" DNA double-strand breaks and activate a diversity of corrective actions. As in AT, frequent chromosomal aberrations at the sites of T-cell receptor and immunoglobulin H rearrangement are observed in lymphocytes of patients with NBS. Treatment and outcome of patients with NBS are similar to patients with AT.

NON-HODGKDIN LYMPHOMA ASSOCIATED WITH AUTOIMMUNE DISEASE

The risk of lymphoma has been increased in patients with autoimmune disease (121). In patients who receive chronic immunosuppressive therapy, the pathogenesis of NHL development is likely the same as other immune deficient states. However, the abnormal immune response and lymphocyte proliferation to chronic antigenic stimulation may also play a role in NHL pathogenesis in some patients. Finally, an inherited defect in apoptosis, i.e., autoimmune lymphoproliferative syndrome (ALPS), has been shown to greatly increase the risk of lymphoma.

Recently, several large metaanalyses (122,123) and a population-based case-control study (124) have better defined the risk and subtypes of lymphoma seen in various autoimmune disorders. As opposed to NHL observed in other immune-deficient hosts, it appears that patients with autoimmune disease when adjusted for comorbidities do as well as patients with immunocompetence when treated with standard chemotherapy regimens (125).

Autoimmune Lymphoproliferative Syndrome

ALPS represents a constellation of genetic apoptosis defects associated with mutations in Fas, Fas ligand, and caspase 8 or 10 genes (126). Most of the cases described have heterozygous, dominant-negative mutations involving Fas. Characteristic clinical features present in early childhood or even at birth. These include chronic multifocal lymphadenopathy, splenomegaly, autoimmune hemolytic anemia (and often other immune cytopenias), with increased proportions of circulating, senescent T cells (CD3+, CD4−, CD8−), so-called double-negative T cells. Many patients experience symptomatic improvement with steroid therapy, and generally, the autoimmune

complications lessen in severity with age. The use of antimetabolite immunosuppression, e.g., mycophenolate mofetil, appears promising to control symptoms in patients that fail corticosteroids (127). The estimated risk of lymphoma in patients with ALPS is around 30%, and some patients having developed more than one lymphoid tumor over time. The risk for developing NHL and HL is 51 and 14-fold, respectively (128). The heterogeneity of lymphomas seen is impressive, with all subtypes of HL, and though there is a predominance of B-cell phenotype, i.e., DLBCL, follicular, marginal zone, and Burkitt, peripheral T-cell lymphoma has also been observed. The median age of diagnosis of ALPS is 5 years, but median age of lymphoma is 25 years (128). Although patients with ALPS tolerate standard therapy, and remissions are common, relapses and new lymphomas are frequent. Allogeneic transplantation has been performed for severe forms of ALPS; whether replacement of the immune system will ultimately reduce risk of lymphomas remains to be determined.

Sjögren Syndrome

Sjögren syndrome has a 6- to 13-fold increased risk of NHL, and is the highest among autoimmune disorders (122,124,129). B-cell NHL, marginal zone, especially extranodal disease of the parotid gland, is most commonly observed, followed by DLBCL and follicular lymphoma (122,124). This risk of NHL is associated with both primary and secondary disease. Of note, neither age nor use of immunosuppressive therapy appears to be associated with increased risk of developing NHL (122,124).

Systemic Lupus Erythematosus

Systemic lupus erythematosus has a 3- to 7-fold increased risk of NHL. The risk appears to be highest in older (>39 years) patients (122,129). Again, B cell, DLBCL, and marginal zone lymphomas predominate, and again the use of immunosuppressive therapy does not appear to increase the risk.

Rheumatoid Arthritis

Studies have shown the risk of NHL in patients with rheumatoid arthritis to be low (129) or not increased over the general population (122). However, the use of immunosuppressive therapy is associated with an increased risk of NHL (122,129). One study suggested that the type of therapy was associated with risk of NHL. This study suggested that use of corticosteroid therapy was associated with the least risk of NHL, followed by cytotoxics (azathioprine, methotrexate, or cyclophosphamide) and biologics, e.g., antitumor necrosis factor monoclonal antibodies were associated with the highest risk of NHL (124,129).

Inflammatory Bowel Disease

Inflammatory bowel disease, consisting of celiac disease, ulcerative colitis, and Crohn disease, overall is not associated with increased risk of NHL (122). However, there is a significant increased incidence of T-cell NHL, enteropathy type T-cell lymphoma in celiac disease (122), and hepatosplenic T-cell lymphoma in Crohn disease (130). The reason for this association is not known; however, it has been speculated that the underlying defect may predispose certain T cells to undergo malignant transformation. Although these are rare complications of the disease, the outcome has been dismal for these types of NHL.

Psoriasis

Psoriasis is not associated with an increased risk of NHL overall. However, there is a weak association with T-cell NHL and anaplastic large cell lymphoma in patients >60 years (122). Of interest, an increased risk of cutaneous lymphoma of any type was not found.

Other Autoimmune Disorders and Non-Hodgkin Lymphoma

Although there are published reports of NHL occurring in numerous autoimmune disorders, at present there is a lack of evidence to say there is an incidence in the following disorders: type 1 diabetes, pernicious anemia, scleroderma, myasthenia gravis, sarcoidosis, multiple sclerosis or polymyositis/dermatomyositis (122).

SUMMARY

There is ample evidence that many patients with immune dysfunction are at increased risk for developing NHL. Defects/deficiencies in T-cell immunity, presumably due to a lack of tumor immunosurveillance, are the most significant risk factor for the development of NHL. Although many of these NHLs are associated with viruses, e.g., EBV, this does not account completely for the increased risk. Patients with abnormalities of their immune system at risk for developing NHL may fall into one of three categories: (a) iatrogenic immunosuppression in the case of transplant recipients or in some cases of autoimmune disease, (b) acquired immunosuppression from HIV, or (c. inherited immunosuppression. There are inherited diseases that may manifest with varying degrees of immunodeficiency, but the pathogenesis of NHL is more likely to be from inability to repair DNA defects than a decrease in tumor immunosurveillance. Additionally, there are patients generally not considered immunodeficient, who can have a significantly increased risk of NHL, presumably due to increased lymphocyte activation from chronic antigenic stimulation, best illustrated in some forms of autoimmune disease. It is unclear to what extent decreased tumor immunosurveillance, defects in DNA repair, and/or chronic antigenic stimulation plays in the pathogenesis of NHL in the immunocompetent host, but further study of these disorders may provide better understanding of the pathogenesis and hopefully, prevention and treatment of all patients with NHL.

REFERENCES

1. Thomas L. *Cellular and humoral aspects of hypersensitivity states.* New York, NY: Hoeber, 1959.
2. Straus SE, Cohen JI, Tosato G, et al. Epstein-Barr virus infections: biology, pathogenesis, and management. *Ann Intern Med* 1993;118:45–58.
3. Thorley-Lawson DA, Gross A. Persistence of the Epstein-Barr virus and the origins of associated lymphomas. *N Engl J Med* 2004;350:1328–1337.
4. Cohen JI. Epstein-Barr virus infection. *New Engl J Med* 2000;343:481–492.
5. Yang J, Tao Q, Flinn IW, et al. Characterization of Epstein-Barr virus-infected B cells in patients with posttransplantation lymphoproliferative disease: disappearance after rituximab therapy does not predict clinical response. *Blood* 2000;96:4055–4063.
6. Tan LC, Gudgeon N, Annels NE, et al. A re-evaluation of the frequency of CD8+ T cells specific for EBV in healthy carriers. *J Immunol* 1999;162:1827–1835.
7. Hislop AD, Annels NE, Gudgeon NH, et al. Epitope-specific evolution of human CD8+ T cell responses from primary to persistent phases of Epstein-Barr virus infection. *J Exp Med* 2002;195:893–905.
8. Gottschalk S, Rooney CM, Heslop HE. Posttransplant lymphoproliferative disorders. *Ann Rev Med* 2005;56:29–44.
9. Penn I, Hammond W, Brettschneider L, et al. Malignant lymphomas in transplantation patients. *Transplant Proc* 1969;1:106–112.
10. Schubach WH, Hackman R, Neiman PE, et al. A monoclonal immunoblastic sarcoma in donor cells bearing Epstein-Barr virus genomes following allogeneic marrow grafting for acute lymphoblastic leukemia. *Blood* 1982;60:180–187.
11. Frizzera G, Hanto DW, Gajl-Peczalska KJ, et al. Polymorphic diffuse B-cell hyperplasias and lymphomas in renal transplant recipients. *Cancer Res* 1981;41:4262–4279.
12. Nalesnik MA, Jaffe R, Starzl TE, et al. The pathology of posttransplant lymphoproliferative disorders occurring in the setting of cyclosporine A-prednisone immunosuppression. *Am J Pathol* 1988;133:173–192.
13. Gross TG, Steinbuch M, DeFor T, et al. B cell lymphoproliferative disorders following hematopoietic stem cell transplantation: risk factors, treatment and outcome. *Bone Marrow Transplant* 1999;23:251–258.
14. WHO. Swerdlow SH, Campo E, Harris NL, et al. *Classification: pathology and genetics of tumours of haematopoietic and lymphoid tissues,* 4th ed. Lyon, France: IARC Press, 2008.
15. Dotti G, Fiocchi R, Motta T, et al. Lymphomas occurring late after solid-organ transplantation: influence of treatment on the clinical outcome. *Transplantation* 2002;74:1095–1102.
16. Opelz G, Dohler B. Lymphomas after solid organ transplantation: a collaborative transplant study report. *Am J Transplant* 2004;4:222–230.
17. Dharnidharka VR, Tejani AH, Ho PL, et al. Post-transplant lymphoproliferative disorder in the United States: young Caucasian males are at highest risk. *Am J Transplant* 2002;2:993–998.
18. Cherikh WS, Kauffman HM, McBride MA, et al. Association of the type of induction immunosuppression with posttransplant lymphoproliferative disorder, graft survival, and patient survival after primary kidney transplantation. *Transplantation* 2003;76:1289–1293.
19. Curtis RE, Travis LB, Rowlings PA, et al. Risk of lymphoproliferative disorders after bone marrow transplantation: a multi-institutional study. *Blood* 1999;94:2208–2216.
20. Cox KL, Lawrence-Miyasaki LS, Garcia-Kennedy R, et al. An increased incidence of Epstein-Barr virus infection and lymphoproliferative disorder in young children on FK506 after liver transplantation. *Transplantation* 1995;59:524–529.
21. Ho M, Jaffe R, Miller G, et al. The frequency of Epstein-Barr virus infection and associated lymphoproliferative syndrome after transplantation and its manifestations in children. *Transplantation* 1988;45:719–727.
22. Dharnidharka VR, Sullivan EK, Stablein DM, et al. Risk factors for post-transplant lymphoproliferative disorder (PTLD) in pediatric kidney transplantation: a report of the North American Pediatric Renal Transplant Cooperative Study (NAPRTCS). *Transplantation* 2001;71:1065–1068.
23. Kowalski R, Post D, Schneider MC, et al. Immune cell function testing: an adjunct to therapeutic drug monitoring in transplant patient management. *Clin Transplant* 2003;17:77–88.
24. Birkeland SA, Hamilton-Dutoit S. Is posttransplant lymphoproliferative disorder (PTLD) caused by any specific immunosuppressive drug or by the transplantation per se? *Transplantation* 2003;76:984–988.
25. Webster AC, Woodroffe RC, Taylor RS, et al. Tacrolimus versus cyclosporin as primary immunosuppression for kidney transplant recipients: meta-analysis and meta-regression of randomised trial data. *BMJ* 2005;331:810.
26. Vaysberg M, Balatoni CE, Nepomuceno RR, et al. Rapamycin inhibits proliferation of Epstein-Barr virus-positive B-cell lymphomas through modulation of cell-cycle protein expression. *Transplantation* 2007;83:1114–1121.
27. Kauffman HM, Cherikh WS, Cheng Y, et al. Maintenance immunosuppression with target-of-rapamycin inhibitors is associated with a reduced incidence of de novo malignancies. *Transplantation* 2005;80:883–889.
28. Dharnidharka VR, Ho PL, Stablein DM, et al. Mycophenolate, tacrolimus and post-transplant lymphoproliferative disorder: a report of the North American Pediatric Renal Transplant Cooperative Study. *Pediatr Transplant* 2002;6:396–399.
29. Adu D, Cockwell P, Ives NJ, et al. Interleukin-2 receptor monoclonal antibodies in renal transplantation: meta-analysis of randomised trials. *BMJ* 2003;326:789–793.

30. Shpilberg O, Wilson J, Whiteside TL, et al. Pre-transplant immunological profile and risk factor analysis of post- transplant lymphoproliferative disease development: the results of a nested matched case-control study: The University of Pittsburgh PTLD Study Group. *Leuk Lymphoma* 1999;36:109–121.

31. Hezode C, Duvoux C, Germanidis G, et al. Role of hepatitis C virus in lymphoproliferative disorders after liver transplantation. *Hepatology* 1999;30:775–778.

32. Cohen AH, Sweet SC, Mendeloff E, et al. High incidence of posttransplant lymphoproliferative disease in pediatric patients with cystic fibrosis. *Am J Respir Crit Care Med* 2000;161:1252–1255

33. Aull MJ, Buell JF, Trofe J, et al. Experience with 274 cardiac transplant recipients with posttransplant lymphoproliferative disorder: a report from the Israel Penn International Transplant Tumor Registry. Transplantation. *Transplantation* 2004;78:1676–1682.

34. Dierksheide JE, Baiocchi RA, Ferketich AK, et al. IFN-gamma gene polymorphisms associate with development of EBV+ lymphoproliferative disease in hu PBL-SCID mice. *Blood* 2005;105:1558–1565.

35. Dhir RK, Nalesnik MA, Demetris AJ, et al. Latent membrane protein expression in posttransplant lymphoproliferative diseases. *Appl Immunohistochem* 1995;3:123–126.

36. Ranganathan S, Jaffe R. Is there a difference between Hodgkin's disease and a Hodgkin's-like post-transplant lymphoproliferative disorder, and why should that be of any interest? *Pediatr Transplant* 2004;8:6–8.

37. Aull MJ, Buell JF, Peddi VR, et al. MALToma: a Helicobacter pylori-associated malignancy in transplant patients: a report from the Israel Penn International Transplant Tumor Registry with a review of published literature. *Transplantation* 2003;75:225–228.

38. Funch DP, Walker AM, Schneider G, et al. Ganciclovir and acyclovir reduce the risk of post-transplant lymphoproliferative disorder in renal transplant recipients. *Am J Transplant* 2005;5:2894–2900.

39. McDiarmid SV, Jordan S, Lee GS, et al. Prevention and preemptive therapy of posttransplant lymphoproliferative disease in pediatric liver recipients. *Transplantation* 1998;66:1604–1611.

40. Opelz G, Volker D, Naujokat C, et al B. Effect of cytomegalovirus prophylaxis with immunoglobulin or with antiviral drugs on post-transplant non-Hodgkin lymphoma: a multicentre retrospective analysis. *Lancet Oncol* 2007;8:212–218.

41. Green M, Michaels MG, Katz BZ, et al. CMV-IVIG for prevention of Epstein-Barr virus disease and posttransplant lymphoproliferative disease in pediatric liver transplant recipients. *Am J Transplant* 2006;6:1906–1912.

42. Humar A, Hebert D, Dele Davies H, et al. A randomized trial of ganciclovir versus ganciclovir plus immune globulin for prophylaxis against Epstein-Barr virus posttransplant lymphoproliferative disorder. *Transplantation* 2006;81:856–861.

43. Lucas KG, Burton RL, Zimmerman SE, et al. Semiquantitative Epstein-Barr virus (EBV) polymerase chain reaction for determination of patients at risk for EBV-induced lymphoproliferative disease after stem cell transplantation. *Blood* 1998;91:3654–3661.

44. Smets F, Lattine D, Bazin H, et al. Ratio between Epstein-Barr viral load and anti-Epstein-Barr virus specific T-cell response as a predictive marker of posttransplant lymphoproliferative disease. *Transplantation* 2002;73:1603–1610.

45. Papadopoulos EB, Ladanyi M, Emanuel D, et al. Infusions of donor leukocytes to treat Epstein-Barr virus-associated lymphoproliferative disorders after allogeneic bone marrow transplantation. *N Engl J Med* 1994;330:1185–1191.

46. Rooney CM, Smith CA, Ng CY, et al. Infusion of cytotoxic T cells for the prevention and treatment of Epstein-Barr virus-induced lymphoma in allogeneic transplant recipients. *Blood* 1998;92:1549–1555.

47. Sherritt MA, Bharadwaj M, Burrows JM, et al. Reconstitution of the latent T-lymphocyte response to Epstein-Barr virus is coincident with long-term recovery from posttransplant lymphoma after adoptive immunotherapy. *Transplantation* 2003;75:1556–1560.

48. Savoldo B, Goss JA, Hammer MM, et al. Treatment of solid organ transplant recipients with autologous Epstein Barr virus-specific cytotoxic T lymphocytes CTLs). *Blood* 2006;108:2942–2949.

49. Haque T, Wilkie GM, Jones MM, et al. Allogeneic cytotoxic T-cell therapy for EBV-positive posttransplantation lymphoproliferative disease: results of a phase 2 multicenter clinical trial. *Blood* 2007;110:1123–1131.

50. Rowe DT, Webber S, Schauer EM, et al. Epstein-Barr virus load monitoring: its role in the prevention and management of post-transplant lymphoproliferative disease. *Transpl Infect Dis* 2001;3:79–87.

51. van Esser JWJ, van der Holt B, Meijer E, et al. Epstein-Barr virus (EBV) reactivation is a frequent event after allogeneic stem cell transplantation (SCT) and quantitatively predicts EBV-lymphoproliferative disease following T-cell-depleted SCT. *Blood* 2001;98:972–978.

52. Meij P, van Esser JW, Niesters HG, et al. Impaired recovery of Epstein-Barr virus (EBV)-specific CD8+ T lymphocytes after partially T-depleted allogeneic stem cell transplantation may identify patients at very high risk for progressive EBV reactivation and lymphoproliferative disease. *Blood* 2003;101:4290–4297.

53. van Esser JW, Niesters HG, van der Holt B, et al. Prevention of Epstein-Barr virus-lymphoproliferative disease by molecular monitoring and preemptive rituximab in high-risk patients after allogeneic stem cell transplantation. *Blood* 2002;99:4364–4369.

54. Ocheni S, Kroeger N, Zabelina T, et al. EBV reactivation and post transplant lymphoproliferative disorders following allogeneic SCT. *Bone Marrow Transplant* 2008;42:181–186.

55. Lee TC, Salvoldo B, Rooney CM, et al. Quantitive EBV viral loads and immunosuppression alterations can decrease PTLD incidence in pediatric liver transplant recipients. *Am J Transpl* 2005;5:2222–2228.

56. Hayashi RJ, Kraus MD, Patel AL, et al. Posttransplant lymphoproliferative disease in children: correlation of histology to clinical behavior. *J Pediatr Hematol Oncol* 2001;23:14–18.

57. Porcu P, Eisenbeis CF, Pelletier RP, et al. Successful treatment of posttransplantation lymphoproliferative disorder (PTLD) following renal allografting is associated with sustained CD8(+) T-cell restoration. *Blood* 2002;100:2341–2348.

58. Perrine SP, Mermine O, Small T, et al. A phase I/II trial of arginine butyrate and ganciclovir in patients with Epstein-Barr virus associated lymphoid malignancies. *Blood* 2007;109:2571–2578.

59. Benkerrou M, Jais JP, Leblond V, et al. Anti-B-cell monoclonal antibody treatment of severe posttransplant B- lymphoproliferative disorder: prognostic factors and long-term outcome. *Blood* 1998;92:3137–3147.

60. Oertel SHK, Verschuuren E, Reinke P, et al Effect of anti-CD 20 antibody rituximab in patients with post-transplant lymphoproliferative disorder (PTLD). *Am J Transpl* 2005;5:2901–2906.

61. Choquet S, Leblond V, Herbrecht R, et al. Efficacy and safety of rituximab in B-cell post-transplantation lymphoproliferative disorders: results of a prospective multicenter phase 2 study. *Blood* 2006;107:3053–3057.

62. Elstrom RL, Andreadis C, Aqui NA, et al. Treatment of PTLD with rituximab or chemotherapy. *Am J Transpl* 2006;6:569–578.

63. Choquet S, Oertel S, Leblond V, et al. Rituximab in the management of post-transplantation lymphoproliferative disorder after solid organ transplantation: proceed with caution. *Ann Hematol* 2007;86:599–607.

64. Pescovitz MD. Rituximab and anti-CD20 monoclonal antibody: history and mechanism of action. *Am J Transpl* 2006;6:859–866.

65. Buell JF, Gross TG, Hanaway MJ, et al. Chemotherapy for PTLD: The Israel Penn International Transplant Tumor Registry Experience. *Transplant Proc* 2005;37:956–957.

66. Choquet S, Trappe R, Leblond V, et al. CHOP-21 for the treatment of post-transplant lymphoproliferative disorders following solid organ transplantation. *Hematologica* 2007;92:273–274.

67. Trappe R, Riess H, Babel N, et al. Salvage chemotherapy for refractory and relapsed posttransplant lymphoproliferative disorders (PTLD) after treatment with single agent rituximab. *Transplantation* 2007;83:912–918.

68. Gross TG, Bucuvalas J, Park J, et al. Low dose chemotherapy for the treatment of refractory post-transplant lymphoproliferative disease in children. *J Clin Oncol* 2005;23:6481–6488.

69. Hanson MN, Morrison VA, Peterson BA, et al. Posttransplant T-cell lymphoproliferative disorders–an aggressive, late complication of solid-organ transplantation. *Blood* 1996;88:3626–3633.

70. Bierman PJ, Vose JM, Langnas AN, et al. Hodgkin's disease following solid organ transplantation. *Ann Oncol* 1996;7:265–270.

71. UNAIDS. *Report on the Global AIDS epidemic, July 2008.* Available at: http://unaids.org/en/.

72. Grulich AE, Wan X, Law MG, et al. B cell stimulation and prolonged immune deficiency are risk factors for non-Hodgkin's lymphoma in people with AIDS. *AIDS* 2000;14:133–140.

73. Reidel DJ, Gonzales-Cuyar LF, Zhao XF, et al. Plasmablastic lymphoma of the oral cavity: a rapidly progressive lymphoma associated with HIV infection. *Lancet Infect Dis* 2008;8:261–267.

74. Mayor AM, Gomez MA, Rios-Olivares E, et al. AIDS-defining neoplasm prevalence in a cohort of HIV-infected patients, before and after highly active antiretroviral therapy. *Ethn Dis* 2008;18(suppl 2):189–194.

75. Carbone A, Gloghini A, Dotti G. EBV-associated lymphoproliferative disorders: classification and treatment. *Oncologist* 2008;13:577–585

76. Blumberg RS, Paradis T, Byington R, et al. Effects of human immunodeficiency virus on the cellular immune response to Epstein-Barr virus in homosexual men: characterization of the cytotoxic response and lymphokine production. *J Infect Dis* 1987;156:877–890

77. van Baarle D, Hovenkamp E, Callan MFC, et al. Dysfunctional Epstein-Barr virus (EBV)-specific CD8+ T lymphocytes and increased EBV load in HIV-1 infected individuals progressing to AIDS-related non-Hodgkin lymphoma. *Blood* 2001;98:146–155

78. Kersten MJ, Klein MR, Holwerda AM, et al. EBV-specific cytotoxic T cell responses in HIV-1 infection: different kinetics in patients progressing to opportunistic infection or non-Hodgkin's lymphoma. *J Clin Invest* 1997;99:1525–1533.

79. Carbone A. AIDS-related non-Hodgkin's lymphomas: from pathology and molecular pathogenesis to treatment. *Hum Pathol* 2003;33, 392–404.

80. Carbone A, Gaidano G, Gloghini A, et al. BCL-6 protein expression in AIDS-related non-Hodgkin's lymphomas: inverse relationship with Epstein-Barr virus encoded latent membrane protein-1 expression. *Am J Pathol* 1997;150:155–165

81. Mounier N, Spina M, Gisselbrecht C. Modern management of non-Hodgkin lymphoma in HIV-infected patients. *Brit J Haematol* 2007;136:685–698.

82. Galicier L, Fieschi C, Borie R. Intensive chemotherapy regimen (LMB86) for St Jude stage IV AIDS-related Burkitt lymphoma/leukemia: a prospective study. *Blood* 2007;110:2846–2854.

83. Lim ST, Levine AM. Recent advances in acquired immunodeficiency syndrome (AIDS)-related lymphoma. *Ca J Clin* 2005;55:229–241.

84. Braaten KM, Betensky RA, de Leval L, et al. BCL-6 expression predicts improved survival in patients with primary central nervous system lymphoma. *Clin Cancer Res* 2003;9:1063–1069.

85. Navarro WH, Kaplan L. AIDS related lymphoproliferative disease. *Blood* 2006;107:13–20.

86. Carbone A, Gloghini A. KSHV/HHV8-associated lymphomas. *Brit J Haematol* 2007;140:13–24.

87. Delecluse H.J, Anagnostopoulos, Dallenbach F, et al. Plasmablastic lymphomas of the oral cavity: a new entity associated with the human immunodeficiency virus infection. *Blood* 1997;89:1413–1420.

88. Dong HY, Scadden DT, de Leval L, et al. Plasmablastic lymphoma in HIV-positive patients: an aggressive Epstein-Barr virus-associated extramedullary neoplasm. *Am J Surg Pathol* 2005;29:1633–1641.

89. Chieng DC, Argosino R, McKenna BJ, et al. Utility of fine-needle aspiration in the diagnosis of salivary gland lesions in patients infected with human immunodeficiency virus. *Diagn Cytopathol* 1999;2:260–264.

90. Ihrler S, Steger W, Riederer A, et al. HIV associated cysts of the parotid glands. A histomorphic and magnetic resonance tomography study of formal pathogenesis. *Laryngorhinootologie* 1996;75:671–676.

91. Boulanger E, Meignin V, Baia M, et al. Mucosa-associated lymphoid tissue lymphoma in patients with human immunodeficiency virus infection. *Brit J Haematol* 2008;140:464–474.

92. Teruya-Feldstein J, Temeck BK, Sloas MM, et al. Pulmonary malignant lymphoma of mucosa-associated lymphoid tissue (MALT) arising in a pediatric HIV-positive patient. *Am J Surg Pathol* 1995;19:357–363.

93. Nador RG, Chadburn A, Gundappa G, et al. Human immunodeficiency virus (HIV)-associated polymorphic lymphoproliferative disorders. *Am J Surg Pathol* 2003;27:293–302.

94. Rezk SA, Weiss LM. Epstein-Barr virus-associated lymphoproliferative disorders. *Hum Pathol* 2007;38:1293–1304.

95. Jaffe ES. Lymphoid lesions of the head and heck: a model of lymphocyte homing and lymphomagenesis. *Mod Pathol* 2002;15:255–263.

96. Navarro WH, Kaplan L. AIDS-related lymphoproliferative disease. *Blood* 2006;107:13–20.

97. Azroo BK, Bu X, Espina BM. T cell lymphoma in HIV-infected patients. *J Acq Immune Defic Syndr* 2004;36:1020–1027.

98. Hegde U, Filie A, Little R, et al. High incidence of occult leptomeningeal disease detected by flow cytometry in newly diagnosed aggressive B-cell lymphomas at risk of central nervous system involvement: the role of flow cytometry. *Blood* 2005;105:496–502.

99. Ortega ME. AIDS-related malignancies—a new approach (hot news). *AIDS Rev* 2008;10:125–126.

100. Seneviratne LC, Espina BM, Nathwani BN, et al. Clinical, immunologic and pathologic correlates of bone marrow involvement in 291 patients with AIDS-related lymphoma. *Blood* 2001;98:2358–2363.

101. Ziegler JL, Beckstead JA, Volberding PA, et al. Non-Hodgkin's lymphoma in 90 homosexual men: relation to generalized lymphadenopathy the acquired immunodeficiency syndrome. *N Engl J Med* 1984;311:565–570.

102. Kaplan LD, Abrams DI, Feigal E, et al. AIDS associated non-Hodgkin's lymphomas in San Francisco. *JAMA* 1989;261:719–724.

103. Filipovich AH, Heinitz KJ, Robison LL, et al. The Immunodeficiency Cancer Registry. A research resource. *Am J Pediatr Hematol Oncol* 1987;9:183–184.

104. Seidemann K, Tiemann M, Henze G, et al. Therapy for non-Hodgkin lymphoma in children with primary immunodeficiency: analysis of 19 patients from the BFM trials. *Med Pediatr Oncol* 1999;33:536–544.

105. Sandoval C, Swift M. Treatment of lymphoid malignancies in patients with ataxia-telangiectasia. *Med Pediatr Oncol* 1998;31:491–497.

106. Hoffman T, Heilman C, Madsen H, et al. Matched unrelated allogeneic bone marrow transplantation for recurrent malignant lymphoma in a patient with X-linked lymphoproliferative disease (XLP). *Bone Marrow Transplant* 1998;22:603–604.

107. Fischer A. Primary immunodeficiency diseases: an experimental model for molecular medicine. *Lancet* 2001;357:1863–1869.

108. Zhu Q, Zhang M, Blaese RM, et al. The Wiskott-Aldrich syndrome and X-linked congenital thrombocytopenia are caused by mutations of the same gene. *Blood* 1995;86:3797–3804.

109. Seemayer TA, Gross TG, Egeler RM, et al. X-linked lymphoproliferative disease: twenty-five years after the discovery. *Pediatr Res* 1995;38:471–478.

110. Sayos J, Wu C, Morra M, et al. The X-linked lymphoproliferative-disease gene product SAP regulates signals induced through the co-receptor SLAM. *Nature* 1998;395:462–469.

111. Wu C, Nguyen KB, Pien GC, et al. SAP controls T cell response to virus and terminal differentiation of TH2 cells. *Nat Immunol* 2001;2:410–414.

112. Okano M, Gross TG. Epstein-Barr virus-associated hemophagocytic syndrome and fatal infectious mononucleosis. *Am J Hematol* 1996;53:111–115.

113. Imashuku S, Kuriyama K, Teramura T, et al. Requirement for etoposide in the treatment of Epstein-Barr virus-associated hemophagocytic lymphohistiocytosis. *J Clin Oncol* 2001;19:2665–273.

114. Lankester A, Visser L, Bredius R, et al. Allogeneic stem cell transplantation in X-linked lymphoproliferative disease in different stages of disease: two cases in one family and review of the literature. *Bone Marrow Transpl* 2005;36:99–105.

115. Sumegi J, Huang D, Lanyi A, et al. Correlation of mutations of the SH2D1A gene and Epstein Barr virus infection with clinical phenotype and outcome in X-linked lymphoproliferative disease. *Blood* 2000;96:3118–3125.

116. Notarangelo LD, Duse M, Ugazio AG. Immunodeficiency with hyper-IgM (HIM). *Immunodefic Rev* 1992;3:101–121.

117. Aghamohammadi A, Pravaneh N, Tirgari F. Lymphoma of mucosa-associated lymphoid tissue in common variable immunodeficiency. *Leuk Lymph* 2006:47:343–346.

118. Shiloh Y, Rotman G. Ataxia-telangiectasia and the ATM gene: linking neurodegeneration, immunodeficiency, and cancer to cell cycle checkpoints. *J Clin Immunol* 1996;16:254–260.

119. Shiloh Y. ATM and related protein kinases: safeguarding genome integrity. *Nat Rev Cancer* 2003;3:155–168.

120. Hecht F, Hecht BK. Chromosome changes connect immunodeficiency and cancer in ataxia-telangiectasia. *Am J Pediatr Hematol Oncol* 1987;9:185–188.

121. Tauchi H, Matsuura S, Kobayashi J, et al. Nijmegen breakage syndrome gene, NBS1, and molecular links to factors for genome stability. *Oncogene* 2002; 21:8967–8980.

122. Ekstrom Smedby K, Valdic CM, Falster M, et al. Autoimmune disorders and risk of non-Hodgkin lymphoma subtypes: a pooled analysis within the InterLymph Consortium. *Blood* 2008;111:4029–4038.

123. Ekstrom Smedby K, Zintzaras E, Voulgarelis M, et al. The risk of lymphoma development in autoimmune disease. *Arch Intern Med* 2005;165:2337–2344.

124. Engels EA, Cerhan JR, Linet MS, et al. Immune-related conditions and immune modulating medications as risk factors for non-Hodgkin's lymphoma: a case-control study. *Am J Epidemiol* 2005;162:1153–1161.

125. Mikuls TR Endo JO, Puumala SE, et al. Prospective study of survival outcomes in non-Hodgkin's lymphoma patients with rheumatoid arthritis. *J Clin Oncol* 2006;24:1597–1602.

126. Rieux-Laucat F, Le DF, Hivroz C, et al. Mutations in Fas associated with human lymphoproliferative syndrome and autoimmunity. *Science* 1995;268:1347–1349.

127. Rao VK, Dugan F, Dale JK, et al. Use of mycophenolate mofetil for chronic, refractory immune cytopenias in children with autoimmune lymphoproliferative syndrome. *Br J Hematol* 2005;129:534–538.

128. Strauss, SE, Jaffe ES, Puck JM, et al. The development of lymphoma in families with autoimmune lymphoproliferative syndrome with germline Fas mutations and defective lymphocyte apoptosis. *Blood* 2001;98:194–220.

129. Zintzaras E, Voulgarelis M, Moutsopoulos HM. The risk of lymphoma development in autoimmune diseases. *Arch Intern Med* 2005;165:2337–2344.

130. Rosh JR, Gross T, Mamula P, et al. Hepatosplenic T-cell lymphoma in adolescents and young adults with Crohn's disease: a cautionary tale. *Inflamm Bowel Dis* 2007;13:1024–1030.

CHAPTER 8 ■ MOLECULAR GENETICS OF LYMPHOMA

RICCARDO DALLA-FAVERA AND LAURA PASQUALUCCI

Many advances have been made in the understanding of the pathogenesis of non-Hodgkin lymphoma (NHL) derived from B cells (B-NHL), whereas, with few exceptions, the molecular basis of T-cell-derived NHL remains relatively undefined. This chapter will focus on: (a) the putative cellular derivation of the various subtypes of NHL; (b) the mechanisms of genetic alteration that are associated with the development of NHL; and (c) the description of the most frequent and biologically important genetic lesions associated with the major subtypes of NHL. Additional details can be found in the chapters describing each NHL subtype.

CELLULAR DERIVATION OF LYMPHOMA

The cellular derivation of NHLs can be identified by comparing the lineage and the differentiation stage of a given type of lymphoma with the features proper of the different maturation stages of normal lymphocytes. To date, the cellular derivation of lymphomas arising from B cells (approximately 85% of the cases) has been sufficiently clarified, whereas it is still relatively undefined in the case of lymphomas originating from T cells (approximately 15% of the cases).

B lymphocytes are generated in the bone marrow as precursor B cells, which first undergo immunoglobulin (Ig) gene rearrangements of the heavy chain locus followed by rearrangements of the light chain loci (1,2). Immature B cells that express a functional surface antibody acting as antigen receptor are positively selected into the peripheral B-cell pool, whereas cells failing to express a functional antigen receptor are eliminated within the bone marrow (1). For many B cells, the subsequent maturation steps are linked to the encounter with the antigen and to the formation of germinal centers (GCs), the sites where B cells are selected based on their affinity to T-cell-dependent antigens (3). The GC is constituted by a dark zone, characterized by rapidly proliferating B cells called centroblasts, and by a light zone, in which B cells cease to proliferate and mature to centrocytes, which are induced to differentiate through interactions with follicular dendritic cells and T-helper cells (Fig. 8.1) (4). Within the GC, antigen-activated B cells accumulate somatic point mutations in the variable region of their rearranged heavy and light chain genes, a phenomenon known as somatic hypermutation, which modifies the affinity of their surface antibody to the antigen (3,5). Only B cells that have acquired mutations leading to high-affinity binding are positively selected and differentiate into memory B cells or plasma cells, whereas the majority of B cells are eliminated by apoptosis within the GC

(6). Thus, the presence of somatic mutations in the IgV genes can be used as a marker of GC transit, allowing the definition of two categories of B-cell lymphoma (7):

1. NHL lacking IgV mutations. This category includes pre-GC-derived NHL, such as most cases of mantle cell lymphoma (MCL). In addition, this category includes tumors deriving from B cells that did not undergo somatic hypermutation in a GC reaction, such as approximately one-third of B-cell chronic lymphocytic leukemia/small lymphocytic lymphoma (B-CLL/SLL) cases (7).
2. NHL with IgV mutations. These tumors are derived from GC or post-GC B cells. Among all NHLs, subtypes associated with Ig somatic hypermutation include Burkitt lymphoma (BL), follicular lymphoma (FL), lymphoplasmacytic lymphoma, mucosa-associated lymphoid tissue (MALT) lymphoma, and diffuse large B-cell lymphoma (DLBCL) (7–15). In addition, B-CLL/SLL is thought to originate from post-GC or GC-independent antigen-experienced B cells (15).

MECHANISMS OF GENETIC LESION IN LYMPHOMA

Similar to most types of cancer, the pathogenesis of lymphoma represents a multistep process that involves the clonal accumulation of multiple genetic lesions affecting protooncogenes and tumor suppressor genes. Nonetheless, several features distinguish the mechanism and type of genetic lesions associated with lymphoma from those associated with solid tumors, especially the ones deriving from epithelial tissues. Cytogenetic studies have shown that the genome of lymphoma cells is relatively stable and is not affected by the massive instability typical of many solid tumors, particularly carcinomas (16). Lymphoma, with the possible exception of MALT lymphoma, appears also devoid of defects in deoxyribonucleic acid (DNA) mismatch repair genes observed in some hereditary cancer predisposition syndromes, as well as, more rarely, in most types of sporadic tumors (17–20). Conversely, the genome of lymphoma cells is characterized by few, sometimes single, nonrandom chromosomal abnormalities, commonly represented by chromosomal translocations (21).

At the molecular level, the genetic lesions identified so far in lymphomas include activation of oncogenes, either by chromosomal translocations or by mutations introduced by the aberrant activity of the somatic hypermutation mechanism, and inactivation of tumor suppressor loci, which can occur by chromosomal deletion and mutation. In addition, the genome of certain lymphoma subtypes can be altered via

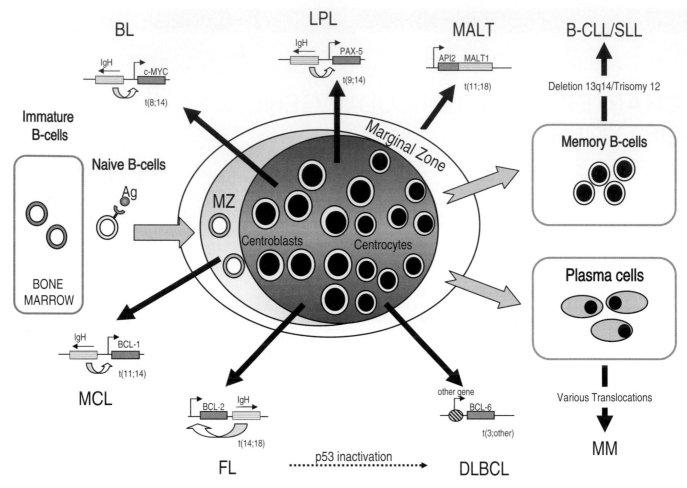

FIGURE 8.1. Model for B-cell NHL histogenesis and pathogenesis. The figure shows a schematic representation of a lymphoid follicle, constituted by the GC and the mantle zone (MZ), along with the surrounding marginal zone. B cells that have successfully rearranged their V(D)J genes in the bone marrow move to peripheral lymphoid organs as naive B cells. Upon encounter with a T-cell dependent antigen, B cells become proliferating centroblasts in the GC and eventually mature into centrocytes. These events are associated with the activation of somatic hypermutation and Ig isotype switch. Only GC B cells with high affinity for the antigen will be positively selected to exit the GC and further differentiate into plasma cells or memory B cells, whereas low-affinity clones are eliminated by apoptosis. Based on the absence or presence of somatically mutated IgV genes, B-cell NHL may be distinguished into two broad histogenetic categories: (a) B-cell NHL derived from pre-GC B cells and devoid of Ig mutations, exemplified in the figure by MCL; and (b) B-cell NHL derived from B cells that have transited through the GC and harbor Ig mutations, exemplified in the figure by FL, lymphoplasmacytoid lymphoma (LPL), MALT lymphoma (MALT), DLBCL, and BL. In B-CLL/SLL, >50% of the cases carry mutated Ig genes, suggesting a derivation from a GC experienced B cell. The genetic lesions most commonly associated with the various lymphoma subtypes are schematically shown for each tumor type. In the case of B-CLL/SLL, as well as in a subset of DLBCL, the relevant cancer-related gene has not been identified.

the introduction of exogenous genes by various types of oncogenic viruses.

Chromosomal Translocations

Chromosomal translocations represent the genetic hallmark of malignancies derived from the hematopoietic system. As in other types of tumors, chromosomal translocations associated with NHL represent reciprocal and balanced recombination events between two specific chromosomes, which are recurrently associated with a given tumor type and clonally represented in each tumor case.

During the past few years, significant advances have been made in the understanding of the mechanisms responsible for chromosomal translocations. Direct experimental evidence has been provided to support the original hypothesis that the translocation process occurs at least in part as a consequence of errors in the mechanisms that mediate the remodeling of antigen-receptor genes during lymphoid cell development, i.e., during Ig and T-cell receptor gene rearrangements in B and T cells, respectively (22,23). In particular, chromosomal translocations may derive from errors of: (a) the variable-diversity-joining (VDJ) recombination machinery, which functions in immature B cells (23); (b) the class-switch recombination mechanism, which functions in mature B cells both within and

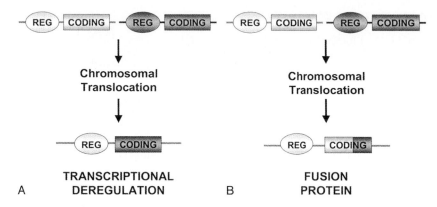

FIGURE 8.2. Molecular consequences of chromosomal translocations. Genes involved in prototypic chromosomal translocations are shown schematically, with their regulatory (REG) and coding sequences. Only one side of the balanced, reciprocal translocations is indicated. Chromosomal translocations may lead to two different outcomes. In the case of transcriptional deregulation (**left** scheme), the normal regulatory sequences of the protooncogene are removed and substituted with regulatory sequences derived from the partner chromosome. The protooncogene coding sequences become, therefore, juxtaposed to heterologous regulatory sequences, resulting in dysregulated expression of the protooncogene. The novel regulatory regions can derive from the Ig loci or from other loci. In the case of fusion proteins (**right** scheme), the coding sequences of the two involved genes are joined in frame into a chimeric transcriptional unit encoding for a novel fusion protein, whose biochemical properties are distinct from the native protein.

outside the germinal centers; and (c) the somatic hypermutation mechanism, which operates in GC B cells (24,25). Because VDJ recombination, class-switch recombination, and, possibly, somatic hypermutation involve double-strand DNA breaks (26–28), translocations likely represent the outcome of illegitimate recombinations that occur between antigen-receptor loci and other loci, or between non-Ig loci. In support of this model, recent evidence indicates that mice defective in their ability to perform class-switch recombination and somatic hypermutation do not develop GC-derived NHL (29).

The common feature of all chromosomal translocations associated with NHL is the presence of a protooncogene in the proximity of the chromosomal recombination sites. In most cases, the structure of the protooncogene, and, in particular, its coding domain, are not affected by the translocation, but the pattern of expression of the involved gene is altered as a consequence of the juxtaposition of heterologous regulatory sequences derived from the partner chromosome (protooncogene deregulation) (Fig. 8.2). Two distinct types of protooncogene deregulation may be distinguished, including homotopic and heterotopic deregulation. Homotopic deregulation occurs when a protooncogene, whose expression is tightly regulated in normal lymphoid cells, becomes constitutively expressed in the lymphoma. Conversely, heterotopic deregulation occurs when the protooncogene, which is normally not expressed in lymphoid cells, undergoes ectopic expression in the tumor cells.

An alternative mechanism of oncogene activation by chromosomal translocation is represented by the juxtaposition of coding sequences derived from the two involved genes, which result in gene fusions coding for a novel chimeric protein (Fig. 8.2). This mechanism, which is common in chromosomal translocations associated with acute leukemias, is rarely associated with NHL. Examples are represented by the t(11;18) of MALT lymphoma and the t(2;5) of T-cell anaplastic lymphoma.

The molecular cloning of the genetic loci involved in the translocations most frequently associated with various NHL subtypes has led to the identification of a number of protooncogenes implicated in lymphomagenesis (Table 8.1).

The structural and functional consequences of each chromosomal translocation associated with NHL will be described in the section dedicated to the molecular pathogenesis of individual NHL subtypes.

Aberrant Somatic Hypermutation

Recently, it has been shown that the process of somatic hypermutation can malfunction and target non-Ig genes in a large fraction of DLBCL cases (30). In normal GC B cells, this process is tightly regulated, and introduces mutations only in the variable region of the Ig genes as well as in 5′ region of a few other genes, including the *BCL6* protooncogene and the CD79 component of the B-cell receptor (31–36). Whereas hypermutation of IgV sequences allows the selection of B cells with increased affinity for the antigen, the role of mutations found in these other genes remains obscure. In over 50% of DLBCL cases and in few other lymphoma types, including, among others, acquired immunodeficiency syndrome-associated B-NHL, primary central nervous system lymphomas, and posttransplant lymphoproliferative disorders (37–40), the somatic hypermutation mechanism appears to function aberrantly and targets the 5′ sequences of a number of additional genes, including several protooncogenes such as: *PIM1*, which encodes a signal transduction molecule with proven oncogenic potential; *MYC*, one of the most frequently altered human oncogenes, encoding a transcription factor involved in the control of cell proliferation and differentiation; *PAX5*, which encodes a transcription factor necessary for B-cell proliferation and whose expression is deregulated by chromosomal translocations in plasmacytic lymphoma; and *RhoH/TTF*, encoding for a small G protein belonging to the RAS superfamily (30). In the case of *PIM1* and *MYC*, due to their genomic configuration, the mutations affect nontranslated as well as coding regions, leading to amino acid changes with potential functional consequences. This abnormal activity may therefore represent a powerful mechanism of malignant transformation because it may have an effect on a multitude

TABLE 8.1

CHROMOSOMAL TRANSLOCATIONS ASSOCIATED WITH NHL

NHL histologic subtype	Translocation	Protooncogene involved	Mechanism of protooncogene activation	Protooncogene function
MCL	t(11;14)(q13;q32)	*BCL1* (cyclinD1)	Transcriptional deregulation	Cell cycle regulator
BL	t(8;14)(q24;q32) t(2;8)(p11;q24) t(8;22)(q24;q11)	c*MYC*	Transcriptional deregulation	Transcription factor regulating cell proliferation and growth
FL	t(14;18)(q32;q21) t(2;18)(p11;q21) t(18;22)(q21;q11)	*BCL2*	Transcriptional deregulation	Negative regulator of apoptosis
MALT lymphoma	t(11;18)(q21;q21) t(1;14)(p22;q32)	API2/MLT BCL10	Fusion protein Transcriptional deregulation	API2 has antiapoptotic activity Antiapoptosis (?)
DLBCL	der(3)(q27)	BCL6	Transcriptional deregulation	Transcriptional repressor required for GC formation
Lymphoplasmacytic lymphoma	t(9;14)(p13;q32)	PAX5	Transcriptional deregulation	Transcription factor regulating B-cell proliferation and differentiation
T-cell ALCL	t(2;5)(p23;q35)	*NPM/ALK*	Fusion protein	*ALK* is a tyrosine kinase

of genes, only part of which have been identified so far. However, a comprehensive characterization of the potentially extensive genetic damage caused by aberrant somatic hypermutation is still lacking.

Other Mechanisms of Protooncogene Alteration

Additional mechanisms can alter the structure and/or the pattern of expression of protooncogenes in NHL. Protooncogene amplification is substantially less common than in epithelial cancers, yet it can be observed in some high-grade NHL, as exemplified by the case of *REL* amplifications in DLBCL (42). Gene amplification may involve many other unknown chromosomal sites, which are likely to be revealed by the extensive use of advanced cytogenetic techniques such as comparative genomic hybridization and high density SNP arrays (43). Point mutations, presumably independent of the somatic hypermutation mechanism, rarely target the *RAS* protooncogenes in NHL, despite the fact that these genes are among the most frequently mutated ones in other types of human cancer (44). More recently, experimental evidence revealed that genes involved in the positive and negative regulation of the nuclear factor-κB (NF-κB) transcription complex can be altered by point mutations in DLBCL, leading to constitutive activation of the antiapoptotic and proproliferative functions of NF-κB (45,46).

Inactivation of Tumor Suppressor Genes

Although deletions and mutations of the *p53* tumor suppressor gene represent the most common genetic alteration in human cancer (46), these lesions are relatively rare in NHL and are restricted to the late stages of FL and BL (47–49). The mechanism of *p53* inactivation in NHL is similar to that detected in other types of tumor, and occurs through point mutation of one allele and chromosomal deletion of the second allele (46).

NHLs are also associated with specific chromosomal deletions, suggesting the loss of tumor suppressor genes, many of which remain unidentified. The most frequent of these deletions involves the long arm of chromosome 6 (6q) (16,50). The observation that 6q deletions may occur as the sole cytogenetic abnormality in some NHL cases (16) and are associated with poor prognosis (21) strongly supports a pathogenetic role for these alterations. Indeed, recent studies have identified the presence of somatic mutations inactivating the PRDM1 gene at chromosomal band 6q21 in approximately 25% of DLBCLs, specifically in the activated B cell (ABC) subtype of the disease (51–53). Furthermore, the PRDM1 protein is not expressed in an additional large fraction of cases, despite expression of the PRDM1 messenger ribonucleic acid (RNA) (53). Given the essential role of PRDM1 in terminal B-cell differentiation, these data suggest that PRDM1 acts as a tumor suppressor gene, whose loss of function may contribute to the pathogenesis of ABC-DLBCL by blocking plasma cell differentiation.

Deletions of chromosome 13q14 represent the most frequent lesion in B-CLL/SLL, occurring in more than 50% of cases (16) and implying the presence of a tumor suppressor gene in the same region (55–60). A micro-RNA mini cluster has been identified in the deleted region, which may represent the critical target of the deletion (61,62).

Finally, tumor suppressor inactivation can occur via epigenetic mechanisms such as transcriptional inactivation by hypermethylation of the promoter region. This mechanism is responsible for the lack of expression of the *p16* tumor suppressor gene in a variety of NHL subtypes (63–67).

Oncogenic Viruses

Oncogenic viruses introduce foreign genes into their target cells and/or alter cellular genes by integrating their genome. At least three viruses are associated with the pathogenesis of specific NHL subtypes: the human T-cell leukemia virus type

1, the Epstein-Barr virus (EBV), and the human herpesvirus-8. Other infectious agents, including human immunodeficiency virus, hepatitis C virus, and *Helicobacter pylori*, have an indirect role in NHL pathogenesis by impairing the immune system and/or providing chronic antigenic stimulation. The role of these infectious agents is described in detail in Chapter 7.

MOLECULAR PATHOGENESIS OF B-CELL NON-HODGKIN LYMPHOMA

Specific genetic lesions have been found associated with distinct B-NHL subtypes classified according to the World Health Organization classification of lymphoid neoplasia (68,69). The following section will focus on well-characterized lesions associated with major B-cell NHL- subtypes, including MCL, DLBCL, FL, BL, and MALT lymphoma. The molecular pathogenesis of other B-NHL types is far less understood.

Mantle Cell Lymphoma

Chromosomal Translocations Involving BCL1. MCL is typically associated with t(11;14)(q13;q32), which can be detected in up to 70% of cases (69–75) (Fig. 8.1 and Table 8.1). The t(11;14)(q13;q32) translocation juxtaposes the BCL1 locus at 11q13 to the IgH locus, leading to homotopic deregulation of BCL1 (also known as CCND1 or PRAD1) (76–78). The BCL1 gene encodes for cyclin D1, a member of the D-type G1 cyclins that regulate the early phases of cell cycle (73,79–82). The consistent and selective clustering of BCL1 expression with NHL carrying t(11;14) strongly suggests that this gene is indeed the critical target of the t(11;14)(q13;q32). By deregulating cyclin D1, t(11;14) is thought to deregulate cell cycle control because this molecule acts primarily as a growth factor sensor integrating extracellular signals with the cell cycle clock (83). The pathogenetic role of BCL1 deregulation in human neoplasia is suggested by the ability of cyclin D1 overexpression to transform cells in vitro and to contribute to B-cell lymphomagenesis in transgenic mice (84–86).

Other Genetic Alterations. Less common genetic lesions, observed in aggressive variants of MCL, include inactivation of the tumor suppressor genes p53 and p16, and mutations of the ataxia telangiectasia mutated (ATM) gene. Mutations of p53 and deletions of the short arm of chromosome 17, frequently associated with p53 overexpression, occur in up to 15% of the cases and represent a marker of poor prognosis (87,88). Inactivation of p16 by deletion, mutation, or hypermethylation can be detected in approximately half of the cases belonging to the aggressive variant of MCL, which is characterized by a blastoid cell morphology (64). Finally, ATM mutations, mainly associated with 11q22-23 deletions, have been identified more recently in this lymphoma subtype (89,90).

Burkitt Lymphoma

Chromosomal Translocations Involving the MYC Protooncogene. BL includes several variants (i.e., sporadic BL, endemic BL, and acquired immunodeficiency syndrome - associated BL) (68,69). All BL cases, including the leukemic variants, are associated with chromosomal translocations involving the MYC locus on chromosome 8q24 and three alternative chromosomal regions, each one containing an Ig locus: IgH, Igκ, or Igλ (91–96) (Table 8.1 and Fig. 8.3). The IgH locus is involved in 80% of the cases, leading to t(8;14)(q24;q32). The remaining cases are characterized by t(2;8)(p11;q24), involving the Igκ locus (15% of cases), and t(8;22)(q24;q11), involving Igλ (5% of cases) (Table 8.1).

Although relatively homogeneous at the microscopic level, these translocations are very heterogeneous at the molecular level. The t(8;14) breakpoints are located 5' and centromeric to MYC, whereas, in t(2;8) and t(8;22), they map 3' to MYC (91–96). Further molecular heterogeneity derives from the exact breakpoint sites on chromosomes 8 and 14 of t(8;14) (Fig. 8.3). In endemic BL, the translocation generally involves sequences on chromosome 8 that are located at undefined distance (>100 kb) 5' to MYC, and sequences on chromosome 14 within or in proximity of the Ig JH region (97,98). In sporadic BL, t(8;14) preferentially involves sequences located within or immediately 5' (<3 kb) to MYC on chromosome 8 and sequences on chromosome 14 mapping within the Ig switch regions.

The common effect of t(8;14), t(2;8), and t(8;22) is the ectopic activation (heterotopic deregulation) of MYC expression in GC B cells, which normally do not express MYC (99,100). Two distinct mechanisms may be responsible for MYC deregulation: (a) juxtaposition of MYC to heterologous enhancers derived from the Ig loci; and (b) structural alterations in the 5' regulatory sequences of the gene, which putatively alter the responsiveness to cell factors regulating its expression. In fact, the MYC exon 1/intron 1 boundary, where MYC regulatory sequences are located, is either decapitated by the translocation or mutated in the translocated alleles (91–96,101) (Fig. 8.3). In addition to heterotopic deregulation, oncogenic conversion of MYC may also be due to amino acid substitutions in the gene exon 2, which encodes the transactivation domain of the MYC protein (102,103). These mutations are thought to affect various aspects of MYC function, including the stability of the protein and its response to p107, a nuclear protein related to RB1 (104,105).

The product of MYC is a ubiquitously expressed nuclear phosphoprotein that functions as a transcriptional regulator involved in the control of DNA replication, cell growth, differentiation, and apoptosis (106–109). In vivo, MYC is found mainly in heterodimeric complexes with the related protein MAX, and such interaction is required for MYC-induced stimulation of transcription and cell proliferation (110–115). Conversely, MAX can form heterodimers with MAD and MXI1, two basic helix-loop-helix/leucine zipper proteins that act as negative regulators of transcription (116,117). In NHL carrying MYC translocations, it is conceivable that constitutive expression of MYC leads to the prevalence of MYC/MAX complexes over MAD/MAX and MXI1/MAX heterodimers, thus inducing positive growth regulation. In fact, expression of MYC regulates transcription of a subset of target genes dynamics, energy metabolism, protein synthesis, and telomere maintenance (109,118). More recent results suggest that deregulated MYC expression contributes to lymphomagenesis by causing genomic instability via stimulating unscheduled DNA replication. Substantial experimental evidence documents that the constitutive expression of MYC can influence the growth of B cells in vitro and in vivo, consistent with a role in B-cell

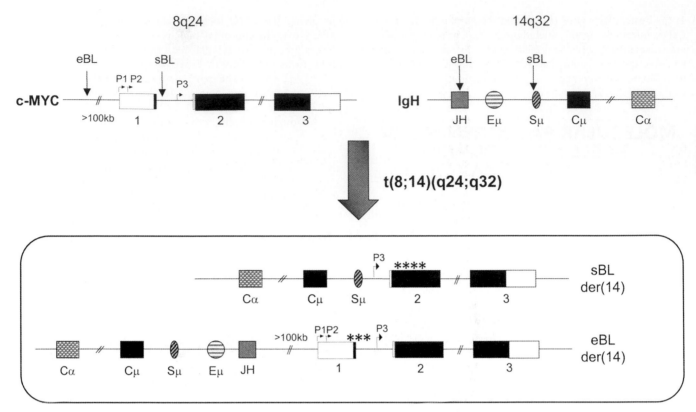

FIGURE 8.3. Schematic representation of chromosomal translocations involving the *MYC* locus. The germline configuration of the *MYC* gene on chromosome 8q24, and the IgH locus on chromosome 14q32 are schematically shown (**top**). In its germline configuration, *MYC* is composed of three exons. Coding regions are indicated by *black boxes*, whereas noncoding regions are indicated by *white boxes*. The two major *MYC* promoters within exon 1 (P1 and P2), and the minor P3 promoter, located 5′ to exon 2, are shown by *arrows*. In the IgH locus, symbols represent the joining (J), switch (S) and constant (C) regions as well as the Ig enhancer (E) (μ, μ region; α, α region). The breakpoint clusters associated with sporadic BL (sBL) and endemic BL (eBL) are indicated for both the 8q24 and the 14q32 chromosomal regions. Two distinct types of translocations can be recognized, which preferentially associate with either sporadic BL or endemic BL. In the case of t(8;14) of sporadic BL, the breakpoints involve sequences within the intron 1 of the MYC locus and sequences in the proximity of the switch μ (Sμ) region on the IgH locus. As a consequence, the MYC gene is decapitated of its first exon. Because the physiologically active promoters of *MYC* are removed, a novel transcriptional initiation site (P3), located within *MYC* intron 1, is utilized in *MYC* alleles affected by this translocation. Notably, although the coding region of the translocated *MYC* alleles is left intact, at the nucleotide level, these alleles frequently harbor point mutations (schematically represented by asterisks) within their exon 2 sequences, which lead to amino acid changes in the MYC protein. The RNA transcribed from t(8;14) of sporadic BL is composed of *MYC* exons 2 and 3, preceded by an abnormally transcribed sequence of intron 1, which starts from the novel transcriptional initiation site. Because the *MYC* coding region remains intact, a normally sized MYC protein is produced. In the case of t(8;14) of endemic BL, the *MYC* breakpoint involves sequences on chromosome 8 located >100 kb 5′ to the gene and sequences on chromosome 14 within or in proximity to the Ig JH region. The genomic configuration of the translocated *MYC* allele is thus apparently preserved. However, *MYC* alleles involved by t(8;14) of endemic BL consistently harbor point mutations clustering around the exon 1-intron 1 border, where *MYC* regulatory regions are located (see asterisks). In addition, and in common with t(8;14) of sporadic BL, mutations within the MYC exon 2 coding sequence are frequently detected in *MYC* alleles affected by t(8;14) of endemic BL. The transcript from t(8;14) of endemic BL includes *MYC* exons 1 through 3 and encodes for a normally sized MYC protein. The functional consequences of t(8;14) on the expression of translocated *MYC* alleles in both sporadic BL and endemic BL are described in detail in the text. Only one side of the balanced, reciprocal translocation t(8;14)(q24;q32) is shown. Variant translocations involving the *MYC* locus and the Ig light chain genes are not shown.

lymphomagenesis. In vitro, the expression of *MYC* oncogenes transfected into EBV immortalized human B cells, a potential natural target for *MYC* activation in EBV-positive BL, leads to their malignant transformation (119). In vivo, the targeted expression of *MYC* oncogenes in the B-cell lineage of transgenic mice leads to the development of B-cell malignancy (120,121).

Other Genetic Alterations. Additional genetic lesions associated with BL include *p53* deletion/mutation, which are found in 30% of the cases (47) (Table 8.2), and deletions of 6q, which are detected in approximately 30% of the cases (50). Inactivation of *p16* has also been reported in a fraction of cases (122). Another lesion that may contribute to the development of this malignancy is monoclonal EBV infection, present in virtually all cases of endemic BL and in approximately 30% of sporadic BL (123–127) (Table 8.2). Because EBV infection in BL displays a latent infection phenotype characterized by the lack of expression of both EBV-transforming antigens, latency membrane protein-1 and Epstein-Barr nuclear antigen-2, the precise pathogenetic role of the virus in these tumors remains unclear.

Follicular Lymphoma

Chromosomal Translocations Involving the BCL2 Protooncogene. The most common chromosomal translocation associated with FL is represented by t(14;18)(q32;q21), which can be detected in 80% to 90% of the cases independent of the cytologic subtype (Table 8.1 and Fig. 8.1) (68,69). In this translocation, the rearrangement joins the *BCL2* gene at its 3′ untranslated region to an Ig JH segment (Fig. 8.4), resulting in homotopic deregulation of BCL2 expression (128–132). Approximately 70% of the breakpoints on chromosome 18 cluster within the major breakpoint region, whereas the remaining 5% to 25% usually map to the more distant minor cluster region. Rearrangements involving the 5′ flanking region of BCL2 have also been reported in a minority of cases (133). The consequence of the translocation is the presence within the cells of constitutively high levels of BCL2 protein, resulting from both enhanced transcription and, possibly, more efficient RNA processing (134,135).

BCL2 is a 26-kDa integral membrane protein that has been localized to mitochondria, endoplasmic reticulum, and perinuclear membrane (136–140). The main function of the BCL2 protein is to control the cell threshold to enter apoptosis or programmed cell death. In the B-cell compartment, BCL2 appears to be important for the emergence of long-living memory cells by promoting survival of antigen-selected GC cells (141). Deregulation of BCL2 expression may contribute to the pathogenesis of FL by preventing apoptosis in GC cells that are normally destined to die (142). Indeed, *BCL2*-Ig transgenic mice develop a pattern of polyclonal hyperplasia characterized by mature, long-lived B cells resting in G0 (143,144). Despite the morphologic similarities, this pattern contrasts with the consistent monoclonality of human FL, indicating that *BCL2* activation is not sufficient for lymphoma development, and that other genetic lesions or host factors are required. In fact, with time and analogous to the human disease, a fraction of the indolent follicular hyperplasia observed in *BCL2*-Ig transgenic mice will progress to aggressive, clonal diffuse large cell lymphomas that have acquired additional genetic lesions (145).

Other Genetic Alterations. Deletions of chromosome 6 are found in approximately 20% of the cases (50), whereas other genes commonly involved in lymphomagenesis, such as *MYC* and *p53*, do not appear to be altered during the development of FL. Over time, FL tends to convert into an aggressive lymphoma with a diffuse large cell architecture (Fig. 8.1) (68,69). This histologic transformation is generally accompanied by the accumulation of *p53* mutations and, in approximately 40% of cases, by inactivation of *p16* (Fig. 8.1) (49,64,146). In rare cases, rearrangements of *MYC* may also occur during transformation of FL in DLBCL (147).

Diffuse Large B-Cell Lymphoma

In contrast with other NHL subtypes, DLBCLs are characterized by a marked biologic, phenotypical, and clinical heterogeneity. Based on the identification of different gene expression profiles and on their highly variable clinical course, it is becoming clear that DLBCL comprises multiple, presently unrecognized disease entities (51,148,149). This marked heterogeneity reflects in part the complex molecular pathogenesis of this disease, which includes specific lesions (i.e., rearrangements of the *BCL6* gene) as well as alterations common to other NHL subtypes.

Alterations Affecting the BCL6 Locus. Chromosomal translocations affecting band 3q27 represent the most common and specific genetic abnormality associated with de novo DLBCL (21,150). These alterations were shown to be "promiscuous" in that they involved balanced, reciprocal recombinations between the 3q27 region, containing the *BCL6* locus, and various alternative chromosomal partners in different DLBCL cases (151–155). The partner sites include, but

TABLE 8.2

FREQUENCY OF GENETIC LESIONS ASSOCIATED WITH B-NHL

NHL subtype	BCL1	BCL2	BCL6	MYC	PAX5	API2/ MLT	BCL10	p53	p16	PRDM1	EBV
B-CLL/SLL	–	–	–	–	–	–	–	10%	–	–	–
MCL	70%	–	–	–	–	–	–	20%[a]	50%[a]	–	–
BL	–	–	–	100%	–	–	–	30%	30%	–	30% to 100%[c]
FL	–	90%	Rare	–	–	–	–	–	–	–	–
MALT lymphoma	–	–	–	–	–	60%	Rare	–	–	–	–
DLBCL	–	30%	35%	20%	–	–	–	30%	30%	20%[b]	–
Lymphoplasmacytic lymphoma	–	–	–	–	50%	–	–	–	–	–	–

–, molecular lesion or viral infection not involved; where present, the percentage of positive cases is indicated.
[a] Fifty percent of the aggressive MCL variant.
[b] Specifically in the ABC type (ABC-DLBCL).
[c] Thirty percent in sporadic BL; 100% in endemic BL.

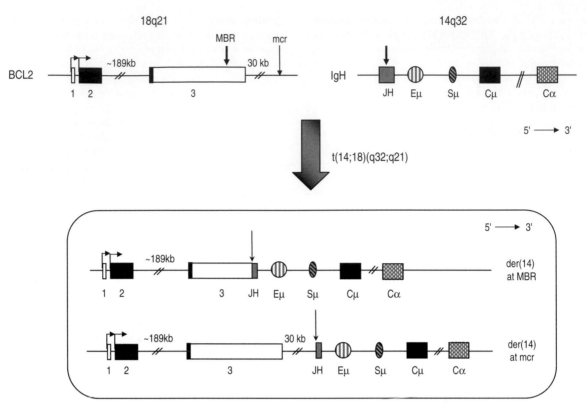

FIGURE 8.4. Schematic representation of *BCL2* translocations. The germline configuration of the *BCL2* gene on chromosome 18q21 and part of the IgH locus on chromosome 14q32 are shown in the figure (*upper panel*, not in scale). In its germline configuration, the *BCL2* gene is composed of three exons separated by a large intron between exon 2 and exon 3. *Black boxes* represent coding regions, whereas *white boxes* represent noncoding regions. Only part of the IgH locus (from the switch region to the constant [C] α region) is schematically shown. *Color-coded symbols* represent the joining (J), switch (S), and constant (C) regions of IgH, as well as the Ig enhancer (E). Alternative transcription initiation sites are indicated by *arrows*. In the majority of cases, t(14;18) breaks cluster within two regions; a major breakpoint region (MBR) in the 3′ untranslated sequences, and a minor cluster region (mcr) located approximately 20 kB downstream of the gene. The 14q32 breakpoint (indicated by a *vertical arrow*) maps within the JH segment. The molecular consequences of t(14;18)(q32;q21), including both the major breakpoint region and minor cluster region type of translocations, are depicted in the **bottom** panel of the figure, with only one side of the reciprocal, balanced translocation being shown. The translocation causes the juxtaposition of an intact *BCL2* coding domain telomeric and in the same transcriptional orientation to the IgH locus. Because the *BCL2* coding region is preserved, the chimeric *BCL2*/IgH transcript gives rise to a wild-type BCL2 protein, whose expression is dysregulated (see Chromosomal Translocations Involving the *BCL2* Protooncogene for a description of the functional consequences of *BCL2* translocations on the transcriptional regulation of *BCL2*).

are not limited to, those harboring the Ig heavy (14q32) or light (2p12, 22q11) chain genes.

The *BCL6* gene encodes for a 95-kDa nuclear phosphoprotein belonging to the POZ/Zinc finger family of transcription factors (156). The BCL6 protein acts as a potent transcriptional repressor of promoter sequences containing its specific DNA recognition motif (157,158). In the B-cell lineage, expression of the BCL6 protein is restricted to GC cells, whereas is absent in pre-GC cells or in their differentiated progenies, such as memory B cells and plasma cells (159,160). Mice deficient for BCL6 are not able to form GCs in response to T-cell dependent antigens and, consequently, completely lack affinity maturation (161,162). Therefore, BCL6 appears to be a master regulator of GC development, where it represses the transcription of genes involved in B-cell activation, differentiation, and apoptotic/cell cycle arrest responses to DNA damage, including ATR, p53, and

p21(163–168). Thus, BCL6 may allow GC B cells to tolerate the physiologic DNA damage associated with Ig gene remodeling processes without eliciting cell cycle arrest and apoptotic responses (164–166,169).

Chromosomal translocations cause rearrangements of the *BCL6* gene in approximately 35% of DLBCL cases and in a minority (5% to 10%) of FL cases (170). These rearrangements juxtapose the intact coding domain of *BCL6* downstream and in the same transcriptional orientation to heterologous sequences derived from the partner chromosome, including IgH (14q23), Igκ(2p12), Igλ(22q11), and at least 20 other chromosomal sites unrelated to the Ig loci (171–173) (Fig. 8.5). Among the genes identified so far in the partner chromosomal site are: *RhoH/TTF* (small GTPase of the RAS superfamily associated with cytoskeleton) (174), *BOB1* (B-cell coactivator) (175), *L-Plastin* (actin-binding protein) (176), *H4* (histone) (177,178), *IKAROS* (179),

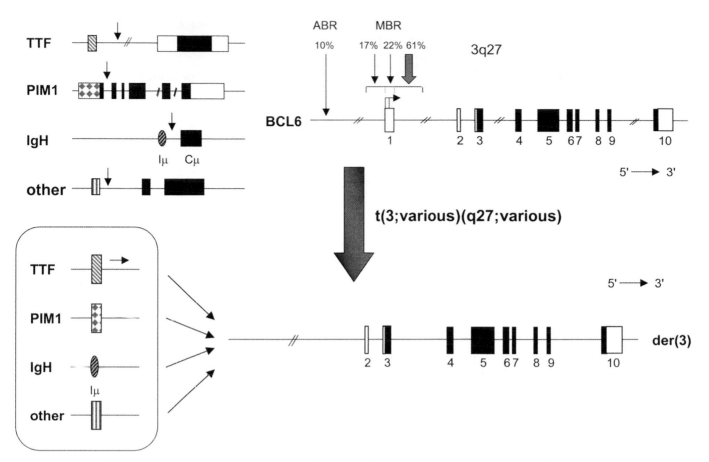

FIGURE 8.5. Schematic representation of chromosomal translocations involving the *BCL6* locus. The germline configuration of the *BCL6* gene on chromosome 3q27 is shown in the **upper-right** panel of the figure, whereas representative *BCL6* translocation partners, including *TTF*, *PIM1*, IgH, and other hypothetical genes (other), are shown in the **upper-left** panel. *BCL6* is composed of ten exons, represented by empty (noncoding) and solid (coding) boxes. *Arrows* indicate the major and minor *BCL6* promoters in exon 1. The distribution and frequency of *BCL6* breaks within the major (MBR) and the alternative (ABR) breakpoint clusters are also shown (*vertical arrows*). **Bottom panel:** Schematic representation of several derivatives on chromosome 3 following t(3q27) chromosomal translocations. Independent of the partner chromosome involved, the translocation decapitates the *BCL6* alleles of variable portions of their 5′ noncoding domain. Novel sequences derived from the partner chromosomes are juxtaposed 5′ to the *BCL6* coding sequences, providing heterologous regulatory sequences with distinct expression patterns, such as the IgH germline transcript promoter Iμ (or Iμ) in the case of t(3;14), the *RhoH/TTF* promoter in the case of t(3;4), and the *PIM1* promoter in the case of t(3;6). Because the genomic configuration of the *BCL6* coding domain downstream to the breakpoint site is preserved, the translocation leads to deregulated expression of a normal BCL6 protein. Only one side of the balanced, reciprocal translocation is shown.

HSP89A (heat shock protein) (180), major histocompatibility complex class II transactivator (*CIITA*), *PIM1* (serine-threonine kinase), eukaryotic initiation factor 4AII (translation factor), and the transferrin receptor (181,182). The majority of these translocations result in a fusion transcript in which the promoter region and the first noncoding exon of Bcl6 are replaced by sequences derived from the partner gene (Fig. 8.5) (171–173). The common denominator of these promoters, when compared with BCL6, is a broader spectrum of activity throughout B-cell development, including expression in the post-GC differentiation stage such as immunoblasts and plasma cells (171). Consequently, the translocation is thought to prevent the down-regulation of BCL6 expression that is normally associated with differentiation into post-GC cells. It is hypothesized that deregulated expression of a normal *BCL6* gene product may play a critical role by enforcing

the proliferative phenotype typical of GC cells. This hypothesis has been partially confirmed by a knock-in mouse model in which deregulated BCL6 expression causes DLBCL (183).

In addition to chromosomal translocations, the 5′ regulatory sequences of *BCL6* can be altered by multiple somatic mutations in up to 75% of DLBCL cases (32,146,184). These mutations, however, are introduced in normal GC B cells and are thought to be generated by the same somatic hypermutation mechanism that targets Ig genes (32,33,36,184). Consistent with their association with the physiologic GC reaction, *BCL6* mutations are found in a fraction of all B-cell tumors carrying mutated IgV sequences and displaying a GC or post-GC phenotype, including B-CLL, BL, FL, MALT lymphoma, and multiple myeloma, as well as DLBCL (32,36,146,184–186). Functional analysis of a number of mutated *BCL6* alleles has shown that some mutations are specifically associated with DLBCL because they are not found in normal GC cells or in other B-cell malignancies (187). These mutations deregulate BCL6 transcription by disrupting an autoregulatory circuit through which the BCL6 protein controls its expression levels via binding to the promoter region of the gene (187,188) or by preventing CD40-induced BCL6 downregulation in post-GC B cells (189). Because the full extent of *BCL6* mutations deregulating gene expression has not been characterized, the fraction of DLBCL cases carrying abnormal BCL6 expression cannot be determined.

Aberrant Somatic Hypermutation. Approximately 50% of DLBCLs are associated with the aberrant activity of the somatic hypermutation mechanism (30). This aberrant activity targets several protooncogenes, including *MYC*, *PIM1*, *PAX5*, and *RhoH/TTF* (see Mechanisms of Genetic Lesion in Lymphoma: Aberrant Somatic Hypermutation). More recently, high-throughput amplification and sequence analysis of over 150 genes, expressed in normal or transformed GC B cells, has led to the identification of an increasing number of target loci (approximately 8% of all genes analyzed) with possible pathogenetic significance in DLBCL. The number and identity of the genes targeted by the aberrant hypermutation mechanism vary in different cases and are still largely undefined. This mechanism may be responsible for the heterogeneity of DLBCL via the alteration of different cellular pathways in different cases.

Other Genetic Lesions. DLBCL can be found associated with mutations and deletions of the *p53* tumor suppressor gene, mostly detectable in cases originating from the transformation of FL and, therefore, associated with chromosomal translocations involving *BCL2* (49). More than 50% of ABC-DLBCL patients carry somatic mutations in multiple genes encoding for NFkB pathway components, including negative (TNFAIP3) and positive (CARD11, TRAF2 among others) regulators of this signaling pathway (ref: Compagno et al., 2009; Kato et al., 2009; Lenz et al., 2008). The TNFAIP3 gene is most frequently involved, with one third of the cases showing biallelic inactivation by mutations and deletions, suggesting that loss of A20 may contribute to lymphomagenesis by inducing prolonged NFkB responses. In addition, up to 25% of ABC-DLBCLs carry biallelic inactivation of the PRDM1 gene due to deletions and truncating mutations (52,53). The PRDM1 gene encodes for a zinc finger transcriptional repressor that is expressed in a subset of GC B cells and in all plasma cells (190,191), and is an essential requirement for plasmacytic differentiation (192). Thus, PRDM1 inactivation may contribute to lymphomagenesis by blocking post-GC B-cell differentiation. Notably, translocations deregulating the BCL6 gene are never found in PRDM1 mutated DLBCLs, suggesting that BCL6 deregulation and PRDM1 inactivation may represent alternative oncogenic mechanisms on the same pathway to promote cell transformation.

Less frequently, DLBCLs are associated with a variety of chromosomal translocations, including those involving the *MYC* and *BCL2* loci; these, however, appear to be mutually exclusive with those involving BCL6 (21). A few sites of amplification have also been identified, including those containing known protooncogenes as *REL*, *MYC*, and *BCL2* (42,193). Finally, deletion or lack of expression of the *p16* tumor suppressor gene and mutations of the *ATM* gene have

been reported in a minority of cases (194,195). Overall, the relative distribution of all these lesions has not been comprehensively assessed in large panels of DLBCL cases.

Mucosa-Associated Lymphoid Tissue Lymphomas

Most cases of gastric MALT lymphomas are associated with *H. pylori* infection (196). It has been suggested that MALT lymphomas may be dependent upon antigen stimulation by *H. pylori* because the malignant lymphoid cells respond to *H. pylori* antigens and because the lymphoma may regress, at least partially, upon eradication of infection (197). The potential role of antigen in MALT lymphoma pathogenesis is further supported by the observation that MALT-lymphoma cells harbor the genotypic hallmark of antigen-experienced B cells, i.e., somatic hypermutation of Ig genes (198–199).

Cytogenetic studies have pointed to several abnormalities specifically associated with these tumors. The most frequent of these abnormalities is t(11;18) (q21; q21) (16), which is observed in approximately 50% of MALT lymphomas, independent of the site of origin (201,202). The genes involved in the t(11;18) are *API2* on 11q21 and *MALT1* (for MALT-lymphoma translocation) on 18q21. *API2* belongs to the family of inhibitor of apoptosis proteins that plays an evolutionary conserved role in regulating programmed cell death in diverse species. The function of *MALT1* appears to be to induce the activation of the NF-κB transcription complex (203). The *API2/MALT1* fusion protein resulting from t(11;18)(q21;q21) appears also to activate the NF-κB complex, with antiapoptotic effects that may contribute to the pathogenesis of MALT lymphomas (201–203).

The second chromosomal abnormality associated with MALT lymphomas is t(1;14)(p22;q32), which occurs in a small fraction of cases and causes alterations of the *BCL10* gene (204,205). *BCL10* encodes an amino-terminal caspase recruitment domain homologous to that found in several apoptotic molecules. The wild-type *BCL10* gene activates the NF-κB signaling cascade and is able to induce apoptosis in different cell types. Interestingly, the BCL10 protein forms a complex and synergizes with the MALT1 protein to activate the NF-κB transcription complex and inhibit apoptosis in normal cells (203). Thus, it is possible that both translocations associated with MALT lymphomas act on the same antiapoptotic pathway with analogous biologic consequences in lymphomagenesis.

Inactivating mutations and deletions of the TNFAIP3 gene have been observed in ~20% of the cases, where they appear to be mutually exclusive with these two chromosomal translocations (new Ref: Novak et al., Blood 2009). MALT lymphomas are less commonly associated with trisomy of chromosome 3, for which no molecular characterization is available (206), and with genetic alterations commonly detected in other lymphoma types, including *BCL6* rearrangements or mutations and *p53* mutations (36,146,207–209).

Small Lymphocytic Lymphoma/B-cell Chronic Lymphocytic Leukemia

Different from other types of malignancies derived from mature B cells, the pathogenesis of B-CLL/SLL is much less understood (Fig. 8.1). Despite initial suggestions, it is now well established that "true" cases of B-CLL/SLL [i.e., CD5+, CD23+, according to the World Health Organization and the Revised European American Lymphoma classification (1,2)], together with hairy cell leukemia (210), are unique among lymphoid neoplasia in that they lack chromosomal translocations (Table 8.2) (211,212). This important difference may be due to the distinct cell of origin of these tumors. Although B-CLL/SLL has been traditionally viewed as a tumor of naive, pre-GC B cells, approximately 50% of the cases have been shown to harbor mutations of Ig and/or *BCL6* genes (15,186,211,213–215), which are well-established markers of GC transit. Furthermore, gene expression profile analysis of B-cell chronic lymphocytic leukemia has suggested that the cases with mutated and germ-line Ig genes both derive from an antigen-experienced B-cell that either has passed the GC or has responded to a T-independent antigen, and may represent a memory/marginal zone B cell (216,217). Because the mechanisms that generate chromosomal translocations (Ig gene rearrangements and hypermutation) are no longer active in memory B cells, these observations may explain the fact that the genome of B-CLL/ SLL is characterized by other types of genetic alterations, including chromosomal deletions, trisomies, and point mutations.

Trisomy 12 is found in approximately 35% of B-CLL/ SLL cases evaluated by interphase fluorescent in situ hybridization and correlates with a poor survival (212,218). Based on karyotypic and deletion mapping studies, it is likely that the 13q14 chromosomal region harbors a novel tumor suppressor gene that is involved at high frequency in B-CLL/ SLL. In fact, deletions of 13q14 occur in approximately 60% of cases when analyzed by sensitive molecular tools (58,59,212). Recent studies have suggested that these deletions target a micro-RNA cluster involved in the control of cell death and proliferation (61,62,219,220). Deletions of 6q define a subset of B-CLL/SLL cases displaying prolymphocytic features (50,212). Mutations of the *p53* gene and loss of heterozygosity in 17p, the *p53* site, are found in a small fraction, 10% to 15%, of cases (47,212,218). A higher frequency of *p53* alterations is observed after transformation of B-CLL/SLL to Richter syndrome, a highly aggressive lymphoma with a poor clinical outcome (47), suggesting that *p53* may be involved in the genetic mechanisms underlying B-CLL/SLL progression. Finally, a small fraction of B-CLL/ SLL harbors mutations of the *ATM* gene (185,221–223). Because these mutations may occur in the patient germline, *ATM* mutations may account, at least in part, for the familial cases of the disease.

MOLECULAR PATHOGENESIS OF T-CELL NON-HODGKIN LYMPHOMA

Only few categories of mature T-cell lymphoid malignancies have been investigated in detail at the molecular level. These include Ki-1+ (CD30)+ anaplastic large cell lymphoma (ALCL), adult T-cell leukemia/lymphoma (ATLL), T-cell prolymphocytic leukemia, and, to a lesser extent, cutaneous T-cell lymphoma (68,69).

T-Cell Anaplastic Large Cell Lymphoma

Conventional karyotyping analysis of ALCL cases have shown a unique translocation involving bands 2p23 and 5q35 in a substantial fraction of cases (16). Molecular characterization of the breakpoints revealed that the t(2;5)(p23;q35) translocation causes the fusion of two genes, the nucleophosmin (NPM) gene encoding for a nucleolar phosphoprotein on chromosome 5, and the anaplastic lymphoma kinase (ALK) gene encoding for a novel orphan receptor tyrosine kinase on chromosome 2 (224). This fusion generates an 80-kDa fusion protein where the amino-terminal portion of NPM is joined to the entire cytoplasmic catalytic portion of ALK (224). NPM-ALK has been shown to have transforming ability in vitro (225,226) and in vivo using retroviral-mediated gene transfer (227,228). Most recently, targeted expression of NPM/ALK in T lymphocytes induced lymphoid malignancies in mice, demonstrating a direct causative role for NPM-ALK in human lymphoma (229). The fusion of NPM to ALK has two distinct consequences, both of which are important in the oncogenic properties of the fusion protein. First, it leads to the ectopic expression of NPM-ALK in T-cells (225). Second, it results in the constitutive activation of ALK activity due to oligomerization mediated by the NPM segment. This activated kinase function, in turn, activates the mitogenic signal transduction pathway through phospholipase Cγ (225,226).

Ten to 20% of ALK-positive ALCLs express ALK-fusion proteins other than NPM-ALK (228,230,231). In these other translocations involving tyrosine kinases, the ALK breakpoints are the same as in the classic (2;5) translocation. Like NPM-ALK, the alternative ALK fusion proteins have functional tyrosine kinase activity (231).

Adult T-Cell Leukemia/Lymphoma

The malignant cells of ATLL are infected by the human T-cell leukemia virus type-1 retrovirus in 100% of cases (232). The retroviral gene Tax has been shown to have a critical role for the pathogenesis of ATLL. Tax can transform T cells both in vitro and in transgenic animals by regulating the expression of cellular genes, including those encoding interleukin-2 and the interleukin-2 receptor (232,233). However, based on the observation of the low incidence of ATLL in patients infected with human T-cell leukemia virus type-1 and the long latency (10 to 30 years) of the disease, it is clear that Tax alone is not sufficient for full-blown malignancy, and additional genetic lesions are required (232). The hypothesis is supported by the observation that p53 is inactivated in 40% of ATLL cases (234).

T-Cell Prolymphocytic Leukemia

T-cell prolymphocytic leukemia is frequently associated with abnormalities of chromosome 11, the most common ones being represented by monosomy 11, partial or terminal deletions of 11q, and unbalanced translocations involving the 11q arm (16). The target gene of these abnormalities has been recently identified as the *ATM* gene, which is also responsible for the hereditary disorder ataxia telangiectasia (235,236). Although

ATM is mutated in the germline of patients with ataxia telangiectasia, in cases of T-cell prolymphocytic leukemia, the mutations are of somatic origin. Mutations of *ATM* in T-cell prolymphocytic leukemia associate with deletion of the second allele, and lead to the absence, premature truncation, or alteration of the *ATM* gene product, consistent with the inactivation model of tumor suppressor genes (235,236). The *ATM* gene is involved in cell cycle regulation and DNA repair, which in fact have been shown to be defective in T-cell prolymphocytic leukemia cells (237).

Cutaneous T-Cell Lymphoma

The most frequent known genetic lesion associated with cutaneous T-cell lymphoma is the rearrangement of the *NFκB2/LYT10* gene, which is present in approximately 15% of cases (238,239). The NFκB2 gene encodes a component of the NF-κB transcription factor complex, which is involved in regulating cell proliferation, differentiation, activation, and apoptosis in response to a variety of extracellular signals (240,241). In NHL, rearrangements cluster within the 3′ terminal ankyrin-coding domain of the NFκB2 gene, resulting in the generation of a protein truncated at its C terminal, which is occasionally fused to heterologous proteins (238). These alterations convert NFκB2 from a repressor to a constitutive transcriptional activator, possibly leading to abnormal expression of genes that enforce proliferation and survival (242).

REFERENCES

1. Burrows PD, Cooper MD. B cell development and differentiation. *Curr Opin Immunol* 1997;9:239–244.
2. Willerford DM, Swat W, Alt FW. Developmental regulation of V(D)J recombination and lymphocyte differentiation. *Curr Opin Genet Dev.* 1996;6:603–609.
3. Rajewsky K. Clonal selection and learning in the antibody system. *Nature* 1996;381:751–758.
4. MacLennan IC. Germinal centers. *Annu Rev Immunol* 1994;12:117–139.
5. Wagner SD, Neuberger MS. Somatic hypermutation of immunoglobulin genes. *Annu Rev Immunol* 1996;14:441–457.
6. McHeyzer-Williams LJ, Driver DJ, McHeyzer-Williams MG. Germinal center reaction. *Curr Opin Hematol* 2001;8:52–59.
7. Küppers R, Klein U, Hansmann ML, et al. Cellular origin of human B-cell lymphomas. *N Engl J Med* 1999;341:1520–1529.
8. Muller-Hermelink HK, Greiner A. Molecular analysis of human immunoglobulin heavy chain variable genes (IgVH) in normal and malignant B cells. *Am J Pathol* 1998;153:1341–1346.
9. Bahler DW, Levy R. Clonal evolution of a follicular lymphoma: evidence for antigen selection. *Proc Natl Acad Sci U S A* 1992;89:6770–6774.
10. Tamaru J, Hummel M, Marafioti T, et al. Burkitt's lymphomas express VH genes with a moderate number of antigen-selected somatic mutations. *Am J Pathol* 1995;147:1398–1407.
11. Bertoni F, Cazzaniga G, Bosshard G, et al. Immunoglobulin heavy chain diversity genes rearrangement pattern indicates that MALT-type gastric lymphoma B cells have undergone an antigen selection process. *Br J Haematol* 1997;97:830–836.
12. Küppers R, Rajewsky K, Hansmann ML. Diffuse large cell lymphomas are derived from mature B cells carrying V region genes with a high load of somatic mutation and evidence of selection for antibody expression. *Eur J Immunol* 1997;27:1398–1405.
13. Sahota SS, Garand R, Bataille R, et al. VH gene analysis of clonally related IgM and IgG from human lymphoplasmacytoid B-cell tumors with chronic lymphocytic leukemia features and high serum monoclonal IgG. *Blood* 1998;91:238–243.
14. Fais F, Gaidano G, Capello D, et al. Immunoglobulin V region gene use and structure suggest antigen selection in AIDS-related primary effusion lymphomas. *Leukemia* 1999;13:1093–1099.
15. Fais F, Ghiotto F, Hashimoto S, et al. Chronic lymphocytic leukemia B cells express restricted sets of mutated and unmutated antigen receptors. *J Clin Invest* 1998;102:1515–1525.
16. Mitelman F, Mertens F, Johansson B. A breakpoint map of recurrent chromosomal rearrangements in human neoplasia. *Nat Genet* 1997;15 Spec No:417–474.
17. Bedi GC, Westra WH, Farzadegan H, et al. Microsatellite instability in primary neoplasms from HIV + patients. *Nat Med* 1995;1:65–68.
18. Eshleman JR, Markowitz SD. Microsatellite instability in inherited and sporadic neoplasms. *Curr Opin Oncol* 1995;7:83–89.
19. Gamberi B, Gaidano G, Parsa N, et al. Microsatellite instability is rare in B-cell non-Hodgkin's lymphomas. *Blood* 1997;89:975–979.
20. Furlan D, Bertoni F, Cerutti R, et al. Microsatellite instability in gastric MALT lymphomas and other associated neoplasms. *Ann Oncol* 1999;10:783–788.
21. Offit K, Wong G, Filippa DA, et al. Cytogenetic analysis of 434 consecutively ascertained specimens of non-Hodgkin's lymphoma: clinical correlations. *Blood* 1991;77:1508–1515.
22. Ramiro AR, Jankovic M, Eisenreich T, et al. AID is required for c-myc/IgH chromosome translocations in vivo. *Cell* 2004;118:431–438.
23. Callen E, Jankovic M, Difilippantonio S, et al. ATM prevents the persistence and propagation of chromosome breaks in lymphocytes. *Cell* 2007;130:63–75.
24. Goossens T, Klein U, Küppers R. Frequent occurrence of deletions and duplications during somatic hypermutation: implications for oncogene translocations and heavy chain disease. *Proc Natl Acad Sci U S A* 1998;95:2463–2468.
25. Küppers R, Dalla-Favera R. Mechanisms of chromosomal translocations in B-cell lymphomas. *Oncogene* 2001;20:5580–5594.
26. Papavasiliou FN, Schatz DG. Cell-cycle-regulated DNA double-stranded breaks in somatic hypermutation of immunoglobulin genes. *Nature* 2000;408:216–221.
27. Bross L, Fukita Y, McBlane F, et al. DNA double-strand breaks in immunoglobulin genes undergoing somatic hypermutation. *Immunity.* 2000;13:589–597.
28. Bross L, Muramatsu M, Kinoshita K, et al. DNA double-strand breaks: prior to but not sufficient in targeting hypermutation. *J Exp Med* 2002;195:1187–1192.
29. Pasqualucci L, Bhagat G, Jankovic M, et al R. AID is required for germinal center-derived lymphomagenesis. *Nat Genet* 2008;40:108–112.
30. Pasqualucci L, Neumeister P, Goossens T, et al. Hypermutation of multiple proto-oncogenes in B-cell diffuse large-cell lymphomas. *Nature* 2001;412:341–346.
31. Klein U, Goossens T, Fischer M, et al. Somatic hypermutation in normal and transformed human B cells. *Immunol Rev* 1998;162:261–280.
32. Pasqualucci L, Migliazza A, Fracchiolla N, et al. BCL-6 mutations in normal germinal center B cells: evidence of somatic hypermutation acting outside Ig loci. *Proc Natl Acad Sci U S A* 1998;95:11816–11821.
33. Shen HM, Peters A, Baron B, et al. Mutation of BCL-6 gene in normal B cells by the process of somatic hypermutation of Ig genes. *Science* 1998;280:1750–1752.
34. Müschen M, Re D, Jungnickel B, et al. Somatic mutation of the CD95 gene in human B cells as a side-effect of the germinal center reaction. *J Exp Med* 2000;192:1833–1840.
35. Gordon MS, Kanegai CM, Doerr JR, et al. Somatic hypermutation of the B cell receptor genes B29 (Igbeta, CD79b) and mb1 (Igalpha, CD79a). *Proc Natl Acad Sci U S A* 2003;100:4126–4131.
36. Peng HZ, Du MQ, Koulis A, et al. Nonimmunoglobulin gene hypermutation in germinal center B cells. *Blood* 1999;93:2167–2172.
37. Vakiani E, Basso K, Klein U, et al. Genetic and phenotypic analysis of B-cell post-transplant lymphoproliferative disorders provides insights into disease biology. *Hematol Oncol* 2008;26:199–211.
38. Montesinos-Rongen M, Van Roost D, Schaller C, et al. Primary diffuse large B-cell lymphomas of the central nervous system are targeted by aberrant somatic hypermutation. *Blood* 2004;103:1869–1875.
39. Gaidano G, Pasqualucci L, Capello D, et al. Aberrant somatic hypermutation in multiple subtypes of AIDS-associated non-Hodgkin lymphoma. *Blood* 2003;102:1833–1841.
40. Deutsch AJ, Aigelsreiter A, Staber PB, et al. MALT lymphoma and extranodal diffuse large B-cell lymphoma are targeted by aberrant somatic hypermutation. *Blood* 2007;109:3500–3504.
41. Houldsworth J, Mathew S, Rao PH, et al. REL proto-oncogene is frequently amplified in extranodal diffuse large cell lymphoma. *Blood.* 1996;87:25–29.
42. Chaganti RS, Nanjangud G, Schmidt H, et al. Recurring chromosomal abnormalities in non-Hodgkin's lymphoma: biologic and clinical significance. *Semin Hematol* 2000;37:396–411.
43. Neri A, Knowles DM, Greco A, et al. Analysis of RAS oncogene mutations in human lymphoid malignancies. *Proc Natl Acad Sci U S A* 1988;85:9268–9272.
44. Lenz G Davis RE, Ngo VN, et al. Oncogenic CARD11 mutations in human diffuse large B cell lymphoma. *Science* 2008;319:1676–1679.
45. Compagno M, Lim WK, Grunn A, et al. Mutations in multiple genes cause deregulate NF-kB pathway in Diffuse Large B cell Lymphoma. *Nature*, 2009; Epub May 3.
46. Kato M, Sanada M, Kato I, et al. Frequent inactivation of A20 in B cell lymphomas. *Nature*, 2009; Epub May 3.

47. Hollstein M, Sidransky D, Vogelstein B, et al. p53 mutations in human cancers. *Science* 1991;253:49–53.

48. Gaidano G, Ballerini P, Gong JZ, et al. p53 mutations in human lymphoid malignancies: association with Burkitt lymphoma and chronic lymphocytic leukemia. *Proc Natl Acad Sci U S A* 1991;88:5413–5417.

49. Ballerini P, Gaidano G, Gong JZ, et al. Multiple genetic lesions in acquired immunodeficiency syndrome-related non-Hodgkin's lymphoma. *Blood* 1993;81:166–176.

50. Lo Coco F, Gaidano G, Louie DC, et al. p53 mutations are associated with histologic transformation of follicular lymphoma. *Blood* 1993;82: 2289–2295.

51. Gaidano G, Hauptschein RS, Parsa NZ, et al. Deletions involving two distinct regions of 6q in B-cell non-Hodgkin lymphoma. *Blood* 1992;80: 1781–1787.

52. Alizadeh AA, Eisen MB, Davis RE, et al. Distinct types of diffuse large B-cell lymphoma identified by gene expression profiling. *Nature* 2000; 403:503–511.

53. Tam W, Gomez M, Chadburn A, et al. Mutational analysis of PRDM1 indicates a tumor-suppressor role in diffuse large B-cell lymphomas. *Blood* 2006;107:4090–4100.

54. Pasqualucci L, Compagno M, Houldsworth J, et al. Inactivation of the PRDM1/BLIMP1 gene in diffuse large B cell lymphoma. *J Exp Med* 2006;203:311–317.

55. Brown AG, Ross FM, Dunne EM, et al. Evidence for a new tumour suppressor locus (DBM) in human B-cell neoplasia telomeric to the retinoblastoma gene. *Nat Genet* 1993;3:67–72.

56. Devilder MC, Francois S, Bosic C, et al. Deletion cartography around the D13S25 locus in B cell chronic lymphocytic leukemia and accurate mapping of the involved tumor suppressor gene. *Cancer Res* 1995;55:1355–1357.

57. Liu Y, Hermanson M, Grander D, et al. 13q deletions in lymphoid malignancies. *Blood* 1995;86:1911–1915.

58. Kalachikov S, Migliazza A, Cayanis E, et al. Cloning and gene mapping of the chromosome 13q14 region deleted in chronic lymphocytic leukemia. *Genomics* 1997;42:369–377.

59. Migliazza A, Bosch F, Komatsu H, et al. Nucleotide sequence, transcription map, and mutation analysis of the 13q14 chromosomal region deleted in B-cell chronic lymphocytic leukemia. *Blood*. 2001;97:2098–2104.

60. Bullrich F, Veronese ML, Kitada S, et al. Minimal region of loss at 13q14 in B-cell chronic lymphocytic leukemia. *Blood* 1996;88:3109–3115.

61. Calin GA, Ferracin M, Cimmino A, et al. A MicroRNA signature associated with prognosis and progression in chronic lymphocytic leukemia. *N Engl J Med* 2005;353:1793–1801.

62. Calin GA, Dumitru CD, Shimizu M, et al. Frequent deletions and down-regulation of micro- RNA genes miR15 and miR16 at 13q14 in chronic lymphocytic leukemia. *Proc Natl Acad Sci U S A* 2002;99:15524–15529.

63. Drexler HG. Review of alterations of the cyclin-dependent kinase inhibitor INK4 family genes p15, p16, p18 and p19 in human leukemia-lymphoma cells. *Leukemia* 1998;12:845–859.

64. Pinyol M, Cobo F, Bea S, et al. p16(INK4a) gene inactivation by deletions, mutations, and hypermethylation is associated with transformed and aggressive variants of non-Hodgkin's lymphomas. *Blood* 1998;91: 2977–2984.

65. Herman JG, Civin CI, Issa JP, et al. Distinct patterns of inactivation of p15INK4B and p16INK4A characterize the major types of hematological malignancies. *Cancer Res* 1997;57:837–841.

66. Martinez-Delgado B, Richart A, Garcia MJ, et al. Hypermethylation of P16ink4a and P15ink4b genes as a marker of disease in the follow-up of non-Hodgkin's lymphomas. *Br J Haematol* 2000;109:97–103.

67. Martinez-Delgado B, Robledo M, Arranz E, et al. Hypermethylation of p15/ink4b/MTS2 gene is differentially implicated among non-Hodgkin's lymphomas. *Leukemia* 1998;12:937–941.

68. Harris NL, Jaffe ES, Diebold J, et al. World Health Organization classification of neoplastic diseases of the hematopoietic and lymphoid tissues: report of the Clinical Advisory Committee meeting-Airlie House, Virginia, November 1997. *J Clin Oncol* 1999;17:3835–3849.

69. Harris NL, Jaffe ES, Stein H, et al. A revised European-American classification of lymphoid neoplasms: a proposal from the International Lymphoma Study Group. *Blood* 1994;84:1361–1392.

70. Berger F, Felman P, Sonet A, et al. Nonfollicular small B-cell lymphomas: a heterogeneous group of patients with distinct clinical features and outcome. *Blood* 1994;83:2829–2835.

71. Fisher RI, Dahlberg S, Nathwani BN, et al. A clinical analysis of two indolent lymphoma entities: mantle cell lymphoma and marginal zone lymphoma (including the mucosa-associated lymphoid tissue and monocytoid B-cell subcategories): a Southwest Oncology Group study. *Blood* 1995;85:1075–1082.

72. Raffeld M, Jaffe ES. bcl-1, t(11;14), and mantle cell-derived lymphomas. *Blood* 1991;78:259–263.

73. Rimokh R, Berger F, Delsol G, et al. Rearrangement and overexpression of the BCL-1/PRAD-1 gene in intermediate lymphocytic lymphomas and in t(11q13)-bearing leukemias. *Blood* 1993;81:3063–3067.

74. Callanan M, Leroux D, Magaud JP, et al. Implication of cyclin D1 in malignant lymphoma. *Crit Rev Oncog* 1996;7:191–203.

75. Campo E, Raffeld M, Jaffe ES. Mantle-cell lymphoma. *Semin Hematol* 1999;36:115–127.

76. Tsujimoto Y, Yunis J, Onorato-Showe L, et al. Molecular cloning of the chromosomal breakpoint of B-cell lymphomas and leukemias with the t(11;14) chromosome translocation. *Science* 1984;224:1403–1406.

77. Tsujimoto Y, Jaffe E, Cossman J, et al. Clustering of breakpoints on chromosome 11 in human B-cell neoplasms with the t(11;14) chromosome translocation. *Nature* 1985;315:340–343.

78. Erikson J, Finan J, Tsujimoto Y, et al. The chromosome 14 breakpoint in neoplastic B cells with the t(11;14) translocation involves the immunoglobulin heavy chain locus. *Proc Natl Acad Sci U S A* 1984;81:4144–4148.

79. Withers DA, Harvey RC, Faust JB, et al. Characterization of a candidate bcl-1 gene. *Mol Cell Biol* 1991;11:4846–4853.

80. Motokura T, Bloom T, Kim HG, et al. A novel cyclin encoded by a bcl1-linked candidate oncogene. *Nature* 1991;350:512–515.

81. Rosenberg CL, Wong E, Petty EM, et al. PRAD1, a candidate BCL1 oncogene: mapping and expression in centrocytic lymphoma. *Proc Natl Acad Sci U S A* 1991;88:9638–9642.

82. Seto M, Yamamoto K, Iida S, et al. Gene rearrangement and overexpression of PRAD1 in lymphoid malignancy with t(11;14)(q13;q32) translocation. *Oncogene* 1992;7:1401–1406.

83. Murakami MS, Strobel MJ, Vande Woude JF. *Cell cycle regulation, oncogenes, and antineoplastic drugs*, vol. 3. Philadelphia, PA: J.B. Lippincott, 1995.

84. Jiang W, Kahn SM, Zhou P, et al. Overexpression of cyclin D1 in rat fibroblasts causes abnormalities in growth control, cell cycle progression and gene expression. *Oncogene* 1993;8:3447–3457.

85. Bodrug SE, Warner BJ, Bath ML, et al. Cyclin D1 transgene impedes lymphocyte maturation and collaborates in lymphomagenesis with the myc gene. EMBO J 1994;13:2124–2130.

86. Lovec H, Grzeschiczek A, Kowalski MB, et al. Cyclin D1/bcl-1 cooperates with myc genes in the generation of B-cell lymphoma in transgenic mice. *EMBO J* 1994;13:3487–3495.

87. Greiner TC, Moynihan MJ, Chan WC, et al. p53 mutations in mantle cell lymphoma are associated with variant cytology and predict a poor prognosis. *Blood* 1996;87:1302–4310.

88. Louie DC, Offit K, Jaslow R, et al. p53 overexpression as a marker of poor prognosis in mantle cell lymphomas with t(11;14)(q13;q32). *Blood* 1995;86:2892–2899.

89. Camacho E, Hernandez L, Hernandez S, et al. ATM gene inactivation in mantle cell lymphoma mainly occurs by truncating mutations and missense mutations involving the phosphatidylinositol-3 kinase domain and is associated with increasing numbers of chromosomal imbalances. *Blood* 2002;99:238–244.

90. Schaffner C, Idler I, Stilgenbauer S, et al. Mantle cell lymphoma is characterized by inactivation of the ATM gene. *Proc Natl Acad Sci U S A* 2000;97:2773–2778.

91. Dalla-Favera R. Chromosomal translocations involving the c-myc oncogene in lymphoid neoplasia. In: Kirsch IR, ed. *The causes and consequences of chromosomal aberrations*. Boca Raton, Fla: CRC Press, 1993:312.

92. Dalla-Favera R, Bregni M, Erikson J, et al. Human c-myc onc gene is located on the region of chromosome 8 that is translocated in Burkitt lymphoma cells. *Proc Natl Acad Sci U S A* 1982;79:7824–7827.

93. Dalla-Favera R, Martinotti S, Gallo RC, et al. Translocation and rearrangements of the c-myc oncogene locus in human undifferentiated B-cell lymphomas. *Science* 1983;219:963–967.

94. Taub R, Kirsch I, Morton C, et al. Translocation of the c-myc gene into the immunoglobulin heavy chain locus in human Burkitt lymphoma and murine plasmacytoma cells. *Proc Natl Acad Sci U S A* 1982;79:7837–7841.

95. Davis M, Malcolm S, Rabbitts TH. Chromosome translocation can occur on either side of the c-myc oncogene in Burkitt lymphoma cells. *Nature* 1984;308:286–288.

96. Hollis GF, Mitchell KF, Battey J, et al. A variant translocation places the lambda immunoglobulin genes 3′ to the c-myc oncogene in Burkitt's lymphoma. *Nature* 1984;307:752–755.

97. Neri A, Barriga F, Knowles DM, et al. Different regions of the immunoglobulin heavy-chain locus are involved in chromosomal translocations in distinct pathogenetic forms of Burkitt lymphoma. *Proc Natl Acad Sci U S A*. 1988;85:2748–2752.

98. Pelicci PG, Knowles DM 2nd, Magrath I, et aR. Chromosomal breakpoints and structural alterations of the c-myc locus differ in endemic and sporadic forms of Burkitt lymphoma. *Proc Natl Acad Sci U S A* 1986; 83:2984–2988.

99. Klein U, Tu Y, Stolovitzky GA, et al. Transcriptional analysis of the B cell germinal center reaction. *Proc Natl Acad Sci U S A* 2003;100:2639–2644.

100. Cesarman E, Dalla-Favera R, Bentley D, et al. Mutations in the first exon are associated with altered transcription of c-myc in Burkitt lymphoma. *Science* 1987;238:1272–1275.

101. Bhatia K, Huppi K, Spangler G, et al. Point mutations in the c-Myc transactivation domain are common in Burkitt's lymphoma and mouse plasmacytomas. *Nat Genet* 1993;5:56–61.

102. Bhatia K, Spangler G, Gaidano G, et al. Mutations in the coding region of c-myc occur frequently in acquired immunodeficiency syndrome-associated lymphomas. *Blood* 1994;84:883–888.

103. Gu W, Bhatia K, Magrath IT, et al. Binding and suppression of the Myc transcriptional activation domain by p107. *Science* 1994;264:251–254.
104. Gregory MA, Hann SR. c-Myc proteolysis by the ubiquitin-proteasome pathway: stabilization of c-Myc in Burkitt's lymphoma cells. *Mol Cell Biol* 2000;20:2423–2435.
105. Lutz W, Leon J, Eilers M. Contributions of Myc to tumorigenesis. *Biochim Biophys Acta* 2002;1602:61–71.
106. Eisenman RN. Deconstructing myc. *Genes Dev* 2001;15:2023–2030.
107. Dominguez-Sola D, Ying CY, Grandori C, et al. Non-transcriptional control of DNA replication by c-Myc. *Nature* 2007;448:445–451.
108. Dang CV. c-Myc target genes involved in cell growth, apoptosis, and metabolism. *Mol Cell Biol* 1999;19:1–11.
109. Amati B, Dalton S, Brooks MW, et al. Transcriptional activation by the human c-Myc oncoprotein in yeast requires interaction with Max. *Nature* 1992;359:423–426.
110. Amati B, Brooks MW, Levy N, et al. Oncogenic activity of the c-Myc protein requires dimerization with Max. *Cell* 1993;72:233–245.
111. Blackwood EM, Eisenman RN. Max: a helix-loop-helix zipper protein that forms a sequence-specific DNA-binding complex with Myc. *Science* 1991;251:1211–1217.
112. Blackwood EM, Luscher B, Eisenman RN. Myc and Max associate in vivo. *Genes Dev* 1992;6:71–80.
113. Kretzner L, Blackwood EM, Eisenman RN. Myc and Max proteins possess distinct transcriptional activities. *Nature* 1992;359:426–429.
114. Gu W, Cechova K, Tassi V, et al. Opposite regulation of gene transcription and cell proliferation by c-Myc and Max. *Proc Natl Acad Sci U S A* 1993;90:2935–2939.
115. Ayer DE, Kretzner L, Eisenman RN. Mad: a heterodimeric partner for Max that antagonizes Myc transcriptional activity. *Cell* 1993;72:211–222.
116. Zervos AS, Gyuris J, Brent R. Mxi1, a protein that specifically interacts with Max to bind Myc-Max recognition sites. *Cell* 1993;72:223–232.
117. Coller HA, Grandori C, Tamayo P, et al. Expression analysis with oligonucleotide microarrays reveals that MYC regulates genes involved in growth, cell cycle, signaling, and adhesion. *Proc Natl Acad Sci U S A* 2000;97:3260–3265.
118. Lombardi L, Newcomb EW, Dalla-Favera R. Pathogenesis of Burkitt lymphoma: expression of an activated c-myc oncogene causes the tumorigenic conversion of EBV-infected human B lymphoblasts. *Cell* 1987;49:161–170.
119. Kovalchuk AL, Qi CF, Torrey TA, et al. Burkitt lymphoma in the mouse. *J Exp Med* 2000;192:1183–1190.
120. Adams JM, Harris AW, Pinkert CA, et al. The c-myc oncogene driven by immunoglobulin enhancers induces lymphoid malignancy in transgenic mice. *Nature* 1985;318:533–538.
121. Klangby U, Okan I, Magnusson KP, et al. p16/INK4a and p15/INK4b gene methylation and absence of p16/INK4a mRNA and protein expression in Burkitt's lymphoma. *Blood* 1998;91:1680–1687.
122. zur Hausen H, Schulte-Holthausen H, Klein G, et al. EBV DNA in biopsies of Burkitt tumours and anaplastic carcinomas of the nasopharynx. *Nature* 1970;228:1056–1058.
123. Neri A, Barriga F, Inghirami G, et al. Epstein-Barr virus infection precedes clonal expansion in Burkitt's and acquired immunodeficiency syndrome-associated lymphoma. *Blood* 1991;77:1092–1095.
124. Pelicci PG, Knowles DM 2nd, Arlin ZA, et al. Multiple monoclonal B cell expansions and c-myc oncogene rearrangements in acquired immune deficiency syndrome-related lymphoproliferative disorders. Implications for lymphomagenesis. *J Exp Med* 1986;164:2049–2060.
125. Hamilton-Dutoit SJ, Pallesen G. A survey of Epstein-Barr virus gene expression in sporadic non-Hodgkin's lymphomas. Detection of Epstein-Barr virus in a subset of peripheral T-cell lymphomas. *Am J Pathol* 1992;140:1315–1325.
126. Carbone A, Gaidano G, Gloghini A, et al. Differential expression of BCL-6, CD138/syndecan-1, and Epstein-Barr virus-encoded latent membrane protein-1 identifies distinct histogenetic subsets of acquired immunodeficiency syndrome-related non-Hodgkin's lymphomas. *Blood* 1998; 91:747–755.
127. Bakhshi A, Jensen JP, Goldman P, et al. Cloning the chromosomal breakpoint of t(14;18) human lymphomas: clustering around JH on chromosome 14 and near a transcriptional unit on 18. *Cell* 1985;41:899–906.
128. Tsujimoto Y, Finger LR, Yunis J, et al. Cloning of the chromosome breakpoint of neoplastic B cells with the t(14;18) chromosome translocation. *Science* 1984;226:1097–1099.
129. Cleary ML, Galili N, Sklar J. Detection of a second t(14;18) breakpoint cluster region in human follicular lymphomas. *J Exp Med* 1986;164:315–320.
130. Cleary ML, Sklar J. Nucleotide sequence of a t(14;18) chromosomal breakpoint in follicular lymphoma and demonstration of a breakpoint-cluster region near a transcriptionally active locus on chromosome 18. *Proc Natl Acad Sci U S A* 1985;82:7439–7443.
131. Cleary ML, Smith SD, Sklar J. Cloning and structural analysis of cDNAs for bcl-2 and a hybrid bcl-2/immunoglobulin transcript resulting from the t(14;18) translocation. *Cell* 1986;47:19–28.
132. Buchonnet G, Jardin F, Jean N, et al. Distribution of BCL2 breakpoints in follicular lymphoma and correlation with clinical features: specific subtypes or same disease? *Leukemia* 2002;16:1852–1856.
133. Ngan BY, Chen-Levy Z, Weiss LM, et al. Expression in non-Hodgkin's lymphoma of the bcl-2 protein associated with the t(14;18) chromosomal translocation. *N Engl J Med* 1988;318:1638–1644.
134. Graninger WB, Seto M, Boutain B, et al. Expression of Bcl-2 and Bcl-2-Ig fusion transcripts in normal and neoplastic cells. *J Clin Invest* 1987; 80:1512–1515.
135. Hockenbery D, Nunez G, Milliman C, et al. Bcl-2 is an inner mitochondrial membrane protein that blocks programmed cell death. *Nature* 1990;348:334–336.
136. Korsmeyer SJ. Bcl-2 initiates a new category of oncogenes: regulators of cell death. *Blood* 1992;80:879–886.
137. Nunez G, Seto M, Seremetis S, et al. Growth- and tumor-promoting effects of deregulated BCL2 in human B-lymphoblastoid cells. *Proc Natl Acad Sci U S A* 1989;86:4589–4593.
138. Chao DT, Korsmeyer SJ. BCL-2 family: regulators of cell death. *Annu Rev Immunol* 1998;16:395–419.
139. Vaux DL, Cory S, Adams JM. Bcl-2 gene promotes haemopoietic cell survival and cooperates with c-myc to immortalize pre-B cells. *Nature* 1988;335:440–442.
140. Nunez G, Hockenbery D, McDonnell TJ, et al. Bcl-2 maintains B cell memory. *Nature* 1991;353:71–73.
141. Smith KG, Light A, O'Reilly LA, et al. bcl-2 transgene expression inhibits apoptosis in the germinal center and reveals differences in the selection of memory B cells and bone marrow antibody-forming cells. *J Exp Med* 2000;191:475–484.
142. McDonnell TJ, Deane N, Platt FM, et al. bcl-2-immunoglobulin transgenic mice demonstrate extended B cell survival and follicular lymphoproliferation. *Cell* 1989;57:79–88.
143. McDonnell TJ, Korsmeyer SJ. Progression from lymphoid hyperplasia to high-grade malignant lymphoma in mice transgenic for the t(14; 18). *Nature* 1991;349:254–256.
144. Dobson CL, Warren AJ, Pannell R, et al. The mll-AF9 gene fusion in mice controls myeloproliferation and specifies acute myeloid leukaemogenesis. *EMBO J* 1999;18:3564–3574.
145. Capello D, Vitolo U, Pasqualucci L, et al. Distribution and pattern of BCL-6 mutations throughout the spectrum of B-cell neoplasia. *Blood* 2000;95:651–659.
146. Yano T, Jaffe ES, Longo DL, et al. MYC rearrangements in histologically progressed follicular lymphomas. *Blood* 1992;80:758–767.
147. Dalla-Favera R, Gaidano G. Molecular biology of lymphomas. In: De Vita VT, Hellman S, Rosenberg SA, eds. *Cancer, principles and practice of oncology*, 6th ed. Philadelphia, PA: Lippincott Williams & Wilkins, 2001:2215–2235.
148. Shipp MA, Ross N, Tamayo P, et al. Diffuse large B-cell lymphoma outcome prediction by gene-expression profiling and supervised machine learning. *Nat Med* 2002;8:68–74.
149. Offit K, Jhanwar S, Ebrahim SA, et al. t(3;22)(q27;q11): a novel translocation associated with diffuse non-Hodgkin's lymphoma. *Blood* 1989;74:1876–1879.
150. Baron BW, Nucifora G, McCabe N, et al. Identification of the gene associated with the recurring chromosomal translocations t(3;14)(q27;q32) and t(3;22)(q27;q11) in B-cell lymphomas. *Proc Natl Acad Sci U S A* 1993;90:5262–5266.
151. Kerckaert JP, Deweindt C, Tilly H, et al. LAZ3, a novel zinc-finger encoding gene, is disrupted by recurring chromosome 3q27 translocations in human lymphomas. *Nat Genet* 1993;5:66–70.
152. Ye BH, Lista F, Lo Coco F, et al. Alterations of a zinc finger-encoding gene, BCL-6, in diffuse large- cell lymphoma. *Science* 1993;262:747–750.
153. Ye BH, Rao PH, Chaganti RS, et al R. Cloning of bcl-6, the locus involved in chromosome translocations affecting band 3q27 in B-cell lymphoma. *Cancer Res* 1993;53:2732–2735.
154. Miki T, Kawamata N, Arai A, et al. Molecular cloning of the breakpoint for 3q27 translocation in B-cell lymphomas and leukemias. *Blood* 1994; 83:217–222.
155. Zollman S, Godt D, Prive GG, et al. The BTB domain, found primarily in zinc finger proteins, defines an evolutionarily conserved family that includes several developmentally regulated genes in Drosophila. *Proc Natl Acad Sci U S A* 1994;91:10717–10721.
156. Chang CC, Ye BH, Chaganti RS, et al. BCL-6, a POZ/zinc-finger protein, is a sequence-specific transcriptional repressor. *Proc Natl Acad Sci U S A* 1996;93:6947–6952.
157. Dalla-Favera R, Migliazza A, Chang CC, et al. Molecular pathogenesis of B cell malignancy: the role of BCL-6. *Curr Top Microbiol Immunol* 1999;246:257–263.
158. Cattoretti G, Chang CC, Cechova K, et al. BCL-6 protein is expressed in germinal-center B cells. *Blood* 1995;86:45–53.
159. Allman D, Jain A, Dent A, et al. BCL-6 expression during B-cell activation. *Blood* 1996;87:5257–5268.
160. Ye BH, Cattoretti G, Shen Q, et al. The BCL-6 proto-oncogene controls germinal-centre formation and Th2- type inflammation. *Nat Genet* 1997; 16:161–170.
161. Dent AL, Shaffer AL, Yu X, et al. Control of inflammation, cytokine expression, and germinal center formation by BCL-6. *Science* 1997;276:589–592.

162. Shaffer AL, Yu X, He Y, et al. BCL-6 represses genes that function in lymphocyte differentiation, inflammation, and cell cycle control. *Immunity* 2000;13:199–212.

163. Ranuncolo SM, Polo JM, Dierov J, et al. Bcl-6 mediates the germinal center B cell phenotype and lymphomagenesis through transcriptional repression of the DNA-damage sensor ATR. *Nat Immunol* 2007;8:705–714.

164. Phan RT, Saito M, Basso K, et al. BCL6 interacts with the transcription factor Miz-1 to suppress the cyclin-dependent kinase inhibitor p21 and cell cycle arrest in germinal center B cells. *Nat Immunol* 2005;6:1054–1060.

165. Phan RT, Dalla-Favera R. The BCL6 proto-oncogene suppresses p53 expression in germinal-centre B cells. *Nature* 2004;432:635–639.

166. Niu H, Cattoretti G, Dalla-Favera R. BCL6 controls the expression of the B7-1/CD80 costimulatory receptor in germinal center B cells. *J Exp Med* 2003;198:211–221.

167. Baron BW, Anastasi J, Thirman MJ, et al. The human programmed cell death-2 (PDCD2) gene is a target of BCL6 repression: implications for a role of BCL6 in the down-regulation of apoptosis. *Proc Natl Acad Sci U S A* 2002;99:2860–2865.

168. Klein U, Dalla-Favera R. Germinal centres: role in B-cell physiology and malignancy. *Nat Rev Immunol* 2008;8:22–33.

169. Lo Coco F, Ye BH, Lista F, et al. Rearrangements of the BCL6 gene in diffuse large cell non-Hodgkin's lymphoma. *Blood* 1994;83:1757–1759.

170. Chen W, Iida S, Louie DC, et al. Heterologous promoters fused to BCL6 by chromosomal translocations affecting band 3q27 cause its deregulated expression during B-cell differentiation. *Blood* 1998;91:603–607.

171. Chang Y, Cesarman E, Pessin MS, et al. Identification of herpesvirus-like DNA sequences in AIDS-associated Kaposi's sarcoma. *Science* 1994;266:1865–1869.

172. Ye BH, Chaganti S, Chang CC, et al. Chromosomal translocations cause deregulated BCL6 expression by promoter substitution in B cell lymphoma. *EMBO J* 1995;14:6209–6217.

173. Dallery E, Galiegue-Zouitina S, Collyn-d'Hooghe M, et al. TTF, a gene encoding a novel small G protein, fuses to the lymphoma- associated LAZ3 gene by t(3;4) chromosomal translocation. *Oncogene* 1995;10:2171–2178.

174. Galieque Zouitina S, Quief S, et al. The B cell transcriptional coactivator BOB1/OBF1 gene fuses to the LAZ3/BCL6 gene by t(3;11)(q27;q23.1) chromosomal translocation in a B cell leukemia line (Karpas 231). *Leukemia* 1996;10:579–587.

175. Galiegue-Zouitina S, Quief S, Hildebrand MP, et al. Nonrandom fusion of L-plastin(LCP1) and LAZ3(BCL6) genes by t(3;13)(q27;q14) chromosome translocation in two cases of B-cell non Hodgkin lymphoma. *Genes Chromosomes Cancer* 1999;26:97–105.

176. Kurata M, Maesako Y, Ueda C, et al. Characterization of t(3;6)(q27;p21) breakpoints in B-cell non-Hodgkin's lymphoma and construction of the histone H4/BCL6 fusion gene, leading to altered expression of Bcl-6. *Cancer Res* 2002;62:6224–6230.

177. Akasaka T, Miura I, Takahashi N, et al. A recurring translocation, t(3;6)(q27;p21), in non-Hodgkin's lymphoma results in replacement of the 5′ regulatory region of BCL6 with a novel H4 histone gene. *Cancer Res* 1997;57:7–12.

178. Hosokawa Y, Maeda Y, Ichinohasama R, et al. The Ikaros gene, a central regulator of lymphoid differentiation, fuses to the BCL6 gene as a result of t(3;7)(q27;p12) translocation in a patient with diffuse large B-cell lymphoma. *Blood* 2000;95:2719–2721.

179. Xu WS, Liang RH, Srivastava G. Identification and characterization of BCL6 translocation partner genes in primary gastric high-grade B-cell lymphoma: heat shock protein 89 alpha is a novel fusion partner gene of BCL6. *Genes Chromosomes Cancer* 2000;27:69–75.

180. Yoshida S, Kaneita Y, Aoki Y, et al M. Identification of heterologous translocation partner genes fused to the BCL6 gene in diffuse large B-cell lymphomas: 5′-RACE and LA - PCR analyses of biopsy samples. *Oncogene* 1999;18:7994–7999.

181. Akasaka T, Ohno H, Mori T, et al. Long distance polymerase chain reaction for detection of chromosome translocations in B-cell lymphoma/leukemia. *Leukemia* 1997;11(suppl 3):316–317.

182. Cattoretti G, Pasqualucci L, Ballon G, et al. Deregulated BCL6 expression recapitulates the pathogenesis of human diffuse large B cell lymphomas in mice. *Cancer Cell* 2005;7:445–455.

183. Migliazza A, Martinotti S, Chen W, et al. Frequent somatic hypermutation of the 5′ noncoding region of the BCL6 gene in B-cell lymphoma. *Proc Natl Acad Sci U S A* 1995;92:12520–12524.

184. Capello D, Carbone A, Pastore C, et al. Point mutations of the BCL-6 gene in Burkitt's lymphoma. *Br J Haematol* 1997;99:168–170.

185. Pasqualucci L, Neri A, Baldini L, et al. BCL-6 mutations are associated with immunoglobulin variable heavy chain mutations in B-cell chronic lymphocytic leukemia. *Cancer Res* 2000;60:5644–5648.

186. Pasqualucci L, Migliazza A, Basso K, et al. Mutations of the BCL6 proto-oncogene disrupt its negative autoregulation in diffuse large B-cell lymphoma. *Blood* 2003;101:2914–2923.

187. Wang X, Li Z, Naganuma A, Ye BH. Negative autoregulation of BCL-6 is bypassed by genetic alterations in diffuse large B cell lymphomas. *Proc Natl Acad Sci U S A* 2002;99:15018–15023.

188. Saito M, Gao J, Basso K, et al. A signaling pathway mediating downregulation of BCL6 in germinal center B cells is blocked by BCL6 gene alterations in B cell lymphoma. *Cancer Cell* 2007;12:280–292.

189. Angelin-Duclos C, Cattoretti G, Lin KI, et al. Commitment of B lymphocytes to a plasma cell fate is associated with Blimp-1 expression in vivo. *J Immunol* 2000;165:5462–5471.

190. Cattoretti G, Angelin-Duclos C, Shaknovich R, et al. PRDM1/Blimp-1 is expressed in human B-lymphocytes committed to the plasma cell lineage. *J Pathol* 2005;206:76–86.

191. Shapiro-Shelef M, Lin KI, McHeyzer-Williams LJ, et al. Blimp-1 is required for the formation of immunoglobulin secreting plasma cells and pre-plasma memory B cells. *Immunity* 2003;19:607–620.

192. Rao PH, Houldsworth J, Dyomina K, et al. Chromosomal and gene amplification in diffuse large B-cell lymphoma. *Blood* 1998;92:234–240.

193. Gronbaek K, Worm J, Ralfkiaer E, et al. ATM mutations are associated with inactivation of the ARF-TP53 tumor suppressor pathway in diffuse large B-cell lymphoma. *Blood* 2002;100:1430–1437.

194. Bai M, Vlachonikolis J, Agnantis NJ, et al. Low expression of p27 protein combined with altered p53 and Rb/p16 expression status is associated with increased expression of cyclin A and cyclin B1 in diffuse large B-cell lymphomas. *Mod Pathol* 2001;14:1105–1113.

195. Parsonnet J, Hansen S, Rodriguez L, et al. Helicobacter pylori infection and gastric lymphoma. *N Engl J Med* 1994;330:1267–1271.

196. Wotherspoon AC, Doglioni C, Diss TC, et al. Regression of primary low-grade B-cell gastric lymphoma of mucosa-associated lymphoid tissue type after eradication of Helicobacter pylori. *Lancet* 1993;342:575–577.

197. Qin Y, Greiner A, Trunk MJ, et al. Somatic hypermutation in low-grade mucosa-associated lymphoid tissue-type B-cell lymphoma. *Blood* 1995;86:3528–3534.

198. Thiede C, Alpen B, Morgner A, et al. Ongoing somatic mutations and clonal expansions after cure of Helicobacter pylori infection in gastric mucosa-associated lymphoid tissue B-cell lymphoma. *J Clin Oncol* 1998;16:3822–3831.

199. Akagi T, Motegi M, Tamura A, et al. A novel gene, MALT1 at 18q21, is involved in t(11;18)(q21;q21) found in low-grade B-cell lymphoma of mucosa-associated lymphoid tissue. *Oncogene* 1999;18:5785–5794.

200. Dierlamm J, Baens M, Wlodarska I, et al. The apoptosis inhibitor gene API2 and a novel 18q gene, MLT, are recurrently rearranged in the t(11;18)(q21;q21) associated with mucosa-associated lymphoid tissue lymphomas. *Blood* 1999;93:3601–3609.

201. Lucas PC, Yonezumi M, Inohara N, et al. Bcl10 and MALT1, independent targets of chromosomal translocation in malt lymphoma, cooperate in a novel NF-kappa B signaling pathway. *J Biol Chem* 2001;276:19012–19019.

202. Willis TG, Jadayel DM, Du MQ, et al. Bcl10 is involved in t(1;14)(p22;q32) of MALT B cell lymphoma and mutated in multiple tumor types. *Cell* 1999;96:35–45.

203. Zhang Q, Siebert R, Yan M, et al. Inactivating mutations and overexpression of BCL10, a caspase recruitment domain-containing gene, in MALT lymphoma with t(1;14)(p22;q32). *Nat Genet* 1999;22:63–68.

204. Ott G, Kalla J, Steinhoff A, et al. Trisomy 3 is not a common feature in malignant lymphomas of mucosa-associated lymphoid tissue type. *Am J Pathol* 1998;153:689–694.

205. Novak U, Rinadi A, Kwee I, et al. The NF-kB negative regulator TNFAIP3 (A20) is commonly inactivated by somatic mutations and genomic deletions in marginal zone B-cell lymphomas. *Blood*, 2009;113:4918–4921.

206. Ott G, Kalla J, Steinhoff A, et al. Trisomy 3 is not a common feature in malignant lymphomas of mucosa-associated lymphoid tissue type. *Am J Pathol* 1998;153:689–694.

207. Du M, Peng H, Singh N, et al L. The accumulation of p53 abnormalities is associated with progression of mucosa-associated lymphoid tissue lymphoma. *Blood* 1995;86:4587–4593.

208. Gaidano G, Volpe G, Pastore C, et al. Detection of BCL-6 rearrangements and p53 mutations in Malt-lymphomas. *Am J Hematol* 1997;56:206–213.

209. Gaidano G, Carbone A, Pastore C, et al. Frequent mutation of the 5′ noncoding region of the BCL-6 gene in acquired immunodeficiency syndrome-related non-Hodgkin's lymphomas. *Blood* 1997;89:3755–3762.

210. Foucar K, Catovsky D. Pathology and genetics of tumours of haematopoietic and lymphoid tissues: World Health Organization Classification of Tumours. In: Jaffe ES, Harris N L, Stein H, et al., eds. Lyon, France: IARC Press, 2001:138–141.

211. Dohner H, Stilgenbauer S, Dohner K, et al. Chromosome aberrations in B-cell chronic lymphocytic leukemia: reassessment based on molecular cytogenetic analysis. *J Mol Med* 1999;77:266–281.

212. Stilgenbauer S, Bullinger L, Lichter P, et al. Genetics of chronic lymphocytic leukemia: genomic aberrations and V(H) gene mutation status in pathogenesis and clinical course. *Leukemia* 2002;16:993–1007.

213. Oscier DG, Thompsett A, Zhu D, et al. Differential rates of somatic hypermutation in V(H) genes among subsets of chronic lymphocytic leukemia defined by chromosomal abnormalities. *Blood* 1997;89:4153–4160.

214. Schroeder HW Jr, Dighiero G. The pathogenesis of chronic lymphocytic leukemia: analysis of the antibody repertoire. *Immunol Today* 1994;15:288–294.

215. Stevenson F, Sahota S, Zhu D, et al. Insight into the origin and clonal history of B-cell tumors as revealed by analysis of immunoglobulin variable region genes. *Immunol Rev* 1998;162:247–259.

216. Rosenwald A, Alizodeh AA, Widhopf G, et al. Relation of gene expression phenotype to immunoglobulin mutation genotype in B cell chronic lymphocytic leukemia. *J Exp Med* 2001;194:1639–1647.

217. Klein U, Tu Y, Stolovitzky GA, et al. Gene expression profiling of B cell chronic lymphocytic leukemia reveals a homogeneous phenotype related to memory B cells. *J Exp Med* 2001;194:1625–1638.

218. Navarro B, Garcia-Marco JA, Jones D, et al. Association and clonal distribution of trisomy 12 and 13q14 deletions in chronic lymphocytic leukaemia. *Br J Haematol* 1998;102:1330–1334.

219. Cimmino A, Calin GA, Fabbri M, et al. miR-15 and miR-16 induce apoptosis by targeting BCL2. *Proc Natl Acad Sci U S A* 2005;102:13944–13949.

220. Calin GA, Cammino A, Fabbri M, et al. MiR-15a and miR-16-1 cluster functions in human leukemia. *Proc Natl Acad Sci U S A* 2008;105:5166–5171.

221. Bullrich F, Rasio D, Kitada S, et al. ATM mutations in B-cell chronic lymphocytic leukemia. *Cancer Res* 1999;59:24–27.

222. Stankovic T, Weber P, Stewart G, et al. Inactivation of ataxia telangiectasia mutated gene in B-cell chronic lymphocytic leukaemia. *Lancet* 1999;353:26–29.

223. Starostik P, Manshouri T, O'Brien S, et al. Deficiency of the ATM protein expression defines an aggressive subgroup of B-cell chronic lymphocytic leukemia. *Cancer Res* 1998;58:4552–4557.

224. Morris SW, Kirstein MN, Valentine MB, et al. Fusion of a kinase gene, ALK, to a nucleolar protein gene, NPM, in non-Hodgkin's lymphoma. *Science* 1994;263:1281–1284.

225. Bischof D, Pulford K, Mason DY, et al. Role of the nucleophosmin (NPM) portion of the non-Hodgkin's lymphoma-associated NPM-anaplastic lymphoma kinase fusion protein in oncogenesis. *Mol Cell Biol* 1997;17:2312–2325.

226. Bai RY, Dieter P, Peschel C, et al. Nucleophosmin-anaplastic lymphoma kinase of large-cell anaplastic lymphoma is a constitutively active tyrosine kinase that utilizes phospholipase C-gamma to mediate its mitogenicity. *Mol Cell Biol* 1998;18:6951–6961.

227. Lange K, Uckert W, Blankenstein T, et al. Overexpression of NPM-ALK induces different types of malignant lymphomas in IL-9 transgenic mice. *Oncogene* 2003;22:517–527.

228. Kuefer MU, Look AT, Pulford K, et al. Retrovirus-mediated gene transfer of NPM-ALK causes lymphoid malignancy in mice. *Blood* 1997;90:2901–2910.

229. Chiarle R, Gong JZ, Guasparri I, et al. NPM-ALK transgenic mice spontaneously develop T-cell lymphomas and plasma cell tumors. *Blood* 2003;101:1919–1927.

230. Falini B, Pulford K, Pucciarini A, et al. Lymphomas expressing ALK fusion protein(s) other than NPM-ALK. *Blood* 1999;94:3509–3515.

231. Hernandez L, Pinyol M, Hernandez S, et al. TRK-fused gene (TFG) is a new partner of ALK in anaplastic large cell lymphoma producing two structurally different TFG-ALK translocations. *Blood* 1999;94:3265–3268.

232. Smith MR, Greene WC. Molecular biology of the type I human T-cell leukemia virus (HTLV-I) and adult T-cell leukemia. *J Clin Invest* 1991;87:761–766.

233. Bex F, Gaynor RB. Regulation of gene expression by HTLV-I Tax protein. *Methods* 1998;16:83–94.

234. Cesarman E, Chadburn A, Inghirami G, et al. Structural and functional analysis of oncogenes and tumor suppressor genes in adult T-cell leukemia/lymphoma shows frequent p53 mutations. *Blood* 1992;80:3205–3216.

235. Vorechovsky I, Luo L, Dyer MJ, et al. Clustering of missense mutations in the ataxia-telangiectasia gene in a sporadic T-cell leukaemia. *Nat Genet* 1997;17:96–99.

236. Stilgenbauer S, Schaffner C, Litterst A, et al. Biallelic mutations in the ATM gene in T-prolymphocytic leukemia. *Nat Med* 1997;3:1155–1159.

237. Westphal CH. Cell-cycle signaling: Atm displays its many talents. *Curr Biol* 1997;7:R789–792.

238. Neri A, Chang CC, Lombardi L, et al. B cell lymphoma-associated chromosomal translocation involves candidate oncogene lyt-10, homologous to NF-kappa B p50. *Cell* 1991;67:1075–1087.

239. Neri A, Fracchiolla NS, Roscetti E, et al. Molecular analysis of cutaneous B- and T-cell lymphomas. *Blood* 1995;86:3160–3172.

240. Siebenlist U, Franzoso G, Brown K. Structure, regulation and function of NF-kappa B. *Annu Rev Cell Biol* 1994;10:405–455.

241. de Martin R, Schmid JA, Hofer-Warbinek R. The NF kappaB/Rel family of transcription factors in oncogenic transformation and apoptosis. *Mutat Res* 1999;437:231–243.

242. Chang CC, Zhang J, Lombardi L, et al. Rearranged NFKB-2 genes in lymphoid neoplasms code for constitutively active nuclear transactivators. *Mol Cell Biol* 1995;15:5180–5187.

SECTION III ■ DIAGNOSIS, STAGING, AND RESPONSE CRITERIA

CHAPTER 9 ■ DIAGNOSIS: DIAGNOSTIC PROCEDURES, HISTOPATHOLOGIC PROBLEMS, IMMUNOPHENOTYPING, AND APPLIED GENETICS

DAVID J. GOOD AND RANDY D. GASCOYNE

Non-Hodgkin lymphomas (NHLs) comprise a wide variety of disorders with varying clinical and biologic features. Correct diagnosis and classification form the basis of clinical patient management. In the past, the diagnosis of lymphoma was based mainly on the cellular composition and histologic appearance of the tumor. However, with increased knowledge of the biologic mechanisms of the various lymphomas, a new approach to classification was developed, beginning with the Revised European American Lymphoma classification (1) and followed by the current World Health Organization classification. These classifications take into account the immunologic characteristics, genetic alterations, and the clinical characteristics of each tumor type. This has led to much more reproducibility than in previous systems and the definition of distinct clinical entities. Nonetheless, the diagnosis of lymphoma still begins with an assessment of the histologic appearance of the biopsied tissue because this is the basis from which a diagnosis is made. However, a morphologic assessment alone is often inadequate for accurate classification because there is often significant overlap between the various entities. Immunophenotyping studies, either by flow cytometry or immunohistochemical (IHC) staining, are often initially done to determine lineage, immunoarchitecture, and clonality. Molecular genetic techniques are of increasing practical importance because they provide an additional level of testing, and are particularly useful in cases where the histology or the immunophenotype are not conclusive, or the biopsy is small, hampering an accurate assessment. As well, molecular genetic testing can detect specific lymphomas that have distinctive molecular abnormalities. Although the ancillary tests are often needed to classify the various lymphomas, they are not without cost and need to be used judiciously. Therefore, based on the histologic findings, appropriate IHC studies and molecular tests are ordered to achieve a diagnosis (Fig. 9.1). This chapter outlines the practical aspects of lymphoma diagnosis, including the procedures for acquiring and processing a representative tissue biopsy, the various ancillary testing that is performed, and common histopathologic problems that arise in routine pathology practice.

DIAGNOSTIC PROCEDURES

Type of Biopsy

There has been considerable debate as to what types of tissue biopsies are adequate for the accurate diagnosis and classification of lymphoma. Because of factors such as the increased demand for operating room time and the advances in ancillary testing for the diagnosis of lymphoma, there has been a movement away from excisional biopsies to needle cores and fine needle aspirates of enlarged lymph nodes. Although these procedures may be easier to perform with less patient discomfort than excisional biopsies, they place pressure on the pathologist to make accurate diagnoses with limited tissue, and eliminate the fundamental principle of tissue architecture in the classification of lymphomas.

Fine needle aspiration cytology (FNAC) has emerged as a diagnostic tool because of its ease of use. It is rapid, relatively painless, inexpensive, does not require anesthetic or hospital admission, and leaves no scar (2). One of the important roles of FNAC of lymph nodes is the exclusion of metastatic carcinoma. The accuracy and utility of FNAC for lymphoma diagnosis remain controversial, with accuracy rates ranging from 12% to 82% in various studies, depending in part on the concurrent use of flow cytometry (3–9).

Probably the most significant disadvantage of FNAC for lymphoma diagnosis is that it does not provide histologic architecture; low-grade B-cell lymphomas, in particular, are often difficult to diagnose even on excisional biopsies, and IHC staining is required. Another problem may arise when the lymphoma only partially involves a lymph node, and the FNAC may only sample the reactive regions, leading to false-negative results. Other factors that influence the diagnostic specificity and sensitivity of FNAC include necrosis in involved nodes, the presence of dual pathology, and sclerosis/fibrosis in involved nodes leading to insufficient diagnostic material.

The concurrent use of flow cytometry, immunohistochemistry, and molecular genetic studies such as polymerase chain reaction (PCR) and fluorescent in situ hybridization (FISH) may significantly increase the diagnostic yield from FNAC. However, the amount of tissue aspirated is often limited, leading to a lack of material for these ancillary studies. Combining FNAC with immunophenotyping using flow cytometry assumes that signature phenotypes are characteristic of most NHLs. Although signature immunophenotypes do exist, for example for classic chronic lymphocytic leukemia (CLL), hairy cell leukemia, and precursor B-lineage acute lymphoblastic leukemia, there are frequent exceptions. For example, follicular lymphomas (FL) often lack expression of CD10, and a sizable minority of mantle cell lymphoma (MCL) cases are CD5 negative. The overutilization of this biopsy strategy and the belief that cytomorphology together with flow cytometric (FC) immunophenotypic data are sufficient to render

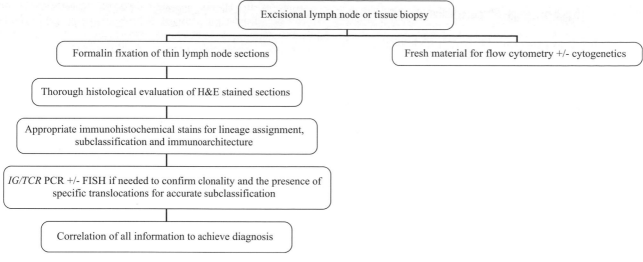

FIGURE 9.1 This algorithm demonstrates the diagnostic pathway for lymphoma from tissue biopsies. There are some important caveats to consider. Histologic assessment is still the gold standard, so if size of the tissue is limited, the priority is formalin fixation. If sufficient tissue is available, it can be divided with some sent for flow cytometry and some to the cytogenetics laboratory if needed. For limited samples, the remaining tissue from flow cytometry can also be forwarded to cytogenetics. To limit cost and save on labor, the cytogenetics laboratory can harvest and culture the cells without proceeding to further cytogenetic analysis. This sample can be maintained at 4°C for months or can be stored indefinitely at −30°C for analysis at a later date. If *IGH/TCR* PCR analysis is required, it can be performed either on fresh tissue or on FFPET. If using fresh tissue, it is important to ensure that the tissue is representative because it may differ from what is seen in the paraffin sections, thus yielding a false-negative result. If using FFPET for FISH analysis, sections can be used and may be suitable for break apart probes. However, nuclei can overlap and be sectioned through, making scoring difficult. Therefore, it is preferable, especially with colocalization probes, to core the area of interest on the paraffin block. This core can then be disaggregated to make a single cell suspension for FISH analysis. An important point to remember is that none of the ancillary tests should be interpreted in isolation. Correlation of all findings, especially with the histologic appearance, is needed to arrive at the correct diagnosis. H&E, hematoxylin and eosin.

accurate diagnoses have followed a similar course to the evaluation of lymphoid disorders involving the peripheral blood. One need only recall the confusion that surrounded the initial descriptions of splenic lymphomas and the recent revelations regarding B-cell prolymphocytic leukemia.

Finally, the use of FNAC approaches results in the loss of archival tissue for clinical research or for additional clinical testing as new markers become available. This is particularly relevant with the emergence of technologies, including genomics and proteomics. Additional smears can be made and stored for future studies, but the suitability of these for molecular genetic analysis is questionable (5).

If the lymphadenopathy is present in an area that cannot be easily subjected to an excisional biopsy or the patient is elderly or has significant comorbidities, a needle core biopsy is often adequate in these situations. Core biopsies can be performed under ultrasound or computed tomography guidance to improve the yield and ensure that the correct pathologic area is being sampled. The single biggest problem with their use is the lack of appreciable architectural features and resulting incorrect diagnosis.

The usefulness of the needle core biopsy technique is limited by several parameters, including the problem of sampling error (partially involved nodes, or variable histology), crush artifact, and small specimen size, resulting in a limited number of possible immunostains as the tissue blocks are rapidly exhausted. This is particularly true for lymphoid processes, such as Hodgkin lymphoma or peripheral T-cell lymphoma, in

which the key cellular subpopulations are in the minority and may be missed or masked by the cellular heterogeneity (10). Moreover, the amount of tissue is important in distinguishing between and grading the various lymphomas of follicle center cell origin (i.e., FL grade 3 vs. diffuse large B-cell lymphoma [DLBCL]), in which tissue architecture is of extreme importance. For lymphomas with a distinct cytologic appearance and immunophenotype (i.e., small lymphocytic lymphoma, MCL), the diagnosis from a needle core biopsy is usually more straightforward. Formalin-fixed needle cores can be used for PCR analysis and for FISH studies if needed. As with FNAC, sending one or more cores for analysis by flow cytometry may improve diagnostic accuracy. Combining FNAC with core biopsy may provide the highest likelihood of a diagnostic specimen.

An excisional lymph node biopsy is still the optimal specimen for the diagnosis of lymphomas. This is especially true when enlarged lymph nodes are present in accessible areas such as the neck, axillary, and inguinal areas. Obtaining an excisional biopsy up front if a diagnosis of lymphoma is expected will often negate the need to have the patient return for a second biopsy and reduce the time to treatment. When patients present with superficial, palpable lymphadenopathy and there is a clinical suspicion of a hematolymphoid tumor, FNAC or needle core biopsies are not indicated. Generous excisional biopsies should be performed. This strategy will virtually always lead to an accurate diagnosis, even in difficult cases.

Specimen Processing

Proper handling and processing of lymph node biopsy specimens are critical in the diagnosis of lymphoma. Biopsies should be sent fresh, intact, and unsectioned to the pathology laboratory, to ensure that optimal histologic sections can be obtained and that the tissue is properly preserved for necessary ancillary studies (11). When received in the laboratory, gross examination includes proper identification of the specimen, a description of how the specimen was received (fresh, in fixative, intact vs. sectioned), and the type of procedure used to obtain the specimen (excisional, incisional, or core biopsy). The specimen is then measured, and a description of its appearance is given. It is then sectioned at 2-mm intervals, to ensure proper fixation. It is preferable to cut sections perpendicular to the long axis of the lymph node to give the best assessment of the architecture.

Different fixatives have their own advantages and disadvantages. The most widely used is formalin because it allows for optimal ancillary studies, including immunohistochemistry and PCR analysis, if needed later on (12). B-5 and other mercury containing fixatives provide excellent cytologic detail but do not allow for the extraction of deoxyribonucleic acid (DNA) for molecular studies and are harmful to the environment. As well, different IHC protocols need to be used for antigen retrieval. For these reasons, formalin fixation is preferred for routine sections. If sufficient tissue is available, further sections can be fixed in B-5 or B-plus. Remaining tissue can also be snap frozen for future molecular studies or to support clinical research activities.

If the lymph node biopsy is of sufficient size, a portion is usually submitted for flow cytometry analysis. The resulting information can be of extreme value, especially in the subtyping of low-grade B-cell lymphomas and the demonstration of B-cell clonality. This sample needs to be fresh because live cells are required. Similar sample requirements are also needed for cytogenetic analysis (see section on conventional cytogenetics).

ANCILLARY TESTING

Immunophenotyping

Immunophenotypic studies are essential for the diagnosis and classification of lymphomas. They are used to rule out non-hematopoietic tumors, to determine cell lineage, to subclassify the lymphoma, and in some cases to detect minimal residual disease. Several approaches may be used for the immunophenotypic analysis of lymphoproliferative disorders, including FC analysis of single cell suspensions from the tissue biopsy specimen and IHC studies of paraffin-embedded tissue sections. Each has advantages and disadvantages, and they are often both used. FC analysis can yield more information because of the greater number of antibodies available and the ability to detect the presence of multiple antigens on the cell surface at the same time. However, no architectural information can be gleaned. IHC analysis on paraffin-embedded tissue allows correlation of the staining pattern with morphologic characteristics, allowing analysis of immunoreactivity in both malignant and reactive cell populations. Often, the combination of both techniques is used, particularly for small B-cell lymphoid neoplasms. An important note is that the antibody staining pattern should always be correlated with the histologic appearance before a diagnosis is made. A diagnosis should never be made on the basis of the immunophenotype alone.

Flow Cytometry

Flow cytometry has become a very important tool in the diagnostic hematopathology laboratory, and is a key ancillary test in the diagnosis and classification of lymphoma. The flow cytometer is able to measure and then analyze multiple physical characteristics of single cells as they flow in single file in a fluid stream through a beam of light. This includes the relative size, relative granularity or internal complexity, and relative fluorescence intensity of the cells. The instrument contains three main systems, including the fluidics, optics, and electronics. The fluidics system moves the cells in a stream so they can pass as individual cells through the laser beam for interrogation. Because flow cytometry requires a single cell suspension, cells from solid tissue samples must be disaggregated before analysis. The optics system uses laser light to illuminate the particles in the sample stream and optical filters to direct the resulting light signals to the appropriate detectors. When particles pass through the laser beam, they scatter the laser light. Before analysis, the cells are incubated with antibodies conjugated to fluorescent labels, which will bind to the cells if the corresponding antigen is present. Fluorescence is produced when the laser light excites electrons of the fluorescent labels from their ground state to higher energy levels with subsequent return of electrons to lower energy levels by emitting light of a longer wavelength. The scattered and fluorescent light is collected by appropriately positioned lenses and steered to the appropriate detectors. The detectors produce electronic signals proportional to the optical signals striking them. The electronics system converts the detected light signals into electronic signals that can be processed by the computer and then analyzed to provide information about subpopulations within the sample.

Immunohistochemistry

IHC is a valuable method for identifying and localizing proteins in cells of a tissue section using the principle of antibodies binding specifically to their corresponding antigens. These antibody-antigen interactions are visualized by conjugating the antibody to an enzyme such as peroxidase that can catalyze a color-producing reaction. Alternatively, the antibody can also be tagged to a fluorophore, such as FITC or Texas Red. This procedure allows the pathologist to directly observe the immunophenotype of specific cells of interest in the tissue section.

There are two strategies used for the IHC detection of antigens in tissue, the direct method and the indirect method. In both cases, antigen retrieval methods (enzymes or heat) are used to reverse changes to antigens brought about by fixation, allowing better detection. The tissue is then treated with blocking agents to inhibit endogenous peroxidases in the tissue from interfering with the color reactions. The direct method is a one-step staining method, and uses a labeled antibody that reacts directly with the antigen in tissue sections. Although this is a simple and rapid method, it has a lower sensitivity due to lower signal amplification. The indirect method is more commonly employed and uses an unlabeled primary antibody that reacts with the tissue antigen, and a labeled secondary antibody that is directed against the primary antibody. The secondary antibody can be labeled with an enzyme or fluorescent dye. There are several secondary antibody reactions with different antigenic sites on the primary antibody, resulting in signal amplification and, therefore, a more sensitive technique. The antibodies used for detection can be either be polyclonal or monoclonal. Polyclonal antibodies are a heterogeneous mix of antibodies, giving them the ability to recognize several epitopes. However, monoclonal antibodies are more commonly used due to their greater specificity. For IHC studies, it is important to know what fixative has been used because the protocols differ depending on the type of fixation.

DEMONSTRATION OF GENETIC ABNORMALITIES

Conventional Cytogenetics

Cytogenetic analysis has been an invaluable method to allow understanding of acquired genetic changes that lead to lymphoma and continues to be a very effective means of surveying the entire genome. Conventional cytogenetics was one of the earliest methods of detecting chromosomal changes. The identification of the chromosomal changes that are associated with specific subtypes of lymphoma has led to our current understanding of how gene dysregulation is involved in the pathogenesis of lymphoma and other malignancies. In the current molecular era, the utility of conventional cytogenetics is often forgotten, but it can still provide very valuable information.

Cytogenetic studies of lymphoma are usually based on analyses of lymph node specimens, but lymphoma cells can be cultured from any site, including bone marrow if it is involved (13). Peripheral blood is generally the most appropriate sample for cytogenetic analysis of the chronic lymphoid leukemias. Because live cells are needed to achieve optimal results, the sample should be transported in sterile tissue culture medium to the cytogenetics laboratory as soon as possible after collection (13,14). If solid tissue-like lymph nodes are submitted for analysis, the cells are disaggregated to produce a single cell suspension, which is then added to culture medium. Some of the chronic B- and T-lymphoid malignancies can be problematic for conventional cytogenetic analysis because these disorders tend to have low mitotic activity and usually do not respond well to most common mitogens, making it difficult to achieve high-quality metaphases. These inherent difficulties of conventional cytogenetic analysis in this group of disorders have largely been overcome by the development of FISH because it allows detection of numerical and structural abnormalities in the majority of cases. FISH techniques also eliminate the need for fresh tissue because they can be effectively applied to formalin-fixed paraffin-embedded tissues (FFPETs).

The primary cytogenetic alterations in lymphomas are typically balanced translocations that are closely associated with specific types of lymphoma [i.e., t(14;18) in follicular lymphoma]. Often, secondary alterations occur and may be whole chromosomal gains or losses, balanced translocations and inversions or unbalanced derivatives of these changes, and simple or complex deletions and duplications.

Southern Blot

Southern blot (SB) analysis was one of the earliest methods to detect immunoglobulin heavy chain (*IGH*) and T-cell receptor (*TCR*) gene rearrangements, and led to the knowledge that the majority of lymphomas contain monoclonal lymphoid populations (15–17). However, SB now has only a limited role in the routine clinical laboratory. It requires large amounts of high-quality DNA, which essentially precludes the use of fixed material. SB has a turnaround time of several days, and is a relatively expensive and labor-intensive procedure. It also involves the use of radioactive materials, although nonradioactive detection systems are available but are not as widely used. It also has a low analytical sensitivity, limiting its utility in lymphomas that have low numbers of monoclonal cells such as T-cell-rich B-cell lymphoma, and in minimal residual disease detection and monitoring (18). As such, SB has now essentially been replaced by PCR-based techniques as the primary molecular diagnostic modality, but it still remains the gold standard in clonality testing, especially in diagnostically difficult cases (19,20).

Fluorescent in Situ Hybridization

FISH has become a very important technique for the detection of both structural and numerical chromosomal abnormalities, even down to the single cell and single gene level (21). The procedure uses labeled DNA probes that hybridize to chromosome-specific target sequences of interest. Many different types of probes can be used, including whole chromosome paints, centromeric probes, and locus-specific probes. Centromeric probes are used for detecting numerical chromosomal anomalies, and locus specific probes are used for detecting translocations, by using single, dual, or triple-color assays (21–23). They are particularly useful in detecting translocations having widely dispersed breakpoints [such as t(11;14) in MCL and t(8;14) or variants in Burkitt lymphoma (BL)] (24–26) because FISH probes are typically large and can span in excess of 100 kb of the genome. The most common FISH methods used are metaphase and interphase FISH. Like conventional cytogenetic analysis, the significant disadvantage of metaphase FISH is that viable cell suspensions are needed, limiting the analysis to fresh tissue. Moreover, its utility is limited in low-grade lymphomas that have a low proliferation rate and a resultant lack of quality metaphases. A further issue is that DNA in metaphase is highly condensed, leading to a relatively low resolution. For these reasons, interphase FISH is more commonly used because it is much more user friendly. The starting material criteria are not so stringent because it can be applied to air-dried smears, paraffin sections, and nuclei isolated from fresh or frozen tissue, or from paraffin sections (22,25,27). It also has a higher resolution than metaphase FISH (18). Interphase FISH is the method of choice to detect translocations where no reverse-transcriptase PCR assays are available, and where breakpoints are widely dispersed. One drawback of interphase FISH that is especially apparent in paraffin sections is that nuclei can overlap or be sectioned through, making it very difficult to accurately score. Therefore, when sufficient tissue is available, it is preferable to core the areas of interest in the paraffin section and disaggregate the cells to produce a single cell suspension that can then be spread on a slide. Cytospin and touch preparations can also be used if available. Two basic FISH strategies are used including colocalization and break-apart assays. Colocalization assays suffer from reduced specificity because there can be false-positive results due to overlapping signals, making this a less optimal technique. Thus, break-apart assays are preferable. This strategy uses two probes, each labeled with a different fluorochrome, that span the region of interest (e.g., *BCL6*). Any disruption of the genetic locus by a translocation will result in a separation of the fused signals and produces an easily identified split signal. This strategy can also be applied to tissue microarray slides and, thus, is highly advantageous for studying large numbers of cases in the clinical research setting.

Polymerase Chain Reaction

PCR-based assays are currently the preferred approach for the molecular diagnosis of lymphomas (28–32). It is not practical to perform in every case, but it is a valuable ancillary test, especially when morphologic and IHC evaluations do not clearly point to a malignant diagnosis (33). PCR assays are not as sensitive as SB or FISH in detecting all chromosomal rearrangements (34). However, PCR has many advantages, including rapid turnaround time, and only small amounts of nucleic acid are required, making it highly useful in the clinical laboratory setting. Many of the PCR procedures can be automated and may also be multiplexed, allowing for analysis of more than one chromosomal aberration. Radioactive materials are not required, improving the safety. One of the significant advantages of PCR-based assays is the less stringent requirements for large amounts of high-quality DNA, allowing for the use of many different specimens. These include small tissue biopsies, fine needle aspiration biopsies, bone marrow aspirates, cells scraped from histologic or cytologic slides, and cells microdissected from fixed tissue specimens (29,35–40). FFPET can also be used for many PCR assays, often with the sensitivity of clonal detection approaching that of fresh specimens (41–43). However, many factors need to be considered when using fixed material because they can affect the sensitivity of the PCR assay. Likely the most important factor is the type of fixative used. The best results are achieved with buffered formalin (44,45). Mercury-based fixatives such as B-5 are not suitable. The average length of preserved and intact DNA for FFPET is typically up to 300 bp in length, although this will vary from case to case and institution to institution. Therefore, successful amplification is most likely to be achieved when the PCR strategies employed have a smaller amplimer than this. As with all PCR assays, appropriate internal controls (housekeeping genes) are always run to avoid false-negative tests secondary to failed amplification of control genes.

Since the advent of PCR techniques, a plethora of assays are available varying in design, complexity, cost, and sensitivity. The choice of what type of assay to use depends on the DNA target being tested, and whether it is being used for primary diagnosis or for minimal residual disease detection. Therefore, each laboratory will need to optimize its assays for its particular needs but also needs to be aware of the sensitivity and limitations of each assay being used (46). For lymphoma diagnosis, DNA-based PCR strategies can be used to detect *IGH/TCR* gene rearrangements, as well as some chromosomal translocations such as t(14;18) and t(11;14). The use of reverse-transcriptase PCR is limited because its role is mainly in the detection of chromosome translocations resulting in novel gene fusions, which are more commonly found in leukemia and myeloproliferative disorders.

The detection of rearranged *IGH/TCR* genes and chromosome aberrations by PCR requires a precise knowledge of the rearranged gene segments to design appropriate primers. To detect all different V, D, and J gene segments for *IGH/TCR* genes, a significant number of different primers would be needed, which is not practical in routine molecular laboratories. As a result, a different strategy is employed. Consensus primers have been designed that are able to recognize most V and J gene segments of the locus under study. Generally, these are optimal for most relevant gene segments. However, other portions show a lower homology to these consensus primers. This can lead to false-negative results, particularly in *IGH/TCR* genes with many different gene segments and families.

For *IGH* PCR, the V region is most commonly targeted. This region contains three framework regions (FRs) and two complementarity determining regions. The FRs are very homologous among the various VH segments, whereas the complementarity determining regions are heterogeneous. The heterogeneity in the complementarity determining regions is in part due to the fact that these are a site for somatic hypermutation in the germinal center reaction. FRs are usually less affected by somatic mutations, but they can be a site for nucleotide substitutions. Some PCR protocols use single *VH* consensus primers, which are able to bind to one of the three FRs, most commonly FR3. The inherent problem with this type of protocol is that the consensus primers are not able to amplify all *VH* segments with the same efficiency. This is partly due to the aforementioned somatic mutations that may occur in FRs, preventing primer annealing and a resultant absence of amplification. Therefore, a significant number of clonal rearrangements cannot be detected by this method, resulting in a false-negative result. This is especially true for FL and some DLBCL cases because these usually contain higher numbers of FR somatic mutations. Attempts have been made to overcome this problem by adding further primers to include the FR2 region as well. The European Biomedicine and Health-2 project has developed and standardized a multiplex PCR strategy, using multiple primers to detect clonally rearranged *IGH*, immunoglobulin light chain and *TCR* genes, and the chromosome aberrations t(11;14) and t(14;18) (32). This has resulted in an extremely high detection rate, even in B-cell malignancies, with an increased load of somatic mutations and those with ongoing mutations (FL).

Other Emerging Methodologies

Newer techniques have been developed that allow for simultaneous evaluation of multiple targets. These include multicolor FISH (47) and spectral karyotyping (48,49). These techniques differ somewhat in methodology and analysis but essentially provide the same information. The end result is color-coded identification of all individual chromosomes within a metaphase spread. Multicolor FISH and spectral karyotyping in particular have some advantages over conventional G-banding (50). Their utility is shown by their ability to detect complex or otherwise unapparent chromosomal rearrangements and translocations that are typically hidden in marker chromosomes. It is not necessary to know which specific probes to use and, thus, provides an advantage over conventional FISH. A drawback is that they are not sensitive enough to detect small intrachromosomal inversions, duplications, and deletions. They also need quality metaphases and come with a high cost, making them impractical for routine clinical use at this time.

Comparative genomic hybridization (CGH) is considered a molecular cytogenetic technique. It is able to detect genome-wide DNA sequence copy number changes, including losses, deletions, gains, and/or amplifications, by using fluorescence-based hybridization techniques. A significant advantage is that this information can be gathered in a single hybridization experiment (51). Balanced structural rearrangements such as inversions or translocations, common to many lymphomas, cannot be detected by this technique, but it is a powerful research tool for detecting unbalanced genomic alterations that might identify candidate genes involved in lymphoma pathogenesis. Two CGH methods are in use, including classic and array CGH. Classic CGH uses metaphase chromosomes for analysis, but the resolution is limited due to condensation of metaphase DNA. Array CGH can overcome this shortcoming because it utilizes hybridization to microarrays of cloned genomic DNA targets or oligonucleotides (52,53). The resolution of this technique is much superior, and it also enables automated analysis (54–56). However, it remains primarily a research tool because the requirement for expensive equipment limits its utility in routine clinical laboratories.

Gene expression profiling or DNA microarray technology is a molecular technique that allows for the simultaneous measurement of messenger ribonucleic acid expression levels of thousands of genes by using an ordered array on a solid support. This results in a profile of gene expression in the particular cell or tumor being analyzed (57,58). The utility of gene expression profiling is that it is able to identify potentially significant genes involved in pathogenesis of lymphoma and those predictive of clinical behavior, yielding valuable information and possible candidate genes that might in the future allow the design of novel targeted therapies (59). It is also beginning to help refine lymphoma subclassification at a molecular level. At this point, gene expression profiling is largely a research tool. However, routine pathology laboratories can play an important part in harvesting and storing of fresh lymphoma tissue and normal blood/tissue control samples because these techniques currently require nondegraded ribonucleic acid.

DEMONSTRATION OF CLONALITY

Flow Cytometry

Clonality analysis in B-cell NHL is usually done by evaluating the expression of immunoglobulin (Ig), kappa (κ), and lambda (λ) light chains in distinct populations, and is generally identified when the $\kappa{:}\lambda$ light chain ratio is greater than 4:1 or less than 1:2 (60). Some cases may show a lower $\kappa{:}\lambda$ ratio, but these cases must be carefully correlated with the histologic appearance to make a diagnosis of lymphoma. Assessment for clonality by FC is most useful when an immunophenotypically abnormal discrete population is present, such as CD10-expressing B cells (Fig. 9.2). The presence of B-cell clonality is also suggested when there is a loss of surface light chain expression because a small number of B-cell NHL cases, especially DLBCL, lack surface expression of both κ and λ light chains (61,62). However, caution needs to be exercised because loss of surface light chain expression is not necessarily diagnostic of lymphoma (63). Again, correlation with histology is needed because other conditions, including precursor B-cell lymphoblastic leukemia and plasma cell neoplasms, can lack surface light chain expression. As well, normal B-cell progenitor cells in the bone marrow (hematogones) and germinal center B cells in rare cases of reactive follicular hyperplasia in a lymph node can produce a subset of cells lacking surface light chain expression.

The determination of clonality in T-cell lymphoproliferative disorders is not as straightforward by FC. In contrast to B-cell NLH cases in which analysis of surface Igs can determine clonality, there are no specific FC markers of T-cell clonality or of malignant T cells. Recently, FC methods using a broad panel of antibodies against the variable region of the $TCR\gamma$ gene have shown it is possible to demonstrate clonality in many T-cell proliferations, although this is not widely in use in routine diagnostic laboratories (64,65). Therefore, the FC analysis of T-cell disorders requires a broad panel of T-cell markers, as well as correlation with morphology and relevant clinical and laboratory data, including molecular studies for TCR gene rearrangement. By FC, there are findings that suggest a clonal T-cell population. These include the complete loss or diminished expression of one or more pan-T antigens (66-68), loss or markedly dim expression of CD45 (69), or CD4/CD8 dual-positive or dual-negative expression. Abnormalities in the CD4:CD8 ratio may suggest a T-cell process, but markedly increased CD4 populations can be seen in Hodgkin lymphoma and in dermatopathic lymphadenitis (69,70). A reversed CD4:CD8 ratio can be present in viral infections, including human immunodeficiency virus (HIV) (71,72). Moreover, the presence of dual CD4/CD8-positive T cells can be commonly seen in nodular lymphocyte-predominant Hodgkin lymphoma and less commonly in related disorders (73).

Immunohistochemistry

As mentioned in the previous section, monotypic Ig light chain expression provides strong evidence of a B-cell lymphoma, although some lymphomas may lack surface Ig expression. IHC in paraffin sections can be used to elucidate this finding. In cells with increased amounts of cytoplasm, including plasma cells in plasma cell dyscrasias and some lymphomas with significant cytoplasmic Ig expression such as lymphoplasmacytic lymphoma, marginal zone lymphoma, and some cases of large B-cell lymphoma, cytoplasmic light chain restriction can be relatively easily demonstrated. The demonstration of surface Ig expression is much more difficult

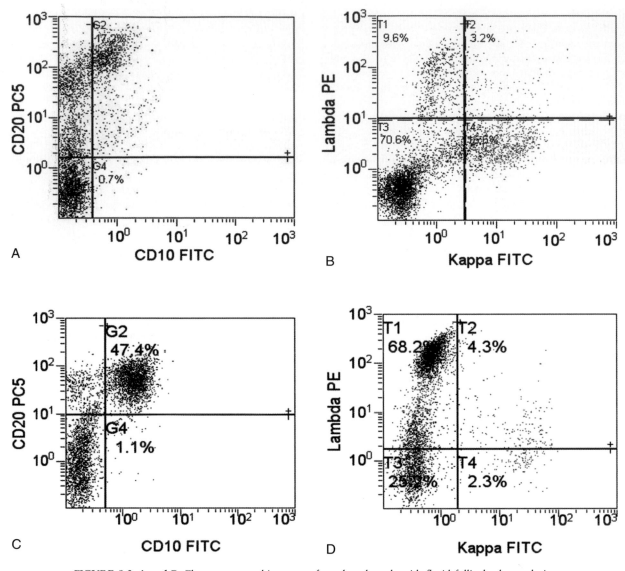

FIGURE 9.2 **A and B:** Flow cytometry histograms for a lymph node with florid follicular hyperplasia. Note the presence of a CD20/CD10-positive population in (**A**). (See also Color Plate 1) However, (**B**) clearly demonstrates polytypic expression of κ and λ light chains. (See also Color Plate 2) **C and D:** The same two histograms for flow cytometry of a lymph node with follicular lymphoma. Note again the presence of a CD20/CD10-positive population in (**C**). (See also Color Plate 3) **D:** Clear λ light chain restriction is demonstrated. FITC, fluorescein isothiocyanate; PE, phycoerythrin; PC5, phycoerythrin-cyanin 5. (See also Color Plate 4)

in fixed tissue, although improved methods, including heat-induced epitope retrieval techniques, have made this possible in some laboratories (74,75). Interpretation of these stains can be quite challenging. It is important to always examine the same areas in the tissue to compare κ and λ expression to confirm that any potential staining is specific and not an artifact. This is especially true when polyclonal antibodies are used. As well, small biopsies such as needle cores and endoscopic biopsies tend to have significant nonspecific background staining, making it necessary to examine the lymphoid areas of interest to look for light chain restriction. It is suggested that a ratio of greater than 10:1 or less than 0.2 for κ:λ is required to be confident of light chain restriction. Importantly, this strategy is underutilized because many laboratories have not optimized their staining methods to detect surface Ig expression in small B cells (Fig. 9.3). One needs to keep in mind, however, that light chain-restricted germinal

centers can also be observed in reactive states. As a result of the immune response and possibly due to an underlying problem in the regulation of the immune response, the germinal centers can have a marked predominance of one light chain over the other (76).

As with FC, it is difficult to establish T-cell clonality by IHC because there are no specific stains analogous to the light chain stains in B-cell lymphomas. Therefore, this necessitates the use of multiple stains, in combination with the histologic appearance, to establish a diagnosis of a T-cell lymphoma. There are some IHC features that point toward a malignancy but are by no means diagnostic. These include aberrant phenotypes such as the coexpression or loss of both CD4 and CD8, the loss of one or more pan T-cell antigens, or the expression of immature markers like CD1a by mature-appearing cells (77,78). However, caution needs to be exercised in the interpretation. The predominance of either CD4-

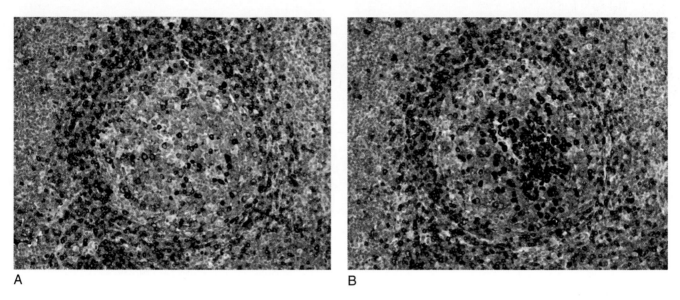

FIGURE 9.3 **A:** IHC staining for κ light chain. (See also Color Plate 5) **B:** λ Light chain staining. These are both from the same lymph node with reactive follicular hyperplasia. These figures demonstrate optimized light chain IHC. Not only are the plasma cells staining but also the small B cells in the mantle zone, confirming polytypic light chain expression in both types of cells. (See also Color Plate 6)

or CD8-positive T cells is not diagnostic of malignancy because many reactive conditions, including viral infections, can lead to the same finding. Cortical thymocytes are CD1a positive, and coexpress CD4 and CD8. $\gamma\delta$ T cells are usually negative for both CD4 and CD8. The loss of pan T-cell antigens such as CD7 can also be seen in reactive or inflammatory lesions, especially in the skin (79,80). Given these inherent problems, in cases that are not obviously malignant by histology or IHC staining, PCR analysis is necessary in establishing a monoclonal T-cell population.

PCR

The majority of lymphoid malignancies contain rearranged *IGH* and/or *TCR* genes not unlike normal lymphoid cells (81). What differs is that they are derived from a single malignantly transformed lymphoid cell, and, therefore, all cells of the malignant population have identically rearranged *IGH/TCR* genes. This provides a very beneficial tool for the detection of malignant populations because the presence of these clonal *IGH/TCR* gene rearrangements can be used to establish evidence of clonality by methods such as PCR (82). They also provide an identification target for molecular monitoring of patients during and after therapy.

Originally, the detection of lymphoid clonality was largely based on SB analysis of predominantly *IGH* genes. This allowed for the detection of partial D-J and complete V(D)J rearrangements, and the presence of somatic hypermutation did not prevent detection of clonal rearrangements. As was mentioned previously, technical restrictions have led to Southern analysis being replaced by PCR and/or FISH-based strategies.

BONE MARROW ASSESSMENT

Examination of the bone marrow is a valuable diagnostic procedure in patients with established or suspected lympho-

proliferative disorders. When a lymphoma diagnosis is known from a previous tissue biopsy, the bone marrow assessment is important both for staging purposes and to evaluate the status of normal bone marrow elements before initiating therapy. It may help to establish a diagnosis of lymphoma in patients clinically suspected to have disease but lacking lymphadenopathy or having no conclusive histologic evidence from other sites. In some lymphoproliferative disorders, such as hairy cell leukemia, it is the primary diagnostic procedure.

Requirements and Processing

The bone marrow procedure for lymphoma consists of the collection of both an aspirate and a biopsy. An adequate aspirate should contain cellular particles to assess the ongoing hematopoiesis and to look for the presence of lymphoid infiltrates. This sample can be used for ancillary studies, including flow cytometry, cytogenetics, and PCR analysis, if needed. The bone marrow biopsy is submitted for fixation and sectioning to assess the bone marrow architecture and cellularity, and to assess for the presence of lymphoid aggregates. There is some debate as to the optimal length of the bone marrow biopsy for lymphoma staging purposes. The National Cancer Institute has attempted to standardize staging procedures and develop methods for assessing response in patients with NHL (83). It recommends a biopsy length of at least 20 mm, although the evidence to support this recommendation is unclear. Other studies have suggested lengths of anywhere from 16 to 20 mm (84–86). The other controversy is whether or not bilateral bone marrow samples are better than unilateral. However, it appears that overall biopsy length may be more important than the number of sites sampled (83,85). As well, assessing more levels of the bone marrow biopsy allows more of the bone marrow to be assessed with no extra morbidity to the patient and may in fact increase the detection of subtle involvement by lymphoma.

Once an adequate biopsy is obtained, the tissue is then fixed, processed, and sectioned to evaluate the histologic findings. Buffered formalin is an adequate fixative, but fixatives containing metals provide much better nuclear detail, including B-5, B-plus, and acetic acid-zinc-formalin (87). The advantage of B-plus and acid-zinc-formalin fixatives is that they are zinc based and do not contain mercury, reducing hazardous waste generation and theoretically providing better preservation of DNA for molecular studies (87,88). To section bone marrow biopsies, the tissue needs to be decalcified. Decalcifying agents include strong acids (hydrochloric, nitric, sulfuric), buffered acids (formic, acetic), and calcium chelators (89,90). Various commercial decalcifying solutions have also been formulated, some having the advantage of better antigen preservation for immunohistochemistry. Typically, the bone marrow core is decalcified after fixation and before processing and embedding into the paraffin block for sectioning.

Lymphoid Aggregates

When the bone marrow is involved by lymphoma and especially by low-grade B-cell lymphomas, aggregates of lymphoid cells are commonly seen. However, not all lymphoid aggregates represent lymphoma because benign lymphoid aggregates may occur in a variety of reactive conditions, including autoimmune diseases and HIV infection, and are also more likely to be found in older individuals (91,92). As well, myeloid disorders such as myelodysplastic syndromes and myeloproliferative diseases can contain lymphoid aggregates in the marrow (93,94).

There are a few morphologic features that can help to distinguish between benign and neoplastic lymphoid aggregates. Benign aggregates tend to be smaller, fewer in number, well circumscribed with minimal infiltration of surrounding marrow, are usually nonparatrabecular, and usually have a polymorphous lymphoid population with occasional germinal center formation (91,95). However, these are not diagnostic features because there is considerable morphologic overlap between benign and neoplastic lymphoid aggregates. Although immunohistochemistry may not always be helpful due to a mixture of B and T cells, an excess of B cells in the aggregate or phenotypic aberrancy, such as abnormal coexpression of CD5 or CD43 in B cells, helps in identifying a neoplastic lymphoid population. In B-cell lymphomas with a plasmacytic component or when light chain staining has been optimized, IHC stains for κ and λ light chains can be very useful in establishing a clonal B-cell population.

In some situations, flow cytometry may be a useful adjunct to morphology in distinguishing between benign or neoplastic lymphoid aggregates. The demonstration of a clonal B-cell population or markedly aberrant T-cell population can help to establish a diagnosis of lymphoma involving bone marrow, but it may not provide definitive classification. However, failure to identify an abnormal lymphoid population by flow cytometry does not necessarily exclude marrow lymphoma because there are many factors that can lead to false-negative results. This includes sampling artifact due to hemodilution because often the sample sent for flow cytometry is the last draw on the bone marrow aspirate, the failure of paratrabecular aggregates to be drawn into the sample due to associated reticulin fibrosis, and loss of lymphoma cells due to poor viability, particularly in large cell lymphoma. Some lymphomas, such as Hodgkin lymphoma, have very few malignant cells, and other lymphomas, including many T-cell lymphomas, do not have a diagnostically abnormal immunophenotype, making flow cytometry of very little value.

Primary Diagnosis of Lymphoma in Bone Marrow

There are some B-cell lymphomas that characteristically involve the bone marrow without involvement of other sites, leading to the necessity of a bone marrow biopsy for the primary diagnosis. To a certain extent, any NHL can present in this fashion, but typically hairy cell leukemia, lymphoplasmacytic lymphoma, and various T-cell lymphoproliferative disorders are restricted to bone marrow with limited peripheral blood involvement. T cell/histiocyte-rich DLBCL frequently involves the bone marrow, and when accompanied by hepatosplenomegaly and minimal lymphadenopathy, may be the primary diagnostic biopsy in this disorder (96).

HISTOPATHOLOGICAL PROBLEMS

As mentioned previously, the diagnosis and classification of lymphoma rely on a thorough histologic evaluation, followed by appropriate ancillary testing for confirmation. A discussion of how this applies to each of the World Health Organization subtypes of lymphoma is beyond the scope of this chapter. Tables 9.1, 9.2, and 9.3 summarize the key diagnostic features in small B-cell lymphomas, intermediate and high-grade B-cell lymphomas, and tissue-based T-cell lymphomas. However, there are some common histopathologic problems that are encountered in day-to-day pathology practice that will serve to highlight the approach.

Distinguishing Between Chronic Lymphocytic Leukemia and Mantle Cell Lymphoma

One of the common pathologic problems in lymphoma diagnosis is the differentiation between CLL and MCL in peripheral blood smears. The distinction in tissue sections is more straightforward. The morphologic appearance in the peripheral blood can suggest a diagnosis but is not infallible. This is due to numerous factors, including the heterogeneity of CLL cells, the technique employed for the blood smear preparation, and the age of the blood specimen arriving at referral hospital laboratories. Typical CLL cells are small, mature lymphocytes with round nuclei, clumped chromatin, and scant amounts of cytoplasm. Occasional cases can show plasmacytoid features with more abundant cytoplasm. Most cases reveal at least some prolymphocytes and, thus, are best described as dimorphic. MCL cells in the peripheral blood typically show more heterogeneity than CLL with a spectrum of morphology. There may be some small lymphocytes resembling CLL cells, but often there are also larger cells with more irregular nuclei, slightly open chromatin, and occasional small nucleoli (Fig. 9.4). Virtually all cases show some immature blast cells, a key distinguishing feature from CLL.

TABLE 9.1

KEY FEATURES OF SMALL B CELL

	FL	CLL/SLL	MCL	SMZL	MALT	LPL
Key histologic findings	High density of follicles Lack of reactive features (starry sky pattern, polarization, mantle zone) Centrocytes and centroblasts	Small round cells with clumped chromatin Growth centers (pseudofollicles) containing prolymphocytes and paraimmunoblasts	Monomorphic small lymphocytes with irregular nuclei and admixed mitotic figures Lack of centroblasts, scattered epithelioid histiocytes Perivascular sclerosis	White pulp expansion with biphasic follicles (prominent marginal zone) Infiltration of red pulp Moderately abundant clear cytoplasm	Small lymphocytes with abundant cytoplasm, plasma cells Monocytoid B cells Colonized follicles Lymphoepithelial lesions	Morphologic spectrum from small lymphocytes to mature plasma cells Primarily involves bone marrow Increased mast cells Russell and Dutcher bodies
Key immunophenotypic findings	CD10+ BCL2+ BCL6+	CD5+ CD23+ FMC-7– dim CD20 dim sIg	CD5+ CD23– FMC-7+ Cyclin-D1+	CD5– CD10– IgD+/– CD43–	CD5– CD10– CD43+/–	Lymphocytes: CD20+ CD10– CD5– (rarely+) Plasma cells: CD138+
Key genetic findings	t(14;18) (q32;q21)	+12, del 11q22-23, del 13q14.3, del 17p13, rare t(14;19)(q32;q13)	t(11;14)(q13;q32)	del 7q31-32	t(11;18)(q21;q21), t(14;18)(q32;q21) t(1;14)(p22;q32), t(3;14)(p14;q32), +3,	Del 6q and 13q

FL, follicular lymphoma; LPL, lymphoplasmacytic lymphoma; MALT, mucosa-associated lymphoid tissue lymphoma; SLL, small lymphocytic lymphoma; SMZL, splenic marginal zone lymphoma.

TABLE 9.2

KEY FEATURES OF INTERMEDIATE AND HIGH-GRADE B CELL LYMPHOMAS

	DLBCL-NOS	T cell/histiocyte rich	ALK+ DLBCL	Primary mediastinal large B-cell lymphoma	Intravascular large B-cell lymphoma	Primary effusion lymphoma	Plasmablastic lymphoma	BL
Key histologic findings	Large pleomorphic cells with diffuse growth pattern Centroblasts or immunoblasts Mitoses and single cell necrosis	Abundant reactive T cells +/– histiocytes <10% large neoplastic B cells Virtual absence of small B cells	Large cells with plasmablastic features May be confused with an epithelial neoplasm Sinus infiltration common	Large cells with moderate amount of clear cytoplasm Fine sclerosis	Large cells growing in the lumina of small blood vessels Can resemble centroblasts or immunoblasts	Plasmablastic or immunoblastic morphology Abundant basophilic cytoplasm	Plasmablastic or immunoblastic morphology without/with plasmacytic differentiation Often present in oral cavity and associated with HIV infection	Monomorphic medium-sized cells Numerous mitoses Starry sky pattern
Key immunophenotypic findings	CD20+ CD79a+ CD10+/– BCL6+/– BCL2+/–	CD20+ CD79a+	CD20– CD79a– CD45+ IgA+/– EMA+ CD138+ CD30– ALK+	CD20+ CD79a+ CD30+/– (weak) CD23+/– Surface Ig– CD15–	CD20+ CD79a+ CD5–/+	Loss of B-cell surface markers CD3+/– CD30+ CD138+ HHV-8+	CD20– CD79a–/+ CD45– CD138+ EBV+/– HHV8–/+	CD20+ CD10+ BCL6+ BCL2– Tdt–
Key molecular findings	*IGH* clonal, *BCL6*, *BCL2*, *MYC*	*IGH* often not clonal due to limited tumor cells	t(2;17)(p23;q23) Rarely other mechanisms that deregulate *ALK*	Gains of 2p GCB-type of DLBCL	Variable	Clonal *IGH*	Variable	t(8;14) or variants – t(2;8) or t(8;22)

ALK, anaplastic lymphoma kinase.

142

TABLE 9.3

KEY FEATURES OF TISSUE-BASED T-CELL LYMPHOMAS

	Peripheral T-cell lymphoma, unspecified	Angioimmunoblastic T-cell lymphoma	Anaplastic large cell lymphoma, ALK+	Extranodal NK/T-cell lymphoma, nasal type	Enteropathy-associated T-cell lymphoma	Subcutaneous panniculitis-like T-cell lymphoma
Key histologic findings	Interfollicular expansion with small to large lymphocytes Heterogeneous cellular composition with frequent inflammatory background Clusters of epithelioid histiocytes (Lennert lymphoma); often eosinophils	Interfollicular expansion with regressed follicles Prominent postcapillary venules with arborization Clusters of lymphoid cells with clear cytoplasm May have large EBV+ B-cell blasts, epithelioid histiocytes, eosinophils	Monomorphic/pleomorphic cells Presence of hallmark cells (horseshoe or wreath shaped nucleus, prominent Golgi region) Preferential involvement of lymph node sinuses; cohesive growth pattern	Small to medium-sized atypical cells Angiocentric and/or angioinvasive growth May be admixture of inflammatory cells Often extensive necrosis	Ulcerating mass in intestine Monomorphic medium to large cells Small cell variant Enteropathy changes in adjacent bowel Eosinophils often numerous	Small to large cells Diffuse infiltrate in subcutaneous tissue with dermal sparing Cells rim around fat cells Necrosis and karyorrhexis
Key immunophenotypic findings	CD4>CD8 Frequent loss of one of the pan-T-cell antigens (CD2, CD3, CD5, CD7)	CD3+ CD4+ CD8− CD10+/− Bcl6+/− CXCR13+ (T cells) CD21+ FDC meshworks EBV+ large B cells	CD30+ CD15− EMA+ ALK+ Loss of many T-cell antigens (e.g., CD3) Cytotoxic markers+	CD2+ CD56+ Surface CD3− Cytoplasmic CD3ε+ EBV+ Cytotoxic markers+	CD3+, CD5− CD4+, CD8+/− CD30 often + Small cell variant CD8+; CD56+	CD3+ CD8+ Cytotoxic markers+
Key genetic findings	Gains of 7q22-31, 1q, 3p, 5p and 8q2ter, losses of 6q22-24 and 10p13pter	Trisomy 5, 21 and gains of 5q, 3q	t(2;5)(p23;q35) and variants	Gains of 2q, 15q, 17q and 22q. Losses of 6q, 8p, 11q, 12q and 13q	Clonal TCR	Clonal TCR

ALK, anaplastic lymphoma kinase; EBV, Epstein-Barr virus; NK, natural killer.

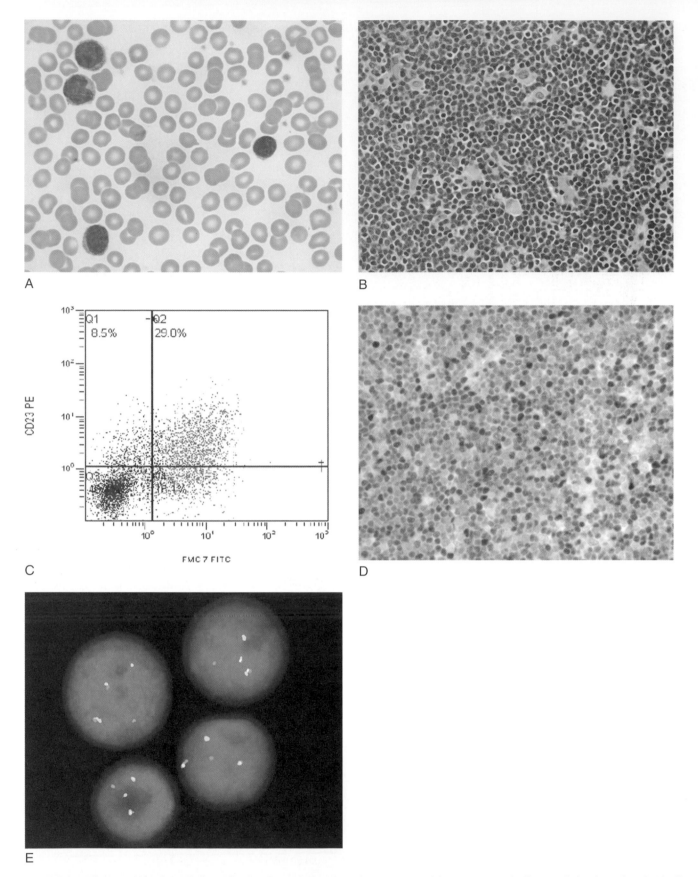

FIGURE 9.4 A: The typical blood morphology of MCL. The nuclei have irregular contours, and there is a range of cell size, including larger lymphoid cells with more immature appearing chromatin. (See also Color Plate 7) **B:** The classic histologic appearance of MCL in a lymph node section. The cells are small and monomorphic with irregular nuclear contours. There are admixed epithelioid histiocytes, and the small blood vessels show fine sclerosis. Scattered mitotic figures are also present. (See also Color Plate 8) **C:** A flow cytometry histogram of CD23 and FMC-7 expression on a lymph node with MCL. This demonstrates the point that every case does not show a classic flow cytometry phenotype because there is clear coexpression of CD23 and FMC-7 in this instance. This diagnostic dilemma can be resolved either by cyclin D1 staining on the tissue section or by FISH analysis for t(11;14) on tissue, bone marrow, or peripheral blood specimens. (See also Color Plate 9) **D:** The same tissue section in (**B**), showing a positive result for an IHC stain for cyclin D1 (CCND1). (See also Color Plate 10) **E:** FISH analysis for t(11;14) using a colocalization assay. A normal signal would show two red probes, localizing to the two alleles of the *CCND1* gene on chromosome 11 and two green probes localizing to the *IGH* gene on chromosome 14. In this case of a t(11;14) translocation, the red and green probes are brought in close proximity. FITC, fluorescein isothiocyanate; PE, phycoerythrin. (See also Color Plate 11)

The distinction between these two entities can often be aided by FC analysis. Both will show coexpression of CD5 on the B–cells, but other antigens and intensity of expression for several antigens are unique. CLL will typically show dim expression of CD20 and surface light chains. These cells typically express CD23 and will be negative for FMC-7. CD11c expression is variable. MCL cells will typically show brighter expression of CD20 and surface light chains, and be positive for FMC-7 but negative for CD23. MCL is typically negative for CD11c. However, not all cases are straightforward, and considerable overlap may be observed.

The most definitive method for differentiating between these entities is analysis for t(11;14), present in MCL but absent in CLL, which can be shown by FISH on smears or by cyclin D1 staining in tissue sections. One caveat is the potential for cyclin D1-negative MCL cases. The existence of such cases has been controversial in the past and remains so. However, gene expression profiling data have proven that this entity does exist and shows the typical gene expression signature of MCL (97,98). Importantly, a confident diagnosis of cyclin D1-negative MCL would require gene expression profiling. Expression of either cyclin D2 or D3 would not suffice.

Nodal Marginal Zone B-Cell Lymphoma versus Follicular Lymphoma

In the relatively uncommon cases of nodal marginal zone B-cell lymphomas (NMZLs), there can often be difficulty in distinguishing this from FL (99). The problem lies in the histologic appearance because NMZL can show a nodular pattern, similar to FL with enlarged, densely packed, malignant appearing follicles. However, there are subtle differences that can help differentiate between the two entities. The nodular pattern in NMZL is a result of malignant marginal zone B cells moving into and colonizing the follicle as opposed to growth of malignant germinal center B cells in FL. The large cells that appear as centroblasts are in fact residual benign germinal center B cells, infiltrated by the marginal zone B cells. These marginal zone B cells colonizing the follicles will lack CD10 and BCL6 expression by immunohistochemistry, with only residual follicle center B cells being positive. In the majority of FL cases, the cells in the follicles will be positive for CD10 and BCL6, although CD10/BCL6-negative FL cases do exist. Many marginal zone B-cell lymphomas will demonstrate overexpression of the BCL2 protein, again mimicking FL by immunohistochemistry because the follicles will be positive. The follicular dendritic cell meshwork pattern is often subtly different as well, because typically the meshwork is much tighter in FL, whereas in MZL it often appears to be disrupted. FISH analysis for the presence of t(14;18) is, therefore, invaluable in these cases because 80% to 90% of FL cases will be positive for this translocation, whereas the NMZL cases will be negative.

Diffuse Large B-Cell Lymphoma versus Burkitt Lymphoma

Occasionally, the histologic distinction between DLBCL and BL can be difficult. However, this distinction is important because of the clinical implications for treatment. Part of the difficulty lies in the heterogeneity of DLBCL morphology. The majority of the malignant cells in DLBCL are large as opposed to intermediate-sized cells in BL. The most common morphologic variant is the centroblast, which has oval to irregular nuclei, vesicular chromatin, and one to three small membrane-bound nuclei. Immunoblasts have a single prominent, centrally located nucleolus. Rarely, the large lymphoid cells can have an anaplastic appearance with very irregular nuclei, occasionally resembling Reed-Sternberg cells. Although some heterogeneity exists in BL, it is much less than that in DLBCL. The classic form shows a monomorphic proliferation of medium-sized cells with round nuclei and multiple small, centrally located basophilic nucleoli. The cytoplasm is deeply basophilic and usually shows multiple vacuoles due to the presence of lipid, often seen better in touch preparations or bone marrow aspirates. In thin sections, the cytoplasm of adjacent cells may appear to square off in BL. The mitotic rate is high, with numerous tingible body macrophages admixed, phagocytosing abundant apoptotic debris, creating a starry sky pattern. In general, the great majority of DLBCLs can be reliably distinguished from BL, and the diagnostic problem occurs in borderline cases composed of small to medium-sized tumor cells with a high proliferation rate, a "starry-sky" appearance, and a cohesive growth pattern.

The immunophenotypic characteristics can be of value in differentiating between DLBCL and BL. BL typically expresses CD10 and BCL6, consistent with a germinal center origin, but lacks expression of BCL2. The proliferation fraction is nearly 100%. In DLBCL, the immunophenotype is much more variable. CD10 and BCL6 are expressed in approximately 30% to 40% and 50% to −90% of cases, respectively (100–102). BCL2 expression is seen in approximately 40% to 75% of cases (103). The proliferation index is usually elevated but not as high as in BL (40% to 90%). A characteristic but underappreciated feature of BL is the virtual absence of infiltrating nonneoplastic T cells, which may be numerous in some cases of DLBCL.

The defining feature of BL is a chromosomal translocation that involves a recombination between the *IGH* locus and the *MYC* oncogene (104–106). The classic t(8;14), observed in nearly 85% of BLs, combines the *MYC* gene on chromosome 8 with the *IGH* gene on chromosome 14. Two variant chromosome translocations, t(2;8) and t(8;22), combining the *MYC* locus with the κ light chain gene on chromosome 2 or the λ light chain gene on chromosome 22, have been observed in approximately 10% to 15% of cases (107,108). However, *MYC* translocations are not exclusive to BL because approximately 5% to 8% of DLBCLs may also harbor this abnormality (109–111). Because DLBCL is so much more common than BL, de novo DLBCL with a *MYC* translocation will be more frequently encountered than BL. On the strength of new data derived from gene expression profiling, IHC surrogates are now being explored that may allow *MYC* translocation-positive cases of DLBCL to be identified (112,113). Importantly, in the current era of therapy with rituximab and cyclophosphamide, doxorubicin, vincristine, and prednisone, the clinical implications of DLBCL harboring a *MYC* translocation are unknown. One could hypothesize that these cases might benefit from the dose-intense strategies used to treat de novo BL.

Another entity to consider in this histologic spectrum is the subgroup of lymphomas containing both t(14;18) and

MYC rearrangements, termed dual translocation or "double hit" lymphomas (114,115). These lymphomas arise by one of two pathways: (a) following a diagnosis of antecedent FL; or (b) de novo, where all metaphases show both translocations (116–118). The histologic features are heterogeneous, taking on many forms, including DLBCL, atypical BL, lymphomas with features intermediate between BL and DLBCL, lymphoblastic lymphoma, surface Ig-positive acute lymphoblastic leukemia, and rarely blastic or blastoid FL. These cases can be distinguished from classic BL by the presence of a t(14;18), a finding that would preclude a diagnosis of classic BL. As well, strong expression of the BCL2 protein is virtually always seen. The diagnosis of dual translocation lymphoma should be considered whenever there is discordance between the morphology and the immunophenotype (e.g., blastoid morphology with cells expressing both surface Ig and nuclear Tdt), particularly in patients with preexisting FL, or in de novo presentations of aggressive lymphomas, when classification is difficult. Based on gene expression-profiling data, dual translocation lymphomas have a molecular signature different than that of BL and constitute a heterogeneous subgroup of high-grade lymphomas (110,111). Most reported cases demonstrate that patients with dual translocation lymphomas have an aggressive clinical presentation and a very poor prognosis, not unexpected based on the molecular consequences of these two translocations (114–116). In any case where this cytogenetic combination is suspected, a G-banded karyotype and/or appropriate locus-specific FISH should be performed.

Some cases fall into a gray zone between classic BL and DLBCL, and cannot be reliably distinguished. Many of the dual translocation cases will meet these criteria. The World Health Organization classification recommends that such cases be diagnosed as B-cell lymphoma unclassifiable, with features intermediate between diffuse large B cell lymphoma and Burkitt lymphoma, accepting that putting such cases into the category of DLBCL only contributes to the existing heterogeneity of this category of lymphomas.

REFERENCES

1. A clinical evaluation of the International Lymphoma Study Group classification of non-Hodgkin's lymphoma. The Non-Hodgkin's Lymphoma Classification Project. *Blood* 1997;89:3909–3918.
2. Buley ID. Fine needle aspiration of lymph nodes. *J Clin Pathol* 1998;51:881–885.
3. Young NA, Al-Saleem TI, Ehya H, et al. Utilization of fine-needle aspiration cytology and flow cytometry in the diagnosis and subclassification of primary and recurrent lymphoma. *Cancer* 1998;84:252–261.
4. Meda BA, Buss DH, Woodruff RD, et al. Diagnosis and subclassification of primary and recurrent lymphoma. The usefulness and limitations of combined fine-needle aspiration cytomorphology and flow cytometry. *Am J Clin Pathol* 2000;113:688–699.
5. Dong HY, Harris NL, Preffer FI, et al. Fine-needle aspiration biopsy in the diagnosis and classification of primary and recurrent lymphoma: a retrospective analysis of the utility of cytomorphology and flow cytometry. *Mod Pathol* 2001;14:472–481.
6. Mourad WA, Tulbah A, Shoukri M, et al. Primary diagnosis and REAL/WHO classification of non-Hodgkin's lymphoma by fine-needle aspiration: cytomorphologic and immunophenotypic approach. *Diagn Cytopathol* 2003;28:191–195.
7. Gong JZ, Snyder MJ, Lagoo AS, et al. Diagnostic impact of core-needle biopsy on fine-needle aspiration of non-Hodgkin lymphoma. *Diagn Cytopathol* 2004;31:23–30.
8. Hehn ST, Grogan TM, Miller TP. Utility of fine-needle aspiration as a diagnostic technique in lymphoma. *J Clin Oncol* 2004;22:3046–3052.
9. Ravinsky E, Morales C. Diagnosis of lymphoma by image-guided needle biopsies: fine needle aspiration biopsy, core biopsy or both? *Acta Cytol* 2005;49:51–57.
10. Farmer PL, Bailey DJ, Burns BF, et al. The reliability of lymphoma diagnosis in small tissue samples is heavily influenced by lymphoma subtype. *Am J Clin Pathol* 2007;128:474–480.
11. Jaffe ES, Banks PM, Nathwani B, et al. Recommendations for the reporting of lymphoid neoplasms: a report from the Association of Directors of Anatomic and Surgical Pathology. *Mod Pathol* 2004;17:131–135.
12. Srinivasan M, Sedmak D, Jewell S. Effect of fixatives and tissue processing on the content and integrity of nucleic acids. *Am J Pathol* 2002;161:1961–1971.
13. Campbell LJ. Cytogenetics of lymphomas. *Pathology* 2005;37:493–507.
14. Juneja S, Lukeis R, Tan L, et al. Cytogenetic analysis of 147 cases of non-Hodgkin's lymphoma: non-random chromosomal abnormalities and histological correlations. *Br J Haematol* 1990;76:231–237.
15. Cleary ML, Chao J, Warnke R, et al. Immunoglobulin gene rearrangement as a diagnostic criterion of B-cell lymphoma. *Proc Natl Acad Sci U S A* 1984;81:593–597.
16. Korsmeyer SJ, Waldmann TA. Immunoglobulin genes: rearrangement and translocation in human lymphoid malignancy. *J Clin Immunol* 1984;4:1–11.
17. Toyonaga B, Mak TW. Genes of the T-cell antigen receptor in normal and malignant T cells. *Annu Rev Immunol* 1987;5:585–620.
18. Spagnolo DV, Ellis DW, Juneja S, et al. The role of molecular studies in lymphoma diagnosis: a review. *Pathology* 2004;36:19–44.
19. Rockman SP. Determination of clonality in patients who present with diagnostic dilemmas: a laboratory experience and review of the literature. *Leukemia* 1997;11:852–862.
20. Kamat D, Laszewski MJ, Kemp JD, et al. The diagnostic utility of immunophenotyping and immunogenotyping in the pathologic evaluation of lymphoid proliferations. *Mod Pathol* 1990;3:105–112.
21. Kearney L. The impact of the new fish technologies on the cytogenetics of haematological malignancies. *Br J Haematol* 1999;104:648–658.
22. Vaandrager JW, Schuuring E, Raap T, et al. Interphase FISH detection of BCL2 rearrangement in follicular lymphoma using breakpoint-flanking probes. *Genes Chromosomes Cancer* 2000;27:85–94.
23. Frater JL, Tsiftsakis EK, Hsi ED, et al. Use of novel t(11;14) and t(14;18) dual-fusion fluorescence in situ hybridization probes in the differential diagnosis of lymphomas of small lymphocytes. *Diagn Mol Pathol* 2001;10:214–222.
24. Haralambieva E, Kleiverda K, Mason DY, et al. Detection of three common translocation breakpoints in non-Hodgkin's lymphomas by fluorescence in situ hybridization on routine paraffin-embedded tissue sections. *J Pathol* 2002;198:163–170.
25. Paternoster SF, Brockman SR, McClure RF, et al. A new method to extract nuclei from paraffin-embedded tissue to study lymphomas using interphase fluorescence in situ hybridization. *Am J Pathol* 2002;160:1967–1972.
26. Martin-Subero JI, Harder L, Gesk S, et al. Interphase FISH assays for the detection of translocations with breakpoints in immunoglobulin light chain loci. *Int J Cancer* 2002;98:470–474.
27. Sanchez-Izquierdo D, Siebert R, Harder L, et al. Detection of translocations affecting the BCL6 locus in B cell non-Hodgkin's lymphoma by interphase fluorescence in situ hybridization. *Leukemia* 2001;15:1475–1484.
28. Arber DA. Molecular diagnostic approach to non-Hodgkin's lymphoma. *J Mol Diagn* 2000;2:178–190.
29. Pan LX, Diss TC, Isaacson PG. The polymerase chain reaction in histopathology. *Histopathology* 1995;26:201–217.
30. Segal GH, Hussey CE, Wittwer CT. PCR for T-cell rearrangements. *Diagn Mol Pathol* 1996;5:297–298.
31. Cairns SM, Taylor JM, Gould PR, et al. Comparative evaluation of PCR-based methods for the assessment of T cell clonality in the diagnosis of T cell lymphoma. *Pathology* 2002;34:320–325.
32. van Dongen JJ, Langerak AW, Bruggemann M, et al. Design and standardization of PCR primers and protocols for detection of clonal immunoglobulin and T-cell receptor gene recombinations in suspect lymphoproliferations: report of the BIOMED-2 Concerted Action BMH4-CT98-3936. *Leukemia* 2003;17:2257–2317.
33. Theriault C, Galoin S, Valmary S, et al. PCR analysis of immunoglobulin heavy chain (IgH) and TcR-gamma chain gene rearrangements in the diagnosis of lymphoproliferative disorders: results of a study of 525 cases. *Mod Pathol* 2000;13:1269–1279.
34. Krafft AE, Taubenberger JK, Sheng ZM, et al. Enhanced sensitivity with a novel TCRgamma PCR assay for clonality studies in 569 formalin-fixed, paraffin-embedded (FFPE) cases. *Mol Diagn* 1999;4:119–133.
35. Inagaki H, Nonaka M, Nagaya S, et al. Monoclonality in gastric lymphoma detected in formalin-fixed, paraffin-embedded endoscopic biopsy specimens using immunohistochemistry, in situ hybridization, and polymerase chain reaction. *Diagn Mol Pathol* 1995;4:32–38.
36. Wan JH, Sykes PJ, Orell SR, et al. Rapid method for detecting monoclonality in B cell lymphoma in lymph node aspirates using the polymerase chain reaction. *J Clin Pathol* 1992;45:420–423.
37. Chen YT, Mercer GO, Chen Y. Polymerase chain reaction-based detection of B-cell monoclonality in cytologic specimens. *Arch Pathol Lab Med* 1993;117:1099–1103.
38. Sukpanichnant S, Vnencak-Jones CL, McCurley TL. Detection of clonal immunoglobulin heavy chain gene rearrangements by polymerase chain reaction in scrapings from archival hematoxylin and eosin-stained

histologic sections: implications for molecular genetic studies of focal pathologic lesions. *Diagn Mol Pathol* 1993;2:168–176.

39. Alkan S, Lehman C, Sarago C, et al. Polymerase chain reaction detection of immunoglobulin gene rearrangement and bcl-2 translocation in archival glass slides of cytologic material. *Diagn Mol Pathol* 1995;4:25–31.

40. Pan LX, Diss TC, Peng HZ, et al. Clonality analysis of defined B-cell populations in archival tissue sections using microdissection and the polymerase chain reaction. *Histopathology* 1994;24:323–327.

41. Wan JH, Trainor KJ, Brisco MJ, et al. Monoclonality in B cell lymphoma detected in paraffin wax embedded sections using the polymerase chain reaction. *J Clin Pathol* 1990;43:888–890.

42. Reed TJ, Reid A, Wallberg K, et al. Determination of B-cell clonality in paraffin-embedded lymph nodes using the polymerase chain reaction. *Diagn Mol Pathol* 1993;2:42–49.

43. Chen YT, Whitney KD, Chen Y. Clonality analysis of B-cell lymphoma in fresh-frozen and paraffin-embedded tissues: the effects of variable polymerase chain reaction parameters. *Mod Pathol* 1994;7:429–434.

44. Greer CE, Lund JK, Manos MM. PCR amplification from paraffin-embedded tissues: recommendations for long-term storage and prospective studies. PCR *Methods Appl* 1991;1:46–50.

45. Greer CE, Peterson SL, Kiviat NB, et al. PCR amplification from paraffin-embedded tissues. Effects of fixative and fixation time. *Am J Clin Pathol* 1991;95:117–124.

46. Hoeve MA, Krol AD, Philippo K, et al. Limitations of clonality analysis of B cell proliferations using CDR3 polymerase chain reaction. *Mol Pathol* 2000;53:194–200.

47. Speicher MR, Gwyn Ballard S, et al. Karyotyping human chromosomes by combinatorial multi-fluor FISH. *Nat Genet* 1996;12:368–375.

48. Schrock E, du Manoir S, Veldman T, et al. Multicolor spectral karyotyping of human chromosomes. *Science* 1996;273:494–497.

49. Bayani JM, Squire JA. Applications of SKY in cancer cytogenetics. *Cancer Invest* 2002;20:373–386.

50. Nordgren A, Sorensen AG, Tinggaard-Pedersen N, et al. New chromosomal breakpoints in non-Hodgkin's lymphomas revealed by spectral karyotyping and G-banding. *Int J Mol Med* 2000;5:485–492.

51. Houldsworth J, Chaganti RS. Comparative genomic hybridization: an overview. *Am J Pathol* 1994;145:1253–1260.

52. Pinkel D, Segraves R, Sudar D, et al. High resolution analysis of DNA copy number variation using comparative genomic hybridization to microarrays. *Nat Genet* 1998;20:207–211.

53. Wessendorf S, Schwaenen C, Kohlhammer H, et al. Hidden gene amplifications in aggressive B-cell non-Hodgkin lymphomas detected by microarray-based comparative genomic hybridization. *Oncogene* 2003;22:1425–1429.

54. Wessendorf S, Fritz B, Wrobel G, et al. Automated screening for genomic imbalances using matrix-based comparative genomic hybridization. *Lab Invest* 2002;82:47–60.

55. de Leeuw RJ, Davies JJ, Rosenwald A, et al. Comprehensive whole genome array CGH profiling of mantle cell lymphoma model genomes. *Hum Mol Genet* 2004;13:1827–1837.

56. Deleeuw RJ, Zettl A, Klinker E, et al. Whole-genome analysis and HLA genotyping of enteropathy-type T-cell lymphoma reveals 2 distinct lymphoma subtypes. *Gastroenterology* 2007;132:1902–1911.

57. Golub TR, Slonim DK, Tamayo P, et al. Molecular classification of cancer: class discovery and class prediction by gene expression monitoring. *Science* 1999;286:531–537.

58. Staudt LM. Molecular diagnosis of the hematologic cancers. *N Engl J Med* 2003;348:1777–1785.

59. Wiestner A, Staudt LM. Towards molecular diagnosis and targeted therapy of lymphoid malignancies. *Semin Hematol* 2003;40:296–307.

60. Kaleem Z, White G, Vollmer RT. Critical analysis and diagnostic usefulness of limited immunophenotyping of B-cell non-Hodgkin lymphomas by flow cytometry. *Am J Clin Pathol* 2001;115:136–142.

61. Kaleem Z, Zehnbauer BA, White G, et al. Lack of expression of surface immunoglobulin light chains in B-cell non-Hodgkin lymphomas. *Am J Clin Pathol* 2000;113:399–405.

62. Li S, Eshleman JR, Borowitz MJ. Lack of surface immunoglobulin light chain expression by flow cytometric immunophenotyping can help diagnose peripheral B-cell lymphoma. *Am J Clin Pathol* 2002;118:229–234.

63. Zhao XF, Cherian S, Sargent R, et al. Expanded populations of surface membrane immunoglobulin light chain-negative B cells in lymph nodes are not always indicative of B-cell lymphoma. *Am J Clin Pathol* 2005;124:143–150.

64. Langerak AW, van Den Beemd R, Wolvers-Tettero IL, et al. Molecular and flow cytometric analysis of the Vbeta repertoire for clonality assessment in mature TCRalphabeta T-cell proliferations. *Blood* 2001;98:165–173.

65. Beck RC, Stahl S, O'Keefe CL, et al. Detection of mature T-cell leukemias by flow cytometry using anti-T-cell receptor V beta antibodies. *Am J Clin Pathol* 2003;120:785–794.

66. Chu PG, Chang KL, Arber DA, et al. Immunophenotyping of hematopoietic neoplasms. *Semin Diagn Pathol* 2000;17:236–256.

67. Jones D, Dorfman DM. Phenotypic characterization of subsets of T cell lymphoma: towards a functional classification of T cell lymphoma. *Leuk Lymphoma* 2001;40:449–459.

68. Jamal S, Picker LJ, Aquino DB, et al. Immunophenotypic analysis of peripheral T-cell neoplasms. A multiparameter flow cytometric approach. *Am J Clin Pathol* 2001;116:512–526.

69. Gorczyca W, Weisberger J, Liu Z, et al. An approach to diagnosis of T-cell lymphoproliferative disorders by flow cytometry. *Cytometry* 2002;50:177–190.

70. Hudnall SD, Betancourt E, Barnhart E, et al. Comparative flow immunophenotypic features of the inflammatory infiltrates of Hodgkin lymphoma and lymphoid hyperplasia. *Cytometry B Clin Cytom* 2008;74:1–8.

71. Ginaldi L, De Martinis M, D'Ostilio A, et al. Altered lymphocyte antigen expressions in HIV infection: a study by quantitative flow cytometry. *Am J Clin Pathol* 1997;108:585–592.

72. Hudnall SD, Patel J, Schwab H, et al. Comparative immunophenotypic features of EBV-positive and EBV-negative atypical lymphocytosis. *Cytometry B Clin Cytom* 2003;55:22–28.

73. Rahemtullah A, Reichard KK, Preffer FI, et al. A double-positive CD4+CD8+ T-cell population is commonly found in nodular lymphocyte predominant Hodgkin lymphoma. *Am J Clin Pathol* 2006;126:805–814.

74. Ashton-Key M, Jessup E, Isaacson PG. Immunoglobulin light chain staining in paraffin-embedded tissue using a heat mediated epitope retrieval method. *Histopathology* 1996;29:525–531.

75. Marshall-Taylor CE, Cartun RW, Mandich D, et al. Immunohistochemical detection of immunoglobulin light chain expression in B-cell non-Hodgkin lymphomas using formalin-fixed, paraffin-embedded tissues and a heat-induced epitope retrieval technique. *Appl Immunohistochem Mol Morphol* 2002;10:258–262.

76. Nam-Cha SH, San-Millan B, Mollejo M, et al. Light-chain-restricted germinal centres in reactive lymphadenitis: report of eight cases. *Histopathology* 2008;52:436–444.

77. Winberg CD. Peripheral T-cell lymphoma. Morphologic and immunologic observations. *Am J Clin Pathol* 1993;99:426–435.

78. Chan JK. Peripheral T-cell and NK-cell neoplasms: an integrated approach to diagnosis. *Mod Pathol* 1999;12:177–199.

79. Murphy M, Fullen D, Carlson JA. Low CD7 expression in benign and malignant cutaneous lymphocytic infiltrates: experience with an antibody reactive with paraffin-embedded tissue. *Am J Dermatopathol* 2002;24:6–16.

80. Alaibac M, Pigozzi B, Belloni-Fortina A, et al. CD7 expression in reactive and malignant human skin T-lymphocytes. *Anticancer Res* 2003;23:2707–2710.

81. Greaves MF. Differentiation-linked leukemogenesis in lymphocytes. *Science* 1986;234:697–704.

82. van Dongen JJ, Wolvers-Tettero IL. Analysis of immunoglobulin and T cell receptor genes. Part II: possibilities and limitations in the diagnosis and management of lymphoproliferative diseases and related disorders. *Clin Chim Acta* 1991;198:93–174.

83. Cheson BD, Horning SJ, Coiffier B, et al. Report of an international workshop to standardize response criteria for non-Hodgkin's lymphomas. NCI Sponsored International Working Group. *J Clin Oncol* 1999;17:1244.

84. Bishop PW, McNally K, Harris M. Audit of bone marrow trephines. *J Clin Pathol* 1992;45:1105–1108.

85. Bain BJ. Bone marrow trephine biopsy. *J Clin Pathol* 2001;54:737–742.

86. Campbell JK, Matthews JP, Seymour JF, et al. Optimum trephine length in the assessment of bone marrow involvement in patients with diffuse large cell lymphoma. *Ann Oncol* 2003;14:273–276.

87. Naresh KN, Lampert I, Hasserjian R, et al. Optimal processing of bone marrow trephine biopsy: the Hammersmith Protocol. *J Clin Pathol* 2006;59:903–911.

88. Bonds LA, Barnes P, Foucar K, et al. Acetic acid-zinc-formalin: a safe alternative to B-5 fixative. *Am J Clin Pathol* 2005;124:205–211.

89. Mullink H, Henzen-Logmans SC, Tadema TM, et al. Influence of fixation and decalcification on the immunohistochemical staining of cell-specific markers in paraffin-embedded human bone biopsies. *J Histochem Cytochem* 1985;33:1103–1109.

90. Mukai K, Yoshimura S, Anzai M. Effects of decalcification on immunoperoxidase staining. *Am J Surg Pathol* 1986;10:413–419.

91. Thiele J, Zirbes TK, Kvasnicka HM, et al. Focal lymphoid aggregates (nodules) in bone marrow biopsies: differentiation between benign hyperplasia and malignant lymphoma—a practical guideline. *J Clin Pathol* 1999;52:294–300.

92. Engels K, Oeschger S, Hansmann ML, et al. Bone marrow trephines containing lymphoid aggregates from patients with rheumatoid and other autoimmune disorders frequently show clonal B-cell infiltrates. *Hum Pathol* 2007;38:1402–1411.

93. Cervantes F, Pereira A, Marti JM, et al. Bone marrow lymphoid nodules in myeloproliferative disorders: association with the nonmyelosclerotic phases of idiopathic myelofibrosis and immunological significance. *Br J Haematol* 1998;70:279–282.

94. Magalhaes SM, Filho FD, Vassallo J, et al. Bone marrow lymphoid aggregates in myelodysplastic syndromes: incidence, immunomorphological characteristics and correlation with clinical features and survival. *Leuk Res* 2002;26:525–30.

95. Hasserjian RP. Reactive versus neoplastic bone marrow: problems and pitfalls. *Arch Pathol Lab Med* 2008;132:587–594.

96. Skinnider BF, Connors JM, Gascoyne RD. Bone marrow involvement in T-cell-rich B-cell lymphoma. *Am J Clin Pathol* 1997;108:570–578.

97. Rosenwald A, Wright G, Wiestner A, et al. The proliferation gene expression signature is a quantitative integrator of oncogenic events that predicts survival in mantle cell lymphoma. *Cancer Cell* 2003;3:185–197.

98. Fu K, Weisenburger DD, Greiner TC, et al. Cyclin D1-negative mantle cell lymphoma: a clinicopathologic study based on gene expression profiling. *Blood* 2005;106:4315–4321.

99. Naresh KN. Nodal marginal zone B-cell lymphoma with prominent follicular colonization—difficulties in diagnosis: a study of 15 cases. *Histopathology* 2008;52:331–339.

100. Pittaluga S, Ayoubi TA, Wlodarska I, et al. BCL-6 expression in reactive lymphoid tissue and in B-cell non-Hodgkin's lymphomas. *J Pathol* 1996;179:145–150.

101. Skinnider BF, Horsman DE, Dupuis B, et al. Bcl-6 and Bcl-2 protein expression in diffuse large B-cell lymphoma and follicular lymphoma: correlation with 3q27 and 18q21 chromosomal abnormalities. *Hum Pathol* 1999;30:803–808.

102. McCluggage WG, Catherwood M, Alexander HD, et al. Immunohistochemical expression of CD10 and t(14;18) chromosomal translocation may be indicators of follicle centre cell origin in nodal diffuse large B-cell lymphoma. *Histopathology* 2002;41:414–420.

103. Gascoyne RD, Adomat SA, Krajewski S, et al. Prognostic significance of Bcl-2 protein expression and Bcl-2 gene rearrangement in diffuse aggressive non-Hodgkin's lymphoma. *Blood* 1997;90:244–251.

104. Taub R, Kirsch I, Morton C, et al. Translocation of the c-myc gene into the immunoglobulin heavy chain locus in human Burkitt lymphoma and murine plasmacytoma cells. *Proc Natl Acad Sci U S A* 1982;79:7837–7841.

105. Hamlyn PH, Rabbitts TH. Translocation joins c-myc and immunoglobulin gamma 1 genes in a Burkitt lymphoma revealing a third exon in the c-myc oncogene. *Nature* 1983;304:135–139.

106. Battey J, Moulding C, Taub R, et al. The human c-myc oncogene: structural consequences of translocation into the IgH locus in Burkitt lymphoma. *Cell* 1983;34:779–787.

107. Emanuel BS, Selden JR, Chaganti RS, et al. The 2p breakpoint of a 2;8 translocation in Burkitt lymphoma interrupts the V kappa locus. *Proc Natl Acad Sci U S A* 1984;81:2444–2446.

108. Hollis GF, Mitchell KF, Battey J, et al. A variant translocation places the lambda immunoglobulin genes 3' to the c-myc oncogene in Burkitt's lymphoma. *Nature* 1984;307:752–755.

109. Ladanyi M, Offit K, Jhanwar SC, et al. MYC rearrangement and translocations involving band 8q24 in diffuse large cell lymphomas. *Blood* 1991;77:1057–1063.

110. Hummel M, Bentink S, Berger H, et al. A biologic definition of Burkitt's lymphoma from transcriptional and genomic profiling. *N Engl J Med* 2006;354:2419–2430.

111. Dave SS, Fu K, Wright GW, et al. Molecular diagnosis of Burkitt's lymphoma. *N Engl J Med* 2006;354:2431–2442.

112. Harris NL, Horning SJ. Burkitt's lymphoma—the message from microarrays. *N Engl J Med* 2006;354:2495–2498.

113. Rodig SJ, Vergilio JA, Shahsafaei A, et al. Characteristic expression patterns of TCL1, CD38, and CD44 identify aggressive lymphomas harboring a MYC translocation. *Am J Surg Pathol* 2008;32:113–122.

114. Macpherson N, Lesack D, Klasa R, et al. Small noncleaved, non-Burkitt's (Burkitt-Like) lymphoma: cytogenetics predict outcome and reflect clinical presentation. *J Clin Oncol* 1999;17:1558–1567.

115. Le Gouill S, Talmant P, Touzeau C, et al. The clinical presentation and prognosis of diffuse large B-cell lymphoma with t(14;18) and 8q24/c-MYC rearrangement. *Haematologica* 2007;92:1335–1342.

116. Kanungo A, Medeiros LJ, Abruzzo LV, et al. Lymphoid neoplasms associated with concurrent t(14;18) and 8q24/c-MYC translocation generally have a poor prognosis. *Mod Pathol* 2006;19:25–33.

117. McDonnell TJ, Korsmeyer SJ. Progression from lymphoid hyperplasia to high-grade malignant lymphoma in mice transgenic for the t(14; 18). *Nature* 1991;349:254–256.

118. Yano T, Jaffe ES, Longo DL, et al. MYC rearrangements in histologically progressed follicular lymphomas. *Blood* 1992;80:758–767.

CHAPTER 10 ■ STAGING AND PROGNOSTIC FACTORS

SUJAATHA NARAYANAN AND KERRY J. SAVAGE

The initial evaluation of the patient with non-Hodgkin lymphoma (NHL) serves to establish the correct diagnosis and extent of disease. Information is assembled through a history, physical examination, relevant radiographic studies, laboratory investigations, and necessary invasive procedures to identify the sites of disease, estimate prognosis, and develop a rational treatment approach. In contrast to the prognostic importance of stage in nonhematologic malignancies, advanced stage in NHL does not always correlate with poor outcome. This is particularly true of indolent lymphomas, which often present with bone marrow involvement but have a long natural history. Nevertheless, a uniform staging system allows for the development of rational treatment strategies and for accurate study comparisons.

ANN ARBOR STAGING SYSTEM

The Ann Arbor staging classification (1), which was originally designed in 1971 for Hodgkin lymphoma, is the recommended staging classification for all NHLs (Table 10.1). This classification emphasizes the number and location of involved nodal and extranodal regions with subcategories based on the presence of B symptoms. The spleen, thymus, Waldeyer ring, appendix, and Peyer patch are all considered lymphoid organs. Localized extralymphatic disease is designated as an "E" lesion; however, diffuse extranodal involvement is indicative of stage IV disease. The Ann Arbor staging originally included pathologic information obtained from invasive procedures such as bone marrow biopsy, staging laparotomy, and splenectomy. Today, only bone marrow biopsies are routinely performed.

Several limitations become apparent when the Ann Arbor classification is applied to NHL. Unlike Hodgkin lymphoma, which has a contiguous pattern of lymphatic involvement, NHLs have a tendency to spread hematogenously and involve noncontiguous lymph node sites (2). In addition, the Ann Arbor staging system does not reflect the unique natural history of specific NHL subtypes or the consequences of lymphomatous involvement of certain extranodal disease sites (e.g., sinus, central nervous system [CNS], testicular) (3–5). In addition, important factors reflecting tumor burden (lactate dehydrogenase [LDH], number of nodal or extranodal sites involved, tumor bulk, β_2-microglobulin, B symptoms) and physiologic reserve of the patient (e.g., age, performance status [PS]) are not included in this conventional staging system.

To more fully incorporate additional relevant prognostic features, more broadly relevant models have been developed in the most common NHLs, diffuse large cell lymphoma (6–15) and follicular lymphoma (FL) (16–21). The most widely utilized model is the International Prognostic Index (IPI), which was originally developed for diffuse large cell lymphoma (22) and will be discussed in more detail later in the chapter. Alternate staging systems have also been adapted in other specific disease entities and sites. For example, in gastrointestinal (GI) NHL, a modified version of the Ann Arbor staging system (23), which distinguishes between local (gastric or mesenteric) and distant (abdominal) nodal disease, has been demonstrated to have prognostic significance (24–26). With the availability of endoscopic ultrasound, a tumor, node, metastasis system has also been used to address the depth of gastric wall invasion. In Burkitt lymphoma, the Ann

---

TABLE 10.1

ANN ARBOR STAGING SYSTEM[a]

Stage	Definition[b]
I	Involvement of a single lymph node or of a single extranodal organ or site (IE)
II	Involvement of two or more lymph node regions on the same side of the diaphragm, or localized involvement of an extranodal site or organ (IIE) and one or more lymph node regions on the same side of the diaphragm
III	Involvement of lymph node regions on both sides of the diaphragm, which may also be accompanied by localized involvement of an extranodal organ or site (IIIE) or spleen (IIIS) or both (IIISE)
IV	Diffuse or disseminated involvement of one or more distant extranodal organs with or without associated lymph node involvement

[a] Fever >38°C, night sweats, and/or weight loss >10% of body weight in the 6 months preceding admission are defined as systemic symptoms.
[b] The spleen is considered nodal.

Arbor classification is less precise because it does not include specific extranodal disease sites.

RECOMMENDED STUDIES FOR INITIAL EVALUATION

The diversity of NHL subtypes and the unique involvement of specific extranodal disease sites make it difficult to apply a uniform method of staging for all patients. Nevertheless, a general strategy can be followed for most patients with NHL with selected additional studies when there are suspicious clinical findings and/or disease-specific characteristics. The National Comprehensive Cancer Network (NCCN) proposed guidelines for staging the most common subtypes of NHL; these recommendations are incorporated here and outlined in Table 10.2 (27).

CLINICAL EVALUATION

A careful history and physical examination are critical in evaluating a new patient with lymphoma to delineate the extent of disease, guide further diagnostic imaging or procedures, and assist in treatment decisions.

History

Approximately two-thirds of patients with NHL present with painless lymph node enlargement. The most frequently involved disease sites include the cervical, supraclavicular, inguinal, and axillary regions. The duration and growth rate of suspected adenopathy should also be noted.

The presence of systemic symptoms, including fever (temperature $>38°C$), night sweats, and unexplained weight loss

---

TABLE 10.2

RECOMMENDED STUDIES FOR INITIAL EVALUATION

Biopsy of lesion with review by an experienced hematopathologist
History: Including B symptoms, PS, duration and growth rate of lymph node enlargement, symptoms to suggest extranodal involvement, risk factors for lymphoma, comorbid illnesses
Physical examination: General examination with attention to node-bearing areas, including Waldeyer ring and liver and spleen span, inspection of skin

Laboratory studies
  Mandatory:
  CBC, differential, peripheral blood smear
  LDH, β_2-microglobulin
  Blood urea nitrogen, creatinine, albumin, serum glutamic-oxaloacetic transmission, total bilirubin, albumin, alkaline phosphatase, calcium, and uric acid (aggressive histologies)
  Serum protein electrophoresis

  In select patients:
  Viral serologies with appropriate risk factors, clinical findings
  Hepatitis B, HIV, HTLV-1
  Hepatitis C (lymphoplasmacytic lymphoma)

Bone marrow aspirate and biopsy

Radiologic studies and Special procedures
  Mandatory:
  Chest radiograph (posteroanterior and lateral)
  CT chest in majority particularly if abnormality in chest radiography
  CT abdomen and pelvis

  In select patients:
  PET scan (optional/study purposes)
  MRI (to detect bone marrow involvement)
  Ear, nose, and throat examination (to detect preauricular, thyroid, GI, testicular involvement)
  Slitlamp examination (to detect CNS and ocular lymphoma)
  Testicular ultrasound (contralateral testis in testicular lymphoma)
  GI evaluation (endoscopy or barium studies; endoscopic ultrasound [study purposes]) for Waldeyer ring involvement or if suggestive symptoms
  Skeletal evaluation (e.g., plain bone radiographs, MRI, bone scan, or PET scan [optional])
  Head CT/MRI if neurologic signs or symptoms
  Lumbar puncture and CSF analysis if neurologic signs or symptoms, high-grade histologies, HIV-associated lymphomas consider in, high-risk extranodal sites (e.g., bone marrow, CNS, ocular, sinus, epidural, testicular, ovary, or bilateral breast [aggressive histology])
  Bilateral mammograms (to detect breast lymphoma)
  Multiple-gated cardiac blood pool or echocardiogram

(>10% of body weight over the past 6 months) (B symptoms), should also be determined. These B symptoms are adverse prognostic factors in patients with aggressive lymphoma, and their resolution is one measure of treatment response. In patients with indolent lymphoma, the onset of B symptoms may indicate transformation into a more aggressive histology.

Focal symptoms may arise from an obstructing nodal mass in the thorax or abdomen. Patients with mediastinal lymphadenopathy can develop cough, chest discomfort, and occasionally, superior vena caval syndrome. Retroperitoneal adenopathy is usually asymptomatic; however, extensive disease may lead to abdominal discomfort, early satiety, and obstructive uropathy. Mesenteric or pelvic adenopathy will rarely result in visceral obstruction or perforation.

Although NHL is primarily a disorder of lymph nodes, extranodal disease often occurs and results in symptoms referable to the particular system (e.g., bone pain, GI complaints, neurologic symptoms, cutaneous involvement, or pulmonary symptoms). In some cases, an extranodal site may be the only area of disease involvement. The skin and GI tract were the most frequent sites of extranodal disease in patients included in the Non-Hodgkin's Classification Project (28).

Several primary extranodal lymphomas involve specific disease sites. For example, over 50% of extranodal marginal zone B-cell lymphomas of mucosa-associated lymphoid tissue (MALT lymphoma) involve the GI tract (29). Less frequent sites of MALT lymphoma include: lung, head and neck, ocular adnexa, skin, thyroid, and breast (30). Gastric MALT lymphoma has been linked to a preceding infection by *Helicobacter pylori*, and patients will often report chronic dyspeptic symptoms (31). In the World Health Organization classification, specific subtypes of peripheral T-cell lymphoma (PTCL) also fall into the primary extranodal category: extranodal natural killer/T-cell lymphoma; nasal and nasal type; enteropathy type T-cell lymphoma; hepatosplenic γδ T-cell lymphoma; and subcutaneous panniculitis-like T-cell lymphoma, as well as the cutaneous T-cell neoplasms (mycosis fungoides, Sézary syndrome, primary cutaneous anaplastic large cell lymphoma [ALCL], lymphomatoid papulosis) (32). Patients will exhibit a spectrum of symptoms specific to these entities.

Rarely, patients present with neurologic symptoms reflecting parenchymal CNS, leptomeningeal, or paraneoplastic disease. Space-occupying masses can result in headache, nausea, vomiting, and focal neurologic deficits. Leptomeningeal involvement may result in multiple cranial nerve palsies, headache, changes in mental status, back or radicular pain, incontinence, lower motor neuron weakness, and/or sensory abnormalities.

Other rare extranodal sites of involvement at presentation most commonly seen in aggressive histologies include the testes, sinus, eye, epidural space, kidney, prostate, bladder, ovary, heart, breast, salivary glands, and adrenal glands.

Risk factors for lymphoma should be reviewed, including a history of human immunodeficiency virus (HIV) infection, immunosuppressive medications, and autoimmune disorders such as rheumatoid arthritis, Hashimoto thyroiditis, and celiac sprue. Inherited disorders such as severe combined immunodeficiency, hypogammaglobulinemia, common variable immunodeficiency, Wiskott-Aldrich syndrome, and ataxia telangiectasia are associated with an increased incidence of lymphoma. Epidemiologic studies suggest that environmental factors may also play an etiologic role in NHL. Thus, an inquiry into potential environmental and occupational exposures should be made (33). Occupations that have been associated with an increased risk of NHL include farmers, pesticide workers, cosmetologists, chemists, workers in the petroleum, rubber, plastics, and synthetics industries, and forestry workers.

Functional capacity based on the Eastern Cooperative Oncology Group (ECOG) PS (Table 10.3) has prognostic value (22). PS reflects the disease's impact on the patient and frequently predicts an individual's tolerance for therapy. Comorbid respiratory, cardiac, neurologic, or renal disease that might influence treatment delivery should also be identified from the initial history.

Physical Examination

The physical examination should include all peripheral (cervical, supraclavicular, axillary, epitrochlear, inguinal, femoral, popliteal) and intra-abdominal (mesenteric, retroperitoneal, pelvic) lymph node-bearing areas. The site and size of all abnormal lymph nodes should be recorded. Waldeyer ring (tonsils, nasopharynx) is best assessed by indirect laryngoscopy or direct fiberoptic examination. This disease site is particularly important in individuals with high neck nodes or thyroid, testicular, or GI involvement. Splenic and hepatic enlargement should be assessed, although this is not always indicative of lymphomatous involvement (34,35). With cutaneous disease, multiple remote areas may be affected simultaneously. Thus, the skin should be thoroughly inspected and any suspicious lesions biopsied. A complete neurologic and cardiorespiratory examination to assess for disease involvement

TABLE 10.3	
ECOG PERFORMANCE STATUS SCALE	
ECOG Scale	**Description**
0	Asymptomatic: Normal activity
1	Symptomatic: Fully ambulatory; able to carry out activities of daily living
2	Symptomatic: In bed less than 50% of the day
3	Symptomatic: In bed greater than 50% of the day
4	Bedridden: May need hospitalization

and the presence of comorbid illnesses that may limit treatment delivery should be undertaken.

LABORATORY STUDIES

Laboratory studies should include a complete blood count (CBC) with examination of the peripheral smear to assess for circulating lymphoma cells. Peripheral blood involvement is seen most commonly with the indolent lymphomas, which have a greater propensity for bone marrow involvement (36). Although abnormalities in the hematologic parameters may reflect bone marrow involvement (37,38), peripheral blood counts are not reliable indicators of bone marrow disease (39). Thrombocytopenia and neutropenia are more consistently associated with bone marrow involvement than anemia (37,40).

LDH and β_2-microglobulin are indirect measurements of tumor burden that have independent prognostic value (41,42). If elevated at presentation, these serologic parameters may also be useful in assessing treatment response. Serum creatinine and uric acid are important in identifying patients at risk for tumor lysis syndrome, particularly in aggressive lymphomas. Impaired renal function may signal ureteral obstruction or rarely indicate lymphomatous kidney involvement. Liver chemistries assess both hepatic function and organ involvement, although abnormalities in liver tests do not correlate well with hepatic infiltration (43,44). An isolated elevation in alkaline phosphatase should prompt an evaluation of the skeletal system. Hypercalcemia can occur in aggressive lymphomas and, in particular, human T-cell lymphotropic virus (HTLV) type-1 associated adult T-cell leukemia/lymphoma. A serum protein electrophoresis may reveal monoclonal gammopathy, most notably in lymphoplasmacytic lymphoma or chronic lymphocytic leukemia/small lymphocytic lymphomas (45,46).

Viral serologies are performed in those patients who are at risk for exposure or who have a compatible clinical picture. Patients with HIV-related lymphomas are more likely to have aggressive B-cell tumors, B symptoms, and advanced stage disease with multiple extranodal sites of involvement (47). Human herpes virus 8 is recovered from virtually all cases of body cavity associated or primary effusion lymphoma (48). HTLV-1 is a retrovirus that is endemic to regions of Southern Japan and the Caribbean basin, and sporadic elsewhere. It is transmitted in intact lymphocytes by blood transfusion, sexual contact, and breast-feeding. Patients infected in infancy can rarely develop a T-cell leukemia/lymphoma associated with peripheral blood involvement, skin and CNS infiltration, and hypercalcemia (49). Epstein-Barr virus is present in almost all cases of Burkitt lymphoma from Africa and in many HIV- or transplant-associated lymphoproliferative disorders. Hepatitis C is seen in approximately 30% of patients with lymphoplasmacytic lymphoma and should be evaluated in this NHL subtype (50). Although hepatitis B virus is not casually related to any of the NHLs, reactivation is a well-recognized complication in patients with chronic hepatitis B virus infection who receive cytotoxic chemotherapy (51). Thus, patients who are in high-risk groups or from endemic areas (Asia, Middle East, Mediterranean) should be screened for chronic infection and strongly considered for prophylactic therapy with lamivudine (52).

RADIOGRAPHIC STAGING

Plain Films, Computed Axial Tomography, and Magnetic Resonance Imaging

A standard posterior-anterior and lateral chest radiograph will detect the majority of abnormalities affecting the mediastinal and hilar lymph nodes, lung parenchyma, and pleura. Pleural effusions are found in approximately 10% of patients, usually in association with mediastinal adenopathy (53). Pathologic verification is required because pleural effusions are often benign. The chest radiograph is less accurate in defining disease extent, detecting adenopathy in the subcarinal and cardiophrenic spaces, and determining chest wall and pericardial involvement (54–56). A computed tomography (CT) of the chest more accurately delineates the extent of mediastinal disease and evaluates the aforementioned regions missed by radiography (57). The NCCN practice guidelines recommend that in the initial staging of a patient with lymphoma, a chest CT is indicated for all patients with aggressive histology as well as the majority of indolent lymphomas (58). Furthermore, a chest CT should be obtained if there are any abnormalities on chest radiograph or further assessment of a poorly visualized region is needed. In addition, if radiotherapy is to be used for mediastinal disease, CT is required for accurate determination of treatment portals. Finally, for patients with disease outside the thorax in whom radiotherapy is being considered as the only mode of therapy (e.g., FL with localized disease), a CT scan may be useful in detecting thoracic lymphadenopathy that is not otherwise appreciated on the standard chest radiograph.

Staging laparotomies were previously performed to provide information regarding intra-abdominal involvement with NHL. With improvements in imaging studies as well as the widespread use of systemic chemotherapy, there are currently no indications for staging laparotomies in NHL. Lymphangiography and ultrasonography were used before CT for the evaluation of intra-abdominal disease. CT has replaced lymphangiography as the preferred method for evaluating disease below the diaphragm because lymphangiographies are difficult to perform and insensitive in certain nodal regions. Abdominal CTs have also replaced ultrasonography because CTs more effectively image continuous lymph node regions.

Lymphomatous involvement of the liver or spleen may be subtle. Although diffuse organ infiltration may not be apparent on CT scan, this pattern is typically associated with subdiaphragmatic lymphadenopathy, and management is unaltered. In a patient with otherwise localized disease, abnormalities in liver function tests or suspicious lesions on imaging are an indication for biopsy. Genitourinary involvement is established by CT, with the exception of testicular masses, which are best assessed by ultrasonography (59,60). Intrinsic GI tract involvement or extension from adjacent nodal disease may occur, particularly with aggressive lymphoma subtypes. In the presence of extensive disease, abnormalities are often apparent on CT, and extraluminal tumor extension can be quantified. However, clinical symptoms suggestive of GI lymphoma should also prompt an endoscopic or barium study because isolated luminal disease may not be detected by CT. The role of endoscopic ultrasound of the stomach may be useful to establish the depth of lymphomatous penetration, but requires prospective validation (61).

Magnetic resonance imaging (MRI) has a limited role in the staging of NHL. Compared with CT scan, MRI is more costly, has limited availability, and a longer imaging time. Nevertheless, MRI is preferable in selected settings. For example, MRI is the modality of choice to characterize bone disease because the technique is more sensitive than bone scintigraphy or conventional radiographs (62,63). MRI can also detect lymphomatous bone marrow involvement (64) and, more specifically, evaluate disease of the chest wall or pericardium. In addition, MRI is superior to CT scan for the detection of CNS disease; when gadolinium is used, meningeal enhancement may indicate leptomeningeal involvement.

Functional Imaging

Gallium-67 Scintigraphy

Gallium-67 (^{67}Ga) scintigraphy was the first whole body, noninvasive imaging modality used for the diagnosis and staging of lymphoma. This technique depends upon the binding of ^{67}Ga to transferrin receptors in the tumor (65) and provides additional information regarding tumor viability (66). Thus, ^{67}Ga scintigraphy can be useful in determining treatment response and evaluating residual masses after therapy.

In aggressive lymphomas, ^{67}Ga scintigraphy can complement CT in identifying initial disease sites (67), assessing response to therapy (68,69), and detecting early recurrences. However, ^{67}Ga scintigraphy has been largely replaced by 2-[fluorine-18]-fluoro-2-deoxy-D-glucose (FDG) positron emission tomography (PET), which has superior sensitivity and specificity.

Positron Emission Tomography

^{18}F-FDG is a glucose analog labeled with a short-lived positron emitter that can be used to image lymphoid neoplasms using PET. ^{18}F-FDG uptake is proportional to the glycolytic metabolic rate of viable tumor cells (70), providing information on the functional status of the tumor (71–73). Malignant lymphocytes have a high metabolic activity and, thus, display avidity for ^{18}F-FDG. Increased ^{18}F-FDG uptake is seen in the kidneys and bladder, as well as tissues with relatively active glucose metabolism such as skeletal and cardiac muscle (66). Physiologic uptake of ^{18}F-FDG occurs in organs such as the thymus following therapy, and in benign disorders such as granulomatous disease (74,75). The combination of PET/CT in which the functional imaging of PET is coregistered with the almost simultaneously acquired anatomic images of CT is widely used, and believed to be more sensitive and specific than either modality in isolation because it allows for anatomic correlation of PET abnormalities (76,77). Attenuation correction is recommended to obtain best results. The use of intravenous contrast-enhanced PET/CT is believed to provide at least equivalent information to contrast-enhanced CT (76,78) and may be an alternative to contrast-enhanced CT posttherapy completion. PET is more sensitive than ^{67}Ga for the staging and restaging of various

lymphomas subtypes, especially FL (79). Also, ^{18}F-FDG PET is easier and quicker to perform than ^{67}Ga scanning, and has, therefore, resulted in widespread use of PET in lymphoma staging.

Limited data indicate that ^{18}F-FDG PET is able to accurately detect splenic, GI, and hepatic disease (73,80). Although physiologic hepatic uptake remains problematic, ^{18}F-FDG PET can detect liver lesions with high glycolytic activity (81). ^{18}F-FDG PET may also be superior to CT or endoscopy at defining the extent of lymphomatous involvement of the stomach (72) or small bowel (82). Furthermore, ^{18}F-FDG PET appears to be superior to bone scan in detecting skeletal lymphomatous lesions (83). ^{18}F-FDG PET has also been useful in distinguishing CNS lymphoma from toxoplasmosis in patients with acquired immunodeficiency syndrome (84).

Avidity to ^{18}F-FDG varies considerably in the different subtypes of NHL. Diffuse large B-cell lymphoma (DLBCL), FL, and mantle cell lymphoma (MCL) are believed to be routinely ^{18}F-FDG avid, whereas extranodal marginal zone, small lymphocytic, and T-cell NHL are variably ^{18}F-FDG avid (85). In the routinely avid NHL, PET detects disease with a sensitivity of 80% and specificity of 90% (86,87), which is superior to CT. PET/CT imaging may also be helpful to guide biopsies for the detection of histologic transformation of indolent lymphoma.

Visual assessment is usually sufficient for interpretation of a PET scan with routine use of standardized uptake value not considered to be necessary. A scan is considered to be positive if there is focal or diffuse FDG uptake above background in a location incompatible with normal anatomy and physiology. However, several exceptions have been noted for the definition of positivity (smaller masses, pulmonary nodules, hepatic and splenic lesions, and residual bone marrow involvement) in a recent recommendation by the Imaging Subcommittee of the International Harmonization Project (IHP) in lymphoma (88). Also, significant interobserver and intraobserver variability remains. The technique for performing and interpreting PET in lymphoma has recently been standardized by the same group.

The Imaging Subcommittee of the International Harmonization Project has recently outlined recommendations on the role of PET scans in staging, response assessment, restaging, and follow-up in patients with lymphoma (Table 10.4) (89). A pretherapy PET is not mandatory for routinely PET-avid lymphomas outside the setting of a clinical trial due to a lack of widespread availability and cost implications because it rarely detects disease at additional sites (approximately 15% to 20%), and a change in therapy occurs in a minority of patients (approximately 10% to 30%) (73,90). However, it is strongly recommended in DLBCL because therapy is usually delivered with curative intent, and a pretherapy PET may aid interpretation of posttherapy PET. Because therapy in FL and MCL is not usually delivered with curative intent and the end point of trials has traditionally been prolongation in progression-free and overall survival (OS), a pretherapy PET is not indicated. However, if response assessment is the end point of a clinical trial, then a pretherapy PET would be appropriate. Similarly, for variably ^{18}F-FDG-avid NHLs, including T-cell lymphomas and extranodal marginal zone lymphoma, a pretherapy PET is recommended only if response is a primary study end point in a clinical trial.

TABLE 10.4

RECOMMENDED TIMING OF PET (PET/CT) SCANS IN LYMPHOMA CLINICAL TRIALS

Histology	Pretreatment	Midtreatment	Response assessment	Posttreatment surveillance
Routinely FDG avid				
DLBCL	Yes[a]	Clinical trial	Yes	No
HL	Yes[a]	Clinical trial	Yes	No
Follicular NHL	No[b]	Clinical trial	No[b]	No
MCL	No[b]	Clinical trial	No[b]	No
Variably FDG avid				
Other aggressive NHLs	No[b]	Clinical trial	No[b,c]	No
Other indolent NHLs	No[b]	Clinical trial	No[b,c]	No

HL, Hodgkin lymphoma.
[a] Recommended but not required pretreatment.
[b] Recommended only if overall response rate/CR is a primary study end point.
[c] Recommended only if PET is positive pretreatment.
Adapted with permission from Cheson BD, Pfistner B, Juweid ME, et al. Revised response criteria for malignant lymphoma. *J Clin Oncol* 2007;25:579–586.

BONE MARROW ASPIRATION AND BIOPSY

Bone marrow disease assessment should include both an aspirate and biopsy. An aspirate maybe useful for morphologic analysis, as well as special studies, such as cytogenetics and flow cytometry; however, it does not replace a biopsy for establishing disease involvement. For optimal accuracy, bone marrow biopsies should be 2.0 cm in aggregate. For the majority of patients, unilateral bone marrow aspirate and biopsy are sufficient.

Bone marrow infiltration varies with histologic subtype. Among indolent lymphomas, small lymphocytic lymphoma/chronic lymphocytic leukemia and FL frequently exhibit bone marrow involvement. MCL commonly involves the bone marrow. In contrast, bone marrow disease is an infrequent occurrence in DLBCL.

The role of routine flow cytometry in detecting bone marrow involvement is not clearly defined, with the majority of studies suggesting that flow cytometry is redundant in most circumstances (91). However, flow cytometry may be more sensitive than morphologic examination for the detection of minimal bone marrow disease (<5%) (92). Disease-specific long-term follow-up studies are required to determine the prognostic significance of bone marrow involvement that is only detected by flow cytometry.

Magnetic Resonance Imaging for Bone Marrow Involvement

Recent studies suggest that MRI may be more sensitive than biopsy in detecting bone marrow infiltration, particularly occult disease (93). On T1-weighted images, fatty marrow is depicted by a homogeneous signal; therefore, lymphomatous involvement is readily detectable. Because MRI is able to readily assess large portions of the bone marrow, it may

direct bone marrow sampling. However, the diagnostic yield of MRI is lower in indolent lymphomas and in younger patients who tend to have a higher proportion of red marrow. Clinical information such as constitutional symptoms, bone pain, and increased alkaline phosphatase may be helpful in selecting patients with normal bone marrow biopsies who should undergo MRI (94). Although MRI may have a role in individual cases, whole body MRI is an impractical and an expensive modality for establishing lymphomatous bone marrow involvement in the majority of patients.

Positron Emission for Bone Marrow Involvement

The utility of ^{18}F-FDG PET to detect bone marrow involvement in NHL is unknown. Abnormal ^{18}F-FDG PET marrow findings include uptake equal to or greater than that in liver, uptake in the distal long bones, and heterogeneous or focal uptake (83,95). A recent metaanalysis estimated the sensitivity and specificity of PET in detecting bone marrow involvement with NHL to be 51% and 91%, respectively, with greater sensitivity in patients with more aggressive NHL (96). Both physiologic uptake and diffuse posttherapy uptake in reactive marrow have been described. Therefore, a positive PET for bone marrow involvement should be confirmed by biopsy.

ADDITIONAL PROCEDURES: SITES OF INVOLVEMENT AND PATTERNS OF PRESENTATION OF NON-HODGKIN LYMPHOMA

Specific procedures, which are not routinely performed in asymptomatic individuals, may be indicated in the presence of specific clinical symptoms. For example, neurologic symptoms should prompt a CT or MRI head imaging, and in the appropriate setting, lumbar puncture and cerebrospinal fluid (CSF) examination. Similarly, complaints of bone pain may warrant additional imaging of the skeletal system. Furthermore, some extranodal disease sites and certain NHL subtypes require additional staging studies because site-specific lymphomatous involvement may alter prognosis and treatment (Table 10.2). The following disease sites deserve special attention due to their predictive pattern of involvement, even in the absence of clinical findings.

Waldeyer Ring

The coexistence of large cell lymphoma of Waldeyer ring and the stomach was first described approximately 25 years ago (97) and repeatedly confirmed thereafter (98,99). Patients with Waldeyer ring involvement are at increased risk for GI tract involvement either at presentation or relapse. Waldeyer ring involvement has also been reported in patients with thyroid, testicular, and preauricular lymph node disease. Thus, patients with Waldeyer ring disease should have an upper GI evaluation with contrast or endoscopic studies, and, conversely, patients with the other aforementioned disease sites should have evaluation of the Waldeyer ring.

Gastrointestinal Tract

The GI tract represents the most frequent extranodal site of NHLs (2). The stomach is the most common site of lymphomatous involvement in the GI tract (100). Gastric lymphomas are typically extranodal marginal zone lymphoma, MALT–type, or DLBCL, most commonly on a background of MALT lymphoma. Endoscopic ultrasound may be helpful to establish the depth of intramural penetration (61,101), although it is suboptimal in distinguishing benign versus malignant lymph nodes (101,102). The development of gastric MALT lymphoma in the presence of *H. pylori* gastritis is well established, and pathologic evaluation should include tests to document underlying infection (103) because eradication of the organism often leads to lymphoma regression of (103,104). In addition to the customary staging evaluation, as described previously, patients with GI lymphomas should also be carefully evaluated for Waldeyer ring involvement (98).

Sinus Lymphoma

The frontal, maxillary, ethmoid, and sphenoid sinuses can all become involved with lymphoma, resulting in local symptoms of pain, nasal obstruction, facial swelling, or rhinorrhea. Sinus lymphomas are usually of aggressive histology (105,106); in North America, the majority are B-cell malignancies (105), whereas in Asia, T- or natural killer-cell tumors predominate (107). Due to the porous nature of the bony sinus walls, there is a high propensity for CNS spread (108,109). Thus, all patients with lymphomatous sinus involvement should have a lumbar puncture and CSF analysis, followed by CNS prophylaxis.

Central Nervous System and Ocular Lymphoma

Primary CNS lymphoma represents 2% of all NHLs (110). CNS lymphomas are frequently multifocal with an increased risk of concomitant leptomeningeal and ocular involvement. Initial analysis should include a CT or MRI (preferred) of the head with gadolinium enhancement, lumbar puncture with analysis of the CSF, and an ophthalmologic evaluation with a slitlamp examination. Although CSF cytology often appears benign, specific immunohistochemical studies may reveal a monoclonal population. Elevation of LDH and/or β_2-microglobulin in the CSF may also provide indirect evidence of lymphomatous involvement (111).

Ocular, as opposed to periorbital, lymphomatous involvement occurs in <1% of patients and is often incorrectly diagnosed as chronic uveitis (112). Lymphomas involving the optic nerve, retina, and vitreous are most often associated with CNS involvement (110). In contrast, lymphoma involving the uveal tract (choroids, ciliary body, and iris) is more commonly associated with visceral involvement (113) A thorough ophthalmologic examination will often identify ocular involvement; however, a vitrectomy is usually required for confirmation. Bilateral ocular involvement is possible, and concurrent brain or leptomeningeal disease is not uncommon. Thus, the initial evaluation of a patient with primary ocular NHL should include a slitlamp examination of the contralateral eye, CT or MRI imaging of the brain, and cytologic examination of the CSF fluid.

Testicular

NHL is the most common cause of a testicular mass in men over the age of 60 years. Testicular lymphomas are almost exclusively aggressive B-cell tumors (114). Approximately 30% to 40% of patients with testicular lymphoma present with advanced-stage disease. Contralateral testicular involvement is common, either at presentation or later in the disease course (115). There is also frequent involvement of the skin and Waldeyer ring, as well as CNS sites, including the meninges, epidural space, and cerebrum (116). Thus, patients with testicular lymphoma should have an ultrasound of the contralateral testis, assessment of Waldeyer ring, and CSF examination for malignant cells in addition to standard staging procedures. Furthermore, with any clinical suspicion of CNS parenchymal disease, a CT or MRI of the head is required.

Other

Patients with diffuse large cell lymphomas with bone marrow involvement may have an increased risk of leptomeningeal disease and require a lumbar puncture as part of their initial staging, and CNS prophylaxis should be considered (117,118). Highly aggressive lymphomas (lymphoblastic lymphoma and small noncleaved-cell lymphoma) and acquired immunodeficiency syndrome-related B-cell lymphomas also have a predilection for leptomeningeal disease. In these NHL subtypes, CSF analysis at diagnosis is mandatory, regardless of the presence of symptoms or other risk factors.

Lymphoma of the bone is not uncommon in advanced disease; however, it represents less than 5% of localized extranodal presentations (119). Bone pain or isolated elevation in alkaline phosphatase should prompt further studies. In addition, approximately 30% of patients with primary lymphoma of the bone will have more than one site involved (120). There does not appear to be a propensity for CNS relapse. A bone scan is highly sensitive in demonstrating bone abnormalities; however, findings are nonspecific, and should be confirmed with either a CT scan or standard radiograph and biopsy. As described, MRI (62,63) or ^{18}F-FDG PET (80) may be superior in detecting lymphoma of the bone and planning additional directed radiation therapy.

In women, lymphomas may infrequently involve the ovaries and breasts. Breast lymphoma can present bilaterally, particularly in younger woman with aggressive NHL subtypes, necessitating evaluation of the contralateral breast (121). Similarly, lymphomas of the ovary are typically aggressive NHL subtypes, and bilateral involvement is common (122).

EVALUATION OF COMORBID DISEASE

In patients with a history of cardiac disease who are scheduled to receive anthracyclines as part of their treatment regimen, baseline cardiac function should be assessed with either a multiple-gated cardiac blood pool scintigraphy or an echocardiogram. Evaluation should also be considered in patients with multiple coronary risk factors, including diabetes mellitus. In patients with a history of respiratory disease who are candidates for thoracic radiotherapy, pulmonary function tests may be needed to identify significant obstructive or restrictive lung pathology.

EVALUATION OF THE RESIDUAL MASS AFTER TREATMENT

A major clinical challenge in the management of patients with lymphoma is the evaluation of residual masses after therapy. Persistent abnormalities are often detected by physical examination, CT scan, or plain radiographs (123). However, these studies cannot reliably distinguish fibrotic or necrotic tissue from active lymphoma. Stability over time provides indirect evidence of fibrosis; nevertheless, it is often advantageous to identify persistent tumor early to optimize further curative treatment. There is poor correlation between the size of a residual mass on CT and risk of relapse (73), and MRI has not proven to be more effective in this setting than CT (124).

[67]Ga scintigraphy has been used to detect persistent viable tumor in patients with a residual mass after therapy (68,125,126). One study evaluating patients with residual mediastinal masses after treatment found the specificity of [18]Ga scintigraphy to be superior (95%) to CT (57%) or chest radiograph (55%) (125). However, reports of the positive and negative predictive value of ^{67}Ga scintigraphy vary between 70% and 80% and 65% and 85%, respectively. A new technique called transmission emission tomography, which simultaneously registers ^{67}Ga uptake with CT findings, appears promising for differentiating residual tissue from active disease (67).

^{18}F-FDG PET is also able to detect viable tumor within a residual mass (73,127,128), with greater accuracy than CT (73,129). The sensitivity and specificity of this technique for posttherapy assessment in aggressive NHL are 72% (95% confidence interval 61% to 82%) and 100% (95% confidence interval 97% to 100%), respectively (130). False positivity at a site of prior disease may be seen with rebound thymic hyperplasia or posttherapy inflammatory change. False positivity outside the site of residual masses may be seen with infection, inflammation, rebound thymic hyperplasia, sarcoidosis (131), or brown fat. Diffuse bone marrow uptake may be observed after treatment due to a bone marrow hyperproliferation (88). However, clearly increased focal marrow uptake should be interpreted as being positive. False-negative results can occur through differences in technique, resolution of equipment, reduced sensitivity for minimal residual disease and variable FDG avidity of the histologic subtypes of NHL.

At present, PET scanning after treatment is only recommended in DLBCL because therapy is usually delivered with curative intent to confirm the attainment of a complete remission (CR) (89) (Table 10.4). Biopsy of PET-positive sites is recommended if further therapy, particularly high-dose chemotherapy and stem cell transplant (SCT), is planned to confirm persistent disease (132). If biopsy is not feasible, then close follow-up with repeat imaging should be considered to monitor for disease progression. As previously discussed, if response rate is the major end point of a clinical trial assessing therapy for FL or MCL, then PET may be performed in the context of a clinical trial (89) for assessment posttherapy completion.

Ideally, posttherapy PET should be performed at least 3 weeks and 8 to 12 weeks following completion of chemotherapy and radiotherapy, respectively (88,89), because posttherapy inflammatory changes may lead to false-positive results (133,134).

There is limited data available on semiquantitative assessment of [18]FDG uptake on a posttherapy PET (78,134). As such, these standardized uptake value cutoffs remain to be validated in large prospective clinical trials and, therefore, are not recommended in routine clinical use (88).

RECOMMENDED STUDIES FOR FOLLOW-UP AFTER TREATMENT

Patient surveillance following treatment of lymphoma should address both long-term complications of therapy and disease recurrence. Long-term effects of therapy depend on the type of treatment and whether radiotherapy was also administered. Radiotherapy to the head and neck region leads to decreased salivation with dental caries; consequently, patients who have received such therapy need careful dental follow-up. Additionally, if the thyroid was included in the radiation field, a large proportion of patients may eventually become hypothyroid. Long-term survivors are also at risk for second malignancies (135,136). In an earlier survey of 6,171 patients with NHL who survived for ≥2 years, second cancers were seen in 541 subjects, with significant excesses for all solid tumors, acute myelogenous leukemia, melanoma, Hodgkin lymphoma, as well as cancers of the lung, brain, kidney, and bladder (137). In addition, following high-dose therapy with autologous bone marrow transplant (ABMT), myelodysplasia and acute leukemia have been reported at an increased frequency (138,139).

However, the greatest risk to patients treated for NHL is relapse of their disease. In aggressive NHL, the majority of recurrences are seen within 2 years of completing therapy; however, late relapses can occur in both limited (140) and advanced-stage disease (141–143). Patients with advanced indolent lymphomas are continuously at risk for relapse, and late relapses are not uncommon.

There is limited information regarding the use of routine imaging in the follow-up of patients with NHL after treatment (67,144,145). Upon completion of treatment, a set of baseline studies is warranted to provide a basis for future comparisons. The value of performing routine surveillance studies rather than responding to new clinical symptoms is not clearly established. Given that the majority (80%) of relapses are detected by patients or their physicians based on the development of new symptoms/signs (145,146), routine surveillance imaging is not currently recommended (145,147). However, in NHL subtypes that can potentially be cured with salvage, high-dose therapy, there is a theoretic advantage to early detection of recurrence (148,149). The role of surveillance abdominopelvic CT in stage I to III FL relative to standard clinical and hematologic studies has been evaluated. Only 14% of relapses were detected solely on the basis of imaging, and only 4% of those patients who achieved a CR benefited from abdominopelvic CT (146).

Current recommendations for the follow-up of patients with DLBCL completing their induction therapy include visits every 3 months for the first 2 years, followed by every 6 months until 5 years, and annually thereafter (150). In patients with indolent histology, follow-up every 3 months for the 2 years followed by every 3 to 6 months indefinitely is recommended. The recommended follow-up evaluation is shown in Table 10.5. At each visit, the following should be performed: a thorough history and physical examination; and laboratory evaluation, including a CBC and LDH. CT scan imaging should be preferred in the event of new symptoms or abnormalities on physical examination. In young patients with high-risk aggressive lymphomas, CT imaging of previously involved diseases sites can be considered. Currently, there is insufficient data to support dynamic imaging (^{18}Ga scintigraphy or ^{67}FDG PET) in the follow up of patients with NHL (89).

RECOMMENDED STUDIES FOR RECURRENT DISEASE

Once a patient is confirmed to have recurrent disease, appropriate restaging, including repeat bone marrow aspirate and biopsy, should be undertaken. Additional investigations should be guided by the presence of any new signs or symptoms. In addition, reevaluation of the cardiorespiratory status, as well as hepatic and renal function should be carried out to assess a patient's suitability for more aggressive salvage therapy.

PROGNOSITC FACTORS IN NON-HODGKIN LYMPHOMA

Introduction

The NHLs are a heterogeneous group of diseases with highly variable clinical behavior and outcome. Over the years, a number of variables have been identified that impact prognosis, including clinical factors, treatment-related variables, and biologic features. Clinical prognostic models such as the IPI have been developed to identify patient groups that are unlikely to be cured with standard therapy. However, these risk models are based on clinical features that are likely surrogate markers of underlying molecular heterogeneity. Recent advances in genetic and molecular analysis have identified specific genes and gene products that influence disease pathogenesis, prognosis, or both. Furthermore, genome-wide approaches based on gene expression profiling (GEP) have characterized the molecular signatures of distinct lymphoid neoplasms and relevant prognostic subgroups. The routine use of immunotherapy along with conventional chemotherapy has also significantly improved outcomes and prompted reevaluation of prognostic factors, particularly in patients with DLBCL. The following section will review prognostic features that have the greatest clinical relevance in NHL, with a focus on DLBCL and FL, and outline recent advances in further elucidating the molecular basis for disease heterogeneity.

Clinical Prognostic Factors

Initial Presenting Clinical Features

As previously described, the Ann Arbor staging system poses many limitations in NHL. For this reason, investigators have attempted to identify clinical prognostic factors that more

---

TABLE 10.5

RECOMMENDED FOLLOW-UP PROCEDURE FOR PATIENTS WITH NHL

History and physical examination: Same as for initial evaluation, including assessment for secondary organ toxicity from treatment
Laboratory studies: CBC and differential, LDH, β_2-microglobulin (optional), thyroid-stimulating hormone (neck radiation)
Imaging: Chest x-ray if initially involved; CT scans of chest, abdomen, pelvis (consider periodic evaluation)
Frequency of surveillance: Every 3 months for 2 yr and every 6 mo to 5 yr for aggressive lymphoma; 3 to 6 monthly for low-grade lymphoma

accurately reflect the behavior of NHLs. A number of pre-treatment clinical features have been associated with the achievement of a CR and long-term survival in patients with NHLs. These factors reflect either tumor burden and invasive potential (LDH, β_2-microglobulin, localized vs. advanced stage, number of nodal and extranodal disease sites, B symptoms, tumor size, bone marrow involvement), the patient's response to the tumor, and the patient's ability to tolerate treatment (PS, bone marrow involvement, age) (6,8,10,12,15,151–154).

Age is a particularly important prognostic factor that has been linked with poor outcome in a number of studies (155–157). Patients over the age of 60 have lower response rates and higher rates of relapse (155,156). The prognosis for patients >70 years of age appears to be worse than those patients 60 to 69 years of age (158). Many factors may contribute to poor outcome in elderly patients, including differences in disease biology, altered drug pharmacokinetics, underlying comorbid disease, and poor PS that may complicate treatment delivery. As a result, dose reductions are often carried out to avoid toxicity. Elderly patients with aggressive lymphoma who receive reduced doses of cyclophosphamide, doxorubicin, vincristine, and prednisone (CHOP)-type chemotherapy have decreased CR and more frequent relapses (159). However, with full-dose treatment, survival of elderly patients approaches that of younger patients (155). Several recent studies have confirmed that the addition of rituximab to CHOP chemotherapy (CHOPR) in DLBCL can be well tolerated in elderly patients (>60 years), and significantly improves response rates and survival (160–162). Once a CR is achieved, the disease-free survival is similar in younger and older patients. Therefore, current protocols attempt to deliver full-dose treatment to older patients with the use of growth factors (granulocyte colony-stimulating factor) if required and diligent management of infectious problems.

International Prognostic Index

The most widely used clinical prognostic model to stratify patients with aggressive NHLs is the IPI (22). Sixteen institutions from the United States, Canada, and Europe all provided information on patients with aggressive lymphomas diagnosed by the Working Formulation, Kiel and Rappaport classifications, and, thus, immunophenotypic information was not available. The purpose was to determine which pretreatment variables predict relapse-free and OS following treatment with doxorubicin-containing combination chemotherapy. Clinical features independently associated with survival were age (≤60 vs. >60), LDH (abnormal vs. normal), PS (<2 vs. ≥2), stage (I/II vs. III/IV), and number of extranodal sites (≤1 vs. >1). Each factor was determined to have an approximately equal impact on outcome, and, thus, the risk for death was estimated by adding up the number of adverse prognostic factors present at diagnosis. Four risk groups were identified: low risk (zero to one factors), low-intermediate risk (two factors), high-intermediate risk (three factors), and high risk (four to five factors). When the model was applied to 2,031 patients with aggressive lymphoma, the four risk groups had 5-year survivals of 73%, 51%, 43%, and 26%, respectively (Table 10.6) (22).

In the same study, 1,274 patients ≤60 years were evaluated using an age-adjusted model with the notion that these patients were more likely to be candidates for experimental therapy. In this simplified age-adjusted model, only stage, LDH, and PS remained independently predictive of survival, and a model based on these three features again identified four risk groups with predicted survivals of 83% (zero factors), 69% (one factor), 46% (two factors), and 32%(three factors). When the age-adjusted IPI is applied to patients >60, clear survival differences are seen in the patients with low and low-intermediate risk, further emphasizing the importance of age in clinical outcome in aggressive NHL (Table 10.6).

TABLE 10.6

IPI

Risk group	Risk factors	Distribution of cases (%)	CR rate (%)	5-yr Overall Survival
All ages				
Low (L)	0,1	35	87	73
Low-intermediate (LI)	2	27	67	51
High-intermediate (HI)	3	22	55	43
High (H)	4,5	16	44	26
Age-adjusted index (≤60)				
Low (L)	0	22	92	83
Low-intermediate (LI)	1	32	78	69
High-intermediate (HI)	2	32	57	46
High (H)	3	14	46	32
Age-adjusted index				
Low (L)	0	18	91	56
Low-intermediate (LI)	1	31	71	44
High-intermediate (HI)	2	35	56	37
High (H)	3	16	36	21

Adapted from Shipp M, Harrington D. A predictive model for aggressive non-Hodgkin's lymphoma: the International NHL Prognostic Factors Project. *N Engl J Med* 1993;329:987–994.

A stage-modified IPI has been developed for limited-stage diffuse large cell lymphomas using age, nonbulky stage II, LDH, and PS to define subgroups that should be treated more aggressively. The 5-year survival in the corresponding risk categories are: 82% (zero to one factor), 71% (two factors), and 48% (three factors) (163).

There are several limitations of the IPI. Given that it is clinically based, it does not highlight disease biology, and it has not been definitively proven that outcome is improved if treatment is altered in patients with high-risk disease. Assignment of some of the risk factors is subjective (e.g., PS), and confusion can arise as to whether a patient should be staged as having "2E" disease if multiple but contiguous extranodal disease sites are encountered or stage IV. Furthermore, the spleen was not considered an extranodal site in the IPI; however, it is often included by some physicians. Despite this, it easy to apply, allows for cross-study comparisons, and remains applicable today.

Therapy for DLBCL remained unchanged for over 2 decades and mainly consisted of CHOP or CHOP-like chemotherapy (164). In recent years, the routine addition of rituximab, a chimeric immunoglobulin (Ig) G1 monoclonal anti-CD 20 antibody, to chemotherapy regimens has resulted in superior progression-free and OS (160–162,165). The initial Groupe d'Etudes des Lymphomes de l'Adulte randomized controlled trial compared CHOP versus CHOPR in elderly (>60 years) patients with newly diagnosed, advanced-stage DLBCL. The addition of rituximab improved the CR rate (76% vs. 63%), and a 5-year update confirmed an improvement in progression-free (54% vs. 30%, p <0.00001) and overall (58% vs. 45%, p <0.0073) survival (166). Similar results were found in the ECOG study of elderly patients (162), in addition to young patients with good prognosis (167) and in a population-based study (165).

In the course of changing the treatment paradigm of DLBCL, the IPI has been reevaluated. The IPI has been applied to 365 patients treated with CHOPR in a population-based setting. The IPI remained an accurate predictor of survival, however, a revised IPI was proposed based on separation into three prognostic groups: "very good," "good," and "poor," with zero, one to two, and three to five IPI risk factors, respectively, and corresponding 4-year OSs were 94%, 79%, and 55% (168). The revised IPI remains to be validated in large prospective clinical trials, but this study does support that the IPI remains a useful prognostic tool in the post-rituximab treatment era.

Although the IPI was originally developed in aggressive lymphomas, numerous retrospective studies have confirmed its usefulness in almost all subtypes of NHL (2,169–172). The Non-Hodgkin's International Classification Project and others have also found the IPI to be prognostic in MCL and Burkitt-like lymphoma (2,28). In contrast, IPI risk categories were less useful in small series of patients with lymphoblastic lymphoma and Burkitt lymphoma.

The IPI has not been rigorously applied to PTCLs due to disease rarity and heterogeneity, and the relatively recent application of routine immunophenotyping. In recent studies of patients with T-cell lymphoma as defined by the Kiel, Revised European-American lymphoma, or World Health Organization classification, IPI-defined risk groups had significantly different outcomes (170,173–176). The IPI also appears to be useful in systemic ALCL (177–179). In more recent larger studies, ALCLs could be stratified into relevant prognostic groups using the IPI. Importantly, even in anaplastic lymphoma kinase-positive ALCL, which has an excellent prognosis, traditional clinical factors remain important in predicting survival (178–180).

The IPI has also been shown to predict survival in some studies of patients with FL (2,28,172), transformed low-grade lymphoma (181), and subtypes of NHL described as small lymphocytic, follicular small cleaved, and follicular mixed lymphoma (Working Formulation) (171). However, the IPI is less useful in FL because few patients present with "high-risk" disease (2,28), thus prompting evaluation of a new prognostic index.

The Follicular Lymphoma International Prognostic Index (FLIPI) is a prognostic index that is based on the pretreatment characteristics of 4,167 patients with FL treated at 27 centers in Europe, the United States, and Asia. Five independent prognostic variables, including age (>60 years vs. ≤60 years), Ann Arbor stage (III to IV vs. I to II), hemoglobin level (<120 g/L vs. ≥120 g/L), number of nodal sites (>4 vs. ≤4), and serum LDH (above normal vs. normal or below), are used to stratify patients into risk groups. This index separates patients based on the number of adverse prognostic variables present at diagnosis into low (zero to one), intermediate (two), and high (three or more) risk groups, with 10-year OSs of 71%, 51%, and 36%, respectively (20). The FLIPI has been found to be a better outcome predictor in patients with FL and is recommended to prognosticate in this group of patients. Because none of the protocols used in the design of FLIPI included rituximab in the treatment regimens, the predictive value of FLIPI has been reassessed in a study of 362 patients with advanced-stage FL treated with up-front CHOPR (182), and 14%, 41%, and 45% were classified as having low, intermediate, and high risk, respectively. The 2-year time to treatment failure was significantly shorter in the high-risk compared with the low and intermediate-risk groups (67% vs. 92% and 90% respectively), confirming the predictive value of FLIPI in the "Rituximab era."

Treatment-Related Prognostic Factors

Time to Achieve Complete Remission and the Residual Mass

In subtypes of NHL that are potentially curable with current induction therapy, the rapidity of response to treatment may have prognostic significance (123,183). In one of the earliest studies to demonstrate the importance of rapidity of response, patients with aggressive lymphomas who failed to achieve a remission by the third cycle of chemotherapy had an inferior outcome (183). In an additional large series of patients with aggressive lymphoma, time to CR was the single most important predictor of OS (184).

Recently, important prognostic information has been attained from ^{18}F-FDG PET in the analysis of tumor response. As described previously, ^{18}F-FDG PET differentiates between fibrosis and active lymphoma by measuring glucose uptake (71) and provides additional information regarding the nature of a residual mass (73,127,185). Several studies have confirmed the prognostic significance of visual normalization of FDG uptake as early as after one to four cycles of chemotherapy (186–188). In representative series evaluating mainly aggressive NHL where therapy was not influenced as a result of the midtreatment PET scan, relapse or disease progression was noted in 71% to 100% of patients with positive midtreatment PET scans with 2-year event-free survival (EFS) was 0% to 35% as opposed to an estimated 2-year EFS of 72% to 93% in patients with a negative midtreatment scan (188). The median time to treatment failure was found to be significantly longer (35 months vs. 1.5 months) in a retrospective study of 70 patients with aggressive NHL with a negative midtreatment (two to four cycles) scan versus a positive one (186). In another study of 90 patients with aggressive NHL where positive midtreatment PET prompted consideration of an autologous SCT, 40% of patients were found to be PET positive after two cycles of therapy. With this therapy modification, the 2-year EFS was 43% versus 82% in patients with a positive and negative midtreatment PET scan, respectively (187). Currently, an ECOG (E3404) study is underway assessing the role of PET after three cycles of CHOPR and treatment modification based on the results. Patients who are PET negative complete therapy with three further cycles of CHOPR, whereas PET-positive patients complete therapy with one additional cycle of CHOPR and four cycles of rituximab, ifosfamide, cisplatin and etoposide. At present, however, there is no clear evidence of improvement in patient outcomes with change in therapy based on midtreatment PET. Also, there is no uniform approach to change in therapy based on these results, and so, at present, the role of midtreatment PET in patient management outside of the setting of a clinical trial is unclear. Therefore, the current recommendation of the Imaging Subcommittee of the International Harmonization Project is for midtreatment PET to be performed in the context of prospective clinical trials (89) (Table 10.4).

Prognostic Factors in Refractory and Relapsed Disease

The management of patients with relapsed lymphoma remains a challenge. Approximately 5% to 10% of patients with aggressive lymphoma fail initial induction, and 20% to 40% who achieve an initial CR develop recurrent disease.

Chemosensitivity to Salvage Therapy

Although at least 50% of patients with relapsed aggressive lymphomas remain chemosensitive, less than 10% have durable remissions with second-line chemotherapy regimens (149,189,190). However, a subset of patients with chemosensitive recurrent disease is cured with high-dose chemotherapy (HDC) and autologous stem cell transplant (SCT) (191–195). Patients who achieve a CR to standard salvage therapy have more favorable outcomes following HDC and SCT (196). In contrast, patients whose relapsed disease is resistant to conventional second-line chemotherapy have a poor outcome to HDC and SCT, with an EFS similar to that observed with salvage regimens (149,192,197).

Failure to Achieve Complete Remission to Induction Therapy

Patients with primary progressive aggressive NHL have a dismal prognosis, faring much worse than those who relapse after attaining a CR (198–200). Clinical features that are associated with shortened OS in NHL are also linked with a lower likelihood of attaining an initial CR (199). However, a small proportion of patients with primary progressive or refractory disease who demonstrate clear chemosensitivity to salvage regimens may benefit from HDC and SCT (195,200,201).

Duration of First Remission

The duration of remission is the single most important predictor of outcome in patients with recurrent aggressive lymphoma (202). Patients with early relapses (<1 year) have a much poorer outcome than those with late relapses (>1 year). The duration of first remission is also related to OS in patients with indolent NHL (203). Patients <60 years of age with a CR or PR of <1 year had a median survival of 2.4 years, whereas those with remissions lasting >1 year had a median survival of 5.9 years.

Clinical Features in Relapsed and Refractory Lymphoma

Factors reflecting tumor burden (bulky disease, advanced stage at relapse, the number of extranodal sites, increased LDH) and patient tolerance for additional therapy (age, PS) are also predictive of outcome in relapsed disease (204,205). The IPI has also been found to be predictive of outcome at relapse. The "second-line" IPI (sIPI) was first analyzed in patients with relapsed aggressive NHL who were randomized to receive additional (dexamethasone, high-dose Ara-C, cisplatin therapy or HDC and ABMT in the Parma trial (206). In patients receiving conventional salvage dexamethasone, high-dose Ara-C, cisplatin therapy, the age-adjusted sIPI was highly correlated with 5-year OS; patients with one, two, or three risk factors had a 5-year OS of 33%, 21%, and 0%, respectively. However, the sIPI did not correlate with 5-year survival in the ABMT arm, suggesting that transplant overcame the poor outcome of patients with one or more risk factors (206). Of interest, patients with zero risk factors who were treated with dexamethasone, high-dose Ara-C, cisplatin or HDT and SCT had comparable outcomes. In a similar study, the predictive value of the sIPI was evaluated in patients who had relapsed or with refractory NHL before receiving ifosfamide, carboplatin, and etoposide, followed by SCT. The sIPI defined two groups: zero to two risk factors, 2.5-year failure-free survival 45%; and three to five risk factors, 2.5-year failure-free survival 9% (207). The same investigators applied the age-adjusted sIPI to a group of patients with primary refractory aggressive NHL, and found that patients with two and three risk factors had poor response rates to salvage treatment (30%) and a dismal 3-yr survival rate (7.4%) (201).

Disease-Related Prognostic Factors

Histopathologic Subtype

The Working Formulation divided NHLs into three groups (or grades) based on growth pattern, cell size, and untreated natural history: (a) low, (b) intermediate, and (b) high grade. The more recent Revised European-American lymphoma and the World Health Organization classifications incorporate more subtle morphologic distinctions, immunophenotypic signatures, and hallmark genetic abnormalities to define several unique biologic entities (32,208) with characteristic natural histories. For example, MCL was recognized as having unique phenotypic (CD5+, CD23-) and genotypic features [t(11;14)(q13;32)], and a natural history characterized by frequent relapses and lack of curative potential. In DLBCL, several disease subtypes are now recognized on the basis of: (a) clinical characteristics and cell of origin (COO) (primary mediastinal large B-cell lymphoma [PMBCL]); (b) histologic appearance (intravascular lymphoma); and (c) viral pathogenesis (primary effusion lymphoma, lymphomatoid granulomatosis). These distinctions are of prognostic relevance because certain newly identified entities have much less favorable natural histories. More recently, GEP has been applied to DLBCL and identified different prognostic subgroups based on a "cell of origin" molecular signature (see below DLBCL).

B- versus T-Cell Phenotype

Approximately 12% to 15% of all NHLs have a T-cell phenotype (2). The T-cell lymphomas are a heterogeneous group of diseases with diverse clinical behavior, immunophenotypic features, and prognosis. The PTCLs are defined as those as being post-thymic in origin. Initial studies failed to reveal a prognostic difference between aggressive B- and T-cell lymphomas (209). However, treatment regimens were nonuniform, and these reports were before the recognition of specific disease entities with unique natural histories. More recent studies support the notion that PTCLs have a worse outcome than DLBCLs (28,174,210–212). In the most common subgroup PTCL subtype, PTCL not otherwise specified that the IPI may identify a low-risk group with a more favorable prognosis (170,175,213,214). In contrast, the T-cell or null-cell ALCLs have a more favorable natural history and additional biologic heterogeneity. Those expressing the t(2;5) anaplastic lymphoma kinase fusion protein have a superior survival compared with those who are anaplastic lymphoma kinase negative (177,178,180), and the IPI also provides additional prognostic information in both types of systemic ALCLs. Many of the rare PTCL subtypes (e.g., enteropathy type, HTLV-1 associated, hepatosplenicγδ) have an extremely poor prognosis, emphasizing the heterogeneity of PTCL and the need to consider these diseases separately.

Biologic Prognostic Factors

The IPI remains the most useful prognostic tool for identification of patients who are unlikely to be cured with standard therapies. However, over the last several years, it has become clear that the clinical features that define "high-risk" disease are likely to be surrogate variables for intrinsic cellular and molecular heterogeneity. Immunophenotypic, cellular, immune, and molecular markers are being increasingly utilized in diagnosis, disease characterization, and initial risk assessment. More recent genome-wide approaches to risk assessment are even more promising.

Molecular Signatures of Prognosis

Molecular analyses of clinical heterogeneity in lymphoid malignancies have largely focused on individual candidate genes, with particular emphasis on genes with known functions in

other malignancies or in normal lymphocyte development. Although some of these candidate genes correlate with outcome, a comprehensive molecular approach to outcome prediction has been lacking. The development of deoxyribonucleic acid (DNA) microarrays provides an opportunity to take a genome-wide approach to predict treatment outcome in specific lymphoid neoplasms. In addition to providing molecular correlates of clinical outcome, genomic approaches may also improve diagnostic accuracy, identify new disease entities, and elucidate novel therapeutic targets.

Two major types of microarray platforms are currently in use: complementary DNA (cDNA) and oligonucleotide microarrays. In brief, cDNA arrays are comprised of polymerase chain reaction-amplified cDNA clones that have been systematically deposited onto glass slides or nitrocellulose filters (215). In the most commonly used protocols, sample and reference ribonucleic acids (RNAs) are used to generate fluorescently labeled cDNAs, which are then simultaneously hybridized to the arrays. In contrast, oligonucleotide microarrays are generated by depositing previously synthesized oligonucleotide probes onto slides or directly synthesizing these probes on the surface of silicon wafers (215). This approach offers the advantage of uniform probe length, more precise information regarding specific splice variants, and the capacity for analyzing approximately 60,000 human genes and expressed sequence tags in a single experiment.

There are two main computational approaches to analyzing the data generated by GEP: unsupervised and supervised learning (Fig. 10.1). Unsupervised learning algorithms (e.g., hierarchical clustering, self-organizing maps) cluster samples according to similarities in their gene expression profiles without a priori assumptions regarding the basis for the designated clusters (215). However, due to the complexity of gene expression profiles, many different relationships may exist in a data set, and an unsupervised learning algorithm may not

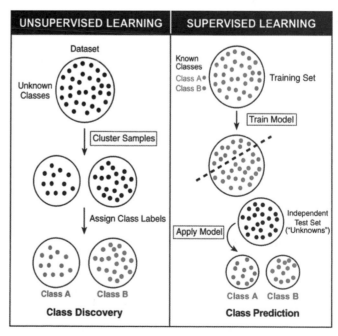

FIGURE 10.1 Unsupervised versus supervised learning. (Adapted from Ramaswamy S, Golub TR. DNA microarrays in clinical oncology. *J Clin Oncol* 2002;20:1932–1941.)

directly address a specific clinical question. In contrast, supervised learning methods (e.g., weighted voting, k-nearest neighbor, support vector machine) can be used to develop gene expression profiles reflective of specific, predetermined differences (i.e., curved vs. fatal/refractory disease) (215).

Diffuse Large B-Cell Lymphoma

DLBCL represents the largest group of NHLs, accounting for 30% to 40% of all lymphoma cases. It has long been recognized that there is significant clinical and biologic heterogeneity within this subgroup, prompting speculation that it may be made of more than one disease. The earliest study of GEP in DLBCL using the lymphochip demonstrated at least two distinct molecular subgroups defined by genes associated with different stages of differentiation through unsupervised learning and hierarchical clustering. One group was called "germinal center B cell" like (GCB) DLBCL, demonstrating a molecular signature reminiscent of normal GCBs (e.g., CD10 and BCL6), and the other was termed "activated B-cell" like (ABC), reminiscent of mitogenically ABCs (216). Importantly, the 5-year survival for the GCB-like DLBCL group was 76% as opposed to 16% for the ABC-like DLBCL group. This model was found to be independent of the IPI, with even low-risk (zero to one risk factors) patients belonging to the ABC-like group having a markedly worse survival outcome compared with the GCB-like group. A further larger retrospective study of lymphoma samples from 240 patients with DLBCL using a revised COO signature using 100 genes that best differentiated these two groups (111) has confirmed the significant survival difference between the GCB and ACB subtypes of DLBCL (59% vs. 34%), and also identified a less well-characterized "Type 3" DLBCL with a similar survival to ACB DLBCL (Fig. 10.2) (217). Subsequently, Cox proportional hazard modeling identified signatures associated with outcome beyond the COO signature. The germinal center (GC), lymph node signature, and major histocompatibility complex (MHC) class II expression were all found to be associated with a more favorable outcome, whereas a proliferation signature and increased expression of bone morphogenetic protein 6 were associated with an aggressive course (217). The lymph node signature and MHC class II expression may represent the host immune response to the lymphoma and thereby influence outcome (218). The COO signature has since been refined and limited to only 27 genes, and uses a Bayes' rule to assign tumor samples to either the GC versus non-GCB phenotypes (219).

Tissue microarrays allow high-throughput study of protein expression, thereby facilitating the identification of prognostic models applicable to clinical practice. The advantages of this technique over GEP include its wider availability and cost-effectiveness with multiple samples being evaluated in a single tissue section (220). Paraffin-embedded formalin-fixed material can be assessed as opposed to fresh tissue as required by GEP. Given the limited ability to apply GEP in clinical practice, an attempt has been made to capture the molecular signature by immunohistochemistry (IHC) using a tissue microarray (220). Cases of newly diagnosed DLBCL treated with anthracycline-based chemotherapy were subclassified using CD10, BCL6, and MUM1 expression into GCB and "non-GCB" subgroups. The 5-year OS for the GCB group was 76% versus 34% for the non-GCB group. The same study also demonstrated the improvement in OS with the individual expression of CD10 and BCL6, and the adverse survival outcomes with the expression of MUM1, cyclin D2, and BCL2. The positive predictive value for accurate classification of DLBCL into GCB type and ABC type was 87% and 73%, respectively, with cDNA microarray classification as the gold standard (220). However, application of the algorithm has been met with mixed findings where some studies have found results consistent with the Hans study (221–223), whereas others have observed conflicting results (224). The reproducibility of this approach can be limited by variations in laboratory techniques, scoring definitions, antibodies used, and interobserver and intraobserver variations; in addition, some cases are negative for all

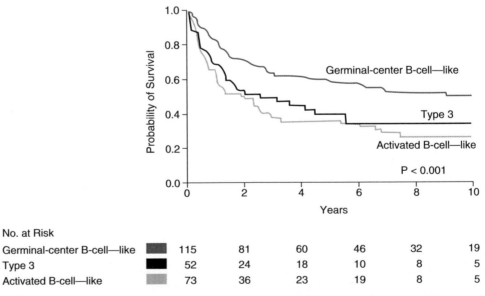

FIGURE 10.2 No., Number. (Adapted from Rosenwald A, Wright G, Chan WC, et al. The use of molecular profiling to predict survival after chemotherapy for diffuse large-B-cell lymphoma. *N Engl J Med* 2002;346:1937–1947.)

markers, and by default, they are assigned to the non-GCB group because there is no unclassified category. The recognition of these limitations has led to an international biomarker consortium to concentrate on the validation and standardization of IHC of prognostic markers in DLBCL (225). In this study, samples were stained for common prognostic and diagnostic markers (e.g., CD20, BCL2, BCL6) according to local methods, and significant variation was seen in the results for almost all markers; particularly BCL6 laboratory variations had a major impact on results along with the inability to assess an individual patient's staining result due to technical artifact or lack of internal control. In view of this significant variability in results, treatment stratification based on these prognostic markers should be limited at present to clinical trials with central pathology review.

A further study (226) described alternative subtypes of DLBCL based on biologically meaningful gene signatures. Using a U133 Affymetrix microarray encompassing all known genes in the human genome, three clusters were identified using a resampling-based method (consensus clustering): OXPHOS group, characterized by increased expression of genes associated with oxidative phosphorylation; B-cell receptor group, with increased expression the B-cell receptor signaling and proliferation genes; and host response group, with increased expression of genes associated with T cells and inflammatory bystander cells. The groups captured by this approach are different from the COO, indicating that the two approaches reflect different aspects of DLBCL biologic heterogeneity; however, there was no correlation with outcome observed in the consensus clusters.

Primary Mediastinal Large B-Cell Lymphoma

PMBCL is clinicopathologic subtype of DLBCL that also appears to have a molecular signature that is distinct from DLBCL (227,228). Two expression profiling studies support that PMBCL has an overlapping gene expression signature with classic Hodgkin lymphoma. High levels of expression of interleukin-13 and downstream effectors (Janus kinase-2, signal transducers and activators of transcription-1), tumor necrosis factor family members, and tumor necrosis factor receptor-associated factor-1 have been found in the PMBCL specimens. In addition, like classic Hodgkin lymphoma, there was evidence of nuclear factor (NF)-κB activation, suggesting the importance of this pathway in both diseases. Using a refined molecular signature, the outcome of PMBCL was favorable (228).

Follicular Lymphoma

A study of GEP in untreated FL has identified two gene signatures that separated patients into distinct prognostic groups (229). The two signatures immune-response 1 and immune-response 2 were separated by the genes expressed by nonmalignant tumor-infiltrating cells. The immune-response 1 signature consisted largely of T-cell-restricted genes and was associated with an improved survival, whereas the immune-response 2 signature included genes preferentially expressed by monocytes, dendritic cells, or both, and was associated with an adverse prognosis. The addition of rituximab to chemotherapy regimens for FL appears to circumvent the negative prognostic value of high tumor-associated macrophage (TAM) content in FL. In patients treated with CHOPR, a high TAM content, determined through IHC,

was associated with a significantly improved progression free compared with patients with low TAM scores ($p = 0.006$) (230). Another more recent study using the same technique found no influence of high TAM count on survival in patients treated with rituximab and anthracycline-containing chemotherapy (231). However, a high tumoral mast cell count appears to continue to correlate to adverse outcomes, even with CHOPR chemotherapy (232).

Single Gene Signatures and Prognosis

In another early profiling study in DLBCL, signatures predictive of outcome (cured vs. fatal/refractory DLBCL) were identified. Using a supervised approach, 13 genes were identified, including those involved in serine/threonine phosphorylation, B-cell receptor signaling, and regulation of apoptosis (233). Protein kinase C β was one of the genes overexpressed in tumors that ultimately resulted in fatal or refractory DLBCL and is under evaluation as a rational therapeutic target in DLBCL (234).

GEP is currently not widely available and is dependent on the availability of frozen biopsy specimens. Lossos et al. (235) have attempted to apply a simplified biologic outcome prediction model in DLBCL, tailored for clinical usage using quantitative reverse-transcriptase polymerase chain reaction to evaluate a condensed set of prognostic markers identified by both the lymphochip and oligonucleotide array platforms in addition to known single prognostic genes. Six genes that had the most striking impact on outcome (BCL6, cyclin D2, BCL2, SCYA3, LMO2, and FN1) were used to develop a prognostic model to differentiate patient groups with significantly different outcome. The model generated separated patients into low, intermediate, and high-risk groups, with a 5-year survival of 65%, 49%, and 15%, respectively, and was predictive of survival independent of the IPI. This approach has some appeal based on a readily available technique, the generation of quantitative data, and a requirement for less RNA. However, by focusing on single prognostic genes across all DLBCLs, this model fails to elucidate deregulated pathways and novel therapeutic targets that may be employed in different DLBCL biologic or prognostic subgroups.

LMO2 is a transcription factor with a significant role in erythropoiesis, angiogenesis, and embryogenesis. The expression of this gene was found to be the best predictor of outcome in a model constructed on the expression of six genes (235). LMO2 has been found to be overexpressed in GC-type DLBCL. A recent study using a tissue microarray established that LMO2 is prognostic in CHOP and CHOPR-treated patients with DLBCL, independent of the IPI (236).

Immune System-Related Prognostic Factors

Major Histocompatibility Molecules

It has been postulated that the absence of MHC-encoded recognition structures may limit the ability of the host to mount an immune response against specific tumor antigens. In earlier studies of patients with aggressive lymphomas, tumors lacking human leukocyte antigen (HLA)-DR were associated with shorter survivals than tumors with intact HLA-DR expression (237). Further tumor expression of class I and class II MHC determinants was found to correlate with the number of CD8+ T-tumor infiltrating lymphocytes in patients with aggressive NHL (238). These results have been confirmed in more recent studies of GEP of MHC class II expression correlated with protein status and tumor-infiltrating lymphocytes (217,239). The 5-year OS was found to be 24%, 37%, 50%, and 55% in patients with the lowest 10%, 10% to 25%, 25% to 50%, and the highest 50% HLA-DR expression. The HLA-DR gene expression correlated with HLA-DR protein expression and the number of CD8+ T cells infiltrating the tumor (239). Together, these reports suggest that an impaired host immune system maybe implicated in both disease pathogenesis and poor response to treatment.

Host Immune Response

The presence of tumor-infiltrating T-lymphocytes has been consistently observed in patients with NHL, suggesting that the host immune response may be a critical factor in determining patient outcome (240–242). This is in keeping with earlier observations correlating the absence of HLA-DR on tumors with an impaired immune response and worse outcome (237). Reports focusing on cytotoxic T cells (CD8+) have suggested that low levels are correlated with patient relapse and/or survival in some lymphoproliferative disorders (243,244). However, helper T-cells (CD4+) levels may be even more critical in determining patient outcome. In a recent study, patients with low levels of tumor infiltrating memory CD4+ cells had a poorer outcome than patients with higher levels of comparable T cells (240). The significance of the percentage of CD4+ infiltration was maintained, along with the IPI, in multivariate analysis (240). More recently, the gene expression profile of T-cell-rich and T-cell poor DLBCL has been evaluated, and >500 genes were differentially expressed in the T-cell-rich group, including certain class II MHC molecules and chemokines. In contrast, adhesion molecules and proliferative markers, such as c-myc, were underrepresented in the T-cell-rich group (245).

Antiapoptosis Proteins

Abnormalities in the balance between cell death and cell viability are critical in the pathogenesis and prognosis of a number of malignancies, including NHL. Many investigators have studied the prognostic significance of proteins that regulate cell cycle (Rb, p27, p21, p53) and apoptosis (p53, bcl-2, survivin, NF-κB) in lymphoid malignancies.

Bcl-2 Bcl-2. was the first described member of a family of apoptosis regulators that homodimerize or heterodimerize. The antiapoptotic protein is widely expressed in both hemopoietic and nonhemopoietic cells; however, it is absent from the GCs of B-cell follicles and from cortical thymocytes (246,247). Bcl-2 overexpression inhibits cell death (248,249), and confers both chemotherapy and radiation resistance (250). Overexpression of bcl-2 occurs in approximately 80% to 90% of FLs, often in association with a t(14;18), which brings the bcl-2 gene under the control of the Ig heavy chain promoter. In diffuse large cell lymphomas, overexpression of the bcl-2 protein is associated with decreased disease-free and OS (251–254). In aggressive B-cell lymphomas, bcl-2 protein is often elevated in the absence of the t(14;18),

suggesting that there are other mechanisms of bcl-2 protein overexpression in these tumors.

In a recent large series of patients treated with CHOP-type chemotherapy with nodal DLBCL, bcl-2 expression was combined with the IPI to increase the predictive value of the IPI (221). Both bcl-2 expression and the IPI were independent poor prognostic factors. Using the IPI alone, only 8% of nodal DLBCLs were identified as being high risk. However, patients in the intermediate-risk group whose tumors expressed high levels of bcl-2- had inferior OSs, comparable to that of the high-risk group.

p53. is a tumor suppressor gene located on chromosome 17, which induces cell cycle arrest and/or apoptosis in response to a variety of stimuli. Mutations in p53 can occur through deletions or rearrangements that lead to loss of function or through dominant-negative mutations (255). p53 mutation can prevent apoptosis, and confer resistance to chemotherapy and radiation treatment (256). Wild-type p53 has a short half-life and is not generally detectable by routine IHC (257). In contrast, mutated p53 has a prolonged half-life, making it detectable by immunostaining techniques. However, p53 immunostaining is complicated by the high frequency of mutations inducing stop codons in the open-reading frame and the occasional detection of background wild-type protein (257).

p53 mutations in NHL appear limited to the late stages of indolent lymphomas (258,259), aggressive lymphoid malignancies (260,261), and relapsed disease (256). In FL, p53 mutations and increased protein expression are associated with higher grades and transformed disease (258,259). MCLs with p53 mutations and immunopositivity have poorer prognoses than those tumors with wild-type P53 (262,263). Mutated p53 has been described more frequently in aggressive lymphomas, with or without abnormalities in 17p; these p53 mutations frequently have been associated with complex karyotypic abnormalities, p53 protein expression, and poor outcome (264). Recent studies suggest that mutations in the DNA-binding codon are associated with poor OS and decreased expression of tumor necrosis factor-related apoptosis-inducing ligand-receptor-2 (265).

Nuclear Factor-κB. NF-κB is a member of the Rel protein family that plays a prominent role in lymphocyte development, activation, and the prevention of apoptosis (266). High levels of NF-κB are required for B-cell proliferation and survival in response to mitogens. NF-κB transcriptional activity is governed by homodimerization and heterodimerization of the NF-κB family members, and by interactions with members of the IκB family of inhibitors that retain (IκB) NF-κB dimers in the cytoplasm (265). Phosphorylation of IkB by IkB kinase targets IkB for ubiquitination and degradation, allowing NF-κB to translocate to the nucleus and activate transcription of a number of targets, including members of the BCL-2 family (e.g., BCL-2, BFL-1/A1,BCL-XL) (266–268). Recent studies suggest that the survival of the malignant cells in the poor-prognosis ABC-like DLBCL is dependent on the constitutive activation of the NF-κB signaling pathway. (266). CARD11 is a cytoplasmic scaffolding protein that is required for the antigen-receptor-induced activation of the NF-κB signaling pathway. Mutations in the coiled-coil domain of CARD11 have been identified in approximately 10% of ABC DLBCL biopsy samples. In lymphoma cell lines, introduction of this mutation resulted in constitutive activation of NF-κB and enhanced response on antigen-receptor stimulation, suggesting a potential therapeutic target in the management of ABC DLBCL (269).

Proliferative Indices

Ki-67 is a nuclear antigen expressed by dividing tumor cells. The percentage of cells expressing Ki-67 reflects the number of cells that are cycling. In patients with aggressive lymphomas, high Ki-67 expression (>80%) has been correlated with poor prognosis (18% survival at 1 year), whereas low Ki-67 expression has been linked with favorable outcome (82% at 1 year) (270,271). However, other studies have failed to confirm the prognostic value of Ki-67 expression in DLBCL (272,273). These differences may be due to the varying definitions of Ki-67 positivity (225) and the relative resistance of tumors with low proliferative rates to chemotherapy because large numbers of malignant cells are in G0/G1 of the cell cycle.

Tumor Invasiveness

A number of factors in NHL have been linked to the invasive potential of the tumor, including overexpression of matrix metalloproteinases, angiogenic peptides, and proteins that influence cellular migration. For example, overexpression of a major matrix metalloproteinase, gelatinase B, has been linked with shortened survival in patients with a subtype of DLBCL (immunoblastic lymphoma) (274).

Tumor angiogenesis is critical for local growth and distant spread of hematologic malignancies(275). In earlier analyses of microvessel densities, aggressive lymphomas had more prominent evidence of a tumor vasculature (276). Vascular endothelial growth factor (VEGF) is a potent angiogenic peptide with demonstrated prognostic significance in multiple tumor types (277–279). Elevated VEGF serum levels in a subset of patients with NHL have been found to correlate with adverse outcome (280). In an additional broad-based analysis of molecular prognostic factors in DLBCL, increased VEGF transcripts were associated with fatal/refractory disease (233). Furthermore, high pretreatment levels of another angiogenic peptide, basic fibroblast growth factor, have also been correlated with inferior survival in DLBCL (281). A recent multi-institutional study has found high tumor vascularity to be predictive of adverse outcomes in de novo DLBCL. As opposed to the aforementioned studies, the same study also found high VEGF and VEGF receptor-1 protein expression by lymphoma cells to correlate with improved progression free and OS, independent of the IPI (282).

In additional recent studies, a novel risk-related gene family, BAL1 and 2 were identified and found to be highly expressed in fatal/refractory DLBCLs (283). Overexpression of cloned BAL 1 cDNAs increased the migratory potential of DLBCL cell lines, suggesting that BAL family members may promote tumor dissemination.

Genetic and Molecular Abnormalities

Hematologic malignancies are characterized by translocations, deletions, and other nonrandom genetic alterations (284–286).

Conventional cytogenetics is limited to the analysis of metaphase chromosomes. Fluorescence in situ hybridization has enabled the detection of chromosomal aberrations in interphase nuclei using probes that span the Ig locus (287). The recent introduction of spectral karyotyping has provided even more precise identification of rearrangements in lymphoid malignancies (288).

t(14;18) and bcl-2

The t(14;18)(q32;q21) translocation is the most common translocation in lymphoid tumors. As a result of the translocation, the Bcl-2 gene on chromosome 18 is juxtaposed to the promoter region of the Ig heavy chain region on chromosome 14, resulting in constitutive expression of the bcl-2 protooncogene. The t(14;18) is found in up to 90% of FLs (289) and approximately 20% to 33 % of aggressive NHLs (251). It is unclear whether the presence of a t(14;18) in DLBCL is a marker of histologic transformation of a previous FL, or reflects an early transforming event in a subset of de novo DLBCL (257). Although a bcl-2 protein expression impacts outcome in DLBCL, patients who harbor a t(14;18) do not appear to have a worse prognosis (251,290). This is in keeping with the observation that t(14;18) travels with the GCB phenotype.

BCL-6

Chromosomal alterations involving the band 3q27 are the most common karyotypic abnormalities in DLBCL (291). Chromosome rearrangements that substitute Ig regulatory elements or alternate promoters upstream of the bcl-6 coding region are found in approximately 40% of DLBCLs, except PMBCL. Subsequent cloning of the 3q27 breakpoints identified the involved gene to be Bcl-6. The Bcl-6 translocation can involve either an Ig or non-Ig partner (292). The Bcl-6 gene encodes a POZ/zinc finger sequence-specific transcriptional repressor, which is specifically expressed in normal GC B cells (293). Although 3q27 translocations are also found in Burkitt lymphoma (291) and a small fraction of FLs (294), they are noticeably absent in other lymphoid neoplasms. Additional somatic point mutations that alter the bcl-6 5' regulatory region, independent of 3q27 translocations, are found in up to 70% of DLBCLs (295), and may accompany transformation of FL to DLBCL (296).

To date, the prognostic significance of bcl-6 rearrangements and mutations is unclear. Although an earlier study suggested that tumors with bcl-6 gene rearrangements were linked with better clinical outcomes (297), the majority of studies have failed to demonstrate this benefit (298,299).

However, more recent studies have correlated the expression of bcl-6 at both the messenger RNA or protein level with an improved OS in patients with DLBCL treated with chemotherapy (220,300). Patients with low or high clinical risk by the IPI were further stratified based on bcl-6 gene expression (300). Bcl-6 mRNA levels were recently compared in DLBCLs with bcl-6 translocations involving Ig or other partner genes. Of interest, bcl-6 transcripts were significantly more abundant in tumors with Ig/bcl-6 translocations, and these tumors were associated with a more favorable prognosis (301).

Prognostic Factors of Diffuse Large B-Cell Lymphoma in the Rituximab-Treatment Era

With the improved outcome of DLBCL with CHOPR chemotherapy, previously defined prognostic factors in DLBCL are under reevaluation. The GCB versus ABC distinction has been reevaluated in 156 patients treated with CHOPR chemotherapy using the Affymetrix U133 array, and both subtypes have a improved outcome in comparison to the historical survival with CHOP, however, the GCBs still retain a more favorable outcome (3 year OS 86% vs. 68%, $p = 0.014$) (302). Furthermore, lymph node and proliferation signatures, but not the MHC class II signature, maintained their prognostic importance in CHOPR-treated patients. In contrast, applying the Hans algorithm to differentiate tumors as GCB versus non-GCB in a group of patients treated with CHOPR, the prognostic distinction was no longer apparent, however, this may also reflect the limitations of immunohistochemical studies, and further studies validating the COO signature at a protein level are needed (303).

The prognostic impact of BCL2 and BCL6 has also been reevaluated in CHOPR-treated patients (304,305). In comparison to CHOP, CHOPR was found to preferentially improve OS in bcl 2+ patients (67% vs. 48%) versus bcl 2- patients (72% vs. 67%) (306). A separate ECOG study evaluated whether the favorable prognostic significance of BCL6 expression is maintained in CHOPR-treated patients. Similarly, only patients who were BCL6- had an improved OS with CHOPR (2 year OS 79% vs. 17%), and there was no apparent benefit in the favorable BCL6 + group (306). Given that interpretation of BCL6 status is subject to the greatest variability and poorest agreement (225), these results need to be validated with standardized testing.

The disparity in results may relate to the limitations of using an IHC-based approach as outlined previously, or the addition of rituximab is altering the impact of established prognostic factors. Further studies are needed to confirm the gene expression results and determine if this translates into differences at a protein level using more stringent IHC criteria for the GCB versus ACB distinction and other prognostic markers. Furthermore, in view of this significant variability in results, treatment stratification based on these prognostic markers should be limited at present to clinical trials with central pathology review (225).

SUMMARY

Accurate staging in patients with lymphoma is critical to ensure the correct therapy is administered. Clinical prognostic models are helpful for study comparisons and estimating the chance of cure with standard therapy but do not provide insight into biology. Gene expression studies in lymphomas have proven useful to elucidate underlying biologic heterogeneity, improve diagnostic accuracy, prognosticate, and are already showing promise for the identification of rational therapeutic targets.

REFERENCES

1. Carbone P, Kaplan H, Musshoff K, et al. Report of the Committee on Hodgkin's disease staging. *Cancer Res* 1971;31:1860–1861.
2. Armitage J. For The Non-Hodgkin's Lymphoma Classification Project. A clinical evaluation of the International Lymphoma Study Group classification of non-Hodgkin's lymphoma. *Blood* 1997;89:3909–3918.
3. d'Amore F, Christensen BE, Brincker H, et al. Clinicopathological features and prognostic factors in extranodal non- Hodgkin lymphomas. Danish LYFO Study Group. *Eur J Cancer* 1991;27:1201–1208.
4. Zucca E, Roggero E, Bertoni F, et al. Primary extranodal non-Hodgkin's lymphomas. Part 1: gastrointestinal, cutaneous and genitourinary lymphomas. *Ann Oncol* 1997;8:727–737.
5. Zucca E, Roggero E, Bertoni F, et al. Primary extranodal non-Hodgkin's lymphomas. Part 2: Head and neck, central nervous system and other less common sites. *Ann Oncol* 1999;10:1023–1033.
6. Fisher R DV, Johnson BL, Simon R, et al. Prognostic factors for advanced diffuse histiocytic lymphoma following treatment with combination chemotherapy. *Amer J Med* 1977;63:177–182.
7. Ferraris AM, Giuntini P, Gaetani GF. Serum lactic dehydrogenase as a prognostic tool for non-Hodgkin lymphomas. *Blood* 1979;54:928–932.
8. Armitage JO DF, Corder MP, Garneau SC, et al. Predicting therapeutic outcome in patients with diffuse histiocytic lymphoma with cyclophosphamide, adriamycin, vincristine and prednisone (CHOP). *Cancer* 1982;50:1695–1702.
9. Fisher RI, Hubbard SM, DeVita VT, et al. Factors predicting long-term survival in diffuse mixed, histiocytic, or undifferentiated lymphoma. *Blood* 1981;58:45–51.
10. Jagannath S, Velasquez W, Tucker S, et al. Tumor burden assessment and its implication for a prognostic model in advanced diffuse large-cell lymphoma. *J Clin Oncol* 1986;4:859–865.
11. Jagannath S, Velasquez WS, Tucker SL, et al. Stage IV diffuse large-cell lymphoma: a long-term analysis. *J Clin Oncol* 1985;3:39–47.
12. Shipp M, Harrington D, Klatt M, et al. Identification of major prognostic subgroups of patients with large-cell lymphoma treated with m-BACOD or M-BACOD. *Ann Intern Med* 1986;104:757–765.
13. Danieu L, Wong G, Koziner B, et al. Predictive model for prognosis in advanced diffuse histiocytic lymphoma. *Cancer Res* 1986;46:5372–5379.
14. Jones S, Miller T, Connors J. Long-term follow-up and analysis for prognostic factors for patients with limited-stage diffuse large-cell lymphoma treated with initial chemotherapy with or without adjuvant radiotherapy. *J Clin Oncol* 1989;7:1186–1191.
15. Hoskins P, Ng V, Spinelli J, et al. Prognostic variables in patients with diffuse large-cell lymphoma treated with MACOP-B. *J Clin Oncol* 1991;9:220–226.
16. Gospodarowicz M, Bush R, Brown T, et al. Prognostic factors in nodular lymphomas: a multivariate analysis based on the Princess Margaret Hospital experience. *Int J Radiat Oncol Biol Phys* 1984;10:489–497.
17. Romaguera J, McLaughlin P, North L, et al. Multivariate analysis of prognostic factors in stage IV follicular low-grade lymphoma: a risk model. *J Clin Oncol* 1991;9:762–769.
18. Soubeyran P, Eghbali H, Bonichon F, et al. Low-grade follicular lymphomas: analysis of prognosis in a series of 281 patients. *Eur J Cancer* 1991;27:1606–1613.
19. Bastion Y, Berger F, Bryon PA, et al. Follicular lymphomas: assessment of prognostic factors in 127 patients followed for 10 years. *Ann Oncol* 1991;2(suppl 2):123–129.
20. Solal-Celigny P, Roy P, Colombat P, et al. Follicular lymphoma international prognostic index. *Blood* 2004;104:1258–1265.
21. Federico M, Vitolo U, Zinzani PL, et al. Prognosis of follicular lymphoma: a predictive model based on a retrospective analysis of 987 cases. Intergruppo Italiano Linfomi. *Blood* 2000;95:783–789.
22. Shipp M, Harrington D, Chairpersons, et al. A predictive model for aggressive non-Hodgkin's lymphoma: The International NHL Prognostic Factors Project. *N Engl J Med* 1993;329:987–994.
23. Musshoff K. Clinical staging classification of non-Hodgkin's lymphomas (author's transl) [in German]. *Strahlentherapie* 1977;153:218–221.
24. Rohatiner A, d'Amore F, Coiffier B, et al. Report on a workshop convened to discuss the pathological and staging classifications of gastrointestinal tract lymphoma. *Ann Oncol* 1994;5:397–400.
25. d'Amore F, Brincker H, Gronbaek K, et al. Non-Hodgkin's lymphoma of the gastrointestinal tract: a population- based analysis of incidence, geographic distribution, clinicopathologic presentation features, and prognosis. Danish Lymphoma Study Group. *J Clin Oncol* 1994;12:1673–684.
26. Gospodarowicz M, Bush R, Brown T, et al. Curability of gastrointestinal lymphoma with combined surgery and radiation. *Int J Radiat Oncol* 1983;9:3–9.
27. Shipp M, Ambinder R, Appelbaum F, et al. NCCN preliminary non-Hodgkin's lymphoma practice guidelines. *Oncology* 1997;11:281–346.

28. Armitage JO, Weisenburger DD. New approach to classifying non-Hodgkin's lymphomas: clinical features of the major histologic subtypes. Non-Hodgkin's Lymphoma Classification Project. *J Clin Oncol* 1998; 16:2780–295.

29. Radaskiewicz T, Brigitte D, Bauer P. Gastrointestinal malignant lymphomas of the mucosa-associated lymphoid tissue: factors relevant to prognosis. *Gastroenterology* 1992;101:1159–1170.

30. Thieblemont C, Bastion Y, Berger F, et al. Mucosa-associated lymphoid tissue gastrointestinal and nongastrointestinal lymphoma behavior: analysis of 108 patients. *J Clin Oncol* 1997;15:1624–1630.

31. Isaacson P. Gastric lymphoma and Helicobacter pylori. *N Engl J Med* 1994;330:1310–1311.

32. Harris NL, Jaffe ES, Diebold J, et al. World Health Organization classification of neoplastic diseases of the hematopoietic and lymphoid tissues: report of the Clinical Advisory Committee meeting-Airlie House, Virginia, November 1997. *J Clin Oncol* 1999;17:3835–3849.

33. Weisenburger DD. Epidemiology of non-Hodgkin's lymphoma: recent findings regarding an emerging epidemic. *Ann Oncol* 1994;5(suppl 1):S19–S24.

34. Chabner B, Johnson R, Devita V, et al Sequential staging in non-Hodgkin's lymphoma. *Cancer Treat Rep* 1977;61:993–997.

35. Moran EM, Ultmann JE, Ferguson DJ, et al. Staging laparotomy in non-Hodgkin's lymphoma. *Br J Cancer* 1975;31(suppl 2_:228–236.

36. McKenna RW, Bloomfield CD, Brunning RD. Nodular lymphoma: bone marrow and blood manifestations. *Cancer* 1975;36:428–440.

37. Bloomfield CD, McKenna RW, Brunning RD. Significance of haematological parameters in the non-Hodgkin's malignant lymphomas. *Br J Haematol* 1976;32:41–46.

38. Conlan MG, Armitage JO, Bast M, et al. Clinical significance of hematologic parameters in non-Hodgkin's lymphoma at diagnosis. *Cancer* 1991;67:1389–1395.

39. Stein RS, Ultmann JE, Byrne GE Jr, et al. Bone marrow involvement in non-Hodgkin's lymphoma: implications for staging and therapy. *Cancer* 1976;37:629–636.

40. Conlan M, Bast M, Armitage J, et al. Bone marrow involvement by non-Hodgkin's lymphoma: the clinical significance of morphologic discordance between the lymph node and bone marrow. *J Clin Oncol* 1990;8:1163–1172.

41. Schneider RJ, Seibert K, Passe S, et al. Prognostic significance of serum lactate dehydrogenase in malignant lymphoma. *Cancer* 1980;46:139–143.

42. Swan F Jr, Velasquez W, Tucker S, et al. A new serologic staging system for large-cell lymphomas based on initial beta 2-microglobulin and lactate dehydrogenase levels. *J Clin Oncol* 1989;7:1518–1527.

43. Chabner BA, Johnson RE, Chretien PB, et al. Percutaneous liver biopsy, peritoneoscopy and laparotomy: an assessment of relative merits in the lymphomata. *Br J Cancer* 1975;31(suppl 2):242–247.

44. Veronesi U, Musumegi R, Pizzetti F, et al. The value of staging laparotomy in non-Hodgkin's lymphomas. *Cancer* 1974;33:446–459.

45. Gandara DR, Mackenzie MR. Differential diagnosis of monoclonal gammopathy. *Med Clin North Am* 1988;72:1155–1167.

46. Kyle RA, Therneau TM, Rajkumar SV, et al. A long-term study of prognosis in monoclonal gammopathy of undetermined significance. *N Engl J Med* 2002;346:564–569.

47. Ioachim HL, Dorsett B, Cronin W, et al. Acquired immunodeficiency syndrome-associated lymphomas: clinical, pathologic, immunologic, and viral characteristics of 111 cases. *Hum Pathol* 1991;22:659–673.

48. Arvanitakis L, Mesri EA, Nador RG, et al. Establishment and characterization of a primary effusion (body cavity- based) lymphoma cell line (BC-3) harboring Kaposi's sarcoma-associated herpesvirus (KSHV/HHV-8) in the absence of Epstein-Barr virus. *Blood* 1996;88:2648–2654.

49. Hollsberg P, Hafler DA. Seminars in medicine of the Beth Israel Hospital, Boston. Pathogenesis of diseases induced by human lymphotropic virus type I infection. *N Engl J Med* 1993;328:1173–1182.

50. Silvestri F, Baccarani M. Hepatitis C virus-related lymphomas. *Br J Haematol* 1997;99:475–480.

51. Lok AS, Liang RH, Chiu EK, et al. Reactivation of hepatitis B virus replication in patients receiving cytotoxic therapy. Report of a prospective study. *Gastroenterology* 1991;100:182–188.

52. Rossi G, Pelizzari A, Motta M, et al. Primary prophylaxis with lamivudine of hepatitis B virus reactivation in chronic HbsAg carriers with lymphoid malignancies treated with chemotherapy. *Br J Haematol* 2001;115:58–62.

53. Celikoglu F, Teirstein AS, Krellenstein DJ, et al. Pleural effusion in non-Hodgkin's lymphoma. *Chest* 1992;101:1357–1360.

54. Castellino RA, Hilton S, O' Brien JP, et al. Non-Hodgkin lymphoma: contribution of chest CT in the initial staging evaluation. *Radiology* 1996;199:129–132.

55. Salonen O, Kivisaari L, Standertskjold-Nordenstam CG, et al. Chest radiography and computed tomography in the evaluation of mediastinal adenopathy in lymphoma. *Acta Radiol* 1987;28:747–750.

56. Romano M, Libshitz HI. Hodgkin disease and non-Hodgkin lymphoma: plain chest radiographs and chest computed tomography of thoracic involvement in previously untreated patients. *Radiol Med* 1998;95:49–53.

57. Khoury MB, Godwin JD, Halvorsen R, et al. Role of chest CT in non-Hodgkin lymphoma. *Radiology* 1986;158:659–662.

58. Zelenetz AD, Hoppe RT. NCCN: Non-Hodgkin's lymphoma. *Cancer Control* 2001;8(6 suppl 2):102–113.

59. Phillips G, Kumari-Subaiya S, Sawitsky A. Ultrasonic evaluation of the scrotum in lymphoproliferative disease. *J Ultrasound Med* 1987;6:169–175.

60. Mazzu D, Jeffrey RB Jr, Ralls PW. Lymphoma and leukemia involving the testicles: findings on gray-scale and color Doppler sonography. *AJR Am J Roentgenol* 1995;164:645–647.

61. Fujishima H, Misawa T, Maruoka A, et al. Staging and follow-up of primary gastric lymphoma by endoscopic ultrasonography. *Am J Gastroenterol* 1991;86:719–724.

62. Hermann G, Klein MJ, Abdelwahab IF, et al. MRI appearance of primary non-Hodgkin's lymphoma of bone. *Skeletal Radiol* 1997;26:629–632.

63. White LM, Schweitzer ME, Khalili K, et al. MR imaging of primary lymphoma of bone: variability of T2-weighted signal intensity. *AJR Am J Roentgenol* 1998;170:1243–1247.

64. Hoane B, Shields A, Porter B, et al. Detection of lymphomatous bone marrow involvement with magnetic resonance imaging. *Blood* 1991; 78:728–738.

65. Nejmeddine F, Caillat-Vigneron N, Escaig F, et al. Mechanism involved in gallium-67 (Ga-67) uptake by human lymphoid cell lines. *Cell Mol Biol (Noisy-le-grand)* 1998;44:1215–1220.

66. Rehm PK. Radionuclide evaluation of patients with lymphoma. *Radiol Clin North Am* 2001;39:957–978.

67. Bar-Shalom R, Mor M, Yefremov N, et al. The value of Ga-67 scintigraphy and F-18 fluorodeoxyglucose positron emission tomography in staging and monitoring the response of lymphoma to treatment. *Semin Nucl Med* 2001;31:177–190.

68. Front D, Israel O, Epelbaum R, et al. Ga-67 SPECT before and after treatment of lymphoma. *Radiology* 1990;175:515–519.

69. Israel O, Front D, Lam M, et al. Gallium 67 imaging in monitoring lymphoma response to treatment. *Cancer* 1988;61:2439–2443.

70. Som P, Atkins HL, Bandoypadhyay D, et al. A fluorinated glucose analog, 2-fluoro-2-deoxy-D-glucose (F-18): nontoxic tracer for rapid tumor detection. *J Nucl Med* 1980;21:670–675.

71. Paul R. Comparison of fluorine-18-2-fluorodeoxyglucose and gallium-67 citrate imaging for detection of lymphoma. *J Nucl Med* 1987;28:288–292.

72. Rodriguez M, Ahlstrom H, Sundin A, et al. [18F] FDG PET in gastric non-Hodgkin's lymphoma. *Acta Oncol* 1997;36:577–584.

73. Jerusalem G, Beguin Y, Fassotte MF, et al. Whole-body positron emission tomography using 18F-fluorodeoxyglucose for posttreatment evaluation in Hodgkin's disease and non-Hodgkin's lymphoma has higher diagnostic and prognostic value than classical computed tomography scan imaging. *Blood* 1999;94:429–433.

74. Bakheet SM, Powe J. Benign causes of 18-FDG uptake on whole body imaging. *Semin Nucl Med* 1998;28:352–358.

75. Vesselle HJ, Miraldi FD. FDG PET of the retroperitoneum: normal anatomy, variants, pathologic conditions, and strategies to avoid diagnostic pitfalls. *Radiographics* 1998;18:805–823.

76. Schaefer NG, Hany TF, Taverna C, et al. Non-Hodgkin lymphoma and Hodgkin disease: coregistered FDG PET and CT at staging and restaging-do we need contrast-enhanced CT? *Radiology* 2004;232:823–829.

77. Tatsumi M, Cohade C, Nakamoto Y, et al. Direct comparison of FDG PET and CT findings in patients with lymphoma: initial experience. *Radiology* 2005;237:1038–1045.

78. Freudenberg LS, Antoch G, Schutt P, et al. FDG-PET/CT in re-staging of patients with lymphoma. *Eur J Nucl Med Mol Imaging* 2004;31:325–329.

79. Kostakoglu L, Leonard JP, Kuji I, et al. Comparison of fluorine-18 fluorodeoxyglucose positron emission tomography and Ga-67 scintigraphy in evaluation of lymphoma. *Cancer* 2002;94:879–888.

80. Moog F, Kotzerke J, Reske SN. FDG PET can replace bone scintigraphy in primary staging of malignant lymphoma. *J Nucl Med* 1999;40:1407–1413.

81. Bangerter M, Moog F, Griesshammer M, et al. Usefulness of FDG-PET in diagnosing primary lymphoma of the liver. *Int J Hematol* 1997;66:517–520.

82. Ullerich H, Franzius CH, Domagk D, et al. 18F-Fluorodeoxyglucose PET in a patient with primary small bowel lymphoma: the only sensitive method of imaging. *Am J Gastroenterol* 2001;96:2497–2499.

83. Moog F, Bangerter M, Kotzerke J, et al. 18-F-fluorodeoxyglucose-positron emission tomography as a new approach to detect lymphomatous bone marrow. *J Clin Oncol* 1998;16:603–609.

84. Hoffman JM, Waskin HA, Schifter T, et al. FDG-PET in differentiating lymphoma from nonmalignant central nervous system lesions in patients with AIDS. *J Nucl Med* 1993;34:567–575.

85. Elstrom R, Guan L, Baker G, et al. Utility of FDG-PET scanning in lymphoma by WHO classification. *Blood* 2003;101:3875–3876.

86. Newman JS, Francis IR, Kaminski MS, et al. Imaging of lymphoma with PET with 2-[F-18]-fluoro-2-deoxy-D-glucose: correlation with CT. *Radiology* 1994;190:111–116.

87. Buchmann I, Reinhardt M, Elsner K, et al. 2-(fluorine-18)fluoro-2-deoxy-D-glucose positron emission tomography in the detection and staging of malignant lymphoma. A bicenter trial. *Cancer* 2001;91:889–899.

88. Juweid ME, Stroobants S, Hoekstra OS, et al. Use of positron emission tomography for response assessment of lymphoma: consensus of the Imaging Subcommittee of International Harmonization Project in Lymphoma. *J Clin Oncol* 2007;25:571–578.

89. Cheson BD, Pfistner B, Juweid ME, et al. Revised response criteria for malignant lymphoma. *J Clin Oncol* 2007;25:579–586.

90. Seam P, Juweid ME, Cheson BD. The role of FDG-PET scans in patients with lymphoma. *Blood* 2007;110:3507–3516.

91. Cheson B, Horning S, Coiffier B, et al. Report of an international workshop to standardize response criteria for non-Hodgkin's lymphomas. *J Clin Oncol* 1999;17:1244.

92. Duggan PR, Easton D, Luider J, et al. Bone marrow staging of patients with non-Hodgkin lymphoma by flow cytometry: correlation with morphology. *Cancer* 2000;88:894–899.

93. Kwee TC, Kwee RM, Verdonck LF, et al. Magnetic resonance imaging for the detection of bone marrow involvement in malignant lymphoma. *Br J Haematol* 2008;141:60–68.

94. Tardivon AA, Munck JN, Shapeero LG, et al. Can clinical data help to screen patients with lymphoma for MR imaging of bone marrow? *Ann Oncol* 1995;6:795–800.

95. Carr R, Barrington SF, Madan B, et al. Detection of lymphoma in bone marrow by whole-body positron emission tomography. *Blood* 1998;91:3340–3346.

96. Pakos EE, Fotopoulos AD, Ioannidis JP. 18F-FDG PET for evaluation of bone marrow infiltration in staging of lymphoma: a meta-analysis. *J Nucl Med* 2005;46:958–963.

97. Banfi A, Bonadonna G, Ricci SB, et al. Malignant lymphomas of Waldeyer's ring: natural history and survival after radiotherapy. *Br Med J* 1972;3:140–143.

98. Gospodarowicz M, Sutcliffe S, Brown T, et al. Patterns of disease in localized extranodal lymphomas. *J Clin Oncol* 1987;5:875–880.

99. Jacobs C, Hoppe R. Non-Hodgkin's lymphomas of head and neck extranodal sites. *Int J Radiat Oncol Biol Phys* 1985;11:357–364.

100. Crump M, Gospodarowicz M, Shepherd FA. Lymphoma of the gastrointestinal tract. *Semin Oncol* 1999;26:324–337.

101. Tio TL, den Hartog Jager FC, Tijrgat GN. Endoscopic ultrasonography of non-Hodgkin lymphoma of the stomach. *Gastroenterology* 1986;91:401–408.

102. Caletti GC, Ferrari A, Bocus P, et al. Endoscopic ultrasonography in gastric lymphoma. *Schweiz Med Wochenschr* 1996;126:819–825.

103. Wotherspoon A, Doglioni C, Diss T, et al. Regression of primary low-grade B-cell gastric lymphoma of mucosa-associated lymphoid tissue type after eradication of Helicobacter pylori. *Lancet* 1993;342:575–577.

104. Bayerdorffer E, Neubauer A, Rudolph B, et al. Regression of primary gastric lymphoma of mucosa-associated lymphoid tissue type after cure of Helicobacter pylori infection. MALT Lymphoma Study Group. *Lancet* 1995;345:1591–1594.

105. Abbondanzo SL, Wenig BM. Non-Hodgkin's lymphoma of the sinonasal tract. A clinicopathologic and immunophenotypic study of 120 cases. *Cancer* 1995;75:1281–1291.

106. Logsdon MD, Ha CS, Kavadi VS, et al. Lymphoma of the nasal cavity and paranasal sinuses; improved outcome and altered prognostic factors with combined modality therapy. *Cancer* 1997;80:477–488.

107. Jaffe E. Classification of natural killer (NK) cell and NK-like T-cell malignancies. *Blood* 1996;87:1207–1210.

108. Johnson CD, Kent DM, Varjabedian GC, et al. Malignant lymphoma of the maxillary sinus. *J Am Osteopath Assoc* 1993;93:252, 255–258.

109. Frierson HF Jr, Mills SE, Innes DJ Jr. Non-Hodgkin's lymphomas of the sinonasal region: histologic subtypes and their clinicopathologic features. *Am J Clin Pathol* 1984;81:721–727.

110. Fine HA, Mayer RJ. Primary central nervous system lymphoma. *Ann Intern Med* 1993;119:1093–1104.

111. Lossos IS, Breuer R, Intrator O, et al. Cerebrospinal fluid lactate dehydrogenase isoenzyme analysis for the diagnosis of central nervous system involvement in hematooncologic patients. *Cancer* 2000;88:1599–1604.

112. Whitcup SM, de Smet MD, Rubin BI, et al. Intraocular lymphoma. Clinical and histopathologic diagnosis. *Ophthalmology* 1993;100:1399–1406.

113. Sutcliffe S, Gospodarowicz M. Primary extranodal lymphomas. In: Canellos GP, Lister TA, Sklar JL, eds. The lymphomas. Philadelphia, PA: Lippincott Williams &, 1998.

114. Ferry J, Harris N, Young R, et al. Malignant lymphoma of the testis, epididymis and spermatic cord: a clinicopathologic study of 69 cases with immunophenotypic analysis. *Cancer* 1994;18:376–390.

115. Seymour JF, Solomon B, Wolf MM, et al. Primary large-cell non-Hodgkin's lymphoma of the testis: a retrospective analysis of patterns of failure and prognostic factors. *Clin Lymphoma* 2001;2:109–115.

116. Tondini C, Ferreri AJ, Siracusano L, et al. Diffuse large-cell lymphoma of the testis. *J Clin Oncol* 1999;17:2854–2858.

117. Bunn PA Jr, Schein PS, Banks PM, et al. Central nervous system complications in patients with diffuse histiocytic and undifferentiated lymphoma: leukemia revisited. *Blood* 1976;47:3–10.

118. Levitt L, Aisenberg A, Harris N, et al. Primary non-Hodgkin's lymphoma of the mediastinum. *Cancer* 1982;50:2486–2492.

119. Rathmell AJ, Gospodarowicz MK, Sutcliffe SB, et al. Localised lymphoma of bone: prognostic factors and treatment recommendations. The Princess Margaret Hospital Lymphoma Group. *Br J Cancer* 1992;66:603–606.

120. Ostrowski ML, Unni KK, Banks PM, et al. Malignant lymphoma of bone. *Cancer* 1986;58:2646–2655.

121. Wong WW, Schild SE, Halyard MY, et al. Primary non-Hodgkin lymphoma of the breast: The Mayo Clinic experience. *J Surg Oncol* 2002;80:19–25.

122. Monterroso V, Jaffe ES, Merino MJ, et al. Malignant lymphomas involving the ovary. A clinicopathologic analysis of 39 cases. *Am J Surg Pathol* 1993;17:154–170.

123. Coiffier B. How to interpret the radiological abnormalities that persist after treatment in non-Hodgkin's lymphoma patients? *Ann Oncol* 1999;10:1141–1143.

124. Zinzani PL, Bendandi M, Martelli M, et al. Anaplastic large-cell lymphoma: clinical and prognostic evaluation of 90 adult patients. *J Clin Oncol* 1996;14:955–962.

125. Israel O, Front D, Epelbaum R, et al. Residual mass and negative gallium scintigraphy in treated lymphoma. *J Nucl Med* 1990;31:365–368.

126. Drossman SR, Schiff RG, Kronfeld GD, et al. Lymphoma of the mediastinum and neck: evaluation with Ga-67 imaging and CT correlation. *Radiology* 1990;174:171–175.

127. Cremerius U, Fabry U, Neuerburg J, et al. Positron emission tomography with 18F-FDG to detect residual disease after therapy for malignant lymphoma. *Nucl Med Commun* 1998;19:1055–1063.

128. Kostakoglu L, Goldsmith SJ. Fluorine-18 fluorodeoxyglucose positron emission tomography in the staging and follow-up of lymphoma: is it time to shift gears? *Eur J Nucl Med* 2000;27:1564–1578.

129. Stumpe KD, Urbinelli M, Steinert HC, et al. Whole-body positron emission tomography using fluorodeoxyglucose for staging of lymphoma: effectiveness and comparison with computed tomography. *Eur J Nucl Med* 1998;25:721–728.

130. Zijlstra JM, Lindauer-van der Werf G, Hoekstra OS, et al. 18F-fluorodeoxyglucose positron emission tomography for post-treatment evaluation of malignant lymphoma: a systematic review. *Haematologica* 2006;91:522–529.

131. de Hemricourt E, De Boeck K, Hilte F, et al. Sarcoidosis and sarcoid-like reaction following Hodgkin's disease. Report of two cases. *Mol Imaging Biol* 2003;5:15–19.

132. Fletcher JW, Djulbegovic B, Soares HP, et al. Recommendations on the use of 18F-FDG PET in oncology. *J Nucl Med* 2008;49:480–508.

133. Spaepen K, Stroobants S, Dupont P, et al. [(18)F]FDG PET monitoring of tumour response to chemotherapy: does [(18)F]FDG uptake correlate with the viable tumour cell fraction? *Eur J Nucl Med Mol Imaging* 2003;30:682–688.

134. Naumann R, Vaic A, Beuthien-Baumann B, et al. Prognostic value of positron emission tomography in the evaluation of post-treatment residual mass in patients with Hodgkin's disease and non-Hodgkin's lymphoma. *Br J Haematol* 2001;115:793–800.

135. Zarrabi MH. Association of non-Hodgkin's lymphoma and second neoplasms. *Semin Oncol* 1990;17:120–132.

136. Travis LB, Gospodarowicz M, Curtis RE, et al. Lung cancer following chemotherapy and radiotherapy for Hodgkin's disease. *J Natl Cancer Inst* 2002;94:182–192.

137. Travis LB, Curtis RE, Glimelius B, et al. Second cancers among long-term survivors of non-Hodgkin's lymphoma. *J Natl Cancer Inst* 1993;85:1932–1937.

138. Travis L, Weeks J, Curtis R, et al. Leukemia following low-dose total body irradiation and chemotherapy for non-Hodgkin's lymphoma. *J Clin Oncol* 1996;14:565–571.

139. Friedberg JW, Neuberg D, Stone RM, et al. Outcome in patients with myelodysplastic syndrome after autologous bone marrow transplantation for non-Hodgkin's lymphoma. *J Clin Oncol* 1999;17:3128–3135.

140. Shenkier TN, Voss N, Fairey R, et al. Brief chemotherapy and involved-region irradiation for limited-stage diffuse large-cell lymphoma: an 18-year experience from the British Columbia Cancer Agency. *J Clin Oncol* 2002;20:197–204.

141. Sanz L, Lopez-Guillermo A, Martinez C, et al. Risk of relapse and clinico-pathological features in 103 patients with diffuse large-cell lymphoma in complete response after first-line treatment. *Eur J Haematol* 1998;61:59–64.

142. Shipp MA, Klatt MM, Yeap B, et al. Patterns of relapse in large-cell lymphoma patients with bulk disease: implications for the use of adjuvant radiation therapy. *J Clin Oncol* 1989;7:613–618.

143. Mead GM, Mackintosh FR, Burke JS, et al. Late relapse from complete remission in nodular and diffuse histiocytic lymphoma. *Cancer* 1983;52:1356–1359.

144. Front D, Bar-Shalom R, Epelbaum R, et al. Early detection of lymphoma recurrence with gallium-67 scintigraphy. *J Nucl Med* 1993;34:2101–2104.

145. Weeks J, Yeop B, Canellos G, et al. Value of follow-up procedures in patients with large-cell lymphoma who achieve a complete remission. *J Clin Oncol* 1991;9:1196–1203.

146. Oh YK, Ha CS, Samuels BI, et al. Stages I-III follicular lymphoma: role of CT of the abdomen and pelvis in follow-up studies. *Radiology* 1999;210:483–486.

147. Elis A, Blickstein D, Klein O, et a. Detection of relapse in non-Hodgkin's lymphoma: role of routine follow- up studies. *Am J Hematol* 2002;69:41–44.

148. Vose J. High-dose chemotherapy and hematopoietic stem cell transplantation for relapsed or refractory diffuse large-cell non-Hodgkin's lymphoma. *Ann Oncol* 1998;9(suppl 1):S1–S3.

149. Velasquez WS, Cabanillas F, Salvador P, et al. Effective salvage therapy for lymphoma with cisplatin in combination with high-dose Ara-C and dexamethasone (DHAP). *Blood* 1988;71:117–122.

150. Zelenetz AD, Advani RH, Buadi F, et al. Non-Hodgkin's lymphoma. Clinical practice guidelines in oncology. *J Natl Compr Canc Netw* 2006;4:258–310.

151. Cabanillas F BJ, Smith TL, Moon ME, et al. Factors predicting for response and survival in adults with advanced non-Hodgkin's lymphoma. *Arch Intern Med* 1978;138:413–418.

152. Coiffier B, Bastion Y, Berger F, et al. Prognostic factors in follicular lymphomas. *Semin Oncol* 1993;20(suppl 5):89–95.

153. Velasquez WS, Fuller LM, Jagannath S, et al. Stages I and II diffuse large cell lymphomas: prognostic factors in long-term results with CHOP-BLEO and radiotherapy. *Blood* 1991;77:942–947.

154. Shipp MA. Prognostic factors in aggressive non-Hodgkin's lymphoma: who has "high-risk" disease? *Blood* 1994;83:1165–1173.

155. Dixon D, Neilan B, Jones S, et al. Effect of age on therapeutic outcome in advanced diffuse histiocytic lymphoma: the southwest oncology group experience. *J Clin Oncol* 1986;4:295–305.

156. Vose J, Armitage J, Weisenburger D, et al. The importance of age in survival of patients treated with chemotherapy for aggressive non-Hodgkin's lymphoma. *J Clin Oncol* 1988;6:1838–1844.

157. d'Amore F, Brincker H, Christensen BE, et al. Non-Hodgkin's lymphoma in the elderly. A study of 602 patients aged 70 or older from a Danish population-based registry. The Danish Lyeo-Study Group. *Ann Oncol* 1992;3:379–386.

158. Effect of age on the characteristics and clinical behavior of non-Hodgkin's lymphoma patients. The Non-Hodgkin's Lymphoma Classification Project. *Ann Oncol* 1997;8:973–978.

159. Coiffier B. What treatment for elderly patients with aggressive lymphoma? *Ann Oncol* 1994;5:873–875.

160. Coiffier B, Lepage E, Briere J, et al. CHOP chemotherapy plus rituximab compared with CHOP alone in elderly patients with diffuse large-B-cell lymphoma. *N Engl J Med* 2002;346:235–242.

161. Pfreundschuh M, Schubert J, Ziepert M, et al. Six versus eight cycles of bi-weekly CHOP-14 with or without rituximab in elderly patients with aggressive CD20+ B-cell lymphomas: a randomised controlled trial (RICOVER-60). *Lancet Oncol* 2008;9:105–116.

162. Habermann TM, Weller EA, Morrison VA, et al. Rituximab-CHOP versus CHOP alone or with maintenance rituximab in older patients with diffuse large B-cell lymphoma. *J Clin Oncol* 2006;24:3121–3127.

163. Miller T, Dahlberg S, Cassady J, et al. Chemotherapy alone compared with chemotherapy plus radiotherapy for localized intermediate- and high-grade non-Hodgkin's lymphoma. *N Engl J Med* 1998;339:21–26.

164. Fisher RI, Gaynor ER, Dahlberg S, et al. Comparison of a standard regimen (CHOP) with three intensive chemotherapy regimens for advanced non-Hodgkin's lymphoma. *N Engl J Med* 1993;328:1002–1006.

165. Sehn LH, Donaldson J, Chhanabhai M, et al. Introduction of combined CHOP plus rituximab therapy dramatically improved outcome of diffuse large B-cell lymphoma in British Columbia. *J Clin Oncol* 2005;23:5027–5033.

166. Feugier P, Van Hoof A, Sebban C, et al. Long-term results of the R-CHOP study in the treatment of elderly patients with diffuse large B-cell lymphoma: a study by the Groupe d'Etude des Lymphomes de l'Adulte. *J Clin Oncol* 2005;23:4117–4126.

167. Pfreundschuh M, Trumper L, Osterborg A, et al. CHOP-like chemotherapy plus rituximab versus CHOP-like chemotherapy alone in young patients with good-prognosis diffuse large-B-cell lymphoma: a randomised controlled trial by the MabThera International Trial (MInT) Group. *Lancet Oncol* 2006;7:379–391.

168. Sehn LH, Berry B, Chhanabhai M, et al. The revised International Prognostic Index (R-IPI) is a better predictor of outcome than the standard IPI for patients with diffuse large B-cell lymphoma treated with R-CHOP. *Blood* 2007;109:1857–1861.

169. Decaudin D, Lepage E, Brousse N, et al. Low-grade stage III-IV follicular lymphoma: multivariate analysis of prognostic factors in 484 patients—a study of the groupe d'Etude des lymphomes de l'Adulte. *J Clin Oncol* 1999;17:2499–2505.

170. Lopez-Guillermo A, Cid J, Salar A, et al. Peripheral T-cell lymphomas: initial features, natural history, and prognostic factors in a series of 174 patients diagnosed according to the R.E.A.L. Classification. *Ann Oncol* 1998;9:849–855.

171. Hermans J, Krol AD, van Groningen K, et al. International Prognostic Index for aggressive non-Hodgkin's lymphoma is valid for all malignancy grades. *Blood* 1995;86:1460–1463.

172. Bastion Y, Coiffier B. Is the International Prognostic Index for aggressive lymphoma patients useful for follicular lymphoma patients? *J Clin Oncol* 1994;12:1340–1342.

173. Gisselbrecht C, Gaulard P, Lepage E, et al. Prognostic significance of T-cell phenotype in aggressive non-Hodgkin's lymphomas. Groupe d'Etudes des Lymphomes de l'Adulte (GELA). *Blood* 1998;92:76–82.

174. Kim K, Kim WS, Jung CW, et al. Clinical features of peripheral T-cell lymphomas in 78 patients diagnosed according to the Revised European-American lymphoma (REAL) classification. *Eur J Cancer* 2002;38:75–81.

175. Savage KJ, Chhanabhai M, Gascoyne RD, et al. Characterization of peripheral T-cell lymphomas in a single North American institution by the WHO classification. *Ann Oncol* 2004;15:1467–1475.

176. Rudiger T, Weisenburger DD, Anderson JR, et al. Peripheral T-cell lymphoma (excluding anaplastic large-cell lymphoma): results from the Non-Hodgkin's Lymphoma Classification Project. *Ann Oncol* 2002;13:140–149.

177. Gascoyne R, Aoun P, Wu D, et al. Prognostic significance of anaplastic lymphoma kinase (ALK) protein expression in adults with anaplastic large cell lymphoma. *Blood* 1999;93:3913–3921.

178. Falini B, Pileri S, Zinzani PL, et al. ALK+ lymphoma: clinico-pathological findings and outcome. *Blood* 1999;93:2697–2706.

179. Savage KJ, Harris NL, Vose JM, et al. ALK− anaplastic large-cell lymphoma is clinically and immunophenotypically different from both ALK+ ALCL and peripheral T-cell lymphoma, not otherwise specified: report from the International Peripheral T-Cell Lymphoma Project. *Blood* 2008;111:5496–5504.

180. Stein H, Foss HD, Durkop H, et al. CD30(+) anaplastic large cell lymphoma: a review of its histopathologic, genetic, and clinical features. *Blood* 2000;96:3681–3695.

181. Micallef IN, Remstein ED, Ansell SM, et al. The International Prognostic Index predicts outcome after histological transformation of low-grade non-Hodgkin lymphoma. *Leuk Lymphoma* 2006;47:1794–1799.

182. Buske C, Hoster E, Dreyling M,. The Follicular Lymphoma International Prognostic Index (FLIPI) separates high-risk from intermediate- or low-risk patients with advanced-stage follicular lymphoma treated front-line with rituximab and the combination of cyclophosphamide, doxorubicin, vincristine, and prednisone (R-CHOP) with respect to treatment outcome. *Blood* 2006;108:1504–1508.

183. Armitage J, Weisenburger D, Hutchins M, et al. Chemotherapy for diffuse large-cell lymphoma-rapidly responding patients have more durable remissions. *J Clin Oncol* 1986;4:160–164.

184. Engelhard M, Meusers P, Brittinger G, et al. Prospective multicenter trial for the response-adapted treatment of high-grade malignant non-Hodgkin's lymphomas: updated results of the COP-BLAM/IMVP-16 protocol with randomized adjuvant radiotherapy. *Ann Oncol* 1991;(suppl 2):177–180.

185. Spaepen K, Mortelmans L. Evaluation of treatment response in patients with lymphoma using [18F]FDG-PET: differences between non-Hodgkin's lymphoma and Hodgkin's disease. *Q J Nucl Med* 2001;45:269–273.

186. Spaepen K, Stroobants S, Dupont P, et al. Early restaging positron emission tomography with (18)F- fluorodeoxyglucose predicts outcome in patients with aggressive non- Hodgkin's lymphoma. *Ann Oncol* 2002;13:1356–1363.

187. Haioun C, Itti F, Rahmouni A, et al. [18F]fluoro-2-deoxy-D-glucose positron emission tomography (FDG-PET) in aggressive lymphoma: an early prognostic tool for predicting patient outcome. *Blood* 2005;106:1376–1381.

188. Kasamon YL, Wahl RL. FDG PET and risk-adapted therapy in Hodgkin's and non-Hodgkin's lymphoma. *Curr Opin Oncol* 2008;20:206–219.

189. Velasquez WS, McLaughlin P, Tucker S et al. ESHAP- an effective chemotherapy in refractory and relapsing lymphoma: a 4 year follow-up study. *JCO* 1994;12(6):1169–76.

190. Cabanillas F, Hagemeister FB, McLaughlin P, et al. Results of mime salvage regimen for recurrent or refractory lymphoma. *J Clin Oncol* 1987;5:407–412.

191. Freedman A, Takvorian T, Anderson K, et al. Autologous bone marrow transplantation in B-cell non-Hodgkin's lymphoma: very low treatment-related mortality in 100 patients in sensitive relapse. *J Clin Oncol* 1990;8:784–791.

192. Philip T, Guglielmi C, Hagenbeek A, et al. Autologous bone marrow transplantation as compared with salvage chemotherapy in relapses of chemotherapy-sensitive non-Hodgkin's lymphoma. *N Engl J Med* 1995;333:1540–1545.

193. Petersen FB, Appelbaum FR, Hill R, et al. Autologous marrow transplantation for malignant lymphoma: a report of 101 cases from Seattle. *J Clin Oncol* 1990;8:638–647.

194. Philips G, Fay J, Herzig R, et al. the treatment of progressive non-Hodgkin's lymphoma with intensive chemotherapy and autologous marrow transplantation. *Blood* 1990;75:831–838.

195. Stiff PJ, Dahlberg S, Forman SJ, et al. Autologous bone marrow transplantation for patients with relapsed or refractory diffuse aggressive non-Hodgkin's lymphoma: value of augmented preparative regimens—a Southwest Oncology Group trial. *J Clin Oncol* 1998;16:48–55.

196. Prince HM, Imrie K, Crump M, et al. The role of intensive therapy and autologous blood and marrow transplantation for chemotherapy-sensitive relapsed and primary refractory non-Hodgkin's lymphoma: identification of major prognostic groups. *Br J Haematol* 1996;92:880–889.

197. Wilson WH, Bryant G, Bates S, et al. EPOCH chemotherapy: toxicity and efficacy in relapsed and refractory non-Hodgkin's lymphoma. *J Clin Oncol* 1993;11:1573–1582.

198. Josting A, Reiser M, Rueffer U, et al. Treatment of primary progressive Hodgkin's and aggressive non-Hodgkin's lymphoma: is there a chance for cure? *J Clin Oncol* 2000;18:332–339.

199. Villela L, Lopez-Guillermo A, Montoto S, et al. Prognostic features and outcome in patients with diffuse large B-cell lymphoma who do not achieve a complete response to first-line regimens. *Cancer* 2001;91:1557–1562.

200. Vose JM, Zhang MJ, Rowlings PA, et al. Autologous transplantation for diffuse aggressive non-Hodgkin's lymphoma in patients never achieving remission: a report from the Autologous Blood and Marrow Transplant Registry. *J Clin Oncol* 2001;19:406–413.

201. Kewalramani T, Zelenetz AD, Hedrick EE, et al. High-dose chemoradiotherapy and autologous stem cell transplantation for patients with primary refractory aggressive non-Hodgkin lymphoma: an intention-to-treat analysis. *Blood* 2000;96:2399–2404.

202. Guglielmi C, Gomez F, Philip T, et al. Time to relapse has prognostic value in patients with aggressive lymphoma enrolled onto the Parma trial. *J Clin Oncol* 1998;16:3264–3269.

203. Weisdorf D, Anderson J, Glick J, et al. Survival after relapse of low-grade non-Hodgkin's lymphoma: implications for marrow transplantation. *J Clin Oncol* 1992;10:942–947.

204. Moskowitz C, Bertino J, Glassman J, et al. Ifosfamide, carboplatin, and etoposide: a highly effective cytoreduction and peripheral-blood progenitor-cell mobilization regimen for transplant-eligible patients with non-Hodgkin's lymphoma. *J Clin Oncol* 1999;17:3776–3785.

205. de Kreuk M, Ossenkoppele GJ, Meijer CJ, et al. Prognostic factors for survival of non-Hodgkin's lymphoma patients treated with high-dose chemotherapy and autologous bone marrow transplantation. *Bone Marrow Transplant* 1996;17:963–971.

206. Blay J, Gomez F, Sebban C, et al. The International Prognostic Index correlates to survival in patients with aggressive lymphoma in relapse: analysis of the PARMA trial. Parma Group. *Blood* 1998;92:3562–3568.

207. Moskowitz CH, Nimer SD, Glassman JR, et al. The International Prognostic Index predicts for outcome following autologous stem cell transplantation in patients with relapsed and primary refractory intermediate-grade lymphoma. *Bone Marrow Transplant* 1999;23:561–567.

208. Harris N, Jaffe E, Stein H, et al. A revised European-American classification of lymphoid neoplasms: a proposal from the International Lymphoma Study Group. *Blood* 1994;84:1361–1392.

209. Kwak LW, Wilson M, Weiss LM, et al. Similar outcome of treatment of B-cell and T-cell diffuse large-cell lymphomas: the Stanford experience. *J Clin Oncol* 1991;9:1426–1431.

210. Armitage J, Greer J, Levine A, et al. Peripheral T-cell lymphoma. *Cancer* 1989;63:158–163.

211. Coiffier B, Brousse N, Peuchmaur M, et al. Peripheral T-cell lymphomas have a worse prognosis than B-cell lymphomas: a prospective study of 361 immunophenotyped patients treated with the LNH-84 regimen. *Ann Oncol* 1990;1:45–50.

212. Morabito F, Gallamini A, Stelitano C, et al. Clinical relevance of immunophenotype in a retrospective comparative study of 297 peripheral T-cell lymphomas, unspecified, and 496 diffuse large B-cell lymphomas: experience of the Intergruppo Italiano Linfomi. *Cancer* 2004;101:1601–1608.

213. Ansell S, Habermann T, Kurtin P, et al. Predictive capacity of the International Prognostic Factor Index in patients with peripheral T-cell lymphoma. *J Clin Oncol* 1997;15:2296–2301.

214. Vose JM. Update on T-cell lymphoma. *Ann Oncol* 2008;19(suppl 4):iv74–iv76.

215. Ramaswamy S, Golub TR. DNA microarrays in clinical oncology. *J Clin Oncol* 2002;20:1932–1941.

216. Alizadeh A, Elsen M, Davis R, et al. Distinct types of diffuse large B-cell lymphoma identified by gene expression profiling. *Nature* 2000;4051:503–511.

217. Rosenwald A, Wright G, Chan WC, et al. The use of molecular profiling to predict survival after chemotherapy for diffuse large-B-cell lymphoma. *N Engl J Med* 2002;346:1937–1947.

218. Rimsza LM, Leblanc ML, Unger JM, et al. Gene expression predicts overall survival in paraffin embedded tissues of diffuse large B cell lymphoma treated with R-CHOP. *Blood* 2008;112:3425–3433.

219. Wright G, Tan B, Rosenwald A, et al. A gene expression-based method to diagnose clinically distinct subgroups of diffuse large B cell lymphoma. *Proc Natl Acad Sci U S A* 2003;100:9991–9996.

220. Hans CP, Weisenburger DD, Greiner TC, et al. Confirmation of the molecular classification of diffuse large B-cell lymphoma by immunohistochemistry using a tissue microarray. *Blood* 2004;103:275–282.

221. Barrans SL, Carter I, Owen RG, et al. Germinal center phenotype and bcl-2 expression combined with the International Prognostic Index improves patient risk stratification in diffuse large B-cell lymphoma. *Blood* 2002;99:1136–1143.

222. van Imhoff GW, Boerma EJ, van der Holt B, et al. Prognostic impact of germinal center-associated proteins and chromosomal breakpoints in poor-risk diffuse large B-cell lymphoma. *J Clin Oncol* 2006;24:4135–4142.

223. Berglund M, Thunberg U, Amini RM, et al. Evaluation of immunophenotype in diffuse large B-cell lymphoma and its impact on prognosis. *Mod Pathol* 2005;18:1113–1120.

224. Veelken H, Vik Dannheim S, Schulte et al. Immunophenotype as prognostic factor for diffuse large B-cell lymphoma in patients undergoing clinical risk-adapted therapy. *Ann Oncol* 2007;18:931–939.

225. de Jong D, Rosenwald A, Chhanabhai M, et al. Immunohistochemical prognostic markers in diffuse large B-cell lymphoma: validation of tissue microarray as a prerequisite for broad clinical applications—a study from the Lunenburg Lymphoma Biomarker Consortium. *J Clin Oncol* 2007;25:805–812.

226. Monti S, Savage KJ, Kutok JL, et al. Molecular profiling of diffuse large B-cell lymphoma identifies robust subtypes including one characterized by host inflammatory response. *Blood* 2005;105:1851–18561.

227. Savage KJ, Monti S, Kutok JL, et al. The molecular signature of mediastinal large B-cell lymphoma differs from that of other diffuse large B-cell lymphomas and shares features with classical Hodgkin lymphoma. *Blood* 2003;102:3871–3879.

228. Rosenwald A, Wright G, Leroy K, et al. Molecular diagnosis of primary mediastinal B cell lymphoma identifies a clinically favorable subgroup of diffuse large B cell lymphoma related to Hodgkin lymphoma. *J Exp Med* 2003;198:851–862.

229. Dave SS, Wright G, Tan B, et al. Prediction of survival in follicular lymphoma based on molecular features of tumor-infiltrating immune cells. *N Engl J Med* 2004;351:2159–2169.

230. Taskinen M, Karjalainen-Lindsberg ML, Nyman H, et al. A high tumor-associated macrophage content predicts favorable outcome in follicular lymphoma patients treated with rituximab and cyclophosphamide-doxorubicin-vincristine-prednisone. *Clin Cancer Res* 2007;13:5784–5789.

231. Canioni D, Salles G, Mounier N, et al. High numbers of tumor-associated macrophages have an adverse prognostic value that can be circumvented by rituximab in patients with follicular lymphoma enrolled onto the GELA-GOELAMS FL-2000 trial. *J Clin Oncol* 2008;26:440–446.

232. Taskinen M, Karjalainen-Lindsberg ML, Leppa S. Prognostic influence of tumor-infiltrating mast cells in patients with follicular lymphoma treated with rituximab and CHOP. *Blood* 2008;111:4664–4667.

233. Shipp MA, Ross KN, Tamayo P, et al. Diffuse large B-cell lymphoma outcome prediction by gene-expression profiling and supervised machine learning. *Nat Med* 2002;8:68–74.

234. Robertson MJ, Kahl BS, Vose JM, et al. Phase II study of enzastaurin, a protein kinase C beta inhibitor, in patients with relapsed or refractory diffuse large B-cell lymphoma. *J Clin Oncol* 2007;25:1741–1746.

235. Lossos IS, Czerwinski DK, Alizadeh AA, et al. Prediction of survival in diffuse large-B-cell lymphoma based on the expression of six genes. *N Engl J Med* 2004;350:1828–1837.

236. Natkunam Y, Farinha P, Hsi ED, et al. LMO2 protein expression predicts survival in patients with diffuse large B-cell lymphoma treated with anthracycline-based chemotherapy with and without rituximab. *J Clin Oncol* 2008;26:447–454.

237. Miller TP, Lippman SM, Spier CM, et al. HLA-DR (Ia) immune phenotype predicts outcome for patients with diffuse large cell lymphoma. *J Clin Invest* 1988;82:370–372.

238. List A, Spier C, Miller T, et al. Deficient tumor-infiltrating T-lymphocyte response in malignant lymphoma: relationship to HLA expression and host immunocompetence. *Leukemia* 1993;7:398–403.

239. Rimsza LM, Roberts RA, Miller TP, et al. Loss of MHC class II gene and protein expression in diffuse large B-cell lymphoma is related to decreased tumor immunosurveillance and poor patient survival regardless of other prognostic factors: a follow-up study from the Leukemia and Lymphoma Molecular Profiling Project. *Blood* 2004;103:4251–4258.

240. Ansell SM, Stenson M, Habermann TM, et al. Cd4+ T-cell immune response to large B-cell non-Hodgkin's lymphoma predicts patient outcome. *J Clin Oncol* 2001;19:720–726.

241. Grogan TM, Miller TP. Immunobiologic correlates of prognosis in lymphoma. *Semin Oncol* 1993;20(suppl 5):58–74.

242. Medeiros L, Picker L, Gelb A, et al. Numbers of host "helper" T cells and proliferating cells predict survival in diffuse small-cell lymphomas. *J Clin Oncol* 1989;7:1009–1017.

243. Lippman SM, Spier CM, Miller TP, et al. Tumor-infiltrating T-lymphocytes in B-cell diffuse large cell lymphoma related to disease course. *Mod Pathol* 1990;3:361–367.

244. Hoppe RT, Medeiros LJ, Warnke RA, et al. CD8-positive tumor-infiltrating lymphocytes influence the long-term survival of patients with mycosis fungoides. *J Am Acad Dermatol* 1995;32:448–453.

245. Chan WC, Huang JZ. Gene expression analysis in aggressive NHL. *Ann Hematol* 2001;80(suppl 3):B38–B41.

246. Pezzella F, Tse A, Cordell J, et al. Expression of the Bcl-2 oncogene protein is not specific for the 14-18 chromosomal translocation. *Am J Pathol* 1990;137:225–32.

247. Fujii Y, Okumura M, Takeuchi Y, et al. Bcl-2 expression in the thymus and periphery. *Cell Immunol* 1994;155:335–344.

248. Hockenbery D, Nunez G, Milliman C, et al. BCL-2 is an inner mitochondrial membrane protein that blocks programmed cell death. *Nature* 1990;(348):334–336.

249. Yang E, Korsmeyer SJ. Molecular thanatopsis: a discourse on the BCL2 family and cell death. *Blood* 1996;88:386–401.

250. Reed JC. Bcl-2 family proteins: regulators of apoptosis and chemoresistance in hematologic malignancies. *Semin Hematol* 1997;34(suppl 5):9–19.

251. Gascoyne R, Adomat S, Krajewski S, et al. Prognostic significance of bcl-2 protein expression and bcl-2 gene rearrangement in diffuse aggressive non-Hodgkin's lymphoma. *Blood* 1997;90:244–251.

252. Hermine O, Haioun C, Lepage E, et al. Bcl-2 protein expression in aggressive non-Hodgkin's lymphoma (NHL). A new adverse prognostic factor? Proceedings of the Fifth International Conference on Malignant Lymphoma. 1993:28.

253. Kramer M, Hermans J, Parker J, et al. Clinical significance of bcl2 and p53 protein expression in diffuse large B-cell lymphoma: a population-based study. *J Clin Oncol* 1996;14:2131–2138.

254. Hill ME, MacLennan KA, Cunningham DC, et al. Prognostic significance of BCL-2 expression and bcl-2 major breakpoint region rearrangement in diffuse large cell non-Hodgkin's lymphoma: a British National Lymphoma Investigation Study. *Blood* 1996;88:1046–1051.

255. Hollstein M, Sidransky D, Vogelstein B, et al. p53 mutations in human cancers. *Science* 1991;253:49–53.

256. Wilson W, Teruya-Feldstein J, Fest T, et al. Relationship of p53, bcl-2, and tumor proliferation to clinical drug resistance in non-Hodgkin's lymphomas. *Blood* 1997;89:601–609.

257. Gascoyne RD. Pathologic prognostic factors in diffuse aggressive non-Hodgkin's lymphoma. *Hematol Oncol Clin North Am* 1997;11:847–862.

258. Sander CA, Yano T, Clark HM, et al. p53 mutation is associated with progression in follicular lymphomas. *Blood* 1993;82:1994–2004.

259. Lo Coco F, Gaidano G, Louie DC, et al. p53 mutations are associated with histologic transformation of follicular lymphoma. *Blood* 1993;82:2289–2295.

260. Ichikawa A, Kinoshita T, Watanabe T, et al. Mutations of the p53 gene as a prognostic factor in aggressive B-cell lymphoma. *N Eng J Med* 1997;337:529–534.

261. Ballerini P, Gaidano G, Gong J, et al. Multiple genetic lesions in AIDS-related non-Hodgkin lymphoma. *Blood* 1993;81:166–176.

262. Louie DC, Offit K, Jaslow R, et al. p53 overexpression as a marker of poor prognosis in mantle cell lymphomas with t(11;14)(q13;q32). *Blood* 1995;86:2892–2899.

263. Hernandez L, Fest T, Cazorla M, et al. p53 gene mutations and protein overexpression are associated with aggressive variants of mantle cell lymphomas. *Blood* 1996;87:3351–3359.

264. Koduru PR, Raju K, Vadmal V, et al. Correlation between mutation in P53, p53 expression, cytogenetics, histologic type, and survival in patients with B-cell non-Hodgkin's lymphoma. *Blood* 1997;90:4078–4091.

265. Young KH, Weisenburger DD, Dave BJ, et al. Mutations in the DNA-binding codons of TP53, which are associated with decreased expression of TRAILreceptor 2, predict for poor survival in diffuse large B-cell lymphoma. *Blood* 2007;110:4396–4405.

266. Davis RE, Brown KD, Siebenlist U, et al. Constitutive nuclear factor kappaB activity is required for survival of activated B cell-like diffuse large B cell lymphoma cells. *J Exp Med* 2001;194:1861–1874.

267. Wang CY, Guttridge DC, Mayo MW, et al. NF-κB induces expression of the Bcl-2 homologue A1/Bfl-1 to preferentially suppress chemotherapy-induced apoptosis. *Mol Cell Biol* 1999;19:5923–5929.

268. Chen C, Edelstein LC, Gelinas C. The Rel/NF-κB family directly activates expression of the apoptosis inhibitor Bcl-x(L). *Mol Cell Biol* 2000;20:2687–2695.

269. Lenz G, Davis RE, Ngo VN, et al. Oncogenic CARD11 mutations in human diffuse large B cell lymphoma. *Science* 2008;319·1676–1679.

270. Miller T, Grogan T, Dahlberg S, et al. Prognostic significance of the Ki-67-associated proliferative antigen in aggressive non-Hodgkin's lymphomas: a prospective Southwest Oncology Group trial. *Blood* 1994;83:1460–1466.

271. Grogan T, Kippman S, Spier C, et al. Independent prognostic significance of a nuclear proliferation antigen in diffuse large cell lymphomas as determined by the monoclonal antibody Ki-67. *Blood* 1988;71:1157–1160.

272. Jerkeman M, Anderson H, Dictor M, e al. Assessment of biological prognostic factors provides clinically relevant information in patients with diffuse large B-cell lymphoma—a Nordic Lymphoma Group study. *Ann Hematol* 2004;83:414–419.

273. Saez AI, Saez AJ. Artiga MJ, et al. Building an outcome predictor model for diffuse large B-cell lymphoma. *Am J Pathol* 2004;164:613–622.

274. Kossakowska A, Urbanski S, Huchcroft S, et al. Relationship between the clinical aggressiveness of large cell immunoblastic lymphomas and expression of 92 kDa gelatinase (type IV collagenase) and tissue inhibitor of metalloproteinases-1 (TIMP-1) RNAs. *Oncol Res* 1992;4:233–240.

275. Salven P. Angiogenesis in lymphoproliferative disorders. *Acta Haematol* 2001;106:184–189.

276. Vacca A, Ribatti D, Iurlaro M, et al. Human lymphoblastoid cells produce extracellular matrix-degrading enzymes and induce endothelial cell proliferation, migration, morphogenesis, and angiogenesis. *Int J Clin Lab Res* 1998;28:55–68.

277. Salven P, Teerenhovi L, Joensuu H. A high pretreatment serum vascular endothelial growth factor concentration is associated with poor outcome in non-Hodgkin's lymphoma. *Blood* 1997;90:3167–3172.

278. Dvorak HF, Sioussat TM, Brown LF, et al. Distribution of vascular permeability factor (vascular endothelial growth factor) in tumors: concentration in tumor blood vessels. *J Exp Med* 1991;174:1275–1278.

279. Yamamoto Y, Toi M, Kondo S, et al. Concentrations of vascular endothelial growth factor in the sera of normal controls and cancer patients. *Clin Cancer Res* 1996;2:821–826.

280. Salven P, Teerenhovi L, Joensuu H. A high pretreatment serum vascular endothelial growth factor concentration is associated with poor outcome in non-Hodgkin's lymphoma. *Blood* 1997;90:3167–3172.

281. Salven P, Teerenhovi L, Joensuu H. A high pretreatment serum basic fibroblast growth factor concentration is an independent predictor of poor prognosis in non-Hodgkin's lymphoma. *Blood* 1999;94:3334–3339.

282. Gratzinger D, Zhao S, Tibshirani RJ, et al. Prognostic significance of VEGF, VEGF receptors, and microvessel density in diffuse large B cell lymphoma treated with anthracycline-based chemotherapy. *Lab Invest* 2008;88:38–47.

283. Aguiar R, Yakushijin Y, Kharbanda S, et al. BAL is a novel risk-related gene in diffuse large B-cell lymphomas which enhances cellular migration. *Blood* 2000;96:4328–4334.

284. Rabbitts TH, Boehm T, Mengle-Gaw L. Chromosomal abnormalities in lymphoid tumours: mechanism and role in tumour pathogenesis. *Trends Genet* 1988;4(11):300–4.

285. Look AT, Downing JR. Molecular biology of leukemia and lymphoma. *Rev Invest Clin* 1994;(suppl):124–134.

286. Willis TG, Dyer MJ. The role of immunoglobulin translocations in the pathogenesis of B-cell malignancies. *Blood* 2000;96:808–822.

287. Taniwaki M, Nishida K, Ueda Y, et al. Interphase and metaphase detection of the breakpoint of 14q32 translocations in B-cell malignancies by double-color fluorescence in situ hybridization. *Blood* 1995;85:3223–3228.

288. Nanjangud G, Rao PH, Hegde A, et al. Spectral karyotyping identifies new rearrangements, translocations, and clinical associations in diffuse large B-cell lymphoma. *Blood* 2002;99:2554–2561.

289. Horsman DE, Gascoyne RD, Coupland RW, et al. Comparison of cytogenetic analysis, southern analysis, and polymerase chain reaction for the detection of t(14; 18) in follicular lymphoma. *Am J Clin Pathol* 1995;103:472–478.

290. Armitage JO, Sanger WG, Weisenburger DD, et al. Correlation of secondary cytogenetic abnormalities with histologic appearance in non-Hodgkin's lymphomas bearing t(14;18)(q32;q21). *J Natl Cancer Inst* 1988;80:576–580.

291. Capello D, Vitolo U, Pasqualucci L, et al. Distribution and pattern of BCl-6 mutations throughout the spectrum of B-cell neoplasia. *Blood* 2000;95:651–659.

292. Ohno H, Fukuhara S. Significance of rearrangement of the BCL6 gene in B-cell lymphoid neoplasms. *Leuk Lymphoma* 1997;27:53–63.

293. Cattoretti G, Chang CC, Cechova K, et al. BCL-6 protein is expressed in germinal-center B cells. *Blood* 1995;86:45–53.

294. Lo Coco F, Ye BH, Lista F, et al. Rearrangements of the BCL6 gene in diffuse large cell non-Hodgkin's lymphoma. *Blood* 1994;83:1757–1759.

295. Pasqualucci L, Migliazza A, Fracchiolla N, et al. BCL-6 mutations in normal germinal center B cells: evidence of somatic hypermutation acting outside Ig loci. *Proc Natl Acad Sci U S A* 1998;95:11816–11821.

296. Lossos IS, Levy R. Higher-grade transformation of follicle center lymphoma is associated with somatic mutation of the 5' noncoding regulatory region of the BCL- 6 gene. *Blood* 2000;96:635–639.

297. Offit K, Lo Coco F, Louie D, et al. Rearrangement of the BCL-6 gene as a prognostic marker in diffuse large-cell lymphoma. *N Engl J Med* 1994;331:74–80.

298. Kramer M, Hermans J, Wijburg E, et al. Clinical relevance of BCL2, BCL6, and MYC rearrangements in diffuse large B-cell lymphoma. *Blood* 1998;92:3152–3162.

299. Shafford EA, Kingston JE, Malpas JS, et al. Testicular function following the treatment of Hodgkin's disease in childhood. *Br J Cancer* 1993;68:1199–1204.

300. Lossos IS, Jones CD, Warnke R, et al. Expression of a single gene, BCL-6, strongly predicts survival in patients with diffuse large B-cell lymphoma. *Blood* 2001;98:945–951.

301. Ueda C, Uchiyama T, Ohno H. Immunoglobulin (Ig)/BCL6 versus non-Ig/BCL6 gene fusion in diffuse large B-cell lymphoma corresponds to a high- versus low-level expression of BCL6 mRNA. *Blood* 2002;99:2624–2625.

302. Lenz GW, Wright G, Dave SS. et al. Stromal gene signatures in large B-cell lymphomas. *NEJM* 2008;359(22):2313–23.

303. Nyman H, Adde M, Karjalainen-Lindsberg ML, et al. Prognostic impact of immunohistochemically defined germinal center phenotype in diffuse large B-cell lymphoma patients treated with immunochemotherapy. *Blood* 2007;109:4930–4935.

304. Mounier N, Briere J, Gisselbrecht C, et al. Rituximab plus CHOP (R-CHOP) overcomes bcl-2–associated resistance to chemotherapy in elderly patients with diffuse large B-cell lymphoma (DLBCL). *Blood* 2003;101:4279–4284.

305. Goethals I, Smeets P, De Winter O, et al. Focally enhanced f-18 fluorodeoxyglucose (FDG) uptake in incidentally detected pulmonary embolism on PET/CT scanning. *Clin Nucl Med* 2006;31:497–498.

306. Winter JN, Weller EA, Horning SJ, et al. Prognostic significance of Bcl-6 protein expression in DLBCL treated with CHOP or R-CHOP: a prospective correlative study. *Blood* 2006;107:4207–4213.

CHAPTER 11 ■ RESTAGING AND RESPONSE CRITERIA

BRUCE D. CHESON

The goal of cancer therapy is to improve the outcome of the patient by reducing the size of or completely eradicating the tumor, or by causing a decrease in disease-related symptoms. In the absence of effective therapy, response criteria are almost irrelevant; however, new advances in treatment have not only increased the number of responding patients but have also resulted in prolongation of survival in several lymphoma subtypes. Restaging as a means of assessing response in patients with non-Hodgkin lymphomas (NHLs) becomes increasingly important with the availability of more effective therapies, especially those administered with curative intent. Therefore, standardized response criteria are essential to accurately gauge response, and to be able to compare results among studies. Assessment of response to treatment is measured in several steps. Staging before treatment provides a baseline against which the effects of treatment can be compared. Restaging of lymphoma is defined as an assessment that is performed following completion of treatment to detect residual tumor or suspected recurrence, or to determine the extent of known recurrence (1). This term is in contrast to monitoring of therapy, which occurs during the course of treatment. However, as risk-adapted treatment strategies evolve, and response evaluation occurs earlier in the course of treatment, the distinction between monitoring and restaging will begin to blur.

Response in patients with lymphomas is most often measured by the extent of regression in the size and number of enlarged lymph nodes or confluent lymph node masses. Thus, agreement on the size of a "normal" lymph node is critical. Before 1999, there was marked variability in the definition of the size of a "normal" lymph node in patients with NHL. Based on computed tomography (CT) scanning and autopsy series, the upper limit of lymph node size in normal individuals is approximately 1.0 cm in the short axis. However, this threshold varies with anatomic location (2–9). The upper limit of normal for mediastinal nodes ranges from 5 to 12 mm in the short axis, with greater variation in the long axis. The size of abdominal nodes on CT scans varies by region from 8 to 11 mm; however, normal nodes in the pelvis may be as large as 15 mm. A lymph node that is either larger than 1 cm in its short transverse diameter or hard to palpation should be considered suspicious for involvement by lymphoma. Moreover, smaller nodes that are more numerous than expected or in usual sites should also be considered suspicious for involvement. Because different radiologists will likely review the pretreatment and posttreatment scans, consistent indicator lesions should be identified and measured to minimize interobserver variability.

Despite the variability among anatomic sites, the criterion of 1.5 cm in transverse diameter as normal was initially established for Hodgkin lymphoma (10). Using the longest transverse diameter appears to provide a more accurate assessment of response than the short axis in patients with NHL (11). Incrementally increasing the bidimensional requirement from 1.0×1.0 cm to 1.5×1.5 cm and to 2.0×2.0 cm does not appear to affect the overall response rate, but it does result in a significant increase in the complete remission (CR) rate (11).

For more than 2 decades, CT scans were the standard method of evaluation for staging and restaging of NHLs. Although CT scans provide relatively high sensitivity and specificity in pretreatment staging (12,13), specificity in response assessment following therapy is relatively low (14–17). One explanation is the inability of the CT to distinguish between scar tissue/fibrosis and viable tumor in patients with a residual mass following therapy. Lymph nodes may be completely or only partially involved by lymphoma. Following effective treatment, a node or mass may decrease in size but persist on CT scan. Because tumor-involved nodes shrink in size following treatment, fibrosis, necrosis, or inflammation results in a persistent enlargement of a node that may be histologically uninvolved by tumor (18). Response assessment of a group of nodes that were initially enlarged and matted together and appeared as a mass, but that broke up into several smaller nodal masses after treatment, may be difficult. Thus, persistence of residual masses following chemotherapy does not necessarily indicate residual disease (15,16,18,19). Fuks et al. (14) treated 100 patients with combination chemotherapy for NHL, resulting in 33 complete and 38 partial remissions (PRs). In 20 of the PRs, whereas clinical evidence suggested a CR, however, lymphangiogram, gallium scan, abdominal CT scan, or ultrasound suggested residual disease. Nevertheless, in only 20% of these cases was persistent disease identified at restaging laparotomy. Surbone et al. (16) reported that of 241 patients with aggressive lymphoma, 30% had an abdominal mass at diagnosis with a residual mass in 40% at clinical CR. Of 22 patients with pathologic evaluations, the specimen was negative in 95%; none of which relapsed at a median follow-up of 31 months.

Attempting to reduce the confusion caused by the presence of residual masses, some investigators classified response retrospectively, depending on the subsequent behavior of the mass (20,21). Other investigators used terms such as "probable CR" (22). In some series, a large abdominal or mediastinal mass that decreased by >50% in size and remained stable for 2 to 4 months was felt to be consistent with a CR in the absence of any other measurable disease (16,19,20,22–24), whereas a cutoff of 75% was used by others (21). In other series, nodes larger than 1 cm were required to be negative by histologic examination to be considered a CR (25).

Before 1999, the considerable variability among clinical trial groups in when and how patients were evaluated, as well as the variable definition of a "normal" sized lymph node, impeded comparisons of study results. Response was sometimes assessed prospectively, other times retrospectively, with disparity as to the size of a "normal" lymph node. The need for standardization was emphasized by an analysis of data from the rituximab pivotal trial in which minor differences in the definition of a normal-sized lymph node resulted in major differences in the percentage of patients considered to have attained a CR (11). To address these issues, an International Working Group (IWG) composed of clinicians, radiologists, and pathologists with expertise in the evaluation and management of patients with lymphoma developed guidelines that standardized the size of a normal lymph node, when and how responses were assessed, and provided response category and end point definitions (26).

These recommendations were widely adopted by international clinical trials groups and regulatory agencies. However, with their application over time, it became clear that revisions were indicated. For example, the IWG criteria relied on physical examination, with its marked interobserver and intraobserver variability, CT scans, and single photon emission CT gallium scans; the latter no longer being widely used.

A major problem with the original IWG criteria was the misinterpretation of the term CR/unconfirmed (CRu). CRu was originally proposed to designate two types of responses. The first was in those patients with curable histologies, such as Hodgkin lymphoma or diffuse large B-cell lymphoma (DLBCL), who, before therapy, had lymphadenopathy that included a large mass and for whom treatment resulted in a disappearance of all detectable tumor except for persistence of that mass, which had decreased by at least 75% on CT scan. In as many as 90% of cases, these lesions are scar tissue or fibrosis rather than active tumor (16,27). Instead, CRu was often applied to situations in which the SPDs of multiple nodes decreased by at least 75%, even in patients with incurable histologies, which would more appropriately be considered partial responses. One consequence has been an artificial inflation of CR rates. The second type of CRu included patients with bone marrow involvement before treatment who fulfilled all of the conditions for a CR following therapy, except that the bone marrow was considered by the pathologist to be morphologically indeterminate. Instead, the term was also assigned to patients who did not undergo a repeat biopsy to confirm response.

The distinction between viable tumor and scar tissue has been largely resolved through the use of metabolic imaging (Fig. 11.1). Gallium scanning has now been replaced by 18-fluoro-deoxyglucose (FDG) positron emission tomography (PET). FDG-PET is a noninvasive metabolic imaging technique that detects FDG labeled with fluorine-18, which, after injection, is taken up by tumor cells. PET scanning has replaced gallium scanning because of its better resolution, increased sensitivity, and shorter procedure time (28,29). PET is more reliable than gallium scanning to monitor disease (30). PET is more accurate for supradiaphragmatic disease than CT scans but may be comparable to CT scans in assessment of subdiaphragmatic disease (31). Overall, FDG-

PET results correlate better with outcome than CT scans (32). The two may be complimentary, and both should be performed. Even with the increasing use of PET-CT scans, an independent contrast-enhanced CT scan may provide additional, clinically meaningful information.

The clinical value of PET scans differs by clinical context, depending on whether the test is used at diagnosis for staging, for restaging after therapy, during treatment, or for detection of early relapse (1,29,32–52).

The frequency of a positive PET scan also varies with the histologic subtype (53–55), with a greater likelihood of aggressive B-cell lymphomas being PET positive than low-grade lymphomas. Most common subtypes of NHL (e.g., diffuse large B-cell NHL, follicular NHL, mantle cell NHL) are routinely FDG–avid, with a sensitivity that exceeds 80% and a specificity of about 90%, which is superior to CT (12,13,31). Extranodal marginal zone NHLs are more likely negative than their nodal counterparts (54), and a low rate of FDG avidity has also been reported for small lymphocytic lymphoma (38). T-cell NHLs are more variably FDG avid than B-cell NHL, and the role of PET in these patients requires further study (54–56).

18-FLUORO-DEOXYGLUCOSE POSITRON EMISSION TOMOGRAPHY IN RESTAGING OF NON-HODGKIN LYMPHOMA

The clearest role for PET is in restaging of patients following completion of therapy (29,32,34,40,41,57,58). PET is more accurate than CT in this setting, largely because of its ability to distinguish viable tumor from necrosis or fibrosis in residual masses. CT-PET is the preferred technique, although the role of an additional contrast-enhanced CT scan is controversial (59). FDG-PET is a strong predictor of patient outcome. Jerusalem et al. (32) prospectively evaluated 54 patients with NHL (n = 35) and Hodgkin lymphoma (n = 19), 24 with residual CT masses. All six patients with a positive PET scan relapsed compared with five of 19 with positive CT/negative PET (26%) and three out of 29 patients with negative CT/negative PET (10%). Spaepen et al. (57) studied 93 patients with various histologies of NHL who underwent PET after treatment and were followed for at least 1 year. Of 67 with a normal study, 56 remained in continuous CR at a median of 653 days. All 26 patients who had a positive PET relapsed at a median of 73 days. Zinzani et al. (40) reported on 44 patients with HL or aggressive NHL presenting with abdominal disease, which was bulky in 41%. Following therapy, none of those with a negative PET and CT relapsed, yet all of those who had a positive CT and PET relapsed. One patient of 24 who was positive by CT but negative by PET, relapsed. The 2-year relapse-free survival for those with a positive PET was 0% compared with 95% for those with negative PET.

PET is most valuable in patients with potentially curable NHL, most notably diffuse large B-cell NHL, where a CR is essential for a successful outcome. In general, PET has a consistently high negative predictive value (NPV), averaging about 85% across studies (29,32,34,40,57,58). The approximate 15% false-negative rate with PET is mostly related to

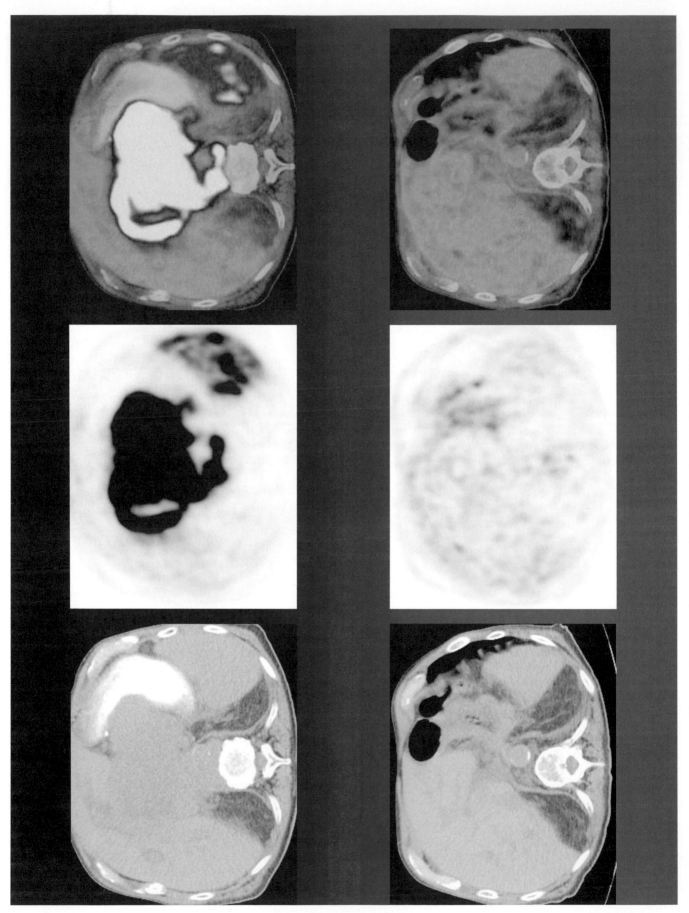

FIGURE 11.1 This patient is a 52-year-old man with DLBCL who was started on therapy with rituximab plus CHOP. A PET/CT scan performed after two cycles demonstrated persistence of the mass on the CT, but no FDG avidity on the PET or fusion scan. The patient remains in CR. (Courtesy of Lale Kostakoglu.) (see also Color Plate 12)

its inability to detect microscopic disease resulting in future relapse. The positive predictive value (PPV) of PET is generally around 85% with NHL (29,32,34,40,57), which is substantially higher than CT, which has a reported PPV in patients with aggressive NHL of about 40% to 50%. The NPV of PET is similar to that of CT, resulting in a considerably higher accuracy of PET for response assessment compared with CT (approximately 80% vs. 50%). Juweid et al. (29) found a PPV of 74% and a NPV of 83% for attenuation-corrected PET scans in patients with aggressive NHL. Older studies used nonattenuation-corrected PET images, where mild FDG-PET uptake, particularly in deep-seated lymph nodes or nodal masses, may have gone undetected because they fail to correct for absorption of photons through body tissues to obtain a true measure of accumulated activity. PET results from recent studies may be more accurate because they utilized currently standard attenuation-corrected PET to evaluate the predictive value of PET.

Thus, although a positive test following therapy is generally considered a strong predictor of failure, such results should be interpreted in conjunction with the history, physical examination, and CT scans. False-positive results have been reported in more than 20% of patients serially studied following therapy as a consequence of infection, inflammation, tumor necrosis, or other causes (60,61) (Fig. 11.2). Because of the substantial PPV, it is important that, in general, a major treatment decision not be based on a single imaging study. Either a biopsy should be performed of the FDG-avid lesion, or the study should be repeated in 2 to 3 months to confirm residual disease.

18-FLUORO-DEOXYGLUCOSE POSITRON EMISSION TOMOGRAPHY IN RESPONSE ASSESSMENT

Juweid et al. (29) were the first to evaluate the impact of integrating PET into the International Response Criteria of

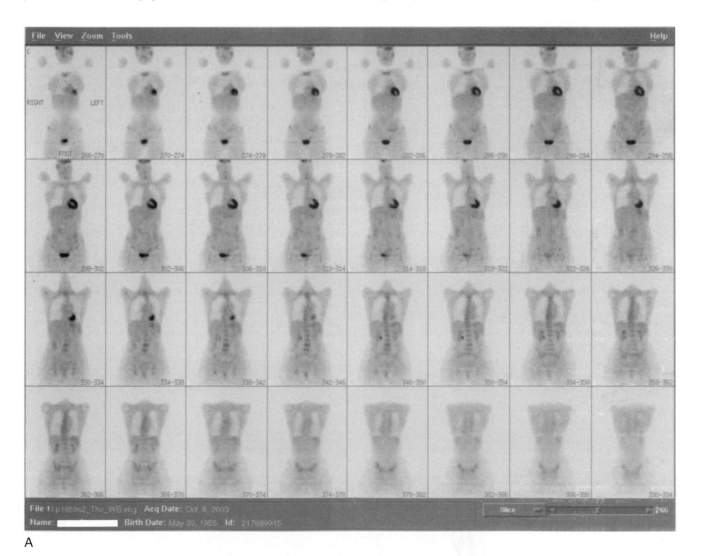

FIGURE 11.2 A: This patient is a 56-year-old woman with stage IIIA DLBCL. (see also Color Plate 13) **B:** A normal CT-PET after completion of six cycles of rituximab plus CHOP. However, several months later, there was an FDG-avid mediastinal mass. Biopsy revealed sarcoidosis. At routine follow-up 4.5 years later, cervical and axillary lymphadenopathy were palpated. (see also Color Plate 14) **C:** CT/PET scan failed to identify either the previous sarcoid or any FDG-avid lymph nodes. The patient remains in a clinical remission. (see also Color Plate 15)

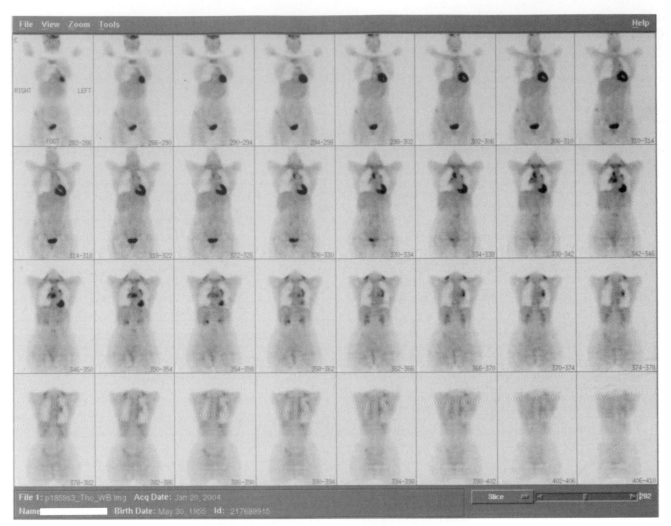

B

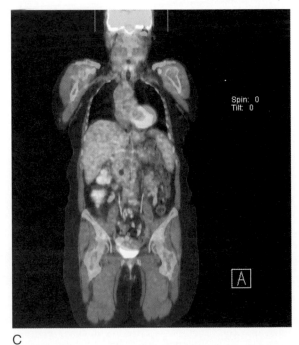

C

FIGURE 11.2 *Continued*

1999. They reported a retrospective analysis of 54 patients with aggressive NHL treated with cyclophosphamide, doxorubicin, vincristine, and prednisone (CHOP)-based chemotherapy who were evaluated by CT and PET, and followed for at least 18 months after treatment. The use of PET increased the number of CRs by converting not only partial responses into complete responses but also by eliminating the subset of patients who would have been considered CRu. The 18-month progression-free survival was similar whether patients were considered as having a CR by CT or PET and CT. However, the major difference was in patients considered as having PR for whom the median progression-free survival was 70% with the International Workshop recommendation and 22% when PET was included.

THE USE OF POSITRON EMISSION TOMOGRAPHY IN CLINICAL TRIALS

After they had been used extensively for several years, a number of issues with the IWG response criteria suggested that a number of modifications were indicated. For example, they were based primarily on physical examination, CT scans, and single photon emission CT scans. However, a major factor in considering revision was the increasing availability of FDG-PET scans. The German Competence Network Malignant Lymphoma facilitated this process by convening the International Harmonization Project (IHP), including an international committee of lymphoma clinical investigators, pathologists, and nuclear medicine physicians to review the IWG and other proposed response criteria (e.g., response evaluation criteria in solid tumors), and to determine how best to clarify and improve on them to ensure transparency among clinical trial groups (62). Assouline et al. (63) had proposed a modified response evaluation criteria in solid tumors criteria for lymphoma using unidimensional measurements of lymph nodes and masses, and reported a high concordance with the IWG criteria; however, the concordance was high only in those studies with low response rates (64).

There were two major outcomes of the IHP. The first of these was a standardization of performance and interpretation of PET in lymphoma clinical trials (50). The recommendation was that PET be performed 6 to 8 weeks following completion of chemotherapy or 8 to 12 weeks after radiation therapy to minimize the possibility of a false-positive result. Patients should be imaged after fasting for at least 4 hours and have a blood glucose not to exceed 200 mg per dL. The study should begin at 60 ± 10 minutes after injection of the radiolabeled glucose. Intravenous and oral contrast facilitates assessment of liver and spleen, and differentiates bowel from other structures. The Working Group defined a positive scan as focal or diffuse FDG uptake above background in a location incompatible with normal anatomy or physiology. Exceptions include mild and diffusely increased FDG uptake at the site of moderate or large-sized masses with an intensity that is lower than or equal to the mediastinal blood pool, hepatic or splenic nodules 1.5 cm with FDG uptake lower than the surrounding liver/spleen uptake, and diffusely increased bone marrow uptake within weeks following treatment (50). Areas of necrosis may be FDG avid within an otherwise negative residual mass, and a follow-up scan in a few months is often indicated to confirm this clinical impression. Residual masses ≥ 2 cm in greatest transverse diameter with FDG activity visually exceeding that of mediastinal blood pool structures are considered PET–positive, whereas residual masses 1.1 to 1.9 cm are considered PET–positive only if their activity exceeds surrounding background activity. Visual assessment is currently considered adequate for determining whether a PET scan is positive. Lin et al. (65) suggested that when the same data set was analyzed, standard uptake value measurements correlated better with outcome than visual assessment. Nevertheless, the correlation between percent reduction in the standard uptake value and response is currently being evaluated in clinical trials (50).

INTERNATIONAL HARMONIZATION PROJECT RECOMMENDATIONS FOR THE USE OF 18-FLUORO-DEOXYGLUCOSE POSITRON EMISSION TOMOGRAPHY IN CLINICAL TRIALS

The IHP also provided modified response criteria incorporating FDG-PET (51). The new recommendations for PET scans in clinical trials took into consideration the variability in FDG avidity among the various lymphoma histologic subtypes, and the relevant end points of clinical trials (Table 11.1). PET was recommended as a standard component of the initial evaluation of patients with routinely FDG-avid, potentially curable lymphomas (e.g., DLBCL, Hodgkin lymphoma) to define the extent of disease and to provide a baseline against which to compare posttreatment (restaging) studies. For the FDG-avid but incurable histologies (e.g., follicular lymphoma, and low-grade and mantle cell lymphoma), PET is indicated only if complete response is a primary end point of the trial because time-dependent end points (e.g., progression-free survival) are generally of greater importance.

Numerous studies have demonstrated that PET scans performed after one or more cycles of chemotherapy predict progression-free and overall survival (34–36,47,66,67). Unfortunately, no available data demonstrate that altering treatment on the basis of PET results improves patient outcome. Moskowitz et al. (68) reported on 87 patients with DLBCL who underwent four cycles of a dose-intense rituximab plus CHOP every 14 days followed by a PET scan. Those with a negative scan received three cycles of ifosfamide, carboplatin, and etoposide (ICE), and observation. Patients with a positive interim PET scan underwent a biopsy. Those with a negative biopsy received three cycles of ICE. Patients with a positive biopsy were to receive ICE for two cycles, rituximab plus ICE for one cycle, and autologous stem cell transplantation. The NPV of the PET scan was 89%. However, the PPV was only 26%. There were four positive biopsies, but 27 were negative, giving an 87% false-positive rate. There was no difference in event-free survival between patients with a positive or negative PET scan.

PET is essential for restaging the potentially curable lymphoma histologies following completion of therapy but

TABLE 11.1

RECOMMENDED TIMING OF PET (PET/CT) SCANS IN LYMPHOMA CLINICAL TRIALS

Histology	Pre-treatment	Mid-treatment	Response Assessment	Post-tx Surveillance
Routinely FDG-Avid				
DLBCL	Yes*	Clinical trial	Yes	No
HL	Yes*	Clinical trial	Yes	No
Follicular NHL	No†	Clinical trial	No†	No
MCL	No†	Clinical trial	No†	No
Variably FDG-Avid				
Other aggressive NHLs	No†	Clinical trial	No‡	No
Other indolent NHLs	No†	Clinical trial	No‡	No

* Recommended but not required pretreatment
† Recommended only if ORR/CR is a primary study endpoint
‡ Recommended only if PET is positive pre-treatment

should not be performed until at least 6 to 8 weeks following completion of therapy to reduce the likelihood of a false-positive result (50). In these patients, a CR is required for cure, and therapeutic intervention is generally indicated if residual disease is present. However, PET is not recommended in the posttreatment assessment of the remaining histologies unless the PET scan was positive before treatment and if complete response rate is a primary end point of a clinical study. A CT scan can usually suffice in these patients.

REVISED RESPONSE CRITERIA

The second major outcome of the IHP was a revision of the IWG response criteria (39) (Table 11.2)
    CR requires:

1. Complete disappearance of all clinical evidence of disease and disease-related symptoms.
2. a. Typically FDG-avid lymphoma. In patients with no pretreatment PET scan or when the FDG-PET scan was positive before therapy, a posttreatment residual mass of any size is permitted as long as it is PET negative.
   b. Variably FDG-avid lymphomas/FDG avidity unknown: In patients without a pretreatment PET scan, or if a pretreatment PET scan was negative, all lymph nodes and nodal masses must have regressed on CT to normal size (≤1.5 cm in their greatest transverse diameter for nodes >1.5 cm before therapy). Previously involved nodes that were 1.1 to 1.5 cm in their long axis and >1.0 cm in their short axis before treatment must have decreased to ≤1.0 cm in their short axis after treatment.
3. The spleen and/or liver, if considered enlarged before therapy on the basis of a physical examination or CT scan should not be palpable on physical examination and should be considered normal size by imaging studies, and nodules related to lymphoma should disappear. However, determination of splenic involvement is not always reliable because a spleen considered normal in size may still contain lymphoma, whereas an enlarged spleen may reflect variations in anatomy, blood volume, the use of hematopoietic growth factors, or other causes rather than lymphoma.

4. If the bone marrow was involved by lymphoma before treatment, the infiltrate must have cleared on repeat bone marrow biopsy. The biopsy sample on which this determination is made must be adequate (with a goal of ≥20 mm unilateral core). If the sample is indeterminate by morphology, it should be negative by immunohistochemistry (Fig. 11.3). A sample that is negative by immunohistochemistry but demonstrating a small population of clonal lymphocytes by flow cytometry will be considered a CR until data become available demonstrating a clear difference in patient outcome.

Complete Remission/Unconfirmed

Using the aforementioned definition for CR and that in the next section for PR eliminates the category of CRu.

Partial Remission Requires All of the Following

1. ≥50% decrease in SPDs of up to six of the largest dominant nodes or nodal masses. These nodes or masses should be selected according to all of the following: (a) they should be clearly measurable in at least two perpendicular dimensions; (b) if possible, they should be from disparate regions of the body; and (c) they should include mediastinal and retroperitoneal areas of disease whenever these sites are involved.
2. No increase in the size of other nodes, liver, or spleen.
3. Splenic and hepatic nodules must regress by ≥50% in their SPD or, for single nodules, in the greatest transverse diameter.
4. With the exception of splenic and hepatic nodules, involvement of other organs is usually evaluable and not measurable disease.
5. Bone marrow assessment is irrelevant for determination of a PR if the sample was positive before treatment. However, if positive, the cell type should be specified, e.g., large cell lymphoma or small neoplastic B cells. Patients who achieve a CR by the aforementioned criteria, but

TABLE 11.2

RESPONSE DEFINITIONS FOR LYMPHOMA

Response	Definition	Nodal Masses	Liver/Spleen	Bone Marrow
Complete Remission (CR)	Disappearance of all evidence of disease	a. FDG-avid or PET+ prior to therapy: mass of any size permitted if PET- b. Variably FDG-avid or PET-: regression to normal size on CT	Not palpable, nodules disappeared	Infiltrate cleared on repeat biopsy, if indeterminate by morphology immunohistochemistry should be negative
Partial Remission (PR)	Regression of measurable disease and no new sites	≥50% decrease in SPD of up to 6 largest dominant masses. No increase in size of other nodes a. FDG-avid or PET+ prior to therapy: one or more PET+ at previously involved site b. Variably FDG-avid or PET-: Regression on CT	≥50% decrease in SPD of nodules (for single nodule in greatest transverse diameter), no increase in size of liver or spleen	Irrelevant if positive prior to therapy, cell type should be specified
Stable Disease (SD)	Failure to attain CR/PR or PD	a. FDG-avid or PET+ prior to therapy: PET+ at prior sites of disease and no new sites on CT or PET b. Variably FDG-avid or PET-: No change in size of previous lesions on CT		
Relapsed/Progressive disease (RD/PD)	Any new lesion or increase by ≥50% of previously involved sites from nadir	Appearance of a new lesion ≥1.5 cm in any axis ≥50% increase in the longest diameter of a previously identifed node >1 cm in short axis or in the SPD of more than one node Lesions PET+ if FDG-avid lymphoma or PET+ prior to therapy	≥50% increase from nadir in the SPD of any previous lesions	New or recurrent involvement

who have persistent morphologic bone marrow involvement, will be considered partial responders.

In cases where the bone marrow was involved before therapy that resulted in a clinical CR, but with no bone marrow assessment following treatment, patients should be considered partial responders.

6. No new sites of disease.
7. Typically FDG-avid lymphoma: For patients with no pretreatment PET scan or if the PET scan was positive before therapy, the posttreatment PET should be positive in at least one previously involved site.
8. Variably FDG-avid lymphomas/FDG-avidity unknown: For patients without a pretreatment PET scan, or if a pretreatment PET scan was negative, CT criteria should be used.

Stable Disease

1. Failing to attain the criteria needed for a CR or PR, but not fulfilling those for progressive disease (see section on Progressive Disease).

2. Typically FGD-avid lymphomas: The FDG-PET should be positive at prior sites of disease with no new areas of involvement on the posttreatment CT or PET.
3. Variably FDG-avid lymphomas/FDG-avidity unknown: For patients without a pretreatment PET scan or if the pretreatment PET was negative, there must be no change in the size of the previous lesions on the posttreatment CT scan.

Relapsed Disease (After Complete Remission)/Progressive Disease (After Partial Remission, Stable Disease)

Lymph nodes should be considered abnormal if the long axis is >1.5 cm, regardless of the short axis. If a lymph node has a long axis of 1.1 to 1.5 cm, it should only be considered abnormal if its short axis is >1.0. Lymph nodes ≤1.0 by ≤1.0 cm will not be considered as abnormal for relapse or progressive disease.

1. Appearance of any new lesion >1.5 cm in any axis during or at the end of therapy, even if others are decreasing in

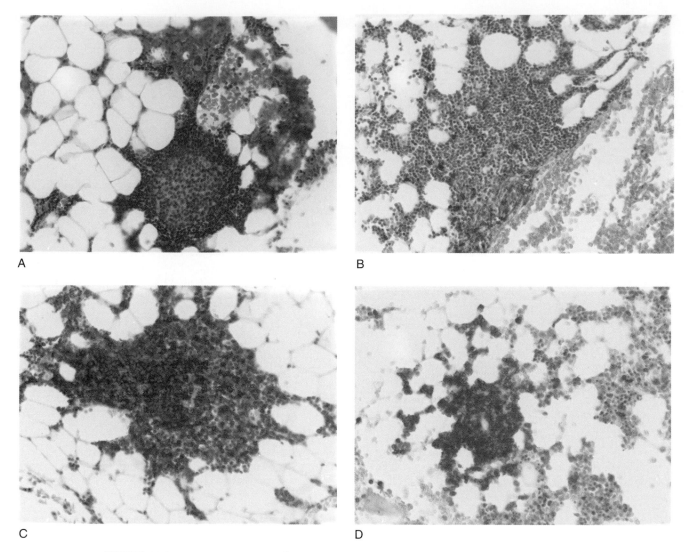

FIGURE 11.3 Bone marrow biopsy of a patient with CLL/SLL following therapy. The residual lymphoid nodule (see also Color Plate 16) (**A**) is demonstrated to represent residual disease because it is negative for CD3 (see also Color Plate 17), (**B**) yet positive for CD20 (see also Color Plate 18) (**C**) and CD 5 (see also Color Plate 19) (**D**).

size. Increased FDG uptake in a previously unaffected site should only be considered relapsed or progressive disease after confirmation with other modalities. In patients with no prior history of pulmonary lymphoma, new lung nodules identified by CT are mostly benign. Thus, a therapeutic decision should not be made solely on the basis of the PET without histologic confirmation.

2. ≥50% increase from nadir in the SPD of any previously involved nodes, or in a single involved node, or the size of other lesions (e.g., splenic or hepatic nodules). To be considered progressive disease, a lymph node with a diameter of the short axis of <1.0 cm must increase by ≥50% and to a size of 1.5 × 1.5 cm or >1.5 cm in the long axis.

3. ≥50% increase in the longest diameter of any single previously identified node >1 cm in its short axis.

4. Lesions should be PET positive if a typical FDG-avid lymphoma or one that was PET positive before therapy unless the lesion is too small to be detected with current PET systems (<1.5 cm in its long axis by CT).

Measurable extranodal disease should be assessed in a manner similar to nodal disease. Disease that is only evaluable (e.g., pleural effusions, bone lesions) is recorded as present or absent only, unless, while an abnormality is still noted by imaging studies or physical examination, it is found to be histologically negative.

In clinical trials where PET is not available to the vast majority of participants, or where PET is deemed neither necessary nor appropriate, response should be assessed as described previously, but only using CT scans. In this setting, residual masses should not be considered a CRu but should be designated as partial responses.

These response criteria have now been adopted internationally by study groups and regulatory agencies. Brepoels et al. (69) attempted to validate the new response criteria in 69 patients with aggressive or indolent NHL. They confirmed that the new response criteria were superior to the IWG criteria alone, although PET was of less value in the incurable, indolent NHL.

FOLLOW-UP EVALUATION

Follow-Up

The manner in which patients are followed after completion of therapy may differ considerably between a clinical trial and clinical practice, by histologic subtype, and whether treatment was initiated with curative or palliative intent.

The most important components of monitoring patients following treatment are a careful history and physical examination, along with complete blood count and serum chemistries, including lactate dehydrogenase and other relevant blood tests. The National Comprehensive Cancer Network published recommendations for follow-up of patients with NHL (70). For patients with a history of follicular or other indolent histology in a CR, the recommendation for follow-up was every 3 months for 1 year, then every 3 to 6 months. For DLBCL, the guidelines proposed assessment every 3 months for 24 months, then every 6 months for 36 months with imaging studies performed when clinically indicated.

Although widely used in clinical practice, there is no evidence to support regular surveillance CT or PET scans, and this practice is discouraged. A number of studies in the pre-PET era demonstrated that the patient or physician identifies the relapse more than 80% of the time (71–74). Weeks et al. (71) assessed the role of conventional screening for relapse in patients with NHL. The authors concluded that follow-up strategies based on standard radiographic procedures and blood tests were not effective in detecting patients with pre-clinical relapse with large cell lymphoma. They recommended that screening studies should not be site–specific, and the frequency of study should be determined by the patient's risk for relapse and whether there is a potentially curative salvage therapy. Oh et al. (72) studied 328 patients with previously untreated stage I follicular NHL, 78 of whom relapsed and were part of the study. They had received a variety of treatments. At a median follow-up of 101 months, only 14% of relapses were identified by CT scans, and just 4.3% benefited from the information provided by the CT. The number of relapses identified by physical examination was similar to CT scans. Minimum testing at follow-up visits should include history, physical examination for lymphadenopathy, abdominal masses or organomegaly, and blood tests, including a complete blood count and serum chemistries, including lactate dehydrogenase. Additional blood tests and imaging studies may be added for relevant clinical indications.

In a clinical trial, uniformity of reassessment is necessary to ensure comparability among studies with respect to the major end points of event-free survival, disease-free survival, and progression-free survival. It is obvious, for example, that a protocol requiring extensive reevaluation every 2 months will produce different apparent intervals for those end points compared with one requiring the same testing annually, even if the true times to events are the same. One recommendation has been to assess patients on clinical trials after completion of treatment at a minimum of every 3 months for 2 years, then every 6 months for 3 years, and then annually for at least 5 years (26). Few recurrences occur beyond that point for patients with large cell NHL. However, there is a continuous risk of relapse for patients with a follicular histology.

These intervals may vary with specific treatments, protocols, or unique drug characteristics.

There is no clear role for surveillance PET scans in the follow-up of patients with NHL. Jerusalem et al. (75) reported a series of 36 patients who underwent PET following therapy and every 4 to 6 months thereafter. There were five events detected by PET, one in a patient with known residual disease. Two of the four patients whose relapse 5 to 24 months following treatment was identified by PET already had developed disease-related symptoms. In addition, there were six false-positive studies. Zinzani et al. (61) conducted a prospective evaluation of 160 patients with Hodgkin lymphoma and 261 patients with indolent or aggressive NHL who underwent PET at 6, 12, 18, and 24 months after therapy, then annually. For the patients with Hodgkin lymphoma, the likelihood of relapse was negligible after 12 months and after 18 months for the aggressive NHLs. Scans were interpreted as positive for relapse, negative for relapse, or inconclusive when they were considered equivocal. All patients with an inconclusive study underwent biopsy; in only 33% was there suspected relapse on CT scan as well. Among the 24 patients who had positive PET/negative CT, there was a 42% false-positive rate. There was a continuous risk of relapse for the indolent NHLs. Patients with suspected relapse underwent biopsy with a 42% false-positive rate of PET scans. The authors concluded that there was no benefit from continued surveillance studies after 18 months.

END POINTS

The major end points of clinical trials should reflect the histology, clinical situation (initial treatment vs. salvage), and objectives of the study (Table 11.3). It is important that consistent definitions of end points are used, and we hope that this document will harmonize the use of those definitions.

End points based on tumor measurements are greatly influenced by response criteria. Overall and complete response rates can usually be accurately assessed in single arm as well as randomized trials. However, response rates do not necessarily impact on other measures of overall clinical benefit or outcome in patients with lymphoma and are not considered as important as other end points. Exceptions are phase II trials of novel new agents where identification of biologic activity is of interest. Durable complete responses, if associated with measures of clinical benefit, may also be relevant.

SUMMARY

The availability of FDG-PET has improved the predictability of restaging and response assessment of patients with NHL. PET is more sensitive and specific than CT, particularly because it better distinguishes fibrosis or scar tissue from metabolically active lymphoma (Fig. 11.1). However, its positive NPV limits its usefulness, especially because of the large number of false-positive results. Whereas interim PET scans are predictive of patient outcome, there are no data that demonstrate that altering therapy on the basis of those results improves survival. Risk-directed studies are needed to validate preliminary observations that suggest that a negative PET may permit a decrease in the amount of chemotherapy or

TABLE 11.3

EFFICACY ENDPOINTS

Primary Endpoints	Patients	Definition	Measured From
Overall survival	All	Death from any cause	Entry onto study
Progression-free survival	All	Disease progression or death from any cause	Entry onto study
Secondary Endpoints			
Event-free survival	All	Failure of treatment or death from any cause	Entry onto study
Time to progression	All	Time to progression or death from lymphoma	Entry onto study
Disease-free survival	In CR	Time to relapse or death from lymphoma or acute toxicity of treatment	Documentation of response
Response duration	In CR or PR	Time to relapse or progression	Documentation of response
Lymphoma-specific survival	All	Time to death from lymphoma	Entry onto study
Time to next treatment	All	Time to new treatment	End of primary treatment

radiation therapy required, especially in patients with limited stage disease that is responding to therapy, or to increase efficacy by altering therapy in patients with less responsive disease (76,77). There are currently no data to support routine surveillance with CT or PET scans. Clearly, PET scans provide additional information regarding the status of activity of lymphoma; however, the impact of this technology on patient management is still being clarified in clinical research trials.

References

1. Juweid M, Cheson BD. Positron emission tomography (PET) in post-therapy assessment of cancer. *N Engl J Med* 2006;354:496–507.
2. Dorfman RE, Alpern MB, Gross BH, et al. Upper abdominal lymph nodes: criteria for normal size determined with CT. *Radiology* 1991;180:319–322.
3. Einstein DM, Singer AA, Chilcote WA, et al. Abdominal lymphadenopathy: spectrum of CT findings. *Radiographics* 1991;11:457–472.
4. Glazer GM, Gross BH, Quint LE, et al. Normal mediastinal lymph nodes: number and size according to American Thoracic Society mapping. *AJR Am J Roentgenol* 1985;144:261–265.
5. Hopper KD, Kasales CJ, Van Slyke MA, et al. Analysis of interobserver and intraobserver variability in CT tumor measurements. *AJR Am J Roentgenol* 1996;187:851–854.
6. Kiyono K, Sone S, Sakai F, et al. The number and size of normal mediastinal lymph nodes: a postmortem study. *AJR Am J Roentgenol* 1988;150:771–776.
7. Steinkamp HJ, Hosten N, Richter C, et al. Enlarged cervical lymph nodes at helical CT. *Radiology* 1994;191:795–798.
8. van den Brekel MW, Castelijns JA, Snow GB. Detection of lymph node metastases in the neck: radiologic criteria. *Radiology* 1994;192:617–618.
9. Genereux GP, Howie JL. Normal mediastinal lymph node size and number: CT and anatomic study. *AJR Am J Roentgenol* 1984;142:1095–1100.
10. Lister TA, Crowther D, Sutcliffe SB, et al. Report of a committee convened to discuss the evaluation and staging of patients with Hodgkin's disease: Cotswolds Meeting. *J Clin Oncol* 1989;7:1630–1636.
11. Grillo-López AJ, Cheson BD, Horning SJ, et al. Response criteria for NHL: importance of "normal" lymph node size and correlations with response rates. *Ann Oncol* 2000;11:399–408.
12. Newman JS, Francis JR, Kaminski MS, et al. Imaging of lymphoma with PET with 2-[F-18]-fluoro-2-deoxy-D-glucose: correlation with CT. *Radiology* 1994;190:111–116.
13. Thill R, Neuerburg J, Fabry U, et al. Comparison of findings with 18-FDG PET and CT in pretherapeutic staging of malignant lymphoma [in German]. *Nuklearmedizin* 1997;36:234–239.
14. Fuks JZ, Aisner J, Wiernik PH. Restaging laparotomy in the management of the non-Hodgkin lymphomas. *Med Pediatr Oncol* 1982;10:429–438.
15. Stewart FM, Williamson BR, Innes DJ, et al. Residual tumor masses following treatment for advanced histiocytic lymphoma. *Cancer* 1985;55:620–623.
16. Surbone A, Longo DL, DeVita VT Jr, et al. Residual abdominal masses in aggressive non-Hodgkin's lymphoma after combination chemotherapy: significance and management. *J Clin Oncol* 1988;6:1832–1837.
17. Stumpe KD, Urbinelli M, Steinert HC, et al. Whole-body positron emission tomography using fluorodeoxyglucose for staging of lymphoma: effectiveness and comparison with computed tomography. *Eur J Nucl Med* 1998;25:721–728.
18. Lewis E, Bernardino ME, Salvador PG, Cabanillas FF, Barnes PA, Thomas JL. Post-therapy CT-detected mass in lymphoma patients: is it viable tissue? *J Computer Assist Tomogr* 1982;6:792–795.
19. Longo DL, DeVita VT, Jr., Duffey PL, et al. Superiority of ProMACE-CytaBOM over ProMACE-MOPP in the treatment of advanced diffuse aggressive lymphoma: Results of a prospective randomized trial. *J Clin Oncol* 1991;9:25–38.
20. Waits TM, Greco FA, Greer JP, et al. Effective therapy for poor-prognosis non-Hodgkin's lymphoma with 8 weeks of high-dose-intensity combination chemotherapy. *J Clin Oncol* 1993;11:943–949.
21. Coiffier B, Gisselbrecht C, Herbrecht R, Tilly H, Bosly A, Brousse N. LNH-84 regimen: a multicenter study of intensive chemotherapy in 737 patients with aggressive malignant lymphoma. *J Clin Oncol* 1989;7:1018–1026.
22. Zuckerman KS, Case DC, Jr., Gams RA, Prasthofer EF. Chemotherapy of intermediate- and high-grade non-Hodgkin's lymphomas with an intensive epirubicin-containing regimen. *Blood* 1993;82:3564–3573.
23. Zuckerman KS, LoBuglio AF, Reeves JA. Chemotherapy of intermediate- and high-grade non-Hodgkin's lymphomas with a high-dose doxorubicin-containing regimen. *J Clin Oncol* 1990;8:248–256.
24. Chopra R, Goldstone AH, Pearce R, et al. Autologous versus allogeneic bone marrow transplantation for non-Hodgkin's lymphoma: A case-controlled analysis of the European Bone Marrow Transplant Group Registry data. *J Clin Oncol* 1992;10:1690–1695.
25. Meyer RM, Quirt IC, Skillings JR, et al. Escalated as compared with standard doses of doxorubicin in BACOP therapy for patients with non-Hodgkin's lymphoma. *New Engl J Med* 1993;329:1770–1776.
26. Cheson BD, Horning SJ, Coiffier B, et al. Report of an International Workshop to standardize response criteria for non-Hodgkin's lymphomas. *J Clin Oncol* 1999;17:1244–1253.
27. Radford JA, Cowan RA, Flanagan M, et al. The significance of residual mediastinal abnormality on the chest radiograph following treatment for Hodgkin's disease. *J Clin Oncol* 1988;6:940–946.
28. Wirth A, Seymour JF, Hicks RJ, et al. Fluorine-18 flurordeoxyglucose positron emission tomography, gallium-67 scintigraphy, and conventional staging for Hodgkin's disease and non-Hodgkin's lymphoma. *Am J Med* 2002;112:262–268.
29. Juweid M, Wiseman GA, Vose JM, et al. Response assessment of aggressive non-Hodgkin's lymphoma by integrated International Workshop criteria (IWC) and 18F-fluorodeoxyglucose positron emission tomography (PET). *J Clin Oncol* 2005;23:4652–4661.
30. Van Den Bossche B, Lambert B, De Winter F, et al. 18FDG PET versus high-dose 67Ga scintigraphy for restaging and treatment follow-up of lymphoma patients. *Nuc Med Comm* 2002;23:1079–1083.
31. Buchmann I, Reinhardt M, Elsner K, et al. 2-(fluorine-18)fluoro-2-deoxy-D-glucose positron emission tomography in the detection and staging of malignant lymphoma. A bicenter trial. *Cancer* 2001;91:889–899.
32. Jerusalem G, Beguin Y, Fassotte MF, et al. Whole-body positron emission tomography using 18F-fluorodeoxyglucose for posttreatment evaluation in Hodgkin's disease and non-Hodgkin's lymphoma has higher diagnostic and prognostic value than classical computed tomography scan imaging. *Blood* 1999;94:429–433.
33. Bangerter M, Moog F, Buchmann I, et al. Whole-body 2-[18F]-fluoro-2-deoxy-D-glucose positron emission tomography (FDG-PET) for accurate staging of Hodgkin's disease. *Ann Oncol* 1998;9:1117–1122.
34. Spaepen K, Stroobants S, Dupont P, et al. Prognostic value of positron emission tomography (PET) with fluorine-18 fluorodeoxyglucose ([¹⁸F]FDG) after first-line chemotherapy in non-Hodgkin's lymphoma: Is [¹⁸F]FDG-PET a valid alternative to conventional diagnostic methods? *J Clin Oncol* 2001;19:414–419.
35. Spaepen K, Stroobants S, Dupont P, et al. Prognostic value of pretransplantation positron emission tomography using fluorine 18-

fluorodeoxyglucose in patients with aggressive lymphoma treated with high-dose chemotherapy and stem cell transplantation. *Blood* 2003;102:53–59.

36. Spaepen K, Stroobants S, Dupont P, et al. Early restaging positron emission tomography with 18F-fluorodeoxyglucose predicts outcome in patients with aggressive non-Hodgkin's lymphoma. *Ann Oncol* 2002;13:1356–1363.

37. Jerusalem G, Beguin Y, Fassotte MF, et al. Whole-body positron emission tomography using 18F-fluorodeoxyglucose compared to standard procedures for staging patients with Hodgkin's disease. *Haematologica* 2001;86:266–273.

38. Jerusalem G, Beguin Y, Najjar F, et al. Positron emission tomography (PET) with 18F-fluorodeoxyglucose (18F-FDG) for the staging of low-grade non-Hodgkin's lymphoma (NHL). *Ann Oncol* 2001;12:825–830.

39. Jerusalem G, Warland V, Najjar F, et al. Whole-body 18F-FDG PET for the evaluation of patients with Hodgkin's disease and non-Hodgkin's lymphoma. *Nucl Med Commun* 1999;20:13–20.

40. Zinzani PL, Magagnoli M, Chierichetti F, et al. The role of positron emission tomography (PET) in the management of lymphoma patients. *Ann Oncol* 1999;10:1141–1143.

41. Weihrauch MR, Re D, Scheidhauer K, et al. Thoracic positron emission tomography using ^{18}F-fluorodeoxyglucose for the evaluation of residual mediastinal Hodgkin disease. *Blood* 2001;98:2930–2934.

42. Naumann R, Vaic A, Beuthien-Baumann B, et al. Prognostic value of positron emission tomography in the evalaution of post-treatment residual mass in patients with Hodgkin's disease and non-Hodgkin's lymphoma. *Br J Haematol* 2001;115:793–800.

43. Kostakoglu L, Leonard JP, Kuji I, Coleman M, Vallabhajosula S, Goldsmith SJ. Comparison of fluorine-18 fluorodeoxyglucose positron emission tomography and Ga-67 scintigraphy in evaluation of lymphoma. *Cancer* 2002;94:879–888.

44. Naumann R, Beuthien-Baumann B, Reiss A, et al. Substantial impact of FDG PET imaging on the therapy decision in patients with early-stage Hodgkin's lymphoma. *Br J Cancer* 2004;90:620–625.

45. Munker R, Glass J, Griffeth LK, et al. Contribution of PET imaging to the initial staging and prognosis of patients with Hodgkin's disease. *Ann Oncol* 2004;15:1699–1704.

46. Mikhaeel NG, Hutchings M, Fields PA, O'Doherty MJ, Timothy AR. FDG PET after two to three cycles of chemotherapy predicts progression-free and overall survival in high-grade non-Hodgkin lymphoma. *Ann Oncol* 2005;16:1514–1523.

47. Haioun C, Itti E, Rahmouni A, et al. ^{18}F-fluoro-2-deoxy-D-glucose positron emission tomography (FDG-PET) in aggressive lymphoma: an early prognostic tool for predicting patient outcome. *Blood* 2005;106:1376–1381.

48. Hutchings M, Loft A, Hansen M, et al. Positron emission tomography with or without computed tomography in the primary staging of Hodgkin's lymphoma. *Haematologica* 2006;91:482–489.

49. Querellou S, Valette F, Bodet-Milin C, et al. FDG-PET/CT predicts outcome in patients with aggressive non-Hodgkin's lymphoma and Hodgkin's disease. *Ann Hematol* 2006;85:759–767.

50. Juweid ME, Stroobants S, Hoekstra OS, et al. Use of positron emission tomography for response assessment of lymphoma: consensus recommendations of the Imaging Subcommittee of the International Harmonization Project in Lymphoma. *J Clin Oncol* 2007;25:571–578.

51. Cheson BD, Pfistner B, Juweid ME, et al. Revised response criteria for malignant lymphoma. *J Clin Oncol* 2007;25:579–586.

52. Seam P, Juweid ME, Cheson BD. The role of FDG-PET scans in patients with lymphoma. *Blood* 2007;110:3507–3516.

53. Najjar F, Hustinx R, Jerusalem G, Fillet G, Rigo P. Positron emission tomography (PET) for staging low-grade non-Hodgkin's lymphomas (NHL). *Cancer Biother Radiopharm* 2001;16:297–304.

54. Hoffmann M, Kletter K, Diemling M, et al. Positron emission tomography with fluorine-18-2-fluoro-2-deoxy-D-glucose (F18-FDG) does not visualize extranodal B-cell lymphoma of the mucosa-associated lymphoid tissue (MALT)-type. *Ann Oncol* 1999;10:1185–1189.

55. Elstrom R, Guan L, Baker G, et al. Utility of FDG-PET scanning in lymphoma by WHO classification. *Blood* 2003;101:3875–3876.

56. Kuo PH, McClennan BL, Carlson K, et al. FDG-PET/CT in the evaluation of cutaneous T-cell lymphoma. *Mol Imaging Biol* 2008;10:74–81.

57. Spaepen K, Stroobants S, Dupont P, et al. Can positron emission tomography with [18F]-fluorodeoxyglucose after first-line treatment distinguish Hodgkin's disease patients who need additional therapy from others in whom additional therapy would mean avoidable toxicity? *Br J Haematol* 2001;115:272–278.

58. Zijlstra JM, Lindauer-van der Werf G, Hoekstra OS, Hooft L, Riphagen II, Huijgens PC. ^{18}F-fluoro-deoxyglucose positron emission tomography for post-treatment evaluation of malignant lymphoma: a systematic review. *Haematologica* 2006;91:522–529.

59. Elstrom RL, Leonard JP, Coleman M, Brown RKJ. Combined PET and low-dose, noncontrast CT scanning obviates the need for additional diagnostic contrast-enhanced CT scans in patients undergoing staging or restaging for lymphoma. *Ann Oncol* 2008;19:1770–1773.

60. Castellucci P, Nanni C, Farsad M, et al. Potential pitfalls of ^{18}F-FDG PET in a large series of patients treated for malignant lymphoma: prevalence and scan interpretation. *Nuc Med Comm* 2005;26:689–694.

61. Zinzani PL, Stefoni V, Tani M, et al. Role of [18F]fluorodeoxyglucose positron emission tomography scan in the follow-up of lymphoma. *J Clin Oncol* 2009;27:1781–1787.

62. Pfistner B, Diehl V, Cheson B. International harmonization of trial parameters in malignant lymphoma. *Eur J Haematol Suppl* 2005;July(66):53–54.

63. Assouline S, Meyer RM, Infante-Rivard C, Connors JM, Belch A, Crump M. Development of adapted RECIST criteria to assess response in lymphoma and their comparison to the International Workshop Criteria. *Leuk Lymphoma* 2007;48:447–448.

CHAPTER 12 ■ LYMPHOBLASTIC LYMPHOMA: PRECURSOR CELL LYMPHOMAS OF B AND T CELLS

JOHN W. SWEETENHAM AND MICHAEL J. BOROWITZ

Precursor B-cell and T-cell lymphoblastic leukemias/lymphoblastic lymphomas are neoplasms of lymphoblasts. The designation of *lymphoblastic lymphoma* has been used previously to describe precursor B- and T-cell tumors with predominantly lymph node-based disease (most commonly affecting the anterior mediastinum). As a consequence, the entity of lymphoblastic lymphoma has been recognized by most classifications of lymphoid neoplasms, including the Kiel and Working Formulation systems. However, the clinical distinction between lymphoblastic lymphoma and lymphoblastic leukemia has been arbitrary, and has varied among different studies and different institutions.

Because it is now recognized that acute lymphoblastic leukemias (ALLs) and lymphoblastic lymphomas represent the same disease entity at the morphologic and immunophenotypic level, the World Health Organization Classification has unified these entities as precursor B- or T-cell lymphoblastic leukemia/lymphoma.

Although the biologic distinction between lymphoblastic leukemia and lymphoma is unclear, the clinical literature describing these entities has been distinct until very recently. Consequently, the treatment approach to lymphoblastic lymphoma, particularly in the adult population, has developed separately from the approach used in ALL. Therefore, although the biology of all lymphoblastic disease is discussed in detail in this chapter, the clinical aspects are confined to the entity designated as lymphoblastic lymphoma. Emerging data from gene expression profiling studies and from T-cell receptor genotyping, reviewed in section headed Molecular Diagnostics, suggest that there may be differences between ALL and lymphoblastic lymphoma at the molecular level, providing a rationale for considering these two entities separately.

FREQUENCY

Lymphoblastic lymphoma is a rare disease that accounts for approximately 2% of all non-Hodgkin lymphomas (1). Approximately 85% to 90% of adult cases are of T-cell phenotype, and occur most frequently in adolescent and young adult males (2–5). B-cell lymphoblastic lymphoma comprises approximately 10% of adult cases of this disease (6). The reported median age for patients with lymphoblastic lymphoma is approximately 20 years, with most series reporting male predominance. There has been no clear evidence for a change in the incidence of lymphoblastic lymphoma in recent years, although in view of the variability in the definition between lymphoblastic lymphoma and ALL, incidence trends may have been obscured.

DIAGNOSIS

The histopathologic and immunophenotypic features of lymphoblastic lymphoma are distinctive, so that diagnosis, if properly approached, is rarely a problem. In many cases, a tissue diagnosis of lymphoblastic lymphoma may be inferred if only peripheral blood, bone marrow, or, in the case of a patient with a mediastinal mass, pleural fluid can be shown to contain lymphoblasts with characteristic immunophenotypic properties. However, the majority of cases of lymphoblastic lymphoma are still diagnosed by tissue examination, coupled with flow cytometric or immunophenotypic analysis.

Histopathologic Findings

Morphologically, lymphoblastic lymphoma is composed of medium-sized cells with finely dispersed chromatin and scant cytoplasm (3) (Color Plate 20). Nucleoli are inconspicuous. The cells may have round nuclei or highly convoluted ones, although this is of no clinical significance. Because it is a high-grade malignancy, mitotic features are invariably present, and there are often numerous apoptotic bodies. These may be phagocytosed by macrophages, thereby imparting a "starry-sky" pattern to the tissue. Although this pattern is often thought of as a characteristic of Burkitt lymphoma, it may be seen in other high-grade lymphomas as well. Morphologic distinction between lymphoblastic and Burkitt lymphoma is easy to accomplish in many cases because the latter tumor has a distinct rim of cytoplasm and multiple nucleoli. However, some caveats are in order. First, the classically described histopathologic findings of lymphoblastic lymphoma correspond to L1 ALL in the French-American-British Classification of ALL. L2 ALL, by contrast, has more cytoplasm and more prominent nucleoli and, thus, can in some cases more closely resemble Burkitt lymphoma in tissue sections (7).

The other concern is that finding the histologic features of lymphoblastic lymphoma is very dependent on optimal tissue fixation and processing. Overstained material can resemble tumors of more mature lymphocytes, whereas the cells of poorly fixed lymphoblastic lymphoma may greatly enlarge and resemble diffuse large cell lymphoma.

Differential diagnostic considerations also include cases of lymphocyte-rich thymoma and, in children, other small round-cell tumors. The latter are readily separated by immunophenotyping studies, particularly if one realizes that CD99, the antigen characteristically present on Ewing sarcoma and peripheral neuroectodermal tumor, is also present in lymphoblastic malignancies (8). Distinction from thymoma is sometimes made more complicated by the fact that lymphoid cells in both tumors have a thymic T-cell phenotype, but the cytology of the cells is generally different, and the characteristic epithelial distribution of thymoma is not present in lymphomas.

Immunophenotypic Analysis

Immunophenotypic analysis almost always allows a diagnosis of lymphoblastic lymphoma to be made with certainty. The great majority of lymphoblastic lymphomas are tumors of precursor T lymphocytes (7,9,10), and finding such a phenotype is essentially pathognomonic of such an entity, although there is no single phenotype associated with precursor T-lymphoblastic lymphoma. CD7, CD5, and CD2 are most commonly expressed, whereas CD3 is often present in the cytoplasm but not on the surface (11). Immunohistochemical staining generally does not allow this distinction. Thus, by immunocytochemistry, most cases are CD3$^+$, whereas the sCD3$^-$/cCD3$^+$ phenotype is best demonstrated by flow cytometry. CD4 and CD8 can be expressed in any combination: one alone, neither, or both together. The best means of distinguishing a T-lymphoblastic lymphoma from a peripheral T-cell lymphoma is by the expression of nonlineage-specific immature markers, such as terminal deoxynucleotidyl transferase or CD99, or in some cases, CD34 (8,12,13). Cytoplasmic CD3 without surface expression is also a relatively specific finding. CD1a, when positive, is also a relatively specific feature. Although coexpression of CD4 and CD8 is a characteristic of normal thymocytes, there is some controversy about the specificity of this expression for lymphoblastic lymphoma because it has also been described in T-cell prolymphocytic leukemia.

The less common precursor B-lymphoblastic lymphomas also generally express immature markers, such as CD99, CD34, and terminal deoxynucleotidyl transferase. They are positive for early expressed pan B markers, including CD79a and CD19, but often lack or show only patchy expression of CD20. CD45 is often negative. By definition, precursor B tumors are surface immunoglobulin negative, but in practice, this is not often the best way to identify them. If only fixed tissue is available, surface immunoglobulin determinations are not reliably done in paraffin sections, and, in addition, some lymphomas of mature B cells also lack surface immunoglobulin. In children, precursor B-lymphoblastic lymphomas often present as cutaneous disease (14).

Molecular Diagnostics

The great majority of T-lymphoblastic lymphomas show clonal rearrangements of T-cell receptor genes, with T-cell receptor δ being the most sensitive (15), but this is not a lineage-specific finding because many B, or even blastic myeloid, tumors may show this as well (16). Thus, gene rearrangement studies play a little role in the diagnosis of this disease. Many precursor T-cell lymphoblastic lymphomas have translocations involving the T-cell receptor gene (17), and although these are important for an understanding of the pathogenesis of the disease (see Pathogenesis), such studies are not particularly important diagnostically or prognostically. Compared with ALL, there is relatively little literature on the role of cytogenetics or molecular analysis of particular translocations. The rare case of precursor B-lymphoblastic lymphoma should probably be screened for the presence of the bcr-abl translocation because of the poor prognosis associated with that abnormality, although specific examples of bcr-abl$^+$ B-lymphoblastic lymphoma have not been described.

PATHOGENESIS

Understanding of the pathogenesis and molecular basis of precursor T-cell lymphoblastic disease has mainly arisen from studies of recurrent chromosomal translocations and chromosomal rearrangements in this disease. Approximately one third of patients have translocations involving the α and δ T-cell receptor loci at 14q11.2, the β locus at 7q35, and the γ locus at 7p14-15 (18). The typical result of these translocations is to juxtapose promoter and enhancer elements producing high levels of T-cell receptor gene expression with transcription factor genes, such as HOX11/TLX1, TAL1/SCL, TAL 2, and LYL 1, resulting in aberrant expression of these genes in the developing thymocyte (19–21).

Recent microarray studies have demonstrated molecular subtypes of precursor T-cell lymphoblastic disease that characterize different stages in thymocyte maturation and may identify prognostic subgroups (22). For example, patients with HOX11 expression show a pattern of gene expression corresponding to the early cortical thymocyte. This subgroup appears to have a more favorable clinical outcome, possibly related to the lower frequency of expression of the antiapoptotic BCL-2 gene. These cells are apparently developmentally arrested at a stage at which they are particularly sensitive to drug-induced apoptosis. In contrast, those samples with gene expression profiles associated with TAL1 or LYL1 expression resemble late cortical and early pro-T thymocytes, respectively, and show more drug resistance and correspondingly higher levels of *bcl-2*.

A classification of lymphoblastic lymphoma based on degree of maturation arrest and expression of specific genes has recently been proposed (23). This describes risk groups for lymphoblastic lymphoma based on T-cell receptor genotype and *HOXA/TLX* expression, which have prognostic significance and which appear to be distinct from those described in ALL. A recent study comparing gene expression profiling between patients with precursor T-cell lymphoblastic disease that is predominantly nodal with that that is predominantly leukemic has identified groups of genes with markedly different levels of expression between these two entities (24). These included genes responsible for the regulation of cell proliferation and apoptosis, transcription factors, and genes involved in tumor cell/microenvironment interactions.

METHODS OF PRESENTATION

Characteristic clinical features of lymphoblastic lymphoma include male predominance, and peak incidence in the second and third decades. Mediastinal involvement at presentation is common, occurring in 60% to 70% of patients, reflecting the thymic origin of the malignant cells in lymphoblastic lymphoma. Mediastinal masses are uncommon in patients with B-cell lymphoblastic lymphoma. Pleural effusions are also a common presenting feature, and pericardial effusions, with resulting cardiac tamponade, may also occur. In addition, symptoms and signs of superior vena caval obstruction may be present.

Peripheral lymph node involvement is present in 60% to 80% of patients at diagnosis, most commonly in cervical, supraclavicular, and axillary regions.

Lymphoblastic lymphoma has a propensity for dissemination to the bone marrow and central nervous system. The frequency of bone marrow involvement at presentation is very difficult to determine from published series in view of the arbitrary and variable distinction between lymphoblastic lymphoma and ALL. In a prospective study from Europe, 21% of adult patients with lymphoblastic lymphoma had bone marrow involvement at presentation (25). Leukemic overspill is also common, but again, the frequency is obscured by inconsistencies in distinction between lymphoblastic lymphoma and ALL.

Central nervous system involvement is uncommon at presentation, occurring in approximately 5% to 10% of patients. Several reports suggest that it is more common in patients with bone marrow involvement at presentation. Typical manifestations of central nervous system involvement include meningeal involvement with a pleocytosis in the cerebrospinal fluid or cranial nerve involvement, characteristically involving ophthalmic or facial nerves. Although central nervous system involvement at presentation is uncommon, it is a frequent site of relapse in the absence of adequate prophylaxis. In one series from Stanford University, central nervous system relapse was reported in 31% of patients (26).

Other less common sites of involvement include the liver, spleen, and subdiaphragmatic lymph nodes, as well as bone, skin, and testes. Presentation in the pharynx and skin is especially typical of precursor B-cell lymphoblastic lymphoma/leukemia in children (27).

In adults, precursor B-cell lymphoblastic leukemia/lymphoma typically presents in an older population, often in the 6th and 7th decades. Transformation from follicular lymphoma is well documented in this population (28). The presentation of precursor B-cell lymphoblastic lymphoma/leukemia in adults is characterized by a high frequency of extranodal disease, including skin, pharynx, and bone (29,30). Mediastinal and bone marrow involvement is less common in this population, and unlike precursor T-cell disease, there is no apparent male predominance. Highly intensive treatment regimens (see in section headed Treatment) are usually tolerated poorly in this population.

UNIQUE ASPECTS OF STAGING

Some centers have adopted the Murphy staging system for lymphoblastic lymphoma in view of the fact that it was devised specifically to address staging of children with non-Hodgkin lymphoma, in whom disseminated, noncontiguous involvement of nodal and extranodal sites is common. In most children with non-Hodgkin lymphoma, the Murphy staging system has been shown to provide more useful prognostic information (4). However, in a comparison of the Ann Arbor and Murphy staging systems in adult lymphoblastic lymphoma, the Ann Arbor system was shown to predict survival more accurately and is, therefore, now used in most centers (26).

The applicability of the International Prognostic Index for aggressive non-Hodgkin lymphomas has now been investigated in three studies. A study from the Non-Hodgkin's Lymphoma Classification Project included a retrospective analysis of a small sample of 26 patients with a median age of 28 years (range, 4 to 65 years) with lymphoblastic lymphoma (31). For the entire group, the 5-year overall and failure-free survival rates were approximately 20%. The number of International Prognostic Index risk factors was not shown to be predictive of overall or failure-free survival in this series. A retrospective series of 62 patients from France also concluded that the International Prognostic Index did not have prognostic significance in adults with lymphoblastic lymphoma (32). The predictive value of the International Prognostic Index was also explored in the context of a European randomized trial in adults with lymphoblastic lymphoma (25). Sixty patients had complete data. The number of International Prognostic Index risk factors was shown to be predictive of overall survival, but this reached significance only for the group with three adverse factors, according to the age-adjusted International Prognostic Index. Larger patient samples are needed to determine whether the International Prognostic Index proves to be a suitable staging and prognostic system for lymphoblastic lymphoma. At present, the Ann Arbor system is still in most widespread use, although because all patients with lymphoblastic lymphoma require intensive systemic therapy (see Treatment below), its relevance is doubtful.

PROGNOSTIC AND PREDICTIVE FACTORS

Identification of prognostic factors in lymphoblastic lymphoma has been variable and inconsistent partly because of the variable criteria used for the distinction between lymphoblastic lymphoma and ALL, and for the distinction between adult and pediatric cases. However, some consistent data, particularly with respect to "biologic" predictors of outcome, have emerged.

"Biologic" Predictive Factors

Various studies have identified phenotypic and genotypic predictors of prognosis. There have been inconsistent reports with respect to the role of B-cell versus T-cell immunophenotype as a prognostic factor. Although there have been reports suggesting a worse outcome for patients with adult lymphoblastic lymphoma with precursor B-cell phenotype, more recent retrospective studies have failed to confirm this, possibly because the number of patients with B-cell immunophenotype is very small.

For patients with T-cell precursor lymphoblastic disease, although genetic abnormalities have been described in approximately 30% of cases, particularly involving α and δ T-cell receptor loci, or deletion of 9p, none of these abnormalities has been shown to have prognostic significance. In adult patients with ALL, expression of T-cell antigens, including CD1, CD2, CD4, and CD5, has been associated with a more favorable prognosis. In the Cancer and Leukemia Group B 8364 study, overall and disease-free survival was shown to correlate with the number of T-cell antigens expressed (33). Similar studies have not been performed in patients with lymphoblastic lymphoma.

For patients with precursor B-cell disease, most prognostic information has been derived from patients classified with ALL.

For example, in childhood B ALL, translocations involving the MLL gene at 11q23 are associated with adverse prognosis (34), as are those involving the t(9;22)(q34;q11.2). Features associated with good prognosis in children include hyperdiploid karyotype, particularly because it is associated with trisomy 4, 10, and 17, and t(12;21)(p13;q22) (35). As in children, adults with B-ALL with 11q23 abnormalities or the t(9;22)(q34;q11.2) translocation have a poor prognosis, although specific studies of these abnormalities as prognostic factors have not been performed in B-lymphoblastic lymphoma.

As mentioned previously, early data from gene expression profiles and T-cell receptor genotyping, performed in relatively small numbers of patients, have identified groups of patients with different outcomes, although these data are very preliminary and require confirmation.

Clinical Predictive Factors

Before the description of the International Prognostic Index, multiple, small retrospective series of patients with lymphoblastic lymphoma identified adverse clinical prognostic factors for overall and disease-free survival (36–38). These have varied in different series, reflecting the small patient numbers and the variable criteria for categorizing ALL and lymphoblastic lymphoma.

Until the description of the International Prognostic Index, the most widely accepted prognostic factors for lymphoblastic lymphoma were those described by Coleman et al. (26) from Stanford University. Patients with Ann Arbor stage less than IV or Ann Arbor stage IV, but without bone marrow or central nervous system involvement, with a serum lactate dehydrogenase level <300 IU per L (normal = 200 IU per L) were considered good risk. This group had a 5-year freedom from relapse rate of 94%. All other patients were considered poor risk. The 5-year freedom from relapse in the poor-risk group was only 19%.

As mentioned previously, the predictive value of the International Prognostic Index has been assessed in three previous studies. Although the numbers of patients in all series are small, the study from Europe represents the only prospectively collected data set in a relatively unselected population of adult patients with lymphoblastic lymphoma (25). This study demonstrated a statistically significant trend for lower overall survival with an increasing number of adverse factors according to the age-adjusted International Prognostic Index ($p = 0.016$). However, although there was a clearly inferior survival in patients with three adverse factors, there was little distinction between those with zero, one, or two factors, and the value of the International Prognostic Index as a prognostic model remains unclear.

Although prognostic factors for ALL have been reasonably well defined in large prospective studies, there are no consistent data for lymphoblastic lymphoma, and, therefore, no clear rationale exists for designing different treatment strategies according to risk group for these patients.

TREATMENT

Early studies of the treatment of lymphoblastic lymphoma were conducted in combined populations of children and adults during the 1970s (3,4,39). These and many of the more recent studies are difficult to interpret because patient numbers in most have been small, and variable criteria have been used to assign patients to protocols for ALL or lymphoblastic lymphoma.

Initial trials in lymphoblastic lymphoma used first- and second-generation chemotherapy regimens initially developed for the treatment of other, less aggressive, types of non-Hodgkin lymphoma (3,4,40–42). Results with these regimens were poor. Nathwani et al. (3) reported results in 95 adult and pediatric patients with lymphoblastic lymphoma treated on a variety of collaborative group protocols, none of which included central nervous system prophylaxis. This series included some patients with leukemic involvement. The complete response (CR) rate was only 24%, and for the 87 patients on whom survival information was available, the median survival was only 17 months, with less than 10% of patients alive and disease free at 5 years. Similar results were reported for other low-intensity chemotherapy regimens.

The introduction of intensive chemotherapy and radiation therapy protocols in childhood lymphoblastic lymphoma produced marked improvements in outcome. Protocols such as the LSA$_2$-L$_2$ regimen combined intensive chemotherapy, comparable to that used in childhood ALL, with central nervous system irradiation (43). Long-term disease-free survival rates between 60% and 80% were reported for children treated with this and similar regimens. A subsequent randomized trial comparing the LSA$_2$-L$_2$ regimen with cyclophosphamide, Oncovin (vincristine), methotrexate, and prednisone demonstrated a 2-year actuarial failure-free survival of 76% for children with lymphoblastic lymphoma receiving LSA$_2$-L$_2$, compared with only 26% for those receiving cyclophosphamide, Oncovin (vincristine), methotrexate, and prednisone ($p = 0.0002$) (44).

Subsequently, chemotherapy/radiotherapy regimens similar in design to LSA$_2$-L$_2$ adapted from those in adult ALL have been applied to adult patients with lymphoblastic lymphoma (26,36,37,43–50). Most of these regimens are characterized by intensive remission-induction chemotherapy, central nervous system prophylaxis, a phase of consolidation chemotherapy, and a prolonged maintenance phase, often lasting for 12 to 18 months. Results from some of these regimens are summarized in Table 12.1.

Most of these studies report long-term disease-free survival rates between 40% and 70%.

For example, the cyclophosphamide, vincristine, doxorubicin, and dexamethasone regimen alternating with high-dose methotrexate and cytosine arabinoside produced a CR rate of 91% and 3-year actuarial overall and progression-free survival rates of 70% and 66%, respectively, in 33 adult patients with lymphoblastic lymphoma (48). Similar results have been obtained with several other regimens, some of which have included high-dose therapy and autologous or allogeneic stem cell transplantation in place of conventional consolidation and maintenance as postremission therapy.

AUTOLOGOUS STEM CELL TRANSPLANTATION IN FIRST REMISSION

Despite the high remission rates reported for first-line therapy in lymphoblastic lymphoma, relapse rates are also

TABLE 12.1

RESULTS OF INTENSIVE COMBINATION CHEMOTHERAPY REGIMENS IN ADULTS WITH LYMPHOBLASTIC LYMPHOMA

First author (reference)	Regimen	No. of patients	Response rate	Failure-free survival (FFS)/relapse-free survival (RFS)	Overall survival (OS)	Comments
Levine (45)	Modified LSA$_2$-L$_2$	15	73% CR; 27% PR	5-y actuarial FFS = 35%	5-y actuarial OS = 40%	Median age = 25 y
Weinstein (46)	APO	21	95% CR	3-y actuarial FFS = 58%	5-y actuarial OS = 69%	Median age = 13 y
Slater (36)	Various ALL protocols	51	80% CR for "nonleukemic"; 77% CR for leukemic	N/A	5-y actuarial OS = 45%	Median age = 22 y. Four successive ALL regimens used. No difference in outcome according to regimen.
Morel (38)	CHOP plus various ALL protocols	80	82% CR	46% at 30 mo FFS	51% at 30 mo	Median age = 33.7 y. No difference in outcome according to induction protocol.
Bernasconi (37)	Various ALL protocols	31	77% OR	3-y RFS = 45%	3-y OS = 59%	Median age = 25 y
Coleman (26)	Two ALL-type protocols with intensified CNS prophylaxis in the second	44	100%	3-y FFS = 56%	—	—
Hoelzer (47)	Two ALL-type protocols, both including CNS and mediastinal irradiation	45	93% CR	7-y actuarial DFS = 62%	7-y actuarial OS = 51%	Median age = 25 y. All patients had T-lymphoblastic lymphoma. No benefit for mediastinal radiotherapy for DFS, OS, or incidence of mediastinal relapse. No prognostic factors identified. Age-adjusted IPI was not predictive of survival.
Thomas (48)	HyperCVAD	33	91%	3-y PFS = 66%	3-y OS = 70%	Median age = 28 y. Twenty Four months cyclical maintenance regimen included
Jabbour (49)	LMT-89 (ALL-type induction regimen derived from LSA$_2$-L$_2$)	27	85% OR	5-y FFP = 44%	5-y OS = 63%	Median age = 31 y
Song (50)	"Hybrid" NHL/ALL regimen plus SCT in first remission	34	100% OR	4-y EFS = 68%	4-y OS = 72%	Median age = 26 y. Intent to treat analysis. Twenty-nine of 34 patients underwent SCT.

APO, Adriamycin (doxorubicin), prednisone, Oncovin (vincristine); CHOP, cyclophosphamide, hydroxydaunomycin, Orcovin (vincristine), prednisone; CNS, central nervous system; DFS, disease-free survival; HyperCVAD, cyclophosphamide, vincristine, Adriamycin (doxorubicin), dexamethasone, cytarabine, methotrexate; IPI, International Prognostic Index; N/A, not available; NHL, non-Hodgkin lymphoma; OR, overall response; PR, partial response; SCT, stem cell transplantation.

relatively high. This has provided a rationale for investigation of the role of high-dose therapy with autologous or allogeneic stem cell transplantation in first remission in an attempt to reduce the incidence of relapse after induction therapy. Most studies to date have explored the role of autologous transplantation in this setting, although some series have also included small numbers of patients receiving sibling-matched allogeneic stem cell transplants (22,42–44).

The results of studies that have investigated this approach are summarized in Table 12.2. Interpretation of most of these studies is difficult because, with a few exceptions, they are not analyzed by intention to treat. For many of these studies, the survivals are calculated from the date of transplant, and pretransplant selection is likely to have occurred. The patient populations included in many of these reports represent patients already in complete or partial remission at the time of inclusion in the study, and they are, therefore, a relatively favorable group.

Three of the listed studies incorporated an intent to treat analysis. The study reported by Jost et al. (51) included adult patients with lymphoblastic lymphoma who received initial induction chemotherapy with methotrexate, Adriamycin (doxorubicin), cyclophosphamide, Oncovin (vincristine), prednisone, and bleomycin or VePesid (etoposide), Adriamycin (doxorubicin), cyclophosphamide, Oncovin (vincristine), prednisone, and bleomycin, followed by high-dose therapy and autologous stem cell transplantation. The 3-year actuarial overall and event-free survival rates were 48% and 31%, respectively.

A more recent study from Song et al. (50) included 34 adults with lymphoblastic lymphoma who received a hybrid induction regimen followed by high-dose therapy and autologous or allogeneic stem cell transplantation in 29. The 4-year overall and event-free survival rates were 72% and 68%, respectively. A study from the Groupe D'Etudes des Lymphomes de l'Adulte included 92 patients treated with standard non-Hodgkin lymphoma-type induction chemotherapy followed by stem cell transplantation in responding patients. The median overall survival was only 32% at 5 years. These results do not appear superior to those reported for conventional dose first-line therapy.

A single, small randomized trial conducted by the European Group for Blood and Marrow Transplantation and the United Kingdom Lymphoma Group has compared the use of high-dose therapy and autologous stem cell transplantation with conventional dose consolidation and maintenance therapy in adult patients with lymphoblastic lymphoma (25).

This study included 119 adult patients who were treated with intensive ALL-type induction chemotherapy, of whom 111 were assessable for response to induction therapy. The overall response rate to induction chemotherapy was comparable to other series at 82%. However, of 98 patients eligible for randomization, only 65 were actually randomized. Reasons for failure to randomize included patient refusal, early disease progression before transplantation, and elective allogeneic transplantation in patients with human leukocyte antigen-matched sibling donors.

Results from this small study are summarized in Figure 12.1. The 3-year actuarial relapse-free survival rate was 24% for patients receiving conventional consolidation and maintenance therapy, compared with 55% for those receiving high-dose therapy and autologous stem cell transplantation

($p = 0.065$). The corresponding values for overall survival were 45% and 56% ($p = 0.71$).

Cross-trial comparisons of outcomes from the various series summarized previously must be interpreted cautiously in view of the variable selection criteria used in these studies. However, the results of the studies summarized previously suggest that the intensity of primary chemotherapy is a more important determinant of long-term survival than the use of stem cell transplantation as consolidation. For example, studies that use "standard dose" induction therapy report relatively disappointing long-term overall and event-free survival rates, despite the use of high-dose therapy in first remission. By contrast, when intensive induction regimens are used, there is no clear survival benefit from stem cell transplant. Stem cell transplantation can, therefore, be considered an alternative approach to postremission therapy compared with standard consolidation and maintenance, which reduces the overall duration of therapy. However, it appears to be equivalent *only* after an intensive ALL-like induction regimen.

Although no direct comparisons have been reported, there is no clear evidence that any high-dose regimen is superior to another before autologous transplantation. Similarly, there is no evidence to suggest that the source of hematopoietic stem cells (peripheral blood vs. bone marrow) has an influence on outcome, and for most centers, peripheral blood progenitors are regarded as the preferred stem cell source.

AUTOLOGOUS STEM CELL TRANSPLANTATION FOR RELAPSED OR REFRACTORY DISEASE

Results of salvage therapy for adult patients with lymphoblastic lymphoma with relapsed or refractory disease are very poor. The use of second-line conventional dose regimens in this situation produces response rates <10%, and median overall survival in these series is only approximately 9 months (26,36–38). High-dose therapy with autologous stem cell rescue has been used increasingly in this situation, either as a component of second-line remission-induction therapy or to consolidate remission after a conventional dose second-line regimen.

Very few published studies have specifically addressed the role of autologous stem cell transplantation in this situation. In a retrospective study from Morel et al. (38), of 37 patients with adult lymphoblastic lymphoma who required salvage therapy, 14 achieved a second complete remission with conventional dose reinduction. Seven of these patients underwent consolidation with autologous stem cell transplantation, of whom three achieved long-term disease-free survival.

In a retrospective study from the European Group for Blood and Marrow Transplantation, 41 patients underwent high-dose therapy and autologous stem cell transplantation in second complete remission (52). The 3-year actuarial progression-free survival and overall survival for this group were 30% and 31%, respectively (Fig. 12.2). This series also included patients in whom high-dose therapy was used before the attainment of second complete remission. As with other types of non-Hodgkin lymphoma, the responsiveness of the disease to conventional dose therapy given before the transplant was predictive of outcome. The 5-year actuarial overall survival for

TABLE 12.2

RECENT RESULTS OF FIRST REMISSION STEM CELL TRANSPLANTATION IN ADULTS WITH LYMPHOBLASTIC LYMPHOMA

First author (reference)	Induction therapy/high-dose regimen/stem cell source	No. of patients	Failure-free surviva/relapse-free survival	Overall survival (OS)	Comments
Jost (51)	MACOP-B or VACOP-B induction/high-dose cyclophosphamide and TBI or CBV/autologous bone marrow	20	3-y EFS = 31%	3-y OS = 48%	Median age = 27 y. Intent-to-treat analysis with survival calculated from start of induction therapy.
Sweetenham (52)	Multiple-induction and high-dose regimens/autologous bone marrow	105	6-y PFS = 63%	6-y OS = 64%	Median age = 25.8 y. Registry based study.
Bouabdallah (32)	Various ALL-type induction regimens/high-dose cyclophosphamide and TBI/12 allogeneic BMT and 18 autologous BMT	62 (30 received BMT in first complete remission)	5-y EFS = 58%	5-y OS = 60%	Apparent advantage to allogeneic vs. autologous transplant.
Le Gouill (53) van Imhoff (54) Song (50)	ACVBP type CHOP-like "Hybrid" NHL/ALL regimen plus SCT in first remission	92 15 34	5-y EFS = 40% 34-mo DFS = 22% 4-y EFS = 68%	5-y OS = 46% 34-mo OS = 32% 4-y OS = 72%	Median age = 26 y. Intent to treat analysis. Twenty-nine of 34 patients underwent SCT.

ACVBP, Adriamycin (doxorubicin), cyclophosphamide, vindesine, bleomycin, prednisone; BMT, bone marrow transplant; CBV, Cytoxan, BCNU, VP-16; CHOP, cyclophosphamide, hydroxydaunomycin, Oncovin (vincristine), prednisone; EFS, event-free survival; MACOP-B, methotrexate, Adriamycin (doxorubicin), cyclophosphamide, Oncovin (vincristine), prednisone, bleomycin; PFS, progression-free survival; NHL, non-Hodgkin lymphoma; TBI, total body irradiation; VACOP-B, VePesid (etoposide), Adriamycin (doxorubicin), cyclophosphamide, Oncovin (vincristine), prednisone, bleomycin.

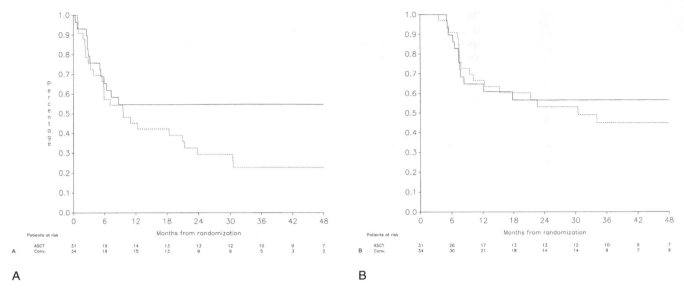

FIGURE 12.1 Results from the United Kingdom Lymphoma Group/European Group for Blood and Marrow Transplantation randomized trial of high-dose therapy and stem cell transplant versus conventional consolidation therapy in adult lymphoblastic lymphoma. **A:** Relapse-free survival. **B:** Overall survival. ASCT, autologous stem cell transplant; Conv., conventional. (Adapted from Sweetenham JW, Santini G, Qian W, et al. High-dose therapy and autologous stem-cell transplantation versus conventional dose consolidation/maintenance therapy as post-remission therapy for adult patients with lymphoblastic lymphoma: results of a randomized trial of the European Group for Blood and Marrow Transplantation and the United Kingdom Lymphoma Group. *J Clin Oncol* 2001;19:2927–2936, with permission.)

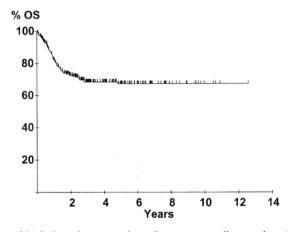

FIGURE 12.2 Results of high-dose therapy and autologous stem cell transplant in adult patients with lymphoblastic lymphoma transplanted in second complete remission. OS, overall survival. (Adapted from Sweetenham JW, Santini G, Pearce R, et al. High-dose therapy and autologous bone marrow transplantation for adult patients with lymphoblastic lymphoma: results from the European Group for Bone Marrow Transplantation. *J Clin Oncol* 1994;12:1358–1365, with permission.)

those with chemosensitive relapse was 31%, compared with 18% for those with chemorefractory disease (Fig. 12.3).

Because patients in chemosensitive relapse have a superior outcome to those with chemorefractory relapse, all patients with relapse should receive conventional dose salvage therapy in an attempt to induce a second remission before high-dose therapy. However, even in those patients with refractory disease, the reported long-term disease-free survival of 18% is superior to that achieved with conventional dose salvage, and these patients should also be offered high-dose therapy.

ALLOGENEIC STEM CELL TRANSPLANTATION

The role of allogeneic stem cell transplantation in adults with lymphoblastic lymphoma is unclear. In view of the relatively young age of adult patients with lymphoblastic lymphoma, it is anticipated that their regimen-related mortality after allogeneic transplantation is likely to be relatively low. If a graft-versus-lymphoma effect exists in this disease, then the low relapse rate observed in patients who survive allogeneic

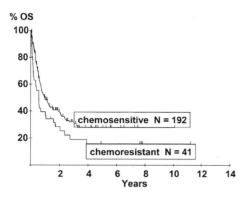

FIGURE 12.3 Results of high-dose therapy and autologous stem cell transplant in adult patients with lymphoblastic lymphoma transplanted in chemosensitive or chemoresistant relapse. OS, overall survival. (Adapted from Sweetenham JW, Santini G, Pearce R, et al. High-dose therapy and autologous bone marrow transplantation for adult patients with lymphoblastic lymphoma: results from the European Group for Bone Marrow Transplantation. *J Clin Oncol* 1994;12:1358–1365, with permission.)

transplantation might result in improved overall survival, compared with autologous transplantation. A retrospective, matched analysis from the European Group for Blood and Marrow Transplantation compared outcomes for 314 patients undergoing allogeneic transplantation for lymphoblastic lymphoma with 1,332 patients who received autologous transplants for this disease (55). Although patients undergoing autologous transplants experienced higher rates of relapse than those receiving allogeneic transplants, this was offset by the higher transplant-related mortality in the allogeneic group. Overall survival was significantly higher for patients receiving autologous transplants. Similar results have been reported from the International Bone Marrow Transplant Registry in a study that compared outcomes for 128 patients receiving autologous transplants, with 76 receiving allogeneic transplants from human leukocyte antigen-identical sibling donors (56). Long-term disease-free and overall survival was comparable in both groups. Relapse rates were higher for autologous recipients, whereas transplant-related mortality was higher in allogeneic recipients. There are currently no convincing data to suggest that allogeneic stem cells are a better stem cell source or that a clinically significant graft–versus-lymphoma effect is active in this disease. Autologous stem cells should still be regarded as the preferred source of hematopoietic rescue in these patients.

UNIQUE COMPLICATIONS

Central Nervous System Relapse

The central nervous system is a frequent site of relapse in lymphoblastic lymphoma when treated with first- and second-generation non-Hodgkin lymphoma regimens (2–4,39–42). Most of these protocols did not include specific central nervous system prophylaxis. The effectiveness of central nervous system prophylaxis in lymphoblastic lymphoma was demonstrated in two sequential studies from Stanford University (26). The first protocol described by this group included intrathecal and moderate-dose systemic methotrexate. The second

protocol introduced the central nervous system prophylaxis phase earlier and used intrathecal methotrexate with cranial irradiation. The incidence of central nervous system relapse in these two relatively small patient groups was reduced from 31% in the first protocol to 3% in the second. Although the effectiveness of this specific protocol in controlling central nervous system disease has been questioned in one series (57), the reported incidence of central nervous system relapse with most ALL-like chemotherapy regimens has been low.

Cranial irradiation was widely used as a component of prophylactic therapy, but concerns for late neuropsychologic effects have limited its use more recently. Pediatric studies have shown that regimens incorporating high-dose systemic agents such as methotrexate and cytarabine result in equivalent rates of central nervous system relapse compared with cranial irradiation. Current protocols, therefore, do not include radiation therapy.

Mediastinal Radiation

In view of the frequent presentation of lymphoblastic lymphoma with bulky mediastinal disease, some centers have incorporated mediastinal irradiation into induction regimens. This approach has not been evaluated prospectively. A series from the M. D. Anderson Cancer Center retrospectively evaluated 43 patients who achieved a complete remission after initial induction chemotherapy, 19 of whom received mediastinal irradiation (58). None of these patients had relapse in the mediastinum. Of the remaining 24 patients who did not receive irradiation, eight had relapse in the mediastinum. The analysis is difficult to interpret because the groups were unbalanced with respect to their induction therapy, that is, almost all of those receiving radiation therapy had cyclophosphamide, vincristine, doxorubicin, and dexamethasone induction. It is, therefore, not clear whether the apparent improvement in disease control is related to the radiation therapy or the chemotherapy. However, no difference in overall or disease-free survival was seen.

A German multicenter group reported favorable results for a regimen that incorporated mediastinal radiation, although mediastinal relapses were observed in patients who received radiation to this site (47).

Overall, current evidence does not support the use of mediastinal irradiation in this disease.

Acute Tumor Lysis Syndrome

Lymphoblastic lymphoma is an extremely chemosensitive disease. All patients with active disease, and especially those with a large tumor burden, are at risk for developing acute tumor lysis after the initiation of chemotherapy. Appropriate prophylactic measures should, therefore, be taken in all patients before chemotherapy.

PROGNOSIS AND MEDIAN SURVIVAL

As summarized in Tables 12.1 and 12.2, for most published series that include adult patients treated with intensive combination chemotherapy protocols with or without the use of stem cell transplantation to consolidate first remission, 5-year overall survival rates of 50% to 65% are typical, with no obvious benefit from stem cell transplantation. Although the International Prognostic Index may provide some prognostic information, there are inadequate data to suggest that patients should have treatment strategies modified according to risk group.

After relapse after first-line chemotherapy, subsequent prognosis is poor, with typical reported median survival rates of 6 to 9 months when conventional chemotherapy is used, although for patients with relapse and primary refractory disease, long-term survival rates of approximately 30% and 20%, respectively, are reported after stem cell transplantation (52).

FUTURE DIRECTIONS

Dose-intensive, multiagent, induction chemotherapy, similar to that used in ALL, has increased response rates and overall survival for adult patients with lymphoblastic lymphoma, compared with standard non-Hodgkin lymphoma-type regimens. Whether further enhancement of dose intensity will improve response rates more is unclear. Recent results have suggested that the relatively T-cell-specific agent, nelarabine, has activity in this disease (59). Nelarabine is a prodrug that is demethylated in T cells to 9-β-D-arabinofuranosyl-guanine. This has now been investigated in a phase II study in relapsed/refractory T-ALL and lymphoblastic lymphoma. An overall response rate of 41% was observed, with a CR rate of 31%. The 1-year overall survival was 20%. Long-term survivors included some patients who were able to proceed to stem cell transplantation after remissions induced by this agent. This represents remarkable activity for a single agent in this disease, and nelarabine should be incorporated into first-line regimens in the near future. Increasing evidence has implicated the *NOTCH* pathway in the pathogenesis of T-cell precursor lymphoblastic disease, suggesting that signaling molecules downstream of *NOTCH* converge on the mammalian target or rapamycin pathway. In vitro studies have shown that simultaneous blockade of mammalian target or rapamycin and *NOTCH* pathways results in synergistic suppression of T-cell ALL growth (60). This pathway is now under active investigation as a potential therapeutic pathway in lymphoblastic disease.

Gene expression profiles and other molecular studies described previously have identified potential new targets for therapy, including *CARD 10*, a caspase recruitment domain family member that is highly expressed in lymphoblastic lymphoma, which is involved in apoptotic signaling via nuclear factor-κB (25). This may prove to be an exploitable target pathway. Molecular studies may also provide a basis for risk stratification in future studies.

References

1. The Non-Hodgkin's Lymphoma Classification Project: a clinical evaluation of the International Lymphoma Study Group classification of non-Hodgkin's lymphomas. *Blood* 1997;89:3909–3918.
2. Rosen PJ, Feinstein DI, Pattengale PK, et al. Convoluted lymphocytic lymphoma in adults: a clinicopathological entity. *Ann Intern Med* 1978;89: 319–324.
3. Nathwani BN, Diamond LW, Winberg CD, et al. Lymphoblastic lymphoma: a clinicopathologic study of 95 patients. *Cancer* 1978;48:2347–2357.
4. Murphy SB. Management of childhood non-Hodgkin's lymphoma. *Cancer Treat Rep* 1977;61:1161–1173.
5. Warnke RA, Weiss LM, Chan JKC, et al. Tumors of the lymph nodes and spleen. In: *Atlas of tumor pathology.* Washington, DC: Armed Forces Institute of Pathology, 1995.
6. Borowitz MJ, Crocker BP, Metzgar RS. Lymphoblastic lymphoma with the phenotype of common acute lymphoblastic leukemia. *Am J Clin Pathol* 1983;79:387–391.
7. Griffith RC, Kelly DR, Nathwani BN, et al. A morphologic study of childhood lymphoma of the lymphoblastic type: the Pediatric Oncology Group experience. *Cancer* 1987;59:1126–1131.
8. Riopel M, Dickman PS, Link MP, et al. MIC analysis in pediatric lymphoma and leukemia. *Hum Pathol* 1994;25:396–399.
9. Cossman J, Chused TM, Fisher RI, et al. Diversity of immunologic phenotypes of lymphoblastic lymphoma. *Cancer Res* 1983;43:4486–4490.
10. Sheibani K, Nathwani BN, Winberg CD, et al. Antigenically defined subgroups of lymphoblastic lymphoma: relationship to clinical presentation and biological behavior. *Cancer* 1987;60:183–190.
11. Link MP, Stewart SJ, Warnke RA, et al. Discordance between surface and cytoplasmic expression of the Leu-4(T3) antigen I thymocytes and in blast cells from childhood T lymphoblastic malignancies. *J Clin Invest* 1985;76:248–253.
12. Chilosi M, Pizzolog G. Review of terminal deoxynucleotidyl transferase: biological aspects, methods of detection, and selected diagnostic applications. *Appl Immunohistochem* 1995;3:209–221.
13. Borowitz MJ. Immunologic markers in childhood acute lymphoblastic leukemia. *Hematol Oncol Clin North Am* 1990;4:743–765.
14. Bernard A, Murphy SM, Melvin S, et al. Non-T, non-B lymphomas are rare in childhood and are associated with cutaneous tumor. *Blood* 1982;59:549–554.
15. Knowles DM. Immunophenotypic and antigen receptor gene rearrangement analysis in T cell neoplasia. *Am J Pathol* 1989;134:761–785.
16. Pilozzi E, Muller-Hermelink HK, Falini B, et al. Gene rearrangements in T cell lymphoblastic lymphoma. *J Pathol* 1999;188:267–270.
17. Kaneko Y, Frizzera G, Shikano T, et al. Chromosomal and immunophenotypic patterns in T cell acute lymphoblastic leukemia and lymphoblastic lymphoma. *Leukemia* 1989;3:886–892.
18. Okuda T, Fisher R, Downing JR. Molecular diagnostics in pediatric acute lymphoblastic leukemia. *Mol Diagn* 1996;1:139–151.
19. Finger LR, Kagan J, Christopher G, et al. Involvement of the TCL5 gene on human chromosome 1 in T-cell leukemia and melanoma. *Proc Natl Acad Sci U S A* 1989;86:5039–5043.
20. Mellentin JD, Smith SD, Cleary ML. Lyl-1, a novel gene altered by chromosomal translocation in T-cell leukemia, codes for a protein with helix-loop-helix DNA binding motif. *Cell* 1989;58:77–83.
21. Xia Y, Brown L, Yang CY, et al. TAL2, a helix-loop-helix gene activated by the t(7;9)(q34;q32) translocation in human T-cell leukemia. *Proc Natl Acad Sci U S A* 1989;88:11416–11420.
22. Ferrando AA, Neuberg D, Staunton J, et al. Gene expression signatures define novel oncogenic pathways in T cell acute lymphoblastic leukemia. *Cancer Cell* 2002;1:75–87.
23. Baleydier F, Decouvelaere AV, Bergeron J, et al. T cell receptor genotyping and HX/TLX1 expression define three T lymphoblastic lymphoma subsets which might affect clinical outcome. *Clin Cancer Res* 2008;14:692–700.
24. Raetz EA, Perkins SL, Bhojwani D, et al. Gene expression profiling reveals intrinsic differences between T-cell acute lymphoblastic leukemia and T-cell lymphoblastic lymphoma. *Pediatr Blood Cancer* 2006;47:130–140.
25. Sweetenham JW, Santini G, Qian W, et al. High-dose therapy and autologous stem-cell transplantation versus conventional dose consolidation/maintenance therapy as post-remission therapy for adult patients with lymphoblastic lymphoma: results of a randomized trial of the European Group for Blood and Marrow Transplantation and the United Kingdom Lymphoma Group. *J Clin Oncol* 2001;19:2927–2936.
26. Coleman CN, Picozzi VJ, Cox RS, et al. Treatment of lymphoblastic lymphoma in adults. *J Clin Oncol* 1986;4:1626–1637.
27. Murphy SB, Fairclough DL, Hutchison RE, et al. Non-Hodgkin's lymphomas of childhood: an analysis of the histology, staging and response to treatment of 338 cases at a single institution. *J Clin Oncol* 1989;7:186–193.
28. Kroft SH, Domiati-Saad R, Finn WG, et al. Precursor B-lymphoblastic transformation of grade 1 follicular lymphoma. *Am J Clin Pathol* 2000;113:411–418.
29. Lin P, Jones D, Dorfman DM, et al. Precursor B-cell lymphoblastic lymphoma—a predominantly extranodal tumor with low propensity for leukemic involvement. *Am J Surg Pathol* 2000;24:1480–1490.
30. Maitra A, McKenna RW, Weinberg AG, et al. Precursor B-cell lymphoblastic lymphoma—a study of nine cases lacking blood and bone marrow involvement and review of the literature. *Am J Clin Pathol* 2001;115:868–875.
31. Armitage JO, Weisenberger DD. New approach to classifying non-Hodgkin's lymphomas: clinical features of the major histologic subtypes. *J Clin Oncol* 1998;16:2780–2795.

32. Bouabdallah R, Xerri L, Bardou VJ, et al. Role of induction chemotherapy and bone marrow transplantation in adult lymphoblastic lymphoma: a report on 62 patients from a single center. *Ann Oncol* 1998;9:619–625.

33. Czuczman MS, Dodge RK, Stewart CC, et al. Value of immunophenotype in intensively treated adult acute lymphoblastic leukemia: Cancer and Leukemia Group B study 8364. *Blood* 1999;93:3931–3939.

34. Secker-Walker LM, Moorman AV, Bain BJ, et al. Secondary acute leukemia and myelodysplastic syndrome with 11q23 abnormalities. EU Concerted Action 11q23 Workshop. *Leukemia* 1998;12:840–844.

35. Raimondi SC. Current status of cytogenetic research in childhood acute lymphoblastic leukemia. *Blood* 1993;81:2237–2251.

36. Slater DE, Mertelsmann R, Koriner B, et al. Lymphoblastic lymphoma in adults. *J Clin Oncol* 1986;4:57–67.

37. Bernasconi C, Brusamolino E, Lazzarino M, et al. Lymphoblastic lymphoma in adult patients; clinicopathological features and response to intensive multi-agent chemotherapy analogous to that used in acute lymphoblastic leukemia. *Ann Oncol* 1990;1:141–160.

38. Morel P, Lepage E, Brice P, et al. Prognosis and treatment of lymphoblastic lymphoma in adults: a report on 80 patients. *J Clin Oncol* 1992;10:1078–1085.

39. Murphy SB. Childhood non-Hodgkin's lymphoma. *N Engl J Med* 1977;299:1446–1448.

40. Voakes JB, Jones SE, McKelvey EM. The chemotherapy of lymphoblastic lymphoma. *Blood* 1981;57:186–188.

41. Colgan JP, Anderson J, Habermann TM, et al. Long-term follow-up of a CHOP-based regimen with maintenance chemotherapy and central nervous system prophylaxis in lymphoblastic non-Hodgkin's lymphoma. *Leuk Lymphoma* 1994;15:291–296.

42. Kaiser U, Uebelacker I, Havemann K. Non-Hodgkin's lymphoma protocols in the treatment of patients with Burkitt's lymphoma and lymphoblastic lymphoma: a report on 58 patients. *Leuk Lymphoma* 1999;36:101–108.

43. Woolner N, Burchenal JH, Liberman PH, et al. Non-Hodgkin's lymphoma in children. A progress report on the original patient treated with the LSA₂-L₂ protocol. *Cancer* 1979;44:1990–1999.

44. Anderson JR, Wilson JF, Jenkin RDT, et al. Childhood non-Hodgkin's lymphoma. The results of a randomized therapeutic trial comparing a 4-drug regimen (COMP) with a 10-drug regimen (LSA₂-L₂). *N Engl J Med* 1983;308:559–565.

45. Levine AM, Forman SJ, Meyer PR, et al. Successful therapy of convoluted T-lymphoblastic lymphoma in the adult. *Blood* 1983;61:92–99.

46. Weinstein HJ, Cassady JR, Levey R. Long-term results of the APO protocol (vincristine, doxorubicin [adriamycin] and prednisone) for the treatment of mediastinal lymphoblastic lymphoma. *J Clin Oncol* 1983;1:537–541.

47. Hoelzer D, Gokbuget N, Digel W, et al. Outcome of adult patients with T-lymphoblastic lymphoma treated according to protocols for acute lymphoblastic leukemia. *Blood* 2002;99:4379–4385.

48. Thomas DA, O'Brien S, Cortes J, et al. Outcome with the hyper-CVAD regimens in lymphoblastic lymphoma. *Blood* 2004;104:1624–1630.

49. Jabbour E, Koscielny S, Cebban C, et al. High survival rate with the LMT-89 regimen in lymphoblastic lymphoma (LL), but not in T-cell acute lymphoblastic leukemia (T-ALL). *Leukemia* 2006;20:814–819.

50. Song KW, Barnett MJ, Gascoyne RD, et al. Primary therapy for adults with T-cell lymphoblastic lymphoma with hematopoietic stem cell transplantation results in favorable outcomes. *Ann Oncol* 2007;18:535–540.

51. Jost LM, Jacky E, Dommann-Scherrer C, et al. Short-term weekly chemotherapy followed by high dose therapy with autologous bone marrow transplantation for lymphoblastic and Burkitt's lymphomas in adult patients. *Ann Oncol* 1995;6:445–451.

52. Sweetenham JW, Santini G, Pearce R, et al. High-dose therapy and autologous bone marrow transplantation for adult patients with lymphoblastic lymphoma: results from the European Group for Bone Marrow Transplantation. *J Clin Oncol* 1994;12:1358–1365.

53. Le Gouill S, Lepretre S, Briere J, et al. Adult lymphoblastic lymphoma: a retrospective analysis of 92 patients under 61 years included in the LNH87/93 trials. *Leukemia* 2003;17:2220–2224.

54. van Imhoff GW, van der Holt B, MacKenzie MA, et al. Short intensive sequential therapy followed by autologous stem cell transplantation in adult Burkitt, Burkitt-like and lymphoblastic lymphoma. *Leukemia* 2005;19:945–952.

55. Peniket AJ, Ruiz de Elvira MC, Taghipour G, et al. An EBMT registry matched study of allogeneic stem cell transplants for lymphoma: allogeneic transplantation is associated with a lower relapse rate but a higher procedure-related mortality rate that autologous transplantation. *Bone Marrow Transplant* 2003;8:667–678.

56. Levine JE, Harris RE, Loberiza FR, et al. A comparison of allogeneic and autologous bone marrow transplantation for lymphoblastic lymphoma. *Blood* 2003;101:2476–2482.

57. Sweetenham JW, Mead GM, Whitehouse JMA. Adult lymphoblastic lymphoma: high incidence of central nervous system relapse in patients treated with the Stanford University protocol. *Ann Oncol* 1992;3:839–841.

58. Dabaja BS, Ha CS, Thomas DA, et al. The role of local radiation therapy for mediastinal disease for adults with T-cell lymphoblastic lymphoma. *Cancer* 2002;94:2738–2744.

59. DeAngelo D, Yu D, Johnson JL, et al. Nelarabine induces complete remissions in adults with relapsed or refractory T-lineage acute lymphoblastic leukemia or lymphoblastic lymphoma: Cancer and Leukemia Group B study 19801. *Blood* 2007;109:5136–5142.

60. Chan SM, Weng AP, Tibshirani R, et al. Notch signals positively regulate activity of the mTOR pathway in T-cell acute lymphoblastic leukemia. *Blood* 2007;109:278–286.

CHAPTER 13 ■ SMALL B-CELL LYMPHOCYTIC LYMPHOMA/CHRONIC LYMPHOCYTIC LEUKEMIA

JOHN G. GRIBBEN, NANCY LEE HARRIS, AND RICCARDO DALLA-FAVERA

DEFINITIONS OF CHRONIC LYMPHOCYTIC LEUKEMIA AND SMALL LYMPHOCYTIC LYMPHOMA

Historically, chronic lymphocytic leukemia (CLL) was believed to be a different disease from B-cell small lymphocytic lymphoma (SLL). In the World Health Organization classification, it is now considered simply as a different clinical manifestation of the same disease (1). B-cell CLL/SLL is a neoplasm of small round B lymphocytes accompanied by larger cell known as prolymphocytes, expressing B-cell antigens and CD5 and CD23. When the disease involves the peripheral blood and bone marrow, it is called CLL, and when lymph nodes or other tissues are infiltrated by cells having the identical morphologic and immunophenotypic features of CLL, but in which there is no leukemic manifestations of the disease, it is called SLL.

Etiology and Epidemiology

It is estimated that 15,110 men and women (8,750 men and 6,360 women) will be diagnosed with and 4,390 men and women will die of CLL/SLL in 2008 (http://seer.cancer.gov/statfacts/html/clyl.html), and there are data to suggest that the incidence may be higher than that reported within the tumor registries (2). Although a higher incidence has been reported for whites compared with African-Americans (3), data from the National Cancer Institute's Surveillance Epidemiology and End Results program data (http://seer.cancer.gov/statistics) now suggest a more similar incidence pattern in these groups. CLL/SLL is considered to be mainly a disease of the elderly, and in the Surveillance Epidemiology and End Results databases, the median at diagnosis for CLL was 72 years of age. The disease is very uncommon in the young: approximately 0.0% were diagnosed <age 20; 0.3% between 20 and 34; 1.8% between 35 and 44; 8.9% between 45 and 54; 19.1% between 55 and 64; 26.8% between 65 and 74; 30.1% between 75 and 84; and 12.9% in those ≥85 years of age. The age-adjusted incidence rate was 4.0 per 100,000 men and women per year. These rates are based on cases diagnosed in 2001 to 2005 from 17 Surveillance Epidemiology and End Results geographic areas. Younger patients do not have a worse prognosis than older patients (4). Although younger and older patients have a similar survival, analysis of the relative survival rates showed that the disease had a greater adverse effect on the expected survival probability of the younger population because the older patients often die of causes unrelated to their CLL. Only 5% of patients with CLL/SLL present with clinical features of SLL without the leukemic component.

The variation in international incidence patterns among the leukemias and lymphomas is most marked for B-cell CLL/SLL, and there is a 26-fold increase in incidence for men in Canada compared with Japan, and a 38-fold increase for women between the United States and Japan (5). Genetic rather than environmental factors most likely explain for these differences because the disease is rare among Japanese-Americans (6).

Although occupational exposures can be linked to an excess occurrence of many cancers, there are no clearly discernible occupational or environmental risk factors that predispose to B-cell CLL/SLL. In particular, there is no evidence linking exposure to ionizing radiation (7). Although there have been reports of increased incidence among farm workers, this has not been substantiated (8). A report from the Institute of Medicine by a panel set up at the request of the Department of Veterans Affairs, reexamined six separate studies on the possible link between Agent Orange and B-cell CLL/SLL, and published its findings in *Committee to Review the Health Effects in Vietnam Veterans of Exposure to Herbicides (Fourth Biennial Update)*. This report supported the idea that people exposed to Agent Orange, a pesticide used for defoliation in Vietnam, have a higher risk of B-cell CLL/SLL. Exposure to petrochemicals does not appear to increase the incidence of CLL/SLL (9). Similarly, whereas exposure to hair dyes has been suggested to be associated with an increased incidence of some types of non-Hodgkin lymphoma, this was not the case for CLL/SLL (10).

Among the strongest risk factors for the development of B-cell CLL/SLL is a family history of this or other lymphoid malignancies. A number of familial clusters of B-cell CLL/SLL has been reported (11). More than 50 years ago, Videbaek (12) reported that in familial cases of leukemia, the incidence of lymphoid leukemias was almost double that of myelogenous leukemias. In a report from the National Cancer Institute Familial Registry, the mean age at diagnosis among familial cases was 58, >12 years younger than the mean age of presentation observed in sporadic cases (13). A higher percentage of second primary tumors (16% vs. 8.8%) were also observed among familial compared with sporadic CLL/SLL cases. Genetic anticipation, the process whereby the median age at onset in a child of a multigenerational family with malignancy is younger than that of the parent generations, has been observed in CLL/SLL (14,15). The risk of transformation to more aggressive non-Hodgkin lymphomas does not appear to be different in familial cases from that reported for sporadic cases. Although there are some differences between familial and sporadic cases, familial cases with CLL do not have a difference in survival from diagnosis compared with nonfamilial cases (16). The repertoire and frequency of immunoglobulin (Ig) heavy chain variable region (IgVH) usage are not significantly different between familial and sporadic CLL (17). There may be an increased frequency of mutated CLL in familial CLL and evidence of intrafamilial concordance in mutation status, but IgVH usage was not correlated between affected members of the same family. These observations provide evidence that familial CLL is essentially indistinguishable from sporadic CLL, favoring a genetic basis to disease development in general rather than a simple environmental etiology. It is highly likely that the study of families with multiple B-cell CLL/SLL cases will aid in delineating the genes and environmental factors that may play a role in the development of both forms of B-cell CLL/SLL.

Diagnosis

Morphology

The diagnosis of B-cell CLL/SLL is made by the detection of a clonal population of small B lymphocytes in the peripheral blood or bone marrow, or by lymph node biopsy showing cells expressing the characteristic morphology and immunophenotype. The diagnostic criteria are shown in Table 13.1. The presence of <5,000 CLL/SLL B-lymphocytes per μL in the absence of lymphadenopathy is defined as "monoclonal B-lymphocytosis." In peripheral blood and bone marrow smears, the cells are monomorphic small round B lymphocytes, with only rare large cells with prominent nucleoli (prolymphocytes) seen. The bone marrow infiltrate may be nodular, interstitial, or diffuse, or may show a combination of these patterns. The lymph node infiltrate of CLL/SLL is

TABLE 13.1
DIAGNOSIS OF CLL
Lymphocytosis (small, mature lymphocytes >5000/μL) for at least 3 months
Bone marrow involvement of >30% lymphocytes ≤55% atypical/immature lymphoid cells in peripheral blood
Clonal expansion of abnormal B lymphocytes
Low density of surface Ig (IgM or IgD) with κ or λ light chains B-cell surface antigens (CD19, CD20 [dim], CD23) CD5 surface antigen

composed of predominantly small lymphocytes with condensed chromatin, round nuclei, and occasionally a small nucleolus (18). Larger lymphoid cells known as prolymphocytes and paraimmunoblasts with more prominent nucleoli and more dispersed chromatin are always present, and are clustered in aggregates known as proliferation centers or pseudofollicles (Fig. 13.1).

Immunophenotype

The cells in B-cell CLL/SLL express CD19, dim CD20, dim CD5, CD23, CD43, CD79a, and weakly express surface IgM and IgD. Immunophenotypic analysis of a case of CLL is shown in Figure 13.2. Cytoplasmic Ig is detectable in approximately 5% of cases. Occasional cases of CLL/SLL lack expression of CD23, and this can lead to a differential diagnosis of mantle cell lymphoma. Dim expression of CD20 and surface Ig is highly characteristic of CLL/SLL, and this can be useful in distinguishing CLL/SLL from mantle cell lymphoma. Expression of CD38 is variable and has been reported to have prognostic significance in this disease (19,20). For this reason, CD38 should continue to be included in the immunophenotypic panel of antigens assessed in this disease. Immunophenotypic features are required to make the diagnosis of B-cell CLL/SLL, and a scoring system has been proposed (21). In difficult cases, particularly those in which there is an atypical immunophenotype, the detection of specific cytogenetic and molecular features can be helpful in making the definitive diagnosis. The immunophenotypic

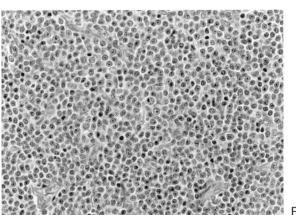

FIGURE 13.1 Lymph node biopsy from a patient with CLL. **A:** At low magnification, there is a vaguely nodular (pseudofollicular) pattern. (see also Color Plate 21) **B:** Higher magnification shows a predominance of small lymphocytes with scattered larger cells known as prolymphocytes and paraimmunoblasts. (see also Color Plate 22).

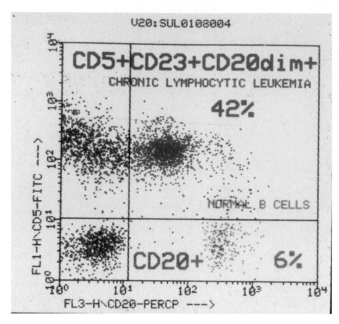

FIGURE 13.2 Flow cytometry of CLL. The cells express dim CD20, dim CD5, and CD23. (see also Color Plate 23) (Courtesy of Dr. Frederick I Preffer, Department of Pathology, Massachusetts General Hospital, Boston, MA.)

and genetic features of B-cell CLL/SLL and other small B-cell neoplasms are shown in Table 13.2.

Pathogenesis

Understanding the pathogenesis of CLL/SLL remains a major challenge. Unlike many of the other low-grade B-cell malignancies, nonrandom reciprocal chromosomal translocations occur rarely in CLL/SLL. However, a number of cytogenetic abnormalities have been identified. Using fluorescent in situ hybridization (FISH) techniques, one or more of these cytogenetic abnormalities can be found in more than 80% of patients with B-cell CLL/SLL and, as described in the Cytogenetic and Molecular Analysis Section, these have important prognostic significance (22).

The most common abnormality is deletion of the long arm of chromosome 13q.14, which occurs in more than 50% of cases. The first report linking micro-ribonucleic acids (RNAs) to cancer was in CLL, where it was demonstrated that two microRNA clusters, mir-15a and mir16-1 (23), were located within the deleted region at 13q14 (24). Considerable interest has also been paid to ultraconserved regions, many of which have altered expression in CLL (25). The next most common cytogenetic abnormality is deletion of the long arm of chromosome 11q, seen in up to 20% of cases of CLL. This deletion is associated with a distinct clinical presentation, including younger age, male sex, bulky lymphadenopathy, and poor prognosis. The ataxia telangiectasia mutated (ATM) gene is located within the minimal region of loss at 11 q23, suggesting that alterations in this gene may be involved in the pathogenesis of the disease. This is further supported by the finding that mutations in the ATM gene are associated with poor prognosis (26). Trisomy 12 occurs in up to 20% of cases of CLL/SLL, but the molecular mechanism by which this genetic abnormality contributes to leukemogenesis is unknown. Although less common and occurring in <10% of patients at diagnosis, deletions in the short arm of chromosome 17p are associated with rapid progression of disease, poor response to therapy, and short survival. The deletion involves the p53 locus at 17p13, and it is clear that mutations in the p53 gene can contribute to disease progression and alter the sensitivity of CLL cells to chemotherapy agents. Although a number of genes, including bcl-2, ATM, and p53, are known to play a role in disease progression, the genes involved in the pathogenesis of the disease remain to be identified.

TABLE 13.2

SMALL B-CELL NEOPLASMS: IMMUNOPHENOTYPIC AND GENETIC FEATURES

Neoplasm	SIg; cIg	CD5	CD10	CD23	CD43	Cyclin D1	Bcl-6 protein[a]	Genetic abnormality	Ig V-region genes
B-cell CLL/SLL	+; –/+	+	–	+	+	–	–	13q deletions (50%), trisomy 12 (20%)	50% unmutated
Lymphoplasmacytic lymphoma	+; +	–	–	–	–/+	–	–	t(9;14)–PAX5R	Mutated
Mantle cell lymphoma	+; –	+	–	–	+	+	–	t(11;14)–BCL1R	Unmutated
Follicle center lymphoma	+; –	–	+	–/+	–	–	+	t(14;18)–BCL2R	Mutated, ongoing
Extranodal and nodal marginal zone lymphoma	+; –/+	–	–	–/+	–/+	–	–	Trisomy 3 t(11;18)–API2/MLT t(1;14)–BCL10R	Mutated, ongoing
Splenic marginal zone lymphoma	+; –/+	–	–	–	–	–	–	Del 7q21-32 (40%)	50% mutated

+, >90% positive; +/–, >50% positive; –/+, <50% positive; –, <10% positive.
[a] Residual germinal center may be positive in marginal zone lymphoma and mantle cell lymphoma.

In addition to the heterogeneity of genetic abnormalities, CLL/SLL is also heterogeneous in its level of differentiation, as evidenced by the status of the Ig genes. CLL/SLL can be divided into two subgroups based upon the presence or absence of IgVH somatic hypermutation (27), and this finding has prognostic significance (19,28). Although this led to the hypothesis of two subsets of B-cell CLL/SLL, based upon different cells of origin, with cases with unmutated IgV regions derived from naive, pregerminal center cells, whereas those that have mutated IgV regions arise from a postgerminal center cell that has encountered antigen. However, gene expression profiling studies have demonstrated that both subtypes of CLL/SLL display a common and distinct gene expression profile, suggesting that both mutated and unmutated groups share a common cell of origin, and these findings do not support the hypothesis of two distinct disease entities arising from different cells of origin. Gene profiling studies did identify a restricted number of genes that are capable of distinguishing IgVH mutated versus unmutated cases (29,30). Most attention has focused on expression of ζ-associated protein (ZAP) 70, which is found in most unmutated but not mutated cases (31,32).

Methods of Presentation

In approximately 25% of cases, B-cell CLL/SLL is diagnosed in the asymptomatic patients at the time of a routine blood count, when a lymphocytosis leads to the subsequent diagnosis. The guidelines for the diagnosis of CLL/SLL require a lymphocytosis with the presence of $>5 \times 10^9$ per L B lymphocytes (33).

In the remaining cases, there is a wide range of initial presenting features. The most consistent physical finding is painless lymphadenopathy, most frequently in the cervical, supraclavicular, or axillary regions, followed by splenomegaly and/or hepatomegaly. Only 5% of patients present with lymphadenopathy without evidence of leukemic infiltration. Although CLL/SLL can involve virtually every tissue, involvement in other organs is rare, particularly at the time of initial diagnosis. Skin is the most commonly involved nonlymphoid organ, but this is present in <5% of cases (34). In contrast to other B-cell malignancies, gastrointestinal involvement is extremely rare in CLL/SLL. Meningeal involvement, although reported, is extremely rare (35,36).

Up to 20% of cases present with "B" symptoms, which are defined as unintentional weight loss of $\geq$10% of body weight over the previous 6 months, fevers >38°C for >2 weeks without evidence of infection, night sweats, or extreme fatigue (Eastern Cooperative Oncology Group [ECOG] performance status $\geq$2) (37). Anemia and thrombocytopenia may be present at the time of initial presentation. In 20% of cases, anemia <11 g per dL and thrombocytopenia <100,000 per μL are present, and are associated with a poor prognosis (see Unique Aspects of Staging below).

Unique Aspects of Staging

The natural history of CLL/SLL is extremely variable, and until the mid 1970s, there were no reliable methods to assess outcome. The two widely used staging systems that are now in place are based upon their prognostic implications for survival (38,39). The Rai staging system (Table 13.3) is based upon the premise that there is a progressive accumulation of neoplastic cells manifested by increasing lymphocytosis, progressive lymphadenopathy, splenomegaly, and hepatomegaly, followed by bone marrow replacement with development of anemia and thrombocytopenia (38). At the time of initial diagnosis, 25% of patients have stage 0 disease, 50% stage I to II, and 25% stage II to IV. The Binet system (Table 13.4) takes into consideration five potential sites of involvement: cervical, axillary, and inguinal lymph nodes (either unilateral or bilateral counts as one site), the spleen, and the liver (39). Patients' disease is staged according to the number of involved sites plus the presence of anemia with hemoglobin <10 g per dL and/or thrombocytopenia with platelets <100,000 per μL. The International Workshop on CLL recommends that in practice, an integrated system using both methods (Table 13.5) should be used for uniformity in reporting clinical trials (40). Although this should be used in reports of clinical trials, it has not been widely accepted by clinicians in their everyday practice, who prefer to use the simpler Rai or Binet systems, and it is often difficult to extract International Workshop on CLL staging in multicenter studies. A number of other staging systems have been proposed but have not received widespread acceptance (41–44).

Prognostic and Predictive Factors

Clinical Stage

A number of prognostic factors have been identified in CLL/SLL. The Rai and Binet staging systems were based upon their prognostic significance, and the stage of disease remains perhaps the most important prognostic factor in CLL/SLL, although there are increasing attempts to correlate prognosis with biologic markers. The median survival from the time of diagnosis based upon the Rai classification was 150 months for stage 0, 71 to 101 months for stages I and II, and 9 months for stages III and IV (38). Although the original Rai staging system comprised five stages (stages 0 through IV), there were only three distinct survival patterns: stage 0,

TABLE 13.3			
RAI CLASSIFICATION OF CLL			
Stage	Simplified three-stage system	Clinical features	Median survival (y)
0	Low risk	Lymphocytosis in blood and marrow only	>10
I	Intermediate risk	Lymphadenopathy	7
II		Splenomegaly +/– hepatomegaly	
III	High risk	Anemia	0.75–4
IV		Thrombocytopenia	

TABLE 13.4

BINET STAGING SYSTEM OF CLL

Group	Clinical features	Median survival (y)
A	<3 areas of lymphadenopathy; no anemia or thrombocytopenia	12
B	>3 involved node areas; no anemia or thrombocytopenia	7
C	Hemoglobin <10 g/dL and/or platelets <100,000/μL	2–4

stages I and II combined, and stages III and IV combined. As a result, a modified Rai staging system recognizes three groups: low risk, Rai stage 0; intermediate risk, Rai stages I and II combined; and high risk, Rai stages III and IV combined (45). The survival of patients using this modified Rai staging system is shown in Figure 13.3. Survival of the three groups within the Binet system is similar to that observed in the three groups of the modified Rai staging system.

The majority of patients with high-risk disease (Rai stages III and IV and Binet stage C) have a rapidly progressive clinical course and short survival, but the course of disease is less uniform in the other groups, with some patients, particularly those with Rai stage 0, Binet stage A, following a benign or "smoldering" course. Therefore, a number of other prognostic factors have been evaluated for their prognostic significance and have shown limited utility in their ability to predict the course of disease (Table 13.6).

Prognostic Markers

Not surprisingly, a lymphocyte doubling time of <12 months in untreated patient predicts a progressive course (46,47). An atypical morphology with increased number of prolymphocytes is also an independent factor associated with an adverse prognosis (48) Bone marrow biopsies are not needed to make the diagnosis of CLL/SLL, but the pattern of bone marrow involvement (diffuse vs. nodular or interstitial) has prognostic significance (49). Several other factors have been used to correlate tumor cell proliferation with clinical outcome, including Ki67 (50), p27 (51), and thymidine kinase (52). Measurement of serum levels of thymidine kinase, an enzyme that reflects cellular division, and elevated serum levels of thymidine kinase have been shown to add independent prognostic information to differentiate progressive from "smoldering" CLL/SLL (52). Smoldering CLL/SLL cases refer to those cases that show little or no evidence of progression over time and that do not appear to affect survival.

β-2 Microglobulin

A number of studies have evaluated the prognostic value of measurement of serum β-2 microglobulin (β2M) in CLL/SLL. In a prospective study of 113 patients with early stage disease, β2M in addition to serum levels of thymidine kinase, performance status and platelet count were independent prognostic factors (53). Reports from the M. D. Anderson Cancer Center have also stressed the important prognostic significance of elevated levels of serum β2M. In 150 patients with CLL/SLL, elevated serum levels of interleukin-6 and interleukin-10 were adverse prognostic factors, and were correlated with serum β2M levels. In a multivariate analysis, serum β2M was the most important independent prognostic factor (54), as demonstrated by the importance of this factor in a nomogram devised to assess risk of progression (55).

Tumor Necrosis Factor

Tumor necrosis factor-α (TNFα) is produced by CLL/SLL cells, and acts as an autocrine and paracrine growth factor in this disease. In 150 patients with CLL/SLL, TNFα levels were measured and correlated with disease characteristics, prognostic factors, and survival (56). Patients having an elevated TNFα level had more advanced Rai and Binet stage disease, higher serum β2M, a greater percentage of cells expressing CD38, and lower hemoglobin and platelet levels. The TNFα level remained predictive of survival in multivariate analysis independent ($p = 0.005$) of Rai staging and β2M, hemoglobin, prior therapy, white cell count, and platelet level (56). Among 41 patients

TABLE 13.5

INTERNATIONAL WORKSHOP ON CLL STAGING SYSTEM AND PROGNOSIS IN CLL

Stage	Description	Median survival (y)
A	Lymphocytosis with clinical involvement of fewer than 3 lymph node groups; no anemia or thrombocytopenia A (0) no nodes enlarged A (I) nodes enlarged A (II) hepatomegaly or splenomegaly	8–2+
B	More than three lymph node groups involved, no anemia or thrombocytopenia B (I) nodes enlarged B (II) hepatomegaly or splenomegaly	5+
C	Anemia or thrombocytopenia regardless of number of lymph node groups involved C (III) anemia C (IV) thrombocytopenia	2.5

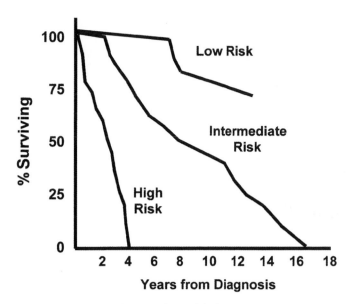

FIGURE 13.3 Survival in CLL by modified Rai stage.

with Binet stage A disease, progression-free survival (PFS) was significantly shorter in those patients whose vascular endothelial growth factor serum concentrations were elevated (57).

Cytogenetic and Molecular Analysis

Conventional cytogenetic analyses only detected chromosome aberrations in 40% to 50% of cases, but newer molecular cytogenetic methods, particularly FISH, have greatly enhanced our ability to detect chromosomal abnormalities in B-cell CLL/SLL. The pattern of cytogenetic abnormalities in CLL/SLL is markedly different form that found in other types of mature B-cell malignancies. In the most comprehensive study published to date, chromosomal abnormalities were detected in >80% of patients with B-cell CLL/SLL studied (22), and this study convincingly demonstrated that genomic aberrations in B-cell CLL/SLL are important independent predictors of disease progression and survival (Figure 13.5). The most frequent changes observed were deletion in 13q,

TABLE 13.6

PROGNOSTIC FACTORS IN CLL

Advanced stage at diagnosis
Diffuse pattern of bone marrow infiltration
Short lymphocyte doubling time
Expression of Ki67, p27
High serum levels of thymideine kinase, β2M, soluble CD23, and TNFα
Poor risk cytogenetics–17p, 11q deletions. and complex abnormralities
IgV mutational status
CD38 expression
ZAP70 expression
MicroRNA expression
Advanced age
Male sex
Response to therapy

TABLE 13.7

CYTOGENETIC ABNORMALITES IN 325 PATIENTS WITH CLL

Abnormality	No. of patients (%)
13q deletion	178 (55)
11q deletion	58 (18)
Trisomy 12	53 (16)
17p deletion	23 (7)

Adapted from Dohner H, Stilgenbauer S, Benner A, et al. Genomic aberrations and survival in chronic lymphocytic leukemia. *N Engl J Med* 2000;343:1910–1916, with permission.

deletion in 11q, trisomy 12q (Fig. 13.4), deletion in 17p. (Table 13.7) The median survival time for patients with 17p deletion was 32 months, 11q deletion 79 months, 12q trisomy 114 months, normal karyotype 111 months, and 13q deletion as the sole abnormality 133 months (Fig. 13.5). Patients in the 17p- and 11q-deletion groups had more advanced disease than those in the other three groups. Patients with 17p deletions had the shortest median treatment-free interval (9 months), and those with 13q deletions had the longest (92 months). Ongoing studies are assessing the impact of specific cytogenetic abnormalities on response to particular therapeutic approaches. However, the presence of 17p deletion predicts for treatment failure with alkylating agents and fludarabine, and short survival times. In multivariate analysis, 11q and 17p deletions provided independent adverse prognostic information. These findings have implications for the design of risk-adapted treatment strategies (58).

Immunoglobulin Gene Mutation Status

An important advance in the understanding of CLL was made with the demonstration that >50% of CLL cases have

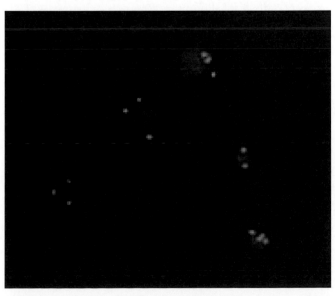

FIGURE 13.4 FISH demonstrating trisomy 12 in CLL. (see also Color Plate 24) (Courtesy of Dr. Randy Gascoyne, British Columbia Cancer Agency, Vancouver, British Columbia, Canada.)

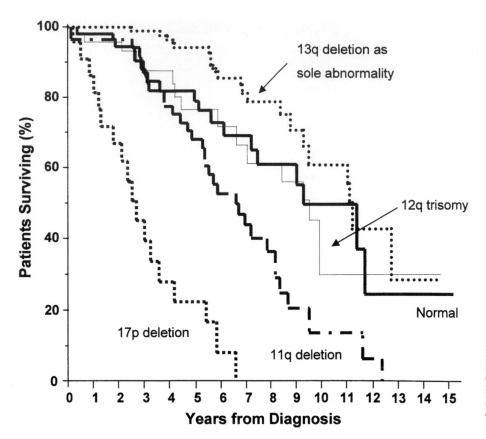

FIGURE 13.5 Survival from time of diagnosis in CLL by cytogenetic abnormalities detected by FISH. (Adapted from Dohner H, Stilgenbauer S, Benner A, et al. Genomic aberrations and survival in chronic lymphocytic leukemia. *N Engl J Med* 2000;343: 1910–1916, with permission.)

IgVH somatic hypermutation and that this has prognostic significance. Patients with CLL/SLL with somatic hypermutation have a more indolent clinical course and longer survival than this without somatic hypermutation (Fig. 13.6) (19,28). The levels of somatic hypermutation are evaluated by comparison of the sequence of the rearranged variable region gene with germline sequences, and guidelines have been reported for analysis of IgVH rearrangements from the Working Group of European Research Initiative in CLL guidelines (59). Sequences with <98% homology to germline are considered to have undergone somatic hypermutation. The finding that CLL cases can be divided into mutated and unmutated groups implied that the two groups may be diseases that arise from different normal cellular counterparts, but as described previously, this was not supported by subsequent gene expression profiling studies (29,30).

Analysis of variable region sequences demonstrated that CLL cells utilize a biased repertoire of V genes characterized by overrepresentation of selected Ig gene segments, in particular *IGHV1-69*, *IGHV4-34*, *IGHV3-7*, and *IGHV3-21* (27,60). Somatic hypermutation does occur uniformly among *IGHV* genes. For example, *IGHV1-69* consistently carries very few mutations as opposed to the typically mutated *IGHV3-7*, *IGHV3-23*, and *IGHV4-34* genes. An apparent exemption to the generalization that mutated CLL cases have good prognosis is in the subgroup of patients with CLL cells that use *IGHV3-21* because these patients have relatively aggressive disease even when the expressed *IGHV3-21* is mutated (61).

Not only is the Ig gene repertoire expressed by CLL cell biased, but it is also notable for the existence of subsets with near identical (stereotyped) B-cell receptors, implying the rec-

ognition of structurally similar epitopes, likely selecting the leukemic clones (62). The nature of the antigens that these B-cell receptors might be recognizing and whether these are important in driving the pathogenesis of CLL remains unknown. The presence of such stereotypic rearrangements may also have prognostic significance (63,64).

Surrogates for Immunoglobulin Heavy Chain Variable Region Mutational Status

CD38 is a surface marker associated with CLL, and easily determined using standard flow cytometric methods. It was initially found to correlate with IgVH mutation status (19), however, the relationship is not absolute, and CD38 expression may vary over time (20,65). The field is somewhat confused by a variety of cutoffs ranging from 5% to 30% being used in different series to define a case as being CD38 (65–67), and it has been suggested that CD38 should be evaluated by its modal expression by flow cytometry, or by antigen density. In multivariate analysis, high levels of expression of CD38 on B-cell CLL/SLL cells were associated with more rapid progression of disease and poor response to therapy (68,69). A multivariate analysis examined the prognostic significance of genetic abnormalities (detected at or shortly after presentation), clinical stage, lymphocyte morphology, CD38 expression, and IGV gene status in 205 patients with CLL/SLL (70). Deletion of chromosome 11q23, absence of a deletion of chromosome 13q14, atypical lymphocyte morphology, and >30% CD38 expression were significantly associated

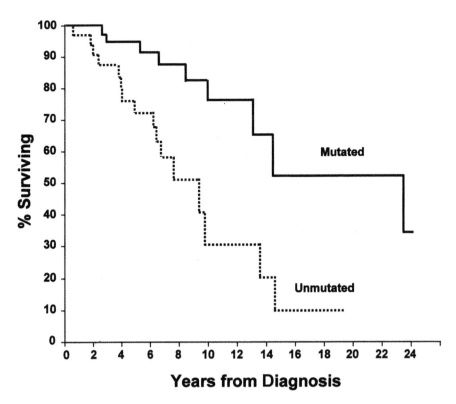

FIGURE 13.6 Survival from time of diagnosis of CLL by presence of mutated versus unmutated Ig gene rearrangements. (Adapted from Hamblin TJ, Davis Z, Gardiner A, et al. Unmutated Ig V(H) genes are associated with a more aggressive form of chronic lymphocytic leukemia. *Blood* 1999;94:1848–1854, with permission.)

with the presence of unmutated IgV genes. Advanced stage, male sex, atypical morphology, >30% CD38 expression, trisomy 12, deletion of chromosome 11q23, loss or mutation of the p53 gene, and unmutated IgV genes were all poor prognostic factors in the univariate analysis in this study. However, IgV gene mutational status, loss or mutation of the p53 gene, and clinical stage retained prognostic significance in a multivariate analysis (70).

When gene expression profiles were analyzed comparing mutated and unmutated cases of CLL (29,30), only a small number of genes were found to be differentially expressed, the most specific being the gene encoding the 70-kDa ζZAP70 (32). Most mutated cases are ZAP70 negative and unmutated cases ZAP70 positive. ZAP70 expression can be measured by a number of methods, including Western blotting, reverse transcriptase-polymerase chain reaction, immunohistochemistry, and flow cytometry (71–74). Levels of expression are higher in T cells and natural killer cells than in CLL cells, and it is important to ensure that effective gating strategies are used to ensure that expression is being measured in the CLL cells. ZAP70 expression appears to be stable over time (73,75). Studies have demonstrated that there is not an absolute relationship between ZAP70 expression and IgVH mutational status, with discrepant cases ranging from 8% to 25%. These discordant cases may have other biologic features with poor prognostic implications such as del 17p, del 11q, or use of *IGHV3-21* (76). Some studies have suggested that ZAP70 status is more useful as a predictor of time to progression than mutation status (73,77), but this remains controversial.

Other surrogates of mutation status have been suggested, including expression of thymidine kinase, activation-induced cytidine deaminase, lipoprotein lipase A, and ADAM29 (78–80). MicroRNA arrays have revealed a 13-gene signature found to correlate with ZAP70 status and unmutated IgVH expression (81), and disease progression (82). This altered microRNA expression regulates expression of genes regulating apoptosis and cell cycle progression (83).

Treatment

In all other leukemias, early treatment is optimal. This is not the case in CLL/SLL for two main reasons. First, a proportion of cases with CLL/SLL have a smoldering clinical course with no difference in survival compared with age-matched controls, and these patients do not merit therapy. Second, the disease remains incurable using standard treatment approaches, and previous trials have demonstrated no survival advantage of early treatment versus an initial "watch and wait" approach. More than 2,000 patients with early disease have been enrolled in trials of immediate versus deferred chemotherapy, all performed using alkylating agents. In a metaanalysis of these studies, there was no statistically significant difference in survival between early versus deferred therapy (84). There was a trend toward a worse outcome for early treatment (10-year survival with immediate chemotherapy was 44% vs. 47% for those whose therapy was deferred). Therefore, the most important treatment decision to be made in CLL/SLL is whether the patient merits therapy at a given time. Guidelines have been established recommending treatment for patients with active disease that recommend treating patients with active progressive disease (33). The traditional goal of therapy of CLL/SLL has been palliation, and patients were usually treated until symptoms resolved. The availability of newer therapies has resulted in an increased awareness of the importance of achieving a complete remission (CR) in CLL/SLL. Formal criteria for achievement of CR and partial remissions (PRs) have been established for CLL/SLL (Table 13.8) (33).

TABLE 13.8

CRITERIA FOR RESPONSE TO THERAPY IN CLL

CR

- Absence of clonal lymphocytosis
- Absence of significant lymphadenopathy
- No hepatosplenomegaly by physical examination
- Absence of constitutional symptoms
- Neutrophils >1,500/μL
- Platelets >100,000/μL
- Hemoglobin >11.0 g/dL untransfused
- Bone marrow free of clonal lymphocytes (in clinical trials only)

CR with incomplete marrow recovery

- As for CR, but with persistent anemia, thrombocytopenia, or neutropenia

PR

- >50% decrease in the number of blood lymphocytes
- >50% decrease in lymph node size in the sum products of up to six lymph nodes, no increase in any lymph node, and no new enlarged lymph nodes
- >50% decrease in the size of hepatosplenomegaly
- One of the following:
  - Neutrophils >1,500/μL or >50% improvement from baseline
  - Platelets >100,000/μL or >50% improvement from baseline
  - Hemoglobin >11.0 g/dL or >50% improvement from baseline

Adapted from Hallek M, Cheson BD, Catovsky D, et al. Guidelines for the diagnosis and treatment of chronic lymphocytic leukemia: a report from the International Workshop on Chronic Lymphocytic Leukemia updating the National Cancer Institute-Working Group 1996 guidelines. *Blood* 2008;111:5446–5456, with permission.

Chemotherapy

Alkylating Agents. The first effective agents used in the treatment of B-cell CLL/SLL were the alkylating agents chlorambucil and cyclophosphamide, with or without corticosteroids. Chlorambucil is rapidly absorbed from the gastrointestinal tract, and peak plasma concentrations occur within 1 hour of ingestion. Metabolism is primarily hepatic and excretion of metabolites via renal clearance. There has been great variability in dosage and schedule of administration, but the two commonly used approaches are low-dose continuous therapy using a continuous dose of 0.08 mg per kg (usual dose 4 to 8 mg orally) or pulsed intermittent dosage of 0.8 mg per kg given (usual dose 40 to 80 mg) in a single oral dose given every 3 to 4 weeks. Chlorambucil is often given in combination with corticosteroids. Results of randomized trials of alkylator alone or with steroids, alkylator dose, and schedule are shown in Table 13.9. There was no difference in survival comparing chlorambucil therapy alone with chlorambucil plus prednisone, but those patients treated with chlorambucil and prednisone had higher CR (20% vs. 9%) and overall response rates (ORRs) (87% vs. 45%) (85). In addition, the hematologic toxicity was less in the combination therapy group. A Cancer and Leukemia Group B study compared prednisone alone with prednisone and chlorambucil, and evaluated two doses of chlorambucil (86). Ninety-six patients with stage III and stage IV CLL were randomized into one of three treatment schedules. Prednisone was given to all patients daily. One group received prednisone plus chlorambucil given as a once-a-month dose of 0.4 to 0.8 mg per kg. A second group also received both drugs, but the chlorambucil was given as a daily dose of 0.08 mg per kg, and the third group received prednisone alone. The ORR was 47% for schedule I, 38% for schedule II, and 11% for schedule III. Patients who responded (complete plus PRs) in each of the treatment schedules survived longer than the nonresponders. There were complete responders in both chlorambucil treatment schedules, but not with the prednisone alone regimen. There was no significant difference in survival time among the three treatment schedules, and toxicity was minimal. Augmentation of the intermittent monthly chlorambucil, even to 1.5 and 2.0 mg per kg, was tolerated without undue marrow toxicity.

A number of randomized trials have compared the efficacy of chlorambucil alone or in combination with prednisone with combinations of cyclophosphamide, vincristine, and prednisone (COP), or with combinations, including hydroxydaunorubicin (CHOP) (Table 13.10). There was no difference in the 5-year survival (48% in both cases) of chlorambucil with or without steroids, compared with combination chemotherapy alone. Six trials involved an anthracycline-containing regimen, but again, there was no difference in overall survival (OS) with chlorambucil compared with anthracycline-containing-based regimens. The CLL-80 trial from the French cooperative compared daily continuous chlorambucil with 12 monthly cycles of COP

TABLE 13.9

SELECTED RANDOMIZED TRIALS OF ALKYLATOR THERAPY ALONE OR WITH STEROIDS

Treatment arm	No. of patients	CR	Overall response (%)	Survival difference	Reference
Chlorambucil	11	9	45	No difference	Han et al. 1973 (85)
Chlorambucil plus prednisone	15	20	87		
I Chlorambucil (qm) plus prednisone	38	8	47	No difference	Sawitsky et al. 1977 (86)
II Chlorambucil (qd) plus prednisone	39	8	38		
III Prednisone	19	0	11		

TABLE 13.10

RANDOMIZED TRIALS OF CHLORAMBUCIL ALONE COMPARED WITH COMBINATION CHEMOTHERAPY

	No. of patients	Survival	Reference
ECOG			71
Chlorambucil plus prednisone	60	48% 5 y	
CVP	62	48% 5 y, no difference	
CLL-80–French Cooperative Group Binet Group B			70
Chlorambucil	151	44% 5 y	
COP	150	43% 5 y, no difference	
CLL-80–French Cooperative Group Binet Group C			73
COP	35	28% 3 y	
CHOP	35	71% 5 y, $p=0.0001$	

CVP, cyclophosphamide, vincristine, and prednisone.

in 291 patients with Binet stage B disease and demonstrated no difference in overall response or survival (87) Similar studies were performed by the ECOG (88) and the Medical Research Council (89). A number of trials, not all of which have been published in peer-reviewed journals, have also compared chlorambucil with CHOP and failed to find any survival advantage, although response rates were generally higher with CHOP. One exception is the CLL-80 trial of the French Cooperative Group, which randomized patients with Binet stage C disease to receive COP versus CHOP (using a low dose of hydroxydaunorubicin) (90). Median survival in the CHOP group was superior at 62 months compared with COP ($p = 0.0005$). However, the outcome of the COP arm in this study was inferior to that seen using COP in an ECOG trial that evaluated COP versus chlorambucil (88). In particular, the outcome of the COP arm in the ECOG study was similar to that seen with CHOP in the CLL-80 study. In a metaanalysis, there was no difference in survival using CHOP in all patients or even when analysis was restricted to patients with Binet stage C disease, the setting where the French study had shown an advantage for CHOP (84).

Together, the trials of alkylator therapy support a conservative treatment strategy for CLL, with no chemotherapy given for the most patients with early stage disease, and single-agent chlorambucil as the first line of treatment for most patients with advanced disease as symptoms appear, with no evidence of benefit from early inclusion of an anthracycline. This strategy will need to be reconsidered as mature results become available from trials of other agents, notably the purine analogs in combination, as discussed below in Purine Analogs.

Purine Analogs

The purine analogs, fludarabine, cladribine, and pentostatin, have major activity against CLL/SLL (Table 13.11). Each of these agents has been used in previously treated (91–100) and previously untreated patients (93,97,101–105). A number of studies that have evaluated cladribine in treatment of alkylator-resistant CLL/SLL have demonstrated response rates of 31% to 67% (96,106,107). In untreated CLL/SLL, cladribine demonstrated responses in 60%, with 25% achieving CR (104). Pentostatin has also demonstrated responses in 16% to 35% of patients with previously treated CLL/SLL (98).

Three large comparative trials have been performed comparing fludarabine with alkylator-based therapies. In a European study, patients were randomized to receive fludarabine (106 patients) or cyclophosphamide, doxorubicin, and prednisone (CAP) (102 patients) (108). This study included both previously treated and untreated patients (Table 13.12). Remission rates were significantly higher after fludarabine than CAP, with ORRs of 60% versus 44%, respectively ($p = 0.023$), with a significantly higher response rate observed with fludarabine in previously treated patients (48% vs. 27%; $p = 0.036$). The response rate with fludarabine was not significantly higher in previously treated patients (71% vs. 60%; $p = 0.26$). However, in the previously untreated patients, the duration of response and OS were significantly longer with fludarabine compared with CAP. The French Cooperative Group evaluated fludarabine versus low-dose CHOP, versus CAP in 938 previously untreated patients, with randomization stratified for patients with Binet stage B and C disease (103). Both CHOP and fludarabine had better response rates than CAP, but no difference in OS was observed. There was, however, an increased CR rate and duration of response noted in patients treated with fludarabine.

In an Intergroup study sponsored by the National Cancer Institute, 544 previously untreated patients with CLL were randomized to receive fludarabine, chlorambucil, or the combination of fludarabine and chlorambucil (102). The combination arm was closed to accrual early because of higher toxicity. In 509 evaluable patients, the CR rate (20% vs. 4%; $p < 0.001$), ORR (63% vs. 37%; $p < 0.001$), and duration of response (25 vs. 14 months; $p < 0.001$) were higher with fludarabine compared with chlorambucil. The response rate to fludarabine of patients who failed chlorambucil was high, most likely explaining the fact that there is no difference in OS among the three arms ($p = 0.21$).

A number of phase II studies have evaluated the combination of fludarabine with cyclophosphamide in previously untreated CLL/SLL, with ORRs of 79% to 100%, with CR rates ranging from 16% in a German multicenter study (109), to 90% to 100% in single center studies (109–111). Three large phase III trials confirmed that the use of combination of fludarabine with cyclophosphamide is associated with improvements in response rates, CR rates, and PFS compared with fludarabine (Table 13.13) (112–114).

Radiation Therapy

Because CLL/SLL is disseminated early in the disease course, radiation therapy is palliative. However, CLL/SLL cells are radiosensitive (115,116), and radiation therapy can provide symptomatic relief for large bulky lymphadenopathy. Splenic

TABLE 13.11

PURINE ANALOGS AS TREATMENT FOR CLL

	No. of patients	CR (%)	Overall response (%)	Reference
Previously treated				
Fludarabine	32	3	13	Grever et al. 1988 (91)
	68	13	57	Keating et al. 1989 (92)
	169[a]	12	52	O'Brien et al. 1993 (93)
	56	5	73	Fenchel et al. 1995 (94)
	68	4	28	Montserrat et al. 1996 (95)
Cladribine (2-CdA)	26	0	31	Tallman et al. 1995 (96)
	184[b]	13	48	Robak et al. 2000 (97)
Pentostatin	26	4	15	Dillman et al. 1989 (98)
	26	0	27	Ho et al. 1990 (99)
	24	8	29	Johnson et al. 1998 (100)
Previously untreated				
Fludarabine	33	33	79	Keating et al. 1991 (101)
	95[a]	30	79	O'Brien et al. 1993 (93)
	170	20	63	Rai et al. 2000 (102)
	341	40	71	Leprrier et al. 2001 (103)
Cladribine (2-CdA)	20	25	85	Saven et al. 1995 (104)
	63	38	75	Juliusson et al. 1996 (105)
	194[c]	45	83	Robak et al. 2000 (97)
Pentostatin	13	0	46	Dillman et al. 1989 (98)

[a] Fludarabine plus prednisone.
[b] One hundred four patients also received prednisone.
[c] One hundred fifty-one patients also received prednisone.

radiation has been used to treat patients with bulky painful splenomegaly and patients with pancytopenia due to hypersplenism (117–119). A number of studies have demonstrated benefit for splenectomy in CLL/SLL (120,121). The role of splenic radiation versus splenectomy has not been evaluated,

TABLE 13.12

RANDOMIZED PHASE II TRIAL OF VERSUS CAP

	Fludarabine[a]	CAP[b]	p value
All			
No. of patients	100	96	
Overall response	60%	44%	0.023
Previously treated			
No. of patients	48	48	
Overall response	48%	27%	0.036
Previously untreated			
No. of patients	52	48	
Overall response	71%	60%	0.26

[a] Fludarabine, 25 mg/m2/d on days 1–5.
[b] Cyclophosphamide, 750 mg/m2 on day 1; doxorubicin, 50 mg/m2 on day 1; and prednisone, 40 mg/m2/d on days 1–5.
Adapted from Johnson S, Smith AG, Loffler H, et al. Multicentre prospective randomised trial of fludarabine versus cyclophosphamide, doxorubicin, and prednisone (CAP) for treatment of advanced-stage chronic lymphocytic leukaemia. The French Cooperative Group on CLL. *Lancet* 1996;347:1432–1438, with permission.

particularly in patients with advanced-stage disease. Low-dose total body irradiation (TBI) has demonstrated efficacy in the treatment of CLL/SLL (122) and was found to be comparable to chlorambucil in patients with advanced-stage CLL/SLL in one study (123). However, in an ECOG study, the response rate to chemotherapy was higher than that observed with TBI (124), and this approach has subsequently been used less frequently. TBI has been used in CLL/SLL but was not found to be superior to chemotherapy in randomized clinical trials (123,124). The toxicity associated with high-dose TBI was high, with 75% of patients experiencing severe thrombocytopenia or neutropenia. Therefore, radiation therapy has a palliative role to play in the management of patients with relapsed and refractory CLL in the management of bulky adenopathy or splenomegaly.

Immune Therapy

Immunotherapy is emerging as an exciting modality with significant potential to advance the treatment of CLL. Immunotherapy includes passive immunotherapy with monoclonal antibodies against antigens on CLL/SLL B–cells, including CD20 and CD52. Active immunotherapy by vaccination tumor antigens or with genetically modified autologous leukemia cells is being evaluated in clinical trials. Humanized monoclonal antibodies have been developed that target antigens on the surface of CLL/SLL cells, and two agents have been approved for the use of CLL/SLL. Rituximab, an anti-CD20 monoclonal antibody, is approved for the use of

TABLE 13.13

RANDOMIZED TRIALS OF FLUDARABINE COMBINATION THERAPY

Study	Treatment	No. of patients	CR (%)	Overall response (%)	PFS (mo)	Reference
GCLLSG CLL4	Fludarabine	180	7	83	20	Eichhorst et al. (112)
	FC	182	24	94	48	
ECOG E2997	Fludarabine	137	5	59	19	Flinn et al. (113)
	FC	141	23	74	32	
LRF CLL4	Chlorambucil	366	7	72	20	Catovsky et al. (114)
	Fludarabine	181	15	80	23	
	FC	182	38	92	43	
GCLLSG CLL8	FC	817 patients recruited	23	85	Significantly	M. Hallek et al. *Blood*
	RFC	to both arms	45	95	prolonged in	2008;112:125,
					RFC arm	Abstr #325)

FC, fludarabine/cyclophosphamide; GCLLSG, German CLL Study Group; LRF, Leukemia Research Fund; RFC, rituximab/fludarabine/cyclophosphamide.

relapsed B-cell non-Hodgkin lymphoma. A number of studies have demonstrated low response rates in patients with CLL/SLL compared with other B-cell lymphomas (125,126). In a study of 28 patients with relapsed or refractory CLL/SLL, the ORR to rituximab therapy was 25%, with no CR noted, and the duration of response was short (127). However, two approaches have demonstrated improvement in response rate by the use of rituximab in CLL/SLL, either by increasing the dose (128) or the frequency (129) of administration of the antibody. Care has to be taken when administering rituximab to patients with CLL/SLL because tumor lysis syndrome and deaths have been reported, likely because of high levels of cytokines released in these patients with high circulating tumor load (127).

There is preclinical evidence that the addition of rituximab to chemotherapeutic agents may increase cell killing, and phase II studies have demonstrated that the addition of rituximab to fludarabine and cyclophosphamide is the most effective combination to date to improve CR and ORR in CLL in previously untreated (130,131) and treated patients (132). In a series of 300 previously untreated patients, ORR was 95%, with CR in 72%, nodular PR in 10%, PR due to cytopenia in 7%, and PR due to residual disease in 6%. At a median follow-up of 6 years, OS was 77% and PFS 51%. This combination has been evaluated in the GCLLSG CLL8 study, and this demonstrated a significant improvement in response rates and duration of response with fludarabine cyclophosphamide and rituximab compared with fludarabine and cyclophosphamide alone.

Alemtuzumab (Campath-1H), an anti-CD52 monoclonal antibody, is approved for patients with CLL/SLL who are fludarabine refractory and may have activity against cases that are unresponsive to chemotherapy due to the presence of p53 mutations (133). Alemtuzumab demonstrated an ORR of 38% in a pilot study in previously treated patients (134). In a subsequent pivotal study of 93 patients with fludarabine refractory CLL/SLL, alemtuzumab demonstrated an ORR of 33% and improved survival in those patients who responded (135). Alemtuzumab has less activity against bulky lymphadenopathy but demonstrates impres-

sive efficacy in clearing the peripheral blood and bone marrow compartments of disease. In previously untreated patients, alemtuzumab has demonstrated increased response rates and has been administered subcutaneously in this clinical setting (136,137). A phase III randomized study evaluated first-line therapy with alemtuzumab compared with chlorambucil in 297 patients with progressive CLL; 149 patients were randomized to receive intravenous alemtuzumab 30 mg three times weekly for up to 12 weeks (138). The results from this study showed significantly superior response rates for alemtuzumab compared with chlorambucil (ORR 83% vs. 56%, p <0.0001; and CR rates 24% vs. 2%, p <0.0001), confirming the efficacy reported in the first-line study with subcutaneous alemtuzumab. Further follow-up is awaited to determine survival outcomes from this study.

Active immunotherapy approaches involve vaccination strategies to induce an immune response in the patient with a tumor. CLL/SLL cells are very poor antigen-presenting cells, but one way to increase their antigen-presenting capacity is to stimulate the cells through their surface receptor CD40 (139). CLL/SLL cells can be made to express recombinant CD40-ligand (CD154) by transduction with a replication-defective adenovirus vector (Ad-CD154). Ad-CD154-transduced and bystander leukemia cells become highly effective antigen-presenting cells that can induce CLL/SLL-specific autologous cytotoxic T lymphocytes in vitro. After a one-time bolus infusion of autologous Ad-CD154-transduced leukemia cells, there was increased or de novo expression of immune accessory molecules on bystander, noninfected CLL/SLL cells in vivo (140). Treated patients also developed high plasma levels of interleukin-12 and interferon-γ. This approach may provide a novel and effective form of gene therapy for patients with this disease, and is currently in phase II trials.

Stem Cell Transplantation for Chronic Lymphocytic Leukemia

Hematopoietic stem cell transplantation (SCT) is not a suitable option for most patients with CLL because most patients are too elderly, and the disease often follows an extremely indolent course. Unlike other hematologic malignancies, where the role of SCT for specific risk groups has been established in prospective studies, there are no studies in CLL that have compared the outcome after standard chemotherapy with either autologous or allogeneic SCT, but encouraging results have been achieved in phase II clinical trials. However, younger patients with CLL will die of their disease, and high-risk patients can be identified using a number of clinical and biologic features. Therefore, it is possible to identify patients who are suitable candidates for enrollment in clinical trials evaluating the role of SCT in CLL. The biggest challenges remain in the decision of which patients are eligible for consideration of SCT and when in their disease course SCT should be offered.

Patient Selection for Stem Cell Transplantation

CLL is an extremely heterogeneous disease, with clinical courses varying from patients who can live for decades in patients who never require therapy despite their disease, to a rapidly progressive and fatal malignancy in others. Considerable work has been performed to identify the clinical and biologic characteristics of this disease, which would allow identification of which patients should merit transplant. Most phase II studies have enrolled younger patients with "high-risk" disease, but this term is rather loosely defined, and it is difficult to determine precisely the risk factors used in each of the reported studies. As described previously, risk factors have changed over time as newer risk factors have been identified. The European Bone Marrow Transplant guidelines outline indications for SCT in CLL (141). Patients requiring treatment who have p53 abnormalities have sufficiently poor prognosis to merit transplantation in first remission because these patients continue to have poor survival. Allogeneic SCT was recommended for young patients with CLL who fail to achieve CR or who have progression within 12 months after purine analogs, those who relapse within 24 months after having achieved a response with purine analog-based combination therapy or prior autologous SCT, or for patients who have become fludarabine refractory. It should be noted that none of these categories requires assessment of biologic risk factors except for cytogenetics for detection of p53 deletions, and ongoing prospective clinical studies will be required to determine the impact of biomarkers, including IgVH mutational status and other cytogenetic abnormalities, to identify patients at sufficiently high risk to merit use of allogeneic SCT in the first CR.

Autologous Stem Cell Transplantation

The role of autologous SCT in the management of CLL remains unclear, and this approach is recommended only in the setting of a clinical trial. A retrospective matched-pair analysis suggested a survival advantage for autologous SCT over conventional therapy (142). In this study a risk-matched comparison was made between 66 patients who had undergone a uniform high-dose therapy and autologous SCT with a database of 291 conventionally treated patients who were matched for risk factors. Survival was significantly longer for the patients who had undergone autologous SCT compared with conventionally treated patients when calculated from diagnosis ($p = 0.03$) or from study entry ($p = 0.006$).

A number of phase II studies have reported outcome following autologous SCT for CLL (143–147). These studies have demonstrated that this approach is feasible in CLL with a transplant-related mortality (TRM) of 1% to 10%, with most toxicity occurring late. Among 115 previously untreated patients with CLL prospectively enrolled in a pilot study to assess the feasibility of performing autologous SCT, only 65 (56%) proceeded to transplant (146). Only one treatment-related mortality (TRM) was seen, and the CR rate after transplantation was 74% (48 of 65). The 5-year estimated OS was 77.5%, and PFS was 51.5%. None of the variables examined at study entry was predictive for OS or PFS, but detectable minimal residual disease (MRD) was highly predictive of disease recurrence. Of concern, five of 65 (8%) patients developed posttransplant acute myeloid leukemia (AML)/myelodysplastic syndrome (MDS), a complication also seen in other series (143). In 137 patients who underwent autologous transplantation at a single center, the 1-year TRM was 4% but rose to 10% when late events were taken into account. At the median follow-up time of 6.5 years, OS was 58% after autologous SCT. There was no TRM among 72 patients autografted in five Finnish centers with median age 57 years (range 38 to 69) and a median of 32 months (range 6 to 181) from diagnosis (147). At a median follow-up of 28 months, 37% had progressed, with a median OS of 95 months and PFS 48 months. In 115 previously untreated patients with CLL prospectively enrolled in a multicenter pilot study to assess the feasibility of performing autologous SCT, only 65 (56%) proceeded to transplant (146).

A number of methods, including multiparameter flow cytometry analysis and polymerase chain reaction, is being used to investigate whether persistence of MRD will predict which patients will relapse following transplant in CLL. Detectable molecular disease after transplant is predictive of clinical recurrence, and patients who achieve CR after autologous SCT will eventually have a relapse (146,148). One approach to increase the likelihood of elimination of MRD after autologous SCT is to attempt to eradicate any residual lymphoma cells ex vivo using monoclonal antibodies (143). Ex vivo purging of stem cells results in stem cell loss that might be overcome by in vivo treatment with alemtuzumab or rituximab. When alemtuzumab was used in the conditioning regimen for autologous SCT in one arm of the German CLL Study Group CLL3 trial, 12 of 16 patients (87%) developed a skin rash between 43 and 601 days after SCT, and in seven of these patients, a biopsy confirmed graft–versus–host disease (GVHD) (149). The trial was discontinued due to the TRM. When alemtuzumab for in vivo purging was used at a lower dose of 10 mg subcutaneously three times per week for 6 weeks in 34 patients who had had a clinical response to a fludarabine-based regimen, the CR rate improved from 35% to 79.5%, with 56% achieving eradication of MRD (150). Peripheral blood stem cell collection was subsequently successfully performed in 92%. Eighteen patients underwent auto-SCT, with 17 remaining in CR at a median follow-up of 14.5 months after SCT.

There are concerns regarding late consequences of high-dose therapy and autologous SCT, especially development of secondary MDS and AML) after autologous SCT. Among 65 newly diagnosed patients treated with fludarabine followed by autologous SCT, eight developed MDS/AML (146), with a 5-year actuarial risk of 12% developing MDS/AML after autologous SCT. Potential causative factors include exposure to fludarabine, low stem cell dose infused, and use of TBI in the conditioning regimen. The study with the longest reported follow-up is from the Dana-Farber Cancer Institute

(143), which reports not only a high incidence of secondary MDS/AML, but also a high incidence of other tumors with longer follow-up. Second (non-CLL) malignancies developed after SCT in 31 (19%) patients.

Allogeneic Stem Cell Transplantation

Allogeneic SCT has significant morbidity and mortality, from regimen-related toxicity, GVHD, and infection, but surviving patients have long-term disease control (143,151–154). In registry data, TRM following allogeneic SCT in patients with CLL was 46%, with mortality from GVHD of 20% (151). Among 14 patients with chemorefractory CLL, 13 (87%) achieved CR after transplant, and nine remained alive and in CR with a median follow-up of 36 months (155), suggesting that allogeneic SCT can induce durable remission even in patients with refractory disease. Of 25 patients with CLL who underwent allogeneic SCT at the Fred Hutchinson Cancer Center (154), grades 2 to 4 acute GVHD were seen in 14 patients, and ten developed clinical extensive chronic GVHD, and estimated OS at 5 years was 32%. No-relapse mortality at day 100 was unacceptably high at 57% for patients conditioned with busulphan and cyclophosphamide compared with 17% for patients conditioned with TBI containing regimens. Among 30 patients (20 related donors and ten unrelated donors) transplanted for CLL between 1989 and 2001 in Vancouver with a median follow-up of 4.3 years, 47% were alive in CR, both estimated OS and disease-free survival at 5 years were 39%. A strong graft versus leukemia (GVL) effect was noted with those developing acute or chronic GVHD having near complete protection from relapse (156).

There are no randomized studies comparing the outcome of autologous versus allogeneic SCT. In a single center phase II study at Dana-Farber Cancer Institute, 162 patients with high-risk CLL were enrolled in a "biologic randomization" in which 25 patients with a human leukocyte antigen-matched sibling donor underwent T-cell-depleted myeloablative allogeneic SCT, whereas 137 with no human leukocyte antigen-matched sibling donor underwent B-cell-purged autologous SCT, with both groups receiving identical conditioning regimen using high-dose cyclophosphamide and TBI (143) The 100-day TRM was 4% after autologous or allogeneic SCT, but later TRM had a major impact on outcome. At the median follow-up of 6.5 years, PFS was significantly longer following autologous than T-cell-depleted allogeneic SCT, but no significant differences were observed in disease recurrence or deaths without recurrence by type of transplant. There was no difference in OS between the two groups, and at the median follow-up time of 6.5 years, OS was 58% after autologous and 55% after allogeneic SCT. The major advantage of the allogeneic SCT is the potential for a GVL effect. There is a decreased risk of relapse in patients with chronic GVHD (156), increased risk of relapse with T-cell depletion (143), and GVL can be generated by donor lymphocyte infusion (143).

Reduced Intensity Conditioning Stem Cell Transplantation for Chronic Lymphocytic Leukemia

Ongoing studies are attempting to exploit maximal GVL effect without concomitant GVHD and decrease the TRM of allogeneic SCT. A major advance in reducing the short-term morbidity and mortality of allogeneic SCT has been the introduction of nonmyeloablative or reduced intensity conditioning (RIC) regimens to allow engraftment of allogeneic stem cells. Several RIC regimens have been developed, and there is wide variation in the regimen components and intensity, GVHD prophylaxis, and timing of the application of donor lymphocyte infusion. RIC regimens allow transplantation in older patients, making this approach more applicable to increased numbers of patients with CLL (157–162). Results from selected studies are shown in Table 13.14. Most reported patients were heavily pretreated and refractory to therapy, but despite this, the majority demonstrated donor engraftment, and there is a high CR rate. The ability of such approaches to eradicate MRD in patients with advanced CLL (163,164) and the observation of late remissions in patients treated with low doses of chemotherapy provide the strongest direct evidence for a powerful GVL effect that can be exploited in the management of CLL. GVHD remains a major concern. GVHD can be decreased using alemtuzumab in the conditioning regimen, but this delays post-SCT immune reconstitution, increases the risk of infective complications, and impairs the GVL effect. In 41 consecutive patients with CLL treated (24 human leukocyte antigen-matched sibling donors and 17 unrelated volunteer donors, including four mismatched), the conditioning regimen alemtuzumab with fludarabine and melphalan had significant antitumor effects, with 100% of patients with chemosensitive disease and 86% with chemorefractory disease responding (160). The TRM rate was 26%, OS 51%, and relapse risk 29% at 2 years. GVHD rates were relatively low, with acute GVHD occurring in 17 (41%) and chronic GVHD in 13 (33%). The unexpectedly high TRM rate was due to a high incidence of fungal and viral infections.

No formal assessment of RIC compared with myeloablative allogeneic SCT has been undertaken, but the outcome after RIC allogeneic SCT of 73 patients who had undergone RIC was compared with that of 82 matched patients who had undergone standard myeloablative conditioning for CLL from the European Bone Marrow Transplant registry database during the same time period. Patients undergoing RIC transplants had significantly reduced TRM, but higher relapse incidence, and there was no significant difference in OS or PFS between these two groups (165).

Unique Complications of Chronic Lymphocytic Leukemia/Small Lymphocytic Lymphoma

CLL/SLL is frequently associated with autoimmune phenomena, the most common being autoimmune hemolytic anemia and immune thrombocytopenia. The direct antiglobulin test (DAT) may be positive in up to one third of cases during the course of disease, and overt autoimmune hemolytic anemia occurs in 11% of cases (166). In a comprehensive report of 1,203 patients with CLL/SLL consecutive cases reported from a single institution, 52 (4.3%) cases of autoimmune hemolytic anemia were observed (167). Nineteen cases were observed at the time of diagnosis and 33 during subsequent follow-up. Ninety percent of the patients with autoimmune hemolytic anemia had active CLL, and 25% occurred when the patient had been treated previously. The autoantibody was IgM in 13% and an IgG in 87% of cases. A lymphocyte count $>60 \times 10^9$ per L ($p < 0.00001$), age >65 years, and

TABLE 13.14

RIC ALLOGENEIC SCT FOR CLL

No. of patients	Age years (range)	Prior regimens (range)	Chemorefractory (%)	Prior auto-SCT	Donor (includes mismatch)	TRM	Acute gd 2–4 GVHD (%)	Chronic extensive GVHD (%)	Survival	Reference
77	54 y (30–66)	3 (0–8)	33	10	81% related	18% 12 mo	34	58	OS 72% 2 y PFS 56%	Dreger et al. 2003 (157)
64	56 y (44–69)	4	53		69% related 31% unrelated	11% at 100 d 22% overall	61	50	OS 60% 2 y PFS 52%	Sorror et al. 2005 (158)
46	53 y (35–67)	5 (1–10)	57	10	33% related 67% unrelated	17% overall	34	43	OS 54% 2 y PFS 34%	Brown et al. 2006 (159)
41	54 y (37–67)	3 (1–8)	27	11	58% related 42% unrelated	5% at 100 d 26% overall	10	33%[a]	OS 51 2 y PFS 45%	Delgado et al. 2006 (160)
39	57 y (34–70)	3 (2–8)	Not stated		90% related 10% unrelated	2% at 100 d	(gd 3–4) 45	58	OS 48% 4 y PFS 44%	Khouri et al. 2006 (161)
30	50 y (12–63)	3 (0–8)	47		50% related 50% unrelated	13% overall	56	21	OS 72% 2 y PFS 67%	Schetelig et al. 2002 (162)

DLI, donor lymphocyte infusion; gd, grade.
[a] GVHD incidence includes incidence after DLI.

male gender emerged as independent factors that correlated significantly with an increased rate of autoimmune hemolytic anemia at CLL diagnosis. Patients previously treated with chlorambucil plus prednisone and with fludarabine showed a similar rate of autoimmune hemolytic anemia (1.8% and 2.5%, respectively). In this study the presence of autoimmune hemolytic anemia was not associated with poor prognosis. In a trial comparing outcome of treatment using chlorambucil, fludarabine, or fludarabine in combination with cyclophosphamide, a positive DAT was found in 14%, and autoimmune hemolytic anemia was detected in 10% (168). For patients receiving the combination of fludarabine and cyclophosphamide, the percentage of DAT-positive individuals fell after treatment, whereas it increased in the fludarabine monotherapy arm. A positive DAT test had poor prognostic significance, even in the absence of autoimmune hemolytic anemia. Autoimmune thrombocytopenia based upon the presence of adequate number so megakaryocytes with a low platelet count in peripheral blood occurs more rarely and is present in 2% to 3% of patients (166). This complication has been reported more frequently following therapy with fludarabine (169). Pure red cell aplasia is rare but may occur early in the disease course. Although the etiology of this disorder is unclear, it has been reported that it responds to therapy with immune modulating agents, including rituximab, fludarabine, and cyclosporin A (170–172). Neutropenia is common, but although agranulocytosis may be encountered, this is rare.

Infections are the major cause of morbidity and mortality in patients with CLL/SLL. Predisposition to infection in CLL/SLL is mediated through various abnormalities, including both the immune defects inherent in the primary disease (impairment in humoral and cellular immunity) and in the further immunosuppression related to the management of CLL/SLL. Hypogammaglobulinemia is probably the most important immune defect in terms of risk of severe bacterial infections, its frequency and severity progressing with the duration of the disease. In a randomized cross-over study among patients with severe hypogammaglobulinemia, the incidence and severity of infections were less in the months when patients received Ig replacement therapy (173). The frequency of infections may also be increased and altered following therapy (174). Although bacterial infections are most common, the purine analogs, especially when used in previously treated patients or in combination, may be associated with a wide spectrum of opportunistic infections, including *Listeria monocytogenes*, *Pneumocystis carinii*, cytomegalovirus, herpes simplex virus, and mycobacteria, because of the resulting T-cell dysfunction (93,175). Long-term follow-up of fludarabine-treated patients suggests that although the purine analogs have an impact on opportunistic infections, complications of infection are more common in those patients with incomplete response to therapy or with progressive disease, suggesting that the disease itself has more impact than the therapy (176). Although opportunistic infections are also seen following therapy with alemtuzumab (135), patients treated with this agent were fludarabine refractory, and serious infectious complications are high in this patient population. Serious infectious complications in patients with fludarabine refractory disease occurred in 89% of patients, with infections being bacterial in 78.5%, viral in 12.5%, fungal in 4.5%, and opportunistic in 4.5% (177).

Future Directions

For many years the treatment of CLL/SLL has been palliative rather than curative and has not resulted in improved survival in patients with CLL/SLL. Over the past decade, there has been considerable progress in development of more effective treatments for CLL, which have moved CR rates from 0% to 4% with chlorambucil, to greater than 70% with fludarabine cyclophosphamide and rituximab. Concomitant with this, there have been major advances in our understanding of CLL pathophysiology and identification of biomarkers of response duration. It, therefore, seems most likely that we will use "risk-adjusted" approaches to manage patients with CLL/SLL. Disease stage remains important, but biologic markers and, in particular, cytogenetics, Ig gene mutation status, CD38 expression, and potentially gene array, may be capable of identifying patients who merit more aggressive therapy. Studies addressing the use of aggressive combination chemoimmunotherapy at the time of diagnosis and reexamining whether the era of "watch and wait" is over for patients with "high risk" disease are underway.

PROLYMPHOCYTIC LEUKEMIA

Prolymphocytic leukemia (PLL) was originally described as a variant of CLL, characterized by its distinct clinical and laboratory features. There is clonal proliferation of medium-sized prolymphocytes involving peripheral blood, bone marrow, and spleen. In this disease, prolymphocytes comprise >55% of the cells in blood and bone marrow, and typically >90% of the neoplastic cells. It is now apparent that this disease represents a separate entity from CLL. PLL can be B cell or T cell in type. Although both of these entities occur with almost equal frequency, the disease is rare and accounts for only 2% of cases with malignant lymphocytosis. Although B-cell and T-cell PLLs are discussed together, they are also distinct diseases based upon their molecular pathogenesis.

B-Cell Prolymphocytic Leukemia

Morphology

In B-cell PLL (B-PLL), prolymphocytes comprise >55% of the cells in blood and bone marrow, and typically >90% of the neoplastic cells. The bone marrow is usually infiltrated with prolymphocytes, most often in an interstitial manner. The spleen shows extensive white and red pulp infiltration by prolymphocytes. Lymph node involvement may demonstrate nodularity, but proliferation centers or pseudofollicles are absent. Peripheral blood prolymphocytes are medium size, and approximately twice the size of small lymphocytes with moderately condensed chromatin and a single prominent vesicular nucleolus. The nucleus is typically round, and the cytoplasm is usually scant to moderate and weakly basophilic.

Immunophenotype

The cells express bright surface IgM and IgD and bright CD20, as well as other B-cell markers, including CD19, CD21, CD22, CD24, and FMC7. In contrast to CLL/SLL, they do not express CD23, and more than two-thirds of cases do not express CD5. The differential diagnosis includes CLL, the leukemic form of mantle cell lymphoma, and other lymphomas. B-PLL may also be confused with hairy cell leukemia variants. The diagnosis requires histologic assessment, extended immunophenotype, with genetic and molecular analysis. Input from expert hematopathologists with experience in these diseases is often required to make a definitive diagnosis.

Genetics

Chromosome abnormalities in B-PLL are often complex, involving a number of different chromosomes. Deletions of 13q14 and 11q23 are frequent chromosome aberrations in B-PLL, and, in contrast to CLL, there is a preferential loss of RB1, suggesting that allelic loss of the RB1 gene may play a role in the pathogenesis of B-PLL (178). More recent data have suggested that many of the cases with 11q23 abnormalities may represent variant cases of mantle cell lymphoma. Staining with cyclin D1 may be important to differentiate mantle cell variants from B-PLL. There is also a very high frequency of p53 mutation (53%) in B-PLL and may be responsible for the frequent resistance to therapy of this disease. In addition, the pattern of p53 mutation was different from that observed in CLL and other hematologic malignancies that may indicate a distinct pathogenesis in this disease (179) B-PLL cells express a skewed repertoire characterized by predominant use of the V3 family members and preferential use of the V3-23 gene. The IgV genes are mutated, suggesting expansion of postgerminal center cells that have undergone antigen-driven selection (180).

Clinical Presentation

Features distinguishing PLL from CLL/SLL include hyperlymphocytosis and massive splenomegaly, although the presenting features can be indistinguishable, and diagnosis depends upon the distinct morphologic and immunophenotypic characteristics of this disease. Patients typically present with a high white count, with one third of patients having a white blood cell count $>200 \times 10^9$ per L. Anemia and thrombocytopenia are common. In contrast to CLL, autoimmune phenomena are rare in B-PLL. Although in some cases the disease can remain stable for months or even years, progression is inevitable. The median survival in a series of 35 patients with B-PLL was 65 months (181). Response to alkylating agents is poor, and addition of anthracyclines appears to offer benefit. Treatment with purine analogs has resulted in responses higher than that seen in historical controls (181,182).

T-Cell Prolymphocytic Leukemia

Morphology

In T-cell PLL (T-PLL), the majority of the circulating cells are prolymphocytes, which are typically smaller than B-PLL cells and have less abundant cytoplasm. In 20% of cases, the cells are small but have the typical immunophenotypic and genetic features in Genetics Section. The pattern of bone marrow infiltration is interstitial and/or diffuse, and often extensive. Histology of the spleen reveals infiltration of both the white and red pulp. Lymph node histology reveals infiltration of the paracortical area with residual follicular centers.

Immunophenotype

Immunologic markers show a post-thymic T-cell phenotype with failure to express terminal deoxynucleotidyl transferase or CD1a. Most cases express CD2 and CD5 but do not express CD3. There is particularly strong expression of CD7. A CD4+ CD8⁻ phenotype is seen in two thirds of cases. CD4 and CD8 are coexpressed in 25%, and a CD4⁻ CD8+ phenotype is rare. All cases exhibit rearrangement of the T-cell receptor α and β genes.

Genetics

T-PLL is characterized by complex karyotypes with recurrent chromosomal abnormalities. The most common abnormality, seen in 75% of cases, includes translocations involving either TCL1 at 14q32.1. Other abnormalities involve the MTCP1 at Xq28, inactivation of the ATM gene by deletion and/or mutation, and isochromosome 8 (183). Deletion of the 11q is frequent, and further analysis has revealed absence, premature truncation, or alteration of the ATM gene product on the other allele, suggesting that ATM functions as a tumor-suppressor gene and has a role in the pathogenesis of T-PLL (184). Deletions at 13q14.3, with additional loss of tumor-suppressor function, could further contribute to the development of overt disease (185).

Diagnosis and Treatment

Differential diagnosis between T-PLL and other T-cell malignancies is based on a constellation of their clinical and laboratory features. Generally, patients with T-PLL are refractory to the therapy used in lymphoid disorders (186). Median survival is short, with a median survival of 7.5 months. Although T-PLL is generally chemotherapy resistant, encouraging results have been observed with alemtuzumab. In a series of 39 patients with T-PLL, all but two were heavily pretreated, and none had achieved a previous CR. Alemtuzumab was administered three times weekly until maximal response (187). The ORR was 76% with 60% CR and 16% PR. The median disease-free survival was 7 months and ranged from 4 to 45 months. Survival was prolonged significantly in patients achieving CR. In another series of 76 patients with T-PLL similarly treated, the ORR was 51%, with 39% achieving CR. The median duration of response was 8.7 months. The median OS was 7.5 months and 14.8 months for patients with CR (188). Alemtuzumab is now being explored as first-line therapy in this disease.

Stem Cell Transplantation for Prolymphocytic Leukemia

A small of number of cases of PLL have been treated by allogeneic hematopoietic stem cell transplantation (187,189). Seven patients who had been treated with alemtuzumab were subsequently treated with high-dose therapy with autologous stem cell support, three of whom remain alive in CR 5, 7, and 15 months after autograft (187). Stem cell harvests in these patients were uncontaminated with T-PLL cells, as demonstrated by dual-color flow cytometry and polymerase chain reaction. Four patients underwent allogeneic stem cell transplants, three from siblings and one from a matched unrelated donor. Two had nonmyeloablative conditioning.

Three are alive in CR up to 24 months after allogeneic stem cell transplant (187).

Future Directions

The treatment of PLL has also been palliative. Better responses are seen with purine analogs, and alemtuzumab is being used increasingly as first-line therapy. Combination therapies, including monoclonal antibodies, are being explored. With more durable responses, stem cell transplant approaches are being used in selected younger patients and may be associated with improved outcome for these previously incurable diseases.

References

1. Harris NL, Jaffe ES, Diebold J, et al. World Health Organization classification of neoplastic diseases of the hematopoietic and lymphoid tissues: report of the Clinical Advisory Committee meeting-Airlie House, Virginia, November 1997. *J Clin Oncol* 1999;17:3835–3849.
2. Zent CS, Kyasa MJ, Evans R, et al. Chronic lymphocytic leukemia incidence is substantially higher than estimated from tumor registry data. *Cancer* 2001;92:1325–1330.
3. Hernandez JA, Land KJ, McKenna RW. Leukemias, myeloma, and other lymphoreticular neoplasms. *Cancer* 1995;75:381–394.
4. Mauro FR, Foa R, Giannarelli D, et al. Clinical characteristics and outcome of young chronic lymphocytic leukemia patients: a single institution study of 204 cases. *Blood* 1999;94:448–454.
5. Parkin DM, Muir CS. Cancer incidence in five continents. Comparability and quality of data. *IARC Sci Publ* 1992;45–173.
6. Haenszel W, Kurihara M. Studies of Japanese migrants. I. Mortality from cancer and other diseases among Japanese in the United States. *J Natl Cancer Inst* 1968;40:43–68.
7. Ron E. Ionizing radiation and cancer risk: evidence from epidemiology. *Radiat Res* 1998;150(suppl):S30–S41.
8. Nanni O, Amadori D, Lugaresi C, et al. Chronic lymphocytic leukaemias and non-Hodgkin's lymphomas by histological type in farming-animal breeding workers: a population case-control study based on a priori exposure matrices. *Occup Environ Med* 1996;53:652–657.
9. Huebner WW, Chen VW, Friedlander BR, et al. Incidence of lymphohaematopoietic malignancies in a petrochemical industry cohort: 1983-94 follow up. *Occup Environ Med* 2000;57:605–614.
10. Zahm SH, Weisenburger DD, Babbitt PA, et al. Use of hair coloring products and the risk of lymphoma, multiple myeloma, and chronic lymphocytic leukemia. *Am J Public Health* 1992;82:990–997.
11. Yuille MR, Matutes E, Marossy A, et al. Familial chronic lymphocytic leukaemia: a survey and review of published studies. *Br J Haematol* 2000;109:794–799.
12. Videbaek A. Familial leukemia. *Acta Medica Scand* 1947;127:26–52.
13. Ishibe N, Sgambati MT, Fontaine L, et al. Clinical characteristics of familial B-CLL in the National Cancer Institute Familial Registry. *Leuk Lymphoma* 2001;42:99–108.
14. Yuille MR, Houlston RS, Catovsky D. Anticipation in familial chronic lymphocytic leukaemia. *Leukemia* 1998;12:1696–1698.
15. Goldin LR, Sgambati M, Marti GE, et al. Anticipation in familial chronic lymphocytic leukemia. *Am J Hum Genet* 1999;65:265–269.
16. Anderson LA, Pfeiffer RM, Rapkin JS, et al. Survival patterns among lymphoma patients with a family history of lymphoma. *J Clin Oncol* 2008;26:4958–4965.
17. Crowther-Swanepoel D, Wild R, Sellick G, et al. Insight into the pathogenesis of chronic lymphocytic leukemia (CLL) through analysis of IgVH gene usage and mutation status in familial CLL. *Blood* 2008;111:5691–5693.
18. Ben-Ezra J, Burke JS, Swartz WG, et al. Small lymphocytic lymphoma: a clinicopathologic analysis of 268 cases. *Blood* 1989;73:579–587.
19. Damle RN, Wasil T, Fais F, et al. Ig V gene mutation status and CD38 expression as novel prognostic indicators in chronic lymphocytic leukemia. *Blood* 1999;94:1840–1847.
20. Hamblin TJ, Orchard JA, Ibbotson RE, et al. CD38 expression and immunoglobulin variable region mutations are independent prognostic variables in chronic lymphocytic leukemia, but CD38 expression may vary during the course of the disease. *Blood* 2002;99:1023–1029.
21. Matutes E, Owusu-Ankomah K, Morilla R, et al. The immunological profile of B-cell disorders and proposal of a scoring system for the diagnosis of CLL. *Leukemia* 1994;8:1640–1645.
22. Dohner H, Stilgenbauer S, Benner A, et al. Genomic aberrations and survival in chronic lymphocytic leukemia. *N Engl J Med* 2000;343:1910–1916.
23. Lagos-Quintana M, Rauhut R, Lendeckel W, et al. Identification of novel genes coding for small expressed RNAs. *Science* 2001;294:853–858.
24. Calin GA, Dumitru CD, Shimizu M, et al. Frequent deletions and down-regulation of micro- RNA genes miR15 and miR16 at 13q14 in chronic lymphocytic leukemia. *Proc Natl Acad Sci U S A* 2002;99:15524–15529.
25. Calin GA, Liu CG, Ferracin M, et al. Ultraconserved regions encoding ncRNAs are altered in human leukemias and carcinomas. *Cancer Cell* 2007;12:215–229.
26. Austen B, Powell JE, Alvi A, et al. Mutations in the ATM gene lead to impaired overall and treatment-free survival that is independent of IGVH mutation status in patients with B-CLL. *Blood* 2005;106:3175–3182.
27. Fais F, Ghiotto F, Hashimoto S, et al. Chronic lymphocytic leukemia B cells express restricted sets of mutated and unmutated antigen receptors. *J Clin Invest* 1998;102:1515–1525.
28. Hamblin TJ, Davis Z, Gardiner A, et al. Unmutated Ig V(H) genes are associated with a more aggressive form of chronic lymphocytic leukemia. *Blood* 1999;94:1848–1854.
29. Klein U, Tu Y, Stolovitzky GA, et al. Gene expression profiling of B cell chronic lymphocytic leukemia reveals a homogeneous phenotype related to memory B cells. *J Exp Med* 2001;194:1625–1638.
30. Rosenwald A, Alizadeh AA, Widhopf G, et al. Relation of gene expression phenotype to immunoglobulin mutation genotype in B cell chronic lymphocytic leukemia. *J Exp Med* 2001;194:1639–1647.
31. Chen L, Widhopf G, Huynh L, et al. Expression of ZAP-70 is associated with increased B-cell receptor signaling in chronic lymphocytic leukemia. *Blood* 2002;100:4609–4614.
32. Wiestner A, Rosenwald A, Barry TS, et al. ZAP-70 expression identifies a chronic lymphocytic leukemia subtype with unmutated immunoglobulin genes, inferior clinical outcome, and distinct gene expression profile. *Blood* 2003;101:4944–4951.
33. Hallek M, Cheson BD, Catovsky D, et al. Guidelines for the diagnosis and treatment of chronic lymphocytic leukemia: a report from the International Workshop on Chronic Lymphocytic Leukemia updating the National Cancer Institute-Working Group 1996 guidelines. *Blood* 2008;111:5446–5456.
34. Cerroni L, Zenahlik P, Hofler G, et al. Specific cutaneous infiltrates of B-cell chronic lymphocytic leukemia: a clinicopathologic and prognostic study of 42 patients. *Am J Surg Pathol* 1996;20:1000–1010.
35. Garicochea B, Cliquet MG, Melo N, et al. Leptomeningeal involvement in chronic lymphocytic leukemia. *Mod Pathol* 1997;10:500–503.
36. Miller K, Budke H, Orazi A. Leukemic meningitis complicating early stage chronic lymphocytic leukemia. *Arch Pathol Lab Med* 1997;121:524–527.
37. Cheson BD, Bennett JM, Rai KR, et al. Guidelines for clinical protocols for chronic lymphocytic leukemia: recommendations of the National Cancer Institute-sponsored working group. *Am J Hematol* 1988;29:152–163.
38. Rai KR, Sawitsky A, Cronkite EP, et al. Clinical staging of chronic lymphocytic leukemia. *Blood* 1975;46:219–234.
39. Binet JL, Auquier A, Dighiero G, et al. A new prognostic classification of chronic lymphocytic leukemia derived from a multivariate survival analysis. *Cancer* 1981;48:198–206.
40. Chronic lymphocytic leukaemia: proposals for a revised prognostic staging system. Report from the International Workshop on CLL. *Br J Haematol* 1981;48:365–367.
41. Rundles RW, Moore JO. Chronic lymphocytic leukemia. *Cancer* 1978;42:941–945.
42. Jaksic B, Vitale B. Total tumour mass score (TTM): a new parameter in chronic lymphocytic leukaemia. *Br J Haematol* 1981;49:405–413.
43. Mandelli F, De Rossi G, Mancini P, et al. Prognosis in chronic lymphocytic leukemia: a retrospective multicentric study from the GIMEMA group. *J Clin Oncol* 1987;5:398–406.
44. Lee JS, Dixon DO, Kantarjian HM, et al. Prognosis of chronic lymphocytic leukemia: a multivariate regression analysis of 325 untreated patients. *Blood* 1987;69:929–936.
45. Rai KR. A critical analysis of staging in CLL. In: Gale RP, Rai KR, eds. *Chronic lymphocytic leukemia: recent progress and future direction: proceedings of a Hyland Laboratories-UCLA symposium held in Napa, California, December 2-5, 1986.* New York, NY: Liss, 1987:253–264.
46. Montserrat E, Sanchez-Bisono J, Vinolas N, et al. Lymphocyte doubling time in chronic lymphocytic leukaemia: analysis of its prognostic significance. *Br J Haematol* 1986;62:567–575.
47. Molica S, Alberti A. Prognostic value of the lymphocyte doubling time in chronic lymphocytic leukemia. *Cancer* 1987;60:2712–2717.
48. Oscier DG, Matutes E, Copplestone A, et al. Atypical lymphocyte morphology: an adverse prognostic factor for disease progression in stage A CLL independent of trisomy 12. *Br J Haematol* 1997;98:934–939.
49. Rozman C, Montserrat E, Rodriguez-Fernandez JM, et al. Bone marrow histologic pattern–the best single prognostic parameter in chronic lymphocytic leukemia: a multivariate survival analysis of 329 cases. *Blood* 1984;64:642–648.
50. Cordone I, Matutes E, Catovsky D. Monoclonal antibody Ki-67 identifies B and T cells in cycle in chronic lymphocytic leukemia: correlation with disease activity. *Leukemia* 1992;6:902–906.
51. Vrhovac R, Delmer A, Tang R, et al. Prognostic significance of the cell cycle inhibitor p27Kip1 in chronic B-cell lymphocytic leukemia. *Blood* 1998;91:4694–4700.

52. Hallek M, Langenmayer I, Nerl C, et al. Elevated serum thymidine kinase levels identify a subgroup at high risk of disease progression in early, non-smoldering chronic lymphocytic leukemia. *Blood* 1999;93:1732–1737.

53. Hallek M, Wanders L, Ostwald M, et al. Serum beta(2)-microglobulin and serum thymidine kinase are independent predictors of progression-free survival in chronic lymphocytic leukemia and immunocytoma. *Leuk Lymphoma* 1996;22:439–447.

54. Fayad L, Keating MJ, Reuben JM, et al. Interleukin-6 and interleukin-10 levels in chronic lymphocytic leukemia: correlation with phenotypic characteristics and outcome. *Blood* 2001;97:256–263.

55. Wierda WG, O'Brien S, Wang X, et al. Prognostic nomogram and index for overall survival in previously untreated patients with chronic lymphocytic leukemia. *Blood* 2007;109:4679–4685.

56. Ferrajoli A, Keating MJ, Manshouri T, et al. The clinical significance of tumor necrosis factor-alpha plasma level in patients having chronic lymphocytic leukemia. *Blood* 2002;100:1215–1219.

57. Molica S, Vitelli G, Levato D, et al. Increased serum levels of vascular endothelial growth factor predict risk of progression in early B-cell chronic lymphocytic leukaemia. *Br J Haematol* 1999;107:605–610.

58. Stilgenbauer S, Bullinger L, Lichter P, et al. Genetics of chronic lymphocytic leukemia: genomic aberrations and V(H) gene mutation status in pathogenesis and clinical course. *Leukemia* 2002;16:993–1007.

59. Ghia P, Stamatopoulos K, Belessi C, et al. ERIC recommendations on IGHV gene mutational status analysis in chronic lymphocytic leukemia. *Leukemia* 2007;21:1–3.

60. Mauerer K, Zahrieh D, Gorgun G, et al. Immunoglobulin gene segment usage, location and immunogenicity in mutated and unmutated chronic lymphocytic leukaemia. *Br J Haematol* 2005;129:499–510.

61. Tobin G, Thunberg U, Johnson A, et al. Somatically mutated Ig V(H)3-21 genes characterize a new subset of chronic lymphocytic leukemia. *Blood* 2002;99:2262–2264.

62. Murray F, Darzentas N, Hadzidimitriou A, et al. Stereotyped patterns of somatic hypermutation in subsets of patients with chronic lymphocytic leukemia: implications for the role of antigen selection in leukemogenesis. *Blood* 2008;111:1524–1533.

63. Stamatopoulos K, Belessi C, Moreno C, et al. Over 20% of patients with chronic lymphocytic leukemia carry stereotyped receptors: pathogenetic implications and clinical correlations. *Blood* 2007;109:259–270.

64. Ghia EM, Jain S, Widhopf GF 2nd, et al. Use of IGHV3-21 in chronic lymphocytic leukemia is associated with high-risk disease and reflects antigen-driven, post-germinal center leukemogenic selection. *Blood* 2008;111:5101–5108.

65. Montillo M, Hamblin T, Hallek M, et al. Chronic lymphocytic leukemia: novel prognostic factors and their relevance for risk-adapted therapeutic strategies. *Haematologica* 2005;90:391–399.

66. Seiler T, Dohner H, Stilgenbauer S. Risk stratification in chronic lymphocytic leukemia. *Semin Oncol* 2006;33:186–194.

67. Boonstra JG, van Lom K, Langerak AW, et al. CD38 as a prognostic factor in B cell chronic lymphocytic leukaemia (B-CLL): comparison of three approaches to analyze its expression. *Cytometry B Clin Cytom* 2006;70:136–141.

68. Del Poeta G, Maurillo L, Venditti A, et al. Clinical significance of CD38 expression in chronic lymphocytic leukemia. *Blood* 2001;98:2633–2639.

69. Ibrahim S, Keating M, Do KA, et al. CD38 expression as an important prognostic factor in B-cell chronic lymphocytic leukemia. *Blood* 2001;98:181–186.

70. Oscier DG, Gardiner AC, Mould SJ, et al. Multivariate analysis of prognostic factors in CLL: clinical stage, IGVH gene mutational status, and loss or mutation of the p53 gene are independent prognostic factors. *Blood* 2002;100:1177–1184.

71. Crespo M, Bosch F, Villamor N, et al. ZAP-70 expression as a surrogate for immunoglobulin-variable-region mutations in chronic lymphocytic leukemia. *N Engl J Med* 2003;348:1764–1775.

72. Orchard JA, Ibbotson RE, Davis Z, et al. ZAP-70 expression and prognosis in chronic lymphocytic leukaemia. *Lancet* 2004;363:105–111.

73. Rassenti LZ, Huynh L, Toy TL, et al. ZAP-70 compared with immunoglobulin heavy-chain gene mutation status as a predictor of disease progression in chronic lymphocytic leukemia. *N Engl J Med* 2004;351:893–901.

74. Carreras J, Villamor N, Colomo L, et al. Immunohistochemical analysis of ZAP-70 expression in B-cell lymphoid neoplasms. *J Pathol* 2005;205:507–513.

75. Bosch F, Muntanola A, Gine E, et al. Clinical implications of ZAP-70 expression in chronic lymphocytic leukemia. *Cytometry B Clin Cytom* 2006;70:214–217.

76. Krober A, Bloehdorn J, Hafner S, et al. Additional genetic high-risk features such as 11q deletion, 17p deletion, and V3-21 usage characterize discordance of ZAP-70 and VH mutation status in chronic lymphocytic leukemia. *J Clin Oncol* 2006;24:969–975.

77. Del Principe MI, Del Poeta G, Buccisano F, et al. Clinical significance of ZAP-70 protein expression in B-cell chronic lymphocytic leukemia. *Blood* 2006;108:853–861.

78. Heintel D, Kroemer E, Kienle D, et al. High expression of activation-induced cytidine deaminase (AID) mRNA is associated with unmutated IGVH gene status and unfavourable cytogenetic aberrations in patients with chronic lymphocytic leukaemia. *Leukemia* 2004;18:756–762.

79. Nuckel H, Huttmann A, Klein-Hitpass L, et al. Lipoprotein lipase expression is a novel prognostic factor in B-cell chronic lymphocytic leukemia. *Leuk Lymphoma* 2006;47:1053–1061.

80. Oppezzo P, Vasconcelos Y, Settegrana C, et al. The LPL/ADAM29 expression ratio is a novel prognosis indicator in chronic lymphocytic leukemia. *Blood* 2005;106:650–657.

81. Calin GA, Liu CG, Sevignani C, et al. MicroRNA profiling reveals distinct signatures in B cell chronic lymphocytic leukemias. *Proc Natl Acad Sci U S A* 2004;101:11755–11760.

82. Calin GA, Ferracin M, Cimmino A, et al. A MicroRNA signature associated with prognosis and progression in chronic lymphocytic leukemia. *N Engl J Med* 2005;353:1793–1801.

83. Calin GA, Cimmino A, Fabbri M, et al. MiR-15a and miR-16-1 cluster functions in human leukemia. *Proc Natl Acad Sci U S A* 2008;105:5166–5171.

84. Chemotherapeutic options in chronic lymphocytic leukemia: a meta-analysis of the randomized trials. CLL Trialists' Collaborative Group. *J Natl Cancer Inst* 1999;91:861–868.

85. Han T, Ezdinli EZ, Shimaoka K, et al. Chlorambucil vs. combined chlorambucil-corticosteroid therapy in chronic lymphocytic leukemia. *Cancer* 1973;31:502–508.

86. Sawitsky A, Rai KR, Glidewell O, et al. Comparison of daily versus intermittent chlorambucil and prednisone therapy in the treatment of patients with chronic lymphocytic leukemia. *Blood* 1977;50:1049–1059.

87. A randomized clinical trial of chlorambucil versus COP in stage B chronic lymphocytic leukemia. The French Cooperative Group on Chronic Lymphocytic Leukemia. *Blood* 1990;75:1422–1425.

88. Raphael B, Andersen JW, Silber R, et al. Comparison of chlorambucil and prednisone versus cyclophosphamide, vincristine, and prednisone as initial treatment for chronic lymphocytic leukemia: long-term follow-up of an Eastern Cooperative Oncology Group randomized clinical trial. *J Clin Oncol* 1991;9:770–776.

89. Catovsky D, Fooks J, Richards S. MRC working party on leukemia in adults. Prognostic factors in chronic lymphocytic leukemia: the importance of age, sex and response to treatment in survival. *Br J Haematol* 1989;72:141–149.

90. Long-term results of the CHOP regimen in stage C chronic lymphocytic leukaemia. French Cooperative Group on Chronic Lymphocytic Leukaemia. *Br J Haematol* 1989;73:334–340.

91. Grever MR, Kopecky KJ, Coltman CA, et al. Fludarabine monophosphate: a potentially useful agent in chronic lymphocytic leukemia. *Nouv Rev Fr Hematol* 1988;30:457–459.

92. Keating MJ, Kantarjian H, Talpaz M, et al. Fludarabine: a new agent with major activity against chronic lymphocytic leukemia. *Blood* 1989;74:19–25.

93. O'Brien S, Kantarjian H, Beran M, et al. Results of fludarabine and prednisone therapy in 264 patients with chronic lymphocytic leukemia with multivariate analysis-derived prognostic model for response to treatment. *Blood* 1993;82:1695–1700.

94. Fenchel K, Bergmann L, Wijermans P, et al. Clinical experience with fludarabine and its immunosuppressive effects in pretreated chronic lymphocytic leukemias and low-grade lymphomas. *Leuk Lymphoma* 1995;18:485–492.

95. Montserrat E, Hallek M. Current strategies for the treatment of CLL. *Leuk Lymphoma* 1996;22(suppl 2):65–68.

96. Tallman MS, Hakimian D, Zanzig C, et al. Cladribine in the treatment of relapsed or refractory chronic lymphocytic leukemia. *J Clin Oncol* 1995;13:983–988.

97. Robak T, Blonski JZ, Kasznicki M, et al. Cladribine with or without prednisone in the treatment of previously treated and untreated B-cell chronic lymphocytic leukemia–updated results of the multicentre study of 378 patients. *Br J Haematol* 2000;108:357–368.

98. Dillman RO, Mick R, McIntyre OR. Pentostatin in chronic lymphocytic leukemia: a phase II trial of Cancer and Leukemia group B. *J Clin Oncol* 1989;7:433–438.

99. Ho AD, Thaler J, Stryckmans P, et al. Pentostatin in refractory chronic lymphocytic leukemia: a phase II trial of the European Organization for Research and Treatment of Cancer. *J Natl Cancer Inst* 1990;82:1416–1420.

100. Johnson SA, Catovsky D, Child JA, et al. Phase I/II evaluation of pentostatin (2'-deoxycoformycin) in a five day schedule for the treatment of relapsed/refractory B-cell chronic lymphocytic leukaemia. *Invest New Drugs* 1998;16:155–160.

101. Keating MJ, Kantarjian H, O'Brien S, et al. Fludarabine: a new agent with marked cytoreductive activity in untreated chronic lymphocytic leukemia. *J Clin Oncol* 1991;9:44–49.

102. Rai KR, Peterson BL, Appelbaum FR, et al. Fludarabine compared with chlorambucil as primary therapy for chronic lymphocytic leukemia. *N Engl J Med* 2000;343:1750–1757.

103. Leporrier M, Chevret S, Cazin B, et al. Randomized comparison of fludarabine, CAP, and ChOP in 938 previously untreated stage B and C chronic lymphocytic leukemia patients. *Blood* 2001;98:2319–2325.

104. Saven A, Lemon RH, Kosty M, et al. 2-Chlorodeoxyadenosine activity in patients with untreated chronic lymphocytic leukemia. *J Clin Oncol* 1995;13:570–574.

105. Juliusson G, Liliemark J. Long-term survival following cladribine (2-chlorodeoxyadenosine) therapy. *Ann Oncol* 1996;7:373–379.

106. Saven A. The Scripps Clinic experience with cladribine (2-CdA) in the treatment of chronic lymphocytic leukemia. *Semin Hematol* 1996;33:28–33.

107. Juliusson G, Liliemark J. High complete remission rate from 2-chloro-2'-deoxyadenosine in previously treated patients with B-cell chronic lymphocytic leukemia: response predicted by rapid decrease of blood lymphocyte count. *J Clin Oncol* 1993;11:679–689.

108. Johnson S, Smith AG, Loffler H, et al. Multicentre prospective randomised trial of fludarabine versus cyclophosphamide, doxorubicin, and prednisone (CAP) for treatment of advanced-stage chronic lymphocytic leukaemia. The French Cooperative Group on CLL. *Lancet* 1996;347:1432–1438.

109. Hallek M, Schmitt B, Wilhelm M, et al. Fludarabine plus cyclophosphamide is an efficient treatment for advanced chronic lymphocytic leukaemia (CLL): results of a phase II study of the German CLL Study Group. *Br J Haematol* 2001;114:342–348.

110. Flinn IW, Byrd JC, Morrison C, et al. Fludarabine and cyclophosphamide with filgrastim support in patients with previously untreated indolent lymphoid malignancies. *Blood* 2000;96:71–75.

111. O'Brien SM, Kantarjian HM, Cortes J, et al. Results of the fludarabine and cyclophosphamide combination regimen in chronic lymphocytic leukemia. *J Clin Oncol* 2001;19:1414–1420.

112. Eichhorst BF, Busch R, Hopfinger G, et al. Fludarabine plus cyclophosphamide versus fludarabine alone in first-line therapy of younger patients with chronic lymphocytic leukemia. *Blood* 2006;107:885–891.

113. Flinn IW, Neuberg DS, Grever MR, et al. Phase III trial of fludarabine plus cyclophosphamide compared with fludarabine for patients with previously untreated chronic lymphocytic leukemia: US Intergroup Trial E2997. *J Clin Oncol* 2007;25:793–798.

114. Catovsky D, Richards S, Matutes E, et al. Assessment of fludarabine plus cyclophosphamide for patients with chronic lymphocytic leukaemia (the LRF CLL4 Trial): a randomised controlled trial. *Lancet* 2007;370:230–239.

115. Thomson AE, Vaughan-Smith S, Peel WE, et al. The intrinsic radiosensitivity of lymphocytes in chronic lymphocytic leukaemia, quantitatively determined independently of cell death rate factors. *Int J Radiat Biol Relat Stud Phys Chem Med* 1985;48:943–961.

116. Thomson AE, Wetherley-Mein G, O'Connor TW, et al. Simplified quantitative estimation in vitro of lymphocyte radiosensitivity applied to patients with chronic lymphocytic leukaemia. *Leuk Res* 1991;15:577–589.

117. Weinmann M, Becker G, Einsele H, et al. Clinical indications and biological mechanisms of splenic irradiation in chronic leukaemias and myeloproliferative disorders. *Radiother Oncol* 2001;58:235–246.

118. Terstappen LW, de Grooth BG, van Berkel W, et al. The effects of splenic irradiation on lymphocyte subpopulations in chronic B-lymphocytic leukemia. *Eur J Haematol* 1988;41:496–505.

119. Chisesi T, Capnist G, Dal Fior S. Splenic irradiation in chronic lymphocytic leukemia. *Eur J Haematol* 1991;46:202–204.

120. Seymour JF, Cusack JD, Lerner SA, et al. Case/control study of the role of splenectomy in chronic lymphocytic leukemia. *J Clin Oncol* 1997;15:52–60.

121. Cusack JC Jr, Seymour JF, Lerner S, et al. Role of splenectomy in chronic lymphocytic leukemia. *J Am Coll Surg* 1997;185:237–243.

122. Johnson RE. Treatment of chronic lymphocytic leukemia by total body irradiation alone and combined with chemotherapy. *Int J Radiat Oncol Biol Phys* 1979;5:159–164.

123. Jacobs P, King HS. A randomized prospective comparison of chemotherapy to total body irradiation as initial treatment for the indolent lymphoproliferative diseases. *Blood* 1987;69:1642–1646.

124. Rubin P, Bennett JM, Begg C, et al. The comparison of total body irradiation vs chlorambucil and prednisone for remission induction of active chronic lymphocytic leukemia: an ECOG study. Part I: total body irradiation-response and toxicity. *Int J Radiat Oncol Biol Phys* 1981;7:1623–1632.

125. McLaughlin P, Grillo-Lopez AJ, Link BK, et al. Rituximab chimeric anti-CD20 monoclonal antibody therapy for relapsed indolent lymphoma: half of patients respond to a four-dose treatment program. *J Clin Oncol* 1998;16:2825–2833.

126. Foran JM, Rohatiner AZ, Cunningham D, et al. European phase II study of rituximab (chimeric anti-CD20 monoclonal antibody) for patients with newly diagnosed mantle-cell lymphoma and previously treated mantle-cell lymphoma, immunocytoma, and small B-cell lymphocytic lymphoma. *J Clin Oncol* 2000;18:317–324.

127. Huhn D, von Schilling C, Wilhelm M, et al. Rituximab therapy of patients with B-cell chronic lymphocytic leukemia. *Blood* 2001;98:1326–1331.

128. O'Brien SM, Kantarjian H, Thomas DA, et al. Rituximab dose-escalation trial in chronic lymphocytic leukemia. *J Clin Oncol* 2001;19:2165–2170.

129. Byrd JC, Murphy T, Howard RS, et al. Rituximab using a thrice weekly dosing schedule in B-cell chronic lymphocytic leukemia and small lymphocytic lymphoma demonstrates clinical activity and acceptable toxicity. *J Clin Oncol* 2001;19:2153–2164.

130. Keating MJ, O'Brien S, Albitar M, et al. Early results of a chemoimmunotherapy regimen of fludarabine, cyclophosphamide, and rituximab as initial therapy for chronic lymphocytic leukemia. *J Clin Oncol* 2005;23:4079–4088.

131. Tam CS, O'Brien S, Wierda W, et al. Long term results of the fludarabine, cyclophosphamide & rituximab regimen as initial therapy of chronic lymphocytic leukemia. *Blood* 2008;112:975–980.

132. Wierda W, O'Brien S, Wen S, et al. Chemoimmunotherapy with fludarabine, cyclophosphamide, and rituximab for relapsed and refractory chronic lymphocytic leukemia. *J Clin Oncol* 2005;23:4070–4078.

133. Stilgenbauer S, Dohner H. Campath-1H-induced complete remission of chronic lymphocytic leukemia despite p53 gene mutation and resistance to chemotherapy. *N Engl J Med* 2002;347:452–453.

134. Osterborg A, Dyer MJ, Bunjes D, et al. Phase II multicenter study of human CD52 antibody in previously treated chronic lymphocytic leukemia. European Study Group of CAMPATH-1H Treatment in Chronic Lymphocytic Leukemia. *J Clin Oncol* 1997;15:1567–1574.

135. Keating MJ, Flinn I, Jain V, et al. Therapeutic role of alemtuzumab (Campath-1H) in patients who have failed fludarabine: results of a large international study. *Blood* 2002;99:3554–3561.

136. Osterborg A, Fassas AS, Anagnostopoulos A, et al. Humanized CD52 monoclonal antibody Campath-1H as first-line treatment in chronic lymphocytic leukaemia. *Br J Haematol* 1996;93:151–153.

137. Lundin J, Kimby E, Bjorkholm M, et al. Phase II trial of subcutaneous anti-CD52 monoclonal antibody alemtuzumab (Campath-1H) as first-line treatment for patients with B-cell chronic lymphocytic leukemia (B-CLL). *Blood* 2002;100:768–773.

138. Hillmen P, Skotnicki AB, Robak T, et al. Alemtuzumab compared with chlorambucil as first-line therapy for chronic lymphocytic leukemia. *J Clin Oncol* 2007;25:5616–5623.

139. Ranheim EA, Kipps TJ. Activated T cells induce expression of B7/BB1 on normal or leukemic B cells through a CD40-dependent signal. *J Exp Med* 1993;177:925–935.

140. Wierda WG, Cantwell MJ, Woods SJ, et al. CD40-ligand (CD154) gene therapy for chronic lymphocytic leukemia. *Blood* 2000;96:2917–2924.

141. Dreger P, Corradini P, Kimby E, et al. Indications for allogeneic stem cell transplantation in chronic lymphocytic leukemia: the EBMT transplant consensus. *Leukemia* 2007;21:12–17.

142. Dreger P, Stilgenbauer S, Benner A, et al. The prognostic impact of autologous stem cell transplantation in patients with chronic lymphocytic leukemia: a risk-matched analysis based on the VH gene mutational status. *Blood* 2004;103:2850–2858.

143. Gribben JG, Zahrieh D, Stephans K, et al. Autologous and allogeneic stem cell transplantation for poor risk chronic lymphocytic leukemia. *Blood* 2005;106:4389–4396.

144. Khouri IF, Keating MJ, Vriesendorp HM, et al. Autologous and allogeneic bone marrow transplantation for chronic lymphocytic leukemia: preliminary results. *J Clin Oncol* 1994;12:748–758.

145. Dreger P, von Neuhoff N, Kuse R, et al. Early stem cell transplantation for chronic lymphocytic leukaemia: a chance for cure? *Br J Cancer* 1998;77:2291–2297.

146. Milligan DW, Fernandes S, Dasgupta R, et al. Results of the MRC pilot study show autografting for younger patients with chronic lymphocytic leukemia is safe and achieves a high percentage of molecular responses. *Blood* 2005;105:397–404.

147. Jantunen E, Itala M, Siitonen T, et al. Autologous stem cell transplantation in patients with chronic lymphocytic leukaemia: the Finnish experience. *Bone Marrow Transplant* 2006;37:1093–1098.

148. Provan D, Bartlett-Pandite L, Zwicky C, et al. Eradication of polymerase chain reaction-detectable chronic lymphocytic leukemia cells is associated with improved outcome after bone marrow transplantation. *Blood* 1996;88:2228–2235.

149. Zenz T, Ritgen M, Dreger P, et al. Autologous graft-versus-host disease-like syndrome after an alemtuzumab-containing conditioning regimen and autologous stem cell transplantation for chronic lymphocytic leukemia. *Blood* 2006;108:2127–2130.

150. Montillo M, Tedeschi A, Miqueleiz S, et al. Alemtuzumab as consolidation after a response to fludarabine is effective in purging residual disease in patients with chronic lymphocytic leukemia. *J Clin Oncol* 2006;24:2337–2342.

151. Michallet M, Archimbaud E, Bandini G, et al. HLA-identical sibling bone marrow transplantation in younger patients with chronic lymphocytic leukemia. European Group for blood and marrow transplantation and the International bone marrow transplant registry. *Ann Intern Med* 1996;124:311–315.

152. Khouri I, Champlin R. Allogenic bone marrow transplantation in chronic lymphocytic leukemia. *Ann Intern Med* 1996;125:780–787.

153. Pavletic ZS, Arrowsmith ER, Bierman PJ, et al. Outcome of allogeneic stem cell transplantation for B cell chronic lymphocytic leukemia. *Bone Marrow Transplant* 2000;25:717–722.

154. Doney KC, Chauncey T, Appelbaum FR. Allogeneic related donor hematopoietic stem cell transplantation for treatment of chronic lymphocytic leukemia. *Bone Marrow Transplant* 2002;29:817–823.

155. Khouri IF, Przepiorka D, van Besien K, et al. Allogeneic blood or marrow transplantation for chronic lymphocytic leukaemia: timing of transplantation and potential effect of fludarabine on acute graft-versus-host disease. *Br J Haematol* 1997;97:466–473.

156. Toze CL, Galal A, Barnett MJ, et al. Myeloablative allografting for chronic lymphocytic leukemia: evidence for a potent graft-versus-leukemia effect associated with graft-versus-host disease. *Bone Marrow Transplant* 2005;36:825–830.

157. Dreger P, Brand R, Hansz J, et al. Treatment-related mortality and graft-versus-leukemia activity after allogeneic stem cell transplantation for chronic lymphocytic leukemia using intensity-reduced conditioning. *Leukemia* 2003;17:841–848.

158. Sorror ML, Maris MB, Sandmaier BM, et al. Hematopoietic cell transplantation after nonmyeloablative conditioning for advanced chronic lymphocytic leukemia. *J Clin Oncol* 2005;23:3819–3829.

159. Brown JR, Kim HT, Li S, et al. Predictors of improved progression-free survival after nonmyeloablative allogeneic stem cell transplantation for advanced chronic lymphocytic leukemia. *Biol Blood Marrow Transplant* 2006;12:1056–1064.

160. Delgado J, Thomson K, Russell N, et al. Results of alemtuzumab-based reduced-intensity allogeneic transplantation for chronic lymphocytic leukemia: a British Society of Blood and Marrow Transplantation Study. *Blood* 2006;107:1724–1730.

161. Khouri IF. Reduced-intensity regimens in allogeneic stem-cell transplantation for non-Hodgkin lymphoma and chronic lymphocytic leukemia. *Hematology Am Soc Hematol Educ Program* 2006:390–397.

162. Schetelig J, Thiede C, Bornhauser M, et al. Reduced non-relapse mortality after reduced intensity conditioning in advanced chronic lymphocytic leukemia. *Ann Hematol* 2002;81(suppl 2):S47–S48.

163. Schetelig J, Thiede C, Bornhauser M, et al. Evidence of a graft-versus-leukemia effect in chronic lymphocytic leukemia after reduced-intensity conditioning and allogeneic stem-cell transplantation: the Cooperative German Transplant Study Group. *J Clin Oncol* 2003;21:2747–2753.

164. Moreno C, Villamor N, Colomer D, et al. Clinical significance of minimal residual disease, as assessed by different techniques, after stem cell transplantation for chronic lymphocytic leukemia. *Blood* 2006;107:4563–4569.

165. Dreger P, Brand R, Milligan D, et al. Reduced-intensity conditioning lowers treatment-related mortality of allogeneic stem cell transplantation for chronic lymphocytic leukemia: a population-matched analysis. *Leukemia* 2005;19:1029–1033.

166. Diehl LF, Ketchum LH. Autoimmune disease and chronic lymphocytic leukemia: autoimmune hemolytic anemia, pure red cell aplasia, and autoimmune thrombocytopenia. *Semin Oncol* 1998;25:80–97.

167. Mauro FR, Foa R, Cerretti R, et al. Autoimmune hemolytic anemia in chronic lymphocytic leukemia: clinical, therapeutic, and prognostic features. *Blood* 2000;95:2786–2792.

168. Dearden C, Wade R, Else M, et al. The prognostic significance of a positive direct antiglobulin test in chronic lymphocytic leukemia: a beneficial effect of the combination of fludarabine and cyclophosphamide on the incidence of hemolytic anemia. *Blood* 2008;111:1820–1826.

169. Leach M, Parsons RM, Reilly JT, et al. Autoimmune thrombocytopenia: a complication of fludarabine therapy in lymphoproliferative disorders. *Clin Lab Haematol* 2000;22:175–178.

170. Ghazal H. Successful treatment of pure red cell aplasia with rituximab in patients with chronic lymphocytic leukemia. *Blood* 2002;99:1092–1094.

171. Ribeiro I, Tsatalas C, Catovsky D. Treatment of red cell aplasia in CLL with fludarabine. *Leukemia* 1999;13:1897.

172. Shimoni A, Shvidel L, Klepfish A, et al. Refractory pure red cell aplasia associated with B-CLL: successful treatment with a combination of fludarabine, cyclosporin A and erythropoietin. *Leukemia* 1999;13:142–143.

173. Griffiths H, Brennan V, Lea J, et al. Crossover study of immunoglobulin replacement therapy in patients with low-grade B-cell tumors. *Blood* 1989;73:366–368.

174. Morrison VA. Update on prophylaxis and therapy of infection in patients with chronic lymphocytic leukemia. *Expert Rev Anticancer Ther* 2001;1:84–90.

175. Morrison VA, Rai KR, Peterson BL, et al. Impact of therapy with chlorambucil, fludarabine, or fludarabine plus chlorambucil on infections in patients with chronic lymphocytic leukemia: Intergroup Study Cancer and Leukemia Group B 9011. *J Clin Oncol* 2001;19:3611–3621.

176. Keating MJ, O'Brien S, Lerner S, et al. Long-term follow-up of patients with chronic lymphocytic leukemia (CLL) receiving fludarabine regimens as initial therapy. *Blood* 1998;92:1165–1171.

177. Perkins JG, Flynn JM, Howard RS, et al. Frequency and type of serious infections in fludarabine-refractory B-cell chronic lymphocytic leukemia and small lymphocytic lymphoma: implications for clinical trials in this patient population. *Cancer* 2002;94:2033–2039.

178. Lens D, Matutes E, Catovsky D, et al. Frequent deletions at 11q23 and 13q14 in B cell prolymphocytic leukemia (B-PLL). *Leukemia* 2000;14:427–430.

179. Lens D, De Schouwer PJ, Hamoudi RA, et al. p53 abnormalities in B-cell prolymphocytic leukemia. *Blood* 1997;89:2015–2023.

180. Davi F, Maloum K, Michel A, et al. High frequency of somatic mutations in the VH genes expressed in prolymphocytic leukemia. *Blood* 1996;88:3953–3961.

181. Shvidel L, Shtalrid M, Bassous L, et al. B-cell prolymphocytic leukemia: a survey of 35 patients emphasizing heterogeneity, prognostic factors and evidence for a group with an indolent course. *Leuk Lymphoma* 1999;33:169–179.

182. Saven A, Lee T, Schlutz M, et al. Major activity of cladribine in patients with de novo B-cell prolymphocytic leukemia. *J Clin Oncol* 1997;15:37–43.

183. Soulier J, Pierron G, Vecchione D, et al. A complex pattern of recurrent chromosomal losses and gains in T-cell prolymphocytic leukemia. *Genes Chromosomes Cancer* 2001;31:248–254.

184. Stilgenbauer S, Schaffner C, Litterst A, et al. Biallelic mutations in the ATM gene in T-prolymphocytic leukemia. *Nat Med* 1997;3:1155–1159.

185. Brito-Babapulle V, Baou M, Matutes E, et al. Deletions of D13S25, D13S319 and RB-1 mapping to 13q14.3 in T-cell prolymphocytic leukaemia. *Br J Haematol* 2001;114:327–332.

186. Matutes E, Brito-Babapulle V, Swansbury J, et al. Clinical and laboratory features of 78 cases of T-prolymphocytic leukemia. *Blood* 1991;78:3269–3274.

187. Dearden CE, Matutes E, Cazin B, et al. High remission rate in T-cell prolymphocytic leukemia with CAMPATH-1H. *Blood* 2001;98:1721–1726.

188. Keating MJ, Cazin B, Coutre S, et al. Campath-1H treatment of T-cell prolymphocytic leukemia in patients for whom at least one prior chemotherapy regimen has failed. *J Clin Oncol* 2002;20:205–213.

189. Collins RH, Pineiro LA, Agura ED, et al. Treatment of T prolymphocytic leukemia with allogeneic bone marrow transplantation. *Bone Marrow Transplant* 1998;21:627–628.

CHAPTER 14 ■ LYMPHOPLASMACYTIC LYMPHOMA/ WALDENSTRÖM MACROGLOBULINEMIA

STEVEN P. TREON AND GIAMPAOLO MERLINI

Waldenström macroglobulinemia (WM) is a distinct clinico-pathologic entity resulting from the accumulation, predominantly in the bone marrow, of clonally related lymphocytes, lymphoplasmacytic cells, and plasma cells that secrete a monoclonal immunoglobulin (Ig) M protein (Fig. 14.1) (1). This condition is considered to correspond to the lymphoplasmacytic lymphoma (LPL) as defined by the Revised European American Lymphoma and World Health Organization classification systems (2,3). Most cases of LPL are WM, with <5% of cases made up of IgA, IgG, and nonsecreting LPL.

EPIDEMIOLOGY AND ETIOLOGY

WM is an uncommon disease, with a reported age-adjusted incidence rate of 3.4 per 1 million among males and 1.7 per million among females in the United States, and a geometric increase with age (4,5). The incidence rate for WM is higher among whites, with African descendants representing only 5% of all patients. Genetic factors appear to be an important factor to the pathogenesis of WM. Approximately 20% of patients with WM have an Ashkenazi (Eastern European) Jewish ethnic background, and there have been numerous reports of familiar disease, including multigenerational clustering of WM and other B-cell lymphoproliferative diseases (6–10). In a recent study, approximately 20% of 257 serial patients with WM presenting to a tertiary referral had a first-degree relative with either WM or another B-cell disorder (7). Frequent familiar association with other immunologic disorders in healthy relatives, including hypogammaglobulinemia and hypergammaglobulinemia (particularly polyclonal IgM), autoantibody (particularly to thyroid) production, and manifestation of hyperactive B cells, have also been reported (9,10). Increased expression of the *bcl-2* gene with enhanced B-cell survival may underlie the increased Ig synthesis in familial WM (9). The role of environmental factors in WM remains to be clarified, but chronic antigenic stimulation from infections, and certain drug and Agent Orange exposures remain suspect. An etiologic role for hepatitis C virus infection has been suggested, though in a recent study examining 100 consecutive patients with WM, no association could be established using both serologic and molecular diagnostic studies for hepatitis C virus infection (11–13).

BIOLOGY

Cytogenetic Findings

Several studies, usually performed on limited series of patients, have been published on cytogenetic findings in WM demonstrating a great variety of numerical and structural chromosome abnormalities. Numerical losses involving chromosomes 17–22, X, and Y have been commonly observed, though gains in chromosomes 3, 4, and 12 have also been reported (7,14–19). Chromosome 6q deletions encompassing 6q21–22 have been observed in up to half of patients with WM, and at a comparable frequency among patients with and without a familial history (7,19). Several candidate tumor suppressor genes in this region are under study, including B-lymphocyte-induced maturation protein-1, a master regulatory gene implicated in lymphoplasmacytic differentiation. Notable, however, is the absence of IgH switch region rearrangements in WM, a finding that may be used to discern cases of IgM myeloma where IgH switch region rearrangements are a predominant feature (20).

Nature of the Clonal Cell

The WM bone marrow B-cell clone shows intraclonal differentiation from small lymphocytes with large focal deposits of surface Igs, to lymphoplasmacytic cells, to mature plasma cells that contain intracytoplasmic Igs (21). Clonal B cells are detectable among blood B lymphocytes, and their number increases in patients who fail to respond to therapy or who have progression (22). These clonal blood cells present the peculiar capacity to differentiate spontaneously, in in vitro

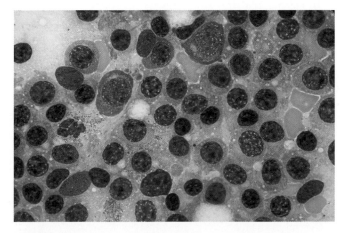

FIGURE 14.1 Aspirate from a patient with WM demonstrating excess mature lymphocytes, lymphoplasmacytic cells, and plasma cells. (See also Color Plate 25) (Courtesy of Marvin Stone, M.D.)

culture, to plasma cells. This is through an interleukin-6-dependent process in IgM monoclonal gammopathy of undetermined significance and mostly an interleukin-6-independent process in patients with WM (23). All these cells express the monoclonal IgM present in the blood, and a variable percentage of them also express surface IgD. The characteristic immunophenotypic profile of the lymphoplasmacytic cells in WM includes the expression of the pan B-cell markers CD19, CD20, CD22, CD79, and FMC7.2 (24–26). Expression of CD5, CD10, and CD23 may be found in 10% to 20% of cases, and does not exclude the diagnosis of WM (27).

The phenotype of lymphoplasmacytic cells in WM cells suggests that the clone is a postgerminal center B cell. This indication is further strengthened by the results of the analysis of the nature (silent or amino acid replacing) and distribution (in framework or complementarity determining regions) of somatic mutations in Ig heavy and light-chain variable regions performed in patients with WM (28,29). This analysis showed a high rate of replacement mutations, compared with the closest germline genes, clustering in the complementarity determining regions and without intraclonal variation. Subsequent studies showed a strong preferential usage of VH3/JH4 gene families, no intraclonal variation, and no evidence for any isotype-switched transcripts (30,31). These data indicate that WM may originate from a IgM$^+$ and/or IgM$^+$ IgD$^+$ memory B cell. Normal IgM$^+$ memory B cells localize in bone marrow, where they mature to IgM-secreting cells (32).

Bone Marrow Microenvironment

Increased numbers of mast cells are found in the bone marrow of patients with WM, wherein they are usually admixed with tumor aggregates (26,33). Recent studies have helped clarify the role of mast cells in WM. Coculture of primary autologous or mast cell lines with WM LPC resulted in dose-dependent WM cell proliferation and/or tumor colony, primarily through CD40 ligand signaling. Furthermore, WM

cells through elaboration of soluble CD27 induced the up-regulation of CD40 ligand on mast cells derived from patients with WM and mast cell lines (34).

CLINICAL FEATURES

The clinical and laboratory findings at diagnosis of WM in one large institutional study (7) are presented in Table 14.1. Unlike most indolent lymphomas, splenomegaly and lymphadenopathy are prominent in only a minority of patients (≤15%). Purpura is frequently associated with cryoglobulinemia and more rarely with AL amyloidosis, whereas hemorrhagic manifestations and neuropathies are multifactorial (see later). The morbidity associated with WM is caused by the concurrence of two main components: tissue infiltration by neoplastic cells; and, more importantly, the physicochemical and immunologic properties of the monoclonal IgM. As shown in Table 14.2, the monoclonal IgM can produce clinical manifestations through several different mechanisms related to its physicochemical properties, nonspecific interactions with other proteins, antibody activity, and tendency to deposit in tissues (35–37).

MORBIDITY MEDIATED BY THE EFFECTS OF IMMUNOGLOBULIN M

Hyperviscosity Syndrome

Blood hyperviscosity is affected by increased serum IgM levels leading to hyperviscosity related complications (38). The mechanisms behind the marked increase in the resistance to blood flow and the resulting impaired transit through the microcirculatory system are rather complex (38–40). The main determinants are: (a) a high concentration of monoclonal IgMs, which may form aggregates and may bind water

---

TABLE 14.1

CLINICAL AND LABORATORY FINDINGS FOR 149 CONSECUTIVE NEWLY DIAGNOSED PATIENTS WITH THE CONSENSUS PANEL DIAGNOSIS OF WM PRESENTING TO THE DANA-FARBER CANCER INSTITUTE

	Median	Range	Institutional normal reference range
Age (y)	59	34–84	NA
Gender (male/female)	85/64		NA
Bone marrow involvement (%)	30	5–95	NA
Adenopathy (%)	16		NA
Splenomegaly (%)	10		NA
IgM (mg per dL)	2,870	267–12,400	40–230
IgG (mg per dL)	587	47–2,770	700–1,600
IgA (mg per dL)	47	8–509	70–400
Serum viscosity (cp)	2.0	1.4–6.6	1.4–1.9
Hct (%)	35.0	17.2–45.4	34.8–43.6
Plt ($\times 10^9$ per L)	253	24–649	155–410
Wbc ($\times 10^9$ per L)	6.0	0.3–13	3.8–9.2
β_2M (mg per dL)	3.0	1.3–13.7	0–2.7
LDH	395	122–1,131	313–618

β_2M, β_2-microglobulin; Hct, hematocrit; LDH, lactate dehydrogenase; NA, not applicable; Plt, platelet; Wbc, white blood cell count.

TABLE 14.2

PHYSICOCHEMICAL AND IMMUNOLOGIC PROPERTIES OF THE MONOCLONAL IGM PROTEIN IN WM

Properties of IgM monoclonal protein	Diagnostic condition	Clinical manifestations
Pentameric structure	Hyperviscosity	Headaches, blurred vision, epistaxis, retinal hemorrhages, leg cramps, impaired mentation, and intracranial hemorrhage.
Precipitation on cooling	Cryoglobulinemia (type I)	Raynaud phenomenon, acrocyanosis, ulcers, purpura, and cold urticaria.
Autoantibody activity to myelin-associated glycoprotein, ganglioside M1, sulfatide moieties on peripheral nerve sheaths	Peripheral neuropathies	Sensorimotor neuropathies, painful neuropathies, ataxic gait, and bilateral footdrop.
Autoantibody activity to IgG	Cryoglobulinemia (type II)	Purpura, arthralgias, renal failure, and sensorimotor neuropathies.
Autoantibody activity to RBC antigens	Cold agglutinins	Hemolytic anemia, Raynaud phenomenon, acrocyanosis, and livedo reticularis.
Tissue deposition as amorphous aggregates	Organ dysfunction	Skin: bullous skin disease, papules, Schnitzler syndrome. Gastrointestinal: diarrhea, malabsorption, bleeding. Kidney: proteinuria, renal failure (light chain component).
Tissue deposition as amyloid fibrils (light chain component most commonly)	Organ dysfunction	Fatigue, weight loss, edema, hepatomegaly, macroglossia, organ dysfunction of involved organs: heart, kidney, liver, peripheral sensory, and autonomic nerves.

through their carbohydrate component; and (b) their interaction with blood cells. Monoclonal IgMs increase red cell aggregation (*rouleaux* formation) and red cell internal viscosity while also reducing deformability. The possible presence of cryoglobulins can contribute to increasing blood viscosity as well as to the tendency to induce erythrocyte aggregation. Serum viscosity is proportional to IgM concentration up to 30 g per L, then increases sharply at higher levels. Plasma viscosity and hematocrit are directly regulated by the body. Increased plasma viscosity may also contribute to inappropriately low erythropoietin production, which is the major reason for anemia in these patients (41). Clinical manifestations are related to circulatory disturbances that can be best appreciated by ophthalmoscopy, which shows distended and tortuous retinal veins, hemorrhages, and papilledema (42) (Fig. 14.2). Symptoms usually occur when the monoclonal IgM concentration exceeds 50 g per L or when serum viscosity is >4.0 centipoises (cp), but there is a great individual variability, with some patients showing no evidence of hyperviscosity even at 10 cp (38). The most common symptoms are oronasal bleeding, visual disturbances due to retinal bleeding, and dizziness that may rarely lead to coma. Heart failure can be aggravated, particularly in the elderly, owing to increased blood viscosity, expanded plasma volume, and anemia. Inappropriate transfusion can exacerbate hyperviscosity and may precipitate cardiac failure.

Cryoglobulinemia

In up to 20% of patients with WM, the monoclonal IgM can behave as a cryoglobulin (type I), but it is symptomatic in ≤5% of the cases (43). Cryoprecipitation is mainly dependent on the concentration of monoclonal IgM; for this

reason, plasmapheresis or plasma exchange is commonly effective in this condition. Symptoms result from impaired blood flow in small vessels and include Raynaud phenomenon, acrocyanosis, and necrosis of the regions most exposed to cold (tip of the nose, ears, fingers, and toes), malleolar ulcers, purpura, and cold urticaria. Renal manifestations may occur but are infrequent.

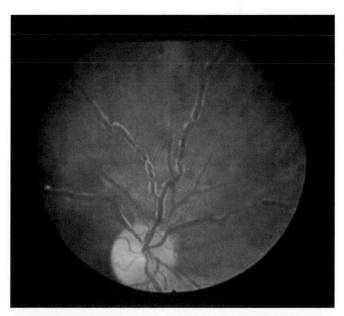

FIGURE 14.2. Funduscopic examination of a patient with WM demonstrating hyperviscosity related changes, including dilated retinal vessels, peripheral hemorrhages, and "venous sausaging." (See also Color Plate 26) (Courtesy of Marvin Stone, M.D.)

Autoantibody Activity

Monoclonal IgM may exert its pathogenic effects through specific recognition of autologous antigens, the most notable being nerve constituents, Ig determinants, and red blood cell (RBC) antigens.

Immunoglobulin M-Related Neuropathy

In a series of 215 patients with WM, Merlini et al. (43) reported the clinical presence of peripheral neuropathy in 24% of patients with WM, although prevalence rates ranging from 5% to 38% have been reported in other series (44,45). An estimated 6.5% to 0% of idiopathic neuropathies are associated with a monoclonal gammopathy, with a preponderance of IgM (60%), followed by IgG (30%) and IgA (10%) [reviewed in (46) and (47)]. In patients with WM, the nerve damage is mediated by diverse pathogenetic mechanisms: IgM antibody activity toward nerve constituents causing demyelinating polyneuropathies; endoneurial granulofibrillar deposits of IgM without antibody activity, associated with axonal polyneuropathy; occasionally by tubular deposits in the endoneurium associated with IgM cryoglobulin; and, rarely, by amyloid deposits or by neoplastic cell infiltration of nerve structures (48). Half of the patients with IgM neuropathy have a distinctive clinical syndrome that is associated with antibodies against a minor 100-kDa glycoprotein component of nerve, myelin-associated glycoprotein (MAG). Anti-MAG antibodies are generally monoclonal IgMκ, and usually also exhibit reactivity with other glycoproteins or glycolipids that share antigenic determinants with MAG (49–51). The anti-MAG-related neuropathy is typically distal and symmetric, affecting both motor and sensory functions; it is slowly progressive with a long period of stability (45,52). Most patients present with sensory complaints (paresthesias, aching discomfort, dysesthesias, or lancinating pains), imbalance, and gait ataxia, owing to lack proprioception, and leg muscle atrophy in advanced stage. Patients with predominantly demyelinating sensory neuropathy in association with monoclonal IgM to gangliosides with disialosyl moieties, such as GD1b, GD3, GD2, GT1b, and GQ1b, have also been reported (53,54). Anti-GD1b and anti-GQ1b antibodies were significantly associated with predominantly sensory ataxic neuropathy. These antiganglioside monoclonal IgMs present core clinical features of chronic ataxic neuropathy with variably present ophthalmoplegia and/or RBC cold agglutinating activity. The disialosyl epitope is also present on RBC glycophorins, thereby accounting for the red cell cold agglutinin activity of anti-Pr2 specificity (55,56). Monoclonal IgM proteins that bind to gangliosides with a terminal trisaccharide moiety, including GM2 and GalNac-GD1A, are associated with chronic demyelinating neuropathy and severe sensory ataxia, unresponsive to corticosteroids (57). Antiganglioside IgM proteins may also cross-react with lipopolysaccharides of *Campylobacter jejuni*, whose infection is known to precipitate the Miller Fisher syndrome, a variant of the Guillain-Barré syndrome (58). This finding indicates that molecular mimicry may play a role in this condition. Antisulfatide monoclonal IgM proteins, associated with sensory/sensorimotor neuropathy, have been detected in 5% of patients with IgM monoclonal gammopathy and neuropathy (59). Motor neuron disease has been reported in patients with WM, and monoclonal IgM with anti-GM1 and sulfoglucuronyl paragloboside activity (60). POEMS (polyneuropathy, organomegaly, endocrinopathy, M protein, and skin changes) syndrome is rarely associated with WM (61).

Cold Agglutinin Hemolytic Anemia

Monoclonal IgM may present with cold agglutinin activity, that is, it can recognize specific red cell antigens at temperatures below physiologic, producing chronic hemolytic anemia. This disorder occurs in <10% of patients with WM (62) and is associated with cold agglutinin titers >1:1,000 in most cases. The monoclonal component is usually an IgMκ and reacts most commonly with I/i antigens, with complement fixation and activation (63,64). Mild chronic hemolytic anemia can be exacerbated after cold exposure, but rarely does hemoglobin drop <70 g per L. The hemolysis is usually extravascular (removal of C3b opsonized cells by the reticuloendothelial system, primarily in the liver) and rarely intravascular from complement destruction of RBC membrane. The agglutination of RBCs in the cooler peripheral circulation also causes Raynaud syndrome, acrocyanosis, and livedo reticularis. Macroglobulins with the properties of both cryoglobulins and cold agglutinins with anti-Pr specificity have been reported. These properties may have as a common basis the immune binding of the sialic acid-containing carbohydrate present on RBC glycophorins and on Ig molecules. Several other macroglobulins with various antibody activity toward autologous antigens (i.e., phospholipids, tissue, and plasma proteins, etc.) and foreign ligands have also been reported.

Tissue Deposition

The monoclonal protein can deposit in several tissues as amorphous aggregates. Linear deposition of monoclonal IgM along the skin basement membrane is associated with bullous skin disease (65). Amorphous IgM deposits in the dermis determine the so-called IgM storage papules on the extensor surface of the extremities, that is, macroglobulinemia cutis (66). Deposition of monoclonal IgM in the lamina propria and/or submucosa of the intestine may be associated with diarrhea, malabsorption, and gastrointestinal bleeding (67,68). It is well known that kidney involvement is less common and less severe in WM than in multiple myeloma, probably because the amount of light chain excreted in the urine is generally lower in WM than in myeloma and because of the absence of contributing factors, such as hypercalcemia, although cast nephropathy has also been described in WM (69). On the other hand, the IgM macromolecule is more susceptible to being trapped in the glomerular loops where ultrafiltration presumably contributes to its precipitation, forming subendothelial deposits of aggregated IgM proteins that occlude the glomerular capillaries (70). Mild and reversible proteinuria may result, and most patients are asymptomatic. The deposition of monoclonal light chain as fibrillar amyloid deposits (AL amyloidosis) is uncommon in patients with WM (71). Clinical expression and prognosis are similar to those of other patients with AL with involvement of heart (44%), kidneys (32%), liver (14%), lungs

(10%), peripheral/autonomic nerves (38%), and soft tissues (18%). However, the incidence of cardiac and pulmonary involvement is higher in patients with monoclonal IgM than with other Ig isotypes. The association of WM with reactive amyloidosis (AA) has been documented rarely (72,73). Simultaneous occurrence of fibrillary glomerulopathy, characterized by glomerular deposits of wide noncongophilic fibrils and amyloid deposits, has been reported in WM (74).

Manifestations Related to Tissue Infiltration by Neoplastic Cells

Tissue infiltration by neoplastic cells can involve various organs and tissues including the bone marrow, lymph nodes, spleen, liver, and more rarely gastrointestinal tract, kidneys, skin, eyes and central nervous system. Pulmonary involvement in the form of masses, nodules, diffuse infiltrate, or pleural effusions is relatively rare with an overall incidence of less than 5% of all WM cases (75–77). Cough is the most common presenting symptom, followed by dyspnea and chest pain. Chest radiographic findings include parenchymal infiltrates, confluent masses, and effusions. Malabsorption, diarrhea, bleeding, or obstruction may indicate involvement of the gastrointestinal tract at the level of the stomach, duodenum, or small intestine (78–81). In contrast to multiple myeloma, infiltration of the kidney interstitium with lymphoplasmacytoid cell has been reported in WM (82), whereas renal or perirenal masses are not uncommon (83). The skin can be the site of dense lymphoplasmacytic infiltrates, similar to that seen in the liver, spleen, and lymph nodes, forming cutaneous plaques and, rarely, nodules (84). Chronic urticaria and IgM gammopathy are the two cardinal features of the Schnitzler syndrome, which is not usually associated initially with clinical features of WM (85), although evolution to WM is not uncommon. Thus, close follow-up of these patients is warranted. Invasion of articular and periarticular structures by WM malignant cells is rarely reported (86). The neoplastic cells can infiltrate the periorbital structures, lacrimal gland, and retro-orbital lymphoid tissues, resulting in ocular nerve palsies (87,88). Direct infiltration of the central nervous system by monoclonal lymphoplasmacytic cells as infiltrates or as tumors constitutes the rarely observed Bing-Neel syndrome, characterized clinically by confusion, memory loss, disorientation, and motor dysfunction [reviewed in (89)].

LABORATORY INVESTIGATIONS AND FINDINGS

Hematologic Abnormalities

Anemia is the most common finding in patients with symptomatic WM and is caused by a combination of factors: mild decrease in red cell survival, impaired erythropoiesis, hemolysis, moderate plasma volume expansion, and blood loss from the gastrointestinal tract. Blood smears are usually normocytic and normochromic, and rouleaux formation is often pronounced. Electronically measured mean corpuscular volume

may be elevated spuriously owing to erythrocyte aggregation. In addition, the hemoglobin estimate can be inaccurate, that is, falsely high, because of interaction between the monoclonal protein and the diluent used in some automated analyzers (90). Leukocyte and platelet counts are usually within the reference range at presentation, although patients may occasionally present with severe thrombocytopenia. As reported previously, monoclonal B lymphocytes expressing surface IgM and late-differentiation B-cell markers are uncommonly detected in blood by flow cytometry. A raised erythrocyte sedimentation rate is almost constantly observed in WM and may be the first clue to the presence of the macroglobulin. The clotting abnormality detected most frequently is prolongation of thrombin time. AL amyloidosis should be suspected in all patients with nephrotic syndrome, cardiomyopathy, hepatomegaly, or peripheral neuropathy. Diagnosis requires the demonstration of green birefringence under polarized light of amyloid deposits stained with Congo red.

Biochemical Investigations

High-resolution electrophoresis combined with immunofixation of serum and urine is recommended for identification and characterization of the IgM monoclonal protein. The light chain of the monoclonal IgM is κ in 75% to 80% of patients. A few patients with WM have more than one M component. The concentration of the serum monoclonal protein is very variable but in most cases lies within the range of 15 to 45 g per L. Densitometry should be adopted to determine IgM levels for serial evaluations because nephelometry is unreliable, and shows large intralaboratory as well as interlaboratory variation. The presence of cold agglutinins or cryoglobulins may affect determination of IgM levels, and, therefore, testing for cold agglutinins and cryoglobulins should be performed at diagnosis. If present, subsequent serum samples should be analyzed under warm conditions for determination of serum monoclonal IgM level. Although Bence Jones proteinuria is frequently present, it exceeds 1 g per 24 hours in only 3% of cases. Whereas IgM levels are elevated in patients with WM, IgA and IgG levels are most often depressed and do not demonstrate recovery even after successful treatment (91). In recent studies by Hunter et al. (92), mutations in the receptor TACI were demonstrated in patients with WM akin to those demonstrated in patients with common variable deficiency disorder, suggesting a possible common variable deficiency disorder background for patients with WM.

Serum Viscosity

Because of its large size (almost 1 million daltons), most IgM molecules are retained within the intravascular compartment and can exert an undue effect on serum viscosity. Therefore, serum viscosity should be measured if the patient has signs or symptoms of hyperviscosity syndrome. Funduscopy remains an excellent indicator of clinically relevant hyperviscosity. Among the first clinical signs of hyperviscosity is the appearance of peripheral and midperipheral dot and blot-like hemorrhages in the retina, which are best appreciated with indirect ophthalmoscopy and scleral depression (42). In more severe cases of hyperviscosity, dot, blot, and flame-shaped hemorrhages can appear in the macular area along with markedly dilated and tortuous veins with focal constrictions, resulting in "venous sausaging," as well as papilledema.

Bone Marrow Findings

The bone marrow is always involved in WM. Central to the diagnosis of WM is the demonstration, by trephine biopsy, of *bone marrow infiltration by a lymphoplasmacytic cell population* constituted by small lymphocytes with evidence of plasmacytoid/plasma cell differentiation (Fig. 14.1). The pattern of bone marrow infiltration may be diffuse, interstitial, or nodular, showing usually an intertrabecular pattern of infiltration. A solely paratrabecular pattern of infiltration is unusual and should raise the possibility of follicular lymphoma (1). The bone marrow infiltration should routinely be confirmed by *immunophenotypic studies* (flow cytometry and/or immunohistochemistry) showing the following profile: sIgM+CD19+CD20+CD22+CD79+ (24–26). Up to 20% of cases may express CD5, CD10, or CD23 (27). In these cases, care should be taken to satisfactorily exclude chronic lymphocytic leukemia and mantle cell lymphoma (1). "Intranuclear" periodic acid-Schiff-positive inclusions (Dutcher-Fahey bodies) (93) consisting of IgM deposits in the perinuclear space, and sometimes in intranuclear vacuoles, may be seen occasionally in lymphoid cells in WM. An increased number of mast cells, usually in association with the lymphoid aggregates, are commonly found in WM, and their presence may help in differentiating WM from other B-cell lymphomas (2,3).

Other Investigations

Magnetic resonance imaging of the spine in conjunction with computed tomography (CT) of the abdomen and pelvis are useful in evaluating the disease status in WM (94). Bone marrow involvement can be documented by magnetic resonance imaging studies of the spine in >90% of patients, whereas CT of the abdomen and pelvis demonstrated enlarged nodes in 43% of patients with WM (94). Lymph node biopsy may show preserved architecture or replacement by infiltration of neoplastic cells with lymphoplasmacytoid, lymphoplasmacytic, or polymorphous cytologic patterns. The residual disease after high-dose chemotherapy with allogeneic or autologous stem cell rescue can be monitored by polymerase chain reaction-based methods using primers specific for the monoclonal Ig variable regions.

PROGNOSIS

WM typically presents as an indolent disease, though considerable variability in prognosis can be seen. The median survival reported in several large series has ranged from 5 to 10 years (95–101). Age is consistently an important prognostic factor (>60 to 70 years) (95,96,98,101), but this factor is often impacted by unrelated morbidities. Anemia that reflects both marrow involvement and the serum level of the IgM monoclonal protein (due to the impact of IgM on intravascular fluid retention) has emerged as a strong adverse prognostic

factor, with hemoglobin levels of <9 to 12 g per dL associated with decreased survival in several series (95–98,101). Cytopenias have also been regularly identified as a significant predictor of survival (96). However, the precise level of cytopenias with prognostic significance remains to be determined (98). Some series have identified a platelet count of <100 to 150 × 10^9 per L and a granulocyte count of <1.5 × 10^9 per L as independent prognostic factors (95,96,98,101). The number of cytopenias in a given patient has been proposed as a strong prognostic factor (96). Serum albumin levels have also correlated with survival in patients with WM in certain but not all studies using multivariate analyses (96,98,99). High β-2 microglobulin levels (>3 to 3.5 g per dL) were shown in several studies (97–101), a high serum IgM M protein (>7 g per dL) (101), as well as a low-serum IgM M protein (<4 g per dL) (99) and the presence of cryoglobulins (95) as adverse factors. A few scoring systems have been proposed based on these analyses (Table 14.3).

TREATMENT OF WALDENSTRÖM MACROGLOBULINEMIA

As part of the Second International Workshops on Waldenström's Macroglobulinemia, a consensus panel was organized to recommend criteria for the initiation of therapy in patients with WM (98). The panel recommended that initiation of therapy should not be based on the IgM level per se because this may not correlate with the clinical manifestations of WM. The consensus panel, however, agreed that initiation of therapy was appropriate for patients with constitutional symptoms, such as recurrent fever, night sweats, fatigue due to anemia, or weight loss. The presence of progressive symptomatic lymphadenopathy or splenomegaly provides additional reasons to begin therapy. The presence of anemia with a hemoglobin value of ≤10 g per dL or a platelet count ≤100 × 10^9 per L owing to marrow infiltration also justifies treatment. Certain complications, such as hyperviscosity syndrome, symptomatic sensorimotor peripheral neuropathy, systemic amyloidosis, renal insufficiency, or symptomatic cryoglobulinemia, may also be indications for therapy (98).

FRONTLINE THERAPY

Although a precise therapeutic algorithm for therapy of WM remains to be defined given the paucity of randomized clinical trials, consensus panels composed of experts who treat WM were organized as part of the International Workshops on Waldenström's Macroglobulinemia, and have formulated recommendations for both frontline and salvage therapy of WM based on the best available clinical trial evidence. Among frontline options, the panels considered alkylator agents (e.g., chlorambucil), nucleoside analogs (cladribine or fludarabine), the monoclonal antibody rituximab, as well as combinations thereof as reasonable choices for the upfront therapy of WM (102,103). Importantly, the panel felt that individual patient considerations, including the presence of cytopenias, need for more rapid disease control, age, and candidacy for autologous transplant therapy, should be taken into account in making the choice of a first-line agent. For patients who are candidates for autologous transplant

TABLE 14.3

PROGNOSTIC SCORING SYSTEMS IN WM

Study	Adverse prognostic factors	Number of groups	Survival
Gobbi et al. (95)	Hb <9 g per dL Age >70 y Weight loss Cryoglobulinemia	0-1 prognostic factors 2–4 prognostic factors	Median: 48 mo Median: 80 mo
Morel et al. (96)	Age $\geq$65 y Albumin <4 g per dL Number of cytopenias: Hb <12 g per dL Platelets <150 × 10^9 per L Wbc <4 × 10^9 per L	0-1 -prognostic factors 2 prognostic factors 3–4 prognostic factors	5 y: 87% 5 y: 62% 5 y: 25%
Dhodapkar et al. (97)	β_2M $\geq$3 g per dL Hb <12 g per dL IgM <4 g per dL	β_2M <3 mg per dL + Hb $\geq$12 g per dL β_2M <3 mg per dL + Hb <12 g per dL β_2M $\geq$3 mg per dL + IgM $\geq$ 4 g per dL β_2M $\geq$3 mg per dL + IgM <4 g per dL	5 y: 87% 5 y: 63% 5 y: 53% 5 y: 21%
Application of International Staging System Criteria for Myeloma to WM Dimopoulos et al. (99)	Albumin $\leq$3.5 g per dL β_2M $\geq$3.5 mg per L	Albumin $\geq$3.5 g per dL + β_2M <3.5 mg per dL Albumin $\leq$3.5 g per dL + β_2M <3.5 or β_2M 3.5–5.5 mg per dL β_2M >5.5 mg per dL	Median: NR Median: 116 mo Median: 54 mo
International Prognostic Scoring System for WM Morel et al. (101)	Age >65 y Hb <11.5 g per dL Platelets <100 × 10^9 per L β_2M >3 mg per L IgM >7 g per dL	0-1 prognostic factors[a] 2 prognostic factors[b] 3–5 prognostic factors Excluding age[a] Or age >65[b]	5 y: 87% 5 y: 68% 5 y: 36%

β_2M, β_2-microglobulin; Hb, hemoglobin; NR, not reached; Wbc, white blood cell count.

therapy, and in whom such therapy is seriously considered, the panel recommended that exposure to alkylator or nucleoside analog therapy should be limited.

Alkylator-Based Therapy

Oral alkylating drugs, alone and in combination therapy with steroids, have been extensively evaluated in the upfront treatment of WM. The greatest experience with oral alkylator therapy has been with chlorambucil, which has been administered on both a continuous (i.e., daily dose schedule) as well as an intermittent schedule. Patients receiving chlorambucil on a continuous schedule typically receive 0.1 mg per kg per day, whereas on the intermittent schedule, patients will typically receive 0.3 mg per kg for 7 days, every 6 weeks. In a prospective randomized study, Kyle et al. (104) reported no significant difference in the overall response rate (ORR) between these schedules, although interestingly the median response duration was greater for patients receiving

intermittent versus continuously dosed chlorambucil (46 vs. 26 months). Despite the favorable median response duration in this study for use of the intermittent schedule, no difference in the median overall survival was observed. Moreover, an increased incidence for development of myelodysplasia and acute myelogenous leukemia with the intermittent (three of 22 patients) versus the continuous (zero of 24 patients) chlorambucil schedule prompted the authors of this study to express preference for use of continuous chlorambucil dosing. The use of steroids in combination with alkylator therapy has also been explored. Dimopoulos and Alexanian (105) evaluated chlorambucil (8 mg per m^2) along with prednisone (40 mg per m^2) given orally for 10 days, every 6 weeks, and reported a major response (i.e., reduction of IgM by >50%) in 72% of patients. Nonchlorambucil-based alkylator regimens employing melphalan and cyclophosphamide in combination with steroids have also been examined by Petrucci (106) and Case (107) et al., producing slightly higher ORRs and response durations, although the benefit of these more complex regimens over chlorambucil remains to be demonstrated. Facon et al. (108) have evaluated parameters predicting for response to alkylator therapy. Their studies in patients receiving single-agent chlorambucil demonstrated that age 60, male sex, symptomatic status, and cytopenias (but, interestingly, not high tumor burden and serum IgM levels) were associated with poor response to alkylator therapy. Additional factors to be taken into account in considering alkylator therapy for patients with WM include necessity for more rapid disease control given the slow nature of response to alkylator therapy, as well as consideration for preserving stem cells in patients who are candidates for autologous transplant therapy.

Nucleoside Analog Therapy

Both cladribine and fludarabine have been extensively evaluated in untreated as well as previously treated patients with WM. Cladribine administered as a single agent by continuous intravenous (IV) infusion, by 2-hour daily infusion, or by subcutaneous bolus injections for 5 to 7 days has resulted in major responses in 40% to 90% of patients who received primary therapy, whereas in the salvage setting, responses have ranged from 38% to 54% (108–115). Median time to achievement of response in responding patients following cladribine ranged from 1.2 to 5 months. The ORR with daily infusional fludarabine therapy administered mainly on 5-day schedules in previously untreated and treated patients with WM has ranged from 38% to 100% and 30% to 40%, respectively (116–121), which are on par with the response data for cladribine. Median time to achievement of response for fludarabine was also on par with cladribine at 3 to 6 months. In general, response rates and durations of responses have been greater for patients receiving nucleoside analogs as first-line agents, although in several of the aforementioned studies wherein both untreated and previously treated patients were enrolled, no substantial difference in the ORR was reported. Myelosuppression commonly occurred following prolonged exposure to either of the nucleoside analogs, as did lymphopenia with sustained depletion of both CD4$^+$ and CD8+ T lymphocytes observed in patients with WM 1 year following initiation of therapy (108,110). Treatment-related mortality due to myelosuppression and/or opportunistic infections attributable to immunosuppression occurred in up to 5% of all treated patients in some series with either nucleoside analog. Factors predicting for response to nucleoside analogs in WM included age at start of treatment (<70 years), pretreatment hemoglobin >95 g per L, platelets >75,000 per mm^3, disease relapsing off therapy, patients with resistant disease within the first year of diagnosis, and a long interval between first-line therapy and initiation of a nucleoside analog in patients with relapse (108,114,120). There are limited data on the use of an alternate nucleoside analog to salvage patients whose disease relapsed or demonstrated resistance off cladribine or fludarabine therapy (122,123). Three of four (75%) patients responded to cladribine to salvage patients who had progression following an unmaintained remission to fludarabine, whereas only one of ten (10%) with disease resistant to fludarabine responded to cladribine (122). However, Lewandowski et al. (123) reported a response in two of six patients (33%) and disease stabilization in the remaining patients to fludarabine, despite an inadequate response or progressive disease following cladribine therapy. The long-term safety of nucleoside analogs in WM was recently examined by Leleu et al. (124) in a large series of patients with WM. A 7-fold increase in transformation to an aggressive lymphoma and a 3-fold increase in the development of acute myelogenous leukemia/myelodysplasia were observed among patients who received a nucleoside analog versus other therapies for their WM.

CD20-Directed Antibody Therapy

Rituximab is a chimeric monoclonal antibody that targets CD20, a widely expressed antigen on lymphoplasmacytic cells in WM (125). Several retrospective and prospective studies have indicated that rituximab, when used at standard dosimetry (i.e., four weekly infusions at 375 mg per m^2), induced major responses in approximately 27% to 35% of previously treated and untreated patients (126–132). Furthermore, it was shown in some of these studies that patients who achieved minor responses (MRs) or even stable disease (SD) benefited from rituximab, as evidenced by improved hemoglobin and platelet counts, and reduction of lymphadenopathy and/or splenomegaly. The median time to treatment failure in these studies was found to range from 8 to 27+ months. Studies evaluating an extended rituximab schedule consisting of four weekly courses at 375 mg per m^2 per week, repeated 3 months later by another 4-week course have demonstrated major response rates of 44% to 48%, with time to progression estimates of 16+ to 29+ months (132,133).

In many patients with WM, a transient increase of serum IgM may be noted immediately following initiation of treatment. Such an increase does not herald treatment failure, and although most patients will return to their baseline serum IgM level by 12 weeks, some continue to show prolonged spiking despite demonstrating a reduction in their bone marrow tumor load (134–136). However, patients with baseline serum IgM levels >50g per dL or serum viscosity >3.5 cp may be particularly at risk for a hyperviscosity related event, and in such patients plasmapheresis should be considered in advance of rituximab therapy (135). Because of the decreased likelihood of response in patients with higher IgM levels, as well as the possibility that serum IgM and viscosity levels may abruptly rise, rituximab monotherapy should not be used as sole therapy for the treatment of patients at risk for hyperviscosity symptoms.

Time to response after rituximab is slow and exceeds 3 months on the average. The time to best response in one study was 18 months (133). Patients with baseline serum IgM levels <60 g per dL are more likely to respond, regardless of the underlying bone marrow involvement by tumor cells (132,133). A recent analysis of 52 patients who were treated with single-agent rituximab has indicated that the objective response rate was significantly lower in patients who had either low serum albumin (<35 g per L) or elevated serum monoclonal protein (>40 g per L M spike). Furthermore, the presence of both adverse prognostic factors was related with a short time to progression (3.6 months). Moreover, patients who had normal serum albumin and relatively low serum monoclonal protein levels derived a substantial benefit from rituximab with a time to progression exceeding 40 months (137).

The genetic background of patients may also be important for determining response to rituximab. In particular, a correlation between polymorphisms at position 158 in the Fc γ RIIIa receptor (CD16), an activating Fc receptor on important effector cells that mediate antibody dependent cell-mediated cytotoxicity, and rituximab response was observed in patients with WM. Individuals may encode either the amino acid valine or phenylalanine at position 158 in the FcγRIIIa receptor. Patients with WM who carried the valine amino acid (either in a homozygous or heterozygous pattern) had a 4-fold higher major response rate (i.e., 50% decline in serum IgM levels) to rituximab versus those patients who expressed phenylalanine in a homozygous pattern (138).

Combination Therapies

Because rituximab is an active and nonmyelosuppressive agent, its combination with chemotherapy has been explored in patients with WM. Weber et al. (139) administered rituximab along with cladribine and cyclophosphamide to 17 previously untreated patients with WM. At least a partial response (PR) was documented in 94% of patients with WM, including a complete response (CR) in 18%. With a median follow-up of 21 months, no patient had relapse. In a study by the Waldenström's Macroglobulinemia Clinical Trials Group (WMCTG), the combination of rituximab and fludarabine was evaluated in 43 patients with WM, 32 (75%) of whom were previously untreated (140). Ninety-one percent of patients demonstrated at least a 25% decrease in serum IgM levels, and response rates were as follows: CR 7%, PR 74.4%, and MR 9.3%. Hematologic toxicity was common with grade III, IV neutropenia observed in 58% of patients. Two deaths occurred in this study, which may have been related to therapy induced immunosuppression. With a median follow-up of 17 months, 34 of 39 (87%) remain in remission. The addition of rituximab to fludarabine and cyclophosphamide has also been explored in the salvage setting by Tam et al. (141), wherein four of five patients demonstrated a response. In another combination study with rituximab, Hensel et al. (142) administered rituximab along with pentostatin and cyclophosphamide to 13 patients with untreated and previously treated WM or LPL. A major response was observed in 77% or patients. In a study by Dimopoulos et al. (143), the combination of rituximab, dexamethasone, and cyclophosphamide was used as primary therapy to treat 72 patients with WM. On an intent to treat basis, at least a major response was observed in 74% of patients. With a median follow-up of 24 months, 67% of patients are progression free. Therapy was well tolerated, though one patient died of interstitial pneumonia.

In addition to nucleoside analog-based trials with rituximab, two studies have examined cyclophosphamide, doxorubicin, vincristine, and prednisone (CHOP) in combination with rituximab. In a randomized frontline study by the German Low Grade Lymphoma Study Group involving 72 patients (71% of whom had LPL), a significantly higher response rate (94% vs. 69%) was observed among patients receiving CHOP in combination with rituximab versus CHOP, respectively (144). Treon et al. (145) have also evaluated CHOP in combination with rituximab in 13 patients with WM, eight and five of whom had relapse or were

refractory to nucleoside analogs and single-agent rituximab, respectively. Among 13 evaluable patients, ten patients achieved a major response (77%), including three CR and seven PR, and two patients achieved a MR.

The addition of alkylating agents to nucleoside analogs has also been explored in WM. Weber et al. (139) administered two cycles of oral cyclophosphamide along with subcutaneous cladribine to 37 patients with previously untreated WM. At least a PR was observed in 84% of patients, and the median duration of response was 36 months. Dimopoulos et al. (146) examined fludarabine in combination with IV cyclophosphamide and observed PRs in six of 11 (55%) patients with WM with either primary refractory disease or who had relapsed on treatment. The combination of fludarabine plus cyclophosphamide was also evaluated in a recent study by Tamburini et al. (147) involving 49 patients, 35 of whom were previously treated. Seventy-eight percent of the patients in this study achieved a response, and median time to treatment failure was 27 months. Hematologic toxicity was commonly observed, and three patients died of treatment-related toxicities. Two interesting findings in this study were the development of acute leukemia in two patients, histologic transformation to diffuse large cell lymphoma in one patient, and two cases of solid malignancies (prostate and melanoma), as well as failure to mobilize stem cells in four of six patients.

In view of the aforementioned data, the consensus panel on therapeutics amended its original recommendations for the therapy of WM to include the use of combination therapy with either nucleoside analogs and alkylator agents, or rituximab in combination with nucleoside analogs, nucleoside analogs plus alkylator agents, or combination chemotherapy such as CHOP as reasonable therapeutic options for the treatment of WM (103).

SALVAGE THERAPY INCLUDING NOVEL AGENTS

For patients in relapse or who have refractory disease, the consensus panels recommended the use of an alternative first-line agent as defined previously, with the caveat that for those patients for whom autologous transplantation was being seriously considered, further exposure to stem–cell-damaging agents (i.e., many alkylator agents and nucleoside analog drugs) should be avoided, and a nonstem cell-toxic agent should be considered if stem cells had not previously been harvested (102,103). Recent studies have also demonstrated activity for several novel agents, including bortezomib, thalidomide alone or in combination, and alemtuzumab can be considered in the treatment of relapsed/refractory WM. Finally, autologous stem cell transplant remains an option for the salvage therapy of WM, particularly among younger patients who have had multiple relapses, or have primary refractory disease.

Proteosome Inhibitor

Bortezomib, a stem cell-sparing agent (148,149), is a proteosome inhibitor that induces apoptosis of primary WM lymphoplasmacytic cells, as well as the WM-WSU WM cell line at pharmacologically achievable levels (150). Moreover, bortezomib may also impact on bone marrow microenvironmental support for lymphoplasmacytic cells (151). In a multicenter study of the WMCTG (152), 27 patients received up to eight cycles of bortezomib at 1.3 mg per m² on days 1, 4, 8, and 11. All but one patient had relapse/or refractory disease. Following therapy, median serum IgM levels declined from 4,660 to 2,092 mg per dL (p <0.0001). The ORR was 85%, with ten and 13 patients achieving a minor (<25% decrease in IgM) and major (<50% decrease in IgM) response, respectively. Responses were prompt and occurred at median age of 1.4 months. The median time to progression for all responding patients in this study was 7.9 (range 3 to 21.4+) months, and the most common grade III/IV toxicities occurring in ≥5% of patients were sensory neuropathies (22.2%), leukopenia (18.5%), neutropenia (14.8%), dizziness (11.1%), and thrombocytopenia (7.4%). Importantly, sensory neuropathies resolved or improved in nearly all patients following cessation of therapy. As part of a National Cancer Institute-Canada study, Chen et al. (153) treated 27 patients with both untreated (44%) and previously treated (56%) disease. Patients in this study received bortezomib utilizing the standard schedule until they either demonstrated progressive disease, or two cycles beyond a CR or SD. The ORR in this study was 78%, with major responses observed in 44% of patients. Sensory neuropathy occurred in 20 patients, five with grade >3, and occurred following two to four cycles of therapy. Among the 20 patients developing a neuropathy, 14 patients had resolution, and one patient demonstrated a 1-grade improvement at 2 to 13 months. In addition to the aforementioned experiences with bortezomib monotherapy in WM, Dimopoulos et al. (154) observed major responses in six of ten (60%) previously treated patients with WM, whereas Goy et al. (155) observed a major response in one of two patients with WM included in a series of patients with relapse or refractory disease with non-Hodgkin lymphoma (NHL). In view of the single-agent activity of bortezomib in WM, Treon et al. (156) have examined the combination of bortezomib, dexamethasone, and rituximab as primary therapy in patients with WM. An ORR of 96% and a major response rate of 78% were observed with the bortezomib, dexamethasone, and rituximab combination. The incidence of grade 3 neuropathy was about 30% in this study but was reversible in most patients following discontinuation of therapy. An increased incidence of herpes zoster was also observed, prompting the prophylactic use of antiviral therapy with bortezomib, dexamethasone, and rituximab. Alternative schedules for administration of bortezomib (i.e., once weekly at higher doses) in combination with rituximab are also being examined by Ghobrial (157) and Agathocleous (158) et al. in patients with WM, with ORRs of 80% to 90%. The impact of these schedules on the development of bortezomib-related peripheral neuropathy remains to be clarified, though in one study appeared diminished (157).

CD52-Directed Antibody Therapy

Alemtuzumab is a humanized monoclonal antibody that targets CD52, an antigen widely expressed on bone marrow LPC in patients with WM, as well as on mast cells that are increased in the bone marrow of patients with WM, and provide growth and survival signals to WM LPC through several tumor necrosis factor family ligands (CD40 ligand, APRIL, BLYS). As part of a WMCTG effort (159), 28 subjects with the Revised European American Lymphoma/World Health Organization clinicopathologic diagnosis of LPL, including 27 patients with IgM (WM) and one with IgA monoclonal gammopathy, were enrolled in this prospective, multicenter study. Five patients were untreated, and 23 were previously treated, all of whom had previously received rituximab. Patients received three daily test doses of alemtuzumab (3, 10, and 30 mg IV), followed by 30 mg alemtuzumab IV three times a week for up to 12 weeks. All patients received acyclovir and Bactrim or equivalent prophylaxis for the duration of therapy plus 8 weeks following the last infusion of alemtuzumab. Among 25 patients evaluable for response, the ORR was 76%, which included eight (32%) major responders, and 11 (44%) minor responders. Hematologic toxicities were common among previously treated (but not untreated) patients, and included grade 3/4 neutropenia 39%, thrombocytopenia 18%, and anemia 7%. Grade 3/4 nonhematologic toxicity for all patients included dermatitis 11%, fatigue 7%, and infection 7%. Cytomegalovirus (CMV) reactivation and infection were commonly seen among previously treated patients and may have been etiologic for one death on study. With a median follow-up of 8.5+ months, 11 of 19 responding patients remain free of progression. High rates of response with the use of alemtuzumab as salvage therapy have also been reported by Owen et al. (160) in a small series of heavily pretreated patients with WM (with a median prior therapies of four) who received up to 12 weeks of therapy (at 30 mg IV three times weekly) following initial dose escalation. Among the seven patients receiving alemtuzumab, five achieved a PR and one a CR. Infectious complications were common, with Cytomegalovirus (CMV) reactivation occurring in three patients requiring ganciclovir therapy, and hospitalization for three patients for bacterial infections. Opportunistic infections occurred in two patients and were responsible for their deaths. An upfront study by the WMCTG examining the role of alemtuzumab in combination with rituximab is anticipated, given the efficacy results of the aforementioned studies.

Thalidomide and Lenalidomide

Thalidomide as a single agent, and in combination with dexamethasone and clarithromycin, has also been examined in patients with WM, in view of the success of these regimens in patients with advanced multiple myeloma. Dimopoulos et al. (161) demonstrated a major response in five of 20 (25%) previously untreated and treated patients who received single-agent thalidomide. Dose escalation from the thalidomide start dose of 200 mg daily was hindered by development of side effects, including the development of peripheral neuropathy in five patients, obligating discontinuation or dose reduction. Low doses of thalidomide (50 mg orally daily) in combination with dexamethasone (40 mg orally once a week) and clarithromycin (250 mg orally twice a day) have also been examined, with ten of 12 (83%) previously treated patients demonstrating at least a major response (162). However, in a follow-up study by Dimopoulos et al. (163) using a higher thalidomide dose (200 mg orally daily) along with dexamethasone (40 g orally once a week) and clarithromycin (500 mg orally twice a day), only two of ten (20%) previously treated patients responded. In a previous study, the immunomodulators thalidomide and its analog lenalidomide significantly augmented rituximab mediated antibody dependent cell-mediated cytotoxicity against lymphoplasmacytic cells (164). Moreover, an expansion of natural killer cells has been observed with thalidomide, which in previous studies have been shown to be associated with rituximab response (165,166). In view of these data, the WMCTG conducted two phase II clinical trials in symptomatic patients with WM, combining thalidomide or lenalidomide with rituximab (167,168). Intended therapy for patients in the phase II study of thalidomide plus rituximab consisted of thalidomide administered at 200 mg daily for 2 weeks, followed by 400 mg daily thereafter for 1 year. Patients received four weekly infusions of rituximab at 375 mg per m^2 beginning 1 week after initiation of thalidomide, followed by four additional weekly infusions of rituximab at 375 mg per m^2 beginning at week 13. Twenty-three of 25 patients were evaluable in this study, and responses included CR ($n = 1$), PR ($n = 15$), MR ($n = 2$), and SD ($n = 1$), for an ORR and a major response rate of 72% and 64% on an intent to treat basis, respectively. Median serum IgM levels decreased from 3,670 (924 to 8,610 mg per dL) to 1,590 (36 to 5,230 mg per dL) ($p < 0.001$), whereas the median hematocrit rose from 33.0 (23.6% to 42.6%) to 37.6 (29.3% to 44.3%) ($p = 0.004$) at best response. The median time to progression (TTP) for evaluable patients in this study was 35 months, and 38 months for responders. Responses were unaffected by FcγRIIIA-158 polymorphism status (81% vs. 71% for VV/FV vs. FF), IgM (78% vs. 80% for <6,000 vs. ≥6,000 mg per dL), and B$_2$M (71% vs. 89% for <3 vs. ≥3 g per dL). Dose reduction of thalidomide occurred in all patients and led to discontinuation in 11 patients. Among 11 patients experiencing grade ≥2 neuro-paresthesias, ten demonstrated resolution to grade 1 ($n = 3$) or complete resolution ($n = 7$) at a median of 6.7 (range 0.4 to 22.5) months.

In a phase II study of lenalidomide and rituximab in WM (168), patients were initiated on lenalidomide at 25 mg daily on a syncopated schedule wherein therapy was administered for 3 weeks, followed by a 1-week pause for an intended duration of 48 weeks. Patients received 1 week of therapy with lenalidomide, after which rituximab (375 mg per m^2) was administered weekly on weeks 2 to 5, then 13 to 16. Twelve of 16 patients were evaluable, and responses included PR ($n = 4$), MR ($n = 4$), SD ($n = 3$), and no response (NR) ($n = 1$), for an overall and major response rate of 50% and 25%, on an intent to treat basis, respectively. The median time to progression (TTP) for responders was 18.9 months in this study. In two patients with bulky disease, significant reduction in node/spleen size was observed. Acute decreases in hematocrit were observed during first 2 weeks of lenalidomide therapy in 13 of 16 (81%) patients with a median hematocrit decrease of 4.4% (1.7% to 7.2%), resulting in hospitalization in four patients. Despite reduction of initiation doses to 5 mg daily, anemia continued to be problematic without evidence of hemolysis or more general myelosuppression. Therefore, the mechanism for pronounced anemia in patients with WM receiving lenalidomide remains to be determined, and the use of this agent among patients with WM remains investigational.

HIGH-DOSE THERAPY AND STEM CELL TRANSPLANTATION

The use of transplant therapy has also been explored in patients with WM. Desikan et al. (169) reported their initial experience of high-dose chemotherapy and autologous stem cell transplant, which has more recently been updated by Munshi and Barlogie (170). Their studies involved eight previously treated patients with WM between the ages of 45 and 69 years, who received either melphalan at 200 mg per m^2 ($n = 7$) or melphalan at 140 mg per m^2 along with total body irradiation. Stem cells were successfully collected in all eight patients, although a second collection procedure was required for two patients who had extensive previous nucleoside analog exposure. There were no transplant-related mortalities, and toxicities were manageable. All eight patients responded, with seven of eight achieving a major response, and one patient achieving a CR with durations of response raging from 5+ to 77+ months. Dreger et al. (171) investigated the use of the dexamethasone, BCNU, etoposide, cytarabine, melphalan regimen followed by myeloablative therapy with cyclophosphamide, and total body irradiation and autologous stem cell transplantation in seven patients with WM, which included four untreated patients. Serum IgM levels declined by >50% following dexamethasone, BCNU, etoposide, cytarabine, and melphalan and myeloablative therapy for six of seven patients, with progression-free survival ranging from 4+ to 30+ months. All three evaluable patients, who were previously treated, also attained a major response in a study by Anagnostopoulos et al. (172), in which patients with WM received various preparative regimens and showed event-free survivals of 26+, 31, and 108+ months. Tournilhac et al. (173) recently reported the outcome of 18 patients with WM in France who received high-dose chemotherapy followed by autologous stem cell transplantation. All patients were previously treated with a median of three (range one to five) prior regimens. Therapy was well tolerated with an improvement in response status observed for seven patients (six PR to CR; one SD to PR), whereas only one patient demonstrated progressive disease. The median event-free survival for all patients without progression was 12 months. Tournilhac et al. (173) have also reported the outcome of allogeneic transplantation in ten previously treated patients with WM (ages 35 to 46) who received a median of three prior therapies, including three patients with progressive disease despite therapy. Two of three patients with progressive disease responded, and an improvement in response status was observed in five patients. The median event-free survival for nonprogressing, evaluable patients was 31 months. Concerning in this series was the death of three patients owing to transplantation-related toxicity. Anagnostopoulos et al. (174) have also reported on a retrospective review of patients with WM who underwent either autologous or allogeneic transplantation, and whose outcomes were reported to the Center for International Blood and Marrow Transplant Research. Seventy-eight percent of patients in this cohort had two or more previous therapies, and 58% of them were resistant to their previous therapy. The relapse rate at 3 years was 29% in the allogeneic group, and 24% in the autologous group. Nonrelapse mortality, however, was 40% in the allogeneic group and 11% in the autologous group in this series. In view of the high rate of nonrelapse mortality

TABLE 14.4

SUMMARY OF UPDATED RESPONSE CRITERIA FROM THE THIRD INTERNATIONAL WORKSHOPS ON WALDENSTRÖM'S MACROGLOBULINEMIA

Complete response	CR	Disappearance of monoclonal protein by immunofixation; no histologic evidence of bone marrow involvement, and resolution of any adenopathy/organomegaly (confirmed by computed tomography scan), along with no signs or symptoms attributable to WM. Reconfirmation of the CR status is required at least 6 weeks apart with a second immunofixation.
Partial response	PR	A ≥50% reduction of serum monoclonal IgM concentration on protein electrophoresis and ≥50% decrease in adenopathy/organomegaly on physical examination or on computed tomography scan. No new symptoms or signs of active disease.
Minor response	MR	A ≥25% but <50% reduction of serum monoclonal IgM by protein electrophoresis. No new symptoms or signs of active disease.
Stable disease	SD	A <25% reduction and <25% increase of serum monoclonal IgM by electrophoresis without progression of adenopathy/organomegaly, cytopenias, or clinically significant symptoms due to disease and/or signs of WM.
Progressive disease	PD	A ≥25% increase in serum monoclonal IgM by protein electrophoresis confirmed by a second measurement or progression of clinically significant findings due to disease (i.e., anemia, thrombocytopenia, leukopenia, bulky adenopathy/organomegaly) or symptoms (unexplained recurrent fever ≥38.4°C, drenching night sweats, ≥10% body weight loss, or hyperviscosity, neuropathy, symptomatic cryoglobulinemia or amyloidosis) attributable to WM.

Adapted from Anagnostopoulos A, Hari PN, Perez WS et al. Autologous or allogeneic stem cell transplantation in patients with Waldenstrom's macroglobulinemia. *Biol Blood Marrow Transplant* 2006;12:845–854, with permission.

associated with high-dose chemotherapy and allogeneic transplantation, Maloney et al. (175) have evaluated the use of nonmyeloablative allogeneic transplantation in five patients with refractory WM. In this series, three of three evaluable patients (all of whom had matched sibling donors) responded with two CR and one in PR at 1 to 3 years after transplant. In view of the aforementioned data, the consensus panel on therapeutics for WM has recommended that autologous transplantation in WM be considered in the relapsed setting, particularly among younger patients who have had multiple relapses or primary refractory disease, whereas allogeneic and mini-allogeneic transplantation should be undertaken ideally in the context of a clinical trial (102,103).

RESPONSE CRITERIA IN WALDENSTRÖM MACROGLOBULINEMIA

Assessment of response to WM treatment has been widely heterogeneous. As a consequence, studies using the same regimen have reported significantly different response rates. As part of the Second and Third International Workshops on Waldenström's Macroglobulinemia, consensus panels developed guidelines for uniform response criteria in WM (176,177). The category of MR was adopted at the Third International Workshops on Waldenström's Macroglobulinemia, given that clinically meaningful responses were observed with newer biologic agents, and is based on a ≥25% to <50% decrease in serum IgM level, which is used as a surrogate marker of disease in WM. In distinction, the term "major response" is used to denote a response of ≥50% in serum IgM levels, and includes partial and CRs (174). Response categories and criteria for progressive disease in WM based on consensus recommendations are summarized in Table 14.4. An important concern with the use of

IgM as a surrogate marker of disease is that it can fluctuate, independent of tumor cell killing, particularly with newer biologically targeted agents such as rituximab and bortezomib (134–136,152,178). Rituximab induces a spike or flare in serum IgM levels that can last for months, whereas bortezomib can suppress IgM levels independent of tumor cell killing in certain patients. In circumstances where the serum IgM levels appear out of context with the clinical progress of the patient, a bone marrow biopsy should be considered to clarify the patient's underlying disease burden. Soluble CD27 is currently being investigated by Ho et al. (34) as an alternative surrogate marker in WM.

References

1. Owen RG, Treon SP, Al-Katib A, et al. Clinicopathological definition of Waldenström's macroglobulinemia: Consensus Panel Recommendations from the Second International Workshop on Waldenström's macroglobulinemia. *Semin Oncol* 2003;30:110–115.
2. Harris NL, Jaffe ES, Stein H, et al. A revised European-American classification of lymphoid neoplasms: a proposal from the International Lymphoma Study Group. *Blood* 1994; 84:1361–1392.
3. Harris NL, Jaffe ES, Diebold J, et al. The World Health Organization classification of neoplastic diseases of the hematopoietic and lymphoid tissues. Report of the Clinical Advisory Committee meeting, Airlie House, Virginia, November, 1997. *Ann Oncol* 1999; 10:1419–1432.
4. Groves FD, Travis LB, Devesa SS, et al. Waldenström's macroglobulinemia: incidence patterns in the United States, 1988–1994. *Cancer* 1998; 82:1078–1081.
5. Herrinton LJ, Weiss NS. Incidence of Waldenström's macroglobulinemia. *Blood* 1993; 82:3148–3150.
6. Bjornsson OG, Arnason A, Gudmunosson S, et al. Macroglobulinaemia in an Icelandic family. *Acta Med Scand* 1978;203:283–288.
7. Treon SP, Hunter ZR, Aggarwal A, et al. Characterization of familial Waldenström's macroglobulinemia. *Ann Oncol* 2006;17:488–494.
8. Renier G, Ifrah N, Chevailler A, et al. Four brothers with Waldenström's macroglobulinemia. *Cancer* 1989;64:1554–1559.
9. Ogmundsdottir HM, Sveinsdottir S, Sigfusson A, et al. Enhanced B cell survival in familial macroglobulinaemia is associated with increased expression of Bcl-2. *Clin Exp Immunol* 1999;117:252–260.
10. Linet MS, Humphrey RL, Mehl ES, et al. A case-control and family study of Waldenström's macroglobulinemia. *Leukemia* 1993;7:1363–1369.

11. Santini GF, Crovatto M, Modolo ML, et al. Waldenström macroglobulinemia: a role of HCV infection? *Blood* 1993; 82:2932.

12. Silvestri F, Barillari G, Fanin R, et al. Risk of hepatitis C virus infection, Waldenström's macroglobulinemia, and monoclonal gammopathies. *Blood* 1996; 88:1125–1126.

13. Leleu X, O'Connor K, Ho A, et al. Hepatitis C viral infection is not associated with Waldenstrom's macroglobulinemia. *Am J Hematol* 2007;82: 83–84.

14. Carbone P, Caradonna F, Granata G, et al. Chromosomal abnormalities in Waldenstrom's macroglobulinemia. *Cancer Genet Cytogenet* 1992;61: 147–151.

15. Mansoor A, Medeiros LJ, Weber DM, et al. Cytogenetic findings in lymphoplasmacytic lymphoma/Waldenström macroglobulinemia. Chromosomal abnormalities are associated with the polymorphous subtype and an aggressive clinical course. *Am J Clin Pathol* 2001;116:543–549.

16. Han T, Sadamori N, Takeuchi J, et al. Clonal chromosome abnormalities in patients with Waldenstrom's and CLL-associated macroglobulinemia: significance of trisomy 12. *Blood* 1983;62:525–531.

17. Rivera AI, Li MM, Beltran G, et al. Trisomy 4 as the sole cytogenetic abnormality in a Waldenstrom macroglobulinemia. *Cancer Genet Cytogenet* 2002;133:172–173.

18. Wong KF, So CC, Chan JC, et al. Gain of chromosome 3/3q in B-cell chronic lymphoproliferative disorder is associated with plasmacytoid differentiation with or without IgM overproduction. *Cancer Genet Cytogenet* 2002;136:82–85.

19. Schop RF, Kuehl WM, Van Wier SA, et al. Waldenström macroglobulinemia neoplastic cells lack immunoglobulin heavy chain locus translocations but have frequent 6q deletions. *Blood* 2002;100:2996–3001.

20. Avet-Loiseau H, Garand R, Lode L, et al. 14q32 translocations discriminate IgM multiple myeloma from Waldenström's macroglobulinemia. *Semin Oncol* 2003;30:153–155.

21. Preud'homme JL, Seligmann M. Immunoglobulins on the surface of lymphoid cells in Waldenström's macroglobulinemia. *J Clin Invest* 1972; 51:701–705.

22. Smith BR, Robert NJ, Ault KA. In Waldenstrom's macroglobulinemia the quantity of detectable circulating monoclonal B lymphocytes correlates with clinical course. *Blood* 1983;61:911–914.

23. Levy Y, Fermand JP, Navarro S, et al. Interleukin 6 dependence of spontaneous in vitro differentiation of B cells from patients with IgM gammopathy. *Proc Natl Acad Sci U S A* 1990; 87:3309–3313.

24. Owen RG, Barrans SL, Richards SJ, et al. Waldenström macroglobulinemia. Development of diagnostic criteria and identification of prognostic factors. *Am J Clin Pathol* 2001;116:420–428.

25. Feiner HD, Rizk CC, Finfer MD, et al. IgM monoclonal gammopathy/Waldenström's macroglobulinemia: a morphological and immunophenotypic study of the bone marrow. *Mod Pathol* 1990;3:348–356.

26. San Miguel JF, Vidriales MB, Ocio E, et al. Immunophenotypic analysis of Waldenström's macroglobulinemia. *Semin Oncol* 2003;30:187–195.

27. Hunter ZR, Branagan AR, Manning R, et al. CD5, CD10, CD23 expression in Waldenström's macroglobulinemia. *Clin Lymphoma* 2005;5:246–249.

28. Wagner SD, Martinelli V, Luzzatto L. Similar patterns of V kappa gene usage but different degrees of somatic mutation in hairy cell leukemia, prolymphocytic leukemia, Waldenström's macroglobulinemia, and myeloma. *Blood* 1994;83:3647–3653.

29. Aoki H, Takishita M, Kosaka M, et al. Frequent somatic mutations in D and/or JH segments of Ig gene in Waldenström's macroglobulinemia and chronic lymphocytic leukemia (CLL) with Richter's syndrome but not in common CLL. *Blood* 1995;85:1913–1919.

30. Shiokawa S, Suehiro Y, Uike N, et al. Sequence and expression analyses of mu and delta transcripts in patients with Waldenström's macroglobulinemia. *Am J Hematol* 2001;68:139–143.

31. Sahota SS, Forconi F, Ottensmeier CH, et al. Typical Waldenström macroglobulinemia is derived from a B-cell arrested after cessation of somatic mutation but prior to isotype switch events. *Blood* 2002;100:1505–1507.

32. Paramithiotis E, Cooper MD. Memory B lymphocytes migrate to bone marrow in humans. *Proc Natl Acad Sci U S A* 1997;94:208–212.

33. Tournilhac O, Santos DD, Xu L, et al. Mast cells in Waldenström's Macroglobulinemia support lymphoplasmacytic cell growth through CD154/CD40 signaling. *Ann Oncol* 2006;17:1275–1282.

34. Ho A, Leleu X, Ciccarelli BT, et al. CD27-CD70 interactions in the pathogenesis of Waldenstrom macroglobulinemia. *Blood* 2008;112:4683–4689.

35. Merlini G, Farhangi M, Osserman EF. Monoclonal immunoglobulins with antibody activity in myeloma, macroglobulinemia and related plasma cell dyscrasias. *Semin Oncol* 1986;13:350–365.

36. Farhangi M, Merlini G. The clinical implications of monoclonal immunoglobulins. *Semin Oncol* 1986;13:366–379.

37. Marmont AM, Merlini G. Monoclonal autoimmunity in hematology. *Haematologica* 1991;76:449–459.

38. Mackenzie MR, Babcock J. Studies of the hyperviscosity syndrome. II. Macroglobulinemia. *J Lab Clin Med* 1975;85:227–234.

39. Gertz MA, Kyle RA. Hyperviscosity syndrome. *J Intensive Care Med* 1995;10:128–141.

40. Kwaan HC, Bongu A. The hyperviscosity syndromes. *Semin Thromb Hemost* 1999;25:199–208.

41. Singh A, Eckardt KU, Zimmermann A, et al. Increased plasma viscosity as a reason for inappropriate erythropoietin formation. *J Clin Invest* 1993;91:251–256.

42. Menke MN, Feke GT, McMeel JW, et al. Hyperviscosity-related retinopathy in Waldenstrom's macroglobulinemia. *Arch Opthalmol* 2006;124: 1601–1606.

43. Merlini G, Baldini L, Broglia C, et al. Prognostic factors in symptomatic Waldenström's macroglobulinemia. *Semin Oncol* 2003; 30:211–215.

44. Dellagi K, Dupouey P, Brouet JC, et al. Waldenström's macroglobulinemia and peripheral neuropathy: a clinical and immunologic study of 25 patients. *Blood* 1983;62:280–285.

45. Nobile-Orazio E, Marmiroli P, Baldini L, et al. Peripheral neuropathy in macroglobulinemia: incidence and antigen-specificity of M proteins. *Neurology* 1987;37:1506–1514.

46. Nemni R, Gerosa E, Piccolo G, et al. Neuropathies associated with monoclonal gammapathies. *Haematologica* 1994;79:557–566.

47. Ropper AH, Gorson KC. Neuropathies associated with paraproteinemia. *N Engl J Med* 1998;338:1601–1607.

48. Vital A. Paraproteinemic neuropathies. *Brain Pathol* 2001;11:399–407.

49. Latov N, Braun PE, Gross RB, et al. Plasma cell dyscrasia and peripheral neuropathy: identification of the myelin antigens that react with human paraproteins. *Proc Natl Acad Sci U S A* 1981; 78:7139–7142.

50. Chassande B, Leger JM, Younes-Chennoufi AB, et al. Peripheral neuropathy associated with IgM monoclonal gammopathy: correlations between M-protein antibody activity and clinical/electrophysiological features in 40 cases. *Muscle Nerve* 1998; 21:55–62.

51. Weiss MD, Dalakas MC, Lauter CJ, et al. Variability in the binding of anti-MAG and anti-SGPG antibodies to target antigens in demyelinating neuropathy and IgM paraproteinemia. *J Neuroimmunol* 1999;95:174–184.

52. Latov N, Hays AP, Sherman WH. Peripheral neuropathy and anti-MAG antibodies. *Crit Rev Neurobiol* 1988;3:301–332.

53. Dalakas MC, Quarles RH. Autoimmune ataxic neuropathies (sensory ganglionopathies): are glycolipids the responsible autoantigens? *Ann Neurol* 1996;39:419–422.

54. Eurelings M, Ang CW, Notermans NC, et al. Antiganglioside antibodies in polyneuropathy associated with monoclonal gammopathy. *Neurology* 2001;57:1909–1912.

55. Ilyas AA, Quarles RH, Dalakas MC, et al. Monoclonal IgM in a patient with paraproteinemic polyneuropathy binds to gangliosides containing disialosyl groups. *Ann Neurol* 1985;18:655–659.

56. Willison HJ, O'Leary CP, Veitch J, et al. The clinical and laboratory features of chronic sensory ataxic neuropathy with anti-disialosyl IgM antibodies. *Brain* 2001;124:1968–1977.

57. Lopate G, Choksi R, Pestronk A. Severe sensory ataxia and demyelinating polyneuropathy with IgM anti-GM2 and GalNAc-GD1A antibodies. *Muscle Nerve* 2002;25:828–836.

58. Jacobs BC, O'Hanlon GM, Breedland EG, et al. Human IgM paraproteins demonstrate shared reactivity between Campylobacter jejuni lipopolysaccharides and human peripheral nerve disialylated gangliosides. *J Neuroimmunol* 1997;80:23–30.

59. Nobile-Orazio E, Manfredini E, Carpo M, et al. Frequency and clinical correlates of antineural IgM antibodies in neuropathy associated with IgM monoclonal gammopathy. *Ann Neurol* 1994;36:416–424.

60. Gordon PH, Rowland LP, Younger DS, et al. Lymphoproliferative disorders and motor neuron disease: an update. *Neurology* 1997;48:1671–1678.

61. Pavord SR, Murphy PT, Mitchell VE. POEMS syndrome and Waldenström's macroglobulinemia. *J Clin Pathol* 1996;49:181–182.

62. Crisp D, Pruzanski W. B-cell neoplasms with homogeneous cold-reacting antibodies (cold agglutinins). *Am J Med* 1982;72:915–922.

63. Pruzanski W, Shumak KH. Biologic activity of cold-reacting autoantibodies (first of two parts). *N Engl J Med* 1977;297:538–542.

64. Pruzanski W, Shumak KH. Biologic activity of cold-reacting autoantibodies (second of two parts). *N Engl J Med* 1977;297:583–589.

65. Whittaker SJ, Bhogal BS, Black MM. Acquired immunobullous disease: a cutaneous manifestation of IgM macroglobulinaemia. *Br J Dermatol* 1996;135:283–286.

66. Daoud MS, Lust JA, Kyle RA, et al. Monoclonal gammopathies and associated skin disorders. *J Am Acad Dermatol* 1999;40:507–535.

67. Gad A, Willen R, Carlen B, et al. Duodenal involvement in Waldenström's macroglobulinemia. *J Clin Gastroenterol* 1995;20:174–176.

68. Case records of the Massachusetts General Hospital. Weekly clinicopathological exercises. Case 3-1990. A 66-year-old woman with Waldenström's macroglobulinemia, diarrhea, anemia, and persistent gastrointestinal bleeding. *N Engl J Med* 1990;322:183–192.

69. Isaac J, Herrera GA. Cast nephropathy in a case of Waldenström's macroglobulinemia. *Nephron* 2002;91:512–515.

70. Morel-Maroger L, Basch A, Danon F, et al. Pathology of the kidney in Waldenström's macroglobulinemia. Study of sixteen cases. *N Engl J Med* 1970;283:123–129.

71. Gertz MA, Kyle RA, Noel P. Primary systemic amyloidosis: a rare complication of immunoglobulin M monoclonal gammopathies and Waldenström's macroglobulinemia. *J Clin Oncol* 1993;11:914–920.

72. Moyner K, Sletten K, Husby G, et al. An unusually large (83 amino acid residues) amyloid fibril protein AA from a patient with Waldenström's macroglobulinaemia and amyloidosis. *Scand J Immunol* 1980;11:549–554.

73. Gardyn J, Schwartz A, Gal R, et al. Waldenström's macroglobulinemia associated with AA amyloidosis. *Int J Hematol* 2001;74:76–78.

74. Dussol B, Kaplanski G, Daniel L, et al. Simultaneous occurrence of fibrillary glomerulopathy and AL amyloid. *Nephrol Dial Transplant* 1998;13:2630–2632.

75. Rausch PG, Herion JC. Pulmonary manifestations of Waldenström macroglobulinemia. *Am J Hematol* 1980;9:201–209.

76. Fadil A, Taylor DE. The lung and Waldenström's macroglobulinemia. *South Med J* 1998;91:681–685.

77. Kyrtsonis MC, Angelopoulou MK, Kontopidou FN, et al. Primary lung involvement in Waldenström's macroglobulinaemia: report of two cases and review of the literature. *Acta Haematol* 2001;105:92–96.

78. Kaila VL, el Newihi HM, Dreiling BJ, et al. Waldenström's macroglobulinemia of the stomach presenting with upper gastrointestinal hemorrhage. *Gastrointest Endosc* 1996;44:73–75.

79. Yasui O, Tukamoto F, Sasaki N, et al. Malignant lymphoma of the transverse colon associated with macroglobulinemia. *Am J Gastroenterol* 1997;92:2299–2301.

80. Rosenthal JA, Curran WJ Jr, Schuster SJ. Waldenström's macroglobulinemia resulting from localized gastric lymphoplasmacytoid lymphoma. *Am J Hematol* 1998;58:244–245.

81. Recine MA, Perez MT, Cabello-Inchausti B, et al. Extranodal lymphoplasmacytoid lymphoma (immunocytoma) presenting as small intestinal obstruction. *Arch Pathol Lab Med* 2001;125:677–679.

82. Veltman GA, van Veen S, Kluin-Nelemans JC, et al. Renal disease in Waldenström's macroglobulinaemia. *Nephrol Dial Transplant* 1997;12:1256–1259.

83. Moore DF Jr, Moulopoulos LA, Dimopoulos MA. Waldenström macroglobulinemia presenting as a renal or perirenal mass: clinical and radiographic features. *Leuk Lymphoma* 1995;17:331–334.

84. Mascaro JM, Montserrat E, Estrach T, et al. Specific cutaneous manifestations of Waldenström's macroglobulinaemia. A report of two cases. *Br J Dermatol* 1982;106:17–22.

85. Schnitzler L, Schubert B, Boasson M, et al. Urticaire chronique, lésions osseuses, macroglobulinémie IgM: Maladie de Waldenström? *Bull Soc Fr Dermatol Syphiligr* 1974;81:363–368.

86. Roux S, Fermand JP, Brechignac S, et al. Tumoral joint involvement in multiple myeloma and Waldenström's macroglobulinemia–report of 4 cases. *J Rheumatol* 1996;23:2175–2178.

87. Orellana J, Friedman AH. Ocular manifestations of multiple myeloma, Waldenström's macroglobulinemia and benign monoclonal gammopathy. *Surv Ophthalmol* 1981;26:157–169.

88. Ettl AR, Birbamer GG, Philipp W. Orbital involvement in Waldenström's macroglobulinemia: ultrasound, computed tomography and magnetic resonance findings. *Ophthalmologica* 1992;205:40–45.

89. Civit T, Coulbois S, Baylac F, et al. Waldenström's macroglobulinemia and cerebral lymphoplasmocytic proliferation: Bing and Neel syndrome. Apropos of a new case [in French]. *Neurochirurgie* 1997;43:245–249.

90. McMullin MF, Wilkin HJ, Elder E. Inaccurate haemoglobin estimation in Waldenström's macroglobulinaemia. *J Clin Pathol* 1995;48:787.

91. Treon SP, Branagan AR, Hunter Z, et al. IgA and IgG hypogammaglobulinemia persists in most patients with Waldenstrom's macroglobulinemia despite therapeutic responses, including complete remissions. *Blood* 2004;104:306b.

92. Hunter Z, Leleu X, Hatjiharissi E, et al. IgA and IgG hypogammaglobulinemia are associated with mutations in the APRIL/BLYS receptor TACI in Waldenstrom's macroglobulinemia (WM). *Blood* 2006;108:228.

93. Dutcher TF, Fahey JL. The histopathology of macroglobulinemia of Waldenström. *J Natl Cancer Inst* 1959;22:887–917.

94. Moulopoulos LA, Dimopoulos MA, Varma DG, et al. Waldenström macroglobulinemia: MR imaging of the spine and CT of the abdomen and pelvis. *Radiology* 1993;188:669–673.

95. Gobbi PG, Bettini R, Montecucco C, et al. Study of prognosis in Waldenström's macroglobulinemia: a proposal for a simple binary classification with clinical and investigational utility. *Blood* 1994;83:2939–2945.

96. Morel P, Monconduit M, Jacomy D, et al. Prognostic factors in Waldenström macroglobulinemia: a report on 232 patients with the description of a new scoring system and its validation on 253 other patients. *Blood* 2000;96:852–858.

97. Dhodapkar MV, Jacobson JL, Gertz MA, et al. Prognostic factors and response to fludarabine therapy in patients with Waldenström macroglobulinemia: results of United States intergroup trial (Southwest Oncology Group S9003). *Blood* 2001;98:41–48.

98. Kyle RA, Treon SP, Alexanian R, et al. Prognostic markers and criteria to initiate therapy in Waldenström's macroglobulinemia: Consensus Panel Recommendations from the Second International Workshop on Waldenström's macroglobulinemia. *Semin Oncol* 2003;30:116–120.

99. Dimopoulos M, Gika D, Zervas K, et al. The international staging system for multiple myeloma is applicable in symptomatic Waldenstrom's macroglobulinemia. *Leuk Lymph* 2004;45:1809–1813.

100. Anagnostopoulos A, Zervas K, Kyrtsonis M, et al. Prognostic value of serum beta 2-microglobulin in patients with Waldenstrom's macroglobulinemia requiring therapy. *Clin Lymphoma Myeloma* 2006;7:205–209.

101. Morel P, Duhamel A, Gobbi P, et al. International prognostic scoring system (IPSS) for Waldenstrom's macroglobulinemia. *Blood* 2006;108:42a.

102. Gertz M, Anagnostopoulos A, Anderson KC, et al. Treatment recommendations in Waldenström's macroglobulinemia: Consensus Panel Recommendations from the Second International Workshop on Waldenström's macroglobulinemia. *Semin Oncol* 2003;30:121–126.

103. Treon SP, Gertz MA, Dimopoulos M, et al. Update on treatment recommendations from the Third International Workshop on Waldenström's Macroglobulinemia. *Blood* 2006;107:3442–3446.

104. Kyle RA, Greipp PR, Gertz MA, et al. Waldenström's macroglobulinaemia: a prospective study comparing daily with intermittent oral chlorambucil. *Br J Haematol* 2000;108:737–742.

105. Dimopoulos MA, Alexanian R. Waldenström's macroglobulinemia. *Blood* 1994;83:1452–1459.

106. Petrucci MT, Avvisati G, Tribalto M, et al. Waldenström's macroglobulinaemia: results of a combined oral treatment in 34 newly diagnosed patients. *J Intern Med* 1989;226:443–447.

107. Case DC Jr, Ervin TJ, Boyd MA, et al. Waldenström's macroglobulinemia: long-term results with the M-2 protocol. *Cancer Invest* 1991;9:1–7.

108. Facon T, Brouillard M, Duhamel A, et al. Prognostic factors in Waldenström's macroglobulinemia: a report of 167 cases. *J Clin Oncol* 1993;11:1553–558.

109. Dimopoulos MA, Kantarjian H, Weber D, et al. Primary therapy of Waldenström's macroglobulinemia with 2-chlorodeoxyadenosine. *J Clin Oncol* 1994;12:2694–2698.

110. Delannoy A, Ferrant A, Martiat P, et al. 2-Chlorodeoxyadenosine therapy in Waldenström's macroglobulinaemia. *Nouv Rev Fr Hematol* 1994;36:317–320.

111. Fridrik MA, Jager G, Baldinger C, et al. First-line treatment of Waldenström's disease with cladribine. Arbeitsgemeinschaft Medikamentose Tumortherapie. *Ann Hematol* 1997;74:7–10.

112. Liu ES, Burian C, Miller WE, et al. Bolus administration of cladribine in the treatment of Waldenström macroglobulinaemia. *Br J Haematol* 1998;103:690–695.

113. Hellmann A, Lewandowski K, Zaucha JM, et al. Effect of a 2-hour infusion of 2-chlorodeoxyadenosine in the treatment of refractory or previously untreated Waldenström's macroglobulinemia. *Eur J Haematol* 1999;63:35–41.

114. Betticher DC, Hsu Schmitz SF, Ratschiller D, et al. Cladribine (2-CDA) given as subcutaneous bolus injections is active in pretreated Waldenström's macroglobulinaemia. Swiss Group for Clinical Cancer Research (SAKK). *Br J Haematol* 1997;99:358–363.

115. Dimopoulos MA, Weber D, Delasalle KB, et al. Treatment of Waldenström's macroglobulinemia resistant to standard therapy with 2-chlorodeoxyadenosine: identification of prognostic factors. *Ann Oncol* 1995;6:49–52.

116. Dimopoulos MA, O'Brien S, Kantarjian H, et al. Fludarabine therapy in Waldenström's macroglobulinemia. *Am J Med* 1993;95:49–52.

117. Foran JM, Rohatiner AZ, Coiffier B, et al. Multicenter phase II study of fludarabine phosphate for patients with newly diagnosed lymphoplasmacytoid lymphoma, Waldenström's macroglobulinemia, and mantle-cell lymphoma. *J Clin Oncol* 1999;17:546–553.

118. Thalhammer-Scherrer R, Geissler K, Schwarzinger I, et al. Fludarabine therapy in Waldenström's macroglobulinemia. *Ann Hematol* 2000;79:556–559.

119. Dhodapkar MV, Jacobson JL, Gertz MA, et al. Prognostic factors and response to fludarabine therapy in patients with Waldenström macroglobulinemia: results of United States intergroup trial (Southwest Oncology Group S9003). *Blood* 2001;98:41–48.

120. Zinzani PL, Gherlinzoni F, Bendandi M, et al. Fludarabine treatment in resistant Waldenström's macroglobulinemia. *Eur J Haematol* 1995;54:120–123.

121. Leblond V, Ben Othman T, Deconinck E, et al. Activity of fludarabine in previously treated Waldenström's macroglobulinemia: a report of 71 cases. Groupe Cooperatif Macroglobulinemie. *J Clin Oncol* 1998;16:2060–2064.

122. Dimopoulos MA, Weber DM, Kantarjian H, et al. 2Chlorodeoxyadenosine therapy of patients with Waldenström macroglobulinemia previously treated with fludarabine. *Ann Oncol* 1994;5:288–289.

123. Lewandowski K, Halaburda K, Hellmann A. Fludarabine therapy in Waldenström's macroglobulinemia patients treated previously with 2-chlorodeoxyadenosine. *Leuk Lymphoma* 2002;43:361–363.

124. Leleu X, Soumerai J, Roccaro A, et al. Increased incidence of Transformation and Myelodysplasia/Acute Leukemia in patients with Waldenstrom's Macroglobulinemia treated with Nucleoside Analogues. *J Clin Oncol* 2009;27:250–5.

125. Treon SP, Kelliher A, Keele B, et al. Expression of serotherapy target antigens in Waldenström's macroglobulinemia: therapeutic applications and considerations. *Semin Oncol* 2003;30:248–252.

126. Treon SP, Shima Y, Preffer FI, et al. Treatment of plasma cell dyscrasias with antibody-mediated immunotherapy. *Semin Oncol* 1999;26(suppl 14):97–106.

127. Byrd JC, White CA, Link B, et al. Rituximab therapy in Waldenstrom's macroglobulinemia: preliminary evidence of clinical activity. *Ann Oncol* 1999;10:1525–527.

128. Weber DM, Gavino M, Huh Y, et al. Phenotypic and clinical evidence supports rituximab for Waldenstrom's macroglobulinemia. *Blood* 1999; 94:125a.

129. Foran JM, Rohatiner AZ, Cunningham D, et al. European phase II study of rituximab (chimeric anti-CD20 monoclonal antibody) for patients with newly diagnosed mantle-cell lymphoma and previously treated mantle-cell lymphoma, immunocytoma, and small B-cell lymphocytic lymphoma. *J Clin Oncol* 2000;18:317–324.

130. Treon SP, Agus DB, Link B, et al. CD20-Directed antibody-mediated immunotherapy induces responses and facilitates hematologic recovery in patients with Waldenstrom's macroglobulinemia. *J Immunother* 2001;24: 272–279.

131. Gertz MA, Rue M, Blood E, et al. Multicenter phase 2 trial of rituximab for Waldenstrom macroglobulinemia (WM): an Eastern Cooperative Oncology Group Study (E3A98). *Leuk Lymphoma* 2004;45:2047–2055.

132. Dimopoulos MA, Zervas C, Zomas A, et al. Treatment of Waldenstrom's macroglobulinemia with rituximab. *J Clin Oncol* 2002;20:2327–2333.

133. Treon SP, Emmanouilides C, Kimby E, et al. Extended rituximab therapy in Waldenström's macroglobulinemia. *Ann Oncol* 2005;16:132–138.

134. Donnelly GB, Bober-Sorcinelli K, Jacobson R, et al. Abrupt IgM rise following treatment with rituximab in patients with Waldenstrom's macroglobulinemia. *Blood* 2001;98:240b.

135. Treon SP, Branagan AR, Anderson KC. Paradoxical increases in serum IgM levels and serum viscosity following rituximab therapy in patients with Waldenstrom's macroglobulinemia. *Blood* 2003;102:690a.

136. Ghobrial IM, Fonseca R, Greipp PR, et al. The initial "flare" of IgM level after rituximab therapy in patients diagnosed with Waldenstrom Macroglobulinemia: an Eastern Cooperative Oncology Group Study. *Blood* 2003;102:448a.

137. Dimopoulos MA, Anagnostopoulos A, Zervas C, et al. Predictive factors for response to rituximab in Waldenstrom's macroglobulinemia. *Clin Lymphoma* 2005;5:270–272.

138. Treon SP, Hansen M, Branagan AR, et al. Polymorphisms in FcγRIIIA (CD16) receptor expression are associated with clinical responses to Rituximab in Waldenstrom's Macroglobulinemia. *J Clin Oncol* 2005;23: 474–481.

139. Weber DM, Dimopoulos MA, Delasalle K, et al. 2-chlorodeoxyadenosine alone and in combination for previously untreated Waldenstrom's macroglobulinemia. *Semin Oncol* 2003;30:243–247.

140. Treon SP, Branagan AR, Ioakimidis L, et al. Long term outcomes to Fludarabine and Rituximab in Waldenstr—m's macroglobulinemia. *Blood* 2009;113:3673–8.

141. Tam CS, Wolf MM, Westerman D, et al. Fludarabine combination therapy is highly effective in first-line and salvage treatment of patients with Waldenstrom's macroglobulinemia. *Clin Lymphoma Myeloma* 2005;6:136–139.

142. Hensel M, Villalobos M, Kornacker M, et al. Pentostatin/cyclophosphamide with or without rituximab: an effective regimen for patients with Waldenstrom's macroglobulinemia/lymphoplasmacytic lymphoma. *Clin Lymphoma Myeloma* 2005;6:131–135.

143. Dimopoulos MA, Anagnostopoulos A, Kyrtsonis MC, et al. Primary treatment of Waldenstrom's macroglobulinemia with dexamethasone, rituximab and cyclophosphamide. *J Clin Oncol* 2007;25:3344–3349.

144. Buske C, Dreyling MH, Eimermacher H, et al. Combined immuno-chemotherapy (R-CHOP) results in significantly superior response rates and time to treatment failure in first line treatment of patients with lymphoplasmacytoid/ic immunocytoma. Results of a prospective randomized trial of the German Low Grade Lymphoma Study Group. *Blood* 2004;104:162a.

145. Treon SP, Hunter Z, Branagan A. CHOP plus rituximab therapy in Waldenström's macroglobulinemia. *Clin Lymphoma Myeloma* 2005;5:273–277.

146. Dimopoulos MA, Hamilos G, Efstathiou E, et al. Treatment of Waldenstrom's macroglobulinemia with the combination of fludarabine and cyclophosphamide. *Leuk Lymphoma* 2003;44:993–996.

147. Tamburini J, Levy V, Chateilex C, et al. Fludarabine plus cyclophosphamide in Waldenstrom's macroglobulinemia: results in 49 patients. *Leukemia* 2005;19:1831–1834.

148. Jagannath S, Durie BG, Wolf J, et al. Bortezomib therapy alone and in combination with dexamethasone for previously untreated symptomatic multiple myeloma. *Br J Haematol* 2005;129:776–783.

149. Oakervee HE, Popat R, Curry N, et al. PAD combination therapy (PS-341/bortezomib, doxorubicin and dexamethasone) for previously untreated patients with multiple myeloma. *Br J Haematol* 2005;129: 755–762.

150. Harousseau JL, Attal M, Leleu X, et al. Bortezomib plus dexamethasone as induction treatment prior to autologous stem cell transplantation in patients with newly diagnosed multiple myeloma. Preliminary results of an IFM Phase II Study. *Blood* 2004;104:416a.

151. Mitsiades CS, Mitsiades N, McMullan CJ, et al. The proteasome inhibitor bortezomib (PS-341) is active against Waldenstrom's macroglobulinemia. *Blood* 2003;102:181a.

152. Treon SP, Hunter ZR, Matous J, et al. Multicenter Clinical Trial of Bortezomib in Relapsed/Refractory Waldenstrom's macroglobulinemia: results of WMCTG Trial 03-248. *Clin Cancer Res* 2007;13:3320–3325.

153. Chen CI, Kouroukis CT, White D, et al. Bortezomib is active in patients with untreated or relapsed Waldenstrom's macroglobulinemia: a phase II study of the National Cancer Institute of Canada Clinical Trials Group. *J Clin Oncol* 2007;25:1570–1575.

154. Dimopoulos MA, Anagnostopoulos A, Kyrtsonis MC, et al. Treatment of relapsed or refractory Waldenstrom's macroglobulinemia with bortezomib. *Haematologica* 2005; 90:1655–1657.

155. Goy A, Younes A, McLaughlin P, et al. Phase II study of proteasome inhibitor bortezomib in relapsed or refractory B-cell non-Hodgkin's lymphoma. *J Clin Oncol* 2005;23:657–658.

156. Treon SP, Ioakimidis L, Soumerai JD, et al. Primary therapy of Waldenstrom's Macroglobulinemia with Bortezomib, Dexamethasone and Rituximab: Results of WMCTG Clinical Trial 05-180. *J Clin Oncol* 2009 in press.

157. Ghobrial IM, Matous J, Padmanabhan S, et al. Phase II Trial of Combination of bortezomib and rituximab in relapsed and/or refractory Waldenstrom Macroglobulinemia. *Blood* 2008;112:832.

158. Agathocleous A, Rule S, Johson P. Preliminary results of a phase I/LL study of weekly or twice weekly bortezomib in combination with rituximab in patients with follicular lymphoma, mantle cell lymphoma, and Waldenstrom's macroglobulinemia. *Blood* 2007;110:754a.

159. Hunter ZR, Boxer M, Kahl B, et al. Phase II study of alemtuzumab in lymphoplasmacytic lymphoma: results of WMCTG trial 02-079. *Proc Am Soc Clin Oncol* 2006;24:427s.

160. Owen RG, Rawstron AC, Osterborg A, et al. Activity of alemtuzumab in relapsed/refractory Waldenstrom's macroglobulinemia. *Blood* 2003;102: 644a.

161. Dimopoulos MA, Zomas A, Viniou NA, et al. Treatment of Waldenström's macroglobulinemia with thalidomide. *J Clin Oncol* 2001;19:3596–3601.

162. Coleman C, Leonard J, Lyons L, et al. Treatment of Waldenström's macroglobulinemia with clarithromycin, low-dose thalidomide and dexamethasone. *Semin Oncol* 2003;30:270–274.

163. Dimopoulos MA, Zomas K, Tsatalas K, et al. Treatment of Waldenström's macroglobulinemia with single agent thalidomide or with combination of clarithromycin, thalidomide and dexamethasone. *Semin Oncol* 2003;30:265–269.

164. Hayashi T, Hideshima T, Akiyama M, et al. Molecular mechanisms whereby immunomodulatory drugs activate natural killer cells: clinical application. *Br J Haematol* 2005;128:192–203.

165. Davies FE, Raje N, Hideshima T, et al. Thalidomide and immunomodulatory derivatives augment natural killer cell cytoxicity in multiple myeloma. *Blood* 2001;98:210–216.

166. Janakiraman N, McLaughlin P, White CA, et al. Rituximab: correlation between effector cells and clinical activity in NHL. *Blood* 1998;92:337a.

167. Treon SP, Soumerai JD, Branagan AR, et al. Thalidomide and rituximab in Waldenstrom macroglobulinemia. *Blood* 2008;112:4452–4457.

168. Treon SP, Soumerai JD, Branagan AR, et al. Lenalidomide and rituximab in Waldenström's macroglobulinemia. *Clin Cancer Res* 2009;15:355–360.

169. Desikan R, Dhodapkar M, Siegel D, et al. High-dose therapy with autologous haemopoietic stem cell support for Waldenström's macroglobulinaemia. *Br J Haematol* 1999;105:993–996.

170. Munshi NC, Barlogie B. Role for high dose therapy with autologous hematopoietic stem cell support in Waldenström's macroglobulinemia. *Semin Oncol* 2003;30:282–285.

171. Dreger P, Glass B, Kuse R, et al. Myeloablative radiochemotherapy followed by reinfusion of purged autologous stem cells for Waldenström's macroglobulinaemia. *Br J Haematol* 1999;106:115–118.

172. Anagnostopoulos A, Dimopoulos MA, Aleman A, et al. High-dose chemotherapy followed by stem cell transplantation in patients with resistant Waldenström's macroglobulinemia. *Bone Marrow Transplant* 2001;27: 1027–1029.

173. Tournilhac O, Leblond V, Tabrizi R, et al. Transplantation in Waldenström's macroglobulinemia – the French Experience. *Semin Oncol* 2003;30:291–296.

174. Anagnostopoulos A, Hari PN, Perez WS, et al. Autologous or allogeneic stem cell transplantation in patients with Waldenström's macroglobulinemia. *Biol Blood Marrow Transplant* 2006;12:845–854.

175. Maloney DG, Sandmaier B, Maris M, et al. The use of non-myeloablative allogeneic hematopoietic cell transplantation for patients with refractory Waldenström's macroglobulinemia: replacing high-dose cytotoxic therapy with graft versus tumor effects. *Proceedings of the Second International Workshop on Waldenström's Macroglobulinemia, Athens, Greece, 2002.* Available at: http://www.wmworkshop.org

176. Weber D, Treon SP, Emmanouilides C, et al. Uniform response criteria in Waldenström's macroglobulinemia: Consensus panel recommendations from the Second International Workshop on Waldenstrom's Macroglobulinemia. *Semin Oncol* 2003;30:127–131.

177. Kimby E, Treon SP, Anagnostopoulos A, et al. Update on recommendations for assessing response from the Third International Workshop on Waldenstrom's Macroglobulinemia. *Clin Lymphoma Myeloma* 2006;6: 380–383.

178. Strauss SJ, Maharaj L, Hoare S, et al. Bortezomib therapy in patients with relapsed or refractory lymphoma: potential correlation of in vitro sensitivity and tumor necrosis factor alpha response with clinical activity. *J Clin Oncol* 2006;24:2105–2112.

CHAPTER 15 ■ EXTRANODAL MARGINAL ZONE B-CELL LYMPHOMA OF MUCOSA-ASSOCIATED LYMPHOID TISSUE (MALT LYMPHOMA)

EMANUELE ZUCCA, FRANCESCO BERTONI, JOACHIM YAHALOM, AND PETER G. ISAACSON

DEFINITION AND CLASSIFICATION

Mucosa-associated lymphoid tissue (MALT) lymphoma is a distinct B-cell lymphoma that develops in extranodal sites and often has an indolent clinical course. It was first recognized as a separate clinical pathological entity by Isaacson and Wright in 1983 (1,2), and was later included in the Revised European American Lymphoma and World Health Organization classifications as a distinct lymphoma entity in the mature B-cell neoplasms category. At present, it is formally classified in the fourth edition of the World Health Organization classification of tumors of lymphoid tissue as the "extranodal marginal zone B-cell lymphoma of mucosa-associated lymphoid tissue (MALT lymphoma)" and defined as follows: "An extranodal lymphoma composed of morphologically heterogeneous small B-cells including marginal zone (centrocyte-like) cells, cells resembling monocytoid cells, small lymphocytes, and scattered immunoblast and centroblast-like cells. There is plasma cell differentiation in a proportion of the cases. The infiltrate is in the marginal zone of reactive B-cell follicles and extends into the interfollicular region. In epithelial tissues the neoplastic cells typically infiltrate the epithelium forming lymphoepithelial lesions" (3). Nodal marginal zone lymphoma and marginal zone lymphoma of the spleen have different clinical and pathologic features than extranodal marginal zone B-cell lymphoma of MALT, and are discussed in other chapters.

INCIDENCE AND EPIDEMIOLOGY

MALT lymphoma is the third most common non-Hodgkin lymphoma, and in a survey of more than 1,400 non-Hodgkin lymphomas from nine institutions in the United States, Canada, the United Kingdom, Switzerland, France, Germany, South Africa, and Hong Kong, this entity represented approximately 8% of the total number of cases (4). The most common and best-studied organ involved by MALT lymphoma is the stomach; up to 40% to 50% of the lymphomas found in the stomach are MALT lymphomas (5–7). Yet, MALT lymphomas may have primary involvement of nearly all organs. Outside the stomach, extranodal marginal zone lymphomas have indeed been described in salivary glands, skin, orbit, conjunctiva, lung, thyroid, larynx, breast, kidney, liver, bladder, prostate, urethra, small intestine, rectum, pancreas, and even in the intracranial dura (8–14). Most cases

occur in adults, with a median age in the 6th decade and a slight female preponderance (4,15). The highest incidence of gastric MALT lymphoma has been reported in northeastern Italy (13.2 per 100,000 per year, 13 times higher than in corresponding communities in the United Kingdom), suggesting the existence of important geographic variations (16). The incidence of primary gastric lymphomas is likely to be related to the rate of *Helicobacter pylori* infection observed in the population. Indeed, a very high prevalence (up to >90% of cases) of *H. pylori* infection has been reported in gastric MALT lymphomas (17,18). There is compelling evidence for a pathogenetic role of this infection in gastric lymphoma. In the United States, the incidence of gastric MALT lymphoma has been estimated as between 1:30,000 and 1:80,000 in the *H. pylori*-infected population (19).

Other infections have been linked to nongastric marginal zone lymphomas: *Borrelia burgdorferi* in cutaneous lymphomas and *Chlamydophila psittaci* in the lymphoma of the ocular adnexa (20,21). There is, however, a great and not completely explained geographic variation in the strength of these associations. A significantly increased risk of developing MALT lymphoma has been reported in individuals affected by autoimmune disorders, especially Sjögren syndrome and systemic lupus erythematosus (22).

A special variant of MALT lymphoma is the immunoproliferative small intestinal disease (IPSID) that occurs mainly in the Middle East, especially in the Mediterranean area where the disease is endemic, affecting young adults of both sexes, but predominantly the males. Other cases have been reported from the Cape region in South Africa and from other subtropic locations. A few cases have been described from industrialized Western countries, usually among immigrants from the endemic areas (23). It was known since the 1970s that in the early phases of IPSID, durable remissions can be obtained with sustained treatment with antibiotics, but only in 2004 Lecuit et al. (24) demonstrated the presence of a specific pathogen, linking this lymphoma to *Campylobacter jejuni*.

PATHOGENESIS OF EXTRANODAL B-CELL MARGINAL ZONE LYMPHOMA

The nomenclature and classification of non-Hodgkin lymphomas have, to a considerable extent, been based on the architectural, cytologic and functional relationships between the various lymphomas and normal lymphoid tissue as exemplified by the peripheral lymph node. The clinicopathologic features of many extranodal B-cell lymphomas are, however, more closely related to the structure and function of MALT than of peripheral lymph nodes (1,2).

The anatomic distribution and structure of lymph nodes are adapted to deal with antigens carried to the node in the afferent lymphatics that drain sites at various distances from the node. Permeable mucosal sites, such as the gastrointestinal (GI) tract, are, however, particularly vulnerable because they are in direct contact with the external environment, and specialized lymphoid tissue, the MALT, has evolved to protect them. MALT contains both B- and T-cell components, and the former comprises the B-cell compartment of Peyer patches, the lamina propria plasma cells, and the B-cell compartment of mesenteric lymph nodes.

Peyer Patches

There are concentrations of organized lymphoid nodules that are distributed throughout the small intestine, appendix, and colorectum. They are concentrated in the terminal ileum where they collectively form the Peyer patches, the generic term applied to this compartment of MALT (25,26). Peyer patches are unencapsulated aggregates of lymphoid and accessory cells that in some respects resemble lymph nodes (Fig. 15.1). Each Peyer patch consists of B- and T-cell areas and associated accessory cells. The B-cell area comprises a germinal center identical to that of reactive lymph nodes. The germinal center is surrounded by a mantle zone of small B lymphocytes that is broadest at the mucosal aspect of the follicle. Surrounding the mantle zone is a broad marginal zone in which most of the cells are small to intermediate-sized B lymphocytes with moderately abundant pale-staining cytoplasm and nuclei with a slightly irregular outline leading to a resemblance to centrocytes. The marginal zone extends toward the mucosal surface, and some marginal zone B cells are present within the overlying "dome" epithelium where they may aggregate in small clusters. These intraepithelial B cells form the lympho-epithelium, which is one of the defining features of MALT. The dome epithelium is a specialized structure containing microfold cells that are thought to sample antigens in the intestinal contents, which then interact with the underlying lymphoid tissue. It is possible, however, that some soluble antigens cross the dome epithelium directly. The immunophenotype of Peyer patches is broadly similar to that of lymph nodes (25–27). The germinal center B cells express immunoglobulin (Ig) M and are surrounded by an IgD-positive, IgM-positive mantle zone that, in turn, is surrounded by the IgM-positive IgD-negative marginal zone. The marginal zone extends toward the dome epithelium wherein CD20-positive, IgM-positive intraepithelial B cells can be seen. Lateral to the serosal aspect of the B-cell follicle, there is a T-cell zone containing prominent high endothelial venules equivalent to the paracortical T zone of the lymph node.

Lamina Propria

Few plasma cells are present in the Peyer patch in contrast to the lamina propria where they comprise the principal

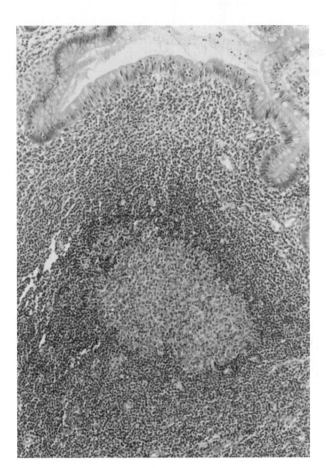

FIGURE 15.1 Section of a Peyer patch showing a central follicle surrounded by a marginal zone. Clusters of marginal zone cells are present in the dome epithelium.

B-cell component. The plasma cells secrete mainly IgA and IgM, and are derived from memory B cells that migrate out of the Peyer patch germinal centers (28,29). These cells leave the intestine via the efferent lymphatics of the Peyer patches, pass through the sinuses of mesenteric lymph nodes, and enter the circulation via the thoracic duct, finally migrating out into the lamina propria from specialized venules. Here, the majority complete their differentiation into plasma cells, whereas a minority persist as small memory B lymphocytes.

Mesenteric Lymph Nodes

The basic structure of mesenteric lymph nodes is the same as that of peripheral lymph nodes, and in the presence of a breach in the intestinal mucosa, these nodes cannot be distinguished from reactive peripheral nodes. In normal circumstances, however, mesenteric nodes are distinguished by small, rather inactive B-cell follicles, which in contrast to peripheral lymph nodes, are usually surrounded by a prominent marginal zone. Mesenteric lymph nodes have a poorly developed paracortex and prominent dilated sinuses containing transformed B blasts, most of which are synthesizing IgA.

THE MUCOSA-ASSOCIATED LYMPHOID TISSUE CONCEPT

In the early 1980s, Isaacson and Wright (1,2) noted that just as low-grade nodal lymphomas exhibited the features of normal lymph nodes, certain low-grade B-cell lymphomas of the GI tract recapitulated features of the MALT of Peyer patches. MALT lymphomas tend to remain localized to their site of origin for long periods, less commonly disseminate to the bone marrow, and frequently respond favorably to local therapeutic measures. Lymphomas exhibiting these features arise at a wide variety of extranodal sites, not only the GI tract. Curiously, MALT lymphomas only rarely arise at sites of concentration of native MALT, such as the terminal ileum or the tonsils. On the contrary, they most commonly arise from "acquired MALT" at sites normally devoid of MALT, such as the stomach, salivary gland, lung, and thyroid (30).

Indeed, MALT lymphomas of the salivary gland and thyroid, organs normally containing no lymphoid tissue, are always preceded respectively by lymphoepithelial (myoepithelial) sialadenitis, usually associated with Sjögren syndrome, and Hashimoto thyroiditis. Histologic and immunohistochemical studies of the heavy lymphoid infiltrate that characterizes these two conditions have shown a remarkable resemblance to MALT. This is most graphically illustrated with reference to lymphoepithelial sialadenitis. In this condition lymphoid tissue accumulates around dilated salivary gland ducts and forms, in effect, small Peyer patches complete with germinal center, mantle, a small marginal zone, and, significantly, collections of intraepithelial B cells (Fig. 15.2). This lymphoid tissue, which has become known as acquired MALT, is also a feature of Hashimoto thyroiditis, and has been identified in fetal and neonatal lung from infants with pulmonary infections of undetermined nature. It is also seen in a condition termed "follicular bronchiolitis," which is associated with various autoimmune disorders, including Sjögren syndrome. Here it is worth emphasizing that MALT of the bronchus is not usually present in normal lung. The absence of lymphoid tissue from normal stomach, the most common site of MALT lymphoma, is well documented, but here, too, MALT is commonly acquired almost always as a result of the reaction to infection with *H. pylori*, which precedes development of most cases of gastric MALT lymphoma (30).

There are certain common factors relating to the acquisition of MALT that may be relevant to development of lymphoma at these sites. In most cases there is a history of chronic inflammatory disorder that leads to the accumulation of lymphoid tissue. In most instances infections and autoimmunity seem to play an important role in the underlying disease. MALT accumulates in relation to columnar epithelium and appears to receive antigenic stimuli either from the epithelium itself or, like physiologic MALT, from antigens that enter the lymphoid tissue across the epithelium rather than from antigens carried in afferent lymphatics. Sequence analysis of the Ig genes expressed by the MALT lymphoma B cells shows a pattern of somatic hypermutation and intraclonal variation, suggesting that the tumor cell has undergone antigen selection in germinal centers, and they continue to be at least partially driven by direct antigen stimulation (31). In the context of this continual antigenic stimulation, abnormal B-cell clones acquiring successive genetic abnormalities can

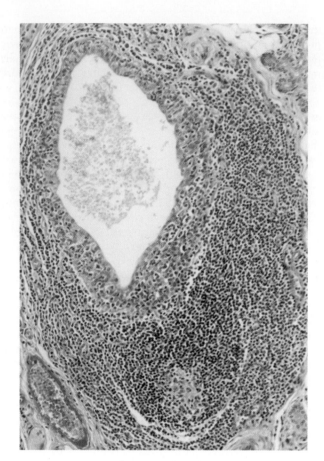

FIGURE 15.2 Section of salivary gland from a case of lymphoepithelial sialadenitis. A lymphoid follicle is adjacent to a dilated salivary duct, which is infiltrated by B cells, resulting in a Peyer patch-like structure.

progressively replace the normal B-cell population of the inflammatory tissue, giving rise to the lymphoma.

The acquisition of MALT, which can be considered the substrate for the development of extranodal marginal zone lymphomas, is induced by a series of agents that are likely different in each organ. Recognition of the driving sources of the antigenic stimulation in different tissues may have important therapeutic implications. Indeed, in addition to *H. pylori* infections that precede gastric MALT lymphoma, other infectious organisms have been found to be possibly implicated in the pathogenesis of extranodal marginal zone lymphomas arising in the skin (*B. burgdorferi*) (20), in the ocular adnexa (*C. psittaci*) (21), and in the small intestine (*C. jejuni*) (24). There is, however, a great variation in the strength of some of these associations that might be related, at least in part, to geographic factors (32).

THE PATHOLOGY OF MUCOSA-ASSOCIATED LYMPHOID TISSUE LYMPHOMA

Macroscopic Appearances

Macroscopically, MALT lymphomas, although sometimes forming obvious tumorous masses, frequently are indistinguishable from the inflammatory lesion that underlies the acquisition of MALT from which the lymphoma arises. Thus, gastric MALT lymphoma, for example, at endoscopy is often indistinguishable from chronic gastritis. Although they may form a single dominant mass, MALT lymphomas are typically multifocal with small, even microscopic foci of lymphoma scattered throughout the organ involved. Each of these foci is clonally identical (33).

Histopathology

MALT lymphomas recapitulate the histologic features of Peyer patches (34). Thus, the neoplastic B lymphocytes infiltrate around reactive B-cell follicles, external to a preserved follicular mantle, in a marginal zone distribution and spread out to form larger confluent areas that eventually overrun some or most of the follicles (Fig. 15.3). Like marginal zone B cells, the neoplastic cells have relatively abundant, pale cytoplasm with small to medium-sized, slightly irregularly shaped nuclei containing moderately dispersed chromatin and inconspicuous nucleoli. The accumulation of more abundant pale-staining cytoplasm may lead to a monocytoid appearance of the lymphoma cells, whereas in some cases the cells more closely resemble small lymphocytes (Fig. 15.4). Large cells resembling centroblasts or immunoblasts are usually present but are in the minority. Plasma cell differentiation

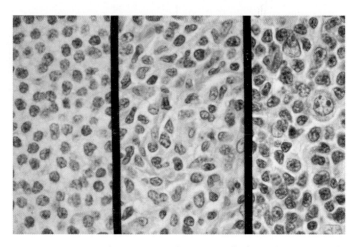

FIGURE 15.4 Neoplastic marginal zone B cells from three cases of gastric MALT lymphoma. In the left-hand panel, the cells resemble small lymphocytes; in the center, they are "centrocyte-like," and in the right-hand panel, they are monocytoid in appearance.

is present in up to a third of cases and tends to be maximal beneath the surface gastric epithelium.

Glandular epithelium is often invaded and destroyed by discrete aggregates of lymphoma cells resulting in the so-called lymphoepithelial lesions (Fig. 15.5). These are defined as aggregates of three or more neoplastic marginal zone lymphocytes within glandular epithelium, preferably associated with distortion or necrosis of the epithelium. In gastric MALT lymphoma, these lesions are often accompanied by eosinophilic degeneration of the epithelium. Lymphoepithelial lesions, although highly characteristic of MALT lymphoma, especially gastric lymphoma, are not pathognomonic.

The lymphoma cells sometimes specifically colonize germinal centers of the reactive follicles (Fig. 15.6). Usually this results in a vaguely nodular or follicular pattern to the lymphoma (35). In some cases the plasma cell differentiation occurs within these reactive germinal centers, and in others the intrafollicular marginal zone cells undergo blast transformation, which can lead to a close resemblance to follicular lymphoma.

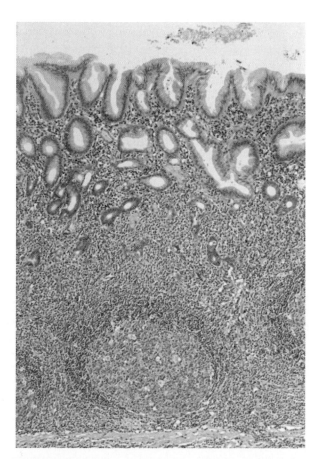

FIGURE 15.3 A case of gastric MALT lymphoma. A reactive B-cell follicle is surrounded by an infiltrate of neoplastic marginal zone B cells that form lymphoepithelial lesions with gastric glands.

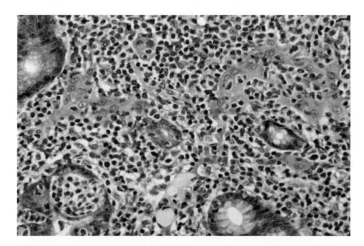

FIGURE 15.5 Neoplastic marginal zone B cells from a case of gastric MALT lymphoma forming lymphoepithelial lesions with gastric glands.

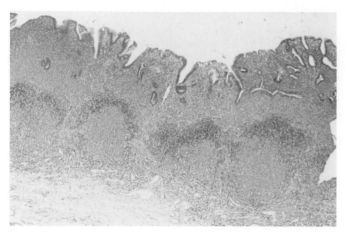

FIGURE 15.6 A case of gastric MALT lymphoma with prominent follicular colonization.

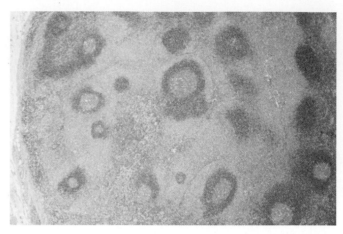

FIGURE 15.8 Infiltration of a gastric lymph node by MALT lymphoma. The pale-staining infiltrate surrounds follicles and expands the interfollicular zones.

Like other low-grade B-cell lymphomas, MALT lymphoma may undergo high-grade transformation (Fig. 15.7). Transformed centroblast or immunoblast-like cells may be present in larger numbers in MALT lymphoma, but only when solid or sheet-like proliferations of transformed cells are present should the lymphoma be considered to have transformed. The result is a tumor that currently cannot reli-

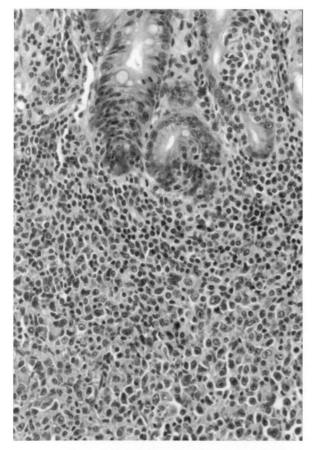

FIGURE 15.7 High-grade transformation in a gastric MALT lymphoma. A typical MALT lymphoma is present in the glandular epithelium, with transformation to a diffuse large cell lymphoma below.

ably be distinguished from other diffuse large B-cell lymphomas, particularly if the preceding MALT lymphoma has been overgrown. Thus, the current recommendation is that such cases are designated as diffuse large B-cell lymphoma and the presence of concurrent MALT lymphoma be documented. The term "high grade MALT lymphoma" should not be used, and the term "MALT lymphoma" should not be applied to a large B-cell lymphoma, even if it has arisen in a MALT site or is associated with lymphoepithelial lesions (3). MALT lymphomas preferentially disseminate to other sites where MALT lymphomas occur. Gastric MALT lymphomas, for example, tend to disseminate to the small intestine, salivary gland, and lung. When MALT lymphomas disseminate to lymphoid tissue, including lymph nodes and spleen, they specifically invade the marginal zone (Fig. 15.8). This can lead to a deceptively benign or reactive appearance, especially in mesenteric lymph nodes in which a marginal zone is normally present. Subsequently, there is interfollicular expansion to form sheets of more obvious lymphoma. Cytologic heterogeneity is still a feature of disseminated disease.

Immunoproliferative Small Intestinal Disease

This condition, previously known as Mediterranean lymphoma or α heavy chain disease, is nowadays considered a special subtype of MALT lymphoma arising in the proximal small intestine, and characterized by malabsorption and protein-losing enteropathy (23,36). IPSID has histologic features similar to other cases of MALT lymphoma but is typically characterized by a diffuse striking plasmacytic infiltrate (3). The distinguishing feature of IPSID is the expression of a monotypic truncated Ig α heavy chain without an associated light chain (24).

Immunohistochemistry

There is no specific marker for MALT lymphoma at present. The tumor cells typically express IgM, less often IgA or IgG, and are usually IgD negative. Their immunophenotype recapitulates that of marginal zone cells. They are CD20, CD79a, CD21, and CD35 positive, and CD5, CD23, and CD10 negative. There is Ig light chain restriction, but this may be difficult to demonstrate in small biopsy samples. Stains for cytokeratin may help identify lymphoepithelial lesions. CD43 is expressed in approximately 30% to 50% of cases, and expression of CD11c is variable. In IPSID both plasma cells and marginal zone cells express α heavy chain without any light chain.

Differential Diagnosis

Because of differences in clinical behavior and management, it is important to differentiate MALT lymphoma from the other small B-cell lymphomas that may present or involve extranodal sites. These include mantle cell lymphoma, lymphocytic lymphoma (chronic lymphocytic leukemia), and follicular lymphoma. The cytologic features of mantle cell lymphoma can closely simulate those of MALT lymphoma, even to the extent that occasional lymphoepithelial lesions may be present. However, the absence of transformed blasts together with expression of CD5, IgD, and, importantly, intranuclear expression of cyclin D1, a consequence of t(11;14), serve to distinguish mantle cell lymphoma. Lymphocytic lymphoma is characterized by small round lymphocytes usually together with peripheral blood lymphocytosis. Expression of CD5, CD23, and IgD without nuclear cyclin D1 provides further distinction from MALT lymphoma. Finally, follicular lymphoma, which may arise extranodally, can be difficult to distinguish from MALT lymphoma with follicular colonization. The transformed MALT lymphoma cells within follicles may closely resemble centroblasts but typically are CD10 and BCL6 (nuclear) negative in contrast to the cells of follicular lymphoma, which usually express both antigens both within and between follicles.

Normal Cell Counterpart

The tumor architecture and cytologic features, together with the immunophenotype, strongly suggest that the MALT lymphomas are related to the postgerminal center marginal zone B cell.

MOLECULAR GENETICS

Chromosomal Translocations

A series of recurrent chromosomal translocations have been described in extranodal marginal zone lymphomas (Table 15.1) (37–42). The translocations show a different anatomic distribution, and they appear mutually exclusive. There are also suggestions that their incidence and distribution have geographic differences, possibly reflecting a different genetic background of the patients or of infectious agents.

Three of them [t(11;18)(q21;q21), t(1;14)(p22;q32), and t(14;18)(q32;q21)] are the most characterized, and, interestingly, they all appear to affect the same signaling pathway, resulting in the activation of nuclear factor-κB (NF-κB), a transcription factor with a central role in immunity, inflammation, and apoptosis (43–45).

The t(11;18)(q21;q21) translocation is the most common translocation, occurring in 15% to 40% of cases (37,43,46–49). It results in the reciprocal fusion of the cellular inhibitor of apoptosis protein 2 (cIAP2) (also known as BIRC3) on 11q21 with MALT1 on 18q21. The creation of a fusion protein encoded by cIAP2-MALT1 on the derivative chromosome 11 is the pathogenetic event. The presence of the t(11;18) is more common in patients with primary gastric marginal zone lymphoma negative for H. pylori, in patients not responding to antibiotics therapy, and in more advanced cases (50–52). Despite these factors associated with a more aggressive disease, the cIAP2/MALT1 predicts a lower risk of transformation to diffuse large B-cell lymphoma (53), and t(11;18)-positive cases seem to have less additional genomic aberrations than negative cases of t(11;18) (54,55).

The t(1;14)(p22;q32) translocation is detected in only 1% to 2% of extranodal marginal zone lymphoma cases, and it determines an overexpression of the BCL10 gene due to the juxtaposition to the promoter region of the Ig heavy chain genes (38). The BCL10 gene codes for an adaptor protein implicated in surface receptor signaling, highly expressed in the nucleus of the neoplastic B cells of extranodal marginal zone lymphomas carrying this translocation. The high nuclear expression occurs also in t(11;18)-positive cases and in other patients without any apparent explanation (52,56–62).

The t(14;18)(q32;q21) translocation, described in approximately 20% of extranodal marginal zone lymphoma cases and cytogenetically identical to the t(14;18)(q32;q21) involving BCL2 in follicular lymphoma, juxtaposes the MALT1 gene to the promoter region of the Ig heavy chain genes with subsequent MALT1 overexpression (39,63).

The t(3;14) determines the juxtaposition of the transcription factor FOXP1 next to the enhancer region of the Ig heavy chain genes (40). The exact role of this translocation is still unclear. High expression of FOXP1 seems to correlate with a poor outcome in both extranodal marginal zone lymphomas and in diffuse large B-cell lymphoma, and, indeed, it carries a higher risk of transformation from marginal zone to high-grade tumors (64,65).

The recurrent t(5;14)(q34;q32) and t(9;14)(9p24;q32) translocations have been described very recently (41). They juxtapose the ODZ2 and the JMJD2C genes, respectively, to the Ig heavy chain gene locus with subsequent overexpression of the two genes. The role in lymphomagenesis is still completely unknown.

Other Genomic Lesions

Extranodal marginal zone B-cell lymphomas, together with the splenic and the nodal subtypes, present gains of chromosome 3/3q and gains of chromosome 18/18q at a frequency higher as compared with other B-cell tumors (66–68). A new recurrent 6q23.3 deletion has been described, which would inactivate the A20/TNFAIP3 gene (68,69). Interestingly, the gene is, again, a member of the NF-κB pathway hit by the t(11;18), t(1;14), and t(14;18) translocations. Thus, A20 inactivation might be another important pathogenetic mechanism of extranodal marginal zone lymphomas.

TABLE 15.1

MAIN CHROMOSOMAL TRANSLOCATIONS DESCRIBED IN EXTRANODAL MARGINAL ZONE LYMPHOMAS OF MALT

Chromosomal translocation	t(11;18)(q21;q21)	t(14;18)(q32;q21)	t(1;14)(p22;q32)	t(3;14)(p14;q32)	t(5;14)(q34;q32)	t(9;14)(9p24;q32)
Consequence	cIAP2-MALT1 fusion protein	Overexpression of MALT1	Overexpression of BCL10	Overexpression of FOXP1	Overexpression of ODZ2	Overexpression of JMJD2C
Frequency (% of cases)	15–40	5–20	<5	5–10	Unknown	Unknown
Main anatomic sites	Stomach, intestine	Ocular adnexa, skin, salivary glands, liver	Stomach, intestine, lung	Skin, thyroid	Skin, ocular adnexa?	Ocular adnexa, salivary glands?
MALT1 expression	Cytoplasmic, weak	Cytoplasmic, strong	Cytoplasmic, weak	Unknown	Unknown	Unknown
BCL10 expression	Nuclear, strong	Cytoplasmic, strong	Nuclear, strong	Unknown	Unknown	Unknown
NF-κB activation	Yes	Yes	Yes	Unknown	Unknown	Unknown
Additional genomic abnormalities	Infrequent	Yes	Yes	Yes	Unknown	Unknown
Histologic transformation	No	Yes	Yes	Yes	Unknown	Unknown

Immunoglobulin Gene Rearrangement

The sequence analysis of the Ig genes expressed by the extranodal marginal zone lymphoma B cells shows a pattern of somatic hypermutation and rearrangement, suggesting that the tumor cell has undergone antigen selection in germinal centers (31,70–72). Moreover, the detection of the so-called ongoing mutations indicates that the expansion of lymphoma cells might still be driven by the antigen stimulation. The expressed Ig genes often show a homology with autoreactive clones. Interestingly, among the three lymphomas believed to derive from marginal zone B cells, extranodal marginal zone lymphoma is the only one to have a unique pattern with somatically mutated IgH genes in all the cases.

Because of the difficulty in distinguishing between acquired MALT and MALT lymphoma, it is has been proposed to use the molecular evidence of monoclonality detected by the polymerase chain reaction for the diagnosis of lymphoma. However, this technique may fail to detect monoclonality in up to 15% of cases of overt lymphoma and, thus, produce false-negative results (73). Moreover, monoclonality can be shown in the context of benign inflammations, such as chronic gastritis, with no evidence of malignancy where there is no histologic evidence (74–76). Thus, MALT lymphoma should not be diagnosed in the absence of clear histologic evidence.

THE PATHOGENESIS OF MUCOSA-ASSOCIATED LYMPHOID TISSUE LYMPHOMA: THE *HELICOBACTER PYLORI* AND GASTRIC MUCOSA-ASSOCIATED LYMPHOID TISSUE LYMPHOMA MODEL

There are several lines of evidence that suggest that gastric MALT lymphoma arises from MALT acquired as a consequence of *H. pylori* chronic infection (Fig. 15.9). *H. pylori* can be demonstrated in the gastric mucosa of the majority of cases of gastric MALT lymphoma. In the first study in which this association was examined, the organism was present in >90% of cases (18). Subsequent studies have shown a lower incidence (17) but also that the density and detectability of *H. pylori* decrease as lymphoma evolves from chronic gastritis (77). A case control study showed an association between previous *H. pylori* infection and the development of primary gastric lymphoma (78). More direct evidence confirming the importance of *H. pylori* in the pathogenesis of gastric lymphoma has been obtained from studies that detected the lymphoma B-cell clone in the chronic gastritis that preceded the lymphoma (77,79) and from a series of in vitro studies showing that lymphoma growth could be stimulated in culture by

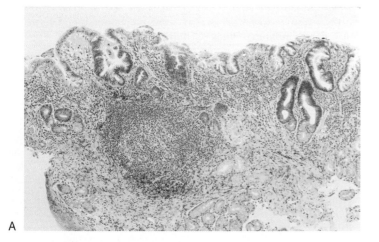

A

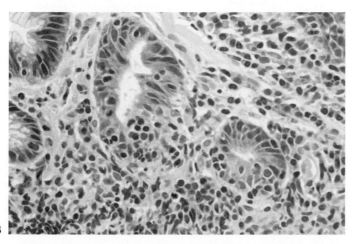

B

FIGURE 15.9 **A:** Gastric mucosa from a case of *H. pylori*-positive chronic gastritis. A B-cell follicle is present, but the mucosal infiltrate is comprised by plasma cells and T lymphocytes. **B:** Two glands adjacent to the B-cell follicle are infiltrated by B cells, resulting in resemblance to a lymphoepithelial lesion.

H. pylori strain-specific T cells when crude lymphoma cultures were exposed to the organism (80). Finally, following the initial study by Wotherspoon et al. (81), several groups have confirmed that eradication of *H. pylori* with antibiotics and proton pump inhibitors results in regression of gastric MALT lymphoma in approximately 75% of cases (19).

Based on the observations described before and on the current knowledge of the genetic lesions of MALT lymphomas, a putative model of the multistage development and progression of gastric lymphoma from the background of a chronic gastritis can be proposed (30,43) (Fig. 15.10). *H. pylori* infection stimulates the formation of lymphocytic infiltration of the gastric mucosa. As a result of direct antigenic stimulation and indirect stimulation (autoantigens and T cells specific for *H. pylori*), B cells proliferate and occasionally can undergo a neoplastic transformation following the acquisition of genetic abnormalities, perhaps facilitated by the presence of free radicals (48,82). The accumulation of genetic abnormalities is associated with both a loss of dependency from antigenic stimulation (with subsequent antibiotic resistance) as well as a possible histologic transformation (43).

CLINICAL FEATURES OF MUCOSA-ASSOCIATED LYMPHOID TISSUE LYMPHOMA

The clinical aspects and presenting symptoms of extranodal marginal zone lymphomas are generally related to the primary location. The most common extragastric MALT lymphoma sites are: salivary glands, skin, orbits and conjunctiva, lung, thyroid, upper airways, breast, other GI sites, and liver (9,11,12,83). Some general characteristics can, however, be described (9,15,19,83,84). Elevated lactate dehydrogenase (LDH) or β-2-microglobulin levels as well as constitutional B symptoms are extremely rare at presentation (15,84). MALT lymphoma can remain localized for a prolonged period within the tissue of origin, but regional lymph nodes can sometimes be infiltrated, and dissemination at multiple sites is not uncommon, occurring in up to one fourth of cases, with either synchronous or metachronous involvement of multiple mucosal sites or nonmucosal sites such as spleen, bone marrow, or liver (9,10). A presentation with disseminated disease appears to be more common in nongastric MALT lymphomas (11,85). Bone marrow involvement is reported in up to 20% of cases (86). Within the stomach, MALT lymphoma is often multifocal, and this may explain the report of relapses in the gastric stump after surgical excision (19). Gastric MALT lymphoma can disseminate to the intestine (87) and to the spleen (88). A concomitant GI and non-GI involvement can be detected in approximately 10% of cases. In a recent survey of Austrian and Dutch patients, site-specific dissemination patterns were seen in paired organs (orbit, lung) and in the GI tract (stomach, colon), and primary pulmonary MALT lymphoma was significantly associated with gastric involvement. These patterns of dissemination were retained in relapsed disease (12). It has been postulated that the dissemination pattern of MALT lymphoma may be due to specific expression of special homing receptors or adhesion molecules on the surface of marginal zone B cells (89,90).

In a retrospective survey from the International Extranodal Lymphoma Study Group (IELSG) of a large series of

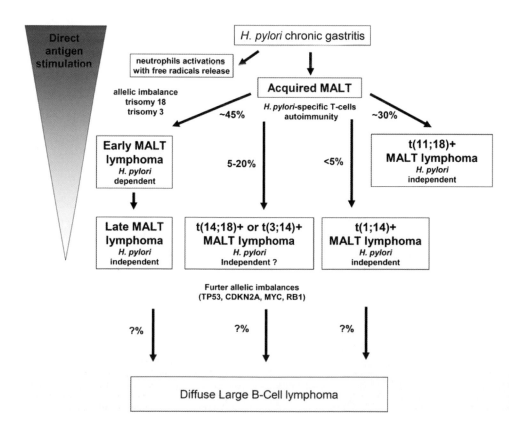

FIGURE 15.10 Schematic model of the multistep development and progression of gastric MALT lymphoma. *H. pylori* infection leads to the formation of acquired MALT in the gastric mucosa. As a result of immunologic stimulation (by autoantigens and *H. pylori*-specific T cells), infiltrating B cells proliferate and can, at times, undergo a neoplastic transformation following the acquisition of genetic abnormalities, perhaps facilitated by the presence of free radicals. MALT lymphomas with t(11;14)(q21;q21)/API2-MALT1 gain autonomous growth ability and do not respond to *H. pylori* eradication, but rarely transform into large cell lymphoma. Lymphomas with t(1;14)(p22;q32)/Ig-BCL10 are probably *H. pylori* independent and might undergo high-grade transformation. MALT lymphomas without these chromosomal translocations, sometimes carrying others genetic alterations, are usually *H. pylori* dependent at early stages but can progress and become *H. pylori* independent, and possibly transform into large cell tumors, following other acquired genetic alterations.

patients who were diagnosed as having nongastric MALT lymphoma, the minority of patients (17%) in the International Prognostic Index intermediate-high or high-risk groups had an inferior progression-free survival. Patients with stage IV disease due to disease at MALT sites plus bone marrow or lymph node involvement, but not those with multiple mucosal localizations only, had a lower overall survival (OS) rate, and the presence of nodal involvement adversely affected cause-specific survival (Fig. 15.11). The IELSG confirmed the indolent course of nongastric MALT lymphomas, despite the fact that one quarter of cases presented with stage IV disease and regardless of treatment type (9). The finding that dissemination to multiple mucosal sites does not change the outcome has also been shown in other series (8,10). Most patients have a favorable outcome (9,10,12), with OS usually >80% at 5 years (Fig. 15.12). The median time to

progression is apparently better for the GI compared with the non-GI lymphomas (9 vs. 5 years, respectively) (83), but no significant differences in OS have been shown. Localization may have prognostic relevance because of organ-specific clinical problems, which result in particular management strategies, but, because different genetic lesions have been reported at different anatomic locations, it may also be possible that different sites have a distinct natural history. In a radiotherapy study from Toronto, gastric and thyroid MALT lymphomas had the best outcome, whereas distant failures were more common for other sites (91). In the multicenter series from the IELSG, the patients with the disease initially presenting in the upper airways appeared to include a higher number of patients with advanced disease and had slightly poorer outcome, but their small number prevented any definitive conclusion (9). In general, despite frequent relapses,

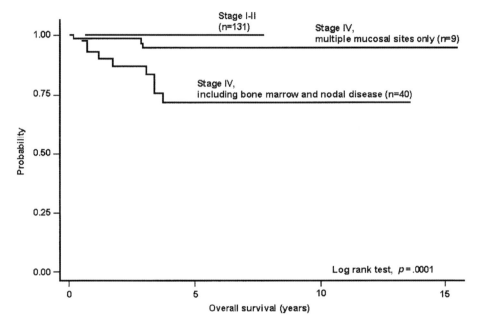

FIGURE 15.11 OS according to the Ann Arbor stage in primary nongastric MALT lymphoma. (From Zucca E, Conconi A, Pedrinis E, et al. Nongastric marginal zone B-cell lymphoma of mucosa-associated lymphoid tissue. *Blood* 2003;101:2489–2495.)

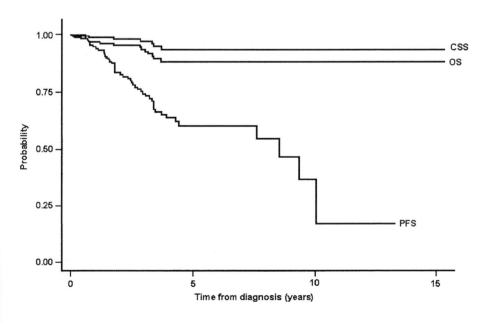

FIGURE 15.12 OS, cause-specific survival (CSS) and progression-free survival (PFS) in primary nongastric MALT lymphoma. (From Zucca E, Conconi A, Pedrinis E, et al. Nongastric marginal zone B-cell lymphoma of mucosa-associated lymphoid tissue. *Blood* 2003;101:2489–2495.)

MALT lymphomas most often maintain an indolent course. Histologic transformation to large cell lymphoma is reported in about 10% of the cases, usually as a late event and independent from dissemination (10,12).

Specific Clinical Aspects of Gastric Mucosa-Associated Lymphoid Tissue Lymphoma

The stomach is the most common organ involved with MALT lymphoma, and clinical aspects of diagnosis, staging, and treatment of gastric MALT lymphoma are discussed separately from all other sites.

The most common presenting symptoms of gastric MALT lymphoma are nonspecific dyspepsia, epigastric pain, nausea, and chronic manifestations of GI bleeding, such as anemia. B symptoms are rare. The upper GI complaints often lead to an endoscopy that usually reveals nonspecific gastritis or peptic ulcer with mass lesions being unusual (84,92). Elevation of LDH is also uncommon (15,84).

Diagnosis and Workup of Gastric Mucosa-Associated Lymphoid TissueLymphoma

The best staging system is still controversial (85,93), and a variety of alternative systems has been proposed. The

modification of the Blackledge staging system known as the "Lugano staging system" (94) has been largely used. However, this system was proposed before the wide use of endoscopic ultrasound and does not accurately describe the depth of infiltration in the gastric wall, a parameter that is highly predictive for the MALT lymphoma response to anti-*Helicobacter* therapy (95–97).

At present, ultrasound endoscopy is strongly recommended. It allows the use of modified Tumor-Node-Metastasis staging systems, such as the recently proposed "Paris staging" (98) that can adequately record the gastric wall infiltration and the involvement of perigastric lymph nodes (Table 15.2).

The initial endoscopic staging should include multiple biopsies from each region of the stomach, duodenum, gastroesophageal junction, and from any abnormal appearing site. Fresh biopsy and washing material should be available for cytogenetic studies in addition to routine histology and immunohistochemistry. The recommended immunophenotyping includes a paraffin panel for CD20, CD3, CD5, CD10, cyclin D1, and κ/λ. A molecular genetic analysis for detection of t(11;18) is recommended for identifying disease that is unlikely to respond to antibiotic therapy (50). The presence of active *H. pylori* infection must determined by histology (Genta stain or Warthin-Starry stain of antral biopsy specimen); serology studies are recommended when the results of histology are negative (99). A repeat endoscopic biopsy is recommended if histology demonstrates atypical lymphoid

---

TABLE 15.2

COMPARISON OF DIFFERENT STAGING SYSTEMS FOR GASTRIC MALT LYMPHOMA

Ann Arbor stage	Lugano staging system for GI lymphomas (94)	Paris staging system for primary GI lymphomas (98)[a]	Lymphoma extension
IE	Confined to GI tract (single primary or multiple, noncontiguous)	T1m N0 M0 T1sm N0 M0 T2 N0 M0 T3 N0 M0	Mucosa Submucosa Muscolaris propria Serosa

II	Extending into abdomen
	    II₁ = local nodal involvement
	    II₂ = distant nodal involvement
		T1–3 N1 M0
		T1–3 N2 M0
			Perigastric lymph nodes
			More distant regional lymph nodes

IIE	Penetration of serosa to involve adjacent organs or tissues	T4 N0 M0	Invasion of adjacent structures
IV	Disseminated extranodal involvement or concomitant supradiaphragmatic nodal involvement	T1–4 N3 M0 T1–4 N0-3 M1 T1–4 N0-3 M2 B0–1	Extra-abdominal lymph nodes on both sides of the diaphragm and/or noncontiguous involvement of separate sites in the GI tract Additional distant non-GI extranodal sites (with or without bone marrow infiltration)

[a] The European Gastro-Intestinal Lymphoma Study Group has proposed in 2003 a novel Tumor-Node-Metastasis–derived system, the "Paris staging system," aimed to improve the accuracy of the description of local tumor extent. The main modifications include the addition of the T1m and T1sm categories to separate the tumors confined to the mucosa from those confined to the submucosa, the definition of N3 as spread to extra-abdominal lymph node, the distinction of M1 referring to noncontiguous involvement of separate sites in the GI tract (e.g., stomach and rectum) from M2, which describes the involvement of non-GI tract tissues (including the serosae) and organs. Moreover, to describe the bone marrow infiltration, the B category was introduced with three subgroups: BX, bone marrow not assessed; B0, bone marrow not involved; and B1, lymphoma infiltration of the bone marrow.

TABLE 15.3

RECOMMENDED STAGING PROCEDURES FOR GASTRIC MALT LYMPHOMA

History (duration and presence of local or systemic symptoms)

Physical examination (careful evaluation of all lymph node regions, inspection of the upper airways and tonsils, clinical evaluation of the size of liver and spleen, detection of any palpable mass)

Laboratory tests, including complete blood counts and peripheral blood smear, LDH, evaluation of renal and liver function

Bone marrow biopsy

Standard posteroanterior and lateral chest radiographs

Abdominal and pelvic CT scan

Gastroduodenal endoscopy with multiple gastric biopsies from all the visible lesions and the noninvolved areas with a complete mapping of the organ

Gastric endoscopic ultrasound

Upper GI series (in selected cases)

---

infiltrates in the presence of *H. pylori*. Other studies should include counts of blood cells, basic biochemical studies (including LDH), computed tomography (CT) of the chest, abdomen, and pelvis, and bone marrow biopsy (Table 15.3).

Although the disease remains usually localized in the stomach, systemic dissemination and bone marrow involvement should be excluded at presentation because prognosis is worse with advanced stage or adverse International Prognostic Index (19). Patients with primary gastric presentation were reported to have a better outcome than patients with MALT lymphoma at other extranodal sites (83,91).

Staging Procedures in Nongastric Mucosa-Associated Lymphoid Tissue Lymphoma

Multiorgan involvement is present in at least a quarter of patients, and presentation with multiple MALT localizations is more frequent in patients with non-GI lymphoma. There-

fore, complete staging procedures with emphasis on all MALT sites at presentation are recommended. Workup studies should include complete blood counts, basic biochemical studies (including LDH and β2-microglobulin, Diagnosis and Workup of Gastric Mucosa-Associated Lymphoid Tissue-Lymphoma), CT of the chest, abdomen, and pelvis, and a bone marrow biopsy. Then, in function of the particular clinical presentation, the investigations should focus on the specific organs suspected of being involved. Additional investigations may include esophagogastroduodenoscopy, small bowel studies, and colonoscopy for intestinal presentation; bronchoscopy and bronchoalveolar lavage in the presence of lung lesions. Particular attention should finally be paid to the demonstration of certain chronic infections that may have a pathogenetic role, i.e., *B. burgdorferi* in cutaneous localizations, *C. psittaci* in the ocular adnexa, and *C. jejuni* in the small intestine.

Treatment of Gastric Mucosa-Associated Lymphoid Tissue Lymphoma

The role of *H. pylori* infection in the pathogenesis of gastric MALT lymphoma has been well established. About 20 studies and several case reports have shown that the cure of *H. pylori* infection is associated with complete remission in approximately 75% of patients with gastric MALT lymphoma in an early clinical stage (100,101). Antibiotic eradication of *H. pylori* is the standard primary treatment for patients with gastric MALT lymphoma and concomitant evidence for the presence of the bacteria in the stomach. Multiple series documented histologic regression of the gastric MALT lymphoma following successful eradication of *H. pylori*, with a response ranging from 35% to 100%. Four relatively large series from Europe and North America documented responses of 50% to 80% (Table 15.4). A treatment algorithm for patients presenting with or without *H. pylori* is outlined in Figure 15.13.

Several effective anti-*H. pylori* programs are available, and the current recommendations (99,102) for frontline anti-*Helicobacter* treatment are summarized in Table 15.5. It is expected that following 10 to 14 days of antibiotic

TABLE 15.4

RESPONSE OF GASTRIC MALT LYMPHOMA TO H. PYLORI ANTIBIOTIC THERAPY

Group	Number of patients with *H. pylori*	CR rate (%)	Number of patients without *H. pylori* / number of CRs	Median follow-up (mo (range))	Relapse rate (%)	Patients with CR remaining monoclonal (%)
GELD (96)	34	56	10/0	6 (2–18)	11	42
MDACC (97)	28	50	6/0	41 (18–70)	0	Not reported
LYO3 (IELSG/GELA/ UKLG) (112)	189	55	Not reported	24 (6–72)	14	44
German MALT Study Group (113)	120	80	Not reported	75 (1.5–116)	17	27

CR, complete remission; GELD, Groupe d'Etude Lymphome Digestif; MDACC, M. D. Anderson Cancer Center; UKLG, United Kingdom Lymphoma Group.

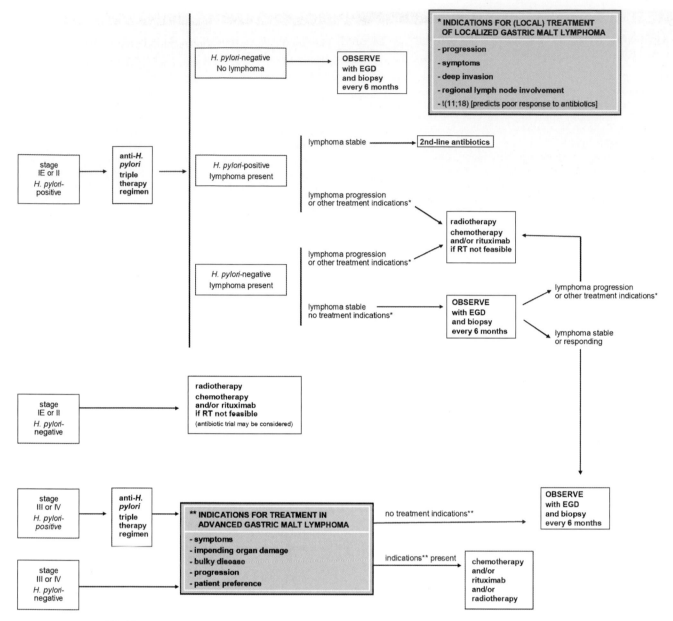

FIGURE 15.13 Recommended treatment algorithm for gastric marginal zone lymphoma. EGD, esophagogastroduodenoscopy; RT, radiotherapy.

treatment, *H. pylori* will be eradicated in 70% to 85% of the patients (103).

In populations with <15% to 20% clarithromycin resistance, the recommended first-choice regimen is triple therapy with a proton pump inhibitor (e.g., lansoprazole 30 mg twice daily, omeprazole 20 mg twice daily, pantoprazole 40 mg twice daily, rabeprazole 20 mg twice daily, or esomeprazole 20 mg twice daily) plus clarithromycin (500 mg twice daily) and amoxicillin (1 g twice daily), or metronidazole (500 mg twice daily). The rationale is that the proton pump inhibitor increases the pH of the stomach and allows the activity of clarithromycin and amoxicillin, which is optimal at neutral pH. The length of treatment is debatable. However, the data from metaanalyses show better results if the treatment is given for 14 days compared with 7 days, whereas the difference is not significant between 7 and 10 days (99,102).

In populations with <40% metronidazole resistance, the combination of proton pump inhibitor plus clarithromycin and metronidazole is preferable (99,102). The most commonly used second-choice treatment in patients with persistent *H. pylori* is bismuth-containing quadruple therapy (103).

The role of "adjuvant" therapy after *H. pylori* eradication in localized MALT lymphoma was investigated in a randomized study (104). Addition of chlorambucil conferred no benefit, with 5-year progression-free survival similar for observed and chlorambucil-treated patients (77% vs. 81%, respectively); OS was also similar (94% vs. 92%). This study, however, did not complete the planned accrual, and its results cannot be taken as conclusive (104).

Several factors predict the likelihood of gastric MALT lymphoma regression following antibiotic therapy (Table 15.6). An obvious prerequisite for expecting a response to antibiotics

TABLE 15.5

STANDARD ANTI-HELICOBACTER TREATMENTS BASED ON CONSENSUS GUIDELINES (99,102,103)

1. The same first choice treatments are recommended worldwide, although different doses may be appropriate.
2. Triple therapy is the recommended first-choice treatment in populations with <15% to 20% clarithromycin resistance (and in populations with <40% metronidazole resistance, proton pump inhibitor-clarithromycin-metronidazole is preferable).
3. Different proton pump inhibitors are equivalent when used in triple therapy, but double dosing is more effective than single dosing.
   Triple therapy
   Proton pump inhibitor (standard dose twice daily)
   Clarithromycin (500 mg twice daily)
   Amoxicillin (1000 mg twice daily) or metronidazole (400 or 500 mg twice daily) for 7, 10, or 14 days (14-day treatment is more effective; a shorter treatment may be acceptable where local studies show that it is adequate).
4. Quadruple therapy is an alternative first-choice treatment in areas with a high prevalence (>15% to 20%) of clarithromycin resistance, or in patients who have previously received a macrolide.
   Quadruple therapy
   Proton pump inhibitor (standard dose twice daily)
   Metronidazole 500 mg three times daily
   Tetracycline 500 mg four times daily
   Bismuth subcitrate 120 mg four times daily for 7, 10, or 14 days
5. Bismuth-containing quadruple treatments remain the best second-choice treatment, if available. Proton pump inhibitor plus amoxicillin or tetracycline and metronidazole are recommended if bismuth is not available.
6. When a third-choice therapy is needed, treatment should be based on antimicrobial susceptibility testing.

TABLE 15.6

PREDICTORS OF REDUCED RESPONSE TO ANTIBIOTIC THERAPY

Absence of *H. pylori* infection (96,97)
Perigastric nodes enlargement (by endoscopy with ultrasound or CT) (96,97,126)
Infiltration beyond the mucosa layers (95,96,129)
Translocation t(11;18) (q21;q21) (50,133)
Translocations involving BCL-10, nuclear localization of BCL-10 protein (52,179).
Proximal location (97,130)
Presence of high-grade lymphoma component (109)
History of autoimmune disease (131)

is evidence of concomitant *H. pylori* infection. Indeed, in two series that included patients with and without *H. pylori*, none of the *H. pylori*-negative lymphomas (16 patients) responded to antibiotic therapy (96,97). Thus, it is highly questionable whether patients with no evidence of active *H. pylori* infection will benefit from a therapeutic trial with antibiotics. Nevertheless, there are anecdotal reports of lymphoma regression following antibiotics also in patients without *H. pylori*(105), and it might be worthwhile to also prescribe an eradication treatment in case of *H. pylori*-negative MALT lymphoma, at least in the cases without the t(11;18) translocation. The reasons are that *H. pylori* may have been missed by the diagnostic tests or that *Helicobacter heilmannii* may be involved. Indeed, the *H. heilmannii* group of microorganisms, which has been found in a few cases of gastric MALT lymphoma, is difficult to diagnose (106) and can be eradicated by the same antibiotic regimens (107).

Posttreatment Histologic Evaluation

The lymphoma may take up to ≥1 years to regress after *H. pylori* eradication (96,108), and it is worthwhile noting that the interpretation of residual lymphoid infiltrate in post-treatment gastric biopsies can be difficult. Indeed, the wide range of the reported remission rates is mainly due to the lack of uniform reproducible criteria in the literature for the definition of histologic remission. The Wotherspoon score (Table 15.7) (81) can be very useful to express the degree of confidence in the MALT lymphoma diagnosis on small gastric biopsies, however, it is difficult to apply in the evaluation of the response to antibiotic therapy, and other criteria have been proposed by German groups (109) and more recently by the French Groupe d'Etudes des Lymphomes de l'Adulte (GELA) (110), with the aim of providing clinically relevant information to the clinician. There are no comparative studies convincingly proving the superiority of any systems in the evaluation of gastric MALT lymphoma course, however, the GELA system (Table 15.7) may become a useful tool if its reproducibility will be confirmed by further testing on larger series (111).

Clinical and Molecular Follow-Up

A number of molecular follow-up studies showed a long-term persistence of monoclonal B cell in almost half of patients that had histologic disappearance of gastric MALT lymphoma following antibiotic therapy (Table 15.4) (112–116), indicating that *H. pylori* eradication suppresses but does not completely obliterate the lymphoma clone. In these cases, watchful waiting is feasible and safe (117). Indeed, most of the patients with molecular residual disease did not have a frank lymphoma relapse nor was histologic

TABLE 15.7

DIFFERENT PROPOSED CRITERIA TO DEFINE THE HISTOLOGIC GASTRIC LYMPHOMA RESPONSE AFTER *H. PYLORI* ERADICATION

Response	Definition	Histologic characteristics
Wotherspoon score (81)		
Score 0	Complete histologic remission	Normal gastric mucosa with scattered plasma cells in LP.
Score 1	Complete histologic remission	Chronic active gastritis with small clusters of lymphocytes in LP, no lymphoid follicles; no LEL
Score 2	Complete histologic remission	Chronic active gastritis with prominent lymphoid follicles with surrounding mantle zone and plasma cells; no LEL
Score 3	Partial histologic remission	Suspicious lymphoid infiltrate, probably reactive with lymphoid follicles surrounded by small lymphocytes that infiltrate diffusely in LP and occasionally into epithelium
Score 4	No change (persistent lymphoma)	Suspicious lymphoid infiltrate, probably lymphoma with lymphoid follicles surrounded by centrocyte-like cells that infiltrate diffusely in LP and into epithelium in small groups
Score 5	No change (persistent lymphoma)	MALT lymphoma with dense diffuse infiltrate of centrocyte-like cells in LP and prominent LEL
German studies (109)		
CR	Complete histologic regression	No remnant lymphoma cells detectable in the posttreatment biopsy specimens and "empty" LP with small basal clusters of lymphocytes and scattered plasma cells
PR	Partial histologic regression	Only partial depletion of atypical lymphoid cells from the LP or focal LEL
NC	No change (low-grade gastric MALT lymphoma)	Unequivocal evidence of LEL and replacement of the gastric glands by uniform centrocyte-like cells
GELA grading system (110)		
CR	Complete histologic remission	Normal or empty LP and/or fibrosis with absent or scattered plasma cells and small lymphoid cells in the LP, no LEL
pMRD	Probable minimal residual disease	Empty LP and/or fibrosis with aggregates of lymphoid cells or lymphoid nodules in the LP/MM and/or SM, no LEL
rRD	Responding residual disease	Focal empty LP and/or fibrosis with dense, diffuse or nodular lymphoid infiltrate, extending around glands in the LP, focal LEL, or absent
NC	No change	Dense, diffuse, or nodular lymphoid infiltrate, LEL usually present

LEL, lymphoepithelial lesions; LP, lamina propria; MM, muscolaris mucosa; SM, submucosa.

transformation documented despite persistent clonality (118), and the clinical relevance of monoclonality detected by polymerase chain reaction methods remains unclear. Even minimal residual microscopic disease detected after macroscopic regression following antibiotics therapy may remain clinically dormant (119–121), and a watch and wait strategy seems safe and could be considered at least for the selected patients agreeable to frequent endoscopies.

On the other hand, cases of lymphoma recurrence following *H. pylori* reinfection have been reported, suggesting that residual dormant tumor cells can be present despite histologic remission (109). Relapses have also been documented in the absence of *H. pylori* reinfection, indicating the presence of B-cell lymphoma clones that may have escaped the antigenic drive (109), and histologic transformation into diffuse large cell lymphoma has also been described in some cases (84,122). A careful long-term follow-up is strongly advisable, and histologic evaluation of repeated biopsies continues to be the fundamental follow-up procedure, despite the reproducibility problems previously discussed. It is recommended to repeat posttreatment endoscopies with multiple biopsies 3

months after treatment (to document *H. pylori* eradication and to exclude early lymphoma progression), then every 6 months for 2 years, and afterward yearly to monitor the histologic regression of the lymphoma.

The projected long-term risk of transformation into aggressive lymphoma seems lower in MALT lymphoma than in other indolent subtypes, at least for the primary gastric presentation (119,120), but it has not been clearly determined as yet. However, several cases have been reported of synchronous or metachronous development of gastric adenocarcinoma in patients with gastric MALT lymphoma. In the German MALT lymphoma trial, three of 120 patients (2.5%) developed early gastric cancer at 4 to 5 years, after complete lymphoma remission following cure of *H. pylori* infection (123). A Dutch nationwide epidemiologic study found 34 cases of gastric adenocarcinoma among 1,419 patients diagnosed with gastric MALT lymphoma (2.4%) (124). Patients with gastric MALT lymphoma had a significantly increased risk (six times higher) for gastric adenocarcinoma in comparison with the general population, and, notably, this risk was >16 times higher in patients younger than 60 years. This may not be surprising because a pathogenetic role of *H. pylori* has been found for both diseases. These findings are a strong argument in favor of regular strict long-term follow-up endoscopies also in patients with complete remission of gastric MALT lymphoma after cure of *H. pylori* infection.

Anti-*Helicobacter* Therapy in Gastric Diffuse Large B-Cell Lymphoma

H. pylori is less frequently detectable in gastric high-grade lymphoma than in MALT lymphoma (17,77). However, *H. pylori* eradication may be of benefit also in some diffuse large B-cell lymphomas of the stomach because in the subset of cases that may have been derived from a MALT lymphoma, proton pump inhibitors in combination with antibiotics may eliminate a residual low-grade component that can be responsible for tumor recurrence following antigen stimulation. Cases of regression of high-grade lesions after anti-*H. pylori* therapy have been reported, suggesting that high-grade transformation is not necessarily associated with the loss of *H. pylori* dependence (56,125). At present, however, the sole antibiotic therapy for gastric large cell lymphoma is strictly investigational and cannot be advised outside clinical trials.

Prediction of Regression of Gastric Mucosa-Associated Lymphoid Tissue Lymphoma Following Eradication of *Helicobacter pylori*

The follow-up of patients with MALT lymphoma following eradication of *H. pylori* is rather complex, requiring repeated gastroscopy, and it would be extremely useful to be able to identify the subset of cases of gastric MALT lymphoma (approximately 25%) that does not respond to eradication of *H. pylori* (Table 15.6).

In addition to the absence of *H. pylori*, other factors have been associated with a low response of gastric MALT lymphoma to antibiotic treatment alone. Studies from the French Groupe d'Etude Lymphome Digestif (96) and M. D. Anderson Cancer Center (97) and other groups (126,127) showed that in patients with *H. pylori*-positive gastric MALT lymphoma, the detection of nodal involvement by echoendoscopy or CT was associated with a significantly lower rate of lymphoma remission. Likewise, penetration of lymphoma beyond the mucosa was also associated with a markedly decreased response. These two features are related because deep involvement is linked to increased risk of nodal involvement (128). Furthermore, the likelihood of *H. pylori* presence is smaller when lymphoma involvement is found beyond the submucosa (17).

Several studies have confirmed that endoscopic ultrasound can be useful to predict the lymphoma response to *H. pylori* eradication, demonstrating that there is a significant difference between the response rates of lymphomas restricted to the gastric mucosa and those with less superficial lesions (95–97,127,129). The response rate is the highest for the mucosa-confined lymphomas (approximately 70% to 90%), and then decreases markedly and progressively for the tumors infiltrating the submucosa, muscularis propria, and serosa.

Tumor location could also be a predictive factor for remission following antibiotic treatment; indeed, *H. pylori* eradication appears more successful in inducing MALT lymphoma remission in the distal stomach compared with proximal disease (97,130).

In a report from a German group, four of six patients whose lymphoma has not regressed following eradication of *H. pylori*, surgical resection showed the presence of high-grade lymphoma in deeper sections that were not appreciated during endoscopy (109). This experience underlines the importance of multiple deep biopsies, particularly if endoscopy with ultrasound indicates deep penetration and/or lymph node enlargement. It also suggests that gastric diffuse large B-cell lymphomas with MALT lymphoma component should be treated as a diffuse large B-cell lymphoma (with chemoimmunotherapy and involved-field radiotherapy).

Patients with preexisting autoimmune disorders have been reported to develop MALT lymphoma significantly earlier in life and to respond poorly to *H. pylori* eradication, even in case of early stage lymphoma (131,132). Their long-term outcome, however, does not appear to be adversely influenced (132). A previously mentioned, the t(11;18)(q21;q21), present in up to 40% of cases, is also strongly associated with failure to respond to eradication of *H. pylori*. Liu et al. (50), in an analysis of biopsy material from 111 patients with *H. pylori*-positive gastric MALT lymphoma, have shown that only two of 48 (4%) patients whose lymphoma completely regressed after *H. pylori* eradication showed t(11;18), whereas 42 of 63 (67%) of the nonresponding patients demonstrated the translocation. Other studies confirmed that t(11;18) translocation can predict the therapeutic response of gastric MALT lymphoma to *H. pylori* eradication (133) and to some extent to chlorambucil (134), but not necessarily to other therapeutic approaches (135,136). Thus, t(11;18) is a powerful indicator of response to *H. pylori* eradication, and its presence at diagnosis may suggest that an alternative treatment (e.g., radiotherapy) might be administered early, rather than waiting for regression with repeated endoscopies. It has been also indicated, however, that tumors that are t(11;18) negative have a higher risk of transformation into diffuse large B-cell lymphoma. Therefore, t(11;18)-negative tumors that have not completely regressed after antibiotics should be closely monitored for early alternative therapeutic intervention.

H. pylori-independent status is often associated with nuclear translocation of BCL10, and gastric MALT lymphomas with strong BCL10 nuclear expression or t(1;14) are also usually resistant to *H. pylori* eradication (52). Indeed, the frequencies of t(11;18)(q21;q21) and BCL10 nuclear expression are significantly higher in the *H. pylori*-negative than *H. pylori*-positive cases (137).

Interestingly, t(11;18) is also associated with nuclear expression of BCL10, albeit more weakly than t(1;14). Moreover, the frequency of both t(11;18)(q21;q21) and nuclear BCL10 expression is significantly higher in tumors that have disseminated beyond the stomach (78% and 93%, respectively) than those confined to the stomach (10% and 38%) (59). These findings in part explain the results based on the use of endoscopic ultrasound, and suggest that both t(11;18)(q21;q21) and BCL10 nuclear expression are associated with failure to respond to *H. pylori* eradication and with more advanced MALT lymphoma. This is in keeping with molecular studies indicating that their oncogenic activities may be related (138).

Treatment of *Helicobacter pylori*-Independent Gastric Mucosa-Associated Lymphoid Tissue Lymphoma

Approximately 30% to 50% of patients with *H. pylori*-positive gastric MALT lymphoma will show persistent or progressing lymphoma even after eradication of *H. pylori* with antibiotic therapy (Table 15.4). Of the complete responders, almost 15% will relapse within 3 years, suggesting that about half of patients with gastric MALT lymphoma will eventually be considered for additional therapies. Most of those will still have disease limited to the stomach. Patients that present with no evidence *H. pylori* infection are unlikely to respond to antibiotics and should be considered for alternative treatments.

There is no consensus for the treatment of patients with gastric MALT lymphoma requiring further treatment beyond *H. pylori* eradication or with extensive disease.

As a local therapy, surgery has been widely used in the past. Cogliatti et al. (139) reviewed 69 cases of low-grade gastric MALT lymphoma, 45 of them treated with surgery alone, the remaining 24 with surgery followed by chemotherapy, radiotherapy, or both. The 5-year OS was 91%, and no significant difference in survival was observed in patients selected for adjuvant therapy following surgery.

In the last decade, the role of surgery in gastric lymphoma has been questioned (19,140–142); gastric MALT lymphoma is a multifocal disease (143), and adequate gastrectomy needs to be quite extensive, severely impairing quality of life, and yet residual disease at the margins may still require additional radiation and/or chemotherapy. Moreover, large German multicenter studies have clearly showed that an organ-preserving approach for early gastric lymphoma is not inferior to primary surgery, showing that patients treated with surgery and radiation or radiation and chemotherapy (six cycles of a cyclophosphamide, vincristine, and prednisone regimen) had similar survival rates (6,144). Aviles et al. (145) reported the results of a three-arm Mexican trial of 241 patients in which event-free survival, but not OS, was significantly inferior in patients treated with radiation or surgery in comparison with those receiving aggressive chemotherapy alone (three cycles of cyclophosphamide, doxorubicin, vincristine, and prednisone, followed by four cycles of cyclophosphamide, vincristine, and prednisone). These results also indicate that organ preservation strategies are not inferior to those based on surgery.

Several institutions reported excellent results using involved-field radiotherapy of the stomach in patients with *H. pylori*-independent gastric MALT lymphoma, who either failed antibiotic therapy or had no evidence for *H. pylori* infection (91,146–151). The last update of the Memorial Sloan-Kettering Cancer Center experience included 51 patients with gastric MALT lymphoma (stage I: 39; stage II: 10; stage IV: 2) who were either without *H. pylori* (30 patients) or remained with persistent lymphoma after antibiotic therapies and adequate observation (21 patients) (152). All patients were treated with radiation to the stomach and perigastric nodes; the median total dose was 30 Gy in 4 weeks. All patients had regular follow-up endoscopic evaluations and biopsies. Forty-nine of 51 (96%) patients obtained a biopsy proven complete response. Of three patients who had relapse, two were salvaged. Three patients died of other malignancies; all second tumors developed outside the radiation field. At a median follow-up of 4 years, freedom from treatment failure, OS, and cause-specific survival were 89%, 83%, and 100%, respectively. Treatment was well tolerated, with no significant acute or chronic side effects. The experience from Toronto and Boston using the same radiation approach was equally successful (91,148,149), supporting the approach that modest dose involved-field radiotherapy is the treatment of choice for patients with persistent gastric MALT lymphoma who have exhausted the antibiotic therapy approach or are unlikely to respond to it (patients without *H. pylori*) (147,153).

The modern development of advanced radiotherapy planning techniques such as three-dimensional conformal radiotherapy and intensity modulated radiotherapy has facilitated the determination of the clinical target volume, reducing the toxicity that is related to the irradiation of normal gastric mucosa and of nontarget organs (especially the left kidney) (147,153,154). Indeed, radiotherapy (30 to 33 Gy) has become a standard treatment, at least in North America, for patients without *H. pylori* with localized disease, and its use in this setting has been recommended by the National Comprehensive Cancer Network Clinical Practice Guidelines in Oncology (155).

Interestingly, in a molecular follow-up study from the Memorial Sloan-Kettering Cancer Center, despite sustained biopsy proven pathologic remission for as long as 10 years after involved-field radiotherapy, the majority of patients remained continuously or intermittently positive by clonotypic polymerase chain reaction. This suggests that residual lymphoma cells remained but were missing a signal essential to the cancer phenotype (156).

Patients with systemic disease should be considered for chemotherapy and/or immunotherapy (anti-CD-20) (117,157). In the presence of disseminated or advanced disease, chemotherapy may be an obvious choice; unfortunately, it has never been adequately evaluated in gastric MALT lymphomas because it was usually not administered, or given after surgery or radiotherapy. Only few compounds have been tested specifically in MALT lymphomas. A nonrandomized study of 24 patients (17 with stage I and seven with stage IV disease, most of them with primary gastric localization) reported that oral alkylating agents (either cyclophosphamide 100 mg per day or chlorambucil 6 mg per day, with a median treatment duration of 1 year) can result in a high rate of disease control with a projected 5-year event-free survival and OS of 50% and 75%, respectively (158). The efficacy of alkylating agents in MALT lymphomas was confirmed by other studies showing a high rate of disease control (126,159). Other phase II studies demonstrated some antitumor activity of the purine analogs fludarabine (160) and cladribine (161), which might, however, be associated with an increased risk of secondary myelodysplastic syndrome (162), and of a combination regimen of chlorambucil/mitoxantrone/prednisone (163). Another potentially active class of anticancer agent drugs is that targeted to the inhibition the NF-κB pathway, the common target of the recurrent translocations in MALT lymphoma. An example of this class is the proteasome inhibitor bortezomib that is currently being investigated in a phase II study by the IELSG (NCT00210327) (164).

Aggressive anthracycline-containing chemotherapy should be reserved for patients with high tumor burden (bulky masses, high International Prognostic Index score) (15,165).

The activity of the anti-CD20 monoclonal antibody rituximab has also been shown in phase II studies, with a response rate of about 70% (135,166,167), and may represent an additional option for the treatment of systemic disease, but the efficacy of its combination with chemotherapy still needs to be explored in this histologic type. Depending on the response to systemic treatment, the presence of bulky lesions and symptoms, selected patients with advanced disease may also benefit from radiation therapy.

Treatment of Nongastric Marginal Zone Lymphomas of the Mucosa-Associated Lymphoid Tissue Type

Nongastric MALT lymphomas have been difficult to characterize because these tumors, numerous when considered together, are distributed so widely throughout the body that it is difficult to assemble an adequate series of any given site. Yet, few large series have addressed the characteristics of nongastric MALT lymphomas. Patients with nongastric MALT lymphoma may have a tendency to have progression more often (83), but whether different sites have a different natural history remains an open question. Location remains an important factor because of organ-specific problems, which result in particular management strategies (9–12). The optimal management of nongastric MALT lymphomas has not yet been clearly established. Retrospective series included patients treated with surgery, radiotherapy, and chemotherapy, alone or in combination (8,9,91,149,153,159). In most patients, good disease control and excellent cause-specific and OS have been demonstrated, independent of the treatment modality selected (9–12). Thus, the treatment choice should be "patient-tailored," taking into account the site, stage, and clinical characteristics of the individual patient. In patients with localized disease, extensive surgery is unnecessary in most sites because marginal zone lymphomas are exquisitely sensitive to relatively low doses of radiation. Specifically, MALT lymphoma in sites such as salivary glands, ocular, conjunctiva, thyroid, breast, and bladder has been successfully eradicated with involved-field radiotherapy encompassing the involved organ alone with a dose of 24 to 36 Gy (91,149,153,168–173). Even unusual sites (such as larynx, base of skull, urethra, prostate) not easily amenable to surgery have been well controlled by involved-field radiotherapy (14,174–176).

There is increasing evidence that antibiotic treatment can be effective in patients with lymphoma of the ocular adnexa (177), despite the evident geographic variability of its association with *C. psittaci* infection and the possibility that other etiopathogenic agents could be involved (32,178).

Patients with extensive lung disease, involvement of multiple sites or the bone marrow are likely to respond to a variety systemic chemotherapy regimens, although no specific chemotherapy regimen has been advocated (15,86). Responses to rituximab have also been reported (166), and the efficacy of the combination of rituximab with chlorambucil in either nongastric or gastric antibiotic-resistant MALT lymphoma is currently being explored in a randomized study by the IELSG (NCT00210353).

Very specific problems are encountered in the management of IPSID; its natural course is usually prolonged, often over many years, including a potentially reversible early phase, when antibiotic treatment may lead to lymphoma regression. However, there is no clear evidence that antibiotics alone are of benefit in the advanced phases. Surgery has diagnostic but no therapeutic role because intestinal involvement is generally diffuse. Early studies reported that aggressive chemotherapy is not well tolerated by patients with advanced disease who then have poor survival rates, however, more recent data suggest that anthracycline-containing regimens, combined with nutritional support plus antibiotics to control diarrhea and malabsorption, may offer the best chance of cure (23).

Future Directions

For a disease that has been defined as a separate entity only in the 1980s, extraordinary progress has been made in understanding the etiology and cellular and molecular pathological events and identifying simply treatable causative bacterial agents. Clinicians have also gathered encouraging experience in eradicating MALT lymphoma disease in sites that are unlikely to respond to antibiotics or in gastric lymphoma that developed or has become independent of *H. pylori*. Modern radiation therapy techniques have been shown to be effective in eradicating MALT lymphoma, allowing organ preservation without a need for surgery. The design of effective chemotherapy regimens and introduction of anti-CD20 therapy for appropriate clinical circumstances are in progress and will expand our treatment options. The establishment of national and international groups to investigate patients with a relatively uncommon disease with involvement of a variety of sites has facilitated our clinical understanding of the disease.

Hopefully, the close collaboration between pathologists, molecular biologists, and clinicians that has characterized the rapid progress in this disease in the last two decades will further advance the understanding of this fascinating lymphoma, better define our treatment strategy, and expand our therapeutic options in the next years.

References

1. Isaacson P, Wright DH. Malignant lymphoma of mucosa-associated lymphoid tissue. A distinctive type of B-cell lymphoma. *Cancer* 1983;52:1410–1416.
2. Isaacson P, Wright DH. Extranodal malignant lymphoma arising from mucosa-associated lymphoid tissue. *Cancer* 1984;53:2515–2524.
3. Isaacson PG, Chott A, Nakamura S, et al. Extranodal marginal zone B-cell lymphoma of mucosa-associated lymphoid tissue (MALT lymphoma). In: Swerdlow S, Campo E, Harris NL, et al., eds. *WHO classification of tumours of haematopoietic and lymphoid tissues*, 4th ed. Lyon, France: IARC, 2008:214–217.
4. A clinical evaluation of the International Lymphoma Study Group classification of non-Hodgkin's lymphoma. The Non-Hodgkin's Lymphoma Classification Project. *Blood* 1997;89:3909–3918.
5. Nakamura S, Matsumoto T, Iida M, et al. Primary gastrointestinal lymphoma in Japan: a clinicopathologic analysis of 455 patients with special reference to its time trends. *Cancer* 2003;97:2462–2473.
6. Koch P, Probst A, Berdel WE, et al. Treatment results in localized primary gastric lymphoma: data of patients registered within the German multicenter study (GIT NHL 02/96). *J Clin Oncol* 2005;23:7050–7059.
7. Shenkier TN, Connors JM. Primary extranodal non-Hodgkin's lymphomas. In: Canellos GP, Lister TA, Young BD, eds. *The lymphomas*, 2nd ed. Philadelphia, PA: Saunders Elsevier, 2006:325–347.

8. Zinzani PL, Magagnoli M, Galieni P, et al. Nongastrointestinal low-grade mucosa-associated lymphoid tissue lymphoma: analysis of 75 patients. *J Clin Oncol* 1999;17:1254.
9. Zucca E, Conconi A, Pedrinis E, et al. Nongastric marginal zone B-cell lymphoma of mucosa-associated lymphoid tissue. *Blood* 2003;101:2489–2495.
10. Thieblemont C, Berger F, Dumontet C, et al. Mucosa-associated lymphoid tissue lymphoma is a disseminated disease in one third of 158 patients analyzed. *Blood* 2000;95:802–806.
11. Raderer M, Wohrer S, Streubel B, et al. Assessment of disease dissemination in gastric compared with extragastric mucosa-associated lymphoid tissue lymphoma using extensive staging: a single-center experience. *J Clin Oncol* 2006;24:3136–3141.
12. de Boer JP, Hiddink RF, Raderer M, et al. Dissemination patterns in non-gastric MALT lymphoma. *Haematologica* 2008;93:201–206.
13. George AC, Ozsahin M, Janzer R, et al. Primary intracranial dural lymphoma of mucosa-associated lymphoid tissue (MALT) type: report of one case and review of the literature. *Bull Cancer* 2005;92:E51–E56.
14. Masuda A, Tsujii T, Kojima M, et al. Primary mucosa-associated lymphoid tissue (MALT) lymphoma arising from the male urethra. A case report and review of the literature. *Pathol Res Pract* 2002;198:571–575.
15. Thieblemont C. Clinical presentation and management of marginal zone lymphomas. *Hematology Am Soc Hematol Educ Program* 2005;307–313.
16. Doglioni C, Wotherspoon AC, Moschini A, et al. High incidence of primary gastric lymphoma in northeastern Italy. *Lancet* 1992;339:834–835.
17. Nakamura S, Yao T, Aoyagi K, et al. Helicobacter pylori and primary gastric lymphoma. A histopathologic and immunohistochemical analysis of 237 patients. *Cancer* 1997;79:3–11.
18. Wotherspoon AC, Ortiz-Hidalgo C, Falzon MR, et al. Helicobacter pylori-associated gastritis and primary B-cell gastric lymphoma. *Lancet* 1991;338:1175–1176.
19. Zucca E, Bertoni F, Roggero E, et al. The gastric marginal zone B-cell lymphoma of MALT type. *Blood* 2000;96:410–419.
20. Roggero E, Zucca E, Mainetti C, et al. Eradication of Borrelia burgdorferi infection in primary marginal zone B-cell lymphoma of the skin. *Hum Pathol* 2000;31:263–268.
21. Ferreri AJ, Guidoboni M, Ponzoni M, et al. Evidence for an association between Chlamydia psittaci and ocular adnexal lymphomas. *J Natl Cancer Inst* 2004;96:586–594.
22. Ekstrom Smedby K, Vajdic CM, Falster M, et al. Autoimmune disorders and risk of non-Hodgkin lymphoma subtypes: a pooled analysis within the InterLymph Consortium. *Blood* 2008;111:4029–4038.
23. Al-Saleem T, Al-Mondhiry H. Immunoproliferative small intestinal disease (IPSID): a model for mature B-cell neoplasms. *Blood* 2005;105:2274–2280.
24. Lecuit M, Abachin E, Martin A, et al. Immunoproliferative small intestinal disease associated with Campylobacter jejuni. *N Engl J Med* 2004;350:239–248.
25. Spencer J, Finn T, Isaacson PG. Human Peyer's patches: an immunohistochemical study. *Gut* 1986;27:405–410.
26. Spencer J, MacDonald TT, Finn T, et al. The development of gut associated lymphoid tissue in the terminal ileum of fetal human intestine. *Clin Exp Immunol* 1986;64:536–543.
27. Spencer J, Finn T, Isaacson PG. Gut associated lymphoid tissue: a morphological and immunocytochemical study of the human appendix. *Gut* 1985;26:672–679.
28. Brandtzaeg P, Bjerke K. Human Peyer's patches: lympho-epithelial relationships and characteristics of immunoglobulin-producing cells. *Immunol Invest* 1989;18:29–45.
29. Brandtzaeg P, Halstensen TS, Kett K, et al. Immunobiology and immunopathology of human gut mucosa: humoral immunity and intraepithelial lymphocytes. *Gastroenterology* 1989;97:1562–1584.
30. Du MQ, Isaacson PG. Gastric MALT lymphoma: from aetiology to treatment. *Lancet Oncol* 2002;3:97–104.
31. Bertoni F, Cazzaniga G, Bosshard G, et al. Immunoglobulin heavy chain diversity genes rearrangement pattern indicates that MALT-type gastric lymphoma B cells have undergone an antigen selection process. *Br J Haematol* 1997;97:830–836.
32. Ferreri AJ, Dolcetti R, Du MQ, et al. Ocular adnexal MALT lymphoma: an intriguing model for antigen-driven lymphomagenesis and microbial-targeted therapy. *Ann Oncol* 2008;19:835–846.
33. Du MQ, Diss TC, Dogan A, et al. Clone-specific PCR reveals wide dissemination of gastric MALT lymphoma to the gastric mucosa. *J Pathol* 2000;192:488–493.
34. Isaacson PG, Spencer J. Malignant lymphoma of mucosa-associated lymphoid tissue. *Histopathology* 1987;11:445–462.
35. Isaacson PG, Wotherspoon AC, Diss T, et al. Follicular colonization in B-cell lymphoma of mucosa-associated lymphoid tissue. *Am J Surg Pathol* 1991;15:819–828.
36. Isaacson PG, Muller-Hermelink HK, Piris MA, et al. Extranodal marginal zone B-cell lymphoma of mucosa-associated lymphoid tissue (MALT lymphoma). In: Jaffe ES, Harris NL, Stein H, et al., eds. *World Health Organization classification of tumours. Pathology and genetics of tumours of haematopoietic and lymphoid tissues*. Lyon, France: IARC Press, 2001:157–160.
37. Dierlamm J, Baens M, Wlodarska I, et al. The apoptosis inhibitor gene API2 and a novel 18q gene, MLT, are recurrently rearranged in the t(11;18)(q21;q21) associated with mucosa- associated lymphoid tissue lymphomas. *Blood* 1999;93:3601–3609.
38. Willis TG, Jadayel DM, Du MQ, et al. Bcl10 is involved in t(1;14)(p22;q32) of MALT B cell lymphoma and mutated in multiple tumor types. *Cell* 1999;96:35–45.
39. Streubel B, Lamprecht A, Dierlamm J, et al. T(14;18)(q32;q21) involving IGH and MALT1 is a frequent chromosomal aberration in MALT lymphoma. *Blood* 2003;101:2335–2339.
40. Streubel B, Vinatzer U, Lamprecht A, et al. T(3;14)(p14.1;q32) involving IGH and FOXP1 is a novel recurrent chromosomal aberration in MALT lymphoma. *Leukemia* 2005;19:652–658.
41. Vinatzer U, Gollinger M, Mullauer, L et al. Mucosa-associated lymphoid tissue lymphoma: novel translocations including rearrangements of ODZ2, JMJD2C, and CNN3. *Clin Cancer Res* 2008;14:6426–6431.
42. Remstein ED, Dogan A, Einerson RR, et al. The incidence and anatomic site specificity of chromosomal translocations in primary extranodal marginal zone B-cell lymphoma of mucosa-associated lymphoid tissue (MALT lymphoma) in North America. *Am J Surg Pathol* 2006;30:1546–1553.
43. Isaacson PG, Du MQ. MALT lymphoma: from morphology to molecules. *Nat Rev Cancer* 2004;4:644–653.
44. Jost PJ, Ruland J. Aberrant NF-{kappa}B signaling in lymphoma: mechanisms, consequences and therapeutic implications. *Blood* 2007;109:2700–2707.
45. Bertoni F, Zucca E. Delving deeper into MALT lymphoma biology. *J Clin Invest* 2006;116:22–26.
46. Farinha P, Gascoyne RD. Molecular pathogenesis of mucosa-associated lymphoid tissue lymphoma. *J Clin Oncol* 2005;23:6370–6378.
47. Murga Penas EM, Hinz K, Roser K, et al. Translocations t(11;18)(q21;q21) and t(14;18)(q32;q21) are the main chromosomal abnormalities involving MLT/MALT1 in MALT lymphomas. *Leukemia* 2003;17:2225–2229.
48. Ye H, Liu H, Attygalle A, et al. Variable frequencies of t(11;18)(q21;q21) in MALT lymphomas of different sites: significant association with CagA strains of H. pylori in gastric MALT lymphoma. *Blood* 2003;102:1012–1018.
49. Hosokawa Y, Suzuki H, Suzuki Y, et al. Antiapoptotic function of apoptosis inhibitor 2-MALT1 fusion protein involved in t(11;18)(q21;q21) mucosa-associated lymphoid tissue lymphoma. *Cancer Res* 2004;64:3452–3457.
50. Liu H, Ye H, Ruskone-Fourmestraux A, et al. T(11;18) is a marker for all stage gastric MALT lymphomas that will not respond to H. pylori eradication. *Gastroenterology* 2002;122:1286–1294.
51. Kuo SH, Chen LT, Yeh KH, et al. Nuclear expression of BCL10 or nuclear factor kappa B predicts Helicobacter pylori-independent status of early-stage, high-grade gastric mucosa-associated lymphoid tissue lymphomas. *J Clin Oncol* 2004;22:3491–3497.
52. Ye H, Gong L, Liu H, et al. Strong BCL10 nuclear expression identifies gastric MALT lymphomas that do not respond to H pylori eradication. *Gut* 2006;55:137–138.
53. Du MQ, Atherton JC. Molecular subtyping of gastric MALT lymphomas: implications for prognosis and management. *Gut* 2006;55:886–893.
54. Starostik P, Greiner A, Schultz A, et al. Genetic aberrations common in gastric high-grade large B-cell lymphoma. *Blood* 2000;95:1180–1187.
55. Zhou Y, Ye H, Martin-Subero JI, et al. Distinct comparative genomic hybridisation profiles in gastric mucosa-associated lymphoid tissue lymphomas with and without t(11;18)(q21;q21). *Br J Haematol* 2006;133:35–42.
56. Chen LT, Lin JT, Tai JJ, et al. Long-term results of anti-Helicobacter pylori therapy in early-stage gastric high-grade transformed MALT lymphoma. *J Natl Cancer Inst* 2005;97:1345–1353.
57. Ye H, Dogan A, Karran L, et al. BCL10 expression in normal and neoplastic lymphoid tissue: nuclear localization in MALT lymphoma. *Am J Pathol* 2000;157:1147–1154.
58. Ye H, Liu H, Dogan A, et al. MALT lymphoma with t(11;18)(q21;q21) express nuclear BCL10 [abstract]. *Blood* 2000;96:468a. Abstract 2014.
59. Liu H, Ye H, Dogan A, et al. T(11;18)(q21;q21) is associated with advanced mucosa-associated lymphoid tissue lymphoma that expresses nuclear BCL10. *Blood* 2001;98:1182–1187.
60. Kuo SH, Chen LT, Wu MS, et al. Differential response to H. pylori eradication therapy of co-existing diffuse large B-cell lymphoma and MALT lymphoma of stomach-significance of tumour cell clonality and BCL10 expression. *J Pathol* 2007;211:296–304.
61. Gallardo F, Bellosillo B, Espinet B, et al. Aberrant nuclear BCL10 expression and lack of t(11;18)(q21;q21) in primary cutaneous marginal zone B-cell lymphoma. *Hum Pathol* 2006;37:867–873.
62. Franco R, Camacho FI, Caleo A, et al. Nuclear bcl10 expression characterizes a group of ocular adnexa MALT lymphomas with shorter failure-free survival. *Mod Pathol* 2006;19:1055–1067.
63. Chng WJ, Remstein ED, Fonseca R, et al. Gene expression profiling of pulmonary mucosa-associated lymphoid tissue lymphoma identifies new biologic insights with potential diagnostic and therapeutic applications. *Blood* 2009;113:635–645.

64. Sagaert X, de Paepe P, Libbrecht L, et al. Forkhead box protein P1 expression in mucosa-associated lymphoid tissue lymphomas predicts poor prognosis and transformation to diffuse large B-cell lymphoma. *J Clin Oncol* 2006;24:2490–2497.

65. Haralambieva E, Adam P, Ventura R, et al. Genetic rearrangement of FOXP1 is predominantly detected in a subset of diffuse large B-cell lymphomas with extranodal presentation. *Leukemia* 2006;20:1300–1303.

66. Dierlamm J, Pittaluga S, Wlodarska, I et al. Marginal zone B-cell lymphomas of different sites share similar cytogenetic and morphologic features. *Blood* 1996;87:299–307.

67. Callet-Bauchu E, Baseggio L, Felman P, et al. Cytogenetic analysis delineates a spectrum of chromosomal changes that can distinguish non-MALT marginal zone B-cell lymphomas among mature B-cell entities: a description of 103 cases. *Leukemia* 2005;19:1818–1823.

68. Novak U, Rinaldi A, Kwee I, et al. The NF-κB negative regulator TNFAIP3 (A20) is inactivated by somatic mutations and genomic deletions in marginal zone lymphomas. *Blood* 2009 May 14;113(20): 4918–21.

69. Honma K, Tsuzuki S, Nakagawa M, et al. TNFAIP3 is the target gene of chromosome band 6q23.3-q24.1 loss in ocular adnexal marginal zone B cell lymphoma. *Genes Chromosomes Cancer* 2008;47:1–7.

70. Bahler DW, Miklos JA, Swerdlow SH. Ongoing Ig gene hypermutation in salivary gland mucosa- associated lymphoid tissue-type lymphomas. *Blood* 1997;89:3335–3344.

71. Du M, Diss TC, Xu C, et al. Ongoing mutation in MALT lymphoma immunoglobulin gene suggests that antigen stimulation plays a role in the clonal expansion. *Leukemia* 1996;10:1190–1197.

72. Qin Y, Greiner A, Trunk MJ, et al. Somatic hypermutation in low-grade mucosa-associated lymphoid tissue- type B-cell lymphoma. *Blood* 1995;86:3528–3534.

73. Diss TC, Pan L. Polymerase chain reaction in the assessment of lymphomas. *Cancer Surv* 1997;30:21–44.

74. Hsi ED, Greenson JK, Singleton TP, et al. Detection of immunoglobulin heavy chain gene rearrangement by polymerase chain reaction in chronic active gastritis associated with Helicobacter pylori. *Hum Pathol* 1996;27:290–296.

75. Hsi ED, Singleton TP, Svoboda SM, et al. Characterization of the lymphoid infiltrate in Hashimoto thyroiditis by immunohistochemistry and polymerase chain reaction for immunoglobulin heavy chain gene rearrangement. *Am J Clin Pathol* 1998;110:327–333.

76. Savio A, Franzin G, Wotherspoon AC, et al. Diagnosis and posttreatment follow-up of Helicobacter pylori- positive gastric lymphoma of mucosa-associated lymphoid tissue: histology, polymerase chain reaction, or both? *Blood* 1996;87:1255–1260.

77. Nakamura S, Aoyagi K, Furuse M, et al. B-cell monoclonality precedes the development of gastric MALT lymphoma in Helicobacter pylori-associated chronic gastritis. *Am J Pathol* 1998;152:1271–1279.

78. Parsonnet J, Hansen S, Rodriguez L, et al. Helicobacter pylori infection and gastric lymphoma. *N Engl J Med* 1994;330:1267–1271.

79. Zucca E, Bertoni F, Roggero E, et al. Molecular analysis of the progression from Helicobacter pylori- associated chronic gastritis to mucosa-associated lymphoid-tissue lymphoma of the stomach. *N Engl J Med* 1998;338:804–810.

80. Hussell T, Isaacson PG, Crabtree JE, et al. The response of cells from low-grade B-cell gastric lymphomas of mucosa- associated lymphoid tissue to Helicobacter pylori. *Lancet* 1993;342:571–574.

81. Wotherspoon AC, Doglioni C, Diss TC, et al. Regression of primary low-grade B-cell gastric lymphoma of mucosa- associated lymphoid tissue type after eradication of Helicobacter pylori. *Lancet* 1993;342:575–577.

82. Rollinson S, Levene AP, Mensah FK, et al. Gastric marginal zone lymphoma is associated with polymorphisms in genes involved in inflammatory response and antioxidative capacity. *Blood* 2003;102:1007–1011.

83. Thieblemont C, Bastion Y, Berger F, et al. Mucosa-associated lymphoid tissue gastrointestinal and nongastrointestinal lymphoma behavior: analysis of 108 patients. *J Clin Oncol* 1997;15:1624–1630.

84. Pinotti G, Zucca E, Roggero E, et al. Clinical features, treatment and outcome in a series of 93 patients with low-grade gastric MALT lymphoma. *Leuk Lymphoma* 1997;26:527–537.

85. Thieblemont C, Coiffier B. MALT lymphoma: sites of presentations, clinical features and staging procedures. In: Zucca E, Bertoni F, eds. *MALT lymphomas*. Georgetown, TX: Landes Bioscience/Eurekah.com, 2004: 60–80.

86. Cavalli F, Isaacson PG, Gascoyne RD, et al. MALT lymphomas. *Hematology Am Soc Hematol Educ Program* 2001:241–258.

87. Du MQ, Xu CF, Diss TC, et al. Intestinal dissemination of gastric mucosa-associated lymphoid tissue lymphoma. *Blood* 1996;88:4445–4451.

88. Du MQ, Peng HZ, Dogan A, et al. Preferential dissemination of B-cell gastric mucosa-associated lymphoid tissue (MALT) lymphoma to the splenic marginal zone. *Blood* 1997;90:4071–4077.

89. Dogan A, Du M, Koulis A, et al. Expression of lymphocyte homing receptors and vascular addressins in low-grade gastric B-cell lymphomas of mucosa- associated lymphoid tissue. *Am J Pathol* 1997;151:1361–1369.

90. Drillenburg P, van der Voort R, Koopman G, et al. Preferential expression of the mucosal homing receptor integrin alpha 4 beta 7 in gastrointestinal non-Hodgkin's lymphomas. *Am J Pathol* 1997;150:919–927.

91. Tsang RW, Gospodarowicz MK, Pintilie M, et al. Localized mucosa-associated lymphoid tissue lymphoma treated with radiation therapy has excellent clinical outcome. *J Clin Oncol* 2003;21:4157–4164.

92. Taal BG, Boot H, van Heerde P, et al. Primary non-Hodgkin lymphoma of the stomach: endoscopic pattern and prognosis in low versus high grade malignancy in relation to the MALT concept. *Gut* 1996;39:556–561.

93. de Jong D, Aleman BM, Taal BG, et al. Controversies and consensus in the diagnosis, work-up and treatment of gastric lymphoma: an international survey. *Ann Oncol* 1999;10:275–280.

94. Rohatiner A, d'Amore F, Coiffier B, et al. Report on a workshop convened to discuss the pathological and staging classifications of gastrointestinal tract lymphoma. *Ann Oncol* 1994;5:397–400.

95. Sackmann M, Morgner A, Rudolph B, et al. Regression of gastric MALT lymphoma after eradication of Helicobacter pylori is predicted by endosonographic staging. MALT Lymphoma Study Group. *Gastroenterology* 1997;113:1087–1090.

96. Ruskone-Fourmestraux A, Lavergne A, Aegerter PH, et al. Predictive factors for regression of gastric MALT lymphoma after anti- Helicobacter pylori treatment. *Gut* 2001;48:297–303.

97. Steinbach G, Ford R, Glober G, et al. Antibiotic treatment of gastric lymphoma of mucosa-associated lymphoid tissue. An uncontrolled trial. *Ann Intern Med* 1999;131:88–95.

98. Ruskone-Fourmestraux A, Dragosics B, Morgner A, et al. Paris staging system for primary gastrointestinal lymphomas. *Gut* 2003;52:912–913.

99. Malfertheiner P, Megraud F, O'Morain, C et al. Current concepts in the management of Helicobacter pylori infection: the Maastricht III Consensus Report. *Gut* 2007;56:772–781.

100. Zucca E, Cavalli F. Are antibiotics the treatment of choice for gastric lymphoma? *Curr Hematol Rep* 2004;3:11–16.

101. Morgner A, Bayerdorffer E, Neubauer A, et al. Malignant tumors of the stomach. Gastric mucosa-associated lymphoid tissue lymphoma and Helicobacter pylori. *Gastroenterol Clin North Am* 2000;29:593–607.

102. Fuccio L, Laterza L, Zagari RM, et al. Treatment of Helicobacter pylori infection. *BMJ* 2008;337:a1454.

103. Chey WD, Wong BC. American College of Gastroenterology guideline on the management of Helicobacter pylori infection. *Am J Gastroenterol* 2007;102:1808–1825.

104. Hancock B, Qian W, Linch D, et al. Chlorambucil versus observation after anti-Helicobacter therapy in gastric MALT lymphomas: results of the international randomised LY03 trial. *Br J Haematol* 2009;144:367–375.

105. Raderer M, Streubel B, Wohrer S, et al. Successful antibiotic treatment of Helicobacter pylori negative gastric mucosa associated lymphoid tissue lymphomas. *Gut* 2006;55:616–618.

106. De Groote D, Van Doorn LJ, Van den Bulck K, et al. Detection of non-pylori Helicobacter species in "Helicobacter heilmannii"-infected humans. *Helicobacter* 2005;10:398–406.

107. Morgner A, Lehn N, Andersen LP, et al. Helicobacter heilmannii-associated primary gastric low-grade MALT lymphoma: complete remission after curing the infection. *Gastroenterology* 2000;118:821–828.

108. Roggero E, Zucca E, Pinotti G, et al. Eradication of Helicobacter pylori infection in primary low- grade gastric lymphoma of mucosa-associated lymphoid tissue. *Ann Intern Med* 1995;122:767–769.

109. Neubauer A, Thiede C, Morgner A, et al. Cure of Helicobacter pylori infection and duration of remission of low-grade gastric mucosa-associated lymphoid tissue lymphoma. *J Natl Cancer Inst* 1997;89:1350–1355.

110. Copie-Bergman C, Gaulard P, Lavergne-Slove A, et al. Proposal for a new histological grading system for post-treatment evaluation of gastric MALT lymphoma. *Gut* 2003;52:1656.

111. Copie-Bergman C, Wotherspoon A. MALT lymphoma pathology, initial diagnosis, and posttreatment evaluation. In: Cavalli F, Stein H, Zucca E, eds. *Extranodal lymphomas pathology and management*. London, UK: Informa Healthcare, 2008:114–123.

112. Bertoni F, Conconi A, Capella C, et al. Molecular follow-up in gastric mucosa-associated lymphoid tissue lymphomas: early analysis of the LY03 cooperative trial. *Blood* 2002;99:2541–2544.

113. Thiede C, Wundisch T, Alpen B, et al. Long-term persistence of monoclonal B cells after cure of Helicobacter pylori infection and complete histologic remission in gastric mucosa-associated lymphoid tissue B-cell lymphoma. *J Clin Oncol* 2001;19:1600–1609.

114. Montalban C, Santon A, Redondo C, et al. Long-term persistence of molecular disease after histological remission in low-grade gastric MALT lymphoma treated with H. pylori eradication. Lack of association with translocation t(11;18): a 10-year updated follow-up of a prospective study. *Ann Oncol* 2005;16:1539–1544.

115. de Mascarel A, Ruskone-Fourmestraux A, Lavergne-Slove A, et al. Clinical, histological and molecular follow-up of 60 patients with gastric marginal zone lymphoma of mucosa-associated lymphoid tissue. *Virchows Arch* 2005; 446:219–224.

116. Begum S, Sano T, Endo H, et al. Mucosal change of the stomach with low-grade mucosa-associated lymphoid tissue lymphoma after eradication of Helicobacter pylori: follow-up study of 48 cases. *J Med Invest* 2000;47:36–46.

117. Zucca E, Dreyling M. Gastric marginal zone lymphoma of MALT type: ESMO clinical recommendations for diagnosis, treatment and follow-up. *Ann Oncol* 2008;(suppl 2):ii70–ii71.

118. Fischbach W, Goebeler-Kolve M, Starostik P, et al. Minimal residual low-grade gastric MALT-type lymphoma after eradication of Helicobacter pylori. *Lancet* 2002;360:547–548.

119. Stathis A, Chini C, Bertoni F, et al. Long-term outcome following *Helicobacter pylori* eradication in a retrospective study of 105 patients with localized gastric marginal zone B-cell lymphoma of MALT type. *Ann Oncol* 2009;20:1086–1093.

120. Fischbach W, Goebeler ME, Ruskone-Fourmestraux A, et al. Most patients with minimal histological residuals of gastric MALT lymphoma after successful eradication of Helicobacter pylori can be managed safely by a watch and wait strategy: experience from a large international series. *Gut* 2007;56:1685–1687.

121. Fischbach W, Goebeler-Kolve ME, Dragosics B, et al. Long term outcome of patients with gastric marginal zone B cell lymphoma of mucosa associated lymphoid tissue (MALT) following exclusive Helicobacter pylori eradication therapy: experience from a large prospective series. *Gut* 2004;53:34–37.

122. Montalban C, Manzanal A, Castrillo JM, et al. Low grade gastric B-cell MALT lymphoma progressing into high grade lymphoma. Clonal identity of the two stages of the tumour, unusual bone involvement and leukemic dissemination. *Histopathology* 1995;27:89–91.

123. Morgner A, Miehlke S, Stolte M, et al. Development of early gastric cancer 4 and 5 years after complete remission of Helicobacter pylori associated gastric low grade marginal zone B cell lymphoma of MALT type. *World J Gastroenterol* 2001;7:248–253.

124. Capelle LG, de Vries AC, Looman CW, et al. Gastric MALT lymphoma: epidemiology and high adenocarcinoma risk in a nation-wide study. *Eur J Cancer* 2008;44:2470–2476.

125. Chen LT, Lin JT, Shyu RY, et al. Prospective study of Helicobacter pylori eradication therapy in stage I(E) high-grade mucosa-associated lymphoid tissue lymphoma of the stomach. *J Clin Oncol* 2001;19:4245–4251.

126. Levy M, Copie-Bergman C, Traulle C, et al. Conservative treatment of primary gastric low-grade B-cell lymphoma of mucosa-associated lymphoid tissue: predictive factors of response and outcome. *Am J Gastroenterol* 2002;97:292–297.

127. Caletti G, Zinzani PL, Fusaroli P, et al. The importance of endoscopic ultrasonography in the management of low-grade gastric mucosa-associated lymphoid tissue lymphoma. *Aliment Pharmacol Ther* 2002;16:1715–1722.

128. Eidt S, Stolte M, Fischer R. Factors influencing lymph node infiltration in primary gastric malignant lymphoma of the mucosa-associated lymphoid tissue. *Pathol Res Pract* 1994;190:1077–1081.

129. Nakamura S, Matsumoto T, Suekane H, et al. Predictive value of endoscopic ultrasonography for regression of gastric low grade and high grade MALT lymphomas after eradication of Helicobacter pylori. *Gut* 2001;48:454–460.

130. Kim JS, Chung SJ, Choi YS, et al. Helicobacter pylori eradication for low-grade gastric mucosa-associated lymphoid tissue lymphoma is more successful in inducing remission in distal compared to proximal disease. *Br J Cancer* 2007;96:1324–1328.

131. Raderer M, Osterreicher C, Machold K, et al. Impaired response of gastric MALT-lymphoma to Helicobacter pylori eradication in patients with autoimmune disease. *Ann Oncol* 2001;12:937–939.

132. Wohrer S, Troch M, Streubel B, et al. MALT lymphoma in patients with autoimmune diseases: a comparative analysis of characteristics and clinical course. *Leukemia* 2007;21:1812–1818.

133. Alpen B, Neubauer A, Dierlamm J, et al. Translocation t(11;18) absent in early gastric marginal zone B-cell lymphoma of MALT type responding to eradication of Helicobacter pylori infection. *Blood* 2000;95:4014–4015.

134. Levy M, Copie-Bergman C, Gameiro C, et al. Prognostic value of translocation t(11;18) in tumoral response of low-grade gastric lymphoma of mucosa-associated lymphoid tissue type to oral chemotherapy. *J Clin Oncol* 2005;23:5061–5066.

135. Martinelli G, Laszlo D, Ferreri AJ, et al. Clinical activity of rituximab in gastric marginal zone non-Hodgkin's lymphoma resistant to or not eligible for anti-Helicobacter pylori therapy. *J Clin Oncol* 2005;23:1979–1983.

136. Streubel B, Ye H, Du MQ, et al. Translocation t(11;18)(q21;q21) is not predictive of response to chemotherapy with 2CdA in patients with gastric MALT lymphoma. *Oncology* 2004;66:476–480.

137. Nakamura S, Matsumoto T, Ye H, et al. Helicobacter pylori-negative gastric mucosa-associated lymphoid tissue lymphoma: a clinicopathologic and molecular study with reference to antibiotic treatment. *Cancer* 2006;107:2770–2778.

138. Lucas PC, Yonezumi M, Inohara N, et al. Bcl10 and MALT1, independent targets of chromosomal translocation in malt lymphoma, cooperate in a novel NF-kappa B signaling pathway. *J Biol Chem* 2001;276:19012–19019.

139. Cogliatti SB, Schmid U, Schumacher U, et al. Primary B-cell gastric lymphoma: a clinicopathological study of 145 patients. *Gastroenterology* 1991;101:1159–1170.

140. Coiffier B, Salles G. Does surgery belong to medical history for gastric lymphomas? *Ann Oncol* 1997;8:419–421.

141. Schechter NR, Yahalom J. Low-grade MALT lymphoma of the stomach: a review of treatment options. *Int J Radiat Oncol Biol Phys* 2000;46:1093–1103.

142. Yoon SS, Coit DG, Portlock CS, et al. The diminishing role of surgery in the treatment of gastric lymphoma. *Ann Surg* 2004;240:28–37.

143. Wotherspoon AC, Doglioni C, Isaacson PG. Low-grade gastric B-cell lymphoma of mucosa-associated lymphoid tissue (MALT): a multifocal disease. *Histopathology* 1992;20:29–34.

144. Koch P, del Valle F, Berdel WE, et al. Primary gastrointestinal non-Hodgkin's lymphoma: II. combined surgical and conservative or conservative management only in localized gastric lymphoma—results of the Prospective German Multicenter Study GIT NHL 01/92. *J Clin Oncol* 2001;19:3874–3883.

145. Aviles A, Nambo MJ, Neri N, et al. Mucosa-associated lymphoid tissue (MALT) lymphoma of the stomach: results of a controlled clinical trial. *Med Oncol* 2005;22:57–62.

146. Schechter NR, Portlock CS, Yahalom J. Treatment of mucosa-associated lymphoid tissue lymphoma of the stomach with radiation alone. *J Clin Oncol* 1998;16:1916–1921.

147. Gospodarowicz M, Tsang R. Radiation therapy of mucosa-associated lymphoid tissue (MALT) lymphomas. In: Zucca E, ed. *MALT lymphomas*. Georgetown, TX: Landes Bioscience/Eurekah.com, 2004:104–129.

148. Fung CY, Grossbard ML, Linggood RM, et al. Mucosa-associated lymphoid tissue lymphoma of the stomach: long term outcome after local treatment. *Cancer* 1999;85:9–17.

149. Hitchcock S, Ng AK, Fisher DC, et al. Treatment outcome of mucosa-associated lymphoid tissue/marginal zone non-Hodgkin's lymphoma. *Int J Radiat Oncol Biol Phys* 2002;52:1058–1066.

150. Vrieling C, de Jong D, Boot H, et al. Long-term results of stomach-conserving therapy in gastric MALT lymphoma. *Radiother Oncol* 2008;87:405–411.

151. Park HC, Park W, Hahn JS, et al. Low grade MALT lymphoma of the stomach: treatment outcome with radiotherapy alone. *Yonsei Med J* 2002;43:601–606.

152. Yahalom J, Gonzales M. H. pylori-independent MALT lymphoma of the stomach: excellent outcome with radiation alone [abstract]. *Blood* 2002;100:160a. Abstract 600.

153. Yahalom J. MALT lymphomas: a radiation oncology viewpoint. *Ann Hematol* 2001;80(suppl 3):B100–B105.

154. Della Biancia C, Hunt M, Furhang E, et al. Radiation treatment planning techniques for lymphoma of the stomach. *Int J Radiat Oncol Biol Phys* 2005;62:745–751.

155. NCCN. National Comprehensive Cancer Network Guidelines V.3.2008—Non-Hodgkin's Lymphoma. Available at: http://www.nccn.org/professionals/physician_gls/PDF/nhl.pdf. Accessed June 11, 2008.

156. Noy A, Yahalom J, Zaretsky L, et al. Gastric mucosa-associated lymphoid tissue lymphoma detected by clonotypic polymerase chain reaction despite continuous pathologic remission induced by involved-field radiotherapy. *J Clin Oncol* 2005;23:3768–3772.

157. Conconi A, Cavalli F, Zucca E. MALT lymphomas: the role of chemotherapy. In: Zucca E, ed. *MALT lymphomas*. Georgetown, TX: Landes Bioscience/Eurekah.com, 2004:99–103.

158. Hammel P, Haioun C, Chaumette MT, et al. Efficacy of single-agent chemotherapy in low-grade B-cell mucosa-associated lymphoid tissue lymphoma with prominent gastric expression. *J Clin Oncol* 1995;13:2524–2529.

159. Ben Simon GJ, Cheung N, McKelvie P, et al. Oral chlorambucil for extranodal, marginal zone, B-cell lymphoma of mucosa-associated lymphoid tissue of the orbit. *Ophthalmology* 2006;113:1209–1213.

160. Zinzani PL, Stefoni V, Musuraca G, et al. Fludarabine-containing chemotherapy as frontline treatment of nongastrointestinal mucosa-associated lymphoid tissue lymphoma. *Cancer* 2004;100:2190–2194.

161. Jager G, Neumeister P, Brezinschek R, et al. Treatment of extranodal marginal zone B-cell lymphoma of mucosa-associated lymphoid tissue type with cladribine: a phase II study. *J Clin Oncol* 2002;20:3872–3877.

162. Jager G, Hofler G, Linkesch W, et al. Occurrence of a myelodysplastic syndrome (MDS) during first-line 2-chloro-deoxyadenosine (2-CDA) treatment of a low-grade gastrointestinal MALT lymphoma. Case report and review of the literature. *Haematologica* 2004;89:ECR01.

163. Wohrer S, Drach J, Hejna M, et al. Treatment of extranodal marginal zone B-cell lymphoma of mucosa-associated lymphoid tissue (MALT lymphoma) with mitoxantrone, chlorambucil and prednisone (MCP). *Ann Oncol* 2003;14:1758–1761.

164. Conconi AR, Lopez-Guillermo A, Martinelli G, et al. Activity of Bortezomib in MALT lymphomas: a IELSG Phase II Study [abstract]. *Ann Oncol* 2008;19 iv191. Abstract 368.

165. Raderer M, Wohrer S, Streubel B, et al. Activity of rituximab plus cyclophosphamide, doxorubicin/mitoxantrone, vincristine and prednisone in patients with relapsed MALT lymphoma. *Oncology* 2006;70:411–417.

166. Conconi A, Martinelli G, Thieblemont C, et al. Clinical activity of rituximab in extranodal marginal zone B-cell lymphoma of MALT type. *Blood* 2003;102:2741–2745.

167. Raderer M, Jager G, Brugger S, et al. Rituximab for treatment of advanced extranodal marginal zone B cell lymphoma of the mucosa-associated lymphoid tissue lymphoma. *Oncology* 2003;65:306–310.

168. Le QT, Eulau SM, George TI, et al. Primary radiotherapy for localized orbital MALT lymphoma. *Int J Radiat Oncol Biol Phys* 2002;52:657–663.

169. Ansell SM, Grant CS, Habermann TM. Primary thyroid lymphoma. *Semin Oncol* 1999;26:316–323.

170. Brogi E, Harris NL. Lymphomas of the breast: pathology and clinical behavior. *Semin Oncol* 1999;26:357–364.

171. Agulnik M, Tsang R, Baker MA, et al. Malignant lymphoma of mucosa-associated lymphoid tissue of the lacrimal gland: case report and review of literature. *Am J Clin Oncol* 2001;24:67–70.

172. Jhavar S, Agarwal JP, Naresh KN, et al. Primary extranodal mucosa associated lymphoid tissue (MALT) lymphoma of the prostate. *Leuk Lymphoma* 2001;41:445–449.

173. Suchy BH, Wolf SR. Bilateral mucosa-associated lymphoid tissue lymphoma of the parotid gland. *Arch Otolaryngol Head Neck Surg* 2000;126:224–226.

174. Estevez M, Chu C, Pless M. Small B-cell lymphoma presenting as diffuse dural thickening with cranial neuropathies. *J Neurooncol* 2002;59:243–247.

175. de Bree R, Mahieu HF, Ossenkoppele GJ, et al. Malignant lymphoma of mucosa-associated lymphoid tissue in the larynx. *Eur Arch Otorhinolaryngol* 1998;255:368–370.

176. Sanjeevi A, Krishnan J, Bailey PR, et al. Extranodal marginal zone B-cell lymphoma of malt type involving the cavernous sinus. *Leuk Lymphoma* 2001;42:1133–1137.

177. Ferreri AJ, Ponzoni M, Guidoboni M, et al. Bacteria-eradicating therapy with doxycycline in ocular adnexal MALT lymphoma: a multicenter prospective trial. *J Natl Cancer Inst* 2006;98:1375–1382.

178. Zucca E, Bertoni F. Chlamydia or not Chlamydia, that is the question: which is the microorganism associated with MALT lymphomas of the ocular adnexa? *J Natl Cancer Inst* 2006;98:1348–1349.

179. Du MQ, Peng H, Liu H, et al. BCL10 gene mutation in lymphoma. *Blood* 2000;95:3885–3890.

CHAPTER 16 ■ SPLENIC MARGINAL ZONE LYMPHOMA

CATHERINE THIEBLEMONT, FRANÇOISE BERGER, PASCALE FELMAN, EVELYNE CALLET-BAUCHU, AND BERTRAND COIFFIER

DEFINITION

Splenic marginal zone lymphoma (SMZL) is a B-cell neoplasm comprised predominantly of small cells, involving the white pulp follicles (surrounding and replacing germinal centers, and involving the mantle and marginal zones) of spleen, splenic hilar lymph nodes, bone marrow, and often the peripheral blood. It is considered as a distinct entity among non-Hodgkin lymphomas (NHLs), after the proposal as a provisional entity in the Revised European American Lymphoma classification (1) and the subsequent recognition as a distinct entity in the World Health Organization classification (2). The relative rarity of these lymphomas, as well as the difficulties in distinguishing them from other low-grade lymphomas, set up crucial issues to conduct epidemiologic surveys, and to describe clinical features and outcomes. The present review displays current data concerning epidemiology, clinical features, staging, and treatment of SMZL (Table 16.1).

EPIDEMIOLOGY

In adults, SMZLs account for <2% of NHLs (3,4). The median age of occurrence for SMZL is 65 years (5,6), although patients as young as 22 years can develop a SMZL (7). There is an equal sex incidence (6).

PHYSIOPATHOLOGY

In the spleen, the SMZL is characterized by a micronodular expansion of small B lymphocytes inside the white pulp, involving both mantle and marginal zones, and often colonizing or replacing germinal centers, associated with variable degree of involvement of the red pulp (Fig. 16.1). The normal counterpart is a mature B cell of unknown differentiation stage, although the presence of somatic hypermutation in a proportion of the cases suggests that it is a memory B cell.

Marginal Zone of Secondary Lymphoid Organs

The marginal zone is located around lymphoid follicles of secondary lymphoid organs, including spleen, and Peyer patches of small intestine, whereas it is rarely identifiable in lymph nodes (8). Marginal zone B cells were initially

TABLE 16.1

COMPARISON OF THE IMMUNOPHENOTYPE BETWEEN SMZL AND LPL/WM

Immunophenotype	SMZL	LPL/WM
CD22	50% strong	100% low
CD25	44%	88%
CD103	40%	0%
CD11c	39%	6%
Bc-l2	0%	70%

Adapted from Gruszka-Westwood AM, Hamoudi RA, Matutes E, et al. p53 abnormalities in splenic lymphoma with villous lymphocytes. *Blood* 2001;97:3552–3558, with permission.

described as postgerminal center-T-dependant memory B cells (9), but recent advances suggest a heterogeneous B-cell composition (10). In mice and humans, a subset of marginal zone memory B cells, although having somatic mutations of their immunoglobulin (Ig) genes, is involved in the T-independent antigenic response, essential against encapsulated bacteria. They provide a fast humoral immune response and play a key role in the eradication of a bacteriemia. Antigens recognized by marginal zone B cells are mainly polysaccharidic antigens of bacterial capsules (11–15).

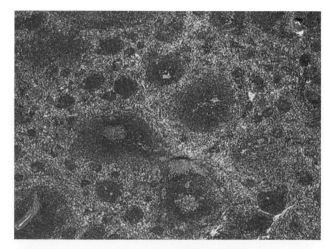

FIGURE 16.1 Microscopic view of SMZL. Micronodular infiltration of the white pulp, with marginal zone differentiation, and involvement of red pulp. (see also Color Plate 27)

Normal Cell Counterpart of Splenic Marginal Zone Lymphoma

The normal cell counterpart of SMZL was originally postulated to be a marginal zone memory B cell. About two-thirds of the cases have somatic hypermutations in Ig heavy chain variable (Ig-VH) region genes (16), suggesting exposure to antigen in the germinal center; however, one-third of the cases are nonmutated (17,18). These lymphomas exhibit a low frequency of somatic mutations concerning several oncogenes (bcl-6, PAX5, PIM1, RHO-H), which are targets non-Ig genes of somatic hypermutations in normal germinal center B cells (19). These findings suggest a particular differentiation pathway, possibly without transit through the germinal center, reflecting the heterogeneity of normal marginal zone B cells (15,16). Interestingly, biased use of VH1-2 04 has been found in these cases, not found in other lymphomas, suggesting an antigen selection-driven process for some SMZL cases (15).

Role of B-Cell Receptor and Chronic Antigenic Stimulation

Survival and selection of B cells depend on the B-cell receptor (BCR), even when they are mature and quiescent. This survival signal is delivered either independently, or secondary to an antigenic stimulation. In many B-cell lymphomas, the BCR signal is also mandatory for B-cell survival, and some of them are antigen-driven proliferations. The best example is gastric mucosa-associated lymphoid tissue lymphoma associated with chronic infection by *Helicobacter pylori*. Other mucosa-associated lymphoid tissue lymphomas are driven by an autoantigen chronic stimulation, such as Sjögren syndrome and Hashimoto thyroiditis.

SMZL pathogenesis may be also associated with a chronic antigenic stimulation (20). A clear relationship has been highlighted between hepatitis C virus (HCV) infection and SMZL (21,22). Since 1994, numerous epidemiologic studies have found a correlation between NHL and HCV infection. Several genotypes of HCV have been identified, and classified in nine groups and 30 subgroups (1a, 1b, 1c ...). Reported genotypes differ according to country, as well as modalities and period of infection. In a given patient, changes in the genomic viral population occur because of mutations in hypervariable regions, providing a failure of the immune system and consequently favoring maintenance of chronic viral infection. In Italy, an association with HCV has been found for lymphoplasmacytic immunocytoma, SMZL, and other nodal or extranodal marginal zone lymphomas (MZLs) (21,22). In the setting of SMZL, the presence of HCV is of major relevance, due to the possible therapeutic implications (23,24). The estradiol glycoprotein of HCV could interact with CD81 in the B cells, and could be responsible for an activation of B cells through BCR signal, leading to their increased proliferation (20). In murine models, MZLs have been described following a chronic stimulation by HCV, and have been associated with mutations of FAS, AP12/ML, and p53 (25). An HCV-associated lymphoplasmacytic lymphoproliferation, usually splenic and hepatic, is correlated with the presence of type II cryoglobulinemia (26). A decrease in lymphoproliferation following antiviral treatments reinforces the data pointing toward a contribution of a chronic antigenic stimulation to the physiopathologic process of HCV-related MZL (24).

Interestingly, SMZL, characterized by splenomegaly and circulating naive CD5-negative villous B lymphocytes, has been described in malaria-endemic areas, here denominated as tropical splenic lymphoma. This is supporting the role of infectious agents on the pathogenesis of SMZL (27).

CLINICAL PRESENTATION

Most of the patients seek medical attention because of an abnormal blood cell count, especially anemia and/or thrombocytopenia, more related to splenic sequestration than to bone marrow infiltration, constantly associated with lymphocytosis. Patients are asymptomatic, but splenomegaly is detectable at clinical examination. In advanced cases of SMZL, the typical clinical presentation is with massive splenomegaly. At this stage, patients complain of asthenia and/or pain of left hypochondrium. Small splenic hilar lymph nodes are frequently associated. Peripheral lymph node involvement, an infrequent phenomenon in SMZL, is generally associated with a poorer outcome (28).

The performance status is usually preserved with a World Health Organization score <2 in 85% of cases (29). General symptoms (fever, weight loss, night sweats) are unusual. This clinical presentation is associated with bone marrow and blood involvement in >90% of patients (29,30). Whereas serum lactate dehydrogenase (LDH) level is usually normal in SMZL, except in case of hemolytic anemia, β2-microglobulin level is increased. A proportion of patients (10% to 40% of cases) have a serum monoclonal paraprotein (M component), mainly of the µ chain (IgM) (3,6,31–33). Autoimmune phenomena are described in 10% to 15% of patients, including autoimmune hemolytic anemia, immune thrombocytopenia, cold agglutinin, circulating anticoagulant (lupic or cardiolipin), acquired von Willebrandt disease, and angioedema due to acquired deficit in C1-esterase inhibitor. Several patterns of neuropathies, including demyelinating polyneuropathy, radiculopathy, or axonal multiple mononeuropathy, may be present and have been shown to precede the lymphoma for up to 4 years (from 1 to 52 months) (34).

SMZL is also associated with autoimmunity. The neoplastic B cells can produce autoantibodies, and a hemolytic autoimmune anemia or autoimmune thrombocytopenia is present in a subset of cases. Splenic lymphomas with numerous basophilic villous cells in the peripheral blood, formerly denominated as splenic lymphoma with villous lymphocytes, are characterized by a peculiar histology with atrophic white pulp and a monomorphic diffuse infiltration of a congested red pulp, reminiscent of HCL variant. Few differences have been found in the clinical presentation, including a significant older age and an absence of immune disorder (6,29). The median age at diagnosis for these patients is 75 years, as compared with 63 years for classic SMZL. Controversies exist in literature about the importance or not to distinguish these two diseases, and about the classification of splenic red pulp lymphoma with villous lymphocytes as a distinct entity (35).

HCV-associated SMZLs are indistinguishable from typical SMZL, except for the presence of HCV viral replication, coexistence of a liver disease, and high frequency of type II cryoglobulinemia (23).

DIAGNOSIS

The diagnosis is based on the study of peripheral blood lymphocytes, bone marrow biopsies, or the study of surgically removed spleens. Most cases of SMZL do not require splenectomy for the diagnosis, which can often be made based on the study of the peripheral blood and bone marrow.

Cytologic Features

The blood infiltration is characterized by small lymphoid cells having a round nucleus with condensed chromatin and basophilic cytoplasm, with frequent short villi (Fig. 16.2). They are frequently associated with small lymphoid cells with or without or lymphoplasmacytoid cells, or with abundant pale cytoplasm. Plasma cells are rare. The degree of blood infiltration by villous lymphocytes is usually low (<20%).

Histologic Features

Histology of the spleen shows a micronodular infiltration of the white pulp, with an inconstant marginal zone differentiation and a variable degree of red pulp involvement. Typically, there is a biphasic pattern of white pulp, with a central zone of small lymphoid cells and an outer zone of medium-sized cells with clear cytoplasm and scattered large cells with large nuclei and prominent nucleoli. Germinal centers may be present, and may be reactive, regressed, or colonized by the tumor cells. In red pulp, both cords and sinuses are usually infiltrated. With some frequency, there is plasmacytic differentiation, with lymphoplasmacytoid cells and plasma cells, both in the marginal zone and the colonized germinal centers. The hilar lymph node histology is characteristic, with a nodular infiltration and preserved sinuses. In the bone marrow, the involvement is initially intrasinusoidal, sometimes subtle, and then nodular. It is always present and better detected after CD20 immunostaining. Intrasinusoidal infiltration is highly typical but nonspecific of SMZL.

Immunophenotypic Data

SMZL B cells express pan-B markers CD19, CD20, CD22 CD79a, and CD79b2. The expression of other markers (CD5, FMC7, CD22 or CD79b, CD23, surface Ig expression), integrated into the Matutes' international score (36), can be helpful for a differential diagnosis between chronic lymphocytic leukemia (CLL) or other small B-cell lymphomas. According to the study of Matutes et al. (36), 87% of CLL present with a four to five score, whereas SMZL is generally below three (usually zero to two), but there is no specific marker. Classically, the immunophenotypic analysis of tumoral cells shows CD19$^+$, CD20$^+$, CD22$^+$, CD24$^+$, CD27$^+$, CD43$^-$, CD76$^{+/-}$, CD79b$^+$, FMC7$^{+/-}$, CD5$^-$, CD10$^-$, CD23$^-$, CD43$^{+/-}$, CD103$^-$, bcl-2$^+$, annexin1$^-$, and cyclin D1$^-$ cells. There is a moderate to strong intensity of IgM and IgD or IgM alone; in rare cases, IgG or IgA. An atypical phenotype is possible, with the expression of CD5 in 15% to 20%, and CD23 in 30% of cases (5). Coexpression of CD5 and CD23 may exist and is rare.

Cytogenetic Data

Cytogenetic abnormalities are present in 80% of cases. The most frequent are complete or partial trisomy 3q (30% to 50% of patients) and gains of 12q (15% to 20% of cases) (37–41). The abnormality considered as typical of SMZL, reported in 40% of cases, consists of deletion or translocation of chromosome 7q32 (42,43). No tumor suppressor genes have been found in this region, and there are good reasons to think that the deletion of a cluster of micro-ribonucleic acids located in this region could contribute to the deregulation of some of the key oncogenes, such as T-cell leukemia 1. Rarer translocations involving CDK6 and cyclin D3 genes with IgH gene have been identified in small subsets of cases (44).

Other chromosomal abnormalities reported at diagnosis include trisomy 18, 17q isochromosome, 13q14 deletion, and structural abnormalities of chromosome 1 (37,38,40,42,44–48). A translocation t(11;14)(q13;q32) combined with a

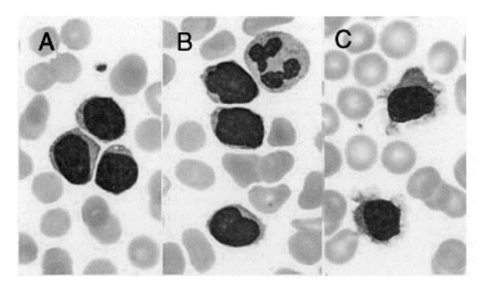

FIGURE 16.2 Different cytologic aspects of blood involvement in SMZL. **A:** Aggregation of three cells with clumped chromatin and small round nucleus. **B:** Cells with notched nucleus. **C:** Typical villous lymphocytes with short cytoplasmic villi (see also Color Plate 28).

rearrangement of bcl-1 and/or the expression of cyclin D1 was described as present in 15% of cases diagnosed as splenic lymphoma with villous lymphocytes, but these cases seem to harbor other morphologic, phenotypic, and cytogenetic features, suggesting a diagnosis of mantle cell lymphoma (49–51). None of the aforementioned cytogenetic abnormalities, with the exception of 7q32 deletion, is considered typical of SMZL, but they may be helpful for the diagnosis. Translocations involving the *MALT 1* gene are not found in SMZL.

Mutational Status of the Immunoglobulin Variable Heavy Chain Gene

Initial analyses of the mutational status of the Ig-VH gene showed the presence of somatic hypermutations in most of cases, suggesting that the precursor cell of MZL was a memory B cell from a postgerminal origin, without pattern of antigen selection (16). However, more recent studies have found a molecular heterogeneity, with an absence of somatic mutations in half of the studied cases. The biased overuse of the VH1.2 gene in both mutated and unmutated cases supports that the tumor derives from a highly selected B-cell population (17,18). Few published cases showed the same VDJ segment usage, including two similar HCDR3 sequences, suggesting the possible selection by a common antigen (18).

Gene Expression Profiling: The Molecular Signature of Splenic Marginal Zone Lymphoma

SMZLs have a specific transcriptional profile compared with other lymphomas, especially small B-cell lymphomas, such as follicular lymphomas, lymphocytic lymphomas, and mantle cell lymphomas (52,53). This specific molecular signature includes genes involved in the signaling cascade of the AKT1 pathway (53), but also the BCR signaling pathway, tumor necrosis factor, and nuclear factor-κB targets (52). To date, gene expression analysis is not routinely available and cannot be applied to the diagnosis.

DIFFERENTIAL DIAGNOSIS

The association of bone marrow involvement and splenomegaly, with or without monoclonal IgM, is not exclusive for SMZL. This clinical presentation may be observed also for CLL, hairy cell leukemia, mantle cell lymphoma, follicular lymphoma, or lymphoplasmacytic lymphoma (LPL). The diagnosis often requires the integration of clinical, histologic, and immunophenotypic data. Cytology as well as expression of CD5 and CD23, with a low CD79b, differentiates SMZL and CLL. The differential diagnosis between SMZL and mantle cell lymphoma is facilitated by the cytology, expression of CD5 and CD43, overexpression of cyclin D1 and GSTpi (54), and loss of p27, even if borderline cases need a detailed study and data integration. The presence of t(11;14), which can be detected by fluorescent in situ hybridization on blood or bone marrow specimens, is specific for mantle cell lymphoma and excludes SMZL (48–50).

Follicular lymphoma may show a pattern of splenic infiltration quite similar to that seen in SMZL, even with marginal zone differentiation, although the expression of CD10, BCL6, or the presence of t(14;18) is useful for the diagnosis (1–3). Hairy cell leukemia is distinguished by the pattern of bone marrow involvement and expression of annexin-1 and CD103.

Differential diagnosis with LPL/Waldenström macroglobulinemia (WM) may have a special difficulty (55). LPL shares numerous characteristics with SMZL with plasmacytic differentiation (1,2,28,56,57), but the clinical presentation is usually different, patients with LPL/WM having a predominant bone marrow involvement, with an IgM paraprotein, and rarely massive splenomegaly. Cytogenetic analysis may be helpful for the diagnosis. More frequent presence of 7q21 deletion, gains of 3q are in favor of SMZL, whereas the presence of 6q deletion is more in favor of LPL/WM (57). However, it may be difficult to distinguish these entities. In this setting, prospective clinical trials could be warranted to evaluate the patient's outcome according to initial diagnosis.

PROGNOSTIC FACTORS AND SURVIVAL

The median overall survival ranges between 5 and 10 years, but in case of aggressive disease, which is the case in roughly one third of patients presenting with a poorer performance status, B symptoms and elevated LDH level, median survival does not reach 4 years (6,29,31,32,58). Treatment is indicated in case of symptomatic splenomegaly, cytopenia, or general symptoms (29,58). Some prognostic factors have been identified. The Italian Intergroup of Lymphomas has developed a prognostic model in 309 patients based on three factors (hemoglobin level <12 g per dL, LDH level greater than normal, and albumin level <3.5 g per dL), the association of the three leading to a prognostic index (29,58,59). This index allowed to separate patients into three groups displaying different 5-year survival rates: 88% in the low-risk group (no risk factor), 73% in the intermediate-risk group (one risk factor), and 50% in the high-risk group (more than one factor) (59). Of note, this index has not been validated by other studies. In this analysis, the International Prognostic Index was found to predict survival, although a multivariate analysis selected the three indicated parameters (59). Other biologic prognostic factors have been described, such as expression of CD38, unmutated Ig-VH gene status, and expression of nuclear factor-κB-activated genes by using gene expression analysis (52).

A histologic transformation into large cell lymphoma remains uncommon, occurring in 10% to 20% of patients. The transformation sets in a median time ranging from 12 to 85 months (60). This situation is associated with the appearance of general symptoms, increase in LDH level, and disseminated lymphoma involvement. After histologic progression, the median survival time is shortened to 26 months (29).

TREATMENT

A treatment is required only in symptomatic patients with large splenomegaly, associated or not with cytopenia due to hypersplenism. Asymptomatic patients may be followed for several years by clinical examinations and blood counts. The absence of treatment does not influence the course of disease, and these patients often have a stable disease, without symptoms for at least 10 years (29,61).

When a treatment is indicated because of the occurrence of clinical symptoms, the recommended first-line therapy is splenectomy (6,29,31,33,58,61,62). The benefit consists of an improvement of performance status in a few months, and a correction of anemia, thrombocytopenia, and neutropenia within 6 months after splenectomy. This improvement is maintained for years with a free of treatment period lasting 8 years in median (6). These patients only have partial response with a persisting bone marrow and blood lymphocytosis; however, such persisting lymphocytosis does not require therapy.

Is there a place for chemotherapy in the management of MZL? Adjuvant chemotherapy to splenectomy provides an increased remission rate without modifying relapse-free and overall survival (29). Chemotherapy may be proposed to patients with contraindications to surgery, to elderly patients, or to those who have progression after surgery. Regimens are based on alkylating agents (chlorambucil, cyclophosphamide), purine analogs (fludarabine), and monoclonal antibody (rituximab) single agent or combined with cytotoxics (63–65). A retrospective study by the M. D. Anderson Cancer Center has reported 88% of response in patients treated with rituximab single agent, 83% in those receiving rituximab plus chemotherapy, and 55% in those receiving chemotherapy alone, with 3-year survival rates of 95%, 100%, and 55%, respectively (66). Rituximab single agent may even yield to a normalization of splenic size of patients (67), and then could be considered as a good therapeutic option for elderly patients and those who could not undergo splenectomy. Efficacy with the association of rituximab and bendamustine has been preliminary reported in the literature and needs confirmation in larger series (68,69). When the MZL is associated with an active HCV infection, the first-line therapy is based on the control of viral infection using interferon-α with or without ribavirin (23).

CONCLUSIONS

SMZLs represent a distinct entity among NHLs. Clinical presentation shows a splenic involvement with bone marrow and blood infiltration, associated with lymph node involvement of the splenic hilum, but usually without peripheral lymph node involvement. No differences in the clinical presentation are clearly detectable between cases denominated in the past as splenic lymphoma with villous lymphocytes with the classic form of the disease. Various immune phenomena (hemolytic anemia, immune thrombocytopenia, acquired coagulation disorders, etc.), and monoclonal serum paraproteinemia, usually IgM, may be associated with SMZL. Splenectomy is an efficient therapy improving performance status and reducing cytopenia. The achievement of a complete response is not considered as a necessary step to extend long-term survival and preserve the quality of life. The association of rituximab and chemotherapy may achieve a high response rate, much better than chemotherapy alone. Novel approaches such as the use of new agents or maintenance therapies with monoclonal antibodies have yet to be documented. The specific association with an active HCV infection is possible, requiring an antiviral therapy inducing tumoral response with the control of the viral infection.

References

1. Harris NL, Jaffe ES, Stein H, et al. A revised European-American Classification of lymphoid neoplasms. A proposal from the International Lymphoma Study Group. *Blood* 1994;84:1361–1392.
2. Jaffe ES, Harris NL, Stein H, et al. Pathology and genetics of tumours of haematopoietic and lymphoid tissues. *Lyon, France: IARC Press*, 2001.
3. Berger F. The different entities and diagnostic problems. Educational program of the European Hematology Association. Roterdam, Netherlands: EHA, 2000:5.
4. Nathwani B, Anderson J, Armitage J, et al. Marginal zone B-cell lymphoma: a clinical comparison of nodal and mucosa-associated lymphoid tissue types. Non-Hodgkin's Lymphoma Classification Project. *J Clin Oncol* 1999;17:2486–2492.
5. Oscier D, Owen R, Johnson S. Splenic marginal zone lymphoma. *Blood Rev* 2005;19:39–51.
6. Thieblemont C, Felman P, Berger F, et al. Treatment of splenic marginal zone B-cell lymphoma: an analysis of 81 patients. *Clin Lymphoma* 2002;3:41–47.
7. Depowski PL, Dunn H, Purdy S, et al T. Splenic marginal zone lymphoma: a case report and review of the literature. *Arch Pathol Lab Med* 2002;126:214–216.
8. Cyster JG. B cells on the front line. *Nat Immunol* 2000;1:9–10.
9. MacLennan IC, Liu YJ, Oldfield S, et al. The evolution of B-cell clones. *Curr Top Microbiol Immunol* 1990;159:37–63.
10. MacLennan IC. B cells: the follicular dimension of the marginal zone. *Immunol Cell Biol* 2008;86:219–220.
11. Kruetzmann S, Rosado MM, Weber H, et al. Human immunoglobulin M memory B cells controlling Streptococcus pneumoniae infections are generated in the spleen. *J Exp Med* 2003;197:939–945.
12. Martin F, Kearney JF. Marginal-zone B cells. *Nat Rev Immunol* 2002;2:323–335.
13. Weller S, Braun MC, Tan BK, et al. Human blood IgM "memory" B cells are circulating splenic marginal zone B cells harboring a prediversified immunoglobulin repertoire. *Blood* 2004;104:3647–3654.
14. Weller S, Faili A, Garcia C, et al. CD40-CD40L independent Ig gene hypermutation suggests a second B cell diversification pathway in humans. *Proc Natl Acad Sci U S A* 2001;98:1166–1170.
15. Weller S, Reynaud CA, Weill JC. Vaccination against encapsulated bacteria in humans: paradoxes. *Trends Immunol* 2005;26:85–89.
16. Zhu DL, Oscier DG, Stevenson FK. Splenic lymphoma with villous lymphocytes involves B cells with extensively mutated Ig heavy chain variable region genes. *Blood* 1995;85:1603–1607.
17. Algara P, Mateo MS, Sanchez-Beato M, et al. Analysis of the IgV(H) somatic mutations in splenic marginal zone lymphoma defines a group of unmutated cases with frequent 7q deletion and adverse clinical course. *Blood* 2002;99:1299–1304.
18. Traverse-Glehen A, Davi F, Ben Simon E, et al. Analysis of VH genes in marginal zone lymphoma reveals marked heterogeneity between splenic and nodal tumors and suggests the existence of clonal selection. *Haematologica* 2005;90:470–478.
19. Traverse-Glehen A, Verney A, Baseggio L, et al. Analysis of BCL-6, CD95, PIM1, RHO/TTF and PAX5 mutations in splenic and nodal marginal zone B-cell lymphomas suggests a particular B-cell origin. *Leukemia* 2007;21:1821–1824.
20. Suarez F, Lortholary O, Hermine O, et al. Infection-associated lymphomas derived from marginal zone B cells: a model of antigen-driven lymphoproliferation. *Blood* 2006;107:3034–3044.
21. Arcaini L, Burcheri S, Rossi A, et al. Prevalence of HCV infection in nongastric marginal zone B-cell lymphoma of MALT. *Ann Oncol* 2007;18:346–350.
22. Arcaini L, Paulli M, Boveri E, et al. Splenic and nodal marginal zone lymphomas are indolent disorders at high hepatitis C virus seroprevalence with distinct presenting features but similar morphologic and phenotypic profiles. *Cancer* 2004;100:107–115.
23. Hermine O, Lefrere F, Bronowicki J, et al. Regression of splenic lymphoma with villous lymphocytes after treatment of hepatitis C virus infection. *N Engl J Med* 2002;11:89–94.
24. Kelaidi C, Rollot F, Park S, et al. Response to antiviral treatment in hepatitis C virus-associated marginal zone lymphomas. *Leukemia* 2004;18:1711–1716.
25. Morse HC, Kearney JF, Isaacson PG, et al. Cells of the marginal zone—origins, function and neoplasia. *Leuk Res* 2001;25:169–178.
26. Saadoun D, Boyer O, Trebeden-Negre H, et al. Predominance of type 1 (Th1) cytokine production in the liver of patients with HCV-associated mixed cryoglobulinemia vasculitis. *J Hepatol* 2004;41:1031–1037.

27. Bates I, Beduaddo G, Rutherford T, et al. Splenic lymphoma with villous lymphocytes in tropical West Africa. *Lancet* 1992;340:575–577.

28. Berger F, Felman P, Thieblemont C, et al. Non-MALT marginal zone B-cell lymphomas: a description of clinical presentation and outcome in 124 patients. *Blood* 2000;95:1950–1956.

29. Thieblemont C, Felman P, Callet-Bauchu E, et al. Splenic marginal-zone lymphoma: a distinct clinical and pathological entity. *Lancet Oncol* 2003;4:95–103.

30. Franco V, Florena A, Stella M, et al. Splenectomy influences bone marrow infiltration in patients with splenic marginal zone cell lymphoma with or without villous lymphocytes. *Cancer* 2001;91:294–301.

31. Chacon J, Mollejo M, Munoz E, et al. Splenic marginal zone lymphoma: clinical characteristics and prognostic factors in a series of 60 patients. *Blood* 2002;100:1648–1654.

32. Parry-Jones N, Matutes E, Gruszka-Westwood AM, et al. Prognostic features of splenic lymphoma with villous lymphocytes: a report on 129 patients. *Br J Haematol* 2003;120:759–764.

33. Troussard X, Valensi F, Duchayne E, et al. Splenic lymphoma with villous lymphocytes: clinical presentation, biology and prognostic factors in a series of 100 patients. Groupe Francais d'Hematologie Cellulaire (GFHC). *Br J Haematol* 1996;93:731–736.

34. Viala K, Behin A, Maisonobe T, et al. Neuropathy in lymphoma: a relationship between the pattern of neuropathy, type of lymphoma and prognosis? *J Neurol Neurosurg Psychiatry* 2008;79:778–782.

35. Traverse-Glehen A, Baseggio L, Bauchu EC, et al. Splenic red pulp lymphoma with numerous basophilic villous lymphocytes: a distinct clinico-pathologic and molecular entity? *Blood* 2008;111:2253–2260.

36. Matutes E, Morilla R, Owusu-Ankomah K, et al. The immunophenotype of splenic lymphoma with villous lymphocytes and its relevance to the differential diagnosis with other B-cell disorders. *Blood* 1994;83:1558–1562.

37. Dierlamm J, Pittaluga S, Wlodarska I, et al. Marginal zone B-cell lymphomas of different sites share similar cytogenetic and morphologic features. *Blood* 1996;87:229–307.

38. Gruszka-Westwood AM, Matutes E, Coignet LJA, et al. The incidence of trisomy 3 in splenic lymphoma with villous lymphocytes: a study by FISH. *Br J Haematol* 1999;104:600–604.

39. Hernandez JN, Garcia JL, Gutierrez NC, et al. Novel genomic imbalances in B-cell splenic marginal zone lymphomas revealed by comparative genomic hybridization and cytogenetics. *Am J Pathol* 2001;158:1843–1850.

40. Sole F, Woessner S, Florensa L, et al. Frequent involvement of chromosomes 1, 3, 7 and 8 in splenic marginal zone B-cell lymphoma. *Br J Haematol* 1997;98:446–449.

41. Wotherspoon A, Doglioni C, Isaacson P. Low-grade gastric B-cell lymphoma of mucosa-associated lymphoid tissue (MALT): a multifocal disease. *Histopathology* 1992;20:29–34.

42. Andersen CL, Gruszka-Westwood A, Atkinson S, et al. Recurrent genomic imbalances in B-cell splenic marginal-zone lymphoma revealed by comparative genomic hybridization. *Cancer Genet Cytogenet* 2005;156:122–128.

43. Mateo M, Mollejo M, Villuendas R, et al. 7q31-32 allelic loss is a frequent finding in splenic marginal zone lymphoma. *Am J Pathol* 1999;154:1583–1589.

44. Corcoran M, Mould S, Orchard J, et al. Dysregulation of cyclin dependent kinase 6 expression in splenic marginal zone lymphoma through chromosome 7q translocations. *Oncogene* 1999;18:6271–6277.

45. Callet-Bauchu E, Baseggio L, Felman P, et al. Cytogenetic analysis delineates a spectrum of chromosomal changes that can distinguish non-MALT marginal zone B-cell lymphomas among mature B-cell entities: a description of 103 cases. *Leukemia* 2005;19:1818–1823.

46. Dierlamm J, Michaux L, Wlodarska I, et al. Trisomy 3 in marginal zone B-cell lymphoma: a study based on cytogenetic analysis and fluorescence in situ hybridization. *Br J Haematol* 1996;93:242–249.

47. Gruszka-Westwood AM, Hamoudi RA, Matutes E, et al. p53 abnormalities in splenic lymphoma with villous lymphocytes. *Blood* 2001;97:3552–3558.

48. Troussard X, Mauvieux L, Radfordweiss I, et al. Genetic analysis of splenic lymphoma with villous lymphocytes: a Groupe Français d'Hématologie Cellulaire (GFHC) study. *Br J Haematol* 1998;101:712–721.

49. Cunco A, Bardi A, Wlodarska I, et al. A novel recurrent translocation t(11;14)(p11;q32) in splenic marginal zone B cell lymphoma. *Leukemia* 2001;15:1262–1267.

50. Jadayel D, Matutes E, Dyer M, et al. Splenic lymphoma with villous lymphocytes: analysis of bcl-1 rearrangements and expression of the cyclin D1 gene. *Blood* 1994;83:3664–3671.

51. Oscier DG, Matutes E, Gardiner A, et al. Cytogenetic studies in splenic lymphoma with villous lymphocytes. *Br J Haematol* 1993;85:487–491.

52. Ruiz-Ballesteros E, Mollejo M, Rodriguez A, et al. Splenic marginal zone lymphoma: proposal of new diagnostic and prognostic markers identified after tissue and cDNA microarray analysis. *Blood* 2005;106:1831–1838.

53. Thieblemont C, Nasser V, Felman P, et al. Small lymphocytic lymphoma, marginal zone B-cell lymphoma, and mantle cell lymphoma exhibit distinct gene-expression profiles allowing molecular diagnosis. *Blood* 2004;103:2727–2737.

54. Thieblemont C, Rolland D, Baseggio L, et al. Comprehensive analysis of GST-pi expression in B-cell lymphomas: correlation with histological subtypes and survival. *Leuk Lymphoma* 2008;49:1403–1406.

55. Berger F, Traverse-Glehen A, Felman P, et al. Clinicopathologic features of Waldenstrom's macroglobulinemia and marginal zone lymphoma: are they distinct or the same entity? *Clin Lymphoma* 2005;5:220–224.

56. Lin P, Bueso-Ramos C, Wilson CS, et al. Waldenstrom macroglobulinemia involving extramedullary sites: morphologic and immunophenotypic findings in 44 patients. *Am J Surg Pathol* 2003;27:1104–1113.

57. Owen RG, Treon SP, Al-Katib A, et al. Clinicopathological definition of Waldenstrom's macroglobulinemia: consensus panel recommendations from the Second International Workshop on Waldenstrom's Macroglobulinemia. *Semin Oncol* 2003;30:110–115.

58. Bertoni F, Zucca E. State-of-the-art therapeutics: marginal-zone lymphoma. *J Clin Oncol* 2005;23:6415–6420.

59. Arcaini L, Lazzarino M, Colombo N, et al. Splenic marginal zone lymphoma: a prognostic model for clinical use. *Blood* 2006;107:4643–4649.

60. Camacho FI, Mollejo M, Mateo MS, et al. Progression to large B-cell lymphoma in splenic marginal zone lymphoma—a description of a series of 12 cases. *Am J Surg Pathol* 2001;25:1268–1276.

61. Catovsky D, Matutes E. Splenic lymphoma with circulating villous lymphocytes/splenic marginal-zone lymphoma. *Semin Hematol* 1999;36:148–154.

62. Mulligan SP, Matutes E, Dearden C, et al. Splenic lymphoma with villous lymphocytes. Natural history and response to therapy in 50 cases. *Br J Haematol* 1991;78:206–209.

63. Bolam S, Orchard J, Oscier D. Fludarabine is effective in the treatment of splenic lymphoma with villous lymphocytes. *Br J Haematol* 1997;99:158–161.

64. Lefrere F, Hermine O, Belanger C, et al. Fludarabine: an effective treatment in patients with splenic lymphoma with villous lymphocytes. *Leukemia* 2000;14:573–575.

65. Paydas S, Yavuz S, Disel U, et al. Successful rituximab therapy for hemolytic anemia associated with relapsed splenic marginal zone lymphoma with leukemic phase. *Leuk Lymphoma* 2003;44:2165–2166.

66. Tsimberidou AM, Catovsky D, Schlette E, et al. Outcomes in patients with splenic marginal zone lymphoma and marginal zone lymphoma treated with rituximab with or without chemotherapy or chemotherapy alone. *Cancer* 2006;107:125–135.

67. Kalpadakis C, Pangalis GA, Dimopoulou MN, et al. Rituximab monotherapy is highly effective in splenic marginal zone lymphoma. *Hematol Oncol* 2007;25:127–131.

68. Manner H, Jung B, Tonassi L, et al. Successful treatment of catastrophic antiphospholipid antibody syndrome (CAPS) associated with splenic marginal-zone lymphoma with low-molecular weight heparin, rituximab and bendamustine. *Am J Med Sci* 2008;335:394–397.

69. Robinson KS, Williams ME, van der Jagt RH, et al. Phase II multicenter study of bendamustine plus rituximab in patients with relapsed indolent B-cell and mantle cell non-Hodgkin's lymphoma. *J Clin Oncol* 2008;26:4473–4479.

CHAPTER 17 ■ NODAL MARGINAL ZONE B-CELL LYMPHOMA

ALEXANDRA TRAVERSE-GLEHEN, FRANÇOISE BERGER, AND GILLES SALLES

DEFINITION

Nodal marginal zone B-cell lymphoma is a primary nodal B-cell lymphoma that shares morphologic, immunophenotypic, and genetic characteristics with extranodal and splenic marginal zone lymphoma, but without those specific localizations at presentation. It was first described as nodal monocytoid B-cell lymphoma in 1986 by Sheibani et al. (1), then as parafollicular B-cell lymphoma by Cousar et al. (2) in 1987. The relationship with marginal zone B cells was established by Piris et al. (3) in 1988. Nodal monocytoid B-cell lymphoma was introduced in the Revised Kiel Classification by Lennert in 1990 (3a). Nodal marginal zone lymphoma with or without monocytoid B cells was considered as a provisional subtype in the Revised European-American Lymphoma Classification, and finally admitted as a distinct entity in the World Health Organization classification in 2001 and 2008. However, few series have been published, and discrepancies remain concerning the morphologic, biologic, and clinical characteristics of this disease (4–17).

FREQUENCY AND EPIDEMIOLOGY

Among other lymphomas, nodal marginal zone lymphoma is rare, representing respectively 1.5% and 1.8% of the cases analyzed within an international study and single-center series (12,18). Two-thirds of the cases of the Southwest Oncology Group study (19) were described as "composite lymphomas" with concomitant follicular lymphoma and may include follicular lymphomas with marginal zone differentiation. Other series probably include cases corresponding to nodal spread of extranodal marginal zone lymphoma or cases disseminated at diagnosis, with peripheral lymph nodes associated with extranodal or splenic involvement. Association with hepatitis C virus infection has been reported essentially in the Italian series but appears rather rare in other settings (17).

DIAGNOSIS

Morphology

Morphologic features of nodal marginal zone lymphoma are very heterogeneous, in terms of both architecture and cytology (9,12,15). The pattern of lymph node infiltration may be perifollicular or "inverse follicular," interfollicular, perisinusoidal, follicular by colonization of reactive follicles (less frequent than in mucosa-associated lymphoid tissue lymphomas), or

diffuse. Those patterns are often associated within the same lymph node. Residual atrophic follicles, rarely hyperplasic, are usually seen. Several cell types can be encountered in varying proportions: small cells with irregular nuclei, clumped chromatin, and clear cytoplasm; cells resembling small lymphocytes, small cells with a plasmacytoid differentiation; plasma cells; and a variable content of medium to large cells centroblast or immunoblast like. Follicular dendritic cells, usually arranged in a nodular meshwork, are always present. "Monocytoid" B cells with more abundant and clear cytoplasm are not usually predominant, and pure monocytoid B-cell lymphomas are less frequent than cases with plasmacytoid or plasmacytic differentiation. Of note, the latter were considered in the past as immunocytoma, and the boundary between nodal marginal zone B-cell lymphoma and lymphoplasmacytic lymphoma (LPL) is still unclear and debated. Unlike extranodal and splenic marginal zone lymphoma, the proportion of large cells is often relatively high (>20%), as is the mitotic index, and questions the classification of nodal marginal zone lymphoma as a low-grade lymphoma.

Differential diagnosis can be difficult with other small B-cell lymphomas, which sometimes have a marginal zone pattern or contain monocytoid B cells, as with LPL, rarely with mantle cell lymphoma. Follicular colonization can also mimic some aspects encountered in follicular lymphoma (20). Immunophenotypic features are helpful to clarify these cases. In fact, because the contingent of large cells is often high, many cases were classified in the past as diffuse mixed in the Working Formulation or polymorphic immunocytoma in the Kiel Classification, and are perhaps sometimes considered among diffuse large B-cell lymphomas. In total, it is likely that this entity is under recognized in routine practice, with cases identified as indolent or as aggressive lymphomas.

IMMUNOPHENOTYPE

The phenotype, usually identical to extranodal marginal zone lymphoma, is an important diagnostic feature that can help distinguish those cases from other small B-cell lymphomas: typically the lymphoma cells are sIgM$^{+/-}$, D/G$^+$, cIg$^{+/-}$, CD19$^+$, CD20$^+$, CD79a$^+$, Oct2$^+$, Pax5$^+$, CD5$^-$, CD10$^-$, CD23$^-$, CD43$^{+/-}$, BCL2$^+$, and cyclinD1$^-$. Few cases have been reported with expression of CD5 and CD23. The expression of immunoglobulin (Ig) D has been reported by Campo et al. (11), who described a splenic type of nodal marginal zone lymphoma. The plasmacytic differentiation is usually associated with the expression of CD38 and MUM1 (13). In cases with follicle colonization, the benign reactive follicle center cells express CD10 and Bcl-6, and are negative for Bcl-2 and MUM1. In contrast, the colonizing marginal zone lymphoma cells express Bcl-2 and often MUM1, and are negative for Bcl-6 and CD10 (20). Ki67 expression is much higher among the residual benign/reactive follicle center cells as compared with the lymphoma cells themselves in most cases.

PATHOGENESIS

Cytogenetic and Molecular Features

Cytogenetics may help recognize the disease (mainly by ruling out other small B-cell lymphomas), but data remain sparse in the literature [only 18 cases reported (21–23)], and it is difficult to establish a characteristic cytogenetic profile. Clonal aberrations are found in the majority of cases, and the karyotype is most frequently complex. Recurrent clonal abnormalities found in the other types of marginal zone lymphoma, such as trisomy 3, trisomy 18, trisomy 7, trisomy 12, or del6q, may contribute to the diagnostic. The presence of trisomy 12 seems to be more frequent than in extranodal or splenic marginal zone lymphoma. The translocation characteristics of mucosa-associated lymphoid tissue have not been reported in nodal marginal zone lymphomas. Rare cases (<10%) of TP53 gene heterozygous deletions detected by fluorescent in situ hybridization were reported (21,24).

Postulated Cell of Origin

The normal counterpart of those lymphoma cells is not well characterized. Normal nodal marginal zones are only seen in mesenteric lymph nodes, and the relationship with monocytoid B cells, observed in reactive lymph nodes (toxoplasmosis lymphadenitis, human immunodeficiency virus infection), remains unclear.

The Ig-heavy chain (IGHV) gene mutational status was investigated in limited series (13,25–29). The majority of cases (87%) presented somatic mutations of the IGHV genes with a biased usage of IGHV4-34 (but also IGHV1-69 in cases associated with hepatitis C virus infection) and evidence of antigen selection in most cases, but without ongoing mutations. No outcome difference was described between mutated and nonmutated cases.

PRESENTATION

Given the recent identification of nodal marginal zone lymphoma, few reports present detailed patients' clinical and outcome data. Only eight clinical series are available with a maximum of 47 cases reported (Table 17.1). The median age is of 50 to 60 years with a slight male predominance. The disease is usually localized in peripheral lymph nodes, mostly cervical, and inguinal, with frequent involvement of other thoracic or abdominal nodes. The clinical stage at diagnosis is variable according to series, but the majority of patients usually present with advanced clinical stage III or IV. The bone marrow infiltration is observed between 19% and 62% of cases, although the peripheral blood involvement is very rare.

PRONOSTIC AND PREDICTIVE FACTORS

Complete response to the first treatment is observed in 50% to 60% of the cases. In the International Lymphoma Study Group, 5-year failure-free survival and overall survival were only 28% and 56%, respectively. This trend toward a poor prognosis was also found for patients with a low or intermediate International Prognostic Index score. Of note, histologic progression toward large cell lymphoma appeared at diagnosis in one out of five patients. In our series, time to progression was 1.3 years, but median overall survival was close to 5 years, indicating that this disease may remain indolent for several years (Fig. 17.1). Given the small numbers of cases reported in these series, no specific prognostic factors were reported for this entity. A poor performance status at diagnosis was the only clinical parameter significantly influencing the outcome, and in the largest series (30), the Follicular Lymphoma International Prognostic Index score identified one-third of patients with a significantly shorter survival. Of note, a higher proportion of large cells in the diagnostic lymph node was not associated with a different outcome (Fig. 17.2). Patients having a complete response to first-line treatment may also have a better prognosis (Fig. 17.3). At the time of relapse, nodal sites are usually predominantly encountered, although splenic or extranodal sites may occur, reminiscent of the other marginal zone lymphoma subtypes. However, histologic progression toward diffuse large cell lymphomas appeared to occur quite frequently, and there was no evidence of plateau on survival curves to suggest that this disease is currently curable.

TREATMENT

There is no standardized treatment for this disease, but patients may be managed according to guidelines established for follicular lymphoma (31,32). Patients with truly localized disease may be considered for localized radiation therapy, with a good tumor control (13–15). Treatment may be delayed in patients with a low tumor burden, or single-agent chemotherapy or immunotherapy can be proposed. In patients with more aggressive features, a standard immunochemotherapy regimen can be proposed, but a substantial proportion of patients does not have a complete response. A more dose-intensive strategy, eventually including autologous bone marrow transplantation, was sometimes applied to younger patients with a high number of large mitotic cells and adverse clinical prognostic factors (33). Radiation therapy may also be considered as a palliative treatment in some cases, using low doses of radiation (34). However, none of these approaches has been prospectively tested. Therefore, no specific therapeutic approach could be recommended at this time, and the clinician may decide based on the morphologic and clinical characteristics of each patient. Monoclonal antibodies directed against the CD20 antigen appeared in some reports to have some efficacy in this setting (15).

CLINICAL CHARACTERISTICS OF NMZL FROM THE LITERATURE DATA

Author	Nathwani et al.	Nathwani et al.	Berger et al.	Camacho et al.	Arcaini et al.	Traverse-Glehen et al.	Oh et al.	Arcaini et al.
Journal and Year	Semin Hematol 1999	J Clin Oncol 1999	Blood 2000	Am J Surg Pathol 2003	Cancer 2004	Histopathology 2006	Ann Hematol 2006	Br J Haematol 2007
Number of patients	20	25	37	22	9	21	36	47
Male (%)	44	64	43	32	44	67	72	36
Median age	59	58	54	62	62	54	50	63
Age range	nd	27–90	nd	26–92	25–74	27–83	13–79	nd
Age >60 y (%)	nd	nd	35	nd	nd	33	nd	64
ECOG score >2 (%)	0	7	12.5	nd	22	14	17	6
B symptoms presence (%)	14	37	13.5	nd	22	10	8	15
Stage III/IV (%)	71	82	68	41	99	76	44	77
Peripheral lymph nodes (%)	100	nd	95	95	100	98	nd	98
Cervical lymph nodes	81	nd	11	nd	nd	71	56	53
Axillary lymph nodes	44	nd	nd	nd	nd	nd	nd	nd
Inguinal lymph nodes	63	nd	nd	nd	nd	33	17	nd
Abdominal and/or chest lymph nodes (%)	85	nd	49	nd	67	48	nd	23
Gastrointestinal involvement	0	5	0	nd	0	0	nd	0
Bone marrow involvement (%)	28	32	43	29	44	62	19	45
Peripheral blood involvement (%)	nd	nd	11	9	11	24	nd	11
Liver involvement (%)	13	nd	5	nd	0	nd	nd	0
Splenomegaly (%)	nd	nd	0	nd	0	0	nd	0
Hb >11g per dl (%)	nd	nd	31	nd	nd	24	36	11
LDH >normal value (%)	36	40	40	43	22	48	19.4	15
$\beta2$-microglobulin >3 mg per L (%)	nd	nd	33	41	33	29	nd	45
M component (%)	nd	nd	8	nd	11	33	nd	15
IPI 1 (%)	57	60	31	48	nd	72	27	37
IPI 2 (%)	36	27	28	47	nd	11		22
IPI 3 (%)	0	0	24	0	nd	11		35
IPI 4 (%)	7	13	17	5	nd	5	8	6
Viral hepatitis C association (%)	nd	nd	nd	20	22	0	2.8	24
Median progression (y)	nd	nd	nd	nd	2.8	1.3	1.3	2.6
Median OS (y)	nd	nd	nd	nd	Not reached		5.5	Not reached
5-y OS (%)	56	57	55	79	nd	64	82.7	69

ECOG, Eastern Cooperative Oncology Group; Hb, hemoglobin; IPI, International Prognostic Index; nd, not determined; OS, overall survival.

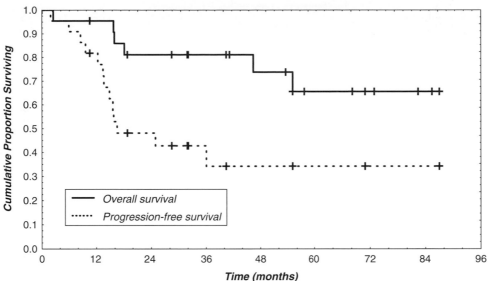

FIGURE 17.1 Progression-free survival and overall survival of patients with nodal marginal zone lymphoma.

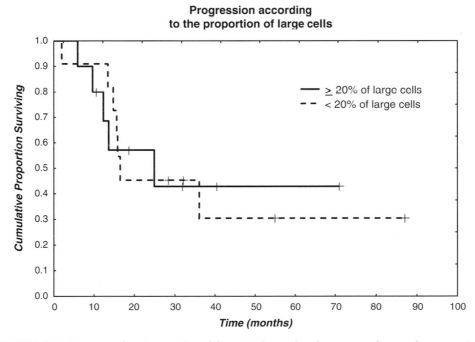

FIGURE 17.2 Outcome of patients with nodal marginal zone lymphoma according to the proportion of large cells at diagnosis.

FUTURE DIRECTIONS

The morphologic and phenotypic description of nodal marginal zone B-cell lymphoma (NMZL) is still incomplete in the literature. There are probably real borderline cases with other types of lymphomas, and the differential diagnosis on morphology and phenotype remains uneasy.

One of the difficult differential diagnoses is with follicular grade 3 with plasmacytic or marginal zone B-cell differentiation. In addition, expression of CD10 has been reported recently in very few cases, but without the coexpression of Bcl-6 protein (a more reliable marker for follicle center cells) (20), and this features needs to be clarified.

The overlap with LPL stays in the center of the debates. LPL is considered in the World Health Organization classification (35) as a lymphoma occurring in adults in the second part of their life, involving bone marrow, and, less frequently (15% to 30%), lymph nodes, spleen, liver, and sometimes peripheral blood. It is often associated with an IgM paraprotein. Waldenström macroglobulinemia is being defined as

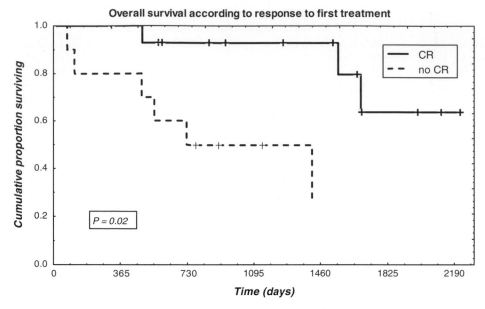

FIGURE 17.3 Outcome of patients with nodal marginal zone lymphoma according to the proportion of large cells at diagnosis. CR, complete response.

LPL with bone marrow involvement and an IgM monoclonal gammopathy. In lymph nodes, the normal architecture is usually preserved, with dilated sinuses and, sometimes, atrophic residual germinal centers. Increased mast cells and hemosiderin are frequent. Other features are, however, possible, and several aspects are shared with NMZL: diffuse or vaguely nodular pattern, plasmacytic differentiation, absence of specific phenotype, trisomy 3, and association with hepatitis C. In addition, literature data concerning LPL are limited and controversial; therefore, the relationship between LPL and MZL needs to be clarified (36). Interestingly, the 6q (21–23) deletion has been described to be recurrent in bone marrow–based LPL but is infrequent in lymph node LPL and was not reported in MZL as a primary alteration. Trisomy 4 also seems to be recurrent in Waldenström macroglobulinemia (37). Additional studies, including a better characterization of the Ig IGHV repertoire in both NMZL and LPL (with only 46 and 53 cases reported, respectively), may help to further decipher these entities in the future. A better recognition of nodal marginal zone lymphoma through new molecular and phenotypic markers may lead to a better identification of those patients to allow meaningful clinical studies.

References

1. Sheibani K, Sohn CC, Burke JS, et al. Monocytoid B-cell lymphoma. A novel B-cell neoplasm. *Am J Pathol* 1986;124:310–318.
2. Cousar JB, McGinn DL, Glick AD, et al. Report of an unusual lymphoma arising from parafollicular B-lymphocytes (PBLs) or so-called "monocytoid" lymphocytes. *Am J Clin Pathol* 1987;87:121–128.
3. Piris MA, Rivas C, Morente M, et al. Monocytoid B-cell lymphoma, a tumour related to the marginal zone. *Histopathology* 1988;12:383–392.
3a. Lennert K, Feller AC. *Histopathologie der non Hodgkin's lymphoma (rach der aktuaPirienton Kiel-klassifikation).* Berlin: Springer Verlag, 1990.
4. Ng CS, Chan JK. Monocytoid B-cell lymphoma. *Hum Pathol* 1987;18:1069–1071.
5. Cogliatti SB, Lennert K, Hansmann ML, et al. Monocytoid B cell lymphoma: clinical and prognostic features of 21 patients. *J Clin Pathol* 1990;43:619–625.

6. Ngan BY, Warnke RA, Wilson M, et al. Monocytoid B-cell lymphoma: a study of 36 cases. *Hum Pathol* 1991;22:409–421.
7. Nizze H, Cogliatti SB, von Schilling C, et al. Monocytoid B-cell lymphoma: morphological variants and relationship to low-grade B-cell lymphoma of the mucosa-associated lymphoid tissue. *Histopathology* 1991;18:403–414.
8. Ortiz-Hidalgo C, Wright DH. The morphological spectrum of monocytoid B-cell lymphoma and its relationship to lymphomas of mucosa-associated lymphoid tissue. *Histopathology* 1992;21:555–561.
9. Nathwani BN, Drachenberg MR, Hernandez AM, et al. Nodal monocytoid B-cell lymphoma (nodal marginal-zone B-cell lymphoma). *Semin Hematol* 1999;36:128–138.
10. Nathwani BN, Anderson JR, Armitage JO, et al. Marginal zone B-cell lymphoma: a clinical comparison of nodal and mucosa-associated lymphoid tissue types. Non-Hodgkin's Lymphoma Classification Project. *J Clin Oncol* 1999;17:2486–2492.
11. Campo E, Miquel R, Krenacs L, et al. Primary nodal marginal zone lymphomas of splenic and MALT type. *Am J Surg Pathol* 1999;23:59–68.
12. Berger F, Felman P, Thieblemont C, et al. Non-MALT marginal zone B-cell lymphomas: a description of clinical presentation and outcome in 124 patients. *Blood* 2000;95:1950–1956.
13. Camacho FI, Algara P, Mollejo M, et al. Nodal marginal zone lymphoma: a heterogeneous tumor: a comprehensive analysis of a series of 27 cases. *Am J Surg Pathol* 2003;27:762–771.
14. Oh SY, Ryoo BY, Kim WS, et al. Nodal marginal zone B-cell lymphoma: analysis of 36 cases. Clinical presentation and treatment outcomes of nodal marginal zone B-cell lymphoma. *Ann Hematol* 2006;85:781–786.
15. Traverse-Glehen A, Felman P, Callet-Bauchu E, et al. A clinicopathological study of nodal marginal zone B-cell lymphoma. A report on 21 cases. *Histopathology* 2006;48:162–173.
16. Arcaini L, Paulli M, Boveri E, et al. Marginal zone-related neoplasms of splenic and nodal origin. *Haematologica* 2003;88:80–93.
17. Arcaini L, Paulli M, Boveri E, et al. Splenic and nodal marginal zone lymphomas are indolent disorders at high hepatitis C virus seroprevalence with distinct presenting features but similar morphologic and phenotypic profiles. *Cancer* 2004;100:107–115.
18. A clinical evaluation of the International Lymphoma Study Group classification of non-Hodgkin's lymphoma. The Non-Hodgkin's Lymphoma Classification Project. *Blood* 1997;89:3909–3918.
19. Fisher RI, Dahlberg S, Nathwani BN, et al. A clinical analysis of two indolent lymphoma entities: mantle cell lymphoma and marginal zone lymphoma (including the mucosa-associated lymphoid tissue and monocytoid B-cell subcategories): a Southwest Oncology Group study. *Blood* 1995;85:1075–1082.
20. Naresh KN. Nodal marginal zone B-cell lymphoma with prominent follicular colonization—difficulties in diagnosis: a study of 15 cases. *Histopathology* 2008;52:331–339.
21. Dierlamm J, Pittaluga S, Wlodarska I, et al. Marginal zone B-cell lymphomas of different sites share similar cytogenetic and morphologic features. *Blood* 1996;87:299–307.

22. Banerjee SS, Harris M, Eyden BP, et al. Monocytoid B cell lymphoma. *J Clin Pathol* 1991;44:39–44.

23. Slovak ML, Weiss LM, Nathwani BN, et al. Cytogenetic studies of composite lymphomas: monocytoid B-cell lymphoma and other B-cell non-Hodgkin's lymphomas. *Hum Pathol* 1993;24:1086–1094.

24. Callet-Bauchu E, Baseggio L, Felman P, et al. Cytogenetic analysis delineates a spectrum of chromosomal changes that can distinguish non-MALT marginal zone B-cell lymphomas among mature B-cell entities: a description of 103 cases. *Leukemia* 2005;19:1818–1823.

25. Tierens A, Delabie J, Pittaluga S, et al. Mutation analysis of the rearranged immunoglobulin heavy chain genes of marginal zone cell lymphomas indicates an origin from different marginal zone B lymphocyte subsets. *Blood* 1998;91:2381–2386.

26. Conconi A, Bertoni F, Pedrinis E, et al. Nodal marginal zone B-cell lymphomas may arise from different subsets of marginal zone B lymphocytes. *Blood* 2001;98:781–786.

27. Traverse-Glehen A, Davi F, Ben Simon E, et al. Analysis of VH genes in marginal zone lymphoma reveals marked heterogeneity between splenic and nodal tumors and suggests the existence of clonal selection. *Haematologica* 2005;90:470–478.

28. Miranda RN, Cousar JB, Hammer RD, et al. Somatic mutation analysis of IgH variable regions reveals that tumor cells of most parafollicular (monocytoid) B-cell lymphoma, splenic marginal zone B-cell lymphoma, and some hairy cell leukemia are composed of memory B lymphocytes. *Hum Pathol* 1999;30:306–312.

29. Kuppers R, Hajadi M, Plank L, et al. Molecular Ig gene analysis reveals that monocytoid B cell lymphoma is a malignancy of mature B cells carrying somatically mutated V region genes and suggests that rearrangement of the kappa-deleting element (resulting in deletion of the Ig kappa enhancers) abolishes somatic hypermutation in the human. *Eur J Immunol* 1996;26:1794–1800.

30. Arcaini L, Paulli M, Burcheri S, et al. Primary nodal marginal zone B-cell lymphoma: clinical features and prognostic assessment of a rare disease. *Br J Haematol* 2007;136:301–304.

31. Salles GA. Clinical features, prognosis and treatment of follicular lymphoma. *Hematology Am Soc Hematol Educ Program* 2007;2007:216–225.

32. Barosi G, Carella A, Lazzarino M, et al. Management of nodal indolent (non marginal-zone) non-Hodgkin's lymphomas: practice guidelines from the Italian Society of Hematology, Italian Society of Experimental Hematology and Italian Group for Bone Marrow Transplantation. *Haematologica* 2005;90:1236–1257.

33. Ghesquières H, Berger F, Felman P, et al. Clinicopathological characteristics and outcome of diffuse large B-cell lymphomas presenting with features of transformed low grade lymphomas at diagnosis. *J Clin Oncol* 2006;24:5234–5241.

34. Luthy SK, Ng AK, Silver B, et al. Response to low-dose involved-field radiotherapy in patients with non-Hodgkin's lymphoma. *Ann Oncol* 2008;19:2043–2047.

35. Swerdlow SH, Berger F, Pileri SA, et al. Lymphoplasmacytic lymphoma. In: Swerdlow SH, Campo E, Harris NL, et al., eds. *WHO classification of tumours of haematopoietic and lymphoid tissues,* 4th ed. Lyon, France: International Agency for Research on Cancer, 2008:194.

36. Berger F, Traverse-Glehen A, Felman P, et al. Clinicopathologic features of Waldenstrom's macroglobulinemia and marginal zone lymphoma: are they distinct or the same entity? *Clin Lymphoma* 2005;5:220–224.

37. Terre C, Nguyen-Khac F, Barin C, et al. Trisomy 4, a new chromosomal abnormality in Waldenstrom's macroglobulinemia: a study of 39 cases. *Leukemia* 2006;20:1634–1636.

CHAPTER 18 ■ FOLLICULAR LYMPHOMA

ARNOLD S. FREEDMAN, JONATHAN W. FRIEDBERG, PETER M. MAUCH, RICCARDO DALLA-FAVERA, AND NANCY LEE HARRIS

DEFINITION

Follicular lymphoma (FL) is defined in the 2008 World Health Organization (WHO) classification (1) as a neoplasm composed of follicle center (germinal center) B cells (typically both centrocytes and centroblasts/large transformed cells), which usually has at least a partially follicular pattern. If diffuse areas of any size comprised predominantly or entirely of blastic cells are present in any case of FL, a diagnosis of diffuse large B-cell lymphoma (DLBCL) is also made. Lymphomas composed of centrocytes and centroblasts with an entirely diffuse pattern in the sampled tissue may be included in this category. Primary cutaneous lymphomas of germinal center cells are considered a distinct category of primary cutaneous follicle center lymphoma (see Chapter 24).

FREQUENCY

FL is the second most common lymphoma in the United States and Western Europe, comprising approximately 20% of all non-Hodgkin lymphomas (NHL), and up to 70% of "low-grade" lymphomas reported in American and European clinical trials (2,3). In contrast, FL is much less common in Asians and Blacks than in whites in Western countries, including the United States, and is uncommon in Asia and developing countries (4). The risk was lower for first-generation migrants from China and Japan than for subsequent-generation migrants (5). Most cases are grade 1 or grade 26. FL most frequently presents in middle-aged individuals and the elderly, with a median age at diagnosis of 60 years and a slight female predominance (6). There are trends showing higher rates of FL in smokers (7). A lower incidence of BCL2 translocations is seen within FLs that occur in Asians as compared to FL in individuals from Western countries (8). This is in spite of similar rates of BCL2 rearrangements detected in normal individuals from either Asian or Western countries. This suggests differences in the pathogenesis of FL in distinct geographic areas. In patients over age 75, the rates of FL increased by 1.8% per year in an analysis of patients diagnosed between 1992 and 2001 (9). FL is extremely rare in childhood (10). The new WHO classification will include an entity of pediatric FL that may have an improved prognosis.

DIAGNOSIS

Morphology

FL is composed of follicle center B cells, usually a mixture of centrocytes (cleaved follicle center cells, "small cells") and centroblasts (large, noncleaved follicle center cells, "large cells"). Centrocytes typically predominate; centroblasts are usually in the minority but always present. Rare cases of FL consist almost entirely of centroblasts. Occasional cases may show plasmacytoid differentiation or foci of marginal zone or monocytoid B cells (11).

Grading

FL has traditionally been graded according to the number of large cells (centroblasts), which roughly correlates with clinical aggressiveness (1). The 2008 WHO classification includes grades 1 to 2 (low grade), defined as having few centroblasts (zero to 15 centroblasts per high-power field [hpf]), and grade 3, in which centroblasts are numerous (>15 centroblasts per hpf) (Table 18.1) (1). Because the clinical behavior and outcome of treatment of FL grades 1 and 2 are similar, and they are generally approached in the same manner, as indolent lymphomas, the decision was made not to separate them (12). In contrast, grade 3 FL is generally approached as an aggressive disease. Grade 3 cases have a morphologic spectrum; most have a background of centrocytes, but with numerous centroblasts, and are a morphologic continuum with low-grade cases, whereas rare cases have solid sheets of centroblasts. The former are classified as grade 3A and the latter as grade 3B (13). Grade 3B cases are often associated with areas of DLBCL. Differences in genetic features and clinical behavior suggest that FL grade 3A may be more indolent and closely related to FL low-grade cases and grade 3B more

---

TABLE 18.1

ORGANIZATION CLASSIFICATION GRADING

Grading	Definition
Grade 1–2 (low grade)	0–15 centroblasts per hpf
1	0–5 centroblasts per hpf
2	6–15 centroblasts per hpf
Grade 3	>15 centroblasts per hpf
3A	Centrocytes present
3B	Solid sheets of centroblasts
Reporting of pattern	**Proportion follicular**
Follicular	>75%
Follicular and diffuse	25–75%[a]
Focally follicular	<25%[b]
Diffuse	0%

[a] Diffuse areas containing >15 centroblasts per hpf are reported as DLBCL with FL (grades 1 to 2, 3A, or 3B).
[b] Gives approximate percentage in report.

closely related to DLBCL; however, these studies have typically included cases of FL grade 3B with DLBCL (14–17).

Pattern

FL reproduces the architecture of normal germinal centers of secondary lymphoid follicles. Neoplastic follicles distort and replace the normal nodal architecture. In contrast to normal follicles, neoplastic follicles often lack mantle zones, and tingible body (debris laden) macrophages are typically absent (18). Neoplastic cells are often present in the interfollicular region. The pattern may be entirely follicular, or diffuse components may be present. FL is reported as "follicular" if the pattern is >75% follicular, follicular and diffuse if it is 25% to 75% follicular, and predominantly diffuse if <25% follicular. Importantly, if a diffuse area contains a sufficient number of centroblasts to be classified as grade 3 (A or B), this is considered to represent DLBCL, a separate diagnosis of DLBCL should be made, with an estimate of the proportion of each (Table 18.1)

Diffuse Follicular Lymphoma

Rare lymphomas composed of centrocytes, with a small proportion of centroblasts (consistent with FL grades 1 to 2), have an entirely diffuse architecture and the same immunophenotype and genetic features as FL. These cases may represent diffuse areas of FL in which the follicular component is not represented in the biopsy. The term *diffuse follicle centel lymphoma* has been used for these cases; the current WHO classification (1) classifies these as "diffuse follicular lymphoma." Although the term sounds internally contradictory, it should be understood that the term "follicular" refers not only to pattern but to cell type, and that these are tumors of the lymphoid follicle, regardless of pattern. If centroblasts predominate (grade 3A or 3B), or if the small cells are T cells, the tumor is classified as DLBCL. The clinical behavior of diffuse FL is not known. This diagnosis cannot be made without immunophenotyping and, if necessary, genetic studies.

Partial Nodal Involvement and Intrafollicular Neoplasia ("in-situ" Follicular Lymphoma)

In some lymph nodes involved by FL, residual nonneoplastic follicles remain, and in some cases, staining for BCL2 protein will reveal partial "colonization" of some of them by neoplastic cells with strong BCL2 expression. Rarely, architecturally normal-appearing lymph nodes may contain one or more follicles that demonstrate BCL2-overexpressing centrocytes and centroblasts, a phenomenon that has been called "in-situ follicular lymphoma." Among 23 reported cases (19), 40% of the patients had FL in other lymph nodes either simultaneously or later, whereas 60% had no evidence of overt lymphoma during follow-up. Thus, in some cases this phenomenon represents colonization of preexisting follicles by neoplastic follicle center cells, whereas in others it may represent the tissue counterpart of circulating clonal B cells with *BCL2* rearrangement, that is a clone of cells that has the translocation but not the other genetic abnormalities to result in overt progressive malignancy, or in some cases it may represent the earliest evidence of a true FL that will progress to overt lymphoma. It is recommended (1) that in such cases a definite diagnosis of FL should not be made; the

pathology report should indicate that the significance of the finding is unknown, and that clinical evaluation for evidence of overt FL elsewhere is suggested.

In the bone marrow, which is involved in 50% to 70% of patients affected, one sees characteristic paratrabecular lymphoid aggregates. Involvement of the peripheral blood is seen in approximately 30% of patients. These circulating malignant cells have nuclear clefts, in contrast to the cells of chronic lymphocytic leukemia.

Hisiologic Progression or Transformation

Over time, a proportion of cases of FL evolve into an aggressive lymphoma, usually DLBCL but occasionally resembling Burkitt lymphoma (BL) or intermediate between BL and DLBCL. The latter cases are often associated with a second translocation involving MYC (20,21). It is recommended that these not be classified as BL, a term that is reserved for de novo cases; the 2008 WHO classification provides a category "High-grade B-cell lymphoma, intermediate between BL and DLBCL" for such cases (1). Recently, development of histiocytic sarcomas has been reported in several patients with FL; in these cases the histiocytic sarcoma had identical immunoglobulin (Ig) H rearranements to the original FL, suggesting a clonal relationship. Switching off of PAX5, a gene that is important in B-lineage commitment, has been suggested as the transforming event in this process (22).

Immunophenotype

The tumor cells typically express monoclonal surface Ig, with 50% to 60% Ig M[+], 40% IgG[+], and rare cases IgA[+] (1). Immunophenotyping studies have provided strong support that FL cells are derived from normal germinal center B cells. Virtually all cases express pan–B-cell antigens (CD19, CD20, CD79a), complement receptors (CD21 and CD35), and CD10 (60%), as well as nuclear bcl-6 (1,23). However, in contrast to normal germinal center B cells, cytoplasmic staining for BCL2 protein in FL cells is typically positive (24). The Ki-67[+] proliferation fraction is lower than that of reactive follicles. Unlike small lymphocytic and mantle cell lymphomas, FL cells lack CD5 and CD43 (most cases); CD23 expression is variable. CD11a/CD18 is more frequently noted on tumor cells at initial diagnosis (60% to 90% of cases) than at relapse. CD4[+] T cells and follicular dendritic cells are present in the malignant follicles in association with malignant B cells. When other tissues, such as liver or skin tissues, are involved, follicular dendritic cells and CD4[+] T cells are generally present along with the FL cells. Rare cases of FL lack CD10. These express MUM-1 and clinically occur in older patients than CD10[+] cases, tend to be grade 3B histology, and lack BCL2/IgH translocations (25).

Genetics

In FL, the Ig heavy and light chain genes are rearranged, and analysis of the Ig variable-region genes shows extensive somatic mutations and a high frequency of intraclonal diversity, indicating ongoing mutations, similar to normal germinal center B cells (26,27).

The genetic hallmark of FL is represented by chromosomal breaks at 18q21 and rearrangements of BCL2, which are detected in 80% to 90% of cases (28,29). In this translocation, the BCL2 gene on chromosome 18 is juxtaposed to the transcriptionally active Ig heavy chain region on chromosome 14, forming the BCL2/IgH rearrangement and up-regulating the BCL2 gene (30,31). Other chromosomal aberrations include gains of 7p, 7q, Xp, 12q, 18q, each occurring in 10% to 20% of patients, and deletions of chromosome 6q occur in 16% to 20% of cases (32). Although FLs with 3q27 (BCL6 gene) abnormalities are rare, the malignant cells express the BCL6 gene and protein, which is a transcription factor involved in normal germinal center development (33).

Over time, a proportion of cases of FL evolve into an aggressive lymphoma, usually DLBCL but occasionally resembling BL. Cytogenetic analysis suggests that patients with FL whose tumor cells have deletions of chromosomes 6p, 17p, and 9p have significantly increased risk of histologic transformation. Specific genes have been identified as being altered in transformation, including deletions of the cyclin-dependent kinase inhibitors p15 and p16, and mutations of p53 and BCL2, as well as of the noncoding regulatory region of the BCL6 gene (34–37). MYC rearrangement may also occur as a secondary abnormality, and in these cases "double hit" with both BCL2 and MYC rearrangements, the morphologic features often resemble those of BL. Such cases are not classified as BL, a term that is reserved for de novo cases; the 2008 WHO classification provides a category "High-grade B-cell lymphoma, intermediate between BL and DLBCL" for such cases (1).

PATHOGENESIS

Chromosomal Translocations Involving BCL2

The t(14;18)(q32;q21) is the most common translocation in human lymphoid malignancies (Color Plate 29). Virtually all FLs and approximately 30% of DLBCLs carry breaks at 18q21. In t(14;18), the rearrangement joins the BCL2 gene at its 3' untranslated region to an IgH J segment, resulting in deregulation of BCL2 expression. The chromosomal breakpoints on BCL2 cluster are at two main regions 3' to the BCL2 coding region. The major breakpoint region is located within the 3' untranslated region, and the minor cluster region is located some 20-kb downstream. Both regions have been cloned and sequenced. The consequence of the translocation is the presence within the cells of constitutively high levels of BCL2 protein, resulting from both enhanced transcription and, possibly, more efficient ribonucleic acid processing (38,39).

The BCL2 gene encodes a 26-kDa integral membrane protein that has been localized to mitochondria, endoplasmic reticulum, and perinuclear membrane (40). In contrast to most protooncogenes of lymphoid neoplasia, BCL2 has little or no ability to promote cell-cycle progression or cell proliferation but rather controls the cellular apoptotic threshold by preventing programmed cell death. In normal cells, the topographic restriction of BCL2 expression to germinal center zones of surviving B cells suggests that BCL2 drives the emergence of long-surviving memory B cells. In fact, BCL2

transgenic animals show markedly protracted secondary immune responses and an extended lifetime for memory B cells in the absence of antigen (41).

BCL2 is only one member of a family of apoptotic regulators, which includes BAX and BCL-X (42,43). BCL2 exists as part of a high-molecular weight complex generated through heterodimerization with bax (44). The inherent ratio of BCL2 to bax determines the functional activity of BCL2. The precise molecular mechanisms by which BCL2 regulates cell death stem from the observation that BCL2 is only one member of a family of opposing regulators of the intrinsic, or mitochondrial pathway, of apoptosis. BCL2, along with BCL-XL and MCL-1 among others, are antiapoptotic family members. Two categories of proapoptotic family members exist, one consisting of multidomain proteins like BAX, and the second consisting of single BH3-domain only proteins like BAD and BID. The single BH3 domain proteins send the signal to trigger death; once activated, they bind to and neutralize the BCL2-like proapoptotic proteins and lead to activation of BAX, which aggregates in the mitochondrial membrane. This aggregation promotes apoptosis by releasing cytochrome c, which leads to the activation of caspase-9, followed by caspase-3, resulting in protein and deoxyribonucleic acid cleavage. When bax is in excess, bax homodimers dominate, and cell death is accelerated. Conversely, when BCL2 is in excess, as in lymphomas carrying BCL2 rearrangements, BCL2/bax heterodimers are the prevalent species, and cell death is repressed (45).

The pathogenetic contribution of BCL2 lesions to FL development is complex (46). The observation that BCL2-transgenic mice develop a pattern of polyclonal hyperplasia of mature, long-lived B cells resting in G0 suggests that BCL2 activation is not sufficient for FL development and that other genetic lesions or host factors are required. Other evidence for this is the observation that complex karyotypic abnormalities are present in 34% of FL grade 1 and 62% of grade 2 cases (32). Chronic antigen stimulation and selection could also synergize with BCL2 in driving FL expansion (47). With time, and analogous to the human disease, a fraction of BCL2-transgenic mice develops aggressive, clonal, large cell lymphomas that have additional genetic lesions, specifically c-myc translocations (48,49). However, these BCL2-transgenic mice do not develop a disease analogous to indolent FL.

Further evidence that the BCL2/IgH translocation alone is not causative for FL is provided by reports that B cells with t(14;18) are present in a substantial number of normal individuals (50). In peripheral blood, t(14;18)+ cells have been reported in 8% to 88% of normal subjects using polymerase chain reaction. The variability of these data is likely due to differing sensitivities of the assays used. Similarly, using fluorescent in situ hybridization techniques, B cells with t(14;18) have been detected in hyperplastic lymphoid tissues (tonsil, lymph nodes) in 12% to 54% of normal individuals (51). The frequency is greatest in IgM+ memory cells. Similar to the risk of FL increasing with age, the detection of t(14;18) in the peripheral blood of normal humans appears to increase with age. One study found that these individuals carry this translocation within a population of atypical germinal center-type B cells that have phenotypic features of FL. These results raise the possibility that the presence of this translocation may represent an early premalignant condition (52). In addition, t(14;18)+ cells have been detected by polymerase chain reaction in the peripheral blood of patients with localized FL who are in long-term remission (>10 years) after radiation therapy (53). One interpretation of this finding is that these cells lack the other genetic changes necessary to develop into recurrent lymphoma. The expression of genes in FL has been compared with normal B cells (54,55). These gene expression profiling studies have provided support for the theory that FLs are derived from normal germinal center B cells; however, a number of genes are clearly differentially expressed. Similarly, IgH/BCL6 translocations have also been identified in germinal center B cells from normal individuals (56). These studies may provide insight into the other genetic events that contribute to the pathogenesis and pathophysiology of FL.

Follicular Lymphoma Variants

Pediatric Follicular Lymphoma

FL is rare in children, and has distinctive clinical and pathologic features. It often presents with early stage disease, involving cervical lymph nodes, Waldeyer ring, or other extranodal sites such as the testis (57–59). Morphologically, they are characterized by large, expansile follicles, with numerous centroblasts (grade 3A). They often express CD43, and lack BCL2 protein expression and t(14;18). Rare cases of florid follicular hyperplasia, particularly in young males, may have clonal populations of CD10$^+$ B cells detected by flow cytometry and molecular analysis; thus, a diagnosis of lymphoma should not be made in the absence of morphologic features of malignancy (60). The prognosis of pediatric FL appears to be good, with the majority of cases disease free at the time of last follow-up. Expression of BCL2 protein may be associated with a higher and worse outcome.

Primary Intestinal Follicular Lymphoma

FL rarely presents in extranodal sites, but one of the most common extranodal presentations is in the gastrointestinal tract, particularly the duodenum (61–64), presenting as multiple small polyps, often as an incidental finding on endoscopy performed for other reasons. The morphology, immunophenotype, and genetic features are similar to those of nodal FLs. Most patients have localized disease (stage IE or IIE), and survival appears to be excellent even without treatment.

CLINICAL PRESENTATION AND STAGING

FL (grades 1 and 2) usually presents in patients with painless peripheral adenopathy in cervical, axillary, inguinal, and femoral regions. Lymph node enlargement has often been present for long periods and is generally slowly progressive. Lymph nodes may wax and wane in size, including complete regressions followed by reappearance. Hilar and mediastinal nodes are often involved, but large mediastinal masses are rare. Some patients present with asymptomatic large abdominal masses with or without evidence of gastrointestinal or urinary tract obstruction. Central nervous system involvement is

exceedingly rare, but peripheral nerve compression and epidural tumor masses causing cord compression may develop.

Although patients may present clinically with one or more sites of nodal disease, staging studies usually demonstrate widely disseminated disease with involvement of the spleen, liver, and bone marrow in 40%, 50%, and 60% to 70% of cases, respectively. Hepatosplenomegaly is diffuse rather than with discrete masses. Very few patients present with extranodal disease besides marrow involvement, and effusions (pleural, pericardial, ascites) are uncommon. Only 10% to 20% of patients present with B symptoms or increased serum concentrations of lactate dehydrogenase (LDH). There are no characteristic laboratory abnormalities specifically associated with FL, although elevation of β2-microglobulin, which is seen in up to 25% of patients, can be a surrogate marker of the extent of disease. In addition to conventional imaging studies with computed tomography scans, positron emission tomography (PET) has been used to evaluate patients with FL. In contrast to aggressive NHLs, there is less evidence that PET scanning is useful in all patients with the disease. Clearly, there is uptake of 18-fluoro-deoxyglucose in FL disease sites (65,66). The revised response criteria for clinical trials in NHL recommend against using PET scans for indolent lymphoma, unless they represent a specific question in a clinical trial (67). There are very limited data on the value of PET scanning after completion of therapy. One study reported two relapses in two patients with FL who had persistently positive PET and two relapses in six patients who had a negative PET scan (68). We do not routinely obtain PET scans in patients with FL, unless they are part of a clinical trial, or unless we suspect histologic transformation, and are using the PET scan to help choose a site with high 18-fluoro-deoxyglucose avidity to subsequently confirm with a biopsy.

FL grade 3 (previously known as *follicular large cell lymphoma*) (12) often presents with larger lymphoid masses and has less frequent bone marrow or peripheral blood involvement than FL grades 1 to 2. The clinical presentation, behavior, and outcome with treatment more closely approximate those of DLBCL, which is considered an aggressive lymphoma (69,70).

Primary cutaneous B-cell lymphomas composed of germinal center cells (centrocytes and centroblasts), with or without a follicular pattern (71), are considered a distinct entity from nodal FL (Chapter 24). Only a minority of cases express BCL2 and have t(14;18) translocations. They tend to occur on the head and trunk, and generally remain localized to the skin. In one study of 122 patients with this disorder, extracutaneous progression was noted in only seven cases (6%), three of which were in the central nervous system (72).

PROGNOSTIC FACTORS

Clinical Prognostic Factors

A large number of pretreatment prognostic factors have been associated with an adverse prognosis in FL. These include age, sex, stage, presence of B symptoms, performance status, serum LDH, serum β2-microglobulin, hemoglobin, bulk disease, and extranodal involvement. Analogous to the International Prognostic Index (IPI) for aggressive lymphomas (73),

TABLE 18.2		
SELECTED PROGNOSTIC AND PREDICTIVE FACTORS FOR FOLLICULAR NHL		
Series	Factors	OS (time)
IPI (74)	Age >60 y, stage III or IV, performance status >2, extranodal sites >2, LDH >normal	Low 73.6% (10 y) Low intermediate 32% (10 y) High intermediate 53.5% (10 y) High 0% (10 y)
FLIPI (75)	Age >60 y, Ann Arbor stage (III-IV), hemoglobin level <120 g per L, no. of nodal areas >4, and serum LDH level above normal	0 or 1 factor 90% (5 y) 2 factors 77% (5 y) ≥3 factors 52% (5 y)

a number of groups have attempted to apply the IPI to patients with FL (Table 18.2). The IPI has been retrospectively applied to patients with FL, and in general the model is predictive for progression-free and overall survival (OS) (74). In one report, the 10-year OSs were 74%, 45%, 54%, and 0% for the four IPI risk groups (low, low-intermediate, high-intermediate, and high-risk). The limitations of the IPI in these patients are that some of the factors are not of prognostic significance and that a low number of patients (between 10% and 20%) are in the higher risk groups (prognostic scores of 3 to 5).

A predictive model based on 4,167 patients with FL diagnosed between 1985 and 1992 has been developed, known as the Follicular Lymphoma IPI (FLIPI) (75). This study identified the following prognostic factors: age >60, stage III/IV, more than four nodal sites, elevated serum LDH concentration, and hemoglobin <12. The 10-year survival rates for patients with zero to one (low risk), two (intermediate risk), or three or more (high risk) of these adverse factors averaged 71%, 51%, and 36%, respectively. Analogous to DLBCL, rituximab therapy has improved outcome for patients with follicular NHL. The FLIPI remains clinically relevant with this improvement in therapy, specifically with the combination of rituximab and cyclophosphamide, doxorubicin, vincristine, and prednisone (CHOP) chemotherapy (76).

Other clinical factors include absolute lymphocyte count (ALC). An ALC >1,000 per μL at the time of diagnosis predicted for a longer OS when compared with those with an initial ALC <1,000 per μL (77) for patients treated before the widespread use of rituximab. This was significant in a multivariable analysis independent of the FLIPI score. More recently, similar associations have been seen for patients treated with rituximab (78–80). In addition to ALC, elevated β2-microglobulin represents a poor prognostic feature in several data sets, and emerged as the most robust prognostic marker in a recent attempt to revise the FLIPI (81).

Histology. The proportion of large cells (centroblasts) has been observed to be an important prognostic factor of clinical behavior and response to therapy (69,70). It is generally agreed that grade 3 FL is an aggressive disease, whereas grade 1 and 2 FL is indolent. The impact of architecture (proportion of the tumor with a follicular pattern) has received attention as a prognostic factor in the literature

(15,82–85). The presence of diffuse areas in FL grades 1 to 2 has been reported in some series as a negative prognostic factor for survival, but in others it has not been found to be significant. In one series from the Eastern Cooperative Oncology Group, patients with a purely follicular pattern, defined as >75% of the cross-sectional area of the tissue examined, had a median survival of 68 months (85). In contrast, patients with a significant diffuse component had a median survival of only 39 months. The impact of a mixed follicular and diffuse architecture was seen in both grades 1 and 2 cases. A similar observation has been reported by Stanford University (84). The presence of sclerosis within the tumor tissue has been associated with a poor prognosis, independent of clinical prognostic factor (86). An analysis of subdividing FL grade 3 (FL3A, FL3B), as suggested by the WHO, and the impact of diffuse architecture has been reported from the University of Nebraska (15). No significant differences were seen in the clinical characteristics or outcome of patients with the different grades of follicular large cell lymphoma. However, patients with a prominent diffuse component (>50%) had a lower OS as compared with patients with a predominantly follicular architecture.

Follicular Lymphoma Microenvironment. Gene expression profiling analysis has been performed of FL tissues. Two major clusters of expressed genes were identified, and referred to as IR-1 and IR-2 (87). The genes in IR-1 had a signature of infiltrating T cells, whereas IR-2 had genes expressed in macrophages and dendritic cells. Patients with an IR-1 signature had a more favorable prognosis than IR-2, suggesting that it is the cells in the neoplastic microenvironment, rather than the FL cells, that predict prognosis. A follow-up study reported that the presence of >15 CD68+ macrophages per hpf was associated with a poor outcome and, in a multivariate analysis, added to the IPI as a predictor of OS in patients with FL (88). Other studies have also related prognosis to presence or absence of normal infiltrating immune cells (89), specifically high levels of CD8+ T cells (90), and high levels of FOXP3+ (Treg) T (91).

Other studies have used gene expression and proteomics to identify factors associated with prognosis. Oligonucleotide arrays have been used to identify expressed genes in FL that are related to prognosis (92). Expression of a number of genes involved in cell cycle regulation, mitosis, or in deoxyribonucleic acid modulation, including CCNB1 (cyclin B1), CDC2, CDKN3A, CKS1B, ANP32E, and KIAA0101, were associated with improved survival (93). In an analysis of proteins involved in apoptotic pathways, high ratios of BCL2/Bak and BCL2/Bax were associated with early death from lymphoma (94).

Clinical Course

The course of FL is quite variable. Some patients have waxing and waning disease for ≥5 years without the need for therapy (95). Others present with more disseminated disease and rapid growth, and require treatment because massive nodal or organ enlargement leads to pain, lymphatic obstruction, or organ obstruction. Historically, the median survival of patients presenting with advanced-stage FL was about 10 years. Over the past decade, several data sets have suggested significant improvements in OS of patients with FL (96,97). Although improved supportive care, refined diagnostic tools, and improved staging may have contributed to the survival improvement, it is likely that most of this improvement is due to routine incorporation of monoclonal antibodies into therapeutic regimens (98).

Histologic transformation of FL from an indolent to a diffuse aggressive lymphoma occurs in 10% to 70% of patients, and is associated with rapid progression of lymphadenopathy, infiltration of extranodal sites, development of systemic symptoms, elevated serum LDH, and often a poor prognosis (99–103). Transformation of FL into diffuse aggressive lymphoma has been investigated with gene expression profiling. One group described two different gene expression profiling signatures in transformed cases that were related to overexpression or underexpression of the c-myc oncogene, supporting the concept of the existence of more than one genetic mechanism for FL transformation (104).

The progression from FL to DLBCL historically occured regardless of whether FL was treated aggressively or conservatively at a rate of approximately 5% to 10% per year, depending on the magnitude of the large cell component (105). A recent series suggested that early anthracycline-based therapy might decrease the risk of transformation over time (106).

At autopsy, up to 95% of patients with FL demonstrate some evidence of DLBCL. Although recent data also suggest improved outcome following histologic transformation, transformation remains a major cause of morbidity and mortality in patients with FL.

TREATMENT

Indications for Treatment

The indolent lymphomas are generally associated with survival measured in years, even if untreated (95,107). However, FL is usually not curable with conventional treatment. Therefore, in contrast to patients with curable aggressive lympho-

mas, in approaching patients with indolent lymphomas, one must consider the indications for treatment. Although the ultimate goal is to cure these diseases, currently the major reason for treatment is to alleviate symptoms. These include local symptoms due to progressive or bulky nodal disease, compromise of normal organ function due to progressive or bulky disease, B symptoms, symptomatic extranodal disease, such as effusions, and cytopenias due to extensive bone marrow infiltration or hypersplenism. Algorithms for management of previously untreated patients and those with relapse are presented in Tables 18.3 and 18.4.

TABLE 18.3

TREATMENT ALGORITHM FOR NEWLY DIAGNOSED FL[a]

Stage I, II
  Locoregional or extended field XRT, or observation in selected cases
Bulky abdominal stage II, stage III, and stage IV
  No indication for therapy[b]
    Observation
  Options if there is indication for therapy
    Local palliative XRT
    Antibody based therapy with or without chemotherapy

XRT, radiation therapy.
[a] Clinical trial participation is always recommended.
[b] Indications for therapy: symptoms, threatened end organ function, cytopenias, massive bulk, rapid progression.

TABLE 18.4

TREATMENT ALGORITHM FOR RELAPSED FOLLICULAR NHL[a]

No indication for treatment
  Observation
Options if there is indication for treatment at first relapse
  Monoclonal antibody based therapy
  Chemotherapy with monoclonal antibody based therapy
Options if there is indication for treatment at second or greater relapse
  Monoclonal antibody based therapy
  Chemotherapy with monoclonal antibody based therapy
  Radioimmunotherapy
  High-dose therapy and autologous or allogeneic SCT
Histologic transformation
  Few prior therapies; localized
    Anthracycline-based combination chemotherapy with rituximab, followed by observation, radiation, radioimmunotherapy, or consideration of high-dose therapy and ASCT
  Options if there is widespread disease and multiple prior therapies
    Anthracycline-based combination chemotherapy with rituximab
    Radioimmunotherapy
    ASCT for responding disease

[a] Clinical trial participation is always recommended.

Therapy for Early Stage Disease

Only 15% to 30% of patients have clinical stage I or II disease, and <10% has pathologic stage I or II disease (108). For this reason, limited studies are available concerning the treatment of early stage indolent lymphoma.

Radiation therapy is the mainstay of treatment for limited-stage follicular grade 1 or 2 lymphoma. Some of the ongoing issues in the treatment of these patients are: (a) What percentage of patients with early stage follicular grade 1 or 2 lymphoma are cured with radiation therapy alone?; (b) What is the frequency of late recurrences (>10 years after diagnosis and complete remission [CR])?; (c) What are the prognostic factors for recurrence?; (d) What are the extent and dose of radiation therapy needed?; (e) What is the role of chemotherapy in early stage low-grade lymphoma?; (f) What is the prognosis in patients who develop recurrent disease?; and (g) What are potential areas for new investigation?

Many published studies have demonstrated the efficacy of radiation therapy in the treatment of clinically staged patients with localized follicular grade 1 to 3 lymphoma. Table 18.5 summarizes data from nine published reports each containing ≥50 patients (109–116). All but one study contains patients with both stage I and stage II disease (in approximately equal frequencies). The 10-year freedom from treatment failure in all nine studies ranged from 41% to 49%. The 10-year OS (all causes) ranged from 43% to 79%, with a median survival of 11.9 to 15.3 years. Nearly all patients were treated with radiation therapy alone, except in the Fondation Bergonie study, in which 70% of patients received some form of systemic treatment (113). The freedom from treatment failure and OS in this combined modality study were no better than in the primary radiation-alone studies. The majority of patients had FL grades 1 and 2; however, FL grade 3 and low-grade diffuse small-cell histologies were included in some of the series. The percentages are noted in Table 18.5 for each study.

Evidence that follicular grade 1 or 2 lymphoma is curable with radiation therapy alone is supported by the nearly 50% freedom from treatment failure (or progression-free, disease-free, or relapse-free survival) results at 10 years in all studies, and by the low rates of recurrence after 10 years in patients who have remained continuously disease free since initial diagnosis and treatment (98,110,111,116). In the Stanford series, for example, only five of 47 patients in continuous remission for ≥10 years have had relapse at longer intervals (111). However, a small series of patients at Stanford who presented with early stage FL and were observed without radiation suggest a similar disease-free interval, with long follow-up, as observed with patients treated with radiation therapy (117). It is clear that there may be a subset of patients with indolent disease who may have very long survivals with no therapy.

Adverse prognostic factors for freedom from treatment failure (or progression-free, disease-free, or relapse-free survival depending on the report) are analyzed by multivariate analysis in many of the studies. Age was the adverse factor most often reported and was seen in five of the nine studies (Table 18.5). Follicular grade 3 histology, extensive clinical stage IIA disease, bulky disease (>2 cm or >3 cm), and extranodal presentations also were reported, but these adverse factors were seen in only one or two of the nine

studies. There appears to be very little difference in outcome between follicular grades 1 and 2 disease. Also, age was the most common significant adverse factor for OS. Because the median age of patients was approximately 60 years in these studies, it is not surprising that age is a significant factor for survival in most of the analyses. Except for FL grade 3, which is treated similarly to DLBCL, and extensive clinical stage II presentations that may be treated similarly to advanced-stage disease, none of the other factors is sufficiently adverse to alter the standard recommendation for curative local radiation therapy as the initial treatment approach for the majority of patients with early stage FL.

One recent study reported on 106 patients with stage I–II, grade 1 to 2 FL treated with radiation therapy (118). With a median follow-up of 12 years, the freedom from treatment failure at 10 years was 46%, and the 10-year survival was 75%. The median survival was 19 years. Despite the long median survival and the median age at diagnosis of 55 years, the leading cause of death remained lymphoma.

The dose and field size of radiation therapy varied greatly within and between studies, and there are no randomized trials to evaluate these parameters. The majority of studies do not report significant differences in the freedom from treatment failure (or progression-free, disease-free, or relapse-free survival) between local/regional and extensive/total nodal fields. In the Stanford series (111), the data reporting the association of larger irradiated field sizes with an increased freedom from recurrence are confounded by the common use of staging laparotomy in the large-field group of patients. Thus, their improved results may be due to the exclusion of patients with stage III and IV disease discovered on surgical staging but not appreciated with clinical staging. In addition, none of the studies that have reported improved freedom from treatment failure results with more aggressive treatment has demonstrated an improvement in survival. Of interest, in the Stanford study, late second tumors were noted in 6.8% of patients who received involved- or extended-field radiation and in 17% of those treated with extensive radiotherapy. In terms of dose, none of the studies shows convincing evidence for improved local control above the 30 to 36 Gy.

We recommend the use of regional radiation therapy fields for patients with clinical stage I or II FL grade 1 or 2. This consists of irradiating the involved nodal region plus one additional uninvolved region on each side of the involved nodes. The recommended dose is 30 to 36 Gy with a boost to areas of initial involvement up to 36 Gy. This approach provides a 40% to 50% probability of cure. Carefully planned local radiation-therapy fields with modest doses can significantly reduce the risk of significant damage to the marrow reserve, the risk of developing a treatment-related malignancy, and the risk of long-term toxicity to the salivary glands, lungs, heart, kidneys, and bowel when in close proximity to the lymphoma. This less toxic approach (compared with larger-field irradiation) preserves the ability to effectively treat patients in whom the same histology later recurs or who have transformation to a higher grade histology. For more than half of all patients, disease will recur at some point in their life, and increasingly, there will be new and more effective approaches for these patients. To maximize cure but reserve the option for effective treatment for relapse, the radiation and medical oncologists must work together to devise an optimum treatment approach.

TABLE 18.5

RADIATION THERAPY FOR EARLY STAGE LOW-GRADE FOLLICULAR NHL (SELECTED TRIALS CONTAINING ≥50 PATIENTS)

Report	No. of patients/ median follow-up time/CT	Stage (%)	10-y FFTF/OS (%)	Median RT dose to the tumor	RT field size (%)	Grade distribution (%)	Adverse prognostic factors (FFTF)
Princess Margaret Hospital (109)	573/10.6 y/27%	I (64) II (36)	48/>60	35 Gy	IF	FG1 (33) FG2 (32) FG3 (35)	Ext CS II >2 cm disease
British National Lymphoma Investigation (110)	208/NA/0%	I (100)	47/64	35 Gy (suggested)	NA	FG1 (39) FG2 (35) FG3 (5) Other (21)	Age ≥50 y
Stanford University (111)	177/7.7 y/5%	I (41) II (59)	44/64	35–50 Gy	IF/RF/EF (77) TLI (23)	FG1 (57) FG2/3 (43)	Age >60 y Extranodal site RT fields < TLI
Foundation Bergonie (112)	103/8.3 y/70%	I (44) II (56)	49/56	35–40 Gy	IF (54) RF (46)	NA	Age >60 y
M. D. Anderson Cancer Center (113)	80/19 y/0%	I (41) II (59)	41/43 at 15 y	40 Gy	IF (9) RF (54)	FG1 (63) FG2 (37)	CS IIA >3 cm disease
Edinburgh (114)	64/5 y/2%	I (58) II (42)	49/78	30–40 Gy (82%) >40 Gy (18%)	EF (37) NA	FG1 (78) FG2 (3) Other (19)	NA
University of Florida (194)	72/8.5 y/7%	I (75) II (25)	46/59	NA	IF (53) EF (43) TNI/WA (4)	NA	NA
NCI (115)	54/9 y/10%	I (50) II (50)	48/69	36 Gy	IF (38) EF (48) TLI/TBI (14)	NA	Age ≥45 y
Royal Marsden Hospital (116)	58/NA/0%	I (69) II (31)	43/79	40 Gy	IF (52) EF (48)	FG1 (64) FG2 (21) Other (15)	Field size not significant for recurrence

CT, chemotherapy; DFS, disease-free survival; EF, extended field radiation (mantle or whole abdominal, inverted Y [Wilder]; mantle, whole abdominal, inverted Y [Pendlebury, McManus]; mantle, inverted Y [Lawrence]); FFTF, freedom from treatment failure; FG, follicular grade; NA, not reported; NCI, National Cancer Institute; Prog, prognostic; RF, regional field radiation (1–3 adjacent nodal regions [Wilder]); RFS, recurrence/relapse -free survival; RT, radiation therapy; TBI, total body irradiation; TLI, total lymphoid irradiation; TNI, total nodal irradiation.

The role of combination chemotherapy in the management of early stage FL is unclear. At least three randomized studies conducted in the 1970s failed to demonstrate that a non–doxorubicin-containing combination chemotherapy regimen plus radiation therapy was superior to radiation therapy alone (119–121). A more recent British National Lymphoma Investigation study randomized 148 patients to receive either radiation therapy alone or radiation therapy plus chlorambucil (122). There were no differences in freedom from recurrence or survival between the groups. A single-arm study of 91 patients with stage I or II disease treated at the M. D. Anderson Cancer Center with cyclophosphamide, vincristine, and prednisone (CVP) or [CHOP and bleomycin chemotherapy in addition to radiation therapy demonstrated an improved freedom from recurrence compared with historical controls but no OS differences (123,124). We do not advocate combined modality therapy for early stage FL, with the exception of localized grade III histology, where it is reasonable to consider approaching the disease as early stage aggressive lymphoma.

There are few data on the outcome of patients who develop recurrent disease after radiation therapy for initial stage I or II presentations. In the Stanford study, most relapses were detected by physical examination (66%), with 76% of patients having stage I or II disease at relapse. Actuarial survival rates 5, 10, 15, and 20 years after relapse were 56%, 35%, 17%, and 17%, respectively (125). The progression-free survival (PFS) rate for the entire group at 5 years was 44%, and remained at 22% 10, 15, and 20 years after relapse. Therefore, approximately one fifth of patients with early stage FL have prolonged survival even after relapse from primary radiation therapy.

In summary, patients with early stage follicular grade 1 or 2 lymphoma have a median survival of nearly 15 years. Local-regional radiation results in cure of approximately 40% of patients. There is a decreasing freedom from recurrence with age and extranodal involvement. There are no treatment outcome differences between patients with grades 1 and 2 disease. There are a number of areas for ongoing investigation. Finally, the roles for adjuvant chemotherapy and immunotherapy need to be better defined.

Therapy of Advanced-Stage Disease

The long natural history of indolent lymphomas and the general lack of symptoms at diagnosis have fostered close observation as the initial approach for some patients. Because up to 23% of patients have spontaneous remissions lasting longer than 1 year, it is recommended that a period of observation is warranted for asymptomatic patients with low-volume disease (95,126,127). The randomized study from the National Cancer Institute in patients with advanced-stage disease provides support for this. In that study, which compared no initial therapy with immediate combined modality treatment with prednisone, methotrexate with leucovorin rescue, Adriamycin, Cytoxan (cyclophosphamide), and etoposide-Mustargen (mechlorethamine), Oncovin (vincristine), procarbazine, and prednisone followed by total lymphoid irradiation, there was no survival advantage to upfront therapy (105).

Withholding therapy in this situation requires an informed and cooperative patient and close follow-up. In a study from Stanford, patients were randomized to either receive therapy

immediately or to defer treatment until the time of progressive symptomatic disease (128). In the latter group, the median time until therapy was administered was 3 years. However, for the three histologic subtypes, the median time to the need for therapy varied significantly, being 16 and 48 months for FL grade 2 (follicular mixed) and FL grade 1 (follicular small cleaved), respectively. Despite this, there was no difference in the 4-year actuarial survival between the two treatment groups.

Recently, the concept of observation rather than active treatment for patients with newly diagnosed FL has again been under scrutiny. Because systemic therapy has become more effective, and evidence that OS can be improved by incorporating rituximab into therapeutic regimens, it has been suggested that early intervention may benefit patients, particularly with high FLIPI scores, or other risk factors. Moreover, the recent suggestion that early anthracycline-based therapy might abrogate risk of transformation has encouraged some physicians to utilize this therapy early in the course of the disease. In addition, nontoxic therapies, such as single-agent rituximab, have lowered the threshold to initiate treatment for even frail, elderly patients. A recent evaluation of the National LymphoCare Study, a large prospective registry of patients with FL in the United States, suggests that observation is still commonly practiced but with a lower threshold to proceed to systemic treatment (129). We still advocate for this approach for carefully selected patients.

Palliative Radiation Therapy

Localized radiation therapy can be very effective palliative treatment for patients with advanced-stage lymphomas. Indications for palliation include: (a) treatment of a resistant localized mass in the setting of other chemotherapy responsive disease to limit the need for additional cytotoxic treatment; (b) prevention or relief of neurologic signs from spinal cord involvement or nerve root compression; (c) relief of a superior vena cava syndrome or obstructive pneumonia; (d) reduction of the risk of fracture in involved weight-bearing bones; (e) relief of venous obstruction from large pelvic adenopathy; (f) alleviation of symptoms of localized involvement in areas such as the orbit or stomach; and (g) cosmetic reasons. The use of radiation therapy in these settings often focuses just on a single area, allowing the use of small fields with a low risk of acute and late effects from treatment. In addition, lower doses (20 to 30 Gy) can be used than otherwise required for curative treatment.

Several studies have advocated using very low doses for palliation, with good results (130–132). Using 4 Gy of involved field radiation therapy, the overall response rate was 92%; and the CR rate was 61% in the study by Haas et al.(130). For the patients with CRs, the median time to progression was 25 (requiring any additional treatment), and the median time to local progression was 42 months. A recent study evaluated the mechanism of this treatment by evaluating the gene expression profile of patients' biopsies taken before and after radiation. In all patients, a major and consistent induction of p53 target genes was seen. Other induced genes revealed genes related to macrophage activation and TH1 immune response (133). This treatment approach, although quite effective, should not be used when a rapid response is needed, such as when there is neurologic compromise or obstructive symptoms.

Systemic Therapy

The initial treatment of choice for patients with indolent NHL who are not eligible for clinical trials has historically included either alkylating-based regimens (single agent or combinations such as CVP), or purine analogs such as fludarabine. Although more aggressive regimens such as CHOP have been used in the initial treatment of FL, there is no evidence that a superior response rate or duration of remission is seen as compared with CVP (134). Other randomized trials have looked at the impact of combination chemotherapy in patients with advanced FL. CHOP with bleomycin was compared with cyclophosphamide alone in patients with FL. There was no difference in disease-free survival or OS for the entire population or the patients with grade 1 FL, but there was a survival advantage for the patients with FL grade 2 (135). Fludarabine-based regimens are highly effective but not superior to CVP in terms of remission duration or OS (136).

The treatment paradigm for treating advanced-stage FL has changed with the use of the anti-CD20 monoclonal antibody rituximab (Table 18.6). Phase III randomized trials have demonstrated a significant improvement in outcome by combining chemotherapy regimens with the anti-CD20 monoclonal antibody rituximab. This has been the major innovation in treating these diseases in the past 3 decades. In an international study of 321 patients randomized to CVP or rituximab plus CVP (CVP-R), the overall (81% vs. 57%) and complete (41% vs. 10%) response rates were higher in the CVP-R treatment arm (137). At a median follow-up of 30 months, the median times to progression (32 vs. 15 months) and treatment failure (27 vs. 7 months) were significantly longer in the CVP-R arm. In long-term follow-up (median 53 months), a survival benefit was observed at 4 years in the CVP-R arm (OS 83% vs. 77%; $p = 0.029$) (138).

Similar findings were observed by the German Low Grade Lymphoma Group, where rituximab was combined with CHOP (CHOP-R) chemotherapy and compared with CHOP alone with improvement in both remission duration and OS (139). Another study using mitoxantrone, chlorambucil, and prednisolone with or without rituximab, saw similar improvement

in response rate, PFS, and a statistically significant improvement in OS (140).

Maintenance rituximab has been demonstrated to improve PFS compared with observation after chemotherapy alone with CVP (141). The efficacy of rituximab maintenance in patients with advanced-stage FL following initial induction with chemotherapy plus rituximab is uncertain at present. The PRIMA (Primary rituximab and maintenance study) study randomized patients to rituximab maintenance or observation following rituximab-containing induction chemotherapy. The trial has enrolled >1,000 patients, and is expected to be reported this year. Given the long PFS reported with rituximab-containing chemotherapy induction, it is anticipated that the benefit of rituximab maintenance will be less after induction therapy, as compared with the relapsed setting. Until the PRIMA (Primary rituximab and maintenance study) trial results have been reported, we do not recommend maintenance rituximab for the majority of patients treated initially with induction chemotherapy combined with rituximab.

Advanced-stage FL grade 3 is generally treated like DLBCL (15,69,70). With combination chemotherapy regimens, the complete-remission rates range from 50% to 75%. The 5- and 10-year failure-free survival rates were 34% and 67%, and the OS rates were 61% and 72%, respectively. The IPI was useful in stratifying these patients, although 71% had either low or low-intermediate prognostic scores (70). The degree of follicularity has been examined by several groups and remains controversial. In a report from the University of Nebraska, the presence of a mixed follicular and diffuse architecture was significantly associated with survival; 3-year survival rates were 47% for patients with purely follicular architecture, and 0% for patients with follicular and diffuse architecture (69). A recent report from Vancouver suggests that there is no significant difference in clinical behavior between FL grades 3A and 3B, and that there does not appear to be a plateau on the PFS curve for either histology (142).

Phase II trials have employed rituximab as initial therapy in patients with indolent lymphoma with overall response rates of 54% and 73% (143–146). At a median follow-up of 30 months, median PFS was 34 months in one of the trials. Moreover, extended rituximab has increased PFS compared with observation (146). The optimal schedule of extended rituximab in this situation remains uncertain. Hainsworth et al.

TABLE 18.6

SELECTED RANDOMIZED THERAPEUTIC STUDIES COMPARING CHEMOTHERAPY WITH CHEMOTHERAPY AND RITUXIMAB FOR FOLLICULAR NHL

Author	Time of prescription	Therapy	Result
Marcus et al. (138)	Induction	CVP vs. CVP-R TTP 34 vs. 15 mo in favor of CVP-R	TTP and OS improved with CVP-R
Hiddemann et al. (139)	Induction	CHOP vs. R-CHOP	Improved TTF and OS with R-CHOP
Herold et al. (140)	Induction	MCP vs R-MCP PFS NR vs. 28 mo in favor of R-MCP	4-y OS 87% vs. 74% in favor of R-MCP
Forstpointer et al. (195)	Relapse	FCM vs. R-FCM PFS 16 vs. 10 mo in favor of R-FCM	OS NR vs. 24 mo median in favor of R-FCM
van Oers et al. (162)	Relapse	R-CHOP vs. CHOP PFS 33 vs. 20 mo in favor of R-CHOP	OS 3 y 83% vs. 72% in favor of R-CHOP

FCM, fludarabine, cyclophosphamide, and mitoxantrone; MCP, mitoxantrone, chlorambucil, and prednisolone; NR, not reached; R-MCP, rituximab, mitoxantrone, chlorambucil, and prednisolone; TTF, time to treatment failure; TTP, time to progression; All results are statistically significant.

(147) performed a randomized phase II study comparing rituximab administered weekly by four every 6 months for 2 years versus rituximab at time of disease progression. The PFS was longer in the scheduled rituximab maintenance arm, however, the primary end point of the study, time of rituximab benefit, was equivalent (147). Prolonged rituximab appears safe in these studies, and is currently under evaluation by the Eastern Cooperative Oncology Group group in the Rituximab Extended Schedule or Re- Treatment trial, which again randomizes patients to scheduled rituximab versus rituximab at the time of progression. Rituximab, therefore, remains a reasonable therapeutic option as initial therapy of low bulk disease.

Radioimmunotherapy has been studied in a limited fashion in previously untreated patients with FL. The overall response rate and CR rate of (147) I tositumomab were 95% and 75%, respectively, and a 5-year PFS of 59% in treatment naive patients (148). Although myelodysplasia has been associated with radioimmunotherapy when used in the relapsed setting, there were no cases of myelodysplasia observed with single-agent iodine-131 tositumomab. The Southwest Oncology Group (SWOG) has performed a pilot trial of iodine-131 tositumomab following standard CHOP chemotherapy. The overall response rate was 91%, including a 69% CR rate. After a median follow-up time of >5 years, the estimated 5-year OS rate was 87%, and the PFS rate was 67%, the best results reported by the SWOG to date for FL (149). Based upon these results, a randomized trial comparing CHOP-R with CHOP followed by iodine-131 tositumomab has been completed by the SWOG. More evidence to the benefit of radioimmunotherapy consolidation after initial chemotherapy comes from the FIT (First-Line Indolent Trial) trial (203), which randomized patients to ibritumomab tiuxetan consolidation versus observation after a variety of chemotherapy induction regimens. A significant benefit in the radioimmunotherapy arm was observed. Most patients in this trial were not treated with rituximab, limiting the applicability to the current practice in the United States.

Autologous Stem Cell Transplantation in First Remission

The absence of a definite plateau in disease-free survival after autologous stem cell transplantation (ASCT) for low-grade lymphoma has led to attempts at transplantation in first remission. At the Dana-Farber Cancer Institute, the actuarial 3-year disease-free survival and OS rates were 63% and 89%, respectively, after autologous bone marrow transplant in first CR or with minimal disease after CHOP chemotherapy (150). Horning et al. (151) at Stanford have reported results for patients transplanted in first complete or partial remission. With a median follow-up of 6.5 years, the estimated OS rates at 5 and 10 years were 92% and 86%, respectively. The estimated 10-year disease-specific survival was 97%, with an OS of 86%. Other reports of ASCT in first remission for low-grade lymphoma have shown a continuous pattern of treatment failure without evidence of cure (152,153). Analogous to studies in patients transplanted after conventional therapy relapse, remission duration is longer after ASCT than after conventional therapy. Whether first remission transplant is superior to transplant for relapsed

disease remains unclear. The OS from diagnosis for patients transplanted in first remission is similar to that seen in patients transplanted in second or greater remission (154). All of these published trials with long-term follow-up enrolled patients who were not treated with rituximab.

There have been three randomized trials comparing conventional therapy to ASCT in first remission. Two of these studies have reported an increased event-free survival (155,156), and one reported no difference (157). In all studies, there was no difference in the OS between conventional induction versus conventional induction followed by ASCT in first remission. These studies have observed higher toxicity in the ASCT arm, and two of three studies reported a higher incidence of second malignancies in the transplant arm, specifically secondary hematologic malignancies, which is the major causative factor in there being no survival advantage to ASCT (156,158).

Treatment of Recurrent Disease

Following relapse, indolent lymphomas continue to be sensitive to single agents and combination chemotherapy, but the median relapse-free survival progressively decreases with each subsequent relapse. A randomized trial compared fludarabine with CVP in previously treated patients with FL. Although the response rates (62% vs. 52%) and 2-year OS (70% vs. 75%) were similar, 2-year PFS was significantly improved with fludarabine (32% vs. 14%) (159). Single-agent rituximab has a 50% to 60% response rate, with 6% CR, in patients with previously treated FL (160). In small lymphocytic lymphoma, the response rate is only about 10%. The median duration of responses is about 11 months. A phase II trial studied the safety and efficacy of retreatment with rituximab in patients with relapsed indolent NHL, all of whom had previously responded to rituximab (161). The overall response rate was 40%, with 11% CRs, and the estimated median time to progression after treatment was 18 months. Rituximab has been combined with other agents (e.g., fludarabine, CVP, CHOP), with encouraging results in patients with relapsed/resistant disease. An international randomized phase III study evaluated the role of rituximab in remission induction as well as maintenance in patients with relapsed FL who had not previously received an anthracycline or rituximab (162). Patients received six cycles of CHOP or CHOP-R. Those patients who acheived complete or partial remission underwent a second randomization to maintenance rituximab (375 mg per m^2 inravenously once every 3 months) for a maximum of 2 years or observation. The overall (85% vs. 72%) and complete (30% vs. 16%) remission rates were significantly higher for CHOP-R than CHOP. The median PFS from first randomization was significantly longer after CHOP-R than after CHOP (33 vs. 20 months). The median PFS from the time of second randomization was longer for those receiving rituximab maintenance (52 vs. 15 months), both after induction with CHOP or CHOP-R. Moreover, maintenance rituximab, as compared with observation, also significantly improved 3-year OS (85% vs. 77%). Because patients with relapsed FL who have not had prior treatment with rituximab are becoming uncommon, it is unclear whether data from this study can be extrapolated to patients with relapsed FL receiving CHOP-R as their initial induction therapy. As previously mentioned, the PRIMA (Primary rituximab and maintenance study) study will definitively answer this question.

TABLE 18.7

COMPARISON OF RADIOIMMUNOCONJUGATES USED IN THE TREATMENT OF FOLLICULAR NHL

	Ibritumomab tiuxetan (Yttrium-90)	Tositumomab (Iodine-131)
Half-life	64 h	192 h
Energy emitter	β (2.30 MeV)	γ (0.36 MeV), β (0.60 MeV)
Path length	χ_{90} 5 mm	χ_{90} 0.8 mm
Nontumor distribution	Bone	Thyroid
Dosing	Based on weight and platelet count	Tracer dose and dosimetry used to customize dose
Administration	Outpatient	Inpatient or restrictions to protect family/environment

Bendamustine is an alkylating agent with unique mechanisms of action (163). Recent trials have suggested high remission rates for patients with relapsed FL when bendamustine is combined with rituximab (164). A phase II trial of single-agent bendamustine enrolled patients with rituximab-refractory disease, and demonstrated a response rate of 76%, including CRs (165). This trial is the only trial of a chemotherapy agent limited to the rituximab-refractory setting. Further studies of chemotherapy combinations, including bendamustine, are underway.

Radioimmunoconjugates are Food and Drug Administration-approved therapies for patients with relapsed follicular NHL. 131-I tositumomab is a murine anti-CD20 monoclonal antibody conjugated to 131-iodine (Table 18.7). The overall response rate in previously treated patients was 65% with 20% CRs (166). The median duration of remission had not been reached by 47 months. A murine anti-CD20 antibody, ibritumomab, conjugated to 90-yttrium has an 82% response rate with 26% CR, and median duration of response of >12 months in patients with relapsed disease (167). In a phase III study of 143 patients with relapsed or refractory low-grade, follicular, or transformed CD20+ NHL, patients were randomized to receive either rituximab or rituximab plus 90-yitrium ibritumomab tiuxetan (168). The overall response rates to rituximab or the rituximab 90-yitrium ibritumomab tiuxetan combination were 56% and 80%, respectively. Long-term follow-up of patients treated with both ibritumomab tiuxetan and iodone-131 tositumomab suggests that a subset of patients have very long response durations, lasting many years (167,169).

Autologous Stem Cell Transplantation for Relapsed Indolent Non-Hodgkin Lymphoma

Long-term follow-up of phase II studies suggests that a subset of patients with relapsed FL, with chemosensitive disease, who undergo high-dose therapy and ASCT, are long-term survivors with a disease-free survival of 48% at 12 years (170) (Table 18.8). A randomized trial compared conventional chemotherapy with ASCT with purged or unpurged bone marrow, referred to as the European CUP (Chemotherapy, unpurged high dose therapy or purged high dose therapy) trial (171). In this study, 89 patients with relapsed or progressive FL received three cycles of CHOP. Those patients who had a CR or PR, and had <20% bone marrow involvement with FL, were randomized to three further cycles of CHOP chemotherapy, or to high-dose therapy and autologous stem cell support with anti-B-cell antibody purging or high-dose therapy and autologous stem cell support without purging. At a median follow-up of 69 months, the overall 5-year survival for all registered patients was 50%, but the median survival had not yet been reached for the subset of patients treated with high-dose therapy and ASCT (either purged or unpurged). Both progression-free and OS favored the transplantation arms, but there was no difference between those patients receiving a purged autograft and those receiving an unmanipulated graft. Importantly, patients in this trial were not treated with rituximab, and it is not clear whether initial therapy with rituximab would impact upon these results.

Several other studies with long-term follow-up suggest meaningful benefit when ASCT is utilized for relapsed FL NHL. For example, in a combined series from the Dana-Farber Cancer Institute and St. Bartholomew's Hospital, 121

TABLE 18.8

STEM CELL TRANSPLANTATION (SCT) IN RELAPSED FOLLICULAR NHL

Study	No. of patients	Stem cell source	Patients with CR at SCT (%)	Patients with BM at SCT (%)	Disease-free survival (%)	OS (%)
Freedman et al., 1999 (196)	153	auto BM	30	47	42 (8 y)	66 (8 y)
Apostolidis et al., 2000 (197)	99	auto BM	38	13	63 (5.5 y)	69 (5.5 y)
Bierman et al., 1997 (198)	100	auto BM/PBSC	9	—	48 (2 y)	65 (4 y)
Bastion et al., 1995 (199)	60	auto BM/PBSC	17	65	53 (2 y)	86 (2 y)
van Besien et al., 1998 (200)	113	allo BM	40	—	49 (3 y)	49 (3 y)
Juckett et al., 1998 (201)	16	allo T-depleted BM	—	—	62 (5 y)	—
Khouri et al., 2001 (202)	20	allo PBSC	60	5	84 (2 y)	84 (2 y)

allo, allogeneic; auto, autologous; BM, bone marrow; PBSC, peripheral blood stem cell.

adults received cyclophosphamide and total body irradiation conditioning supported by antibody purged autologous bone marrow transplantation. Fifty-seven patients are alive, 41 without progression between 9 and 19 years. There was an apparent plateau on the remission duration curve at 48% at 12 years. Myelodysplasia and secondary acute leukemia were major morbidities of this procedure (170). Preliminary reports of other ASCT series conducted in the prerituximab era also suggest a plateau on the PFS curve (172).

Allogeneic Stem Cell Transplantation in Relapsed Follicular Lymphoma

In 176 patients with FL, 67% of whom had chemosensitive disease at the time of transplantation, estimates of treatment-related mortality, recurrence rates, and OS at 5 years following allogeneic bone marrow transplantation were 30%, 21%, and 51%, respectively. During this same period, 597 patients with FL received unpurged autologous transplantation; 82% were chemosensitive at the time of transplant. The estimates of treatment-related mortality, recurrence rates, and OS at 5 years following unpurged autologous bone marrow transplantation were 8%, 58%, and 55%, respectively (173). To have lower treatment-related mortality and to exploit the graft versus lymphoma effect of allogeneic transplantation, nonmyeloablative allogeneic transplants have been studied actively in indolent NHLs, with encouraging results to date.

Long-term follow-up of selected series of patients treated with allogeneic transplantation has recently been published. These series suggest prolonged cures in a majority of patients who survive the initial toxicity of the transplant procedure. For example, 47 patients at M. D. Anderson Cancer Center were treated with a conditioning regimen of fludarabine (30 mg per m^2 daily for 3 days), cyclophosphamide (750 mg per m^2 daily for 3 days), and rituximab (375 mg per m^2 for 1 day plus 1,000 mg per m^2 for 3 days) (174). All patients experienced CR, with only two relapses. With a median follow-up time of 60 months (range 19–94), the estimated survival and PFS rates were 85% and 83%, respectively. The Blood and Marrow Transplant-Clinical Trials Network group in collaboration with the SWOG has initiated a national trial to confirm these very promising results. Results from Seattle are similarly promising; in a series of patients treated with low-dose total body irradiation and fludarabine conditioning, the estimated OS and PFS rates were 52% and 43%, respectively, for patients with indolent lymphoma (175). Finally, a series of patients treated at Dana-Farber Cancer Institute, with busulfan and fludarabine conditioning, demonstrated a 3-year OS of 81%, and 3-year PFS of 59% (176). Thus, the results of this procedure in experienced centers appear very favorable. Clearly, this is only applicable for a minority of patients with reasonable disease control, and no significant comorbid medical problems.

HISTOLOGIC TRANSFORMATION

The prognosis for patients following histologic transformation of indolent NHL is generally poor (177). The median survival of a large series of patients with follicular NHL undergoing histologic conversion was 11 months (102). In a report from Stanford, the median survival for the entire group of patients was only 22 months, except for patients

who had a CR with treatment who had an actuarial survival of 75% at 5 years (99). There have been several reports of ASCT in patients with chemosensitive disease and a good performance status after histologic transformation for FL. In the series from Dana-Farber Cancer Institute, where 21 patients have undergone anti-B-cell purged autologous bone marrow transplantation for transformed FL, the estimate of the percentage of patients alive and disease free at 5 years is 46%, with follow-up from 12 to 120+ months (178). When pathology at relapse was available, all patients had recurrence with DLBCL. Similar results were reported from St. Bartholomew's Hospital, Stanford University, and the European Bone Marrow Transplant Registry (179–182). Aggressive therapy with ASCT is a reasonable treatment option for selected patients who have chemosensitive disease. In the rituximab era, the outcome of histologic transformation may be improving (183). The Vancouver group has demonstrated that the addition of rituximab to anthracycline-based chemotherapy has dramatically improved the outcome of histologic transformation (184).

UNIQUE COMPLICATIONS

The major unique complication of FL is histologic transformation. It is well recognized that an integral part of the natural history of indolent lymphoma is progression to a higher grade histologic subtype, such as DLBCL (95,105). However, the implications of histologic conversion for prognosis are controversial because there are many associated variables, such as prior disease stage and treatment and length of survival before transformation, as well as the response of the transformed disease to more aggressive therapy. Armitage et al. (103) compared the response of patients who had histologic conversion with DLBCL with a similarly treated group of patients who developed DLBCL de novo. They found no instances of prolonged CR in the former group, along with a significantly shorter median survival of 12 versus 40 months, respectively. The median survival of a large series of patients with FL undergoing histologic conversion was 11 months (102). An update from Stanford suggests that patients who were never treated had a better prognosis, as did patients with limited disease (99). Although the median survival for the entire group was only 22 months, patients who had a CR after histologic transformation had an actuarial survival of 75% at 5 years.

In a series from St. Bartholomew's Hospital, with a median follow-up of 15 years, biopsy proven transformation occurred in 88 of 325 patients with FL. The risk of transformation in this series was higher in patients with advanced-stage, high-risk FLIPI, and expectant management (as opposed to treatment being initiated at diagnosis). The median survival from transformation was 1.2 years. There appeared to be a subgroup of patients in whom histologic transformation does not occur with very prolonged follow-up (106).

PROGNOSIS

Historically, the median survival from diagnosis for patients with FL was approximately 9 years; as previously mentioned, this appears to be significantly improving in the rituximab era. The median survival after relapse is 4.5 years (102). Weisdorf et al. (185) reported that for patients <60 years, the median survival after relapse was 5.9 years if the first CR was >1.0 year, 4.2 years for patients whose first partial remission was >1.0 year, and 2.4 years for patients whose initial remission was <1.0 year. The survival rates for patients who attained a second complete or partial remission were 53% and 28% at 10 years, respectively. The median survival for patients after histologic transformation ranged from 11 (102) to 22 (99) months. If patients attained a CR with combination therapy, the median survival was 81 months after transformation (102).

NEW TREATMENT APPROACHES

Significant improvements have been made in the treatment of FL, with the major impact due to monoclonal antibody therapy, however, the majority of patients are not cured. There are a vast number of new agents that are undergoing evaluation, many of which go under the auspices of rational targets. These include new monoclonal antibodies focused on antigens besides CD20, and improved antibodies targeting CD20 with enhanced cytotoxicity. Several small molecules developed to antagonize BCL2, kinases, or pathways involved in cell survival, are also in clinical trials. Further ways to enhance host immunity against the patients' own tumor cells have involved vaccination studies with the Ig idiotype to induce specific immunotherapy against residual tumor cells, although recent results of randomized trials suggest that vaccination with idiotype vaccine does not appear to change PFS (186). Other drugs with demonstrated activity in FL include the proteasome inhibitor bortezomib and the immunomodulatory agent lenalidomide (187–189). Finally, several novel antibodies are under development targeting CD20 (190), CD80 (191,192), and CD22 (193), which have demonstrated significant clinical activity in patients with FL.

References

1. *WHO classification of tumours of haematopoietic and lymphoid systems*, 4th ed. Lyon, France: IARC, 2008.
2. Glass AG, Karnell LH, Menck HR. The National Cancer Data Base report on non-Hodgkin's lymphoma. *Cancer* 1997;80:2311–2320.
3. A clinical evaluation of the International Lymphoma Study Group classification of non-Hodgkin's lymphoma. The Non-Hodgkin's Lymphoma Classification Project. *Blood* 1997;89:3909–3918.
4. Groves FD, Linet MS, Travis LB, et al. Cancer surveillance series: non-Hodgkin's lymphoma incidence by histologic subtype in the United States from 1978 through 1995. *J Natl Cancer Inst* 2000;92:1240–1251.
5. Herrinton LJ, Goldoft M, Schwartz SM, et al. The incidence of non-Hodgkin's lymphoma and its histologic subtypes in Asian migrants to the United States and their descendants. *Cancer Causes Control* 1996;7:224–230.
6. Armitage JO, Weisenburger DD. New approach to classifying non-Hodgkin's lymphomas: clinical features of the major histologic subtypes. Non-Hodgkin's Lymphoma Classification Project. *J Clin Oncol* 1998;16:2780–2795.
7. Herrinton LJ, Friedman GD. Cigarette smoking and risk of non-Hodgkin's lymphoma subtypes. *Cancer Epidemiol Biomarkers Prev* 1998;7:25–28.
8. Biagi JJ, Seymour JF. Insights into the molecular pathogenesis of follicular lymphoma arising from analysis of geographic variation. *Blood* 2002;99:4265–4275.
9. Morton LM, Wang SS, Devesa SS, et al. Lymphoma incidence patterns by WHO subtype in the United States, 1992-2001. *Blood* 2006;107:265–276.
10. Lorsbach RB, Shay-Seymore D, Moore J, et al. Clinicopathologic analysis of follicular lymphoma occurring in children. *Blood* 2002;99:1959–1964.
11. Nathwani BN, Anderson JR, Armitage JO, et al. Clinical significance of follicular lymphoma with monocytoid B cells. Non-Hodgkin's Lymphoma Classification Project. *Hum Pathol* 1999;30:263–268.
12. Harris NL, Jaffe ES, Diebold J, et al. World Health Organization classification of neoplastic diseases of the hematopoietic and lymphoid tissues: report of the Clinical Advisory Committee meeting-Airlie House, Virginia, November 1997. *J Clin Oncol* 1999;17:3835–3849.
13. Bosga-Bouwer AG, van Imhoff GW, Boonstra R, et al. Follicular lymphoma grade 3B includes 3 cytogenetically defined subgroups with primary t(14;18), 3q27, or other translocations: t(14;18) and 3q27 are mutually exclusive. *Blood* 2003;101:1149–1154.
14. Bosga-Bouwer AG, van den Berg A, Haralambieva E, et al. Molecular, cytogenetic, and immunophenotypic characterization of follicular lymphoma grade 3B; a separate entity or part of the spectrum of diffuse large B-cell lymphoma or follicular lymphoma? *Hum Pathol* 200637:528–533.
15. Hans CP, Weisenburger DD, Vose JM, et al. A significant diffuse component predicts for inferior survival in grade 3 follicular lymphoma, but cytologic subtypes do not predict survival. *Blood* 2003;101:2363–2367.
16. Ott G, Katzenberger T, Lohr A, et al. Cytomorphologic, immunohistochemical, and cytogenetic profiles of follicular lymphoma: 2 types of follicular lymphoma grade 3. *Blood* 2002;99:3806–3812.
17. Katzenberger T, Ott G, Klein T, et al. Cytogenetic alterations affecting BCL6 are predominantly found in follicular lymphomas grade 3B with a diffuse large B-cell component. *Am J Pathol* 2004;165:481–490.
18. Stein H, Gerdes J, Mason DY. The normal and malignant germinal centre. *Clin Haematol* 1982;11:531–559.
19. Cong P, Raffeld M, Teruya-Feldstein J, et al. In situ localization of follicular lymphoma: description and analysis by laser capture microdissection. *Blood* 2002;99:3376–3382.
20. Lee JT, Innes DJ Jr, Williams ME. Sequential bcl-2 and c-myc oncogene rearrangements associated with the clinical transformation of non-Hodgkin's lymphoma. *J Clin Invest* 1989;84:1454–1459.
21. Yano T, Jaffe ES, Longo DL, et al. MYC rearrangements in histologically progressed follicular lymphomas. *Blood* 1992;80:758–767.
22. Feldman AL, Arber DA, Pittaluga S, et al. Clonally related follicular lymphomas and histiocytic/dendritic cell sarcomas: evidence for transdifferentiation of the follicular lymphoma clone. *Blood* 2008;111:5433–5439.
23. Flenghi L, Bigerna B, Fizzotti M, et al. Monoclonal antibodies PG-B6a and PG-B6p recognize, respectively, a highly conserved and a formol-resistant epitope on the human BCL-6 protein amino-terminal region. *Am J Pathol* 1996;148:1543–1555.
24. Pittaluga S, Ayoubi TA, Wlodarska I, et al. BCL-6 expression in reactive lymphoid tissue and in B-cell non-Hodgkin's lymphomas. *J Pathol* 1996;179:145–150.
25. Karube K, Guo Y, Suzumiya J, et al. CD10-MUM1+ follicular lymphoma lacks BCL2 gene translocation and shows characteristic biologic and clinical features. *Blood* 2007;109:3076–3079.
26. Cleary ML, Meeker TC, Levy S, et al. Clustering of extensive somatic mutations in the variable region of an immunoglobulin heavy chain gene from a human B cell lymphoma. *Cell* 1986;44:97–106.
27. Bahler DW, Campbell MJ, Hart S, et al. Ig VH gene expression among human follicular lymphomas. *Blood* 1991;78:1561–1568.
28. Bloomfield CD, Arthur DC, Frizzera G, et al. Nonrandom chromosome abnormalities in lymphoma. *Cancer Res* 1983;43:2975–2984.
29. Rowley JD. Chromosome studies in the non-Hodgkin's lymphomas: the role of the 14;18 translocation. *J Clin Oncol* 1988;6:919–925.
30. Cleary ML, Smith SD, Sklar J. Cloning and structural analysis of cDNAs for bcl-2 and a hybrid bcl-2/immunoglobulin transcript resulting from the t(14;18) translocation. *Cell* 1986;47:19–28.
31. Cleary ML, Galili N, Sklar J. Detection of a second t(14;18) breakpoint cluster region in human follicular lymphomas. *J Exp Med* 1986;164:315–320.
32. Viardot A, Moller P, Hogel J, et al. Clinicopathologic correlations of genomic gains and losses in follicular lymphoma. *J Clin Oncol* 2002;20:4523–4530.
33. Skinnider BF, Horsman DE, Dupuis B, et al. Bcl-6 and Bcl-2 protein expression in diffuse large B-cell lymphoma and follicular lymphoma: correlation with 3q27 and 18q21 chromosomal abnormalities. *Hum Pathol* 1999;30:803–808.
34. Lo Coco F, Gaidano G, Louie DC, et al. p53 mutations are associated with histologic transformation of follicular lymphoma. *Blood* 1993;82:2289–2295.
35. Matolcsy A, Casali P, Warnke RA, et al. Morphologic transformation of follicular lymphoma is associated with somatic mutation of the translocated Bcl-2 gene. *Blood* 1996;88:3937–3944.
36. Tilly H, Rossi A, Stamatoullas A, et al. Prognostic value of chromosomal abnormalities in follicular lymphoma. *Blood* 1994;84:1043–1049.
37. Elenitoba-Johnson KS, Gascoyne RD, Lim MS, et al. Homozygous deletions at chromosome 9p21 involving p16 and p15 are associated with histologic progression in follicle center lymphoma. *Blood* 1998;91:4677–4685.
38. Graninger WB, Seto M, Boutain B, et al. Expression of Bcl-2 and Bcl-2-Ig fusion transcripts in normal and neoplastic cells. *J Clin Invest* 1987;80:1512–1515.

39. Ngan BY, Chen-Levy Z, Weiss LM, et al. Expression in non-Hodgkin's lymphoma of the bcl-2 protein associated with the t(14;18) chromosomal translocation. *N Engl J Med* 1988;318:1638–1644.

40. Korsmeyer SJ. Bcl-2 initiates a new category of oncogenes: regulators of cell death. *Blood* 1992;80:879–886.

41. Nunez G, Hockenbery D, McDonnell TJ, et al. Bcl-2 maintains B cell memory. *Nature* 1991;353:71–73.

42. Boise LH, Gonzalez-Garcia M, Postema CE, et al. bcl-x, a bcl-2-related gene that functions as a dominant regulator of apoptotic cell death. *Cell* 1993;74:597–608.

43. Oltvai ZN, Milliman CL, Korsmeyer SJ. Bcl-2 heterodimerizes in vivo with a conserved homolog, Bax, that accelerates programmed cell death. *Cell* 1993;74:609–619.

44. Yin XM, Oltvai ZN, Korsmeyer SJ. BH1 and BH2 domains of Bcl-2 are required for inhibition of apoptosis and heterodimerization with Bax. *Nature* 1994;369:321–323.

45. Cory S, Adams JM. Killing cancer cells by flipping the Bcl-2/Bax switch. *Cancer Cell* 2005;8:5–6.

46. Staudt LM. A closer look at follicular lymphoma. *N Engl J Med* 2007;356:741–742.

47. Zelenetz AD, Chen TT, Levy R. Clonal expansion in follicular lymphoma occurs subsequent to antigenic selection. *J Exp Med* 1992;176:1137–1148.

48. McDonnell TJ, Deane N, Platt FM, et al. bcl-2-immunoglobulin transgenic mice demonstrate extended B cell survival and follicular lymphoproliferation. *Cell* 1989;57:79–88.

49. McDonnell TJ, Korsmeyer SJ. Progression from lymphoid hyperplasia to high-grade malignant lymphoma in mice transgenic for the t(14; 18). *Nature* 1991;349:254–256.

50. Hirt C, Dolken G, Janz S, et al. Distribution of t(14;18)-positive, putative lymphoma precursor cells among B-cell subsets in healthy individuals. *Br J Haematol* 2007;138:349–353.

51. Aster JC, Kobayashi Y, Shiota M, et al. Detection of the t(14;18) at similar frequencies in hyperplastic lymphoid tissues from American and Japanese patients. *Am J Pathol* 1992;141:291–299.

52. Roulland S, Navarro JM, Grenot P, et al. Follicular lymphoma-like B cells in healthy individuals: a novel intermediate step in early lymphomagenesis. *J Exp Med* 2006;203:2425–2431.

53. Price CG, Meerabux J, Murtagh S, et al. The significance of circulating cells carrying t(14;18) in long remission from follicular lymphoma. *J Clin Oncol* 1991;9:1527–1532.

54. Alizadeh AA, Eisen MB, Davis RE, et al. Distinct types of diffuse large B-cell lymphoma identified by gene expression profiling. *Nature* 2000;403:503–511.

55. Husson H, Carideo EG, Neuberg D, et al. Gene expression profiling of follicular lymphoma and normal germinal center B cells using cDNA arrays. *Blood* 2002;99:282–289.

56. Yang X, Lee K, Said J, et al. Association of Ig/BCL6 translocations with germinal center B lymphocytes in human lymphoid tissues: implications for malignant transformation. *Blood* 2006;108:2006–2012.

57. Finn LS, Viswanatha DS, Belasco JB, et al. Primary follicular lymphoma of the testis in childhood. *Cancer* 1999;85:1626–1635.

58. Pinto A, Hutchison RE, Grant LH, et al. Follicular lymphomas in pediatric patients. *Mod Pathol* 1990;3:308–313.

59. Swerdlow SH. Pediatric follicular lymphomas, marginal zone lymphomas, and marginal zone hyperplasia. *Am J Clin Pathol* 2004;122(suppl):S98–S109.

60. Kussick SJ, Kalnoski M, Braziel RM, et al. Prominent clonal B-cell populations identified by flow cytometry in histologically reactive lymphoid proliferations. *Am J Clin Pathol* 2004;121:464–472.

61. Misdraji J, Fernandez del Castillo C, Ferry JA. Follicle center lymphoma of the ampulla of Vater presenting with jaundice: report of a case. *Am J Surg Pathol* 1997;21:484–488.

62. Sato Y, Ichimura K, Tanaka T, et al. Duodenal follicular lymphomas share common characteristics with mucosa-associated lymphoid tissue lymphomas. *J Clin Pathol* 2008;61:377–381.

63. Shia J, Teruya-Feldstein J, Pan D, et al. Primary follicular lymphoma of the gastrointestinal tract: a clinical and pathologic study of 26 cases. *Am J Surg Pathol* 2002;26:216–224.

64. Yoshino T, Miyake K, Ichimura K, et al. Increased incidence of follicular lymphoma in the duodenum. *Am J Surg Pathol* 2000;24:688–693.

65. Wohrer S, Jaeger U, Kletter K, et al. 18F-fluoro-deoxy-glucose positron emission tomography (18F-FDG-PET) visualizes follicular lymphoma irrespective of grading. *Ann Oncol* 2006;17:780–784.

66. Elstrom R, Guan L, Baker G, et al. Utility of FDG-PET scanning in lymphoma by WHO classification. *Blood* 2003;101:3875–3876.

67. Cheson BD, Pfistner B, Juweid ME, et al. Revised response criteria for malignant lymphoma. *J Clin Oncol* 2007;25:579–586.

68. Spaepen K, Stroobants S, Dupont P, et al. Prognostic value of positron emission tomography (PET) with fluorine-18 fluorodeoxyglucose ([18F]FDG) after first-line chemotherapy in non-Hodgkin's lymphoma: is [18F]FDG-PET a valid alternative to conventional diagnostic methods? *J Clin Oncol* 2001;19:414–419.

69. Anderson JR, Vose JM, Bierman PJ, et al. Clinical features and prognosis of follicular large-cell lymphoma: a report from the Nebraska Lymphoma Study Group. *J Clin Oncol* 1993;11:218–224.

70. Rodriguez J, McLaughlin P, Hagemeister FB, et al. Follicular large cell lymphoma: an aggressive lymphoma that often presents with favorable prognostic features. *Blood* 1999;93:2202–2207.

71. Willemze R, Jaffe ES, Burg G, et al. WHO-EORTC classification for cutaneous lymphomas. *Blood* 2005;105:3768–3785.

72. Bekkenk MW, Postma TJ, Meijer CJ, et al. Frequency of central nervous system involvement in primary cutaneous B-cell lymphoma. *Cancer* 2000;89:913–919.

73. A predictive model for aggressive non-Hodgkin's lymphoma. The International Non-Hodgkin's Lymphoma Prognostic Factors Project. *N Engl J Med* 1993;329:987–994.

74. Lopez-Guillermo A, Montserrat E, Bosch F, et al. Applicability of the International Index for aggressive lymphomas to patients with low-grade lymphoma. *J Clin Oncol* 1994;12:1343–1348.

75. Solal-Celigny P, Roy P, Colombat P, et al. Follicular lymphoma international prognostic index. *Blood* 2004;104:1258–1265.

76. Buske C, Hoster E, Dreyling M, et al. The Follicular Lymphoma International Prognostic Index (FLIPI) separates high-risk from intermediate- or low-risk patients with advanced-stage follicular lymphoma treated frontline with rituximab and the combination of cyclophosphamide, doxorubicin, vincristine, and prednisone (R-CHOP) with respect to treatment outcome. *Blood* 2006;108:1504–1508.

77. Siddiqui M, Ristow K, Markovic SN, et al. Absolute lymphocyte count predicts overall survival in follicular lymphomas. *Br J Haematol* 2006;134:596–601.

78. Ghielmini M, Rufibach K, Salles G, et al. Single agent rituximab in patients with follicular or mantle cell lymphoma: clinical and biological factors that are predictive of response and event-free survival as well as the effect of rituximab on the immune system: a study of the Swiss Group for Clinical Cancer Research (SAKK). *Ann Oncol* 2005;16:1675–1682.

79. Behl D, Ristow K, Markovic SN, et al. Absolute lymphocyte count predicts therapeutic efficacy of rituximab therapy in follicular lymphomas. *Br J Haematol* 2007;137:409–415.

80. Porrata LF, Ristow K, Witzig TE, et al. Absolute lymphocyte count predicts therapeutic efficacy and survival at the time of radioimmunotherapy in patients with relapsed follicular lymphomas. *Leukemia* 2007;21:2554–2556.

81. Federico M, Guglielmi C, Luminari S, et al. Prognostic relevance of serum beta2 microglobulin in patients with follicular lymphoma treated with anthracycline-containing regimens. A GISL study. *Haematologica* 20;92:1482–1488.

82. Warnke RA, Kim H, Fuks Z, et al. The coexistence of nodular and diffuse patterns in nodular non-Hodgkin's lymphomas: significance and clinicopathologic correlation. *Cancer* 1977;40:1229–1233.

83. Colby TV, Hoppe RT, Burke JS. Nodular lymphoma: clinicopathologic correlations of parafollicular small lymphocytes and degree of nodularity. *Cancer* 1980;45:2364–2367.

84. Hu E, Weiss LM, Hoppe RT, et al. Follicular and diffuse mixed small-cleaved and large-cell lymphoma—a clinicopathologic study. *J Clin Oncol* 1985;3:1183–1187.

85. Ezdinli EZ, Costello WG, Kucuk O, et al. Effect of the degree of nodularity on the survival of patients with nodular lymphoma. *J Clin Oncol* 1987;5:413–418.

86. Klapper W, Hoster E, Rolver L, et al. Tumor sclerosis but not cell proliferation or malignancy grade is a prognostic marker in advanced-stage follicular lymphoma: the German Low Grade Lymphoma Study Group. *J Clin Oncol* 2007;25:3330–3336.

87. Dave SS, Wright G, Tan B, et al. Prediction of survival in follicular lymphoma based on molecular features of tumor-infiltrating immune cells. *N Engl J Med* 2004;351:2159–2169.

88. Farinha P, Masoudi H, Skinnider BF, et al. Analysis of multiple biomarkers shows that lymphoma-associated macrophage (LAM) content is an independent predictor of survival in follicular lymphoma (FL). *Blood* 2005;106:2169–2174.

89. Alvaro T, Lejeune M, Salvado MT, et al. Immunohistochemical patterns of reactive microenvironment are associated with clinicobiologic behavior in follicular lymphoma patients. *J Clin Oncol* 2006;24:5350–5357.

90. Wahlin BE, Sander B, Christensson B, et al. CD8+ T-cell content in diagnostic lymph nodes measured by flow cytometry is a predictor of survival in follicular lymphoma. *Clin Cancer Res* 2007;13:388–397.

91. Carreras J, Lopez-Guillermo A, Fox BC, et al. High numbers of tumor-infiltrating FOXP3-positive regulatory T cells are associated with improved overall survival in follicular lymphoma. *Blood* 2006;108:2957–2964.

92. Glas AM, Kersten MJ, Delahaye LJ, et al. Gene expression profiling in follicular lymphoma to assess clinical aggressiveness and to guide the choice of treatment. *Blood* 2005;105:301–307.

93. Bjorck E, Ek S, Landgren O, et al. High expression of cyclin B1 predicts a favorable outcome in patients with follicular lymphoma. *Blood* 2005;105:2908–2915.

94. Gulmann C, Espina V, Petricoin E 3rd, et al. Proteomic analysis of apoptotic pathways reveals prognostic factors in follicular lymphoma. *Clin Cancer Res* 2005;11:5847–5855.

95. Horning SJ, Rosenberg SA. The natural history of initially untreated low-grade non-Hodgkin's lymphomas. *N Engl J Med* 1984;311:1471–1475.

96. Swenson WT, Wooldridge JE, Lynch CF, et al. Improved survival of follicular lymphoma patients in the United States. *J Clin Oncol* 2005;23:5019–5026.

97. Fisher RI, LeBlanc M, Press OW, et al. New treatment options have changed the survival of patients with follicular lymphoma. *J Clin Oncol* 2005;23:8447–8452.

98. Horning SJ. Follicular lymphoma, survival, and rituximab: is it time to declare victory? *J Clin Oncol* 2008;26:4537–4538.

99. Yuen AR, Kamel OW, Halpern J, et al. Long-term survival after histologic transformation of low-grade follicular lymphoma. *J Clin Oncol* 1995;13:1726–1733.

100. Bastion Y, Sebban C, Berger F, et al. Incidence, predictive factors, and outcome of lymphoma transformation in follicular lymphoma patients. *J Clin Oncol* 1997;15:1587–1594.

101. Gallagher CJ, Gregory WM, Jones AE, et al. Follicular lymphoma: prognostic factors for response and survival. *J Clin Oncol* 1986;4:1470–1480.

102. Johnson PW, Rohatiner AZ, Whelan JS, et al. Patterns of survival in patients with recurrent follicular lymphoma: a 20-year study from a single center. *J Clin Oncol* 1995;13:140–147.

103. Armitage JO, Dick FR, Corder MP. Diffuse histiocytic lymphoma after histologic conversion: a poor prognostic variant. *Cancer Treat Rep* 1981;65:413–418.

104. Lossos IS, Alizadeh AA, Diehn M, et al. Transformation of follicular lymphoma to diffuse large-cell lymphoma: alternative patterns with increased or decreased expression of c-myc and its regulated genes. *Proc Natl Acad Sci U S A* 2002;99:8886–8891.

105. Longo DL. What's the deal with follicular lymphomas? *J Clin Oncol* 1993;11:202–208.

106. Montoto S, Davies AJ, Matthews J, et al. Risk and clinical implications of transformation of follicular lymphoma to diffuse large B-cell lymphoma. *J Clin Oncol* 2007;25:2426–2433.

107. Portlock CS, Rosenberg SA. No initial therapy for stage III and IV non-Hodgkin's lymphomas of favorable histologic types. *Ann Intern Med* 1979;90:10–13.

108. Anderson T, Chabner BA, Young RC, et al. Malignant lymphoma. 1. The histology and staging of 473 patients at the National Cancer Institute. *Cancer* 1982;50:2699–2707.

109. Tsang RW, Gospodarowicz MK. Radiation therapy for localized low-grade non-Hodgkin's lymphomas. *Hematol Oncol* 2005;23:10–17.

110. Vaughan Hudson B, Vaughan Hudson G, MacLennan KA, et al. Clinical stage 1 non-Hodgkin's lymphoma: long-term follow-up of patients treated by the British National Lymphoma Investigation with radiotherapy alone as initial therapy. *Br J Cancer* 1994;69:1088–1093.

111. Mac Manus MP, Hoppe RT. Is radiotherapy curative for stage I and II low-grade follicular lymphoma? Results of a long-term follow-up study of patients treated at Stanford University. *J Clin Oncol* 1996;14:1282–1290.

112. Soubeyran P, Eghbali H, Bonichon F, et al. Localized follicular lymphomas: prognosis and survival of stages I and II in a retrospective series of 103 patients. *Radiother Oncol* 1988;13:91–98.

113. Wilder RB, Jones D, Tucker SL, et al. Long-term results with radiotherapy for Stage I-II follicular lymphomas. *Int J Radiat Oncol Biol Phys* 2001;51:1219–1227.

114. Taylor RE, Allan SG, McIntyre MA, et al. Low grade stage I and II non-Hodgkin's lymphoma: results of treatment and relapse pattern following therapy. *Clin Radiol* 1988;39:287–290.

115. Lawrence TS, Urba WJ, Steinberg SM, et al. Retrospective analysis of stage I and II indolent lymphomas at the National Cancer Institute. *Int J Radiat Oncol Biol Phys* 1988;14:417–424.

116. Pendlebury S, el Awadi M, Ashley S, et al. Radiotherapy results in early stage low grade nodal non-Hodgkin's lymphoma. *Radiother Oncol* 1995;36:167–171.

117. Advani R, Rosenberg SA, Horning SJ. Stage I and II follicular non-Hodgkin's lymphoma: long-term follow-up of no initial therapy. *J Clin Oncol* 2004;22:1454–1459.

118. Guadagnolo BA, Li S, Neuberg D, et al. Long-term outcome and mortality trends in early-stage, Grade 1-2 follicular lymphoma treated with radiation therapy. *Int J Radiat Oncol Biol Phys* 2006;64:928–934.

119. Monfardini S, Banfi A, Bonadonna G, et al. Improved five year survival after combined radiotherapy-chemotherapy for stage I-II non-Hodgkin's lymphoma. *Int J Radiat Oncol Biol Phys* 1980;6:125–134.

120. Landberg TG, Hakansson LG, Moller TR, et al. CVP-remission-maintenance in stage I or II non-Hodgkin's lymphomas: preliminary results of a randomized study. *Cancer* 1979;44:831–838.

121. Toonkel LM, Fuller LM, Gamble JF, et al. Laparotomy staged I and II non-Hodgkin's lymphomas: preliminary results of radiotherapy and adjunctive chemotherapy. *Cancer* 1980;45:249–260.

122. Kelsey SM, Newland AC, Hudson GV, et al. A British National Lymphoma Investigation randomised trial of single agent chlorambucil plus radiotherapy versus radiotherapy alone in low grade, localised non-Hodgkins lymphoma. *Med Oncol* 1994;11:19–25.

123. McLaughlin P, Fuller L, Redman J, et al. Stage I-II low-grade lymphomas: a prospective trial of combination chemotherapy and radiotherapy. *Ann Oncol* 1991;2(suppl 2):137–140.

124. Seymour JF, McLaughlin P, Fuller LM, et al. High rate of prolonged remissions following combined modality therapy for patients with localized low-grade lymphoma. *Ann Oncol* 1996;7:157–163.

125. Mac Manus MP, Rainer Bowie CA, Hoppe RT. What is the prognosis for patients who relapse after primary radiation therapy for early-stage low-grade follicular lymphoma? *Int J Radiat Oncol Biol Phys* 1998; 42:365–371.

126. Gattiker HH, Wiltshaw E, Galton DA. Spontaneous regression in non-Hodgkin's lymphoma. *Cancer* 1980;45:2627–2632.

127. Krikorian JG, Portlock CS, Cooney P, et al. Spontaneous regression of non-Hodgkin's lymphoma: a report of nine cases. *Cancer* 1980;46:2093–2099.

128. Hoppe RT, Kushlan P, Kaplan HS, et al. The treatment of advanced stage favorable histology non-Hodgkin's lymphoma: a preliminary report of a randomized trial comparing single agent chemotherapy, combination chemotherapy, and whole body irradiation. *Blood* 1981;58:592–598.

129. Friedberg W, Taylor MD, Cerhan JR, et al. Follicular lymphoma in the United States: first report of the national LymphoCare study. *J Clin Oncol* 2009;27:1202–1208.

130. Haas RL, Girinsky T. HOVON 47/EORTC 20013: chlorambucil vs 2x2 Gy involved field radiotherapy in stage III/IV previously untreated follicular lymphoma patients. *Ann Hematol* 2003;82:458–462.

131. Haas RL, Poortmans P, de Jong D, et al. High response rates and lasting remissions after low-dose involved field radiotherapy in indolent lymphomas. *J Clin Oncol* 2003;21:2474–2480.

132. Luthy SK, Ng AK, Silver B, et al. Response to low-dose involved-field radiotherapy in patients with non-Hodgin's lymphoma. *Ann Oncol* 2008;19:2043–2047.

133. Knoops L, Haas R, de Kemp S, et al. In vivo p53 response and immune reaction underlie highly effective low-dose radiotherapy in follicular lymphoma. *Blood* 2007;110:1116–1122.

134. Jones SE, Grozea PN, Metz EN, et al. Improved complete remission rates and survival for patients with large cell lymphoma treated with chemoimmunotherapy. A Southwest Oncology Group Study. *Cancer* 1983;51:1083–1090.

135. Peterson BA, Petroni GR, Frizzera G, et al. Prolonged single-agent versus combination chemotherapy in indolent follicular lymphomas: a study of the cancer and leukemia group B. *J Clin Oncol* 2003;21:5–15.

136. Hagenbeek A, Eghbali H, Monfardini S, et al. Fludarabine compared with CVP chemotherapy in newly diagnosed patients with stages III and IV low grade malignant non-Hodgkin's lymphoma. Final analysis of a prospective randomized phase III intergroup trial of 381 patients. *Blood* 2001;98:843a.

137. Marcus R, Imrie K, Belch A, et al. CVP chemotherapy plus rituximab compared with CVP as first-line treatment for advanced follicular lymphoma. *Blood* 2005;105:1417–1423.

138. Marcus R, Imrie K, Solal-Celigny P, et al. Phase III study of R-CVP compared with cyclophosphamide, vincristine, and prednisone alone in patients with previously untreated advanced follicular lymphoma. *J Clin Oncol* 2008;26:4579–4586.

139. Hiddemann W, Kneba M, Dreyling M, et al. Frontline therapy with rituximab added to the combination of cyclophosphamide, doxorubicin, vincristine, and prednisone (CHOP) significantly improves the outcome for patients with advanced-stage follicular lymphoma compared with therapy with CHOP alone: results of a prospective randomized study of the German Low-Grade Lymphoma Study Group. *Blood* 2005;106: 3725–3732.

140. Herold M, Haas A, Srock S, et al. Rituximab added to first-line mitoxantrone, chlorambucil, and prednisolone chemotherapy followed by interferon maintenance prolongs survival in patients with advanced follicular lymphoma: an East German Study Group Hematology and Oncology Study. *J Clin Oncol* 2007;25:1986–1992.

141. Hochster H, Weller E, Gascoyne RD, et al. Maintenance rituximab after CVP results in superior clinical outcome in advanced follicular lymphoma. Results of the El496 phase III trial. *Blood* 2005;106:349a.

142. Shustik J, Quinn M, Connors JM, et al. Follicular non-Hodgin lymphoma grade #A and 3B subtypes have similar outcome and appear incurable with anthracycline-based therapy. *Ann Oncol* 2008;19:180.

143. Hainsworth JD, Litchy S, Barton JH, et al. Single-agent rituximab as first-line and maintenance treatment for patients with chronic lymphocytic leukemia or small lymphocytic lymphoma: a phase II trial of the Minnie Pearl Cancer Research Network. *J Clin Oncol* 2003;21:1746–1751.

144. Colombat P, Salles G, Brousse N, et al. Rituximab (anti-CD20 monoclonal antibody) as single first-line therapy for patients with follicular lymphoma with a low tumor burden: clinical and molecular evaluation. *Blood* 2001;97:101–106.

145. Witzig TE, Vukov AM, Habermann TM, et al. Rituximab therapy for patients with newly diagnosed, advanced-stage, follicular grade I non-Hodgkin's lymphoma: a phase II trial in the North Central Cancer Treatment Group. *J Clin Oncol* 2005;23:1103–1108.

146. Ghielmini M, Schmitz SF, Cogliatti SB, et al. Prolonged treatment with rituximab in patients with follicular lymphoma significantly increases event-free survival and response duration compared with the standard weekly x 4 schedule. *Blood* 2004;103:4416–4423.

147. Hainsworth JD, Litchy S, Shaffer DW, et al. Maximizing therapeutic benefit of rituximab: maintenance therapy versus re-treatment at progression in patients with indolent non-Hodgkin's lymphoma—a randomized

phase II trial of the Minnie Pearl Cancer Research Network. *J Clin Oncol* 2005;23:1088–1095.

148. Kaminski MS, Tuck M, Estes J, et al. 131I-tositumomab therapy as initial treatment for follicular lymphoma. *N Engl J Med* 352:441–449.

149. Press OW, Unger JM, Braziel RM, et al. Phase II trial of CHOP chemotherapy followed by tositumomab/iodine I-131 tositumomab for previously untreated follicular non-Hodgkin's lymphoma: five-year follow-up of Southwest Oncology Group Protocol S9911. *J Clin Oncol* 2006;24:4143–4149.

150. Brown JR, Feng Y, Gribben JG, et al. Long-term survival after autologous bone marrow transplantation for follicular lymphoma in first remission. *Biol Blood Marrow Transplant* 2007;13:1057–1065.

151. Horning SJ, Negrin RS, Hoppe RT, et al. High-dose therapy and autologous bone marrow transplantation for follicular lymphoma in first complete or partial remission: results of a phase II clinical trial. *Blood* 2001;97:404–409.

152. Morel P, Laporte JP, Noel MP, et al. Autologous bone marrow transplantation as consolidation therapy may prolong remission in newly diagnosed high-risk follicular lymphoma: a pilot study of 34 cases. *Leukemia* 1995;9:576–582.

153. Haas R, Moos M, Mohle R, et al. High-dose therapy with peripheral blood progenitor cell transplantation in low-grade non-Hodgkin's lymphoma. *Bone Marrow Transplant* 1996;17:149–155.

154. Seyfarth B, Kuse R, Sonnen R, et al. Autologous stem cell transplantation for follicular lymphoma: no benefit for early transplant? *Ann Hematol* 2001;80:398–405.

155. Lenz G, Dreyling M, Schiegnitz E, et al. Myeloablative radiochemotherapy followed by autologous stem cell transplantation in first remission prolongs progression-free survival in follicular lymphoma: results of a prospective, randomized trial of the German Low-Grade Lymphoma Study Group. *Blood* 2004;104:2667–2674.

156. Deconinck E, Foussard C, Milpied N, et al. High-dose therapy followed by autologous purged stem-cell transplantation and doxorubicin-based chemotherapy in patients with advanced follicular lymphoma: a randomized multicenter study by GOELAMS. *Blood* 2005;105:3817–3823.

157. Sebban C, Mounier N, Brousse N, et al. Standard chemotherapy with interferon compared with CHOP followed by high-dose therapy with autologous stem cell transplantation in untreated patients with advanced follicular lymphoma: the GELF-94 randomized study from the Groupe d'Etude des Lymphomes de l'Adulte (GELA). *Blood* 2006;108:2540–2544.

158. Lenz G, Dreyling M, Schiegnitz E, et al. Moderate increase of secondary hematologic malignancies after myeloablative radiochemotherapy and autologous stem-cell transplantation in patients with indolent lymphoma: results of a prospective randomized trial of the German Low Grade Lymphoma Study Group. *J Clin Oncol* 2004;22:4926–4933.

159. Klasa RJ, Meyer RM, Shustik C, et al. Randomized phase III study of fludarabine phosphate versus cyclophosphamide, vincristine, and prednisone in patients with recurrent low-grade non-Hodgkin's lymphoma previously treated with an alkylating agent or alkylator-containing regimen. *J Clin Oncol* 2002;20:4649–4654.

160. McLaughlin P, Grillo-Lopez AJ, Link BK, et al. Rituximab chimeric anti-CD20 monoclonal antibody therapy for relapsed indolent lymphoma: half of patients respond to a four-dose treatment program. *J Clin Oncol* 1998;16:2825–2833.

161. Davis TA, Grillo-Lopez AJ, White CA, et al. Rituximab anti-CD20 monoclonal antibody therapy in non-Hodgkin's lymphoma: safety and efficacy of re-treatment. *J Clin Oncol* 2000;18:3135–3143.

162. van Oers MH, Klasa R, Marcus RE, et al. Rituximab maintenance improves clinical outcome of relapsed/resistant follicular non-Hodgkin lymphoma in patients both with and without rituximab during induction: results of a prospective randomized phase 3 intergroup trial. *Blood* 2006;108:3295–3301.

163. Leoni LM, Bailey B, Reifert J, et al. Bendamustine (Treanda) displays a distinct pattern of cytotoxicity and unique mechanistic features compared with other alkylating agents. *Clin Cancer Res* 2008;14:309–317.

164. Rummel MJ, Al-Batran SE, Kim SZ, et al. Bendamustine plus rituximab is effective and has a favorable toxicity profile in the treatment of mantle cell and low-grade non-Hodgkin's lymphoma. *J Clin Oncol* 2005;23:3383–3389.

165. Friedberg JW, Cohen P, Chen L, et al. Bendamustine in patients with rituximab-refractory indolent and transformed non-Hodgkin's lymphoma: results from a phase II multicenter, single-agent study. *J Clin Oncol* 2008;26:204–210.

166. Kaminski MS, Estes J, Zasadny KR, et al. Radioimmunotherapy with iodine (131)I tositumomab for relapsed or refractory B-cell non-Hodgkin lymphoma: updated results and long-term follow-up of the University of Michigan experience. *Blood* 2000;96:1259–1266.

167. Gordon LI, Molina A, Witzig T, et al. Durable responses after ibritumomab tiuxetan radioimmunotherapy for CD20+ B-cell lymphoma: long-term follow-up of a phase 1/2 study. *Blood* 2004;103:4429–4431.

168. Witzig TE, Gordon LI, Cabanillas F, et al. Randomized controlled trial of yttrium-90-labeled ibritumomab tiuxetan radioimmunotherapy versus rituximab immunotherapy for patients with relapsed or refractory low-grade, follicular, or transformed B-cell non-Hodgkin's lymphoma. *J Clin Oncol* 2002;20:2453–2463.

169. Fisher RI, Kaminski MS, Wahl RL, et al. Tositumomab and iodine-131 tositumomab produces durable complete remissions in a subset of heavily pretreated patients with low-grade and transformed non-Hodgkin's lymphomas. *J Clin Oncol* 2005;23:7565–7573.

170. Rohatiner AZ, Nadler L, Davies AJ, et al.: Myeloablative therapy with autologous bone marrow transplantation for follicular lymphoma at the time of second or subsequent remission: long-term follow-up. *J Clin Oncol* 2007;25:2554–2559.

171. Schouten HC, Qian W, Kvaloy S, et al. High-dose therapy improves progression-free survival and survival in relapsed follicular non-Hodgkin's lymphoma: results from the randomized European CUP trial. *J Clin Oncol* 2003;21:3918–3927.

172. Safar V, Gastinne T, Milpied N, et al. Very long term follow-up of autologous stem cell transplantation in follicular lymphoma: a retrospective single-institution experience. *Ann Oncol* 2008;19:183.

173. van Besien K, Loberiza FR Jr, Bajorunaite R, et al. Comparison of autologous and allogeneic hematopoietic stem cell transplantation for follicular lymphoma. *Blood* 2003;102:3521–3529.

174. Khouri IF, McLaughlin P, Saliba RM, et al. Eight-year experience with allogeneic stem cell transplantation for relapsed follicular lymphoma after nonmyeloablative conditioning with fludarabine, cyclophosphamide, and rituximab. *Blood* 2008;111:5530–5536.

175. Rezvani AR, Storer B, Maris M, et al. Nonmyeloablative allogeneic hematopoietic cell transplantation in relapsed, refractory, and transformed indolent non-Hodgkin's lymphoma. *J Clin Oncol* 200826:211–217.

176. Armand P, Kim HT, Ho VT, et al. Allogeneic transplantation with reduced-intensity conditioning for Hodgkin and non-Hodgkin lymphoma: importance of histology for outcome. *Biol Blood Marrow Transplant* 2008;14:418–425.

177. Freedman AS. Biology and management of histologic transformation of indolent lymphoma. *Hematology Am Soc Hematol Educ Program* 2005:314–320.

178. Friedberg JW, Neuberg D, Gribben JG, et al. Autologous bone marrow transplantation after histologic transformation of indolent B cell malignancies. *Biol Blood Marrow Transplant* 1999;5:262–268.

179. Foran JM, Apostolidis J, Papamichael D, et al. High-dose therapy with autologous haematopoietic support in patients with transformed follicular lymphoma: a study of 27 patients from a single centre. *Ann Oncol* 1998;9:865–869.

180. Williams CD, Harrison CN, Lister TA, et al. High-dose therapy and autologous stem-cell support for chemosensitive transformed low-grade follicular non-Hodgkin's lymphoma: a case-matched study from the European Bone Marrow Transplant Registry. *J Clin Oncol* 2001;19:727–735.

181. Chen CI, Crump M, Tsang R, et al. Autotransplants for histologically transformed follicular non-Hodgkin's lymphoma. *Br J Haematol* 2001;113:202–208.

182. Cao TM, Horning S, Negrin RS, et al. High-dose therapy and autologous hematopoietic-cell transplantation for follicular lymphoma beyond first remission: the Stanford University experience. *Biol Blood Marrow Transplant* 2001;7:294–301.

183. Tan D, Rosenberg SA, Lavori P, et al. Improved prognosis after histologic transformation of follicular lymphoma: the Stanford experience. *Ann Oncol* 2008;19:111.

184. Al-Tourah A, Kerry J, Savage K, et al. Addition of rituximab to CHOP chemotherapy significantly improves survival of patients with transformed lymphoma. *Blood* 2007;110:790a.

185. Weisdorf DJ, Andersen JW, Glick JH, et al. Survival after relapse of low-grade non-Hodgkin's lymphoma: implications for marrow transplantation. *J Clin Oncol* 1992;10:942–947.

186. Levy R, Robertson M, Leonard J, et al. Results of a phase 3 trial evaluating safety and efficacy of specific immunotherapy, recombinant idiotype conjugated to KLH with GM-CSF, compared to non-specific immunotherapy, KLH with GM-CSF, in patients with follicular non-Hodgin's lymphoma. *Ann Oncol* 2008;19:101.

187. Wiernik PH, Lossos IS, Tuscano JM, et al. Lenalidomide monotherapy in relapsed or refractory aggressive non-Hodgkin's lymphoma. *J Clin Oncol* 2008;26:4952–4957.

188. Strauss SJ, Maharaj L, Hoare S, et al. Bortezomib therapy in patients with relapsed or refractory lymphoma: potential correlation of in vitro sensitivity and tumor necrosis factor alpha response with clinical activity. *J Clin Oncol* 2006;24:2105–2112.

189. Goy A, Younes A, McLaughlin P, et al. Phase II study of proteasome inhibitor bortezomib in relapsed or refractory B-cell non-Hodgkin's lymphoma. *J Clin Oncol* 2005;23:667–675.

190. Hagenbeek A, Gadeberg O, Johnson P, et al. First clinical use of ofatumumab, a novel fully human anti-CD20 monoclonal antibody in relapsed or refractory follicular lymphoma: results of a phase 1/2 trial. *Blood* 2008;111:5486–5495.

191. Leonard JP, Friedberg JW, Younes A, et al. A phase I/II study of galiximab (an anti-CD80 monoclonal antibody) in combination with rituximab for relapsed or refractory, follicular lymphoma. *Ann Oncol* 2007;18:1216–1223.

192. Czuczman MS, Thall A, Witzig TE, et al. Phase I/II study of galiximab, an anti-CD80 antibody, for relapsed or refractory follicular lymphoma. *J Clin Oncol* 2005;23:4390–4398.

193. Leonard JP, Coleman M, Ketas J, et al. Combination antibody therapy with epratuzumab and rituximab in relapsed or refractory non-Hodgkin's lymphoma. *J Clin Oncol* 2005;23:5044–5051.

194. Kamath SS, Marcus RB Jr, Lynch JW, et al. The impact of radiotherapy dose and other treatment-related and clinical factors on in-field control in stage I and II non-Hodgkin's lymphoma. *Int J Radiat Oncol Biol Phys* 1999;44:563–568.

195. Forstpointner R, Unterhalt M, Dreyling M, et al. Maintenance therapy with rituximab leads to a significant prolongation of response duration after salvage therapy with a combination of rituximab, fludarabine, cyclophosphamide, and mitoxantrone (R-FCM) in patients with recurring and refractory follicular and mantle cell lymphomas: results of a prospective randomized study of the German Low Grade Lymphoma Study Group (GLSG). *Blood* 2006;108:4003–4008.

196. Freedman AS, Neuberg D, Mauch P, et al. Long-term follow-up of autologous bone marrow transplantation in patients with relapsed follicular lymphoma. *Blood* 94:3325—3333.

197. Apostolidis J, Gupta RK, Grenzelias D, et al. High-dose therapy with autologous bone marrow support as consolidation of remission in follicular lymphoma: long-term clinical and molecular follow-up. *J Clin Oncol* 2000;18:527–536.

198. Bierman PJ, Vose JM, Anderson JR, et al. High-dose therapy with autologous hematopoietic rescue for follicular low-grade non-Hodgkin's lymphoma. *J Clin Oncol* 1997;15:445–450.

199. Bastion Y, Brice P, Haioun C, et al. Intensive therapy with peripheral blood progenitor cell transplantation in 60 patients with poor-prognosis follicular lymphoma. *Blood* 1995;86:3257–3262.

200. van Besien K, Sobocinski KA, Rowlings PA, et al. Allogeneic bone marrow transplantation for low-grade lymphoma. *Blood* 1998;92:1832–1836.

201. Juckett M, Rowlings P, Hessner M, et al. T cell-depleted allogeneic bone marrow transplantation for high-risk non-Hodgkin's lymphoma: clinical and molecular follow-up. *Bone Marrow Transplant* 1998;21: 893–899.

202. Khouri IF, Saliba RM, Giralt SA, et al. Nonablative allogeneic hematopoietic transplantation as adoptive immunotherapy for indolent lymphoma: low incidence of toxicity, acute graft-versus-host disease, and treatment-related mortality. *Blood* 2001;98:3595–3599.

203. Morschhauser F, Radford J, Van Hoof A, et al. Phase III Trial of Consolidation Therapy With Yttrium-90–Ibritumomab Tiuxetan Compared With No Additional Therapy After First Remission in Advanced Follicular Lymphoma. *J Clin Oncol* 2008;26:5156–5164.

CHAPTER 19 ■ MANTLE CELL LYMPHOMA

JASMINE ZAIN, GOVIND BHAGAT, AND OWEN A. O'CONNOR

One of the major liabilities of older lymphoma classification schemes is that they relied heavily on morphology and nodal architecture, coupled in some cases to the clinical history. As a result, mantle cell lymphoma (MCL) was admixed with other distinctly different types of lymphoma because of its cytologic and morphologic resemblance to other types of low-grade non-Hodgkin lymphomas (NHLs) (Table 19.1 and Fig. 19.1). MCL has moved rapidly from being a poorly described disease entity, to now being the subject of many basic and clinical research endeavors. These new data have made MCL a target for novel drugs targeting basic pathogenetic mechanisms. Although the disease is rare, it has become a model of cancer cell biology, providing insights that are now affecting many areas of cancer research.

EPIDEMIOLOGY AND CLINICAL FEATURES

MCL is a disease of the elderly. The median age of patients with MCL is estimated to be 58 years. Like most other lymphoproliferative malignancies, MCL has a higher incidence in males, with a gender ratio of approximately 2:1. Despite the collection of robust data sets on "lymphoma" (i.e., NHL and Hodgkin lymphoma), the present Surveillance Epidemiology and End Results databases do not report the incidence or prevalence of the different NHL subtypes, making it difficult to obtain firm estimates for any given type of NHL, let alone MCL (1). Nonetheless, it is generally estimated that MCL represents approximately 6% of all NHL cases (2), giving an incidence of nearly 4,000 cases per year. The prevalence of the disease, calculated by multiplying the incidence by the median survival (assume range of 3 to 5 years), is estimated to range between 15,000 and 20,000 cases. These estimates make MCL a true orphan disease (i.e., a disease with a prevalence of <200,000 cases per year).

Interestingly, a Surveillance Epidemiology and End Results summary of changes in cancer mortality from 1950 to 2005, based on 5-year relative survival rates, suggests that the annual percent change in NHL mortality was +1.4% (i.e., a 1.4% increase in mortality), which is worse than virtually every other malignancy, including breast cancer, leukemia, melanoma, and even brain tumors. Although significant progress has been made in treating many forms of lymphoma, these data suggest that more attention is required for those subtypes associated with markedly inferior outcomes. Despite the aforementioned statistics, there is a paucity of information regarding the incidence, prevalence, and changes in mortality for the discrete NHL subtypes.

One recently reported experience from Zhou et al. (3) examined data from all patients with MCL diagnosed between 1992 and 2004 in 13 geographic areas across the United States. They found 87,166 patients with NHL during that 13-year period, of which 2.8% had confirmed MCL. The overall incidence of MCL was 0.55, which increased with age (0.07 in patients <50 years, 2.97 for patients aged 70 to 79, and 2.78 in patients >80 years). The age-adjusted incidence rate increased from 0.27/100,000 in 1992 to 0.69/100,000 in 2004, reflecting a 5.87% change (p <0.05). The median age at diagnosis was 68 years, and the disease was 2.5 times more prevalent in males than females. MCL was also more common in whites (0.61/100,000) than African-Americans (0.32/100,000), and nearly 75% of all patients diagnosed presented with advanced stage 3 or 4 disease. Strikingly, there was a significant geographic variation in the disease, with the lowest incidence occurring in Alaska natives (0.1/100,000), and the highest incidence occurring in residents of Seattle near the Puget Sound (0.67/100,000).

TABLE 19.1

DECIPHERING THE DIAGNOSIS BY IMMUNOHISTOCHEMISTRY—THE SMALL LYMPHOCYTIC LYMPHOMAS

Surface marker	MCL	Follicular lymphoma	Small lymphocytic lymphoma	Marginal zone lymphoma
CD5	++	−	++	−
Surface Ig	++	+++	+	+
CD19	++	++	++	++
CD20	+++	++	+ (weak)	++
CD10	−	+ (80%)	−	−
CD23	−	+/−	+	−
Cyclin D1	+++	−	−	−
Cytogenetics	t(11:14)	t(14:18)	−	t(11:18)

(+), weakly positive; (++), moderately positive; (+++), strongly positive; (−), negative.

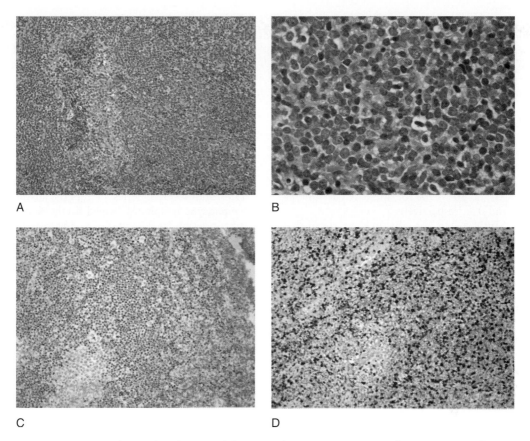

A   B

C   D

FIGURE 19.1 Mantle zone lymphoma, nodular ("Mantle zone") pattern; a small reactive germinal center is seen surrounded by a markedly expanded mantle zone (Panel A, Hematoxylin & Eosin stain, original magnification 100X). The neoplastic lymphocytes have predominantly ovoid or irregular nuclear contours, fine chromatin, indistinct or small nucleoli, and scant cytoplasm (Panel B, Hematoxylin & Eosin stain, original magnification 400X). Cyclin D1 expressing lymphocytes are largely confined to the mantle zone (Panel C, original magnification 100X) and these cells show a moderately elevated proliferation index (approximately 30%), as assessed with a stain for Ki-67 (Panel D, original magnification 100X). (See also Color Plates 30-33).

Like other lymphoproliferative malignancies, patients with MCL can present with a very broad spectrum of clinical presentations (2,4–13). Staging for MCL typically follows the Cotswald staging system for all NHLs. The overwhelming majority of patients present with advanced-stage disease (stage III–IV), with estimates ranging from 70% to 95% (3,6,8,12). Approximately 70% to 90% of patients present with generalized lymphadenopathy above and below the diaphragm. Bone marrow involvement is also felt to be very common, being seen in 50% to 80% of patients, though some specialists in the field believe virtually every patient is likely to have marrow involvement at the time of diagnosis. These data are based on unilateral bone marrow biopsies that are likely to underestimate the true rate of involvement. After these features, most other presentations are relatively less common. For example, gastrointestinal tract involvement is considered to be relatively more common in patients with MCL compared with other subtypes of NHL, typically being found in 15% to 25% of cases. Patients with Waldeyer ring involvement have a significantly higher risk of gastrointestinal tract involvement, and the presence of MCL at this location is an absolute indication for upper endoscopy and colonoscopy. Enlargement of the spleen and liver can be seen in 35% to 81% and 18% to 35% of patients, respectively. Lymphocytosis has been reported in between 10% and 69%

of patients with MCL. A recent study by Ferrer et al. (14) documented peripheral blood involvement or leukemic disease in 92% ($n = 44$) of patients by flow cytometry. Twenty-five of 44 patients (56%) presented with a lymphocyte count of $>5 \times 10e9$ per L.

In general, central nervous system involvement by MCL is considered unusual. In one report (15), cerebrospinal fluid sampling was performed on 25 of 108 patients who exhibited some neurologic sign or symptom prompting lumbar puncture. Ten of the 25 patients sampled had evidence of cerebrospinal fluid involvement. Other signs and symptoms of MCL include "B" symptoms in 35% to 55% of patients, elevated lactate dehydrogenase (LDH) in 30% to 50% of patients, and elevated β_2-microglobulin in roughly 50% of patients.

The clinical separation of MCL from the other subtypes of lymphoma with which it was often lumped was reported in an initial Southwest Oncology Group (SWOG) report, which was based upon an analysis of patient tissue obtained from three sequential randomized clinical trials conducted between 1972 and 1983 (2). These data reevaluated the tissue diagnosis from >376 patients with Working Formulation diagnoses encompassing categories A through E. They reported that six of 70 patients with small lymphocytic/diffuse, well-differentiated lymphoma (category A), nine of 171 patients with follicular small cleaved/nodular poorly differentiated lymphoma (category B), and 21 of 66 patients with diffuse small cleaved/diffuse poorly differentiated lymphoma (category E) had MCL. The analysis demonstrated that the failure-free survival (FFS) and overall survival (OS) of patients with MCL were significantly worse than that for patients with Working Formulation diagnoses from categories A and E ($p = 0.0001$ and 0.0001, respectively), lymphomas that would today be classified as indolent. In fact, the OS at 10 years for patients with MCL was only 8% compared with 35% for the Working Formulation categories A through E. In addition, separating the different histologic variants of MCL into nodular, diffuse, and blastic demonstrated that the OSs at 10 years for these MCL subtypes were 14%, 10%, and 0%, respectively.

Based on the SWOG data set, the median survival of patients with MCL has been considered to be about 3 to 4 years, and the median FFS from up-front conventional cyclophosphamide, doxorubicin, vincristine, and prednisone (CHOP)-based treatment is only 15 to 18 months. Since this publication, however, there are now a number of more recent data sets that appear to suggest that depending upon the treatment, survival is significantly more variable, and possibly more favorable, than that originally reported by SWOG. These data will be addressed below under the sections on conventional treatment.

DISTINGUISHING PATHOLOGIC AND CLINICAL FEATURES OF MANTLE CELL LYMPHOMA

Historically, MCL had been referred to as "lymphocytic lymphoma of intermediate differentiation" in the American literature, and "centrocytic lymphoma" in the European literature. These descriptions were based on the observation that some of the cells had well-rounded nuclei (as seen in small noncleaved cell lymphomas), whereas others appeared to have indented or cleaved nuclei like those of small-cleaved cell lymphoma. In 1982, Weisenburger (16) and Palutke (17) et al. described a distinctive type of "follicular lymphoma" characterized by the proliferation of atypical small lymphoid cells in the wide mantle zones around benign or reactive germinal centers (18). Believing that this represented the follicular counterpart of diffuse intermediate lymphocytic lymphoma, they coined the term *mantle zone* lymphoma to describe this entity. In the early 1990s, it became evident that there was a subset of diffuse-small cleaved cell lymphomas and small lymphocytic lymphomas (SLLs) that behaved very differently from other diseases with similar morphology. These patients often carried a worse prognosis with a distinctly different natural history. The development of new monoclonal antibodies used for phenotypic characterization by immunohistochemistry, coupled with new techniques in cytogenetics, allowed pathologists to make important distinctions between these disease subtypes that transcended simple morphologic descriptors. As a result, in the early 1990s, Raffeld and Jaffe (19) and Banks et al. (20) coined the term "mantle cell lymphoma" to describe a subset of SLLs that carried a unique translocation that results in the transpositioning of the B-cell lymphoma-1 (BCL1) gene (11q13) to a site downstream of the immunoglobulin (Ig) heavy chain gene promoter (14q32). The BCL1 gene, also known as PRAD1 because it was first identified in parathyroid adenomas, encodes the protein cyclin D1. This balanced translocation, t(11;14)(q13:q32), leads to the constitutive up-regulation or overproduction of BCL1 due to "promoter substitution."

The linkage of lymphocytic lymphoma of intermediate differentiation with cyclin D1 rearrangement clearly changed our understanding of the disease. The t(11:14)(q13:q32) translocation was originally reported as early as 1979 and 1984 as being a recurring cytogenetic abnormality in lymphoproliferative malignancies (21,22). However, between 1990 and 1991, a series of reports linking the t(11:14) to lymphocytic lymphoma helped firmly establish this particular genetic lesion as essentially pathognomonic for MCL (23–29). Given the rarity of this lesion outside of MCL, it, coupled with the distinct immunophenotype, helped lay the basis for making a "definitive" pathologic diagnosis.

The nodal architecture is characterized by a nodular or diffuse infiltration by small to medium-sized lymphocytes that have round or indented nuclei, sometime with elements of each. Focal areas of nodularity are evident in about 30% of cases on initial presentation. In *nodular MCL*, some of the nodules may consist of follicles with reactive germinal centers surrounded by broad expansile mantles of neoplastic lymphocytes, also referred to as the "mantle zone" pattern (16,30). As the disease progresses, there is a gradual invasion and obliteration of the interfollicular/nodular areas by the neoplastic cells, leading to a diffuse pattern of growth, a variant known as *diffuse MCL*. In about 20% of cases, the neoplastic cells of MCL are larger than those typically seen in the nodular variant, and the nuclei have finely dispersed chromatin and prominent nucleoli. These cases have been referred to as the "blastic variant" or "anaplastic centrocytic" form of MCL. The blastic variants are often associated with a higher mitotic rate, more aggressive clinical course, and an unfavorable natural history. Histologic progression from a nodular pattern to a diffuse pattern may be evident in repeat biopsy specimens obtained from the same patient, as may progression from the predominantly small lymphocytic forms to blastic MCL. Some reports suggest that histologic transformation to blastic cytology on rebiopsy can occur in up to 17% of cases, and may be as high as 70% at autopsy. Histologic transformation of MCL to diffuse large B-cell lymphoma, like that seen in patients with follicular lymphoma or SLL, is not seen (18).

MCL (Table 19.1) is characterized by the expression of pan B-cell antigens (CD20+, CD22+, though typically CD23-), with monotypic Ig (IgM+D+ often λ+) and coexpression of the T-cell antigen CD5, and nuclear expression of cyclin D1 (31). These phenotypic and cytogenetic features help to distinguish it from other small B-cell lymphomas, including chronic lymphocytic leukemia/SLL, marginal zone lymphoma, and follicular lymphoma.

GENETIC FEATURES OF MANTLE CELL LYMPHOMA

These data have established that there are a number of recurring genetic abnormalities associated with MCL that go well beyond the t(11:14)(q13;q32) translocation. Table 19.2

TABLE 19.2

SELECT MOLECULAR DEFECTS DESCRIBED IN MCL

Molecular gene defect	Biologic consequence	Comments	Reference
Cyclin D1 gene expression	Increases cellular proliferation.	The ratio of cyclin D1 to D3 has predictive value in diagnosing MCL.	(22, 24, 26)
Loss of cyclin-dependent kinase inhibitor (CDK1) ■ p27 ■ p21 ■ p16 INK 4 ■ p15 INK 4	Impairs ability of cell to inhibit proliferation.	Loss of p27 may be attributed to: (a) Increased proteasome mediated degradation due to increased activity of p27^{Kip1} ubiquitin ligases and loss of p16/15 due to methylation of promotor. (b) Sequestration by cyclin D1.	(32) (33, 38)
Mutated p53	Chemotherapy resistance impaired induction of apoptosis. Loss of cell cycle control.	More common in blastic MCL, less common in other MCL variants.	(35)
ATM	Inability to repair double-strand DNA damage.	Twenty percent to 40% of MCL cases have defects in ATM, which correlated with more DNA damage but does not appear to correlate with OS.	(39)
Bcl-2/MCL-1 family	inhibits induction of apoptosis	Contributes to chemotherapy resistance and high proliferative state.	(31)
BCL-6	Overexpression and/or dysregulation leads to impaired differentiation and apoptosis.	Small subset of MCL with BCL-6 dysregulation. BCL-6 derangements more common in germinal center lymphomas like follicular and diffuse large B-cell lymphomas. MCL is considered a naive pregerminal center lymphoma.	(31)

---

summarizes some of the major molecular aberrations seen in MCL.

The constitutive overexpression of cyclin D1 serves to enhance or "accelerate" the cycling of cells from resting states into active states of proliferation. However, many lines of evidence are beginning to demonstrate that MCL is a disease also characterized by the loss of "functional brakes." The loss of cell cycle-dependent kinase (cdk) inhibitors like p27, p21, and p16 create the situation where proliferation signals can continue unopposed. Among the cdk inhibitors lost, p27 has emerged as one commonly encountered defect.

Clinically, there is a strong correlation between the overexpression of p53 and/or loss of p27 in MCL. Patients with both of these cytogenetic defects show a statistically significant reduction in OS (32), which is inferior to patients with only one or none of these defects. Although the mechanism of p27 loss is not entirely clear, two major mechanisms have been advanced, including: (a) sequestration of p27 with the abundant cyclin D1, and (b) increased proteolytic degradation of p27. Interestingly, increased levels of Skp2, a component of the p27^{Kip1} ubiquitin ligase, may be important in explaining this observation in select subtypes of NHL (33). The basis for the Skp2 involvement pertains to the observation that Skp2 levels correlate with greater ubiquitin ligase (E3) activity and, therefore, greater proteasome-mediated degradation of the target protein (i.e., p27), establishing an inverse relationship between the two proteins. In aggressive lymphomas and blastic MCL, Skp2 levels are associated with low levels of p27^{Kip1} protein, suggesting increased proteasome-mediated degradation of p27^{Kip1} in these diseases (33). Loss of p27 identified the worse outcome among the

p53-negative cases and established this pathway as an important high-risk marker in patients with MCL. Further evidence in support of the importance of the ubiquitin-proteasome pathways in MCL was recently presented by Bogner et al. (34). These authors demonstrated that treatment of MCL cell lines (Granta 519 and NCEB) with the proteasome inhibitor lactacystin failed to result in cyclin D1 or cdk4 accumulation, despite the overexpression already mediated by the t(11:14) translocation. Interestingly, cell cycle arrest and induction of apoptosis were accompanied by accumulation of the cdk inhibitor p21 and p27 in both cell lines, suggesting enhanced sensitivity linked to the reconstitution of p27.

Although derangements in cyclin D1 and cdk inhibitors may explain some of the molecular defects in MCL, it is also clear that there are a variety of other abnormalities that revolve around p53, p16, and the ataxia telangiectasia mutated (ATM) gene as well (Table 19.2). Louie et al. (35) demonstrated that mutation of p53 was associated with a significantly worse prognosis compared with cases where p53 was not mutated. Cases with wild-type p53 were associated with a median survival of 63 months, whereas cases with mutant p53 were associated with a median survival of only 12 months. These observations have been confirmed by others as well (36–38).

Approximately 20% to 40% of MCL cases have demonstrable inactivation of the ATM gene, which is located at 11q22–23, near the critical BCL1 locus at 11q13. The ATM gene encodes for a serine-threonine kinase belonging to the phosphatidylinositol-3 kinase family, and plays a central role in signaling pathways activated by double-strand deoxyribonucleic acid (DNA) damage. Interestingly, ATM gene alterations, while common, were not related to the histologic variant of the tumor, p53 status, survival, or other clinico-pathologic features but did lead to a marked increase in chromosomal imbalances (39).

Rosenwald et al. (40) from the National Cancer Institute reported on the use of gene expression profiling in patients with MCL. This experience established the fact that not all patients with MCL have the same prognosis, and helped further support the importance of cell cycle dysregulation as a critical determinant of the disease. This experience established that the tumor cell "proliferation signature" accurately risk stratified patients into favorable (reduced proliferation index) and unfavorable (elevated proliferation index) risk groups. For example, those patients in the first quartile with respect to high proliferative rates had an estimated OS of <1 year, whereas that group with the slowest growing disease exhibited a median survival of >5 years. Although these techniques cannot be applied in real time for patients with MCL today, it does offer an explanation for the possible enrichment for favorable or unfavorable subtypes of the disease in various studies.

PROGNOSTIC FACTORS IN MANTLE CELL LYMPHOMA

The risk stratification of patients with any form of cancer represents a potentially important strategy for identifying relatively favorable and unfavorable populations, which could create opportunities for individualizing treatment. The optimal features of any prognostic score would ideally: (a) allow separation of favorable, intermediate, and high-risk groups; (b) allocate uniformly equivalent fractions of the patient population across all prognostic subgroups; and (c) show reproducible correlation with overall response, progression-free survival (PFS), and OS. Given the sometimes subtle differences among many lymphoproliferative malignancies, it is not surprising that many new prognostic models are being generated in a very disease-specific context.

To date, the International Prognostic Index (IPI), originally developed for aggressive lymphomas, represents one of the longest and most robustly studied models used to risk stratify patients with MCL. The IPI identifies five adverse prognostic factors, including: age >60; performance status >2; LDH level above normal; extranodal sites more than one, and stage III or IV disease. Application of the IPI to MCL has been criticized for the inability to separate the two intermediate risk groups, which comprise approximately two thirds of all MCL cases. The Follicular Lymphoma International Prognostic Index (FLIPI) was developed based on data from patients with follicular lymphoma, and has also been applied to patient populations with MCL. The FLIPI takes into account five prognostic factors, including: number of nodal sites more than four, LDH above normal, age >60, stage >III/IV, and hemoglobin <12 g per dL. The FLIPI has been found to poorly separate the low and intermediate-risk groups, with an exceptionally large number of patients being represented in the high-risk group, which appears to exhibit a relatively good outcome. Moller et al. (41) conducted an analysis on 93 patients, formally comparing the IPI to the FLIPI, and concluded that the FLIPI identified three risk

groups with markedly different outcomes, with 5-year survival rates of 65%, 42%, and 8%, respectively. The high-risk group, however, contained 53% of the patients. In contrast, the IPI allocated only 16% of cases to the high-risk group and produced a lower overall predictive capacity. In multivariate analyses, only the FLIPI in the Moller study correlated well with OS.

Given the imperfect application of the IPI and FLIPI, Hoster et al. (42) recently described a new prognostic index for patients with MCL called the MCL International Prognostic Index (MIPI). Based on data from three consecutive randomized trials conducted in Germany and Europe, the clinical and pathologic features of 455 patients with MCL were analyzed by multiple Cox regression analyses. Four independent prognostic factors for OS were identified, including: age, Eastern Cooperative Oncology Group performance status, LDH, and white blood cell count (WBC). Patients were assigned points depending upon the measurement of these variables, as described in Table 19.3. According to the MIPI, patients were classified into low-risk (44% of patients, median OS not reached), intermediate-risk (35% of patients, median OS 51 months), and high-risk groups (21% of patients, median OS 29 months). For example, patients with age <50, Eastern Cooperative Oncology Group 0 or 1, LDH <0.67 × upper limit of normal, and a WBC <6.7 × 10e9 per L are assigned zero points. In contrast, one to three points are assigned depending on the unfavorable nature of the following parameters: age >70, LDH >1.5 upper limit of normal (ULN), and WBC >15,00010e9 per L, all worth three points each. At 3 years, approximately 50%, 70%, and >95% of patients with high, intermediate and low risk disease, respectively, were still alive. Table 19.4 compares and contrasts the available prognostic modes commonly used in patients with MCL.

Besides clinical prognostic factors, a variety of biologic prognostic factors have emerged as critical in MCL. For example, the Ki-67 proliferation index, in many ways a surrogate for the proliferation index defined by gene expression profiling, has emerged as being strongly correlated with OS in patients with MCL. Based on data from 134 patients with MCL, and a median follow-up of 24 months, Katzenberger et al. (43) divided the "proliferation" groups into those with a Ki-67 index of: (a) ≤20%, (b) 21% to 40%, (c) 41% to 60%, or (d) >60%. A Kaplan-Meier analysis revealed dramatically different survival curves, with median survivals of

TABLE 19.3				
MIPI				
Points	Age (y)	Performance status (ECOG)	LDH (× upper limit of normal)	WBC (×10e9 per L)
0	<50	0–1	<0.67	<6.7
1	50–59	–	0.67–0.99	6.7–9.9
2	60–69	2–4	1–1.49	10–14.9
3	>70	–	>1.5	>15

ECOG, Eastern Cooperative Oncology Group. Patients with zero to three points are at low risk, with four to five points at intermediate risk, and patients with six to 11 points are at high risk.

TABLE 19.4

COMPARISON OF PROGNOSTIC SCORES IN PATIENTS WITH MCL

Time (mo)	International Prognostic Index (n = 93)				FLIPI (n = 93)			MIPI (n = 220)		
	Low	Low-intermediate	High-intermediate	High	Low	Intermediate	High	Low	Intermediate	High
0	20 (22%)	38 (41%)	20 (22%)	15 (16%)	21 (23%)	23 (25%)	49 (53%)	62 (28%)	103 (47%)	55 (25%)
36	16 (17%)	22 (24%)	8 (9%)	3 (3%)	17 (18%)	16 (17%)	16 (17%)	38 (17%)	41 (19%)	18 (8%)
72	5 (5%)	5 (5%)	3 (3%)	0	5 (5%)	5 (5%)	3 (3%)	7 (3%)	7 (3%)	1 (<1%)
108 (96 for MIPI)	0	2 (2%)	2 (2%)	0	0	2 (2%)	2 (2%)	2 (1%)	4 (2%)	0

53, 33, 19, and 13 months from the low to high proliferation group, respectively. Interestingly, to develop a combined biologic and clinical index (MIPIb), Hoster et al. (42) found high prognostic relevance of Ki-67 independent from the MIPI, though the combined biologic and clinical index did reveal a low-risk group with a very favorable prognosis. However, given that the Ki-67 data were available on only 50% of the population used for the clinical prognostic score, the conclusion of the authors was to limit the application of the combined biologic and clinical index until additional data become available. The significance of the Ki-67 index was further validated in a subsequent study. Determann et al. (44) demonstrated that in >249 patients receiving rituximab with CHOP (R-CHOP)-based chemotherapy, those patients with elevated Ki-67 experienced significantly shorter Overall Survivals compared with patients with more indolent disease.

More recent biologically based prognostic models have identified enriched gene sets that appear to predict clinical outcome. In one such experience, Hartmann et al. (45) evaluated the expression of 33 genes with potential prognostic and pathogenetic significance in MCL using quantitative reverse-transcription polymerase chain reactions (PCRs) in 73 patients. They found that the optimized survival predictor was composed of five genes: (a) RAN, a guanosine triphosphate binding protein required for nuclear ribonucleic acid and protein transport; (b) myc, a transcription factor that plays a key role in cell cycle progression and apoptosis; (c) TNFRSF10B, a member of the tumor necrosis factor receptor superfamily that triggers an apoptotic signal on activation by the cytokine tumor necrosis factor–related apoptosis inducing ligand; (d) POLE2, a DNA polymerase that plays a role in DNA replication and repair; and (e) SLC29A2, a member of the SLC29 family of nucleoside carriers that transport a broad range of purine and pyrimidine nucleosides. These five genes were reported to be superior to immunohistochemical staining for Ki-67.

The overwhelming preponderance of available data suggests that some of the most important prognostic factors in MCL revolve around the proliferative rate of the disease. Although clinical prognostic factors are surely important, it will likely be that the best future prognostic models incorporate some aspects of the clinical and biologic data. These prognostic models also offer a potentially paradigm-changing opportunity to risk stratify our patients based upon the nature of their disease, so chemotherapy approaches can be tailored to specific subtypes of MCL.

CONVENTIONAL TREATMENT STRATEGIES FOR MANTLE CELL LYMPHOMA

Because patients with MCL demonstrate some of the poorest long-term survivals of all lymphoma subtypes, up-front treatment is typically indicated for most patients. Despite this, there does appear to exist a small fraction of elderly patients whose MCL can assume a more indolent course, justifying in these otherwise frail and elderly patients a closely monitored "watch-and-wait" approach. In general, the up-front care of patients with MCL usually revolves around several basic questions: (a) Which combination chemotherapy regimen offers the patient the best chance for a durable remission of his/her disease?; (b) Is an anthracycline-based treatment regimen necessary?; (c) What are the benefits of high-dose chemotherapy and autologous stem cell transplant (ASCT) in first remission?; (d) Is there a benefit to some consolidation or maintenance-based therapy in the form of rituximab, a course of radioimmunotherapy (RIT), or possibly even a novel small molecule with promising activity?; and (e) Is there any strategy presently in development that might hold the promise of curative intent? To date, although many studies are actively addressing these issues, the jury is still largely adjourned regarding the definitive answers to these questions. We will address the data pertaining to each issue below.

Alkylator-based anthracycline-containing regimens have become the cornerstone of up-front MCL therapy, despite conflicting evidence regarding the real benefits of the anthracycline component (Table 19.5). Complete response rates from 13% to 51% for standard CHOP-based chemotherapy have been published in a number of series (2,4–6,13,46). To date, one randomized study comparing cyclophosphamide, vincristine, and prednisone (n = 37) versus CHOP (n = 26) has been reported in MCL (46). This study did not demonstrate any statistically significant difference between the two arms with regard to complete (41% vs. 58%) or partial remission (PR) (43% vs. 31%), median OS (32 vs. 37 months), relapse-free survival (10 vs. 7 months), rates of relapse (73% vs. 67%), or death. One of the first studies exploring the

TABLE 19.5

SUMMARY OF ALKYLATOR-BASED CHEMOTHERAPY REGIMEN IN THE TREATMENTS OF MCL

Regimen	Evaluable patients (n)	Response (n)			Duration of response (mo)	Comments	Reference
		CR (%)	PR (%)	ORR (%)			
R-CHOP	40	48	48	96	16.6	First line. No benefit in patients having molecular CR	(47)
CHOP vs.	122	7	68	75	TTF 14 mo	First-line treatment. No difference to PFS.	(48)
R-CHOP		34	60	94	TTF 21 mo		
FCM vs.	48	0	46	46	PFS 4 mo	Patients with relapsed or refractory disease.	(49)
R-FCM		29	29	58	PFS 8 mo		
R-HyperCVAD	97	89	11	100	At 3 y, FFS is 65%, and OS is 79%	First-line therapy with a median follow-up 40 mo. β_2-microglobulin strongly predictive of prolonged survival.	(50–53)
HyperCVAD	25	68	24	92	At a median of 17 mo, the FFS was 15 mo	First-line therapy patients	(50)

TTF, Time to Treatment Failure.

merits of combining rituximab was performed by Howard et al. (47). Of 40 patients enrolled in the study, 48% achieved a complete remission (CR) or unconfirmed complete remission (Cru), whereas another 48% experienced a PR, which suggests that the CR rate may be higher with the addition of rituximab. The median PFS was about 16 months, which is not dramatically different from CHOP alone. Surprisingly though, nine of 25 patients who achieved molecular remissions (i.e., no evidence of PCR-detectable BCL1/IgH or clonal IgH products) of their disease in peripheral blood or bone marrow had a median PFS that was not statistically different from those patients who did not achieve a molecular remission (18.8 vs. 16.5 months; $p = 0.51$).

A follow-up study to test the importance of rituximab was reported by Lenz et al. (48). A randomized phase II study of CHOP versus R-CHOP in previously untreated patients with MCL concluded that the addition of rituximab improved the overall response rate (ORR) and CR from 75% and 7%, to 94% and 34%, respectively (48). Collectively, these data demonstrated that R-CHOP was superior to CHOP in terms of ORR, CR rate, and time to treatment failure, though, surprisingly, it had absolutely no impact on OS. Although these data strongly suggest an important role for the use of rituximab in the up-front combination chemotherapy program in patients with MCL, it leaves open many questions regarding precisely how to employ it in the longer term treatment of MCL. What remains frustrating is the continual observation that the integration of additional drugs may improve ORRs, perhaps even molecular responses, but do not appear to markedly change the OS.

The HyperCVAD regimen (fractionated cyclophosphamide with doxorobicin, vincristine, steroids methotrexate, cytorabine) has gained a lot of attention in the up-front treatment of MCL, though there are only limited published data on the regimen for this disease (49–52). HyperCVAD is a complex, *hyper*fractionated, inpatient combination chemotherapy regimen originally developed for patients with leukemia. It consists of repeat cycles of cyclophosphamide, doxorubicin, vincristine, and dexamethasone (essentially the same drugs as in CHOP) alternating with methotrexate and cytarabine (Ara-C). Rather than administering all the drugs on the same day, it administers the drugs over successive days, leading to a marked increase in both the dose intensification and toxicity of the regimen. In one of the earlier reports, Romaguera et al. (50) reported on the use of the regimen in 25 patients >65 who received HyperCVAD followed by methotrexate/cytarabine. They reported an ORR of 92% and a CR rate of 68%. At a median follow-up of 17 months, the FFS was 15 months. The addition of rituximab (375 mg per m^2 preceding each of the first six cycles of therapy by 24 hours) into the HyperCVAD regimen was reported on 92 patients with a median age of 61 (52). Again, rituximab markedly improved both the response rate, now nearly 100%, and improved the complete response rate to 91%. Of the 92 evaluable patients, three deaths due to toxicity were noted. For those patients younger than age 65, the median FFS at 2 years was 80%, compared with 50% for patients >65 years of age. Trying to exploit the merits of this chemotherapy program, Khouri et al. (49,50) employed HyperCVAD as a cytoreductive regimen before ASCT. They reported that at 3 years, the OS and event-free survival (EFS) for previously untreated patients were 92% and 72%, respectively. For those patients who were previously treated, the results were significantly worse, with the OS and EFS falling to only 25% and 17%, respectively. Based on the very short follow-up of these studies, these authors concluded that the addition of rituximab to the HyperCVAD-MTX/Ara-C regimen produced results nearly identical to that seen with HyperCVAD followed by a consolidative ASCT. These results have been recently validated in a multi-institutional phase II SWOG study (53). Based on 40 patients who have been evaluated for response, the ORR was 88%, including 58% of patients who were in CR or CRu. Although the median follow-up of this SWOG study was short (1.6 years), the 1 and 2-year PFSs were 89% and 63%, respectively. In addition, there was one death attributed to the study treatment, and 87% of patients experienced a grade 4 hematologic toxicity. The investigators of this cooperative group study concluded that while the regimen is active, there is a definite pattern of continued relapse within the period of follow-up, and the toxicity of the regimen is significant.

Based on the available data for the HyperCVAD-MTX/Ara-C regimen, a variety of HyperCVAD-like regimens have been developed. These have mostly included omitting the MTX/Ara-C to make the treatment program less toxic, and adding maintenance-type rituximab. These modifications, although generating a likely more favorable toxicity profile, are also not significantly different from classic R-CHOP–based chemotherapy regimens. The integration of the synergistic antimetabolites following the cytoreduction has strong cytokinetic rationale, and may exploit the sensitivity of MCL to cytidine analogs as discussed previously. Nonetheless, in one such study (54), 22 patients were treated with a modified HyperCVAD regimen every 28 days for four cycles, followed by maintenance rituximab every 6 months for 2 years. The ORR was 77% with a CR rate of 64%, both inferior to what has been seen with traditional HyperCVAD containing the antimetabolites. With a median follow-up of 37 months, the median PFS was approximately 3 years, whereas the OS has not yet been reached at the time of the most recent report. In addition, two of the 22 patients (nearly 10%) died during the treatment program.

Table 19.6 presents a summary of studies evaluating the merits of purine analog based treatment programs. In general, as a single agent, fludarabine has minimal activity,

though the studies conducted to date have been small (55, 57). Combination of fludarabine with cyclophosphamide, an anthracycline and rituximab appear more promising (58–60). For example, R-FCM (rituximab, fludarabine, cyclophosphamide, mitoxantrone) regimen produced an overall response rate of nearly 60% in patients with relapsed or refractory disease, half of which were complete remission (58). In addition, these responses were durable, and superior to those patient who did not receive rituximab with the FCM. While these regimens appear to be effective in patients with relapses disease, concerns regarding stem cell toxicity and myelosuppression have limited their use in the upfront setting.

Although modified HyperCVAD regimens may have some theoretic advantages in terms of reduced toxicity, strategies of this type are orienting the field toward the major problem in MCL. In general, cytoreduction in MCL is not the major barrier to successful treatment. The major problem is inevitable relapse, and our inability to eradicate the final clone and effectively treat minimal residual disease (MRD). New evolving concepts regarding cancer stem cells may shed light on the unique natural history of MCL. Although there may be some drugs that are more active than others, the major question is whether adding additional new drugs to existing treatment programs will overcome the hurdles of the disease. Given the history, it is possible that this may not be the correct approach. Rather, refocusing our strategies to adopt a more acute lymphoblastic leukemia-type treatment strategy may be a more effective way forward. Employing a cytoreduction phase (R-CHOP, HyperCVAD) followed by a consolidation phase (ASCT, bortezomib-containing regimen) and eventually a maintenance phase (rituximab, bortezomib, mammalian target of rapamycin [mTOR] inhibitors, etc.) could help overcome the major hurdle in MCL, persistent MRD. Thus, concepts like the ones represented in the modified HyperCVAD protocol could shift our focus from

TABLE 19.6

SUMMARY OF PURINE ANALOG-BASED CHEMOTHERAPY REGIMENS FOR THE TREATMENT OF MCL

Regimen	Evaluable patients (n)	Response (n)			Duration of response (mo)	Comments	Reference
		CR (%)	PR (%)	ORR (%)			
FLU single agent	15	0	33	33	Range 4–8 mo	13 of 15 patients treated previously	(55)
FLU single agent	17	29	12	41	PFS 13 mo	First line. No difference in OS in patients with CR or PR.	(56)
FLU vs. FLU/ idarubicin	29	27 45	33 28	72 61	NR[a]	First line. No difference in OS idarubicin	(59)
Cyclophos/phamide and FLU	30	30	33	63	The median FFS was 4.8 and the OS 17.5	33% Untreated retrospective study	(60, 61)
FCM vs. R-FCM	48	0 29	46 29	46 58	PFS 4/OS 11 PFS 8/OS NR[a] (p = 0.38)	OS (p = 0.0042)	(58)
Cladribine	18	33% (a) 56% (b)	67% (a) 44% (b)	100% (a) 100% (b)	24 mo 68% alive at 36 mo	9 treated (a) 9 relapsed (b)	(57)

FLU, fludarabine; R, rifuximab; NR[a] - Not reached; FCM, fludarabine, cyclophosphamide, mitoxantron; PFS, progression free survival; OS, overall survival; CR, complete remission; PR, partial remission; FFS, Failure Free Survival.

cytoreduction to MRD. It is in this particular setting that the role of stem cell transplantation and novel new drugs could help us begin to change the natural history of MCL.

THE ROLE OF AUTOLOGOUS STEM CELL TRANSPLANTATION

High-dose chemotherapy with ASCT rescue has been incorporated into a variety of different treatment strategies for MCL. The Nebraska group was among the first to report on the role of high-dose chemotherapy and stem cell transplant in nine patients with relapsed MCL, observing a 2-year survival of 34%. Despite several early relapses, the authors concluded that stem cell transplant had merit but needed to be incorporated into the front-line treatment of patients with MCL. Since that report, there have been a number of studies that have looked at the value of ASCT in MCL. These studies reflect significant differences in patient selection, induction, disease

status at the time of transplant, and myeloablative regimen. Although the degree of benefit varies from study to study, it is clear that ASCT should not be considered curative at this time because there is no plateau seen on any of the survival curves. Similar to most studies in MCL, there appears to be a pattern of continual late relapses. A summary of the published experiences of ASCT in MCL is presented in Table 19.7.

TIMING OF AUTOLOGOUS STEM CELL TRANSPLANT

The optimal timing for high-dose chemotherapy and ASCT in MCL is a matter of considerable debate, though increasingly many believe it may be most effective in first remission after induction therapy. Dreyling et al. (62) presented data on the results of their study exploring the merits of up-front ASCT in patients with MCL following a standard CHOP-based induction regimen. Following induction chemotherapy,

TABLE 19.7

SUMMARY OF AUTOLOGUS STEM CELL TRANSPLANT STUDIES IN MANTLE CELL LYMPHOMA

Conditioning Regimen	n	Disease status at transplant	Median Follow Up (months)	Progression Free Survival	Overall Survival	Comments	Ref
Rituximab + high dose therapy	28	CR1	35	79% at 4.5 yrs	89% at 4.5 yrs	Molecular CR seen in 95% pts.	(77)
Registry Data	195	59% in CR1	47	33% at 5 yrs	50% at 5 yrs	Registry data. Disease status at transplant affected survival	(65)
TBI/CTX after HyperCVAD	33	PR/CR1	49	43% at 5 yr	77% at 5 yrs	Hyper CVAD induction improved outcome	(49,50)
Cy + BCUNU + VP16, R maintenance	20	CR1/PR1	25	89% at 3 yrs	88% at 3 yrs	Improved results with R maintenance	(67)
TBI in 26 pts R prior to conditioning	34	85% first line, 41% in CR, 56% PR	30	70% at 3 yrs	87% at 3 yrs	Pre transplant R followed by high dose therapy improved outcome	(74)
ASCT after CHOP/R or after HyperCVAD/R	48 vs 32		38	At 3 yrs, 55% vs 78%	At 3 yrs, 68% vs 98%	HyperCVAD induction improves survival	(63)
Cy/TBI	29	29% CR1, 59% PR1	48	92 months vs 21 months if MRD +	NR vs 44 months	Molecular MRD in PB or BM predictive of PFS and OS	(75)
Cy/TBI + R after Ara-C containing mobilization	34	CR1/PR1	90 vs 33 for historical controls	At 4 yrs 83% vs 47%	At 4 yrs 87% vs 77%	Rituximab improves outcome by improving molecular remission	(72)
Yttrium-90(^{90}Y) + BEAM	13		18.4	68.4 months at 2 yrs	84.6% at 2 yrs	Feasible	(78)
BEAM / BEAC after augmented CHOP followed by high dose Ara-C + R	160	CR1/PR1		63% at a median follow up 3.8 yrs. — 63%, 67% if molecular remission	81% at 4 yrs	High dose Ara-C and R improved molecular response and outcome	(62)

CHOP, Cyclophosphamide, Adriamycin, Oncovin, Prednisone; ICE, Ifosfamide, Carboplatin, Etoposide; BEAM, Carmustine, Etoposide, Cytarabine, Melphalan; BEAC, Carmustine, Etoposide, Cytatabine, Cyclophosphamide R, Rituximab; CR1, First remission; PR1, First partial Remission; MRD, minimal residual disease; NR, not reached; EFS, Event free survival; Yrs, years; TBI, Total Body Irradiation, Cy, Cytoxan; ASCT, Autologous stem cell transplant; PB, peripheral blood; BM, Bone marrow, IFN-α = alpha interferon; Ara-C, Cytarabine;

they randomized patients to receive consolidative treatment with either an ASCT or conventional α-interferon maintenance. They demonstrated that the PFS at 2 years for patients undergoing the ASCT was 73% compared with 43% for those patients receiving maintenance α-interferon. After a follow-up of nearly 7 years (median follow-up 2.8 years), the 3-year survival after ASCT was 83% compared with 77% with α-interferon maintenance. Subgroup analysis demonstrated that those patients who were transplanted in CR did better than those who were transplanted in PR at the time of transplant. This is a recurring theme through many transplant studies in lymphoma in general. Further support for the use of ASCT in the up-front setting has been established by many other centers. The University of Nebraska reported on its experience of ASCT in MCL (63) and found that the 2-year EFS was 45% for patients who received less than three prior therapies versus 0%. In the Johns Hopkins' experience, having one or more relapses before transplant and primary refractory disease was associated with an inferior EFS (64). Collectively, these data suggest that ASCTs may provide their best benefit when used in first remission (65).

These and other smaller studies have established that high-dose chemotherapy and ASCT are best performed in the frontline setting in first remission. These trials have now established that cytoreduction followed by an ASCT in first remission is an accepted treatment paradigm for patients with MCL. Other risk factors that predict for better outcomes with ASCT include normal β_2-microglobulin, either at diagnosis or transplant (66). The recently published prospective series by the Nordic Lymphoma group (67) have reported that the Ki-67 index is the best single predictor of EFS in patients with MCL. On the other hand, bone marrow involvement, IPI score, or even the subtype of MCL has not been found to be of prognostic significance (68). Thus, chemotherapy sensitive disease and transplant in first remission may be the optimal strategies for incorporating ASCT in the treatment paradigm for patients with MCL (65,69).

Induction and Conditioning Regimens

The use of intensive regimens like HyperCVAD as initial induction therapy for MCL may improve the outcome of ASCT. Khouri et al. (66) reported impressive results with ASCT following HyperCVAD induction with a 5-year follow-up showing an OS and EFS of 77% and 43%, respectively. Historical comparisons between HyperCVAD and CHOP-like induction regimens have been reported by Vose et al. (68). For example, HyperCVAD ± rituximab before the transplant led to a PFS and OS of 78% and 98% at 3 years compared with 55% and 78%, respectively, with CHOP (± rituximab).

Perhaps some of the best results reported to date regarding the up-front treatment of MCL, though still early, come from the Nordic Lymphoma Group. Geisler et al. (67) recently reported that more intensive up-front programs containing high-dose cytarabine (HiDAC) were associated with superior PFS and OS. They compared their more recent results with a historical trial (MCL-1, 1996 to 2000) that administered four cycles of Maxi-CHOP (cyclophosphamide 1,200 g per m², doxorubicin 75 mg per m² on day 1, vincris-

tine 2 mg on day 1, and prednisone 100 mg on days 1–5), followed by stem cell harvest, and a BEAM (carmustine, etoposide, cytarabine, melphalan)/BEAC (carmustine, etoposide, cytarabine, cyclophosphamide)-based myeloablation and stem cell rescue. This approach resulted in a 50% EFS with continued relapses beyond 5 years. The MCL-1 Trial (2000 to 2006) alternated HiDAC (3 g per m²) after each cycle of MaxiCHOP, delivering now a total of three cycles each of MaxiCHOP and HiDAC, with rituximab built into the latter cycles of chemotherapy before ASCT. Once the cytoreduction was completed, patients underwent stem cell harvest, BEAM/BEAC myeloablation, and stem cell infusion. In MCL-2, 160 patients with MCL were treated in the study. With a median follow-up of 3.8 years, the EFS and OS were 61%, and 81%, respectively. These results, significantly better than other reported approaches, compelled the authors to conclude that this approach has potentially curative intent in patients with MCL, a concept not previously felt to be possible with standard cytotoxic chemotherapy approaches. Although promising, the results need to be viewed cautiously, given the nature of MCL to relapse late. Longer term follow-up will be essential before firm conclusions regarding the curability of the approach can be made. This important study also highlights the value of including rituximab in the initial regimen for MCL, and possibly underscores earlier concepts regarding the importance of HiDAC (67,70).

To date, there is no evidence for the superiority of one conditioning regimen over any other. Generally, total body irradiation (TBI)-based conditioning regimens are associated with better disease control in NHL, though there is more short- and long-term toxicity associated with radiation, particularly the risk of secondary malignancies. In MCL, only one study has suggested improved results with a TBI-containing regimen (71), whereas a subsequent analysis of the registry data where 43% of the patients had radiation as part of their conditioning did not show any difference in outcome (65). The experience at Johns Hopkins also failed to show a benefit in EFS of cyclophosphamide and total body irradiation (Cy/TBI) over busulfan-cyclophosphamide (Bu/Cy) conditioning in 58 patients with MCL. Of course, many of these studies employ a diversity of patients, including differences in disease state, which could conceivably alter the results.

The incorporation of rituximab into the initial therapy improves the likelihood of achieving a state of MRD measured by molecular methods, and may, improve the outcome of the subsequent transplant. Dreger et al. (72) reported a prospective trial of 34 patients with MCL who received CHOP induction followed by cytarabine, rituxan mobilization, and a TBI/Cy-based ASCT. The results were compared with historical controls in the same center treated on the same regimen except they did not receive rituximab. These results unequivocally demonstrated a benefit in favor of rituximab, with a 4-year EFS of 83% (plus rituximab) compared with 47% (no rituximab), and an OS of 87% versus 77% in favor of the rituximab-containing regimen. Other investigators have also confirmed that the addition of rituximab in the conditioning regimen improves the outcome not merely by enhancing the efficacy of the cytotoxic therapy, but also by providing some degree of in vivo purging (73,74). Data regarding the use of rituximab maintenance are limited, though some data suggest that it may improve disease-free survival (DFS) after ASCT. A randomized trial will be required to definitively establish the merits of maintenance rituximab, though one study reported >89% EFS at 3 years (73) in patients receiving maintenance therapy.

Minimal Residual State and Purging

The use of PCR has allowed the evaluation of MRD states in MCL. Achievement of MRD has become an important goal to improve the outcome of patients with MCL. Pott et al. (75) have reported on the MRD kinetics by quantitative PCR performed on blood or bone marrow within the first year after ASCT. They found that for patients who had a state of MRD negativity, the EFS was 92 months, and the median OS had not been reached. In contrast, patients who had detection of MRD within the first year exhibited an EFS and OS of 21 and 44 months, respectively. Reinfusion of tumor cells in the contaminated stem cell product is thought to be a likely cause of relapse after ASCT. This is based on the observation that a PCR-negative stem cell product at the time of infusion may lead to a better DFS. During the 1990s, ex vivo immunologic purging was used in an attempt to achieve a clean product, though this collective experience indicates that most patients still had a PCR-positive bone marrow or peripheral blood stem cell product (76) at the time of transplant. The incorporation of rituximab in the mobilization and conditioning regimen increases the probability of achieving a PCR-negative stem cell product. Several groups (67,72,77) have shown superior results of ASCT in their series and have demonstrated that the addition of rituximab improves molecular remissions.

Future Directions

Other strategies to improve the outcome of ASCT in MCL have included the use of tandem transplants (77), and the use of RIT (yttrium 90 or I tositumomab) in the conditioning regimen. The latter is particularly attractive because it incorporates radiation in the treatment program, which exploits the radiosensitivity of MCL. These approaches, however, have been reported to have less long-term effects of myelodysplasia and secondary leukemias, even though follow-up of these studies is short. Thus far, feasibility studies integrating both standard-dose and high-dose RIT into conditioning regimens have been performed (78). Sixteen patients with relapsed or refractory MCL were treated with the high-dose I131-tositumomab followed by etoposide, cyclophosphamide, and stem cell infusion (79). There were no treatment-related deaths, and with 19 months of follow-up, the 3-year PFS was 61% in this high-risk cohort.

In conclusion, for a young otherwise healthy patient, dose-intense induction chemotherapy followed by ASCT should be considered as up-front therapy with a goal to achieve a state of MRD. Randomized clinical trials are needed to answer important questions regarding the optimal chemotherapy and conditioning regimens. Additionally, newer active agents like bortezomib, and mTOR and histone deacetylase inhibitors will continue to be incorporated into conditioning regimens and stem cell infusion trials.

THE ROLE OF ALLOGENIC STEM CELL TRANSPLANTATION

Nonmyeloablative Transplants

Because ASCTs are not curative in MCL, the management of a patient with relapsed disease represents a major clinical challenge. For young otherwise healthy patients, allogeneic transplants have been explored as a therapeutic option to exploit the graft versus lymphoma effect for disease control. They are typically conducted in the setting of relapsed disease, usually after failing more conventional therapies or ASCT. In some cases, up-front allogeneic transplants have been attempted after the initial induction therapy, however, this tends to be restricted to cases where stem cell mobilization and collection have not been possible, or the patient had primary refractory disease. The literature consists of small single institution series that vary in patient characteristics, conditioning regimens, disease status, and other clinical variables. An attempt to understand the role of an allogeneic transplant in MCL requires one to analyze the available data with the following perspectives in mind.

Are Allogeneic Transplants Effective in Mantle Cell Lymphoma?

Certainly, this approach has been used in patients with MCL who have failed prior therapies, resulting in PFS and OS rates of around 50% at 3 years (as described in Table 19.8). Compared with these results, ASCT resulted in only 17% DFS at 3 years in patients with relapsed disease. However, an allogeneic stem cell transplant comes with a high treatment-related mortality rate of around 40% at 2 years. This therapy is also limited to patients who are under the age of 60, and have otherwise adequate cardiac, renal, and pulmonary functions due to the associated toxicities of a fully ablative regimen. Most of the patients reported in these series had either relapsed or primary refractory disease.

Is There a Graft versus Mantle Cell Lymphoma Effect?

The establishment of a graft versus MCL (GVL) effect requires the following elements: (a) a therapeutic benefit can be seen with a reduced intensity conditioning (RIC) regimen (80), (b) presence of graft versus host disease correlates with a decreased likelihood of disease relapse, (c) T-cell depleted transplants result in a high likelihood of relapse, and (d) that biopsy proven-relapsed disease can be successfully treated with withdrawal of immunosuppression and/or donor lymphocyte infusion. Although fully ablative allogeneic transplants have been performed in MCL (some of which are described in Table 19.8), there has been a shift toward RIC allogeneic transplants for MCL in the recent years. Khouri et al. (81) have reported an excellent EFS and OS of >80% at 3 years using a minimally intensive fludarabine-containing conditioning regimen in 22 patients. These patients experienced no up-front complications, with 0% mortality at day 100. All patients failed prior therapy, including five who had a prior ASCT. Out of the three patients who had disease progression, donor lymphocyte infusion was given to two patients, of whom one went into a

TABLE 19.8

SUMMARY OF REDUCED INTENSITY ALLOGENIC STEM CELL TRANSPLANTS FOR MCL

Preparative regimen	IMS	Patients (n)	Acute GvHD III–IV	Chronic GvHD	Transplant-related mortality	Relapse rated	PFS at 2 y	Reference
Fludarabine/CY/R and CYS/fludarabine/AraC	Tacro MTX	18	0%	36%	1/18	3/18	82%	(122)
TBI 200 cGy fludarabine plus	CSA MMF	33	30%	64%	24%	16%	60%	(69)
BEAM plus Alemtuzumab	CSA	5	0%	17%	12%	68%	18%	(131)
Fludarabine 150 Melphalan 140 Alemtuzumab	CSA	10	5%	7%	20%	50%	34%	(69)

BEAM (carmustine, etoposide, cytanabire, melphalan); CSA, cyclosporin; GvHD, graft versus host disease; IMS, immunosuppression.

complete sustained molecular remission, whereas the other experienced stable disease for >1 year. These observations illustrate the immunologic effects of the donor T cells, supporting the contention that a GVL effect is potentially therapeutic. More importantly, 66% of the patients were demonstrated to be in a molecular remission by PCR. This approach resulted in a graft versus host disease incidence of 35% and a mortality ratio of 13%.

Subsequently, Maris et al. (82) reported on the outcome of 33 patients with relapsed MCL using RIC. They reported a 2-year EFS and OS of 65% with a plateau in the survival curve, though the overall mortality was 24% at 2 years. Further proof of a GVL effect for MCL comes from registry data reported by Robinson et al. (83) from the European Group for Blood and Bone Marrow transplantation, in which 22 patients underwent a RIC allogeneic transplant. Most of the patients received in vivo T-cell depletion with alemtuzumab or antithymocyte globulin, and resulted in a PFS of 0% at 2 years. The lack of an immunologic response was attributed to disease progression in the majority of cases. Although rigorous data in the form of randomized trials are lacking, RIC is considered the preferred approach for a patient who is being considered for an allergenic transplant with a diagnosis of MCL. This strategy has the additional benefit of allowing this therapy to be considered for patients who are older than age 60 and may otherwise not qualify for a fully ablative allogeneic transplant.

Autologous versus Allogenic Stem Cell Transplant for Mantle Cell Lymphoma

For a young healthy patient with relapsed disease, a RIC-based allogenic transplant from a human leukocyte antigen identical donor is clearly the better option. There is no randomized trial comparing ASCT with allogeneic transplants in MCL. Some centers have reported their results with both autologous and allogeneic stem cell transplants in a comparative manner to clarify the various risks and benefits of these therapies. The transplant group at the University of Nebraska compared 17 patients undergoing ASCT with 17 patients who had a Cy/TBI-based allogeneic transplant. There was an increased percentage of patients with refractory disease in the group undergoing allogeneic transplant (65% vs. 44%), though the estimated 5-year relapse EFS and OS were similar in both the allogeneic and ASCT groups (44% vs. 39%) and (49% vs. 47%), respectively. The relapse rate was higher in the autologous group (56% vs. 21%), whereas the allogeneic group experienced a higher treatment-related mortality. The group at Johns Hopkins reported similar results when it presented the outcome of its ASCT versus its allogencic experience for MCL (64). More patients with relapsed or refractory disease were transplanted with an allogeneic donor, and this group exhibited a higher mortality of 58% compared with 26% in the ASCT group. The OS was 59% for both groups at 3 years. Although a direct comparison was never made between the two cohorts of patients, the benefit of both types of transplant was more evident in first remission. Thirty-three percent of the patients undergoing an allogeneic transplant received a T-cell-depleted graft.

Together, these results indicate that there is a GVL effect in MCL, and that there is high rate of mortality and morbidity associated with this approach. A fully ablative conditioning regimen is not needed, and even though there is no consensus on the best regimen, a reduced intensity approach seems adequate. If considered, these transplants should be performed early in the course of the disease.

Continued studies will need to explore and control for very specific features of these transplants to clarify the best ways to integrate allogeneic transplantation into the treatment of MCL. Clearly, despite what would be considered very aggressive therapy, curative intent may not yet be possible for patients with MCL. For this reason, new strategies that seek to exploit some of the unique biology underlying MCL are warranted.

Future Directions

Better understanding of the immunologic mechanisms involved in evoking the GVL effect will lead to improved therapeutic results with an allogeneic transplant. This could be a platform to further exploit the immunologic effects of some of the newer targeted agents that have shown activity in MCL, like histone deacetylase and mTOR inhibitors.

NONTRANSPLANT-RELATED TREATMENTS FOR RELAPSED OR REFRACTORY DISEASE

The treatment of relapsed or refractory MCL poses even more significant treatment dilemmas compared with sorting out the frontline treatment options. Needless to say, there is virtually no consensus on the optimal treatment program, though a number of general venues should be considered:

1. Novel drugs on clinical trial. Although certainly not an option for every patient, or physician, it is recommended that a clinical trial be considered the first option for all patients with relapsed or refractory MCL. Presently, there are now a number of promising new agents with clinically significant activity in MCL, many of which are moving into various up-front treatment programs.
2. Autologous stem cell or allogeneic stem cell transplant.
3. Conventional combination chemotherapy regimens, including, for example: ifosfamide, carboplatin, and etoposide; cyclophosphamide, etoposide, procarbazine, and prednisone; infusional therapy; fludarabine-containing regimens (fludarabine, cyclophosphamide, and mitoxantrone [FCM] with rituximab [R-FCM]); low-dose oral chemotherapy (PEP-C); and most recently, gemcitabine-based chemotherapy regimens.

Although it is difficult to proclaim that any one of these approaches is superior to any other, there are some new regimens that have not yet become part of the usual portfolio. Cytidine analogs are known to be active in the treatment NHL, especially MCL, either as a single agent or in combination. Exploratory phase II studies of gemcitabine in smaller phase II trials of patients with MCL have suggested activity across a panel of different lymphomas, including MCL. With these data as a basis, one phase II study evaluated the merits of adding cisplatin(P) to a regimen of gemcitabine(G) and dexamethasone (O)(PDG vs. DG) (1,000 mg per m^2 of gemcitabine on days 1 and 8; 40 mg per m^2 dexamethasone on days 1–4) with and without cisplatin (100 mg per m^2 on day 1). The ORR was 36% with DG and 44% with PDG, with a median PFS of 3 and 8.5 months, respectively. Overall, the regimen was felt to be well tolerated, with thrombocytopenia being the most common toxicity. In a similar study, Rodriguez et al. (84) reported an 85% ORR, with 64% CR, in patients with MCL receiving rituximab, gemcitabine (1,000 mg per m^2 on day 1 every 2 weeks) and oxaliplatin (100 mg per m^2 on day 1 every 2 weeks). With a median follow-up of 11 months, the OS and PFS at 12 months were 58% and 45%, respectively. These data, although based on small numbers of patients, suggest that the combination of gemcitabine and a platinum analog may be associated with very good response rates and PFS in patients with relapsed MCL.

In contrast to using conventional intravenous doses of active agents, Chao et al. (85) have employed a metronomic multidrug strategy for patients with MCL. They adapted the agents from the cyclophosphamide, etoposide, procarbazine, and prednisone-based regimen (CEPP), which includes these drugs being administered at a fixed 50-mg dose (except prednisone used at 20 mg). These medications were taken daily until the white blood count dropped to <3.0 × 10e9 per L. Based on a retrospective chart review of this experience in 22 patients, they reported an 82% ORR with a 46% CR rate. The median time on therapy was 17 months. Although no data were provided on PFS or OS, these data suggested that oral metronomic dosing of chemotherapy can obtain disease control and may be a highly effective palliative strategy. Studies investigating the molecular basis for the activity of this regimen in patients who have achieved frankly resistant disease are now focused on understanding the impact of metronomic therapy on angiogenesis.

Clearly, there are a host of treatments available for the patient with relapsed or refractory disease. The goals of therapy need to be carefully defined with each patient. Selection of an optimal treatment program must be tailored to the patients' comorbidities, and use of a regimen with the optimal potential for efficacy with the most favorable safety profile. Where possible, the choice of therapy should first consider enrollment in a clinical trial where feasible. Presently, there are enormous novel agents with promising activity in MCL, many of which we will address below.

NOVEL AGENTS IN DEVELOPMENT FOR MANTLE CELL LYMPHOMA

Over the last several years, there has been an explosion in the number of new drugs being tested in early phase clinical trials for patients with lymphoma. Several of these agents have already shown promising activity in MCL, justifying more detailed advanced-phase studies. Although there are many agents that deserve attention here, we can only discuss those compounds that are the most mature.

Proteasome Inhibitors: Bortezomib

The proteasome is one component of a larger intracellular pathway responsible for the degradation of >90% of all cytoplasmic protein, a pathway commonly referred to as the ubiquitin-proteasome pathway. The first step in the degradation of such proteins involves the highly regulated and coordinated cascade of enzymatic reactions that leads to the polyubiquitination of intracellular proteins targeted for degradation. The second major component of the pathway is the proteasome proper. The proteasome itself is composed of two components, one commonly referred to as the 20S proteasome, the second referred to as the 19S regulatory subunit. Collectively, they combine to form the 26S proteasome, which internally houses a number of different proteases responsible for degrading proteins into smaller irrelevant fragments (86).

Many theories abound regarding the potential mechanisms by which proteasome inhibition may lead to cell death or cell cycle arrest (87). One line of evidence has shown that inhibition of the proteasome leads to the accumulation of several cell cycle regulatory proteins, including the cyclins, and cdk inhibitors p21 and p27 (88). Another potentially important mechanism pertains to the potential for direct induction of apoptosis through the modulation of antiapoptotic and proapoptotic proteins, namely *bax* and *bik* (89,90). To date, the most extensively studied mechanism revolves around the inhibition of nuclear factor-κB (NF-κB) (91). Many investigators have demonstrated that inhibitors of the proteasome can block the activation of the transactivating transcription factor NF-κB by inhibiting the degradation of its cognate inhibitor, IκB. In normally quiescent cells, NF-κB exists in an inactivated form bound to IκB. In malignant cells, and in cells stimulated or stressed through exposure to various cytokines, cytotoxic drugs, viruses, oxidative triggers, or other mitogenic factors, IκB is phosphorylated by IκB kinase. This phosphorylation event then leads to ubiquitylation, leading to its eventual degradation, and liberation of active-free NF-κB. Free NF-κB then leads to a number of cellular effects that can include increased proliferation and inhibition of programmed cell death.

Bortezomib is a first in the class of drugs capable of inhibiting the proteasome, which has been recently approved by the US Food and Drug Administration for the treatment of multiple myeloma. In the phase I study of bortezomib in patients with advanced hematologic malignancies, one heavily treated patient with MCL achieved a durable PR (92). Subsequently, at least four single-agent phase II studies (93–97) with significant experiences in MCL have been reported. In the first of these studies, eligible patients were required to have either indolent or MCL (93). All patients were treated with a dose of 1.5 mg per m^2 on the typical day 1, 4, 8, and 11 schedule. Based on an update of the original data set (94), >26 evaluable patients with MCL had been treated, with an ORR of 54% (five with CR/CRu and nine patients with PR). The median PFS for these patients was nearly 1 year, despite the fact that these patients had received a median of three prior cytotoxic chemotherapy regimens (94). Several patients were induced into a second durable major remission on retreatment. A second study (95) designed in exactly the same way, save a broader set of inclusion criteria that allowed essentially all subtypes of NHL, reported on 29 evaluable patients with MCL, 12 of whom had a major response to bortezomib (41% response rate). Interestingly, six of these patients had a CR, six had a PR, and six attained stable disease. Although the follow-up in both studies was short, the median duration of response (DOR) thus far was approximately 6 months, in what would be considered a very heavily treated population of patients.

In addition to these phase II experiences, another study conducted by the National Cancer Institute of Canada in patients with untreated and relapsed MCL was reported (96). Of 28 evaluable patients, the ORR was 46%, which was identical in both arms. One patient had a CRu. The National Cancer Institute of Canada study differed from the previous studies in that it employed a lower dose of bortezomib (1.3 mg per m^2). Among those patients having a PR, the median time to response was about two cycles, with a duration of remission that ranged from 2.4 to 6.7 months (as of this report, and with unclear period of follow-up, the median DOR had not been attained). One European study in patients with both NHL and Hodgkin disease reported on 18 patients with MCL, of which one had a CR and

six PR following treatment with bortezomib at a dose of 1.3 mg per m^2 (97).

Based on the reproducible activity seen with bortezomib in MCL, a pivotal study of the agent was performed in a multicenter phase II study in 141 assessable patients (98). The ORR was 33%, which included 8% CR. The median DOR and time to progression were 9.2 and 6.2 months, respectively. After a follow-up period of 13.4 months, the median OS had not yet been reached. The toxicity profile was nearly identical to what has been published previously. These data supported the US Food and Drug Administration approval for bortezomib as the first drug ever approved specifically for the treatment of MCL. Presently, there are numerous studies exploring the merits of combining bortezomib with both conventional and novel therapies. Most recently, bortezomib has been found to mathematically synergize Bcl-2-targeted agents in MCL (99,100), which may offer a unique platform to integrate this platform regimen into the conventional treatment paradigms for MCL.

Mammalian Target of Rapamycin Inhibitors

The phosphoprotein kinase target of rapamycin is an important downstream component of the phosphoinositol-3 kinase/Akt pathway, playing an important role in the regulation of protein translation. Following mitogenic stimulation, activation of these kinases leads to the proliferation of both T and B cells. In fact, increased phosphatidylinositol-3 kinase activity in transgenic mice induces a T-cell lymphoproliferative disorder that leads to the early development of T-cell lymphoma (101–103). Constitutive activation of the Akt pathway has been described in many cell lines, including lymphomas, multiple myeloma, and solid tumors. The importance of this pathway is underscored by the spectrum of activity that various mTOR inhibitors (i.e., the rapamycin analogs, RAD-001) have against T and B cells. Rapamycin, temsirolimus (CCI-779), and everolimus (RAD-001) bind the FK506-binding protein-12 and interact with mTOR, inhibiting its phosphorylation capability, and halting the translation of proteins important for proliferation and survival.

One of the first reported experiences with an mTOR inhibitor in lymphoma was published by Witzig et al. (104). This single-agent phase II study of the rapamycin analog temsirolimus (CCI-779) was conducted in 35 patients with relapsed or refractory MCL. They administered the drug at a dose of 250 mg intravenously weekly. The median age of the study population was 70, and the median number of prior therapies was three (range one to 11). The ORR was 38%, including one complete response, whereas the median time to progression and DOR were 6.5 and 6.9 months, respectively. The most common toxicities were hematologic, including 71% of patients experiencing grade 3 and 11% experiencing grade 4 hematologic toxicities. A transient thrombocytopenia was the most frequent cause for dose reduction. Because of the significant hematologic toxicity, the trial was redesigned with a lower dose of temsirolimus (25 mg intravenously weekly). Of 29 patients enrolled, 28 were evaluable for efficacy. This patient population was remarkably similar to the earlier experience. The ORR at the lower dose level was 41%, with one

CR (105). The median time to progression and median DOR were 6 months. However, the incidence of hematologic toxicities was greatly reduced, now with only 50% of patients experiencing a grade 3 event, and 4% experiencing a grade 4 toxicity. These data demonstrated that a one-log reduction in the dose could appreciably reduce the hematologic toxicity without compromising the overall efficacy.

In addition to temsirolimus, everolimus (RAD001) has emerged as another mTOR inhibitor that has demonstrated important activity against MCL in both in vitro and in vivo assays of the disease (106). Early phase I and II experiences have established a safe dose of 10 mg once daily continuously in patients with hematologic malignancies. Interestingly, no dose-limiting toxicities were observed, though grade 3 toxicities potentially related to the study drug included hyperglycemia (22%), hypophosphatemia (7%), fatigue (7%), and anorexia and diarrhea in 4% of patients. Phase II studies of everolimus in MCL are now underway.

The "IMids" Thalidomide and Revlimid

Thalidomide, originally developed as a sedative in the 1950s, was found to have marked teratogenic properties when administered to pregnant women, which eventually restricted its general use and study. Over the past decade, the drug has been resurrected based on its promising activity in both multiple myeloma and in combination with clarithromycin (Biaxin) and dexamethasone in Waldenström macroglobulinemia (107). Thalidomide is an immunomodulatory agent whose exact mechanism of action in both liquid and solid tumors remains to be clarified. It is known to have a number of pleotrophic effects on cells, ranging from antiangiogenic to anti-inflammatory properties, presumably by altering cytokine production. One of the properties that may explain its efficacy in multiple myeloma revolves around its potential to modify the stromal environment in the bone marrow, leading to a perturbation in the signaling pathways responsible for plasma cell survival. Damaj et al. (108) published a case report on two patients with very heavily pretreated MCL who achieved major durable PRs on thalidomide, which in both cases was maintained for >1 year on maintenance therapy. Kaufmann et al. (109) conducted a phase II study of rituximab (375 mg per m^2 intravenously weekly times four weekly doses) given concomitantly with thalidomide (thalidomide 200 mg by mouth daily, with incremental dose increases to 400 mg on day 15). The therapy was administered until progression or relapse. Interestingly, 13 patients (81%) experienced an objective response, with five complete responses (31%). The median PFS was 20.4 months, and the estimated 3-year survival was 75%. In those patients attaining a response, the PFS after rituximab plus thalidomide was longer than that achieved with the preceding chemotherapy. Overall, the regimen was well tolerated, and the major adverse effects included two thromboembolic events and one grade 4 neutropenia. Of importance, however, is the fact that most of these patients were rituximab naive. Future studies exploring this strategy will need to understand the activity in patients who have already been treated with rituximab as part of their initial therapy.

Based on the anticancer properties of thalidomide, a significant research effort has been dedicated to the generation of new small molecules that are structurally similar though functionally distinct from thalidomide. These novel molecules, known as IMiDs, are orally bioavailable compounds with a safety profile that so far seems more favorable compared to thalidomide. One of these compounds, lenalidomide, has now completed phase I/II evaluation in multiple myeloma. These studies have demonstrated that lenalidomide is not associated with the same spectrum of toxicities associated with thalidomide (sedation, thromboembolic events, constipation, neuropathy), and has produced significant responses in patients with myeloma (110).

Over the past 2 years, an array of new phase II studies has begun to clarify the role of lenalidomide in patients with relapsed or refractory NHL. In one phase II study, patients were treated with 25 mg daily on days 1 through 21 of a 28-day cycle for 52 weeks or until disease progression (111). Forty-nine patients with a median age of 65 were treated on study, including 26 patients with diffuse large B-cell lymphoma, 15 with MCL, five with follicular NHL, and three with transformed NHL. Although the numbers are small, the ORR in MCL was 53%, among the highest for any subtype of NHL reported in the series. The median times to PR or CR were 1.9 and 4.3 months, respectively, whereas the estimated DOR was 6.2 months, and the median PFS was 4 months. Recently, several factors have emerged as critically important determinants of lenalidomide response (112). These include tumor burden, time from before rituximab, and absolute lymphocyte count (ALC). For example: (a) patients whose tumor burden was <50 cm^3 has an ORR of 32% compared with 21% for those with more tumor volume, (b) those whose time from prior rituximab was >230 days had a response rate of 40% compared with 16% of those who prior exposure was <230 days, and (c) those with an ALC >0.6e9 per L had an ORR of 35% compared with 6% for those whose ALC was <0.6e9 per L. These data suggest that the optimal patient population for these types of immunomodulatory treatments should have a relative smaller tumor burden and a more functional immune system, at least based on ALC and time from prior rituximab exposure. Clearly, the IMiDs are a class of molecules that warrant further attention in patients with MCL, especially in combination with other active agents like proteasome inhibitors, mTOR inhibitors, and perhaps even as a maintenance program following more traditional chemotherapy programs.

Cell Cycle-Dependent Kinase Inhibitors

Flavopiridol

One promising class of agents in development, which make perfect sense in targeting a disease characterized by gross dysregulation of a cyclin, are new drugs targeting cell cycle-specific biology. A number of new agents like PD-0332991, Roscovitine, AZ-703, and flavopiridol all have the potential to complement other MCL active drugs by directly addressing the intrinsic cell cycle regulatory defects associated with MCL (113–116). Flavopiridol is a large multicyclic compound originally derived from a plant indigenous to India known as *Dysoxylum binectariferum*. Flavopiridol is a pan cdk inhibitor that binds directly to the adenosine 5c-triphosphate-binding site at nanomolar concentrations of most cdks (117). It is a potent inhibitor of the cyclin D1, D2, D3-cdk4/6 complex, the cyclin E/cdk2 complex, the cyclin B/cdk1 complex, and the cyclin A/cdk 1complex. These properties have led it to be referred to as a pan-specific cdk inhibitor, which can potently induce apoptosis when used in combination with traditional chemotherapy drugs in a schedule-dependent manner (118–119).

Kouroukis et al. (120) published their experience with a phase II study of flavopiridol in 30 patients with MCL, of whom 11 had no prior therapy. The response rate was about 11% (three of 28 patients), with a median DOR of only about 3 months (range 3 to 13 months). Although these data suggested only modest activity, it is clear from the solid tumor experience to date that the merit of flavopiridol may not exist in its use as a single agent, but rather when combined rationally, and in a schedule-dependent manner, with other chemotherapeutic agents with known single-agent activity (117–118). These preclinical experiences suggest that flavopiridol has potent, schedule-dependent activity across many kinds of cancer. In addition, recent reports have suggested that the administration of the drug is very dependent on how the drug is infused, owing to it significant protein binding, and the need to achieve higher free concentrations in plasma (121).

New Derivatives of Familiar Drugs

Bendamustine

Although new to the United States, bendamustine is hardly a new drug. The agent is a novel compound consisting of a mechlorethamine group (nitrogen mustard), a benzimidazole ring, and a butyric acid side chain. Preclinical studies have demonstrated that bendamustine is capable of inducing DNA cross-linkings and double-strand breaks. In addition to the DNA damage similar to what more traditional alkylating agents are capable of mediating, bendamustine is capable of inhibiting mitotic checkpoints and inducing mitotic catastrophe. These features likely account for the drug's ability to induce apoptosis in relatively chemotherapy resistant cell lines.

A number of recent clinical studies have established the activity of bendamustine across a diverse range of lymphoid malignancies. In one single-agent phase II study, 76 patients received bendamustine at a dose of 120 mg per m^2 intravenously on days 1 and 2 of a 21-day cycle (122). Despite the heavily treated nature of this patient population, the ORR was 77%, including 34% CR or Cru. The median DOR was 6.7 months, though in 36% of the patients, the DOR exceeded 1 year. Although encouraging, none of these patients had MCL. In a subsequent study, Robinson et al. (123) conducted a phase II trial of bendamustine plus rituximab in patients with relapsed indolent B-cell and MCL. In this study, rituximab was administered at its usual dose on day 1, whereas bendamustine was given at a dose of 90 mg per m^2 on days 2 and 3 of a 28-day cycle. The ORR was 92%, which included 55% CR/Cru. The median DOR was 21 months, and the median PFS was 23 months. What was encouraging from this study was the fact that of the 12 patients with MCL, 92% of them responded to the combination, with none of the 12 experiencing progression of disease. Clearly, while early, and with only small numbers of patients treated thus far, there is a strong sense that bendamustine and rituximab may be a valuable regimen for the treatment of patients with relapsed or refractory MCL. Clearly, bendamustine and rituximab could form the backbone of future combinations in MCL. One trial is now evaluating the integration of bortezomib with bendamustine and rituximab in MCL. In addition, several reports combining bendamustine with mitoxantrone or cyclophosphamide, vincristine and prednisone have also shown promising activity across a variety of NHL subtypes, including small numbers of patients with MCL.

Pixantrone (BBR 2778)

Anthracyclines are among the most active drugs in the treatment of aggressive large cell lymphoma. These compounds as a class are known to inhibit topoisomerase II and intercalate into DNA. Unfortunately, however, anthracyclines are often associated with significant cardiotoxicity, especially when used in high cumulative doses. In preclinical models, pixantrone, a novel aza-anthracenedione, has demonstrated greater potency against P388 and L1210 leukemia cell lines compared with mitoxantrone and doxorubicin, and an in vivo murine model (124,125). These studies reported a more favorable therapeutic index with less cardiotoxicity. A small phase II experience in lymphoma was published on 33 patients with either diffuse large B-cell lymphoma ($n = 24$), MCL ($n = 7$), and two patients with transformed lymphoma (126). The ORR in this heavily treated population of patients was 27%. Of the seven patients with MCL, one patient had a CR that was durable for over 15 months. Five of the seven patients experienced a transient tumor reduction of >50%, which was unfortunately not durable. Although pixantrone may have some activity in MCL, its most promising venue for development may reside in the treatment of aggressive lymphomas, where biomarkers of activity like glutathione S-transferase-π and topoisomerase IIα levels may favor enhanced activity.

Recent reports have shown that topoisomerase IIα (topoIIα) correlated very strongly with OS in patients with MCL (127). Patients with low topoisomerase IIα expression (i.e., 0% to 10%) had a median OS of 49 months, whereas those patients with levels >10% had a median survival of only 17 months. A multivariate Cox regression analysis revealed that the expression of topoIIα was one of the most important prognostic factors in MCL ($p < 0.001$), superior to the IPI. In many ways, topoIIα can be viewed as yet another surrogate marker of proliferation, being most highly expressed in cells in the S phase of the cell cycle. Thus, these observations are not surprising, though do yield a potentially important rationale for using drugs of this class in MCL. In addition, Bennaceur-Griscelli et al. (128) reported that the level of glutathione-S-transferase-π expression in MCL was significantly higher than that typically seen in diffuse large B-cell lymphoma or follicular lymphoma. Interestingly, glutathione-S-transferase-π is located at 11q13 and is coamplified with the cyclin D1 gene in the same amplicon, which may account for some of the intrinsic chemotherapy resistance in MCL. Given that pixantrone produces its cytotoxic effects through the inhibition of topoisomerase II by inducing double-strand breaks and intercalating into DNA, interpreting these results in the context of these important prognostic molecular markers may afford new opportunities to tailor some of these new drugs to an individual's particular subtype of MCL.

Radioimmunotherapy

The development of monoclonal antibodies armed with a radioisotope offer yet another new and promising opportunity to impact on the natural history of MCL. Integral to this effort is the widely recognized belief that MCL is among one of the most radiosensitive lymphomas. Although the experiences to date in MCL with RIT are still limited, several studies have begun to establish at least feasibility. For example, one study in heavily pretreated patients ($n = 15$) treated with ^{90}Y-ibritumomab tiuxetan (Zevalin) showed an ORR of approximately 33%, which included three CRs (129). Another study seeking to integrate ^{131}I-tositumomab into standard CHOP-based chemotherapy gave the RIT first followed by the chemotherapy (130). The ORR to the RIT alone was about 75%, including about 38% CRs ($n = 16$). After the CHOP (11 evaluable), 91% of patients had achieved a major remission, including 73% CRs. Although this experience is small, future efforts will focus on the optimal way of integrating RIT into the conventional treatment paradigms for MCL.

FUTURE DIRECTIONS

In a relatively short period of time, MCL has gone from a state of relative anonymity to a state of unprecedented attention. In parallel, new developments in understanding the unique biology that defines MCL have been accompanied by new breakthroughs in identifying new agents with promising activity. Interestingly, it has been the empirical observations from early phase clinical trials that have helped identify what biologic processes in MCL deserve more focused attention, as has been shown with drugs that target the proteasome and mTOR. As with most developments in cancer medicine, promising observations made in patients with relapsed and refractory disease begin to form the basis for moving these therapies gradually into the frontline treatment programs. For example, if peripheral blood stem cell transplants in first remission prolong the PFS of patients, then how will the integration of potentially active drugs with novel mechanisms of action change that natural history, either by using the agents together, or in sequential fashion? Likewise, if the available evidence suggests a true GVL effect in the allogeneic transplant setting, how can these T-cell-based approaches be exploited earlier to raise our hopes of therapies with even greater promise? Clearly, the strategy in treating challenging diseases like MCL requires a careful, methodic approach that emerges gradually with time. Identify the most promising approaches, then begin to integrate them logically into the available treatment paradigms with the most promise. Unquestionably, however, it is the parallel commitment to understanding the unique biology of MCL, coupled with a commitment to focusing our early drug discovery and development efforts on the disease, that will lead to the new breakthroughs that will offer our patients the greatest hope.

References

1. Jemal A, Murray T, Ward E, et al. Cancer statistics, 2005. CA Cancer J Clin 2005;55:10–30.
2. Fisher RI, Dahlberg S, Nathwani BN, et al. A clinical analysis of two indolent lymphoma entities: mantle cell lymphoma and marginal zone lymphoma (including the mucosa-associated lymphoid tissue and monocytoid B-cell subcategories): a Southwest Oncology Group study. Blood 1995;85:1075–1082.
3. Zhou Y, Wang H, Fang W , et al. Incidence trends of mantle cell lymphoma in the United States between 1992 and 2004. Cancer 2008;113:791–798.
4. Zucca E, Roggero E, Pinotti G, et al. Patterns of survival in mantle cell lymphoma. Ann Oncol 1995;6:257–262.
5. Teodorovic I, Pittaluga S, Kluin-Nelemans JC, et al, Efficacy of four different regimens in 64 mantle-cell lymphoma cases: clinicopathologic comparison with 498 other non-Hodgkin's lymphoma subtypes. European Organization for the Research and Treatment of Cancer Lymphoma Cooperative Group. J Clin Oncol 1995;13:2819–2826.
6. Bosch F, Lopez-Guillermo A, Campo E, et al. Mantle cell lymphoma: presenting features, response to therapy, and prognostic factors. Cancer 1998;82:567–575.
7. Matutes E, Parry-Jones N, Brito-Babapulla V, et al. The leukemic presentation of mantle-cell lymphoma: disease features and prognostic factors in 58 patients. Leuk Lymphoma 2004;45:2007–2015.
8. Berger F, Felman P, Sonet A, et al. Nonfollicular small B-cell lymphomas: a heterogeneous group of patients with distinct clinical features and outcome. Blood 1994;83:2829–2835.
9. Norton AJ, Mattews J, Pappa V, et al. Mantle cell lymphoma: natural history defined in a serially biopsied population over a 20-year period. Ann Oncol 1995;6:249–256.
10. Pittaluga S, Wlodarska I, Stul MS, et al. Mantle cell lymphoma: a clinicopathological study of 55 cases. Histopathology 1995;26:17–24.
11. Velders GA, Kluin-Nelemans JC, De Boer CJ, et al. Mantle-cell lymphoma: a population-based clinical study. J Clin Oncol 1996;14:1269–1274.
12. Majlis A, Pugh WC, Rodriguez MA, et al. Mantle cell lymphoma: correlation of clinical outcome and biologic features with three histologic variants. J Clin Oncol 1997;15:1664–1671.
13. Hiddemann W, Unterhalt M, Herrmann R, et al. Mantle-cell lymphomas have more widespread disease and a slower response to chemotherapy compared with follicle-center lymphomas: results of a prospective comparative analysis of the German Low-Grade Lymphoma Study Group. J Clin Oncol 1998;16:1922–1930.
14. Ferrer A, Salaverria I, Bosch F, et al. Leukemic involvement is a common feature in mantle cell lymphoma.. Cancer 2007;109:2473–2480.
15. Valdez R, Kroft SH, Ross CW, et al. Cerebrospinal fluid involvement in mantle cell lymphoma. Mod Pathol 2002;15:1073–1079.
16. Weisenburger DD, Kim H, Rappaport H, et al. Mantle-zone lymphoma: a follicular variant of intermediate lymphocytic lymphoma. Cancer 1982;49:1429–1438.
17. Palutke M, Eisenberg L, Mirchandani I, et al. Malignant lymphoma of small cleaved lymphocytes of the follicular mantle zone. Blood 1982;59:317–322.
18. Weisenburger DD, Armitage JO, et al. Mantle cell lymphoma—an entity comes of age. Blood 1996;87:4483–4494.
19. Raffeld M, Jaffe ES. bcl-1, t(11;14), and mantle cell-derived lymphomas. Blood 1991;78:259–263.
20. Banks PM, Chan J, Cleary ML, et al. Mantle cell lymphoma. A proposal for unification of morphologic, immunologic, and molecular data. Am J Surg Pathol 1992;16:637–640.
21. Van Den Berghe H, Parloir C, David G, et al. A new characteristic karyotypic anomaly in lymphoproliferative disorders. Cancer 1979;44:188–195.
22. Tsujimoto Y, Yunis J, Onorato-Showe L, et al. Molecular cloning of the chromosomal breakpoint of B-cell lymphomas and leukemias with the t(11;14) chromosome translocation. Science 1984;224:1403–1406.
23. Weisenburger DD, Sanger WG, Armitage JO, et al. Intermediate lymphocytic lymphoma: immunophenotypic and cytogenetic findings. Blood 1987;69:1617–1621.
24. Vandenberghe E, De Wolf-Peeters C, Van Krieken JH, et al. Translocation (11;14): a cytogenetic anomaly associated with B-cell lymphomas of non-follicle centre cell lineage. J Pathol 1991;163:13–18.
25. Medeiros LJ, Van Krieken JH, Jaffe ES, et al. Association of bcl-1 rearrangements with lymphocytic lymphoma of intermediate differentiation. Blood 1990;76:2086–2090.
26. Williams ME, Meeker TC, Swerdlow SH. Rearrangement of the chromosome 11 bcl-1 locus in centrocytic lymphoma: analysis with multiple breakpoint probes. Blood 1991;78:493–498.
27. Williams ME, Westermann CD, Swerdlow SH. Genotypic characterization of centrocytic lymphoma: frequent rearrangement of the chromosome 11 bcl-1 locus. Blood 1990;76:1387–1391.
28. Rimokh R, Berger F, Cornillet P, et al. Break in the BCL1 locus is closely associated with intermediate lymphocytic lymphoma subtype. Genes Chromosomes Cancer 1990;2:223–226.
29. Leroux D, Le Marc'Hadour F, Gressin R, et al. Non-Hodgkin's lymphomas with t(11;14)(q13;q32): a subset of mantle zone/intermediate lymphocytic lymphoma? Br J Haematol 1991;77:346–353.
30. Duggan MJ, Weisenburger DD, Ye YL, et al. Mantle zone lymphoma. A clinicopathologic study of 22 cases. Cancer 1990;66:522–529.
31. Barista I, Romaguera JE, Cabanillas F, et al. Mantle-cell lymphoma. Lancet Oncol 2001;2:141–148.

32. Chiarle R, Budel LM, Skolink J, et al. Increased proteasome degradation of cyclin-dependent kinase inhibitor p27 is associated with a decreased overall survival in mantle cell lymphoma. *Blood* 2000;95:619–626.

33. Lim MS, Adamson A, Lin Z, et al. Expression of Skp2, a p27(Kip1) ubiquitin ligase, in malignant lymphoma: correlation with p27(Kip1) and proliferation index. *Blood* 2002;100:2950–2956.

34. Bogner C, Ringshausen I, Schneller F, et al. Inhibition of the proteasome induces cell cycle arrest and apoptosis in mantle cell lymphoma cells. *Br J Haematol* 2003;122:260–268.

35. Louie DC, Offit K, Jaslow R, et al. p53 overexpression as a marker of poor prognosis in mantle cell lymphomas with t(11;14)(q13;q32). *Blood* 1995;86:2892–2899.

36. Greiner TC, Moynihan MJ, Chan WC, et al. p53 mutations in mantle cell lymphoma are associated with variant cytology and predict a poor prognosis. *Blood* 1996;87:4302–4310.

37. Hernandez L, Fest T, Cazorla M, et al. p53 gene mutations and protein overexpression are associated with aggressive variants of mantle cell lymphomas. *Blood* 1996;87:3351–3359.

38. Gronbaek K, Nedergaard T, Andersen MK, et al. Concurrent disruption of cell cycle associated genes in mantle cell lymphoma: a genotypic and phenotypic study of cyclin D1, p16, p15, p53 and pRb. *Leukemia* 1998;12:1266–1271.

39. Camacho E, Hernandez L, Hernandez S, et al. ATM gene inactivation in mantle cell lymphoma mainly occurs by truncating mutations and missense mutations involving the phosphatidylinositol-3 kinase domain and is associated with increasing numbers of chromosomal imbalances. *Blood* 2002;99:238–244.

40. Rosenwald A, Wright G, Wiestner A, et al. The proliferation gene expression signature is a quantitative integrator of oncogenic events that predicts survival in mantle cell lymphoma. *Cancer Cell* 2003;3:185–197.

41. Moller MB, Pedersen NT, Christensen BE. Mantle cell lymphoma: prognostic capacity of the Follicular Lymphoma International Prognostic Index. *Br J Haematol* 2006;133:43–49.

42. Hoster E, Dreyling M, Klapper W, et al. A new prognostic index (MIPI) for patients with advanced-stage mantle cell lymphoma. *Blood* 2008;111:558–565.

43. Katzenberger T, Petzoldt C, Holler S, et al. The Ki67 proliferation index is a quantitative indicator of clinical risk in mantle cell lymphoma. *Blood* 2006;107:3407.

44. Determann O, Hoster E, Ott G, et al. Ki-67 predicts outcome in advanced-stage mantle cell lymphoma patients treated with anti-CD20 immunochemotherapy: results from randomized trials of the European MCL Network and the German Low Grade Lymphoma Study Group. *Blood* 2008;111:2385–2387.

45. Hartmann E, Fernandez V, Moreno V, et al. Five-Gene Model to Predict Survival in Mantle-Cell Lymphoma Using Frozen or Formalin-Fixed, Paraffin-Embedded Tissue. *J Clin Oncol* 2008.

46. Meusers P, Engelhard M, Bartels H, et al. Multicentre randomized therapeutic trial for advanced centrocytic lymphoma: anthracycline does not improve the prognosis. *Hematol Oncol* 1989;7:365–380.

47. Howard OM, Gribben JG, Neuberg DS, et al. Rituximab and CHOP induction therapy for newly diagnosed mantle-cell lymphoma: molecular complete responses are not predictive of progression-free survival. *J Clin Oncol* 2002;20:1288–1294.

48. Lenz G, Dreyling M, Hoster E, et al. Immunochemotherapy with rituximab and cyclophosphamide, doxorubicin, vincristine, and prednisone significantly improves response and time to treatment failure, but not long-term outcome in patients with previously untreated mantle cell lymphoma: results of a prospective randomized trial of the German Low Grade Lymphoma Study Group (GLSG). *J Clin Oncol* 2005;23:1984–1992.

49. Khouri IF, Romaguera J, Kantarjian H, et al. Hyper-CVAD and high-dose methotrexate/cytarabine followed by stem-cell transplantation: an active regimen for aggressive mantle-cell lymphoma. *J Clin Oncol* 1998;16:3803–3809.

50. Khouri IF, Saliba R, Hosing C, et al. Long-term follow-up of autologous stem cell transplantation in first remission in patients with diffuse mantle cell lymphoma. *Ann Oncol* 2002;13.

51. Romaguera JE, Khouri IF, Kantarjian HM, et al. Untreated aggressive mantle cell lymphoma: results with intensive chemotherapy without stem cell transplant in elderly patients. *Leuk Lymphoma* 2000;39:77–85.

52. Romaguera J, Cabanillas F, Dang NH, et al. Mantle cell lymphoma (MCL)—high rates of complete remission (CR) and prolonged failure-free survival (FFS) with Rituxan-HyperCVAD (R-HCVAD) without stem cell transplant (SCT) 2001;98:726a [Abstract 3030].

53. Epner EM, Unger J, Miller T, et al. A multi center trial of hyperCVAD+rituxan in patients with newly diagnosed mantle cell lymphoma. *Blood* 2007;110:. Abstract 387.

54. Kahl BS, Longo WL, Eickhoff JC, et al. Maintenance rituximab following induction chemoimmunotherapy may prolong progression-free survival in mantle cell lymphoma: a pilot study from the Wisconsin Oncology Network. *Ann Oncol* 2006;17:1418–1423.

55. Decaudin D, Bosq J, Tertian G, et al. Phase II trial of fludarabine monophosphate in patients with mantle-cell lymphomas. *J Clin Oncol.* 1998;16:579–583.

56. Foran JM, Rohatiner AZ, Coiffer B, et al. Multicenter phase II study of fludarabine phosphate for patients with newly diagnosed lymphoplasmacytoid lymphoma, Waldenstrom's macroglobulinemia, and mantle-cell lymphoma. *J Clin Oncol.* 1999;17:546–553.

57. Rummel MJ, Chow KU, Karakas T, et al. Reduced-dose cladribine (2-CdA) plus mitoxantrone is effective in the treatment of mantle-cell and low-grade non-Hodgkin's lymphoma. *Eur J Cancer.* 2002;38:1739–1746.

58. Forstpointner R, Dreyling M, Repp R, et al. The addition of rituximab to a combination of fludarabine, cyclophosphamide, mitoxantrone (FCM) significantly increases the response rate and prolongs survival as compared with FCM alone in patients with relapsed and refractory follicular and mantle cell lymphomas: results of a prospective randomized study of the German Low-Grade Lymphoma Study Group. *Blood.* 2004;104:3064–3071.

59. Zinzani PL, Magagnoli M, Moretti L, et al. Randomized trial of fludarabine versus fludarabine and idarubicin as frontline treatment in patients with indolent or mantle-cell lymphoma. *J Clin Oncol.* 2000;18:773–779.

60. Cohen BJ, Moskowitz C, Straus D, et al. Cyclophosphamide/fludarabine (CF) is active in the treatment of mantle cell lymphoma. *Leuk Lymphoma.* 2001;42:1015–1022.

61. Forstpointner R, Unterhalt M, Dreyling M, et al. Maintenance therapy with rituximab leads to a significant prolongation of response duration after salvage therapy with a combination of rituximab, fludarabine, cyclophosphamide, and mitoxantrone (R-FCM) in patients with recurring and refractory follicular and mantle cell lymphomas: Results of a prospective randomized study of the German Low Grade Lymphoma Study Group (GLSG). *Blood.* 2006;108:4003–4008.

62. Dreyling M, Lenz G, Hoster E, et al. Early consolidation by myeloablative radiochemotherapy followed by autologous stem cell transplantation in first remission significantly prolongs progression-free survival in mantle cell lymphoma—results of a prospective randomized trial of the European MCL network. *Blood* 2004.

63. Vose JM, Bierman PJ, Weisenburger DD, et al. Autologous hematopoietic stem cell transplantation for mantle cell lymphoma. *Biol Blood Marrow Transplant* 2000;6:640–645.

64. Kasamon YL, Jones RJ, Diehl LF, et al. Outcomes of autologous and allogeneic blood or marrow transplantation for mantle cell lymphoma. *Biol Blood Marrow Transplant* 2005;11:39–46.

65. Vandenberghe E, Ruiz de Elvira C, Loberiza F, et al. Outcome of autologous transplantation for mantle cell lymphoma: a study by the European Blood and Bone Marrow Transplant and Autologous Blood and Marrow Transplant Registries. *Br J Haematol* 2003;120:793–800.

66. Khouri IF, Saliba RM, Okoroji GJ, et al. Long-term follow-up of autologous stem cell transplantation in patients with diffuse mantle cell lymphoma in first disease remission: the prognostic value of beta2-microglobulin and the tumor score. *Cancer* 2003;98:2630–2635.

67. Geisler CH, Elonen E, Kolstad A, et al. Mantle Cell Lymphoma Can Be Cured by Intensive Immunochemotherapy With In-Vivo Purged Stem-Cell Support; Final Report Of The Nordic Lymphoma Group MCL2 Study. *Blood* 2007;110: Abstract LB1.

68. Vose J, Loberiza F, Bierman P, et al. Mantle cell lymphoma (MCL): induction therapy with HyperCVAD/high dose methotrexate and cytarabine (M-C) (±rituximab) improves results of autologous stem cell transplant in first remission.. *Journal of Clinical Oncology, 2006 ASCO Annual Meeting Proceeding* 2006; Part I. 24,: Abstract 7511.

69. Popplewell LL, Nademanee A, Carter N, et al. Autologous vs allogeneic cell transplantation for mantle cell lymphoma (MCL): outcomes over a 10-year period at City of Hope. *Blood* 2004;104:. Abstract 894.

70. Lefrere F, Delmer A, Suzan F, et al. Sequential chemotherapy by CHOP and DHAP regimens followed by high-dose therapy with stem cell transplantation induces a high rate of complete response and improves event-free survival in mantle cell lymphoma: a prospective study. *Leukemia* 2002;16:587–593.

71. Milpied N, Gaillard F, Moreau P, et al. High-dose therapy with stem cell transplantation for mantle cell lymphoma: results and prognostic factors, a single center experience. *Bone Marrow Transplant* 1998;22:645–650.

72. Dreger P, Rieger M, Seyfarth B, et al. Rituximab-augmented myeloablation for first-line autologous stem cell transplantation for mantle cell lymphoma: effects on molecular response and clinical outcome. *Haematologica* 2007;92:42–49.

73. Mangel J, Leitch HA, Connors JM, et al. Intensive chemotherapy and autologous stem-cell transplantation plus rituximab is superior to conventional chemotherapy for newly diagnosed advanced stage mantle-cell lymphoma: a matched pair analysis. *Ann Oncol* 2004;15:283–290.

74. Thieblemont C, Antal D, Lacotte-Thierry L, et al. Chemotherapy with rituximab followed by high-dose therapy and autologous stem cell transplantation in patients with mantle cell lymphoma. *Cancer* 2005;104:1434–1441.

75. Pott C, Schrader C, Gesk S, et al. Quantitative assessment of molecular remission after high-dose therapy with autologous stem cell transplantation predicts long-term remission in mantle cell lymphoma. *Blood* 2006;107:2271–2278.

76. Anderson JE, Gooley TA, Schoch G, et al. Stem cell transplantation for secondary acute myeloid leukemia: evaluation of transplantation as initial therapy or following induction chemotherapy. *Blood* 1997;89:2578–2585.

77. Gianni AM, Magni M, Martelli M, et al. Long-term remission in mantle cell lymphoma following high-dose sequential chemotherapy and in vivo rituximab-purged stem cell autografting (R-HDS regimen). *Blood* 2003;102:749–755.

78. Krishnan A, Nademanee A, Fung HC, et al. Phase II trial of a transplantation regimen of yttrium-90 ibritumomab tiuxetan and high-dose chemotherapy in patients with non-Hodgkin's lymphoma. *J Clin Oncol* 2008;26:90–95.

79. Gopal AK, Rajendran JG, Petersdorf SH, et al. High-dose chemo-radio-immunotherapy with autologous stem cell support for relapsed mantle cell lymphoma. *Blood* 2002;99:3158–3162.

80. Butcher BW, Collins RH Jr, The graft-versus-lymphoma effect: clinical review and future opportunities. *Bone Marrow Transplant* 2005;36:1–17.

81. Khouri IF, Lee MS, Saliba RM, et al. Nonablative allogeneic stem-cell transplantation for advanced/recurrent mantle-cell lymphoma. *J Clin Oncol* 2003;21:4407–4412.

82. Maris MB, Sandmaier BM, Storer BE, et al. Allogeneic hematopoietic cell transplantation after fludarabine and 2 Gy total body irradiation for relapsed and refractory mantle cell lymphoma. *Blood* 2004;104:3535–3542.

83. Robinson SP, Goldstone AH, Mackinnon S, et al. Chemoresistant or aggressive lymphoma predicts for a poor outcome following reduced-intensity allogeneic progenitor cell transplantation: an analysis from the Lymphoma Working Party of the European Group for Blood and Bone Marrow Transplantation. *Blood* 2002;100:4310–4316.

84. Rodriguez J, Gutierrez A, Palacios A, et al. Rituximab, gemcitabine and oxaliplatin: an effective regimen in patients with refractory and relapsing mantle cell lymphoma. *Leuk Lymphoma* 2007;48:2172–2178.

85. Chao NJ, Rosenberg SA, Horning SJ. CEPP(B): an effective and well-tolerated regimen in poor-risk, aggressive non-Hodgkin's lymphoma. *Blood* 1990;76:1293–1298.

86. O'Connor OA. The emerging role of bortezomib in the treatment of indolent non-Hodgkin's and mantle cell lymphomas. *Curr Treat Options Oncol* 2004;5:269–281.

87. Paoluzzi L O'Connor OA. Mechanistic rationale and clinical evidence for the efficacy of proteasome inhibitors against indolent and mantle cell lymphomas. *BioDrugs* 2006;20:13–23.

88. Pagano M, Tam SW, Theodoras AM, et al. Role of the ubiquitin-proteasome pathway in regulating abundance of the cyclin-dependent kinase inhibitor p27. *Science* 1995;269:682–685.

89. Marshansky V, Wang X, Bertrand R, et al. Proteasomes modulate balance among proapoptotic and antiapoptotic Bcl-2 family members and compromise functioning of the electron transport chain in leukemic cells. *J Immunol* 2001;166:3130–3142.

90. Ling YH, Liebes L, Ng B, et al. PS-341, a novel proteasome inhibitor, induces Bcl-2 phosphorylation and cleavage in association with G2-M phase arrest and apoptosis. *Mol Cancer Ther* 2002;1;841–849.

91. Palombella VJ, Conner EM, Fuseler JW, et al. Role of the proteasome and NF-kappaB in streptococcal cell wall-induced polyarthritis. *Proc Natl Acad Sci U S A* 1998;95:15671–15676.

92. Orlowski RZ, Stinchcombe TE, Mitchell BS, et al. Phase I trial of the proteasome inhibitor PS-341 in patients with refractory hematologic malignancies. *J Clin Oncol* 2002;20:4420–4427.

93. O'Connor OA, Wright J, Moskowitz C, et al. Phase II clinical experience with the novel proteasome inhibitor bortezomib in patients with indolent non-Hodgkin's lymphoma and mantle cell lymphoma. *J Clin Oncol* 2005;23:676–684.

94. O'Connor OA, Moskowitz, C., Portlock, C. et al. Patients with chemotherapy-refractory mantle cell lymphoma experience high response rates and identical progression-free survivals compared with patients with relapsed disease following treatment with single agent bortezomib: results of a multicentre Phase 2 clinical trial. *Br. J. Hematology* 2009;145:34–39.

95. Goy A, Younes, A., McLaughlin, P., et al. Phase II study of proteasome inhibitor bortezomib in relapsed or refractory B-cell non-Hodgkin's lymphoma. *J. Clin. Oncol.* 2005;23:667–675.

96. Belch A, Kouroukis, C.T., Crump, M, et al. A Phase II study of bortezomib in mantle cell lymphoma. *Ann. Oncol.* 2007;18: 116–121.

97. Strauss S, Maharaj. L., Hoare, S. Bortezomib therapy in patients with relapsed or refractory lymphoma: potential correlation of in vitro sensitivity and tumor necrosis factor alpha response with clinical activity. *J. Clin. Oncol.* 2006;24: 2105–2112.

98. Fisher RI, Bernstein SH, Kahl BS, et al. Multicenter phase II study of bortezomib in patients with relapsed or refractory mantle cell lymphoma. *J Clin Oncol* 2006;24:4867–4874.

99. Paoluzzi L, Gonen M, Gardner JR, et al. Targeting Bcl-2 family members with the BH3 mimetic AT-101 markedly enhances the therapeutic effects of chemotherapeutic agents in in vitro and in vivo models of B-cell lymphoma. *Blood* 2008.

100. Perez-Galan P, Roue G, Villamor N, et al. The BH3-mimetic GX15-070 synergizes with bortezomib in mantle cell lymphoma by enhancing Noxa-mediated activation of Bak. *Blood* 2007;109:4441–4449.

101. Podsypanina K, Lee RT, Politis C, et al. An inhibitor of mTOR reduces neoplasia and normalizes p70/S6 kinase activity in Pten+/- mice. *Proc Natl Acad Sci U S A* 2001;98:10320–10325.

102. Cantley LC. The phosphoinositide 3-kinase pathway. *Science* 2002;296:1655–1657.

103. Sekulic A, Hudson CC, Homme JL, et al. A direct linkage between the phosphoinositide 3-kinase-AKT signaling pathway and the mammalian target of rapamycin in mitogen-stimulated and transformed cells. *Cancer Res* 2000;60:3504–3513.

104. Witzig TE, Geyer SM, Ghobrial I, et al. Phase II trial of single-agent temsirolimus (CCI-779) for relapsed mantle cell lymphoma. *J Clin Oncol* 2005;23:5347–5356.

105. Ansell SM, Inwards DJ, Rowland KM, Jr., et al. Low-dose, single-agent temsirolimus for relapsed mantle cell lymphoma: a phase 2 trial in the North Central Cancer Treatment Group. *Cancer* 2008;113:508–514.

106. Haritunians T, Mori A, O'Kelly J, et al. Antiproliferative activity of RAD001 (everolimus) as a single agent and combined with other agents in mantle cell lymphoma. *Leukemia* 2007;21:333–339.

107. Coleman M, Leonard J, Lyons L, et al. Treatment of Waldenstrom's macroglobulinemia with clarithromycin, low-dose thalidomide, and dexamethasone. *Semin Oncol* 2003;30:270–274.

108. Damaj G, Lefrere F, Delarue R, et al. Thalidomide therapy induces response in relapsed mantle cell lymphoma. *Leukemia* 2003;17:1914–1915.

109. Kaufmann H, Raderer M, Woehrer S, et al. Anti-tumor activity of rituximab plus thalidomide in patients with relapsed/refractory mantle cell lymphoma. *Blood* 2004;104:2269–2271.

110. Rajkumar SV, Hayman SR, Lacy MQ, et al. Combination therapy with lenalidomide plus dexamethasone (Rev/Dex) for newly diagnosed myeloma. *Blood* 2005;106:4050–4053.

111. Wiernik PH, Lossos IS, Tuscano JM, et al. Lenalidomide monotherapy in relapsed or refractory aggressive non-Hodgkin's lymphoma. *J Clin Oncol* 2008.

112. Czuczman MS, Reeder CB, Polikoff J, et al. International study of lenalidomide in relapsed/refractory aggressive non-Hodgkin's lymphoma. *J Clin Oncol* 2008;26:. abstr 8509.

113. Marzec M, Kasprzycka M, Lai R, et al. Mantle cell lymphoma cells express predominantly cyclin D1a isoform and are highly sensitive to selective inhibition of CDK4 kinase activity. *Blood* 2006;108:1744–1750.

114. Cai D, Byth KF, Shapiro GI. AZ703, an imidazo[1,2-a]pyridine inhibitor of cyclin-dependent kinases 1 and 2, induces E2F-1-dependent apoptosis enhanced by depletion of cyclin-dependent kinase 9. *Cancer Res* 2006;66:435–444.

115. Fry DW, Harvey PJ, Keller PR, et al. Specific inhibition of cyclin-dependent kinase 4/6 by PD 0332991 and associated antitumor activity in human tumor xenografts. *Mol Cancer Ther* 2004;3:1427–1438.

116. Lacrima K, Valentini A, Lambertini C, et al. In vitro activity of cyclin-dependent kinase inhibitor CYC202 (Seliciclib, R-roscovitine) in mantle cell lymphomas. *Ann Oncol* 2005;16:1169–1176.

117. Kaur G, Stetler-Stevenson M, Sebers S, et al. Growth inhibition with reversible cell cycle arrest of carcinoma cells by flavone L86-8275. *J Natl Cancer Inst* 1992;84:1736–1740.

118. Motwani M, Jung C, Sirotnak FM, et al. Augmentation of apoptosis and tumor regression by flavopiridol in the presence of CPT-11 in Hct116 colon cancer monolayers and xenografts. *Clin Cancer Res* 2001;7:4209–4219.

119. Motwani M, Rizzo C, Sirotnak F, et al. Flavopiridol enhances the effect of docetaxel in vitro and in vivo in human gastric cancer cells. *Mol Cancer Ther* 2003;2:549–555.

120. Kouroukis CT, Belch A, Crump M, et al. Flavopiridol in untreated or relapsed mantle-cell lymphoma: results of a phase II study of the National Cancer Institute of Canada Clinical Trials Group. *J Clin Oncol* 2003;21:1740–1745.

121. Byrd JC, Lin TS, Dalton JT, et al. Flavopiridol administered using a pharmacologically derived schedule is associated with marked clinical efficacy in refractory, genetically high-risk chronic lymphocytic leukemia. *Blood* 2007;109:399–404.

122. Friedberg JW, Cohen P, Chen L, et al. Bendamustine in patients with rituximab-refractory indolent and transformed non-Hodgkin's lymphoma: results from a phase II multicenter, single-agent study. *J Clin Oncol* 2008;26:204–210.

123. Robinson KS, Williams ME, van der Jagt RH, et al. Phase II multicenter study of bendamustine plus rituximab in patients with relapsed indolent B-cell and mantle cell non-Hodgkin's lymphoma. *J Clin Oncol* 2008.

124. Beggiolin G, Crippa L, Menta E, et al. Bbr 2778, an aza-anthracenedione endowed with preclinical anticancer activity and lack of delayed cardiotoxicity. *Tumori* 2001;87:407–416.

125. Bertazzoli C, Bellini O, Magrini U, et al. Quantitative experimental evaluation of adriamycin cardiotoxicity in the mouse. *Cancer Treat Rep* 1979;63:1877–1883.

126. Borchmann P, Morschhauser F, Parry A, et al. Phase-II study of the new aza-anthracenedione, BBR 2778, in patients with relapsed aggressive non-Hodgkin's lymphomas. *Haematologica* 2003;88:888–894.

127. Schrader C, Meusers P, Brittinger G, et al. Topoisomerase IIalpha expression in mantle cell lymphoma: a marker of cell proliferation and a prognostic factor for clinical outcome. *Leukemia* 2004;18:1200–1206.

128. Bennaceur-Griscelli A, Bosq J, Koscielny S, et al. High level of glutathione-S-transferase pi expression in mantle cell lymphomas. *Clin Cancer Res* 2004;10:3029–3034.

129. Oki Y, Pro, B., Delpassand, E., et al. A phase II study of yttrium 90 (90Y) Ibritumomab Tiuxetan (Zevalin) for Treatment of Patients with relapsed and Refractory Mantle Cell Lymphoma (MCL). American Society of Hematology. 2004.

130. Zelenetz AD, Noy, A., Pandit-Taskar, N., et al., Sepuential radioimmunotherapy with tositumomab/Iodine I131 tositumomab followed by CHOP for mantle cell lymphoma demonstrates RIT can induce molecular remissions. Journal of Clinical Oncology. 2006;24:Abstract 7560.

CHAPTER 20 ■ DIFFUSE LARGE B-CELL LYMPHOMA

JAMES O. ARMITAGE, PETER M. MAUCH, NANCY LEE HARRIS, RICCARDO DALLA-FAVERA, AND PHILIP J. BIERMAN

DEFINITION

Diffuse large B-cell lymphoma (DLBCL) is defined in the fourth edition of the World Health Organization (WHO) classification (1) as a neoplasm of large B-lymphoid cells with nuclear size equal to or exceeding normal macrophage nuclei, or more than twice the size of a normal lymphocyte, which has a diffuse growth pattern. Within this broad definition, morphologic variants, molecular and immunophenotypic subgroups, and distinct disease entities are recognized (Table 20.1). Many cases remain that are probably biologically heterogeneous but for which there are no clear and accepted criteria for further subclassification. These are classified as DLBCL, not otherwise specified (NOS). DLBCL, NOS comprises all DLBCL cases that do not belong to specific subtypes or disease entities described in Table 20.1 and discussed in other chapters.

DLBCL may be primary, or may arise secondarily from indolent B-cell lymphomas, such as small lymphocytic lymphoma/chronic lymphocytic leukemia, lymphoplasmacytic lymphoma, extranodal or splenic marginal zone lymphoma, lymphocyte predominant Hodgkin lymphoma, or follicular lymphoma, a phenomenon that is often called a *transformed DLBCL*.

TABLE 20.1

DLBCL, VARIANTS AND SUBTYPES

DLBCL, NOS
   Common morphologic variants
      Centroblastic
      Immunoblastic
      Anaplastic
   Immunohistochemical subgroups
      CD5-positive DLBCL
      GCB
      Non-GCB
DLBCL, subtypes
   T-cell/histiocyte-rich large B-cell lymphoma
   Primary DLBCL of the CNS
   Primary cutaneous DLBCL, leg type
   EBV-positive DLBCL of the elderly
Other large B-cell lymphomas
   Primary mediastinal (thymic) large B-cell lymphoma
   Intravascular large B-cell lymphoma
   DLBCL associated with chronic inflammation
   Lymphomatoid granulomatosis
   ALK-positive large B-cell lymphoma
   Plasmablastic lymphoma
   Large B-cell lymphoma arising in human herpesvirus
      8-associated multicentric Castleman disease
   Primary effusion lymphoma

DLBCLs can arise in nodal or extranodal sites. DLBCLs that occur in sites where low-grade lymphomas of mucosa-associated lymphoid tissue are often found should be called *DLBCL* rather than *transformed* or *high-grade mucosa-associated lymphoid tissue lymphoma* to avoid confusion in therapeutic decisions.

FREQUENCY AND ETIOLOGY

DLBCL is the most common type of non-Hodgkin lymphoma, representing approximately one-third of all non-Hodgkin lymphomas in most parts of the world (2). Geographic differences in the incidence rate of DLBCL are not as large as the differences observed between other histologic subtypes (3). The increase in non-Hodgkin lymphoma incidence that has been observed over the last 50 to 60 years is largely due to an increase in the incidence of DLBCL, although the rate of increase of this histology has declined in recent years (4). DLBCL is more common in whites than other races and is more common in men than women. DLBCL is most commonly diagnosed in patients in their 7th decade of life, and the incidence of this histology increases steadily with age (4). However, it is also one of the more common lymphomas of childhood.

The etiology of most individual cases of DLBCL is unknown, despite our increasing understanding of lymphoma pathogenesis. The incidence of non-Hodgkin lymphoma, including DLBCL, is increased in patients with inherited and acquired immune deficiency disorders such as rheumatoid arthritis (5,6). Lymphomas in these situations are often associated with Epstein-Barr virus (EBV) infection, although this virus is associated with approximately 10% of other cases of DLBCL. Exposure to a variety of environmental agents, such as herbicides, has been associated with an increased risk of DLBCL. An increased risk of lymphoma, including DLBCL, has also been observed among first-degree relatives of patients with lymphoma. DLBCL often arises in patients with preexisting small lymphocytic lymphoma, mucosa-associated lymphoid tissue lymphoma, and follicular lymphoma. The multiple genetic and morphologic subtypes of DLBCL suggest that there are likely to be multiple, as yet unidentified, etiologic factors leading to developing this lymphoma.

PATHOLOGY

Morphology

DLBCLs are typically composed of large cells (three times the size of normal lymphocytes) that resemble either the proliferating cells of the germinal center (centroblasts/large non-cleaved cells) or immunoblasts, most often with a mixture of the two (Color Plate 34). Several morphologic variants can be recognized, but their clinical significance is debated. The *centroblastic type* (80% of the cases) is composed of cells resembling centroblasts, with one to three peripheral nucleoli and a narrow rim of basophilic cytoplasm, often with a variable admixture of immunoblasts. Some cases have multilobated centroblasts. The *immunoblastic type* (10% of the cases) has >90% immunoblasts, with a prominent central nucleolus and abundant, basophilic cytoplasm, often with plasmacytoid differentiation. These cases are more common in patients with immunosuppression. In patients without immunosuppression, they have been reported in some studies to have a worse prognosis, whereas others have failed to confirm this (7,8). In the *anaplastic type*, the cells are morphologically similar to those of T/null-anaplastic large cell lymphoma, with pleomorphic nuclei, abundant cytoplasm and sinusoidal growth pattern, and CD30 expression. Although these have been called *B-anaplastic large cell lymphoma*, they do not have the same distinctive clinical or genetic features of T-cell anaplastic large cell lymphoma and are considered a morphologic variant of large B-cell lymphoma.

Bone marrow involvement in DLBCL may take two forms. In approximately 10% of cases, there is large cell lymphoma in the marrow. However, a slightly higher proportion may show so-called discordant marrow involvement, that is, aggregates of small atypical lymphoid cells consistent with involvement of low-grade lymphoma, particularly follicular lymphoma. Several studies have shown that discordant marrow involvement is not associated with a worse prognosis than are cases without marrow involvement (9,10); however, these patients may be at risk for late relapses (11).

Immunophenotype

DLBCLs express one or more B-cell–associated antigens (CD19, CD20, CD22, CD79a, PAX5), as well as CD45, and often surface immunoglobulin (Ig). They may coexpress CD5 (10%) or CD10 (30% to 60%) (12,13). Some cases with plasmablastic differentiation may lack CD20 and PAX5, and express only CD79a; expression of CD138 is rare. Twenty-five percent to 80% of cases in various studies express BCL2 protein, and this may be associated with a worse prognosis (14–18). Approximately 60% to 90% express BCL6 protein (17,18), independent of BCL6 gene rearrangement. Postgerminal center markers such as IRF4/MUM1 are expressed in 35% to 50% of the cases, often together with Bcl-6. Proliferation fraction as estimated by Ki67 staining is usually >40% and may be >90%.

A panel of antibodies has been used to stratify DLBCL-NOS into germinal center B-cell (GCB) and non-GCB types (19), but its correlation with prognosis is controversial. Expression of CD10 by >30% of the cells is considered diagnostic of GCB type; CD10-cases that express of BCL6 without IRF4/MUM1 are considered GCB, whereas those that express BCL6 and IRF4/MUM1 are considered non-GCB.

Genetic Features

Ig genes are rearranged, and most have somatic hypermutation in the variable-region genes (20,21). The BCL2 gene is rearranged in 15% to 30%; it is associated with disseminated nodal disease but not with either a worse prognosis or bcl-2 protein expression (14). The MYC gene is rearranged in 5% to 15% (22,23); the BCL6 gene is rearranged in 20% to 40% of cases (23,24) and shows mutations in the 5′ noncoding region in 70% (25,26). Both the 5′ noncoding mutations of the BCL6 gene (27,28) and the Ig variable-region gene somatic hypermutation are found in normal germinal center cells (29); their presence in DLBCL is consistent with a germinal center or postgerminal center stage of differentiation.

The postulated normal counterpart is peripheral B cells of germinal center or postgerminal center (activated B cell) stage.

Diffuse Large B-Cell Lymphoma Subtypes

Primary DLBCL of the central nervous system (CNS) is covered in a separate chapter. Other subtypes are described briefly below.

T-Cell/Histiocyte-Rich Large B-Cell Lymphoma

These cases have a minority of neoplastic large B cells in a prominent background of reactive T cells and, typically, epithelioid histiocytes, often with a vaguely nodular pattern in lymph nodes and spleen. They may resemble Hodgkin lymphoma of nodular lymphocyte predominant or lymphocyte-rich classic type (30,31); this diagnosis should not be made in a patient with Hodgkin lymphoma of nodular lymphocyte predominant in the same or another lymph node either synchronously or metachronously. The neoplastic cells may resemble centroblasts, immunoblasts, or the Reed-Sternberg cell variants of either LP (LP cells) or classic HL. They express B-cell-associated antigens (CD20, CD79a), and often both Bcl6 and IRF4/MUM1, but typically lack CD15 and CD30 and are EBV-. The background lymphocytes are CD3+ T cells; by definition small B cells and B-cell follicles with CD21/23+ follicular dendritic cells are absent. No specific genetic abnormalities have been reported. Patients typically present with disseminated disease involving lymph nodes, liver, spleen, and bone marrow. They may respond to aggressive therapy for large cell lymphoma.

Primary Cutaneous Diffuse Large B-Cell Lymphoma

Rare cases of primary cutaneous lymphoma are composed of solid sheets of large transformed B cells (centroblasts or immunoblasts). They typically have strong expression of bcl-2 as well as IRF4/MUM1, in addition to pan-B antigens. They have genetic features similar to nodal DLBCL, often with translocations of MYC, BCL6, and IgH genes. They most commonly occur on the lower legs in elderly women ("leg type"), and are associated with a high frequency of nodal and systemic spread and an aggressive clinical course. They may occur at other sites (trunk, arms, head) and must be distinguished from primary cutaneous follicle center lymphoma, which contain predominantly large centrocytes, are typically bcl-2 negative, and have an indolent clinical course (see Chapter 24).

Epstein-Barr Virus-Positive Diffuse Large B-Cell Lymphoma

EBV+ DLBCL of the elderly is defined in the World Health Organization classification as an EBV+ clonal lymphoproliferation that occurs in patients >50 years of age, without known immunodeficiency or prior lymphoma (1). Similar cases may rarely occur in younger patients. Cases of lymphomatoid granulomatosis and other EBV+ specific types of DLBCL are excluded (DLBCL associated with chronic inflammation, plasmablastic lymphoma, primary effusion lymphoma). These cases have been primarily reported in Asia but clearly also occur in Western countries; their frequency is 8% to 10% of DLBCLs in Asian countries. The proportion of DLBCLs that are EBV+ increases with age.

Other Lymphomas of Large B Cells

Several specific types of large B-cell lymphomas are covered in separate chapters: primary mediastinal large B-cell lymphoma (see Chapter 21); and plasmablastic lymphoma, large B-cell lymphoma in human herpesvirus 8+ multicentric Castleman disease, and primary effusion lymphoma (see Chapters 35 and 37). Others are described briefly below.

Intravascular Large B-Cell Lymphoma

This is a disseminated intravascular proliferation of large B cells involving small blood vessels, without an obvious extravascular tumor mass or leukemia (32,33). This tumor has also been variously known as *intravascular lymphomatosis*, *angiotropic lymphoma*, and *malignant angioendotheliomatosis*. The neoplastic lymphoid cells are mainly lodged in the lumina of small vessels in many organs, most commonly the CNS, kidney, and lung; in Asian patients there is an increased frequency of involvement of liver, spleen, and bone marrow sinuses. Rare cases are localized to the skin. The tumor cells may resemble centroblasts or immunoblasts and express B-cell–associated antigens; coexpression of CD5, 10, or both may be seen (34). The cells may lack homing receptors that permit them to leave blood vessels (35). No specific genetic abnormality has been reported. Peripheral blood involvement is uncommon but may occur, particularly in Asian-type cases and CD5+ cases. Patients present with symptoms of organ dysfunction secondary to vascular occlusion. Because the diagnosis is difficult, many reported cases were diagnosed at autopsy. If a timely diagnosis is made and combination chemotherapy instituted, many patients achieve complete remission, and long-term survival appears to be possible (33,36). Cutaneous cases may be indolent.

Diffuse Large B-Cell Lymphoma Associated with Chronic Inflammation

This is a subtype of EBV+ DLBCL that occurs in a setting of chronic inflammation (1). The prototype is pyothorax-associated DLBCL involving the pleural cavities of patients with artificial pneumothorax for the treatment of tuberculosis (37). It may also occur in association with chronic osteomyelitis, adjacent to prosthetic implants, or chronic skin ulcers (38). The cells resemble centroblasts or immunoblasts, and there is often extensive necrosis or an angiocentric growth pattern. They typically express CD20 and CD79a but may have plasmacytoid differentiation and express only IRF4/

Mum1 and CD138, with or without CD30. EBV-Epstein-Barr-encoded ribonucleic acid is detected by in situ hybridization. The tumor is aggressive but may respond to treatment for DLBCL.

Lymphomatoid Granulomatosis

Lymphomatoid granulomatosis is an EBV-positive large B-cell lymphoma with a T-cell–rich background (39–42). Patients typically present with extranodal disease, most commonly involving the lung, CNS, or kidneys. Evidence of past or present immunosuppression may be found. The infiltrates show extensive necrosis, often with only a few EBV+ large B cells in a background of small T lymphocytes; the infiltrate may be both angiocentric and angioinvasive. Lymphomatoid granulomatosis is graded according to the number of large B cells (grades 1 to 3). The large cells express CD20 and may be CD30+, but CD15 is negative. Ig genes are clonally rearranged; no specific genetic abnormality has been described. The lower-grade cases are not typically treated as lymphoma; grade 3 cases fulfill the criteria for large B-cell lymphoma.

Anaplastic Lymphoma Kinase-Positive Diffuse Large B-Cell Lymphoma

This is a rare DLBCL with immunoblastic or plasmablastic morphology, with a translocation involving the anaplastic lymphoma kinase (ALK) protein that results in cytoplasmic expression of ALK protein (43,44). It affects males more than females and can occur in any age group. Most cases involve lymph nodes, but it may present as a mediastinal mass or in extranodal sites (45). The tumor cells typically involve lymph node sinuses and are monomorphic large immunoblast-like cells that may have a plasmacytoid appearance. The cohesive growth pattern and sinus involvement may resemble a metastatic carcinoma. The tumor cells may lack CD45 and are typically CD20- CD79a-; they express plasma-cell-associated antigens such as EMA and CD138, and may have cytoplasmic Ig, usually IgA or IgG. CD4, CD57, and/or CD43 may be expressed. They are typically CD30- but may express the cytotoxic protein perforin. The differential diagnosis includes nonlymphoid tumors, plasmablastic lymphoma, and anaplastic large cell lymphoma, ALK+; a high index of suspicion and extensive immunophenotyping are required to establish the diagnosis. The tumor cells have a translocation involving the ALK gene on chromosome 2, most commonly a t(2;17)(p23;q23) involving the clathrin gene and resulting in a clathrin heavy polypeptide-ALK fusion protein (44). The tumor is aggressive but may respond to chemotherapy, and long survival has been reported, particularly in children.

PATHOGENESIS

Although biologically and clinically heterogeneous, all DLBCLs derive from GCBs, as documented by the presence of somatic mutations in their Ig variable genes, by their expression of germinal center-related markers, and by the lack of expression of markers typical of plasma-cell differentiation. Recently, the genome-wide analysis of the pattern of expression of thousands of genes by deoxyribonucleic acid array technology has identified distinct subsets of DLBCLs that may correspond to distinct stages of germinal center development or to different mechanisms of malignant transformation (46,47). Together, these studies clearly indicate that DLBCLs comprise a heterogeneous group of tumors with distinct and still largely unknown biologic features.

The molecular pathogenesis of DLBCL is complex and involves several mechanisms of genetic lesion: chromosomal translocations; the recently identified aberrant somatic hypermutation mechanism; and other mechanisms common to all malignancies, such as gene amplifications and deletions.

Chromosomal Translocations

Cytogenetic studies of non-Hodgkin lymphoma have demonstrated that chromosomal alterations affecting band 3q27 are a frequent recurrent abnormality in B-lineage diffuse large cell lymphoma (48,49). These alterations are represented by reciprocal translocations between the 3q27 region and several alternative partner chromosomes, including, although not restricted to, the sites of the Ig genes at 14q32 (Ig$_H$), 2p11 (Igκ), and 22q11 (Igγ) (48,49). The variability of the partner chromosomes juxtaposed to 3q27 in B-lineage diffuse large cell lymphoma translocations suggests that these abnormalities belong to the group of "promiscuous" translocations, which involve a fixed chromosomal breakpoint on one side and, on the other side, different chromosomal partners in different cases. These translocations juxtapose heterologous promoters derived from different partner chromosomes to the coding region of the BCL6 gene, thereby leading to its deregulated expression by a mechanism called *promoter substitution* (50,51). The BCL6 gene encodes a transcription factor that binds the specific deoxyribonucleic acid sequences located in the promoter region of its target genes and represses their transcription (52). In the B-cell lineage, the bcl-6 protein is expressed only in germinal center cells, but not in pregerminal center cells, e.g., the mantle zone cells, or postgerminal center cells, such as immunoblasts and plasma cells (53). Mice deficient for bcl-6 are not capable of forming germinal centers and show a complete lack of affinity maturation (54,55). Therefore, bcl-6 appears to be a pivotal regulator of germinal center development.

Chromosomal translocations involving the BCL6 gene can be detected in approximately 35% of DLBCLs and in a minority (5% to 10%) of follicular lymphomas (56). The majority of these translocations give rise to a fusion transcript in which exon1 and the promoter of BCL6 are replaced by the partner gene sequences (51). These fusion transcripts are initiated from the heterologous promoters, and they contain the intact coding exons of BCL6. Compared with the BCL6 promoter, these promoters demonstrate a broader spectrum of activity in B-cell development, including expression in the postgerminal center differentiation stage, such as immunoblasts and plasma cells (57). Consequently, they can prevent the normal down-regulation of BCL6 expression that occurs during differentiation into postgerminal center cells. The constitutive expression of BCL6 is thought to contribute to lymphomagenesis by repressing the transcription of genes, inducing cell-cycle arrest, apoptosis,

and differentiation (58). In vivo studies in transgenic mice are necessary to confirm this hypothesis.

Besides promoter substitution, BCL6 gene can also be altered by somatic hypermutation of its 5′ noncoding region. Hypermutation of BCL6 can be found in normal germinal center cells (27,59), and it is also found in many non-Hodgkin lymphomas, most frequently in DLBCL (73%) independent of BCL6 rearrangement (25,59). Functional analysis of BCL6 promoter-containing mutations indicates that some mutations associated with DLBCL but not from normal germinal center cells may deregulate the basal level of BCL6 transcription by interfering with its physiologic mechanism of negative feedback regulation (60). Given the occurrence of BCL6 mutations in normal B cells and their frequency and heterogeneity, further studies are needed to identify the full spectrum of mutations, which have a pathogenetic significance.

In addition to translocations involving BCL6, DLBCL displays a variety of other translocations, including those whose target gene has not yet been identified, as well as those involving the BCL2 gene. Based on the genetic configuration of BCL6 and BCL2, DLBCL can be separated into three categories (22,26,61,62). The first one, accounting for approximately 40% of the cases, associates with rearrangement of BCL6 without other known genetic lesions. The second category contains BCL2 rearrangement with or without the presence of p53 alterations. This type probably presents DLBCL evolving from clinical or subclinical follicular lymphoma. The third category contains germline BCL2 and BCL6, and, therefore, includes cases with mutated BCL6 as well as those with other types of translocations.

Aberrant Somatic Hypermutation

It has been recently shown that the process of somatic hypermutation, which normally engenders antibody diversity in GCBs by mutating the variable region of Ig genes, malfunctions and aberrantly targets on Ig genes in the majority of DLBCLs. As a consequence, the protooncogenes, PIM1, cMYC, PAX5, and RhoH/TTF, are hypermutated in >50% of DLBCLs (63). In the case of PIM1 and cMYC, the mutations affect nontranslated as well as coding regions, leading to amino acid changes, with potential functional consequences. This mechanism may represent a powerful mechanism of malignant transformation because it may have an effect on multiple genes, with consequences in part analogous to deoxyribonucleic acid mismatch-repair defects in colon carcinogenesis. Although a comprehensive characterization of the potentially extensive genetic damage caused by aberrant somatic hypermutation is still lacking, this mechanism also provides a plausible explanation for the biologic and clinical heterogeneity of DLBCL.

METHODS OF PRESENTATION AND PROGNOSTIC FACTORS

The most common presentation of patients with DLBCL is rapidly enlarging lymphadenopathy. However, as many as 40% of patients can have presentation in extranodal sites, with gastrointestinal involvement being most common.

Patients with primary nodal DLBCL with disease in the chest or abdomen can present with symptoms related to those sites (e.g., shortness of breath with mediastinal nodes, pain with retroperitoneal nodes). Primary extranodal DLBCLs often present with symptoms related to dysfunction at the site of origin (e.g., neurologic symptoms with brain lymphomas, pain or digestive symptoms with stomach or bowel lymphomas, pain with bone lymphomas). Approximately one-third of patients have B symptoms at the time of diagnosis.

Unusual presentations are seen with some uncommon subtypes of DLBCL. Intravascular large B-cell lymphoma often presents with a confusing system complex that reflects organ dysfunction secondary to vascular occlusion or systemic symptoms such as unexplained fever (36,64). Although the most common presentation is neurologic dysfunction, also reported are endocrine dysfunction, syndrome of inappropriate secretion of antidiuretic hormone, disseminated intravascular coagulopathy, atypical skin lesions, anasarca, and thrombotic thrombocytopenic purpura.

Pleural cavity lymphoma has frequently been associated with tuberculosis and pyothorax but is also seen in patients infected with human immunodeficiency virus. Unless new symptoms in a patient with preexisting effusion are investigated aggressively or this unusual diagnosis is considered in a patient at risk with a new effusion, the diagnosis will be missed.

Plasmablastic lymphoma has recently been described and is frequently seen as a mass in the oral cavity in a patient infected with human immunodeficiency virus. The tumor is most likely to involve extranodal sites. In addition to the oral cavity, these include the sinus, orbit, skin, bone, soft tissue, and gastrointestinal tract. This lymphoma is distinct from anaplastic transformations of myeloma that might have similar tumor cells.

Another recently recognized subtype of DLBCL is primary cutaneous DLBCL, leg type. This reflects a clinical observation that cutaneous tumors that appear to be DLBCL on biopsy are more likely to pursue an aggressive course if they occur below the umbilicus than above it. These patients are typically elderly, with a female predominance, who present with cutaneous lesions involving the lower extremities that frequently disseminate to other sites.

Approximately 40% to 50% of patients with DLBCL have disease that is stage I/II. Approximately 20% of patients have truly localized, or stage I, disease. Very bulky (i.e., >10 cm) tumor masses are seen in one-quarter to one-third of patients. A reduced performance status is present in approximately one-quarter of patients. The most common sites of extranodal disease are the gastrointestinal tract or bone marrow, although any site in the body can be involved. Bone marrow involvement is seen in approximately 15% of patients with DLBCL. However, in many of these patients, bone marrow is infiltrated by smaller cells rather than large cells. Large cell involvement of the marrow carries an ominous prognosis, but the same is not true for minimal involvement by small-cleaved B lymphocytes (9,65).

Approximately 35% of patients with DLBCL have an International Prognostic Index (IPI) (Table 20.2) score of zero or one. Forty-five percent have an IPI score of two to three, and approximately 20% have an IPI score of four to five. The IPI was developed by studying patients with DLBCL and accurately predicts the survival of patients with

TABLE 20.2
FACTORS INDEPENDENTLY PROGNOSTIC OF OVERALL SURVIVAL IN THE IPI

All patients ($n = 1,385$)
  Age ($\leq$60 y vs. >60 y)
  Serum LDH ($\leq$1 × normal vs. >1 × normal)
  Performance status (0 or 1 vs. 2–4)
  Stage (I or II vs. III or IV)
  Extranodal involvement ($\leq$1 site vs. >1 site)
Patients $\leq$60 y old ($n = 885$)
  Stage (I or II vs. III or IV)
  Serum LDH ($\leq$1 × normal vs. >1 × normal)
  Performance status (0 or 1 vs. 2–4)

From A predictive model for aggressive non-Hodgkin's lymphoma. The International Non-Hodgkin's Lymphoma Prognostic Factors Project. *N Engl J Med* 1993;329:987–994, with permission.

this disease (66) (Table 20.3). However, the specific prognosis for patients with any particular IPI subgroup seems to have changed with the addition of rituximab. Patients with any particular IPI score have a better prognosis when rituximab is included in the treatment (67–69). Sehn et al. (70) have proposed that patients with an IPI score of zero should be classified as having a "very good" prognosis. Those with an IPI score of one or two having a "good" prognosis, and the "poor" prognosis group would be those having three to five risk factors (Table 20.4). However, with rituximab in combination with cyclophosphamide, doxorubicin, Oncovin (vincristine), and prednisone (R-CHOP), the 4-year overall survival for the "poor" group still was better than 50%. Other factors proposed to predict treatment outcome for patients with DLBCL include large tumor masses, serum β_2-microglobulin level, tumor growth fraction, and genetics.

The rapidity of response to chemotherapy has been found to be prognostic in at least one study, in which patients achieving a complete remission in three cycles had a better chance for long-term disease-free survival than did patients who took longer to achieve a complete remission (71). Functional imaging as performed by 18-fluoro-deoxyglucose-positron emission tomography (PET) scans has become important in the initial evaluation of patients with DLBCL. A negative scan after treatment has become a key step in documenting complete remission. PET scans have also been used to look for a rapid response to therapy and hope this would be associated with a good outcome. In a study of 90 patients who received an anthracycline-containing regimen with or without rituximab, a negative PET scan after two cycles predicted an event-free survival at 2 years of 82% versus 43% for the patients who had not responded quickly (72). Other studies have reported similar results (73,74). Whether treatment can be modified based on the results of an early PET scan is still an unanswered question.

The host immune response to the presence of DLBCL has been studied as a prognostic factor. Patients with T-cell-rich B-cell lymphoma do not have a better survival than do patients with other subtypes of DLBCL. The absence of expression of human leukocyte antigen-DR has been associated with a poor response to treatment (75,76). A higher number of circulating natural killer cells has been found to

TABLE 20.3

OUTCOME ACCORDING TO RISK GROUP DEFINED BY THE IPI AND THE AGE-ADJUSTED IPI

Index	Risk group	No. of risk factors	Distribution of patients (%)	Complete response rate (%)	2-y relapse-free survival rate (%)	5-y relapse-free survival rate (%)	2-y survival rate (%)	5-y survival rate (%)
International index, all patients (n = 2,031)	Low	0 or 1	35	87	79	79	84	73
	Low intermediate	2	27	67	66	50	66	51
	High intermediate	3	22	55	59	49	54	43
	High	4 or 5	16	44	58	40	34	26
Age-adjusted index, patients ≤60 y (n = 1,274)	Low	0	22	92	88	86	90	83
	Low intermediate	1	3	78	74	66	79	69
	High intermediate	2	32	57	62	53	59	46
	High	3	14	46	61	58	37	32
Age-adjusted index, patients >60 y (n = 761)	Low	0	18	91	75	46	80	56
	Low intermediate	1	31	71	64	45	68	44
	High intermediate	2	35	56	60	41	48	37
	High	3	16	36	47	37	31	21

From A predictive model for aggressive non-Hodgkin's lymphoma. The International Non-Hodgkin's Lymphoma Prognostic Factors Project. *N Engl J Med* 1993;329:987–994, with permission.

TABLE 20.4

A REVISED IPI IS BETTER WHEN R-CHOP IS GIVEN FOR DLBCL

Group	No. of factors	Percentage of Patients	Percentage of 4-y overall survival
Standard IPI	0, 1	28	86
	2	27	81
	3	21	54
	4, 5	24	58
Revised IPI	0	10	92
	1, 2	45	82
	3–5	45	58

From Sehn LH, Berry B, Chhanabhai M, et al. The revised International Prognostic Index (R-IPI) is a better predictor of outcome than the standard IPI for patients with diffuse large B-cell lymphoma treated with R-CHOP. *Blood* 2007;109:1857–1861, with permission.

be associated with an improved prognosis (77). As has been found to be true in follicular lymphoma, the infiltrating immune cells in the tumor itself might have prognostic significance. Another study found that infiltrating mast cells were associated with a better prognosis (78). A higher number of infiltrating CD4+ T cells in patients with DLBCL was found to be associated with an improved prognosis (79). One study found that small numbers of T-cell–restricted intracellular antigen-1+ cytoxic T cells were associated with a good prognosis, but there was no impact of the number of FOXP3+ regulatory T cells on outcome (80), whereas another found that an increased number of FOXP3+ cells favorably impacted survival in germinal center-type DLBCL but had a negative impact on survival with nongerminal center-type DLBCL (81).

A number of other biomarkers have been proposed to have prognostic significance in DLBCL. Patients with evidence of EBV positivity in tumor cells seem to have a poorer treatment outcome (82). A number of specific biologically active molecules have been found to have an impact on treatment outcome (83). Studies of the cell cycle regulatory molecules TP53, P27, and cyclin D have been reported. All found that a poorer treatment outcome was associated with alterations in expression with an adverse impact of mutations in TP53, and an adverse outcome associated with a higher level of expression of P27 and cyclin D. Expression by the tumor cells of CD5, FOXP1, and protein kinase C-β has been associated with a poorer treatment outcome. In contrast, expression of CD21 was associated with a better outcome. Elevated levels of circulating ICAM-1, CD44, endostatin, and vascular endothelial growth factor have all been associated with a poorer treatment outcome.

Overexpression of BCL2 protein in the tumor cells of DLBCL is seen in approximately 50% of patients, but only a minority of these have the overexpression of the protein related to the t(14;18). The prognostic impact of BCL2 protein overexpression has been controversial (14,23,84,85). At least one report has suggested that any adverse impact of BCL2 protein expression in DLBCL can be overcome with the use of rituximab (86). More recently, it appears that the impact of BCL2 protein expression on outcome in DLBCL may depend on the genetic subtype of the tumor, with the adverse impact only in the nongerminal center subtype (87).

BCL6 protein is of germinal center derivation and a predictor of outcome in DLBCL, with elevated levels of BCL6 protein expression associated with a good outcome (88). There is evidence that the poorer outcome seen with lack of BCL6 protein expression can be overcome by the addition of rituximab to the treatment regimen (89).

Increasingly, genetic characteristics of DLBCL have been associated with treatment outcome. For example, patients with MYC rearrangements have been found to have a poorer treatment outcome as have those whose lymphomas have both the t(14;18) and MYC rearrangements (90). However, the most important advances have been related to the results of gene expression profiling. Initial reports of gene expression profiling in DLBCL found that the lymphoma could be divided into at least two subtypes based on the pattern of gene expression (46). A superior survival was associated with a gene expression pattern that resembled normal GCBs and an inferior outcome associated with DLBCLs that had a gene expression pattern reminiscent of postgerminal center, activated B cells. Subsequent studies have confirmed this outcome (47,91). A minority of patients with DLBCL has tumors that do not fit easily into these two subgroups. Subsequent studies have suggested that patterns of protein expression as measured by immunohistochemistry can predict the molecular subgroup (19), but this has been imperfect, and attempts are underway to develop a better algorithm. There is increasing evidence that the use of rituximab in treatment regimens does not eliminate the adverse impact of a nongerminal center cell phenotype but improves the outcome in both germinal center and nongerminal center subtypes (92,93).

New prognostic factors have the potential to change the way patients with DLBCL are managed. It is possible that early functional imaging (i.e., currently performed with 18-fluoro-deoxyglucose-PET scans) will make it possible to shorten treatment in rapidly responding patients and change treatment early in those destined to have failure. Patients with specific genetic or protein expression patterns might well be found to benefit from particular treatment regimens, and treatment might be driven more by these findings than stage or other characteristics.

THERAPY

Early Stage Diffuse Large B-Cell Lymphoma

Radiation Therapy and Results of Early Clinical Trials

Before 1980, radiation therapy alone was often used as the primary treatment for patients with localized diffuse large cell lymphoma. Approximately 50% of patients with stage I and 20% of patients with stage II disease were alive without recurrence 5 years after treatment (94,95). These results were even better in small series, in which selected patients with stage I and II disease with a negative staging laparotomy were treated with extended-field irradiation alone. One series reported a 5-year survival of approximately 80% (96). Another study reported a 10-year actuarial relapse-free survival of 91% in patients with stage I disease and 35% with stage II disease (97).

The relationship between radiation dose (and field size) and probability of tumor control has been the subject of numerous reports extending back to the early 1970s. A number of factors probably affect the relationship between dose and tumor control in diffuse large cell lymphoma, including tumor size, use of chemotherapy before radiation therapy, and responsiveness to chemotherapy. However, there are no randomized trials evaluating the dose of radiation therapy in the management of diffuse large cell lymphoma.

Two of the earliest retrospective papers on dose were published by Stanford University and the Princess Margaret Hospital in Toronto. Both series evaluated patients with early stage diffuse large cell lymphoma. In the 1973 Stanford study, Fuks and Kaplan (98) reported that local control rates were 70% to 80%, regardless of the dose of radiotherapy delivered (from 20 to 50 Gy). The lack of a dose response in this study may be misleading because patients with larger tumors probably received higher doses. In the Princess Margaret Hospital study, the bulk of disease and patterns of relapse were evaluated (99,100). Patients with diffuse large cell lymphoma had local or local-plus-distant recurrence rates of nearly 30%. Patients with medium- or large-bulk disease, defined as 2.5 to 5.0 cm in size and >5 cm, respectively, had higher local or local-plus-distant recurrence rates (>45%) than did patients with smaller-bulk disease (<20%). The dose-regional-control curve for diffuse large cell lymphoma treated with radiation alone in patients with medium- or large-bulk disease showed 50% and 80% local control rates with 25 and 40 Gy, respectively, with a plateau in the local-control curve after 40 Gy (99).

Several other retrospective studies using radiation therapy alone helped to establish early standards for the technical use of radiation therapy, including guidelines for dose and field size. These studies used a median dose of 50 Gy to the initial sites of involvement, and two of the retrospective studies treated extended fields to cover adjacent sites of disease (96,97,101,102).

Several randomized trials published from 1979 to 1982 helped to improve the outcome of patients with early stage diffuse large cell lymphoma. The trials compared radiation therapy alone with radiation therapy followed by cyclophosphamide, vincristine, and prednisone (CVP) or bleomycin, Adriamycin (doxorubicin), cyclophosphamide, Oncovin (vincristine), and prednisone chemotherapy (103–105). The addition of chemotherapy to radiation therapy resulted in a disease-free and overall survival advantage for combining the two regimens compared with radiation therapy alone. The trials somewhat reduced the dose of radiation therapy compared with previous reports without chemotherapy but continued to give prophylactic radiation therapy to uninvolved adjacent lymph node regions. In the Italian trial, 40 to 50 Gy was delivered to clinically involved areas, and proximal uninvolved lymph node-bearing areas received 35 to 45 Gy

(103). Similar field sizes were used in the Danish trial, with the tumor receiving 37 to 43 Gy, with higher doses given for persistent disease (104). Data suggested that the addition of chemotherapy to radiation therapy not only reduced the incidence of distant relapse, but it also made the radiation therapy more effective for control of initial sites of involvement. In addition, approximately 10% of patients developed distant recurrences while on radiation therapy before chemotherapy was initiated. This suggested that the combination of the two modalities might be more effective with the chemotherapy given first. Results from these trials dramatically changed the treatment of localized large cell lymphoma. Staging laparotomy and large-field radiation therapy became obsolete because combination chemotherapy with or without radiation therapy produced disease-free and overall survival rates equivalent to or better than those seen in even the most selective studies reporting results with radiation therapy alone.

Clinical Stage I and II Diffuse Large B-Cell Lymphoma Treated with Combined Doxorubicin-Based Chemotherapy and Radiation Therapy

With the use of the more effective doxorubicin-based regimens, a number of retrospective trials reported good data using smaller radiation fields limited to the initial regions of involvement and given at somewhat reduced doses in patients with diffuse large cell lymphoma. Table 20.5 shows selected retrospective studies using doxorubicin-based chemotherapy regimens and radiation therapy (106–114). The first six series used six to eight cycles of chemotherapy (106,107,109–111,115); the last three series gave three to four cycles (112–114). Two of the three series using three to four cycles of chemotherapy excluded patients with bulky disease (>10 cm). The median radiation doses range from 36 to 45 Gy in the first six studies and 35 to 40 Gy in the last three studies, except for some patients in the Rotterdam study who received 26 Gy. In one study, a greater number of cycles of chemotherapy was used for patients not achieving a complete remission (109). The M. D. Anderson Cancer Center study used 40 Gy for patients in complete remission after chemotherapy and 50 Gy for a partial response (PR) or remission (111). Another study used a higher dose of radiation therapy (40 Gy) with three to four cycles of chemotherapy versus a lower dose (36 Gy) with six to eight cycles of chemotherapy. Most of the studies use involved-field irradiation; in two series, approximately one-half of the patients were treated to larger fields (109,110). The majority of patients in the studies had diffuse large cell lymphoma, although diffuse undifferentiated, follicular large cell, and diffuse poorly differentiated small-cleaved cell lymphomas were included in many of the series. Recurrences within or on the edge of the radiation field as the only site of relapse were rare (0% to 7%). Although the range of median doses was small, no differences in local control were seen in the different studies within this dose range. Similarly, no differences in local control were seen in studies that used six to eight cycles of chemotherapy versus four cycles. All the trials used multiagent chemotherapy before the routine addition of rituximab to the chemotherapy regimen. It is not known if the use of rituximab would allow a somewhat lower dose of radiation in patients receiving adjuvant radiation therapy.

Four prospective randomized trials have further evaluated the role of radiation therapy in patients with early stage DLBCL (Table 20.6). The Eastern Cooperative Oncology Group randomized 352 patients with bulky stage I (mediastinal or retroperitoneal involvement or masses >10 cm), stage IE, stage II, or stage IIE disease to eight cycles of cyclophosphamide, doxorubicin, Oncovin (vincristine), and prednisone (CHOP) chemotherapy with or without radiation therapy. Patients with no response or progression to chemotherapy were removed from the study. Patients in complete remission were randomized to 30-Gy involved-field radiation therapy (to sites of initial involvement) or no further treatment. Patients in partial remission received 40 Gy to the site or sites of pretreatment involvement plus radiation to contiguous uninvolved regions. In patients randomized after complete remission, the 5-year disease-free survival (73% vs. 58%; $p = 0.03$), freedom from recurrence (73% vs. 58%; $p = 0.04$), and survival (84% vs. 70%; $p = 0.06$) all favored the patients who received adjuvant involved-field irradiation (116). At 10 years, the disease-free survival continues to favor the addition of radiation therapy (57% vs. 46%; $p = 0.04$), but the survival differences no longer are statistically significant (117). In the patients who achieved a partial remission, 28% converted to a complete remission with the addition of 40 Gy of radiation therapy.

The Southwest Oncology Group (SWOG) 8736 trial randomized 401 patients with stage I and nonbulky stage II disease to receive either three cycles of CHOP and involved-field irradiation (40 to 55 Gy) or eight cycles of CHOP alone. The 5-year progression-free survival (77% vs. 64%; $p = 0.03$) and overall survival (82% vs. 72%; $p = 0.02$) favored the CHOP and involved-field radiation therapy treatment arm (118). This trial demonstrated that the addition of radiation therapy allowed the use of three cycles instead of eight cycles of CHOP, and that combined modality therapy using abbreviated chemotherapy and radiation therapy resulted in a better outcome than a prolonged course of chemotherapy alone. The updated results of this trial (119), reported at the 2001 American Society of Hematology meetings, showed that at 7 to 9 years, there were no longer differences in failure-free survival and overall survival between the two arms. This was largely due to late relapses and lymphoma deaths beyond 5 years in all but the most favorable patients who received abbreviated chemotherapy followed by radiation therapy. These findings suggest that three cycles of CHOP are inadequate systemic therapy for most patients with early stage diffuse large cell lymphoma. Of note, a subanalysis of the SWOG 8736 trial revealed that patients without any stage-adjusted IPI risk factors had a 5-year overall survival of 94% after three cycles of CHOP and radiation therapy (120). However, in those with one or more risk factors, the 5-year overall survival was only 70% after the same treatment, suggesting that more extensive chemotherapy is needed for this subgroup before adjuvant radiation therapy. This has been confirmed in a recent phase II SWOG trial using three cycles of R-CHOP followed by involved-field irradiation, in patients with limited-stage aggressive lymphoma with at least one modified risk factor. The study revealed a progression-free survival at 4 years of 88% and a 4-year survival of 92% compared with historical controls of 78% and 88% at 4 years (taken from patients in the 8736 trial that received CHOP without rituximab) (121). As a result of these data, combination chemotherapy and adjuvant radiation therapy have become the standard care in many centers for patients with stage I or II DLBCL.

TABLE 20.5

MULTIAGENT CHEMOTHERAPY AND LOCAL RADIATION THERAPY FOR STAGES I AND II INTERMEDIATE- OR HIGH-GRADE LYMPHOMAS: SELECTED RETROSPECTIVE TRIALS

Institution (reference)	No. of patients	Stage	Median RT dose (Gy)	Type and median number of CT cycles	RT field size	MM/IF recur only	Freedom from recurrence (%)	Survival (%) (y)
University of Florida (211)	121	I/II	NA	Nearly all ABR; ≥4 cycles	NA	5/121 (4%)	63 (10 y)	44 (10)
Institute Gustave-Roussy (107)	96	I/II	45	CHVmP; NA	NA	7/95 (7%)	NA	77 (5)
Stanford University (108)	23	I	40	ABR (85%); 6 cycles	IF (86%)	6/94 (6%)	78	81 (5)
Milan (109)	71	II	40–44	CHOP ∞ 4 cycles (CR) or 6 cycles (PR)	IF (41%) REG (59%)	9/183 (3%)	70	72 (5)
	183	I/II					—	83 (5)
The Netherlands Multicenter Trial (110)	94	I/IE	36 (6–8 cycles CT)	92% ABR; 3–8 cycles	IF (53%)	0/94, 3/94 local and distant	NA	70 (10)
			40 (3–4 cycles CT)		EF (47%)			
M. D. Anderson Cancer Center (111)	57	I	40 (CR)	CHOP-Bleo; 8 cycles	Gross disease + margin	5/147 (3%)	—	72 (10)
Rotterdam (112)	90	II	50 (PR)		IF	5/74 (7%)	—	43 (10)
	74	I/II	26 (CR)	CHOP; 4 cycles		1/20 (5%)	69 (DFS)	76 (5)
	20		40 (CR)			2/34 (6%)	90	100 (5)
	34		40 (PR)				75	75 (5)
British Columbia (113)	308	I/II	30/10 fx	ABR; 3 cycles	IF	7/308 (2%)	—	80 (5)
National Cancer Institute (212)	47	I	35/20 fx 40	ProMACE-MOPP; 4 cycles	IF	2/47 (4%) 0/45 (CR)	96	63 (10)
								94 (5)

ABR, Adriamycin-based regimens; Bleo, bleomycin; CHVmP, cyclophosphamice, doxorubicin, teniposide, and prednisone; CR, complete response; CT, chemotherapy; DFS, disease-free survival; EF, extended field; fx, fraction; IF, involved field; MM/IF recur only, recurrences limited to within or on the edge of the radiation field; NA, information not available; ProMACE-MOPP, prednisone, procarbazine, doxorubicin, cyclophosphamide, etoposide-mechlorethamine, vincristine, procarbazine and prednisone; REG, regional radiation, usually the involved region and immediately adjacent uninvolved regions; RT, radiation therapy.

TABLE 20.6

CHEMOTHERAPY VERSUS COMBINED MODALITY THERAPY FOR STAGES I AND II INTERMEDIATE- OR HIGH-GRADE LYMPHOMA: PROSPECTIVE RANDOMIZED TRIALS

Reference	No. of evaluable patients	Stage	Chemotherapy	Radiation therapy dose (Gy)	CR or PR (%)	Failure-free survival (%)	Survival (%) (y)
Eastern Coopera- tive Oncology Group (116)	345	CS I (B) and all CS II	CHOP ∞ 8 (CR)	—	61% (CR)	58	70 (6)
			CHOP ∞ 8 (CR)	30 (IF)		73[a]	84 (6)[a]
			CHOP ∞ 8	40 (IF)	28% (PR)	60	64 (6)
SWOG (118)	401	CS I/IE (B/NB) and CS II (NB)	CHOP ∞ 8	—	73	64	72 (5)
			CHOP ∞ 3	40–55	75	77[b]	82 (5)[b]
GELA (213)	518	IPI 0, 1	CHOP ∞ 4	—	—	69	78
		CS I-II	CHOP ∞ 4	40	—	64	70
GELA (214)	631	CS I-II	ACVBP	—	—	83[c]	89[c]
		Low risk	CHOP ∞ 3	30–40	—	74	80

B, bulky disease; CR, complete response; CS, clinical stage; IF, involved field; NB, no bulky disease.
[a] Significant difference between radiation therapy and no radiation therapy.
[b] Borderline significant difference between radiation and no radiation therapy ($p = 0.06$).
[c] Significantly better result with ACVBP.

Two additional, more recent European randomized trials have been published. The Groupe d'Etudes des Lymphomes de l'Adulte (GELA) LNH 93-1 trial, conducted in patients with stage I to II mostly low-risk aggressive lymphoma (122), had a similar design to the SWOG trial comparing aggressive chemotherapy alone with abbreviated chemotherapy followed by radiation therapy. Patients in this trial were all aged <60 with normal lactate dehydrogenase (LDH) and performance status, and two-thirds of the patients had stage I disease. The comparison arms were dose-intensified doxorubicin, cyclophosphamide, vindesine, bleomycin, and prednisone (ACVBP) plus sequential consolidation (an aggressive regimen originally developed for patients with poor-risk disease), compared with three cycles of CHOP plus involved-field radiation therapy. Patients randomized to receive ACVBP, which has a theoretical dose intensity of at least 150% of that delivered by three cycles of CHOP, had significantly higher 5-year event-free and overall survival rates. Although the addition of radiation therapy after three cycles of CHOP reduced relapses at initial sites of disease, it was not enough to overcome the increased risk of distant relapse after the abbreviated therapy.

The GELA LNH 93-4 trial studied patients over the age of 60 with localized aggressive lymphoma with a normal LDH (vs. 20% with an abnormal LDH in the SWOG trial) and performance status. Two-thirds of the patients had stage I disease, and 8% had bulky disease. Patients were randomized at diagnosis to four cycles of CHOP alone or four cycles of CHOP followed by radiation therapy to 40 Gy (123). At a median follow-up of 7 years, there were no significant differences in 5-year event-free survival (64% vs. 61%, respectively) and 5-year overall survival (68% vs. 72%, respectively) between the two arms. An intriguing finding in this trial is that the chemotherapy alone arm, which utilized only four cycles of CHOP, yielded very similar survival as that following eight cycles of CHOP in the SWOG 8736 study, both of which had a 5-year overall survival rate of 72%. This highlights the heterogeneity of this disease and the importance of careful patient selection for reduced treatment.

An early report from British Columbia looked at the use of PET scores to guide the therapy of patients with localized DLBCL. Patients received three cycles of R-CHOP and then had a PET scan. If the PET scan was negative, the patients received only one more cycle of chemotherapy, and if positive, they received radiotherapy. The 2-year progression-free survival was 83% for patients with a positive PET and 97% for patients with a negative PET scan (124), suggesting that an early negative PET scan might select for patients who could avoid radiotherapy.

In summary, The ECOG trial and GELA LNH 93-4, which used the same systemic therapy on both arms, showed that the addition of radiation therapy reduced the percentage of isolated relapse at initial sites from 48% (15 of 31 relapse) to 17% (three of 17 relapses), and from 47% (37 of 79 relapses) to 21% (14 of 66 relapses), respectively. However, data from the four trials overall suggest that the benefit of improved local control with the addition of radiation therapy will only translate into a disease-free and overall survival improvement when it is combined with effective systemic therapy that allows for the eradication of occult distant disease. The results of the SWOG 8736 and GELA LNH 93-1 trials show that radiation therapy cannot be used to replace inferior and inadequate chemotherapy, and that there may be a role for radiation therapy when additional chemotherapy is employed. There also is a subgroup of patients for whom three cycles of CHOP chemotherapy followed by radiation therapy may be adequate, namely, patients with a stage-adjusted IPI of zero (age <60, normal LDH, performance status of zero to one, and stage I disease). Finally, R-CHOP is considered the standard systemic therapy for DLBCL; all four of the trials used CHOP without rituximab in the combined modality therapy arm. The recent phase II R-CHOP trial with three cycles of chemotherapy and involved-field irradiation suggested that this approach gives superior results compared with CHOP alone with involved-field irradiation.

What can we conclude regarding the dose and field size of radiation therapy when combined with chemotherapy based on these retrospective and prospective trials? For diffuse large cell lymphoma, radiation therapy alone is associated with a high-distant failure rate as well as a 20% infield recurrence rate despite doses of ≥45 Gy. The infield recurrence rates appear to be higher for bulky disease than for patients with less bulky disease. In contrast, using involved-field radiation therapy to doses of 30 to 45 Gy after a complete response to four to eight cycles of CHOP is associated with a low infield or margin of the field recurrence rate (0% to 7%, Table 20.5). Exactly what doses to recommend for patients with initial bulk disease is still unclear, but after a complete remission after CHOP, data suggest that doses of 36 Gy should be sufficient (125). Less data are available on what doses to use in patients who have a PR to chemotherapy or who have refractory localized disease.

Based on all the aforementioned data and our own personal experience, we recommend the following for diffuse large cell lymphoma treated with combined modality therapy:

1. Use of involved fields.
2. After a complete remission after eight cycles of CHOP or R-CHOP: 36 Gy if initial bulky disease; 30 to 36 Gy for the remainder of patients. Patients with paranasal sinus disease or primary bone involvement should receive 40 Gy.
3. After a partial remission: 40 Gy.
4. Localized refractory disease to chemotherapy: 44 to 55 Gy, depending on bulk of disease and location. For rapidly growing tumors, consider twice a day irradiation (126).

In the studies reported previously, the definitions of *complete* or *partial remission* are not always consistent, especially because nuclear medicine imaging was not available for the majority of patients in these reports. Residual masses are common on computed tomography after chemotherapy, especially in patients with bulky mediastinal or abdominal disease. We do not have data on the success of radiation therapy (or on the doses or field sizes needed) after a PR based on PET scans. The data that are available, using a variety of methods to define PR, suggest that radiation therapy alone after a partial remission to chemotherapy can yield long-term survival (106,116,127).

In a study by Zinzani et al. (127), 50 patients with primary mediastinal large B-cell lymphoma were prospectively treated with methotrexate, Adriamycin (doxorubicin), cyclophosphamide, Oncovin (vincristine), prednisone, and bleomycin, followed by radiation therapy. Computed tomography and gallium-67-citrate single-photon emission scans (GaSPECTs) were obtained at diagnosis, at the end of chemotherapy, and 3 months after radiation therapy. Three patients with progressive disease during chemotherapy were excluded from the analysis. After chemotherapy, 31 of 47 patients (66%) had a positive GaSPECT. Among these 31 patients, 22 had a negative GaSPECT after radiation therapy. None of the patients with a negative GaSPECT after treatment had a relapse at a median follow-up of 39 months.

Disseminated Diffuse Large B-Cell Lymphoma

The first convincing reports of the curability of diffuse aggressive lymphoma (i.e., the majority of which would be called DLBCL today) with chemotherapy appeared in 1972 (128) and 1975 (129). In both of these reports, the majority of patients who achieved a complete remission at the end of the initial treatment did not have relapse, despite no further therapy. It was originally thought that patients staying in remission for 2 years were cured. We now know that late relapses, even after 10 years, can occur, especially in patients with good-risk, low-stage disease (130). The next important advance was the incorporation of the anthracycline doxorubicin into the treatment of patients with diffuse aggressive lymphomas. The most widely used of these regimens was developed in the United States in the 1970s and has always been referred to as CHOP. Although drugs in CHOP have not always been administered in the same doses and sequence, the most popular way has been, and remains, cyclophosphamide 750 mg per m² intravenously on day 1, doxorubicin 50 mg per m² intravenously on day 1, vincristine 1.4 mg per m² with a maximum dose of 2 mg intravenously on day 1, and prednisone 100 mg orally daily for 5 days. The regimen has been typically administered at 21-day intervals. Once again the majority of patients who achieve a complete remission appear to be cured (71,131).

Because the ultimate cure rate for patients with disseminated diffuse aggressive lymphoma using the CHOP regimen was <50%, numerous attempts have been made to improve the treatment outcome. A large number of different regimens were tested in randomized trials (132). Investigators in different countries favored different approaches. For example, in France the ACVBP regimen (i.e., containing doxorubicin, cyclophosphamide, vindesine, bleomycin, methylprednisolone, and intrathecal methotrexate followed by a consolidative phase incorporating high-dose methotrexate, ifosfamide, etoposide, L-asparaginase, and cytarabine) became the standard approach for younger patients with diffuse aggressive lymphoma. When compared with CHOP in patients 60 to 69 years of age, the event-free survival (i.e., 45% vs. 33%; *p* = 0.004) favored ACVBP (133). However, there was a significant treatment-related death rate with the ACVBP regimen, and its use was largely confined to patients <60 years of age.

Investigators in Germany carried out an important trial comparing CHOP administered at 14- or 21-day intervals with or without the addition of etoposide in patients of all ages (134,135). This study showed a significant improvement in outcome in patients >60 years of age with CHOP administered at 14-day intervals, but not with the addition of etoposide. In contrast, in younger patients the addition of etoposide to CHOP administered at 21-day intervals led to the best outcome.

In the United States during the 1980s, a number of new regimens were developed (i.e., often called "third generation" regimens) that appeared to be more intensive than CHOP, and in phase II trials reported a failure-free survival that seemed to be approximately 50% greater than what had been reported with CHOP. The most popular of these regimens were methotrexate, bleomycin, doxorubicin, cyclophosphamide, vincristine, and dexamethasone, prednisone, procarbazine, doxorubicin, cyclophosphamide, etoposide, cytarabine, bleomycin, vincristine, and methotrexate, and methotrexate, doxorubicin, cyclophosphamide, vincristine, prednisone, and bleomycin (136–138). Over the objections of some who felt that the results with the new regimens were clearly superior to CHOP, a comparative clinical trial was carried out. In this landmark study, CHOP was found to be equivalent to the newer regimens with long-term, disease-free survival in 35% to 40% of the patients regardless of treatment (139). The apparent discrepancy between the results of the phase II trials and the randomized trial is probably explained by selection of patients with more favorable IPI scores and patients with stage II disease for participation in the phase II trials.

A number of new approaches have been tested in an attempt to improve the results for patients with disseminated DLBCL. The use of high-dose therapy and autologous transplantation is addressed in *Hematopoietic Stem Cell Transplantation as Part of Primary Therapy*. The use of infusional chemotherapy in the etoposide, prednisone, vincristine, cyclophosphamide, and doxorubicin plus rituximab regimen has reported excellent results in phase II trials (140) and is currently in a randomized trial in the United States. However, the most important new advance has been the incorporation of immunotherapy using the monoclonal antibody rituximab into the initial treatment of patients with DLBCL (Table 20.7). In 2002, investigators from France reported a trial of CHOP versus R-CHOP in initial treatment of patients with DLBCL who were >60 years of age (67). A highly significant advantage in complete remission rate, failure-free survival, and overall survival was found in favor of the group that received rituximab. A subsequent report of the results with a median follow-up of 5 years showed that relapse remained

significantly less frequent in the patients treated with rituximab (i.e., 20% vs. 34%), a higher proportion of patients who received rituximab remained event free (i.e., 48% vs. 28%), and the overall survival favored receiving rituximab (58% vs. 45%) (141).

In the United States a trial of CHOP with or without rituximab was also carried out in patients >60 years of age (69). In this trial there was a two-part randomization with patients receiving induction with CHOP or R-CHOP followed by a randomization to receive or not receive rituximab maintenance therapy. Patients treated initially with R-CHOP had a superior 3-year failure-free survival (53% vs. 46%). The impact of maintenance rituximab was seen only in the group of patients who did not receive rituximab in induction therapy. The 2-year failure-free survival from second randomization was 77% for R-CHOP without maintenance, 79% for R-CHOP with maintenance, 74% for CHOP with maintenance rituximab, and 45% for CHOP alone. The conclusion from this study was that rituximab is an important component in the treatment of patients with DLBCL that does not need to be administered both during induction and maintenance therapy, at least in patients who achieve an initial complete remission.

An international study was carried out in patients <60 years of age who had none or one adverse risk factor in the age-adjusted IPI (i.e., risk factors included elevated LDH, high stage, and poor performance status) and at least stage II disease with the exception that patients who had stage I disease with tumor bulk were able to be enrolled. The patients were randomly assigned to receive six cycles of a "CHOP-like" regimen with or without rituximab. In most of the participating countries, the patients received CHOP, but in Germany, because of the studies noted previously in this section, the patients received CHOP plus etoposide. The 3-year

---

TABLE 20.7

COMPARATIVE TRIALS OF THE ADDITIONS OF RITUXIMAB TO THE TREATMENT OF PATIENTS WITH DLBCL

Reference	Patient characteristics	Regimen	No. of patients	CR (%)	EFS	OS
(67,141)	Age 60–80	CHOP ×8	197	63	28% (5 y)	45% (5 y)
	Stage II–IV	R-CHOP ×8	202	75	48% (5 y)	58% (5 y)
(69)[a]	Age 60–92	CHOP ×8	85	–	34% (2 y)	–
	Stage I–IV	CHOP ×8→maintenance R	94	–	56% (2 y)	–
		R-CHOP ×8	93	–	59% (2 y)	–
		R-CHOP ×8 →maintenance R	80	–	61% (2 y)	–
(68)[b]	Age 18–60	"CHOP-like" ×6	411	68	59% (3 y)	84% (3 y)
	Stage II–IV Age adjusted IPI 0–1	"CHOP-like" +R ×6	413	86	79% (3 y)	93% (3 y)
(142)[b]	Age 61–80	CHOP-14 ×6	307	68	47% (3 y)	68% (3 y)
	Stage I–IV	CHOP-14 ×8	305	72	53% (3 y)	66% (3 y)
		R-CHOP-14 ×6	306	78	67% (3 y)	78% (3 y)
		R-CHOP-14 ×8	304	76	63% (3 y)	73% (3 y)
(143)	Any age	"CHOP-like" before approval of	140	–	51% (2 y PFS)	52% (2 y)
	Any age	rituximab in British Columbia	152	–		78% (2 y)
		"CHOP-like" after approval of rituximab in British Columbia			69% (2 y PFS)	

CR, complete response; OS, overall survival; PFS, progression-free survival.
[a] Event-free survival (EFS) is from initiation of induction therapy, not from second randomization.
[b] Radiotherapy was permitted for sites of bulk.

event-free survival favored chemotherapy plus rituximab (i.e., 79% vs. 59%), and the 3-year overall survival also favored receiving rituximab (93% vs. 84%) (68).

The German study group carried out a trial of CHOP administered at 14-day intervals in patients >60 years of age with a double randomization (142). Patients received either six or eight cycles of CHOP at 14-day intervals with or without rituximab. Once again, the outcome favored receiving rituximab. For patients who received no rituximab, the 3-year event-free survival was 47% after six cycles of CHOP at 14-day intervals and 53% for patients who received eight cycles. In contrast, patients who received rituximab in addition to CHOP at 14-day intervals had a 3-year event-free survival of 67% for six cycles of therapy and 63% for eight cycles. There was a hint in this study that patients >70 years of age did less well when they received eight cycles rather than six cycles of chemotherapy.

Although not a randomized trial, an important observation was made by investigators from British Columbia by measuring the impact of the introduction of rituximab into the treatment of patients with DLBCL (143). In Canada, anticancer drugs are made available without cost after they are approved by a central agency. Investigators were able to identify all patients treated for DLBCL in British Columbia 18 months before and 18 months after rituximab was approved for use. One hundred forty patients were treated in the pre-rituximab group and 152 in the post-rituximab group. The only variable in the study was the date that the drug was approved, and 10% of the patients in the preapproval group actually received rituximab, and 14% of the patients in the postapproval group did not receive rituximab. All patients did receive CHOP-like regimens. The results improved dramatically after the drug was generally available, with a 2-year progression free-survival improvement from 51% to 69% and an improvement of 2-year overall survival from 52% to 78%.

There is no doubt that the single most important recent advance in the treatment of patients with DLBCL has been the introduction of rituximab into induction therapy. However, it is not necessarily the case that R-CHOP is the superior treatment approach. In the international trial of a "CHOP-like" regimen with or without rituximab, it was possible to analyze patients who received CHOP plus etoposide versus those who received CHOP alone, in both cases with or without rituximab. There was an advantage to the addition of etoposide to CHOP in patients who did not receive rituximab, but the advantage disappeared when rituximab was administered (68). However, this does not mean that all chemotherapy regimens plus rituximab would be equivalent to R-CHOP. For example, studies are underway comparing the infusional regimen etoposide, prednisone, vincristine, cyclophosphamide, and doxorubicin plus rituximab with R-CHOP, and another trying to estimate the extent of contribution of rituximab to treatment with ACVBP.

Patients with certain presentations of DLBCL can be at risk for relapse in sanctuary sites. For example, patients with testicular DLBCL have a high risk to have relapse in the opposite testicle if these do not receive scrotal radiation as part of their initial treatment (144). However, the most frequent issue is which patients with DLBCL are at risk for CNS relapse. A number of factors have been proposed as risk factors,, including epidural presentation, sinus presenta-

tion, testicular presentation, bone marrow involvement, bone involvement, peripheral blood involvement, breast involvement, adrenal involvement, elevated serum LDH level and others (145–147). To prevent central nervous relapse, intrathecal methotrexate and/or cytarabine administered with each chemotherapy treatment and systemic high-dose methotrexate have both been utilized. In the absence of a randomized trial documenting the efficacy of CNS prophylaxis, most groups treat patients that they consider to be at high risk with intrathecal chemotherapy administered with each chemotherapy cycle or, as in the ACVBP regimen, high-dose methotrexate in the consolidation phase of treatment in addition to intrathecal methotrexate. Patients presenting with primary CNS DLBCL present a special problem that is dealt with in Chapter 37. These patients must have high-dose methotrexate as part of their initial treatment, and some patients can be cured (148).

Patients with disseminated DLBCL who present with a large tumor mass and achieve an initial complete remission as documented by PET scan often have residual imaging abnormalities at the site of the large mass. Many physicians would treat these patients with involved-field radiotherapy to the site of the original large mass, although this remains a point for debate. This dilemma is frequently encountered in patients with mediastinal DLBCL (Chapter 21). In the international study comparing a "CHOP-like" regimen with or without rituximab, a retrospective analysis was done to determine the impact of maximum tumor bulk at presentation. The presence of a 10-cm mass did predict an eventual worse prognosis (142). This was despite the fact that patients with bulky disease received radiotherapy as part of their treatment. However, the results might have been worse in the absence of the radiotherapy.

It is likely that our treatments will continue to improve for patients with widespread diffuse large B-cell lymphoma. New classes of agents that are becoming available, for example, proteosome inhibitors, might benefit subsets of patients with this disease. This is a radiosensitive tumor, and it may well be that some patients will benefit from adjuvant radioimmunotherapy. New scientific observations about the disease might guide treatment advances. For example, recent observations that stromal cells in DLBCL effect treatment outcome might offer a therapeutic opportunity for a subset of patients (149). One of the gene signatures identified was associated with a poorer prognosis and reflected increased tumor blood vessel density. These are patients that might benefit from antiangiogenesis agents such as bevacizumab. It is likely that treatments will be increasingly chosen based on the biologic characteristics of the patient's tumor as well as the clinical characteristics of the patient.

Hematopoietic Stem Cell Transplantation as Part of Primary Therapy

Pretreatment prognostic factors can be used to identify patients with DLBCL who are less likely to attain a remission with primary therapy and more likely to have relapse. The results of treatment for these patients may potentially be improved by incorporation of autologous hematopoietic stem cell transplantation into primary therapy. The use of this type of "upfront" transplant requires the ability to accurately identify patients with poor prognosis, as well as the ability to perform transplants with low morbidity and mortality. One of the earliest attempts at using up-front transplantation for non-Hodgkin lymphoma was reported by investigators at Memorial Sloan-Kettering Cancer Center (150). Fourteen patients with large cell lymphoma with poor-prognosis characteristics received high-dose therapy followed by autologous hematopoietic stem cell transplantation in first complete or partial remission. The overall survival of this cohort was significantly improved when compared with a historical control group with similar characteristics that refused early transplantation. Subsequent phase II trials demonstrated that approximately 60% to 80% of patients with high-risk aggressive lymphoma could achieve long-term progression-free survival following autologous hematopoietic stem cell transplantation in first remission (151–153). Although results from these series were encouraging, potential advantages of up-front transplantation were overestimated because survival curves were often reported only for those patients who were able to proceed to transplant, rather than for all patients from the time of diagnosis. Therefore, these reports led to several randomized trials of early hematopoietic stem cell transplantation for aggressive lymphomas.

A large number of prospective randomized trials of up-front transplantation have been reported. Although some have demonstrated survival advantages with this approach (154–156), others have failed to show significant differences in outcome, and some showed inferior results (157). These differences are likely due to the wide variation in study design related to inclusion criteria, extent of primary therapy before transplantation, and differences in the transplant regimen itself. Furthermore, some studies randomized all patients at the time of diagnosis, whereas others only randomized patients who demonstrated a response to initial therapy. The use of up-front transplantation for DLBCL has been evaluated in metaanalyses and a systematic review (158–160). These analyses noted the heterogeneity of trial designs and conflicting results, and concluded that there is no definite survival advantage associated with up-front transplantation as compared with conventional chemotherapy. Patients without adverse prognostic factors clearly do not benefit from this approach, although subgroup analyses did show suggestive evidence for survival advantages associated with up-front transplantation for patients with high-intermediate and high-risk IPI groups treated with a full course of primary therapy before transplantation.

Encouraging results of novel tandem dose-intensive chemotherapy regimens followed by up-front transplantation have been reported (161). Other investigators have evaluated the role of high-dose sequential chemotherapy regimens in an attempt to improve treatment outcomes. These regimens consist of an initial induction or debulking phase. This is followed by administration of high doses of noncross-resistant single agents at intervals of 1 to 3 weeks to prevent the emergence of resistant clones. This phase is followed by collection and infusion of autologous hematopoietic stem cells. Recent randomized trials have failed to show survival benefits when high-dose sequential chemotherapy regimens were compared with conventional therapy (162,163), despite earlier promising results with this approach (155).

Interpretation of up-front transplantation trials is also difficult because they were performed before the routine use of rituximab with primary therapy, and before the use of new strategies such as 14-day treatment cycles. As results of primary therapy improve, the potential benefits of additional high-dose therapy may diminish, and these innovations have made it more difficult to identify candidates with poor risk for up-front transplantation. The North American intergroup S9704 trial was amended to allow the use of rituximab with primary therapy. In this trial for patients with high-intermediate and high-risk IPI groups, eight cycles of CHOP or R-CHOP are being compared with six cycles of CHOP or R-CHOP, followed by autologous hematopoietic stem cell transplantation. Accrual has been completed, and results are pending. Encouraging results have been reported with rituximab-containing primary treatment regimens that utilize repeated infusions of autologous hematopoietic stem cells (164). The German High-Grade non-Hodgkin's lymphoma Study Group trial 2002-1 is conducting a phase III trial with the MegaCHOEP regimen (165), which utilizes repeated up-front stem cell transplantations for high-risk aggressive non-Hodgkin lymphoma.

The role of up-front transplantation for patients with poor prognosis remains controversial. It is hoped that new technologies such as gene expression profiling or interim PET scanning may identify patients who are appropriate candidates for early transplantation. Patients with DLBCL in first remission may be appropriate candidates for trials involving autologous hematopoietic stem cell transplantation according to National Comprehensive Cancer Network guidelines. Up-front transplantation is felt to be indicated for high-intermediate and high-risk IPI groups according to a position statement from the American Society for Blood and Marrow Transplantation executive committee (166).

Trials of Chemotherapy in Elderly Patients

Elderly patients present unique problems when they are diagnosed with DLBCL. Although some elderly patients are at least as healthy as younger adults and can be treated with the same regimens, this is not always true. Also, age is an important prognostic factor in the IPI. There are multiple potential explanations for a poor outcome in elderly patients. These include comorbid illnesses, altered metabolism of the chemotherapeutic agents, diagnosis later in the course of the disease, and different disease biology. Older patients sometimes are less willing to accept very intensive and potentially more toxic regimens, even if they are apparently able to tolerate them. One trial found that regimens optimal in younger patients might not be the same as those that would have optimal activity in elderly patients (142). Elderly patients seemed to benefit more by shortening the treatment interval and increasing the dose intensity of CHOP, whereas younger patients benefited more from the addition of an extra drug to the CHOP regimen, with the drugs administered at 3-week intervals.

A number of other randomized trials have been carried out specifically addressing the care of elderly patients with diffuse large cell lymphoma in which most or all of the patients had DLBCL (Table 20.8). One of the most influential clinical trials ever carried out in the treatment of patients with lymphoma was a trial of CHOP versus CHOP plus the monoclonal anti-CD20 antibody rituximab in elderly patients (i.e., ages 60 to 80 years), all of whom had DLBCL (67). This trial of 399 patients found a superior complete

TABLE 20.8

RANDOMIZED THERAPEUTIC TRIALS IN ELDERLY PATIENTS WITH DLBCL

Reference	Comparison	No. of patients	Patient characteristics	Significant differences
(67)	CHOP vs. CHOP + rituximab	399	Age 60–80 y Stage II–IV All DLBC	CR: CHOP, 63%; R-CHOP, 76% ($p = 0.005$) 2-y event-free survival: CHOP, 38%; R-CHOP, 57% ($p = 0.001$) 2-y overall survival: CHOP, 57%; R-CHOP, 70% ($p = 0.007$)
(167)	CVP vs. CTVP	453	Age ε70 y Stage I–IV	CR: CVP, 32%; CTVP, 47% ($p = 0.0001$) 5-y survival: CVP, 19%; CTVP, 26% ($p = 0.05$)
(215)	CHOP vs. ACVBP	635	Age 60–69 y Age-adjusted IPI 1–3	Event-free survival: CHOP, 33%; ACVBP, 45% ($p = 0.004$)
(216)	ACVBP vs. alternating VIMMM/ACVBP	810	Age 55–69 y Stage I–IV	CR: ACVBP, 58%; Alternating regimen, 48% ($p = 0.003$) 5-y event-free survival: ACVBP, 33%; alternating regimen, 28% ($p = 0.03$)
(217)	CHOP vs. VMP	120	Age >70 y Stage II–IV	Progression-free survival: CHOP, 55%; VMP, 30% ($p = 0.004$)
(168)	CHOP vs. CHOP + filgrastim vs. CNOP vs. CNOP + filgrastim	455	Age 60–86 y Stage II–IV	CR: CHOP + filgrastim, 60%; CNOP + filgrastim, 43% ($p < 0.001$) 5-y overall survival: CHOP + filgrastim, 48%; CNOP + filgrastim, 26% ($p < 0.001$)
(169)	CHOP vs. CNOP	148	Age ε60 y Stage II–IV	CR: CHOP, 49%; CNOP, 31% ($p = 0.03$) 3-y overall survival: CHOP, 42%; CNOP, 26% ($p = 0.03$)
(218)	CHOP q 21 d vs. weekly CHOP	38	Age ε65 y Stage I–IV	None
(219)	VNCOP-B ∞ 12 wk vs. VNCOP-B ∞ 8 wk	306	Age ε60 y Stage II–IV	None

CR, complete remission; CTVP, cyclophosphamide, pirarubicin (THP-doxorubicin), teniposide (VM-26), and prednisone; CVP, cyclophosphamide, teniposide (VM-26), and prednisone; VIMMM, teniposide (VM-26), ifosfamide, mitoxantrone, methylgag, and methotrexate; VMP, VePesid (etoposide), mitoxantrone, prednimustine; VNCOP-B, VePesid (etoposide), Novantrone (mitoxantrone), cyclophosphamide, Oncovin (vincristine), prednisone, and bleomycin.

remission rate (76% vs. 63%; $p = 0.005$), 2-year event-free survival (57% vs. 38%; $p = 0.001$), and 2-year overall survival (70% vs. 57%; $p = 0.007$), in each case favoring the combination of R-CHOP. In this trial, the rituximab was administered at a dose of 375 mg per m^2 on day 1 of each treatment cycle, the same day as the cyclophosphamide, doxorubicin, and vincristine were administered. Although this trial was restricted to elderly patients, this treatment approach has been broadly accepted in the United States, and currently, essentially all new patients with DLBCL receive R-CHOP. The approach is supported by an intergroup trial that also showed the advantage of rituximab and found that maintenance therapy had no further benefit when rituximab was given in the initial remission induction (69).

A German study carried out in patients >60 years of age compared CHOP at 14-day intervals administered with or without rituximab for six or eight total cycles of therapy (142). Patients who received rituximab did better than those who did not, and eight cycles of therapy did not show an advantage over six cycles. However, when only patients >70 years of age were analyzed, it appeared that the additional two cycles of therapy might provide a therapeutic disadvantage and lower overall survival. A similar finding came from a French trial (123) in which patients >60 years of age

received four cycles of CHOP without rituximab and were randomized to receive or not receive radiotherapy after the chemotherapy. There was no difference overall between the two groups but a hint that the patients >70 years of age did less well if they received the additional radiotherapy. It may well be that in very elderly patients, there is a narrow therapeutic "window" to achieve the optimal result.

Another study from France compared a regimen not containing an anthracycline (i.e., cyclophosphamide, teniposide, and prednisone) versus the same drugs plus the anthracycline epirubicin in 453 patients with diffuse aggressive non-Hodgkin lymphoma >70 years of age (167). Both the complete remission rate (47% vs. 32%; $p = 0.0001$) and the 5-year survival (26% vs. 19%; $p = 0.05$) favored the anthracycline-containing regimen. This study reinforces the importance of including an anthracycline or anthracenedione in the treatment of patients of any age with diffuse large cell lymphoma when cure is the goal.

Three studies in elderly patients have compared CHOP with alternate regimens incorporating the anthracenedione mitoxantrone rather than the anthracycline doxorubicin. A Scandinavian study compared CHOP plus or minus filgrastim with Cytoxan (cyclophosphamide), Novantrone (mitoxantrone), Oncovin (vincristine), and prednisone (CNOP) plus or minus filgrastim in 455 patients aged 60 to 86 years (168). The dose of doxorubicin in this study was 50 mg per m^2 and the dose of mitoxantrone 10 mg per m^2. Both the complete remission rate (60% vs. 43%; p <0.001) and the 5-year survival (48% vs. 26%; p <0.001) favored the CHOP regimen. In a Dutch study of 148 patients, CHOP was compared with CNOP (169); once again, the doxorubicin dose was 50 mg per m^2, and the mitoxantrone dose was 10 mg per m^2. In this study, both the complete remission rate (49% vs. 31%; p = 0.03) and the 3-year overall survival (42% vs. 26%; p = 0.03) favored the CHOP regimen. Because the equitoxic dose of mitoxantrone to 50 mg per m^2 of doxorubicin is probably 12 mg per m^2, not 10 mg per m^2, these studies leave open the question of the results if the higher dose of mitoxantrone had been used. In one historically controlled study, the results with doxorubicin at 50 mg per m^2 and mitoxantrone at 12 mg per m^2 were similar (170).

Elderly patients with DLBCL should not be denied potentially curative therapy simply because of their age. Long-term, disease-free survival free from relapse is possible for both localized and disseminated disease. However, the poor clinical condition of some patients, or their unwillingness to accept very toxic therapy, might make a less intensive therapy that is unlikely to be curative the best choice. In these patients, radiotherapy to symptomatic areas, single-agent rituximab, or lower doses of various chemotherapeutic drugs can be used to eliminate or ameliorate unpleasant symptoms. In patients unwilling to accept any of these approaches, involvement of the hospice team can be the best approach.

Recurrent and Refractory Diffuse Large B-Cell Lymphoma

Conventional Treatment

At least 30% to 40% of patients with advanced-stage DLBCL will fail to attain a remission with primary therapy or will have relapse after achieving a remission. Occasional asymptomatic patients can be managed with a watch and wait approach if they are not candidates for aggressive therapy. Selected patients may experience prolonged remissions with involved-field radiation therapy. However, the vast majority of patients will require second-line (salvage) chemotherapy.

A large number of drugs have single-agent activity for patients with relapsed and refractory aggressive non-Hodgkin lymphoma (171). Response rates average 20% to 30%, although response rates >50% have been reported. The duration of response with single agents is usually brief, and few patients have long progression-free survival. Commonly used salvage regimens include mitoxantrone, ifosfamide, and etoposide (172), dexamethasone, cytarabine, and cisplatin (DHAP) (173), etoposide, methylprednisolone, cytarabine, and cisplatin (174), and ifosfamide, carboplatin, and etoposide (ICE) (60). Other regimens, including etoposide, vincristine, doxorubicin, cyclophosphamide, and prednisone and cyclophosphamide, doxorubicin, and etoposide, utilize continuous infusion of agents as a means of overcoming drug resistance (175,176). Use of these salvage regimens result in overall response rates of 50% to 70%, although prior therapy often makes it difficult to administer repeated cycles,

and few patients experience prolonged progression-free survival. The prognostic factors for patients treated with these salvage regimens are similar to the prognostic factors that are important for primary treatment regimens. These regimens are frequently used only briefly to reduce tumor burden before administration of high-dose therapy followed by autologous hematopoietic stem cell transplantation.

Approximately one third of patients with relapsed or refractory DLBCL will respond to rituximab alone (177). In current practice, conventional salvage regimens are almost always administered in combination with rituximab (178,179). Response rates may be lower for patients who received rituximab with primary treatment (180). When compared with historical controls, the response rate for refractory DLBCL was improved when rituximab was added to ICE salvage chemotherapy (181), and the addition of rituximab increased the response to DHAP in a matched-pair analysis (182). In a prospective trial, the overall response rate and ability to proceed to transplant were significantly higher when rituximab was added to the DHAP and etoposide, ifosfamide, and methotrexate salvage regimens (183). Rituximab has been added to combinations of newer agents, such as gemcitabine and oxaliplatin (184,185). Few comparisons of salvage regimens have been performed, although response rates following ICE were higher than DHAP in a retrospective analysis (186). DHAP plus rituximab is being compared with ICE plus rituximab in the phase III international CORAL trial (187).

A wide variety of other agents display single-agent activity for patients with relapsed and refractory DLBCL and have also been used in salvage regimens (171). Patients may occasionally respond to treatment with interferon-α (188). Radiolabeled antibodies have not been extensively studied in DLBCL. The response to ^{131}I-tositumomab among patients with aggressive lymphomas was poor when compared with patients with low-grade or transformed lymphomas (189). In another trial, the overall response rate exceeded 50% for patients with relapsed or refractory DLBCL who were treated with ^{90}Y-ibritumomab tiuxetan, although response rates were considerably lower for patients who had previously received rituximab (190). Liposomal-encapsulated anthracyclines may be used alone or in combination for patients who cannot receive additional anthracyclines (191,192), and a liposomal vincristine formulation may improve efficacy and reduce toxicity (193). Modest response rates with newer agents such as bendamustine (194), and lenalidomide (195), have been described for patients with relapsed and refractory DLBCL. A number of new monoclonal antibodies and agents directed at targets such as protein kinase C (enzastaurin), vascular endothelial growth factor (bevacizumab), mammalian target of rapamycin (temsirolimus, everolimus), and SYK (tamatinib) are being evaluated.

High-Dose Therapy

The poor results of treatment with conventional salvage chemotherapy regimens for DLBCL led to the increasing use of high-dose therapy followed by autologous hematopoietic stem cell transplantation for patients with relapsed and refractory disease. The first large series of autologous transplantation for aggressive lymphoma validated the observation that transplant outcome was related to the response to conventional salvage chemotherapy administered before

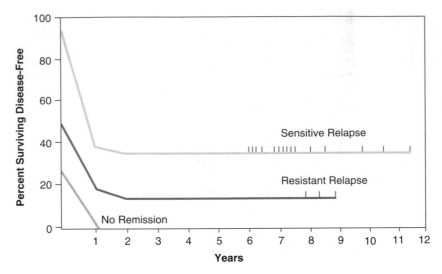

FIGURE 20.1 Late follow-up from study by Thomas et al. (5), showing that patients still chemotherapy sensitive after relapse from complete remission have a better outcome than those that are chemotherapy resistant or never achieved an initial remission. The *tic marks* indicate patients in remission at that interval. (From Philip T, Armitage JO, Spitzer G, et al. High-dose therapy and autologous bone marrow transplantation after failure of conventional chemotherapy in adults with intermediate-grade or high-grade non-Hodgkin's lymphoma. *N Engl J Med* 1987;316:1493–1498, with permission.)

transplant (196) (Fig. 20.1). Approximately 40% of patients achieved long-term remissions following transplantation if they responded to conventional salvage chemotherapy before receiving high-dose therapy (sensitive relapse). The long-term disease-free survival was approximately 15% for patients who did not respond to conventional salvage chemotherapy (resistant relapse), and there were no long-term survivors among patients with primary refractory disease.

After this a large number of phase II trials evaluated the role of autologous hematopoietic transplantation for aggressive lymphomas (197–199) (Table 20.9). These studies demonstrated that long-term progression-free survival could be observed following transplantation. These studies also confirmed the prognostic significance of chemotherapy sensitivity before transplant, and most patients receive conventional chemotherapy to test sensitivity and reduce tumor burden before transplantation. Other factors associated with improved transplant outcomes include good performance status, younger age, absence of tumor bulk, less extensive prior therapy, and low IPI score at the time of relapse.

The value of autologous hematopoietic transplantation for DLBCL was not conclusively demonstrated until the landmark PARMA trial was performed (200). In this trial, patients with relapsed aggressive lymphoma were treated with two cycles of DHAP salvage chemotherapy. Patients with sensitive disease were then randomized to receive treatment with four additional cycles of DHAP, or to treatment with high-dose therapy followed by autologous hematopoietic stem cell transplantation. The actuarial 5-year event-free survival was 46% for patients randomized to transplant, as compared with 12% for patients who received DHAP (*p* = 0.001). The actuarial 5-year overall survival rates were 53% and 32%, respectively (*p* = 0.038) (Fig. 20.2). Follow-up studies demonstrated that survival advantages were only seen for patients with an IPI score of more than zero, and that prognosis was better for patients with a longer duration of

initial remission (201,202). Since then, the use of autologous hematopoietic stem cell transplantation has become accepted therapy for first chemotherapy sensitive relapse of patients with DLBCL (166). Although transplantation is unlikely to benefit patients who are truly refractory to primary therapy, some patients with a PR to primary chemotherapy will obtain sustained remissions, especially if they have a continued response to additional salvage chemotherapy. Reports from North American and Spanish registries demonstrate

---

TABLE 20.9

SELECTED SERIES OF AUTOLOGOUS HEMATOPOIETIC STEM CELL TRANSPLANTATION FOR AGGRESSIVE NON-HODGKIN LYMPHOMA

Reference	No. of patients	Early mortality (%)	Outcome
(196)	100	21	19% actuarial 3-y DFS
(220)	101	21	11% actuarial 5-y EFS
(221)	158	NS	29% actuarial 3-y FFS
(222)	107	7	35% actuarial 5-y PFS
(223)	221	10	55% CCR (median 2.4 y)
(224)	112	3	71% actuarial 3-y DFS (for intermediate grade)
(225)	136	4.4	34% actuarial 5-y EFS
(226)	94	10.6	33% actuarial 3-y PFS
(227)	90	NS	40% actuarial 4-y DFS

CCR, continuous complete remission; DFS, disease-free survival; EFS, event-free survival; FFS, failure-free survival; NS, not stated; PFS, progression-free survival.

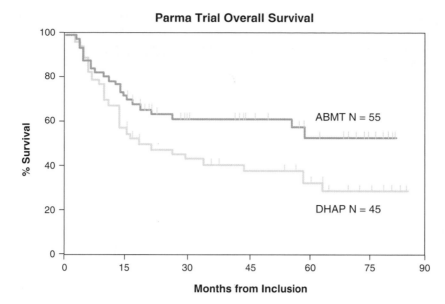

FIGURE 20.2 Overall survival of patients with chemotherapy sensitive relapsed aggressive lymphoma who were randomly allocated to autologous transplant or further standard dose chemotherapy and radiotherapy. ABMT, autologous bone marrow transplant; Parma, (From Philip T, Guglielmi C, Hagenbeek A, et al. Autologous bone marrow transplantation as compared with salvage chemotherapy in relapses of chemotherapy-sensitive non-Hodgkin's lymphoma. *N Engl J Med* 1995;333:1540–1545, with permission.)

that 5-year survival rates are approximately 40% for these patients (203,204).

It is important to note that the majority of studies evaluating the role of autologous hematopoietic stem cell transplantation for DLBCL were performed before the routine use of rituximab with primary therapy. Rituximab may improve the efficacy of salvage chemotherapy and allow more patients to proceed to transplantation (181,183). In a retrospective analysis, both disease-free survival and overall survival were significantly longer for patients with intermediate-grade lymphomas who received rituximab with salvage chemotherapy within 3 months of the transplant date (205). Alternatively, it is possible that the use of rituximab with primary therapy might make it less likely for patients to respond to salvage chemotherapy and proceed to transplant (180,187). Nevertheless, virtually all investigators would recommend adding rituximab to pretransplant chemotherapy if this improves the response rate. Ongoing trials are evaluating whether transplant results will be improved when radiolabeled antibodies are added to high-dose chemotherapy preparative regimens. It is also hoped that trials using PET scan-based risk-adapted strategies may identify the best candidates for transplant.

There is less experience with allogeneic hematopoietic stem cell transplantation for DLBCL. Transplant-related mortality is higher with this approach, and trials comparing autologous and allogeneic transplantation have generally failed to show survival advantages associated with allogeneic transplantation, despite lower rates of relapse (206,207). Allogeneic transplantation using reduced intensity conditioning may also benefit some patients with DLBCL, especially those who have had a prior autologous transplant (208–210). Relapse rates appear to be higher when patients transplanted with these regimens are compared with patients with indolent lymphoma, and results are inferior for patients with resistant disease and a significant tumor burden. There is little consensus on which patients are candidates for allogeneic transplantation and whether reduced-intensity or myeloablative conditioning should be utilized.

FUTURE DIRECTIONS

The subtype of non-Hodgkin lymphoma that we refer to as *DLBCL* is clearly a heterogeneous entity. We have known for many years that some patients could be cured with available therapies, whereas others go on to die of their disease. The chances for a good survival have been found to be better with low stage, fewer symptoms, less bulky disease, low LDH levels, no involvement of the liver or CNS, and other factors. The use of gene arrays has demonstrated that patients with this disease can be subdivided based on gene expression patterns. Patients with a gene expression pattern that resembles normal GCBs have a better outcome than do those whose gene expression pattern resembles activated postgerminal center B lymphocytes, even with rituximab-containing therapy regimens. It is likely that further understanding of gene expression and protein expression patterns in DLBCLs will eventually lead to more specific treatments for individual subgroups. In fact, whether DLBCL can be usefully further subdivided depends not only on our ability to find diagnostic tests to subcategorize the illness but also on the development of specific therapies that make these subdivisions clinically important. It is likely that, to some degree, this will happen. DLBCL is one of the chemotherapy curable malignancies and can be cured in a significant proportion of patients. Hopefully, a better understanding of the biology of this lymphoma will see an increased cure rate.

References

1. Swerdlow SH. *WHO classification of tumours of haematopoietic and lymphoid tissues*, 4th ed. Lyon, France: International Agency for Research on Cancer, 2008.
2. A clinical evaluation of the International Lymphoma Study Group classification of non-Hodgkin's lymphoma. The Non-Hodgkin's Lymphoma Classification Project. *Blood* 1997;89:3909–3918.
3. Anderson JR, Armitage JO, Weisenburger DD. Epidemiology of the non-Hodgkin's lymphomas: distributions of the major subtypes differ by geographic locations. Non-Hodgkin's Lymphoma Classification Project. *Ann Oncol* 1998;9:717–720.
4. Morton LM, Wang SS, Devesa SS, et al. Lymphoma incidence patterns by WHO subtype in the United States, 1992-2001. *Blood* 2006;107:265–276.
5. Thomas E, Brewster DH, Black RJ, et al. Risk of malignancy among patients with rheumatic conditions. *Int J Cancer* 2000;88:497–502.
6. Mikuls TR, Endo JO, Puumala SE, et al. Prospective study of survival outcomes in Non-Hodgkin's lymphoma patients with rheumatoid arthritis. *J Clin Oncol* 2006;24:1597–1602.
7. Engelhard M, Brittinger G, Huhn D, et al. Subclassification of diffuse large B-cell lymphomas according to the Kiel classification: distinction of centroblastic and immunoblastic lymphomas is a significant prognostic risk factor. *Blood* 1997;89:2291–2297.
8. Armitage JO, Weisenburger DD. New approach to classifying non-Hodgkin's lymphomas: clinical features of the major histologic subtypes. Non-Hodgkin's Lymphoma Classification Project. *J Clin Oncol* 1998;16:2780–2795.
9. Fisher DE, Jacobson JO, Ault KA, et al. Diffuse large cell lymphoma with discordant bone marrow histology. Clinical features and biological implications. *Cancer* 1989;64:1879–1887.
10. Velasquez WS, Jagannath S, Tucker SL, et al. Risk classification as the basis for clinical staging of diffuse large-cell lymphoma derived from 10-year survival data. *Blood* 1989;74:551–557.
11. Cabanillas F, Velasquez WS, Hagemeister FB, et al. Clinical, biologic, and histologic features of late relapses in diffuse large cell lymphoma. *Blood* 1992;79:1024–1028.
12. Stein H, Lennert K, Feller AC, et al. Immunohistological analysis of human lymphoma: correlation of histological and immunological categories. *Adv Cancer Res* 1984;42:67–147.
13. Doggett RS, Wood GS, Horning S, et al. The immunologic characterization of 95 nodal and extranodal diffuse large cell lymphomas in 89 patients. *Am J Pathol* 1984;115:245–252.
14. Gascoyne RD, Adomat SA, Krajewski S, et al. Prognostic significance of Bcl-2 protein expression and Bcl-2 gene rearrangement in diffuse aggressive non-Hodgkin's lymphoma. *Blood* 1997;90:244–251.
15. Kramer MH, Hermans J, Parker J, et al. Clinical significance of bcl2 and p53 protein expression in diffuse large B-cell lymphoma: a population-based study. *J Clin Oncol* 1996;14:2131–2138.
16. Sanchez E, Chacon I, Plaza MM, et al. Clinical outcome in diffuse large B-cell lymphoma is dependent on the relationship between different cell-cycle regulator proteins. *J Clin Oncol* 1998;16:1931–1939.
17. Skinnider BF, Horsman DE, Dupuis B, et al. Bcl-6 and Bcl-2 protein expression in diffuse large B-cell lymphoma and follicular lymphoma: correlation with 3q27 and 18q21 chromosomal abnormalities. *Hum Pathol* 1999;30:803–808.
18. De Leval L, Shipp M, Neuberger D, et al. Diffuse large B-cell lymphomas are tumors of germinal center origin. *Blood.* In press.
19. Hans CP, Weisenburger DD, Greiner TC, et al. Confirmation of the molecular classification of diffuse large B-cell lymphoma by immunohistochemistry using a tissue microarray. *Blood* 2004;103:275–282.
20. Kuppers R, Rajewsky K, Hansmann ML. Diffuse large cell lymphomas are derived from mature B cells carrying V region genes with a high load of somatic mutation and evidence of selection for antibody expression. *Eur J Immunol* 1997;27:1398–1405.
21. Klein U, Goossens T, Fischer M, et al. Somatic hypermutation in normal and transformed human B cells. *Immunol Rev* 1998;162:261–280.
22. Yunis JJ, Mayer MG, Arnesen MA, et al. bcl-2 and other genomic alterations in the prognosis of large-cell lymphoma [see comments]. *N Engl J Med* 1989;320:1047–1054.
23. Kramer MH, Hermans J, Wijburg E, et al. Clinical relevance of BCL2, BCL6, and MYC rearrangements in diffuse large B-cell lymphoma. *Blood* 1998;92:3152–3162.
24. Bastard C, Deweindt C, Kerckaert JP, et al. LAZ3 rearrangements in non-Hodgkin's lymphoma: correlation with histology, immunophenotype, karyotype, and clinical outcome in 217 patients. *Blood* 1994;83:2423–2427.
25. Migliazza A, Martinotti S, Chen W, et al. Frequent somatic hypermutation of the 5' noncoding region of the BCL6 gene in B-cell lymphoma. *Proc Natl Acad Sci U S A* 1995;92:12520–12524.
26. Vitolo U, Gaidano G, Botto B, et al. Rearrangements of bcl-6, bcl-2, c-myc and 6q deletion in B-diffuse large-cell lymphoma: clinical relevance in 71 patients. *Ann Oncol* 1998;9:55–61.
27. Shen HM, Peters A, Baron B, et al. Mutation of BCL-6 gene in normal B cells by the process of somatic hypermutation of Ig genes. *Science* 1998;280:1750–1752.
28. Peng HZ, Du MQ, Koulis A, et al. Nonimmunoglobulin gene hypermutation in germinal center B cells. *Blood* 1999;93:2167–2172.
29. Kuppers R, Zhao M, Hansmann ML, et al. Tracing B cell development in human germinal centres by molecular analysis of single cells picked from histological sections. *EMBO J* 1993;12:4955–4967.
30. Delabie J, Vandenberghe E, Kennes C, et al. Histiocyte-rich B-cell lymphoma. A distinct clinicopathologic entity possibly related to lymphocyte predominant Hodgkin's disease, paragranuloma subtype. *Am J Surg Pathol* 1992;16:37–48.
31. McBride JA, Rodriguez J, Luthra R, et al. T-cell-rich B large-cell lymphoma simulating lymphocyte-rich Hodgkin's disease. *Am J Surg Pathol* 1996;20:193–201.
32. Ferry JA, Harris NL, Picker LJ, et al. Intravascular lymphomatosis (malignant angioendotheliomatosis). A B- cell neoplasm expressing surface homing receptors. *Mod Pathol* 1988;1:444–452.
33. Ponzoni M, Ferreri AJ, Campo E, et al. Definition, diagnosis, and management of intravascular large B-cell lymphoma: proposals and perspectives from an international consensus meeting. *J Clin Oncol* 2007;25:3168–3173.
34. Murase T, Yamaguchi M, Suzuki R, et al. Intravascular large B-cell lymphoma (IVLBCL): a clinicopathologic study of 96 cases with special reference to the immunophenotypic heterogeneity of CD5. *Blood* 2007;109:478–485.
35. Ponzoni M, Arrigoni G, Gould VE, et al. Lack of CD 29 (beta1 integrin) and CD 54 (ICAM-1) adhesion molecules in intravascular lymphomatosis. *Hum Pathol* 2000;31:220–226.
36. DiGiuseppe JA, Nelson WG, Seifter EJ, et al. Intravascular lymphomatosis: a clinicopathologic study of 10 cases and assessment of response to chemotherapy. *J Clin Oncol* 1994;12:2573–2579.
37. Nakatsuka S, Yao M, Hoshida Y, et al. Pyothorax-associated lymphoma: a review of 106 cases. *J Clin Oncol* 2002;20:4255–4260.
38. Copie-Bergman C, Niedobitek G, Mangham DC, et al. Epstein-Barr virus in B-cell lymphomas associated with chronic suppurative inflammation. *J Pathol* 1997;183:287–292.
39. Guinee D Jr, Jaffe E, Kingma D, et al. Pulmonary lymphomatoid granulomatosis. Evidence for a proliferation of Epstein-Barr virus infected B-lymphocytes with a prominent T-cell component and vasculitis. *Am J Surg Pathol* 1994;18:753–764.
40. Haque AK, Myers JL, Hudnall SD, et al. Pulmonary lymphomatoid granulomatosis in acquired immunodeficiency syndrome: lesions with Epstein-Barr virus infection. *Mod Pathol* 1998;11:347–356.
41. Katzenstein AL, Peiper SC. Detection of Epstein-Barr virus genomes in lymphomatoid granulomatosis: analysis of 29 cases by the polymerase chain reaction technique. *Mod Pathol* 1990;3:435–441.
42. Myers JL, Kurtin PJ, Katzenstein AL, et al. Lymphomatoid granulomatosis. Evidence of immunophenotypic diversity and relationship to Epstein-Barr virus infection. *Am J Surg Pathol* 1995;19:1300–1312.
43. Delsol G, Lamant L, Mariame B, et al. A new subtype of large B-cell lymphoma expressing the ALK kinase and lacking the 2; 5 translocation. *Blood* 1997;89:1483–1490.
44. Gascoyne RD, Lamant L, Martin-Subero JI, et al. ALK-positive diffuse large B-cell lymphoma is associated with Clathrin-ALK rearrangements: report of 6 cases. *Blood* 2003;102:2568–2573.
45. Reichard KK, McKenna RW, Kroft SH. ALK-positive diffuse large B-cell lymphoma: report of four cases and review of the literature. *Mod Pathol* 2007;20:310–319.
46. Alizadeh AA, Eisen MB, Davis RE, et al. Distinct types of diffuse large B-cell lymphoma identified by gene expression profiling. *Nature* 2000;403:503–511.
47. Shipp MA, Ross KN, Tamayo P, et al. Diffuse large B-cell lymphoma outcome prediction by gene-expression profiling and supervised machine learning. *Nat Med* 2002;8:68–74.
48. Offit K, Jhanwar S, Ebrahim SA, et al. t(3;22)(q27;q11): a novel translocation associated with diffuse non- Hodgkin's lymphoma. *Blood* 1989;74:1876–1879.
49. Bastard C, Tilly H, Lenormand B, et al. Translocations involving band 3q27 and Ig gene regions in non-Hodgkin's lymphoma. *Blood* 1992;79:2527–2531.
50. Ye BH, Lista F, Lo Coco F, et al. Alterations of a zinc finger-encoding gene, BCL-6, in diffuse large- cell lymphoma. *Science* 1993;262:747–750.
51. Ye BH, Chaganti S, Chang CC, et al. Chromosomal translocations cause deregulated BCL6 expression by promoter substitution in B cell lymphoma. *EMBO J* 1995;14:6209–6217.
52. Chang CC, Ye BH, Chaganti RS, et al. BCL-6, a POZ/zinc-finger protein, is a sequence-specific transcriptional repressor. *Proc Natl Acad Sci U S A* 1996;93:6947–6952.
53. Cattoretti G, Chang CC, Cechova K, et al. BCL-6 protein is expressed in germinal-center B cells. *Blood* 1995;86:45–53.
54. Dent AL, Shaffer AL, Yu X, et al. Control of inflammation, cytokine expression, and germinal center formation by BCL-6. *Science* 1997;276:589–592.

55. Ye BH, Cattoretti G, Shen Q, et al. The BCL-6 proto-oncogene controls germinal-centre formation and Th2- type inflammation. *Nat Genet* 1997;16:161–170.
56. Lo Coco F, Ye BH, Lista F, et al. Rearrangements of the BCL6 gene in diffuse large cell non-Hodgkin's lymphoma. *Blood* 1994;83:1757–1759.
57. Chen W, Iida S, Louie DC, et al. Heterologous promoters fused to BCL6 by chromosomal translocations affecting band 3q27 cause its deregulated expression during B-cell differentiation. *Blood* 1998;91:603–607.
58. Shaffer AL, Yu X, He Y, et al. BCL-6 represses genes that function in lymphocyte differentiation, inflammation, and cell cycle control. *Immunity* 2000;13:199–212.
59. Pasqualucci L, Migliazza A, Fracchiolla N, et al. BCL-6 mutations in normal germinal center B cells: evidence of somatic hypermutation acting outside Ig loci. *Proc Natl Acad Sci U S A* 1998;95:11816–11821.
60. Pasqualucci L, Migliazza A, Basso K, et al. Mutations of the BCL6 proto-oncogene disrupt its negative autoregulation in diffuse large B-cell lymphoma. *Blood* 2003;101:2914–2923.
61. Dalla-Favera R, Ye BH, Lo Coco F, et al. Identification of genetic lesions associated with diffuse large-cell lymphoma. *Ann Oncol* 1994;5(suppl 1):55–60.
62. Tang SC, Visser L, Hepperle B, et al S. Clinical significance of bcl-2-MBR gene rearrangement and protein expression in diffuse large-cell non-Hodgkin's lymphoma: an analysis of 83 cases. *J Clin Oncol* 1994;12:149–154.
63. Pasqualucci L, Neumeister P, Goossens T, et al. Hypermutation of multiple proto-oncogenes in B-cell diffuse large-cell lymphomas. *Nature* 2001;412:341–346.
64. Fredericks RK, Walker FO, Elster A, et al. Angiotropic intravascular large-cell lymphoma (malignant angioendotheliomatosis): report of a case and review of the literature. *Surg Neurol* 1991;35:218–223.
65. Conlan MG, Bast M, Armitage JO, et al. Bone marrow involvement by non-Hodgkin's lymphoma: the clinical significance of morphologic discordance between the lymph node and bone marrow. Nebraska Lymphoma Study Group. *J Clin Oncol* 1990;8:1163–1172.
66. A predictive model for aggressive non-Hodgkin's lymphoma. The International Non-Hodgkin's Lymphoma Prognostic Factors Project. *N Engl J Med* 1993;329:987–994.
67. Coiffier B, Lepage E, Briere J, et al. CHOP chemotherapy plus rituximab compared with CHOP alone in elderly patients with diffuse large-B-cell lymphoma. *N Engl J Med* 2002;346:235–242.
68. Pfreundschuh M, Trumper L, Osterborg A, et al. CHOP-like chemotherapy plus rituximab versus CHOP-like chemotherapy alone in young patients with good-prognosis diffuse large-B-cell lymphoma: a randomised controlled trial by the MabThera International Trial (MInT) Group. *Lancet Oncol* 2006;7:379–391.
69. Habermann TM, Weller EA, Morrison VA, et al. Rituximab-CHOP versus CHOP alone or with maintenance rituximab in older patients with diffuse large B-cell lymphoma. *J Clin Oncol* 2006;24:3121–3127.
70. Sehn LH, Berry B, Chhanabhai M, et al. The revised International Prognostic Index (R-IPI) is a better predictor of outcome than the standard IPI for patients with diffuse large B-cell lymphoma treated with R-CHOP. *Blood* 2007;109:1857–1861.
71. Armitage JO, Weisenburger DD, Hutchins M, et al. Chemotherapy for diffuse large-cell lymphoma—rapidly responding patients have more durable remissions. *J Clin Oncol* 1986;4:160–164.
72. Haioun C, Itti E, Rahmouni A, et al. [18F]fluoro-2-deoxy-D-glucose positron emission tomography (FDG-PET) in aggressive lymphoma: an early prognostic tool for predicting patient outcome. *Blood* 2005;106:1376–1381.
73. Spaepen K, Stroobants S, Dupont P, et al. Early restaging positron emission tomography with (18)F-fluorodeoxyglucose predicts outcome in patients with aggressive non-Hodgkin's lymphoma. *Ann Oncol* 2002;13:1356–1363.
74. Mikhaeel NG, Hutchings M, Fields PA, et al. FDG-PET after two to three cycles of chemotherapy predicts progression-free and overall survival in high-grade non-Hodgkin lymphoma. *Ann Oncol* 2005;16:1514–1523.
75. Miller TP, Lippman SM, Spier CM, et al. HLA-DR (Ia) immune phenotype predicts outcome for patients with diffuse large cell lymphoma. *J Clin Invest* 1988;82:370–372.
76. Swan F, Huh Y, Katz R, et al. Beta-2-microglobuin and HLA-DR cellular expression in relapsing large cell lymphoma (LCL): relationship to survival and serum Beta-2-microglobulin levels [abstract] 1489. *Blood* 1990;76:375a. Abstract 1489.
77. Plonquet A, Haioun C, Jais JP, et al. Peripheral blood natural killer cell count is associated with clinical outcome in patients with aaIPI 2-3 diffuse large B-cell lymphoma. *Ann Oncol* 2007;18:1209–1215.
78. Hedstrom G, Berglund M, Molin D, et al. Mast cell infiltration is a favourable prognostic factor in diffuse large B-cell lymphoma. *Br J Haematol* 2007;138:68–71.
79. Ansell SM, Stenson M, Habermann TM, et al. Cd4+ T-cell immune response to large B-cell non-Hodgkin's lymphoma predicts patient outcome. *J Clin Oncol* 2001;19:720–726.
80. Hasselblom S, Sigurdadottir M, Hansson U, et al. The number of tumour-infiltrating TIA-1+ cytotoxic T cells but not FOXP3+ regulatory T cells predicts outcome in diffuse large B-cell lymphoma. *Br J Haematol* 2007;137:364–373.
81. Tzankov A, Meier C, Hirschmann P, et al. Correlation of high numbers of intratumoral FOXP3+ regulatory T cells with improved survival in germinal center-like diffuse large B-cell lymphoma, follicular lymphoma and classical Hodgkin's lymphoma. *Haematologica* 2008;93:193–200.
82. Park S, Lee J, Ko YH, et al. The impact of Epstein-Barr virus status on clinical outcome in diffuse large B-cell lymphoma. *Blood* 2007;110:972–978.
83. Lossos IS, Morgensztern D. Prognostic biomarkers in diffuse large B-cell lymphoma. *J Clin Oncol* 2006;24:995–1007.
84. Hill ME, MacLennan KA, Cunningham DC, et al. Prognostic significance of BCL-2 expression and bcl-2 major breakpoint region rearrangement in diffuse large cell non-Hodgkin's lymphoma: a British National Lymphoma Investigation Study. *Blood* 1996;88:1046–1051.
85. Hermine O, Haioun C, Lepage E, et al. Prognostic significance of bcl-2 protein expression in aggressive non- Hodgkin's lymphoma. Groupe d'Etude des Lymphomes de l'Adulte (GELA). *Blood* 1996;87:265–272.
86. Mounier N, Briere J, Gisselbrecht C, et al. Rituximab plus CHOP (R-CHOP) overcomes bcl-2-associated resistance to chemotherapy in elderly patients with diffuse large B-cell lymphoma (DLBCL). *Blood* 2003;101:4279–4284.
87. Iqbal J, Neppalli VT, Wright G, et al. BCL2 expression is a prognostic marker for the activated B-cell-like type of diffuse large B-cell lymphoma. *J Clin Oncol* 2006;24:961–968.
88. Lossos IS, Jones CD, Warnke R, et al. Expression of a single gene, BCL-6, strongly predicts survival in patients with diffuse large B-cell lymphoma. *Blood* 2001;98:945–951.
89. Winter JN, Weller EA, Horning SJ, et al. Prognostic significance of Bcl-6 protein expression in DLBCL treated with CHOP or R-CHOP: a prospective correlative study. *Blood* 2006;107:4207–4213.
90. Le Gouill S, Talmant P, Touzeau C, et al. The clinical presentation and prognosis of diffuse large B-cell lymphoma with t(14;18) and 8q24/c-MYC rearrangement. *Haematologica* 2007;92:1335–1342.
91. Rosenwald A, Wright G, Chan WC, et al. The use of molecular profiling to predict survival after chemotherapy for diffuse large-B-cell lymphoma. *N Engl J Med* 2002;346:1937–1947.
92. Fu K, Weisenburger DD, Choi WW, et al. Addition of rituximab to standard chemotherapy improves the survival of both the germinal center B-cell-like and non-germinal center B-cell-like subtypes of diffuse large B-cell lymphoma. *J Clin Oncol* 2008;26:4587–4594.
93. Lenz G, Wright G, Dave SS, et al. Gene expression signatures predict survival in diffuse large B cell lymphoma following rituximab and CHOP-like chemotherapy [abstract]. *Ann Oncol* 2008;19(suppl 4):033. Abstract 034.
94. Chen MG, Prosnitz LR, Gonzalez-Serva A, et al. Results of radiotherapy in control of stage I and II non-Hodgkin's lymphoma. *Cancer* 1979;43:1245–1254.
95. Reddy S, Saxena VS, Pellettiere EV, et al. Early nodal and extra-nodal non-Hodgkin's lymphomas. *Cancer* 1977;40:98–104.
96. Levitt SH, Lee CK, Bloomfield CD, et al. The role of radiation therapy in the treatment of early stage large cell lymphoma. *Hematol Oncol* 1985;3:33–37.
97. Hallahan DE, Farah R, Vokes EE, et al. The patterns of failure in patients with pathological stage I and II diffuse histiocytic lymphoma treated with radiation therapy alone. *Int J Radiat Oncol Biol Phys* 1989;17:767–771.
98. Fuks Z, Kaplan HS. Recurrence rates following radiation therapy of nodular and diffuse malignant lymphomas. *Radiology* 1973;108:675–684.
99. Bush R, Gospodarowicz M. The place of radiation therapy in the management of patients with localized non-Hodgkin's lymphoma. Rosen SA, Kaplan HS, eds. In: *Malignant Lymphoma*. Orlando: Academic Press, 1982:485–502.
100. Gospodarowicz M, Bush R, et al. *Role of Radiation in Treatment of Patients with Localized Intermediate and High Grade Non-Hodgkin's Lymphoma: Proceedings of the American Society of Clinical Oncology,* 1984;3:235. Abstract C-922.
101. Mauch P, Leonard R, Skarin A, et al. Improved survival following combined radiation therapy and chemotherapy for unfavorable prognosis stage I-II non-Hodgkin's lymphomas. *J Clin Oncol* 1985;3:1301–1308.
102. Vokes EE, Ultmann JE, Golomb HM, et al. Long-term survival of patients with localized diffuse histiocytic lymphoma. *J Clin Oncol* 1985;3:1309–1317.
103. Monfardini S, Banfi A, Bonadonna G, et al. Improved five year survival after combined radiotherapy-chemotherapy for stage I-II non-Hodgkin's lymphoma. *Int J Radiat Oncol Biol Phys* 1980;6:125–134.
104. Nissen NI, Ersboll J, Hansen HS, et al. A randomized study of radiotherapy versus radiotherapy plus chemotherapy in stage I-II non-Hodgkin's lymphomas. *Cancer* 1983;52:1–7.
105. Landberg TG, Hakansson LG, Moller TR, et al. CVP-remission-maintenance in stage I or II non-Hodgkin's lymphomas: preliminary results of a randomized study. *Cancer* 1979;44:831–838.
106. Kamath SS, Marcus RB Jr, Lynch JW, et al. The impact of radiotherapy dose and other treatment-related and clinical factors on in-field control

in stage I and II non-Hodgkin's lymphoma. *Int J Radiat Oncol Biol Phys* 1999;44:563–568.

107. Munck JN, Dhermain F, Koscielny S, et al. Alternating chemotherapy and radiotherapy for limited-stage intermediate and high-grade non-Hodgkin's lymphomas: long-term results for 96 patients with tumors > 5 cm. *Ann Oncol* 1996;7:925–931.

108. Prestidge BR, Horning SJ, Hoppe RT. Combined modality therapy for stage I-II large cell lymphoma. *Int J Radiat Oncol Biol Phys* 1988;15:633–639.

109. Tondini C, Giardini R, Bozzetti F, et al. Combined modality treatment for primary gastrointestinal non-Hodgkin's lymphoma: the Milan Cancer Institute experience. *Ann Oncol* 1993;4:831–837.

110. van der Maazen RW, Noordijk EM, Thomas J, et al. Combined modality treatment is the treatment of choice for stage I/IE intermediate and high grade non-Hodgkin's lymphomas. *Radiother Oncol* 1998;49:1–7.

111. Velasquez WS, Fuller LM, Jagannath S, et al. Stages I and II diffuse large cell lymphomas: prognostic factors and long-term results with CHOP-bleo and radiotherapy. *Blood* 1991;77:942–947.

112. Krol AD, Berenschot HW, Doekharan D, et al. Cyclophosphamide, doxorubicin, vincristine and prednisone chemotherapy and radiotherapy for stage I intermediate or high grade non-Hodgkin's lymphomas: results of a strategy that adapts radiotherapy dose to the response after chemotherapy. *Radiother Oncol* 2001;58:251–255.

113. Shenkier TN, Voss N, Fairey R, et al. Brief chemotherapy and involved-region irradiation for limited-stage diffuse large-cell lymphoma: an 18-year experience from the British Columbia Cancer Agency. *J Clin Oncol* 2002;20:197–204.

114. Longo DL, Glatstein E, Duffey PL, et al. Treatment of localized aggressive lymphomas with combination chemotherapy followed by involved-field radiation therapy. *J Clin Oncol* 1989;7:1295–1302.

115. Schlembach PJ, Wilder RB, Tucker SL, et al. Impact of involved field radiotherapy after CHOP-based chemotherapy on stage III-IV, intermediate grade and large-cell immunoblastic lymphomas. *Int J Radiat Oncol Biol Phys* 2000;48:1107–1110.

116. Glick J, Kim K, Earle J, et al. *An ECOG Randomized Phase III Trial of CHOP vs. CHOP + Radiotherapy for Intermediate Grade Early Stage Non-Hodgkin's Lymphoma: Proceedings of the American Society of Clinical Oncology,* 1995;14:391. Abstract 1221.

117. Horning SJ, Weller E, Kim K, et al. Chemotherapy with or without radiotherapy in limited-stage diffuse aggressive non-Hodgkin's lymphoma: Eastern Cooperative Oncology Group study 1484. *J Clin Oncol* 2004;22:3032–3038.

118. Miller TP, Dahlberg S, Cassady JR, et al. Chemotherapy alone compared with chemotherapy plus radiotherapy for localized intermediate- and high-grade non-Hodgkin's lymphoma. *N Engl J Med* 1998;339:21–26.

119. Miller TP, Leblanc M, Spier CM, et al. CHOP alone compared to CHOP plus radiotherapy for early stage aggressive non-Hodgkin Lymphomas: update from the Southwest Oncology Group (SWOG) Randomized Trial [abstract]. *Blood* 2001;98:724a. Abstract 3024.

120. Fisher RI, Miller TP, O'Connor OA. Diffuse aggressive lymphoma. *Hematology Am Soc Hematol Educ Program* 2004:221–236.

121. Persky DO, Unger JM, Spier CM, et al. Phase II study of rituximab plus three cycles of CHOP and involved-field radiotherapy for patients with limited-stage aggressive B-cell lymphoma: Southwest Oncology Group study 0014. *J Clin Oncol* 2008;26:2258–2263.

122. Reyes F, Lepage E, Ganem G, et al. ACVBP versus CHOP plus radiotherapy for localized aggressive lymphoma. *N Engl J Med* 2005;352:1197–1205.

123. Bonnet C, Fillet G, Mounier N, et al. CHOP alone compared with CHOP plus radiotherapy for localized aggressive lymphoma in elderly patients: a study by the Groupe d'Etude des Lymphomes de l'Adulte. *J Clin Oncol* 2007;25:787–792.

124. Sehn LH, Savage KJ, Hoskins P, et al. Limited-stage DLBCL patients with a negative PET scan following three cycles of R-CHOP have an excellent outcome following abbreviated immuno-chemotherapy alone [abstract]. *Ann Oncol* 2008;19(suppl 4):099. Abstract 052.

125. Roy I, Yahalom J. Excellent local control with involved-field radiotherapy following CHOP chemotherapy: analysis of 145 patients with early-stage intermediate-grade non-Hodgkin's lymphoma [abstract]. *Int J Radiat Oncol Biol Phys* 2001;51:362a–363a. Abstract.

126. Martens C, Hodgson DC, Wells WA, et al. Outcome of hyperfractionated radiotherapy in chemotherapy-resistant non-Hodgkin's lymphoma. *Int J Radiat Oncol Biol Phys* 2006;64:1183–1187.

127. Zinzani PL, Martelli M, Magagnoli M, et al. Treatment and clinical management of primary mediastinal large B-cell lymphoma with sclerosis: MACOP-B regimen and mediastinal radiotherapy monitored by (67)Gallium scan in 50 patients. *Blood* 1999;94:3289–3293.

128. Levitt M, Marsh JC, DeConti RC, et al. Combination sequential chemotherapy in advanced reticulum cell sarcoma. *Cancer* 1972;29:630–636.

129. DeVita VT Jr, Canellos GP, Chabner B, et al. Advanced diffuse histiocytic lymphoma, a potentially curable disease. *Lancet* 1975;1:248–250.

130. Vose JM, Weisenburger DD, Loberiza FR, et al. Late relapse in patients with diffuse large B-cell lymphoma. Submitted.

131. Armitage JO, Fyfe MA, Lewis J. Long-term remission durability and functional status of patients treated for diffuse histiocytic lymphoma with the CHOP regimen. *J Clin Oncol* 1984;2:898–902.

132. Armitage JO, Mauch P, Harris N, et al. Diffuse large B-cell lymphoma. In: Mauch PM, Armitage JO, Coiffier B, et al., eds. *Non-Hodgkin's lymphomas.* Baltimore, Md: Lippincott Williams & Wilkins, 2003:427–453.

133. Tilly H, Lepage E, Coiffier B, et al. Intensive conventional chemotherapy (ACVBP regimen) compared with standard CHOP for poor-prognosis aggressive non-Hodgkin lymphoma. *Blood* 2003;102:4284–4289.

134. Pfreundschuh M, Trumper L, Kloess M, et al. Two-weekly or 3-weekly CHOP chemotherapy with or without etoposide for the treatment of elderly patients with aggressive lymphomas: results of the NHL-B2 trial of the DSHNHL. *Blood* 2004;104:634–641.

135. Pfreundschuh M, Trumper L, Kloess M, et al. Two-weekly or 3-weekly CHOP chemotherapy with or without etoposide for the treatment of young patients with good-prognosis (normal LDH) aggressive lymphomas: results of the NHL-B1 trial of the DSHNHL. *Blood* 2004;104:626–633.

136. Longo DL, DeVita VT Jr, Duffey PL, et al. Superiority of ProMACE-CytaBOM over ProMACE-MOPP in the treatment of advanced diffuse aggressive lymphoma: results of a prospective randomized trial [published erratum appears in *J Clin Oncol* 1991;9:710]. *J Clin Oncol* 1991;9:25–38.

137. Klimo P, Connors JM. MACOP-B chemotherapy for the treatment of diffuse large-cell lymphoma. *Ann Intern Med* 1985;102:596–602.

138. Shipp MA, Yeap BY, Harrington DP, et al. The m-BACOD combination chemotherapy regimen in large-cell lymphoma: analysis of the completed trial and comparison with the M-BACOD regimen. *J Clin Oncol* 1990;8:84–93.

139. Fisher RI, Gaynor ER, Dahlberg S, et al. Comparison of a standard regimen (CHOP) with three intensive chemotherapy regimens for advanced non-Hodgkin's lymphoma. *N Engl J Med* 1993;328:1002–1006.

140. Wilson WH, Dunleavy K, Pittaluga S, et al. Phase II study of dose-adjusted EPOCH and rituximab in untreated diffuse large B-cell lymphoma with analysis of germinal center and post-germinal center biomarkers. *J Clin Oncol* 2008;26:2717–2724.

141. Feugier P, Van Hoof A, Sebban C, et al. Long-term results of the R-CHOP study in the treatment of elderly patients with diffuse large B-cell lymphoma: a study by the Groupe d'Etude des Lymphomes de l'Adulte. *J Clin Oncol* 2005;23:4117–4126.

142. Pfreundschuh M, Schubert J, Ziepert M, et al. Six versus eight cycles of bi-weekly CHOP-14 with or without rituximab in elderly patients with aggressive CD20+ B-cell lymphomas: a randomised controlled trial (RICOVER-60). *Lancet Oncol* 2008;9:105–116.

143. Sehn LH, Donaldson J, Chhanabhai M, et al. Introduction of combined CHOP plus rituximab therapy dramatically improved outcome of diffuse large B-cell lymphoma in British Columbia. *J Clin Oncol* 2005;23:5027–5033.

144. Zucca E, Conconi A, Mughal TI, et al. Patterns of outcome and prognostic factors in primary large-cell lymphoma of the testis in a survey by the International Extranodal Lymphoma Study Group. *J Clin Oncol* 2003;21:20–27.

145. Haioun C, Lepage E, Gisselbrecht C, et al. Survival benefit of high-dose therapy in poor-risk aggressive non-Hodgkin's lymphoma: final analysis of the prospective LNH87-2 protocol—a groupe d'Etude des lymphomes de l'Adulte study. *J Clin Oncol* 2000;18:3025–3030.

146. Bashir RM, Bierman PJ, Vose JM, et al. Central nervous system involvement in patients with diffuse aggressive non-Hodgkin's lymphoma. *Am J Clin Oncol* 1991;14:478–482.

147. Hollender A, Kvaloy S, Nome O, et al. Central nervous system involvement following diagnosis of non-Hodgkin's lymphoma: a risk model. *Ann Oncol* 2002;13:1099–1107.

148. Batchelor T, Loeffler JS. Primary CNS lymphoma. *J Clin Oncol* 2006;24:1281–1288.

149. Lenz G, Wright G, Dave SS, et al. Stromal gene signatures in large-B-cell lymphomas. *N Engl J Med* 2008;359:2313–2323.

150. Gulati SC, Shank B, Black P, et al. Autologous bone marrow transplantation for patients with poor-prognosis lymphoma. *J Clin Oncol* 1988;6:1303–1313.

151. Chim CS, Choy C, Liang R, et al. Isolated uterine relapse of nasal T/Nk cell lymphoma. *Leuk Lymphoma* 1999;34:629–632.

152. Kato N, Yasukawa K, Onozuka T, et al. Nasal and nasal-type T/NK-cell lymphoma with cutaneous involvement. *J Am Acad Dermatol* 1999;40(pt 2):850–856.

153. Au WY, Chan AC, Kwong YL. Scrotal skin ulcer in a patient with a previous tonsillectomy because of natural killer cell lymphoma. *Am J Dermatopathol* 1998;20:582–585.

154. Liang R, Todd D, Chan TK, et al. Treatment outcome and prognostic factors for primary nasal lymphoma. *J Clin Oncol* 1995;13:666–670.

155. Han JY, Seo EJ, Kwon HJ, et al. Nasal angiocentric lymphoma with hemophagocytic syndrome. *Korean J Intern Med* 1999;14:41–46.

156. Milpied N, Deconinck E, Gaillard F, et al. Initial treatment of aggressive lymphoma with high-dose chemotherapy and autologous stem-cell support. *N Engl J Med* 2004;350:1287–1295.

157. Kwong YL, Chan AC, Liang R, et al. CD56+ NK lymphomas: clinicopathological features and prognosis. *Br J Haematol* 1997;97:821–829.

158. Strehl J, Mey U, Glasmacher A, et al. High-dose chemotherapy followed by autologous stem cell transplantation as first-line therapy in aggressive non-Hodgkin's lymphoma: a meta-analysis. *Haematologica* 2003;88:1304–1315.

159. Greb A, Bohlius J, Trelle S, et al. High-dose chemotherapy with autologous stem cell support in first-line treatment of aggressive non-Hodgkin lymphoma - results of a comprehensive meta-analysis. *Cancer Treat Rev* 2007;33:338–346.

160. Greb A, Bohlius J, Schiefer D, et al. High-dose chemotherapy with autologous stem cell transplantation in the first line treatment of aggressive Non-Hodgkin Lymphoma (NHL) in adults. *Cochrane Database Syst Rev* 2008;23:CD004024.

161. Stewart DA, Bahlis N, Valentine K, et al. Upfront double high-dose chemotherapy with DICEP followed by BEAM and autologous stem cell transplantation for poor-prognosis aggressive non-Hodgkin lymphoma. *Blood* 2006;107:4623–4627.

162. Olivieri A, Santini G, Patti C, et al. Upfront high-dose sequential therapy (HDS) versus VACOP-B with or without HDS in aggressive non-Hodgkin's lymphoma: long-term results by the NHLCSG. *Ann Oncol* 2005;16:1941–1948.

163. Betticher DC, Martinelli G, Radford JA, et al. Sequential high dose chemotherapy as initial treatment for aggressive sub-types of non-Hodgkin lymphoma: results of the international randomized phase III trial (MISTRAL). *Ann Oncol* 2006;17:1546–1552.

164. Tarella C, Zanni M, Di Nicola M, et al. Prolonged survival in poor-risk diffuse large B-cell lymphoma following front-line treatment with rituximab-supplemented, early-intensified chemotherapy with multiple autologous hematopoietic stem cell support: a multicenter study by GITIL (Gruppo Italiano Terapie Innovative nei Linfomi). *Leukemia* 2007;21:1802–1811.

165. Glass B, Kloess M, Bentz M, et al. Dose-escalated CHOP plus etoposide (MegaCHOEP) followed by repeated stem cell transplantation for primary treatment of aggressive high-risk non-Hodgkin lymphoma. *Blood* 2006;107:3058–3064.

166. Hahn T, Wolff SN, Czuczman M, et al. The role of cytotoxic therapy with hematopoietic stem cell transplantation in the treatment of diffuse large cell B-cell non-Hodgkin's lymphoma. *Biol Blood Marrow Transplant* 2003;9:667.

167. Bastion Y, Blay JY, Divine M, et al. Elderly patients with aggressive non-Hodgkin's lymphoma: disease presentation, response to treatment, and survival—a Groupe d'Etude des Lymphomes de l'Adulte study on 453 patients older than 69 years. *J Clin Oncol* 1997;15:2945–2953.

168. Bjorkholm M, Osby E, Hagberg H, et al. Randomized trial of r-metHu granulocyte colony-stimulating factor (G-CSF) as adjunct to CHOP or CNOP treatment of elderly patients with aggressive non-Hodgkin's lymphoma. *Blood* 1999;94:599a.

169. Sonneveld P, de Ridder M, van der Lelie H, et al. Comparison of doxorubicin and mitoxantrone in the treatment of elderly patients with advanced diffuse non-Hodgkin's lymphoma using CHOP versus CNOP chemotherapy. *J Clin Oncol* 1995;13:2530–2539.

170. Vose JM, Weisenburger DD, Lynch JC, et al. CNOP for diffuse aggressive non-Hodgkin's lymphoma: the Nebraska lymphoma study group experience. *Leuk Lymphoma* 2002;43:799–804.

171. Webb MS, Saltman DL, Connors JM, et al. A literature review of single agent treatment of multiply relapsed aggressive non-Hodgkin's lymphoma. *Leuk Lymphoma* 2002;43:975–982.

172. Salhany KE, Macon WR, Choi JK, et al. Subcutaneous panniculitis-like T-cell lymphoma: clinicopathologic, immunophenotypic, and genotypic analysis of alpha/beta and gamma/delta subtypes. *Am J Surg Pathol* 1998;22:881–893.

173. Parisi M, McNutt N. Subcutaneous panniculitis-like T-cell lymphoma associated with a hemophagocytic syndrome in a patients with polycythemia vera and interferon-alpha therapy [abstract]. *J Cutan Pathol* 1998;25:580. Abstract.

174. Velasquez WS, McLaughlin P, Tucker S, et al. ESHAP–an effective chemotherapy regimen in refractory and relapsing lymphoma: a 4-year follow-up study. *J Clin Oncol* 1994;12:1169–1176.

175. Gutierrez M, Chabner BA, Pearson D, et al. Role of a doxorubicin-containing regimen in relapsed and resistant lymphomas: an 8-year follow-up study of EPOCH. *J Clin Oncol* 2000;18:3633–3642.

176. Sparano JA, Wiernik PH, Leaf A, et al. Infusional cyclophosphamide, doxorubicin, and etoposide in relapsed and resistant non-Hodgkin's lymphoma: evidence for a schedule-dependent effect favoring infusional administration of chemotherapy. *J Clin Oncol* 1993;11:1071–1079.

177. Coiffier B, Haioun C, Ketterer N, et al. Rituximab (anti-CD20 monoclonal antibody) for the treatment of patients with relapsing or refractory aggressive lymphoma: a multicenter phase II study. *Blood* 1998;92:1927–1932.

178. Jermann M, Jost LM, Taverna C, et al. Rituximab-EPOCH, an effective salvage therapy for relapsed, refractory or transformed B-cell lymphomas: results of a phase II study. *Ann Oncol* 2004;15:511–516.

179. Witzig TE, Geyer SM, Kurtin PJ, et al. Salvage chemotherapy with rituximab DHAP for relapsed non-Hodgkin lymphoma: a phase II trial in the North Central Cancer Treatment Group. *Leuk Lymphoma* 2008;49:1074–1080.

180. Martin A, Conde E, Arnan M, et al. R-ESHAP as salvage therapy for patients with relapsed or refractory diffuse large B-cell lymphoma: the influence of prior exposure to rituximab on outcome. A GEL/TAMO study. *Haematologica* 2008;93:1829–1836.

181. Kewalramani T, Zelenetz AD, Nimer SD, et al. Rituximab and ICE as second-line therapy before autologous stem cell transplantation for relapsed or primary refractory diffuse large B-cell lymphoma. *Blood* 2004;103:3684–3688.

182. Mey UJ, Olivieri A, Orlopp KS, et al. DHAP in combination with rituximab vs DHAP alone as salvage treatment for patients with relapsed or refractory diffuse large B-cell lymphoma: a matched-pair analysis. *Leuk Lymphoma* 2006;47:2558–2566.

183. Vellenga E, van Putten WL, van 't Veer MB, et al. Rituximab improves the treatment results of DHAP-VIM-DHAP and ASCT in relapsed/progressive aggressive CD20+ NHL: a prospective randomized HOVON trial. *Blood* 2008;111:537–543.

184. El Gnaoui T, Dupuis J, Belhadj K, et al. Rituximab, gemcitabine and oxaliplatin: an effective salvage regimen for patients with relapsed or refractory B-cell lymphoma not candidates for high-dose therapy. *Ann Oncol* 2007;18:1363–1368.

185. Lopez A, Gutierrez A, Palacios A, et al. GEMOX-R regimen is a highly effective salvage regimen in patients with refractory/relapsing diffuse large-cell lymphoma: a phase II study. *Eur J Haematol* 2008;80:127–132.

186. Abali H, Urun Y, Oksuzoglu B, et al. Comparison of ICE (ifosfamide-carboplatin-etoposide) versus DHAP (cytosine arabinoside-cisplatin-dexamethasone) as salvage chemotherapy in patients with relapsed or refractory lymphoma. *Cancer Invest* 2008;26:401–406.

187. Hagberg H, Gisselbrecht C. Randomised phase III study of R-ICE versus R-DHAP in relapsed patients with CD20 diffuse large B-cell lymphoma (DLBCL) followed by high-dose therapy and a second randomisation to maintenance treatment with rituximab or not: an update of the CORAL study. *Ann Oncol* 2006;17(suppl 4):iv31–iv32.

188. Armitage JO, Coiffier B. Activity of interferon-alpha in relapsed patients with diffuse large B-cell and peripheral T-cell non-Hodgkin's lymphoma. *Ann Oncol* 2000;11:1–3.

189. Kaminski MS, Estes J, Zasadny KR, et al. Radioimmunotherapy with iodine (131)I tositumomab for relapsed or refractory B-cell non-Hodgkin lymphoma: updated results and long-term follow-up of the University of Michigan experience. *Blood* 2000;96:1259–1266.

190. Morschhauser F, Illidge T, Huglo D, et al. Efficacy and safety of yttrium-90 ibritumomab tiuxetan in patients with relapsed or refractory diffuse large B-cell lymphoma not appropriate for autologous stem-cell transplantation. *Blood* 2007;110:54–58.

191. Tulpule A, Rarick MU, Kolitz J, et al. Liposomal daunorubicin in the treatment of relapsed or refractory non- Hodgkin's lymphoma. *Ann Oncol* 2001;12:457–462.

192. Macpherson N, Belch A, Taylor M, et al. Liposomal encapsulated doxorubicin (Caelyx) in the treatment of relapsed aggressive non-Hodgkin's lymphoma: a phase II study. *Leuk Lymphoma* 2006;47:1327–1332.

193. Boehlke L, Winter JN. Sphingomyelin/cholesterol liposomal vincristine: a new formulation for an old drug. *Expert Opin Biol Ther* 2006;6:409–415.

194. Weidmann E, Kim SZ, Rost A, et al. Bendamustine is effective in relapsed or refractory aggressive non-Hodgkin's lymphoma. *Ann Oncol* 2002;13:1285–1289.

195. Wiernik PH, Lossos IS, Tuscano JM, et al. Lenalidomide monotherapy in relapsed or refractory aggressive non-Hodgkin's lymphoma. *J Clin Oncol* 2008;26:4952–4957.

196. Philip T, Armitage JO, Spitzer G, et al. High-dose therapy and autologous bone marrow transplantation after failure of conventional chemotherapy in adults with intermediate-grade or high-grade non-Hodgkin's lymphoma. *N Engl J Med* 1987;316:1493–1498.

197. Hamlin PA, Zelenetz AD, Kewalramani T, et al. Age-adjusted International Prognostic Index predicts autologous stem cell transplantation outcome for patients with relapsed or primary refractory diffuse large B-cell lymphoma. *Blood* 2003;102:1989–1996.

198. Caballero MD, Perez-Simon JA, Iriondo A, et al. High-dose therapy in diffuse large cell lymphoma: results and prognostic factors in 452 patients from the GEL-TAMO Spanish Cooperative Group. *Ann Oncol* 2003;14:140–151.

199. Vose JM, Rizzo DJ, Tao-Wu J, et al. Autologous transplantation for diffuse aggressive non-Hodgkin lymphoma in first relapse or second remission. *Biol Blood Marrow Transplant* 2004;10:116–127.

200. Philip T, Guglielmi C, Hagenbeek A, et al. Autologous bone marrow transplantation as compared with salvage chemotherapy in relapses of chemotherapy-sensitive non-Hodgkin's lymphoma. *N Engl J Med* 1995;333:1540–1545.

201. Blay J, Gomez F, Sebban C, et al. The International Prognostic Index correlates to survival in patients with aggressive lymphoma in relapse: analysis of the PARMA trial. Parma Group. *Blood* 1998;92:3562–3568.

202. Guglielmi C, Gomez F, Philip T, et al. Time to relapse has prognostic value in patients with aggressive lymphoma enrolled onto the Parma trial. *J Clin Oncol* 1998;16:3264–3269.

203. Vose J, Zhang MJ, Rowlings P, et al. Autologous transplantation for diffuse aggressive non-Hodgkin's lymphoma in patients never achieving remission: a report from the autologous blood and marrow transplant registry. *J Clin Oncol* 2001;19:406–413.

204. Rodriguez J, Caballero MD, Gutierrez A, et al. Autologous stem-cell transplantation in diffuse large B-cell non-Hodgkin's lymphoma not achieving complete response after induction chemotherapy: the GEL/TAMO experience. *Ann Oncol* 2004;15:1504–1509.

205. Hoerr AL, Gao F, Hidalgo J, et al. Effects of pretransplantation treatment with rituximab on outcomes of autologous stem-cell transplantation for non-Hodgkin's lymphoma. *J Clin Oncol* 2004;22:4561–4566.

206. Peniket AJ, Ruiz de Elvira MC, Taghipour G, et al. An EBMT registry matched study of allogeneic stem cell transplants for lymphoma: allogeneic transplantation is associated with a lower relapse rate but a higher procedure-related mortality rate than autologous transplantation. *Bone Marrow Transplant* 2003;31:667–678.

207. Aksentijevich I, Jones RJ, Ambinder RF, et al. Clinical outcome following autologous and allogeneic blood and marrow transplantation for relapsed diffuse large-cell non-Hodgkin's lymphoma. *Biol Blood Marrow Transplant* 2006;12:965–972.

208. Robinson SP, Goldstone AH, Mackinnon S, et al. Chemoresistant or aggressive lymphoma predicts for a poor outcome following reduced-intensity allogeneic progenitor cell transplantation: an analysis from the Lymphoma Working Party of the European Group for Blood and Bone Marrow Transplantation. *Blood* 2002;100:4310–4316.

209. Kahl C, Storer BE, Sandmaier BM, et al. Relapse risk in patients with malignant diseases given allogeneic hematopoietic cell transplantation after nonmyeloablative conditioning. *Blood* 2007;110:2744–2748.

210. Corradini P, Dodero A, Farina L, et al. Allogeneic stem cell transplantation following reduced-intensity conditioning can induce durable clinical and molecular remissions in relapsed lymphomas: pre-transplant disease status and histotype heavily influence outcome. *Leukemia* 2007;21:2316–2323.

211. Qin Y, Greiner A, Trunk MJ, et al. Somatic hypermutation in low-grade mucosa-associated lymphoid tissue- type B-cell lymphoma. *Blood* 1995;86:3528–3534.

212. Isaacson PG. Gastrointestinal lymphoma. *Hum Pathol* 1994;25:1020–1029.

213. Fillet G, Bonnet C. Radiotherapy is unnecessary in elderly patients with localized aggressive non-Hodgkin's lymphoma: results of the GELA LNH 93-4 study [abstract]. *Blood* 2002;100:92a. Abstract 337.

214. Reyes F, Lepage E, Munck J, et al. Superiority of chemotherapy alone with the ACVBP regimen over treatment with three cycles of CHOP plus radiotherapy in low risk localized aggressive lymphoma: the LNH93-1 GELA study [abstract]. *Blood* 2002;100:93a. Abstract 343.

215. Tilly H, Lepage E, Coiffier B, et al. A randomized comparison of ACVBP and CHOP in the treatment of advanced aggressive non-Hodgkin's lymphoma: the LNH93-5 study. *Blood* 2000;96:832a.

216. Bosly A, Lepage E, Coiffier B, et al. Outcome is not improved by the use of alternating chemotherapy in elderly patients with aggressive lymphoma. *Hematol J* 2001;2:279–285.

217. Tirelli U, Errante D, Van Glabbeke M, et al. CHOP is the standard regimen in patients > or = 70 years of age with intermediate-grade and high-grade non-Hodgkin's lymphoma: results of a randomized study of the European Organization for Research and Treatment of Cancer Lymphoma Cooperative Study Group. *J Clin Oncol* 1998;16:27–34.

218. Meyer RM, Browman GP, Samosh ML, et al. Randomized phase II comparison of standard CHOP with weekly CHOP in elderly patients with non-Hodgkin's lymphoma. *J Clin Oncol* 1995;13:2386–2393.

219. Zinzani PL, Gherlinzoni F, Storti S, et al. Randomized trial of 8-week versus 12-week VNCOP-B plus G-CSF regimens as front-line treatment in elderly aggressive non-Hodgkin's lymphoma patients. *Ann Oncol* 2002;13:1364–1369.

220. Petersen FB, Appelbaum FR, Hill R, et al. Autologous marrow transplantation for malignant lymphoma: a report of 101 cases from Seattle. *J Clin Oncol* 1990;8:638–647.

221. Vose JM, Anderson JR, Kessinger A, et al. High-dose chemotherapy and autologous hematopoietic stem-cell transplantation for aggressive non-Hodgkin's lymphoma. *J Clin Oncol* 1993;11:1846–1851.

222. Mills W, Chopra R, McMillan A, et al. BEAM chemotherapy and autologous bone marrow transplantation for patients with relapsed or refractory non-Hodgkin's lymphoma. *J Clin Oncol* 1995;13:588–595.

223. Stockerl-Goldstein KE, Horning SJ, Negrin RS, et al. Influence of preparatory regimen and source of hematopoietic cells on outcome of autotransplantation for non-Hodgkin's lymphoma. *Biol Blood Marrow Transplant* 1996;2:76–85.

224. Caballero MD, Rubio V, Rifon J, et al. BEAM chemotherapy followed by autologous stem cell support in lymphoma patients: analysis of efficacy, toxicity and prognostic factors. *Bone Marrow Transplant* 1997;20:451–458.

225. Rapoport AP, Lifton R, Constine LS, et al. Autotransplantation for relapsed or refractory non-Hodgkin's lymphoma (NHL): long-term follow-up and analysis of prognostic factors. *Bone Marrow Transplant* 1997;19:883–890.

226. Stiff PJ, Dahlberg S, Forman SJ, et al. Autologous bone marrow transplantation for patients with relapsed or refractory diffuse aggressive non-Hodgkin's lymphoma: value of augmented preparative regimens—a Southwest Oncology Group trial. *J Clin Oncol* 1998;16:48–55.

227. Popat U, Przepiork D, Champlin R, et al. High-dose chemotherapy for relapsed and refractory diffuse large B-cell lymphoma: mediastinal localization predicts for a favorable outcome. *J Clin Oncol* 1998;16:63–69.

CHAPTER 21 ■ PRIMARY MEDIASTINAL LARGE B-CELL LYMPHOMA

PIER LUIGI ZINZANI, NANCY LEE HARRIS, PETER M. MAUCH, AND RICCARDO DALLA M. FAVERA

DEFINITION

Primary mediastinal large B-cell lymphoma (PMBL) was first described in the 1980s (1,2). It is an uncommon but not rare clinicopathologic entity with a worldwide distribution, and was recently recognized in both the Revised European-American Lymphoma and World Health Organization classifications (3–5). This localized malignancy is characterized by aggressive and invasive behavior in an unusual site in a cohort of young adult females in whom large cell lymphoma is infrequent. Although it resembles nodal diffuse large B-cell lymphoma (DLBCL), it has distinct morphologic, immunophenotypic, and genetic features. PMBL is a DLBCL that arises in the thymus from a putative thymic peripheral B cell.

EPIDEMIOLOGY

In a review of 1,400 cases of non-Hodgkin lymphomas from nine centers all over the world, PMBL was found to account for 2% of all cases (6). It was the only tumor type for which clinical data were essential for its recognition (6). The disease is most common in young women, with a male to female ratio of 1:2 and a median age in the 4th decade (6–8). Table 21.1 summarizes the clinical features of PMBL compared with nodal DLBCL PMBL.

No risk factors have been clearly identified for the development of PMBL.

TABLE 21.1

COMPARISON OF DLBCL AND PMBL

	Nodal DLBCL	PMBL
Median age (yr)	55	35
Nodal/extranodal presentation (%)	65/35	0/100
Sex distribution (M:F)	1.2:1	1:2
Stage I–II/III–IV (%)	40/60	80/20
Bulky disease (%)	30	60–70

F, female; M, male.

DIAGNOSIS

Morphology

The tumor usually evokes fibrosis with compartimentalization (9–13) and shows a wide morphologic/cytologic spectrum (11). Tumor cells are medium- to large-sized with abundant pale cytoplasm and more or less regular round or ovoid nuclei (Fig. 21.1). At times they appear more pleomorphic with multiplobated nuclei or Reed-Stemberg-like features. The latter may raise suspicion of classic Hodgkin lymphoma (CHL) (11,14). Rare "grey zone" borderline cases combine features of both PMBL and CHL or cases of

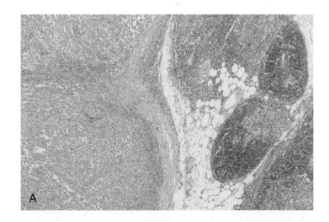

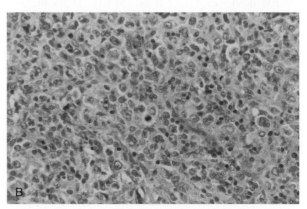

FIGURE 21.1 Histopathology of PMBL. **A:** At low magnification, there is a focus of normal thymus (**right**) and a large mass of tumor cells (**left**). (See also Color Plate 35) **B:** At high magnification, the cells are large and range from round to oval to multiolobated, with moderately abundant, pale cytoplasm (hematoxylin and eosin stain) (See also Color Plate 36) (Courteously by S.A. Pileri).

composite PMBL and CHL (14). These borderline cases are now given a separate category in the World Health Organization classification (B-cell lymphoma with features intermediate between DLBCL and CHL) (5).

Immunophenotype

Tumor cells are as a rule immunoglobulin (Ig) negative but express B-cell-associated antigens (CD19, CD20, CD22, CD79a) and CD45 (12,13,15). CD30 staining occurs in >80% of the cases, being usually weaker and more heterogeneous than in CHL (13,16). CD15 is usually negative (17); if positive, it usually results in placement in the borderline category. Tumor cells are often positive for IRF4, MAL, Bcl-6, CD23, CD54, and CD95, but seldom express CD10 (8% to 32%) (13,18–20). They coexpress TRAF1 and nuclear c-REL (21), and can lack human leukocyte antigen class I and/or class II molecules (22).

Genetic Features

Ig genes are clonally rearranged with a high load of stable (i.e., not ongoing) somatic hypermutations (17). Comparative genomic hybridization studies demonstrated gains in chromosome 9p24, 2p15, Xp11.4–21 (33%), and Xq24–26 (33%) (23–26). Candidate genes include REL and BCL11A (at chromosome 2p) (27,28), and Janus kinase 2, PDL1, and PDL2 (at chromosome 9p) (25,29,30). Nuclear accumulation of REL protein is common (20,28) but does not perfectly correlate with REL amplification and REL transcript abundance (28,31).

PMBL has a unique gene signature but shares features with CHL (30,32), including constitutive activation of the nuclear factor-κB (31) and Janus kinase-signal transduction and activator of transcription signaling pathways (29,33) often related to inactivating mutations of supresor of cytokine signaling 1 (29,34).

Rearrangements of BCL2, BCL6, and MYC genes are occasionally detected (32,35,36), whereas inactivation of p16INK4A and p53 genes has been reported (36).

The discordant expression of CD79a and Ig is characteristic of PMBL (13,15,37). It does not depend on the lack of functional Ig gene rearrangements nor to a defect in the transcription machinery (i.e., BOB.1, OCT-2, and PU.1) (13,37) but, else, to a down-regulation of the intronic heavy chain enhancer (38) or posttranscriptional blockage (37).

Postulated Normal Counterpart

The postulated normal counterpart is the thymic medullary B cell.

Differential Diagnosis

PMBL must be distinguished from other lymphomas that can present with anterior mediastinal masses, including Hodgkin lymphoma, nodal-type DLBCL, anaplastic large cell lymphoma, anaplastic lymphoma kinase (ALK)+ or ALK−, and thymic mucosa-associated lymphoid tissue lymphoma, as well as thymoma, particularly type B3. Knowledge of the clinical features, adequate tissue for morphologic analysis, complete immunophenotyping (T-cell and B-cell antigens, CD15, ALK-1), and assessment of proliferation fraction are all helpful in differential diagnosis. Cases with morphologic features of PMBL but with an immunophenotype that suggests CHL (absence of CD20, strong expression of CD30 and CD15) or with morphologic features of CHL but with an immunophenotype that suggests PMBL (expression of the complete B-cell program [OCT.2, BOB.1, CD20, Cd79a], and lack of CD15) may be best classified in the borderline category (5).

CLINICAL FEATURES AND STAGING

PMBL is a distinct clinicopathologic entity, characterized by a locally invasive anterior mediastinal mass that originates in the thymus and frequently compromises the airway, causing superior vena cava syndrome (2,39). In fact, 30% to 50% of patients have signs and symptoms of superior vena cava syndrome, thoracic and neck vein distension, facial edema, conjunctival swelling, and occasionally arm edema. At the time of diagnosis, the stage of disease is I or II in 80% of the patients. The mediastinal tumor is >10 cm (bulky mass) in 60% to 70% of patients, infiltrating lung, chest wall, pleura, and pericardium (39,40). Figure 21.2 shows a chest x-ray illustrating a typical patient with this presentation. Pleural or pericardial effusions are present in one-third of cases (41,42). The invasive neoplasm results in cough, chest pain, dyspnea, or complaints resulting from caval obstruction.

Despite the local invasiveness, distant spread is infrequent at the outset; even spread to the supraclavicular nodes is unusual at the time of presentation, although the upper border of the tumor can often be palpated at the base of the neck.

The duration of symptoms oscillates between 6 weeks and 3 months. Systemic symptoms, mainly fever or weight loss, are present in <20% of cases.

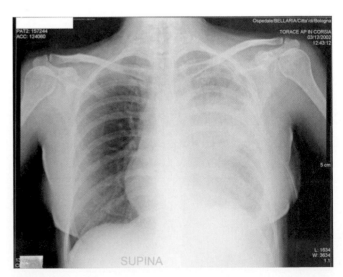

FIGURE 21.2 Chest x-ray showing a typical presentation of the PMBL (Courteously by P.L. Zinzani).

Spread to peripheral lymph nodes is infrequent, and marrow or cerebrospinal fluid involvement is unusual. Distant relapses tend to be extranodal, including liver, gastrointestinal tract, kidneys, ovaries, adrenal glands, pancreas, and central nervous system (43–45). Moderate to high lactate dehydrogenase levels are observed in 70% to 80% of patients.

The complete staging workup for PMBL is the same as that routinely used for nodal lymphoma. It includes an accurate physical examination, complete hematologic and biochemical examinations, abdomen ultrasonography, total body computerized tomography, and bone marrow biopsy. A diagnostic tissue sample is obtained by mediastinoscopy, biopsy of the tumor mass through the supraclavicular fossa, or anterior mediastinotomy or minithoracotomy. Formal thoracotomy is infrequently required, and total excision is rarely an option. Gallium-67 scanning is a meaningful procedure for staging, response and relapse assessment, and follow-up. It is the most useful adjunctive test also to assess cure (42,46,47). [18F]-2-fluoro-2-deoxyglucose-positron emission tomography has demonstrated an excellent usefulness in residual-mass assessment considering the elevated tracer uptake that characterizes this lymphoma, but a longer experience is necessary.

The standard staging system used for PMBL is the same as that proposed for Hodgkin disease at the Ann Arbor conference in 1971 (48). This system is currently used for all lymphomas, even if other staging systems are used in some extranodal lymphomas with particular biologic behavior. Concerning molecular analysis of minimal residual disease, no reliable molecular markers are available for monitoring minimal residual disease in PMBL.

PROGNOSIS: NATURAL HISTORY AND PROGNOSTIC FACTORS

Recurrence is almost exclusively observed in the first 2 years of follow-up. Most early publications on PMBL described an aggressive disease with poor prognosis (49,50). Further published series showed a 5-year survival of 65% with a cyclophosphamide, hydroxydaunorubicin, Oncovin (vincristine),

and prednisone (CHOP) regimen followed by radiation therapy (39). Similar results have been obtained with third-generation regimens followed by radiation therapy, and some authors have suggested that the CHOP regimen is insufficient in patients with larger masses resulting from more aggressive lymphomas (44,51,52).

PROGNOSTIC FACTORS

Features associated with poor prognosis in PMBL are poor performance status, pericardial effusion, bulky disease, and high-serum lactate dehydrogenase. A compromised dose intensity of anthracycline and cyclophosphamide predicted a nonresponse to frontline chemotherapy, which is the major important predictor of survival in PMBL (39,41,53). The age-adjusted International Prognostic Index did not provide a useful subdivision of PMBL (41).

TREATMENT

Frontline Therapy

The results of most series on PMBL are reported in Table 21.2. Reported approaches to the treatment of this entity range from first-generation (39,43,53–60) to third-generation (6,40,41,44,47,51,52,61,62) chemotherapy protocols. Early studies suggesting that PMBLs were unusually aggressive, with a poorer prognosis with respect to other large cell lymphomas, have been contradicted by more recent reports. Complete response (CR) rates of 53% to 80% have been reported after initial therapy, with a 50% to 65% overall survival (OS) rate at 5 years (5,39,41,46,51,52,55,61). Regarding the use of different chemotherapeutic regimens (CHOP or CHOP-like vs. third-generation regimens), a report by Fisher et al. (63) showed that CHOP and intensive third-generation regimens produce equivalent results. This observation may limit discussion about the use of more aggressive protocols for PMBL.

TABLE 21.2

IMMUNOPHENOTYPING IN DIFFERENTIAL DIAGNOSIS OF PMBL

Antigen	PMBL	CHL	DLBCL-NOS	ALCL ALK+
CD20	+	+	+	−
CD79a	+	−	+	−
Pax5	+	+ weak	+	−
Oct.2, Bob.1	+	−	+	−
CD45	+	−	+	+
CD30	+ weak	+ strong	−/+	+ strong
Pan-T antigens	−	−	−	+ variable
IRF4/Mum1	+	+	+/−	+
MAL	+	−	−	−
ALK	−	−	−	+
Bcl6	+	−	+/−	−
EBV-EBER	−	−/+	−/+	−

ALCL, anaplastic large cell lymphoma; EBV-EBER, Epstein-Barr virus-Epstein-Barr-encoded ribonucleic acid; NOS, not otherwise specified.

TABLE 21.3

STUDIES ON TREATMENT AND OUTCOME OF PATIENTS WITH PMBL

Author (reference)	No. of patients	Regimen (no. of patients)	Local RT	PR (%)	CR (%)	FFS (%)
Jacobson et al., 1988 (39)	30	CHOP/CHOP-like (22), C-MOPP (2)	Yes		80	59 (5 y)
Haioun et al., 1989 (43)	20	CHOP (4) or variants (16)	Yes	55	45	40 (2 y)
Todeschini et al., 1990 (52)	21	CHOP-B (6), MACOP-B (12), m-BACOD (3)	Yes	25	64	52 (3 y)
Bertini et al., 1991 (51)	18	MACOP-B	Yes	6	89	73 (2 y)
Kim et al., 1993 (53)	57	M/m-BACOD (38), CHOP (10), other (9)	Yes	39	53	45 (5 y)
Lazzarino et al., 1993 (44)	30	CHOP (14), MACOP-B or VACOP-B (16)	Yes		55	38 (3 y)
Rodriguez et al., 1994 (55)	18	Doxorubicin regimens	Yes	12	67	45 (2 y)
Falini et al., 1995 (40)	18	MACOP-B (7), F-MACHOP (11)	No	61	33	61 (2 y)
Zinzani et al., 1996 (42)	22	MACOP-B (20), F-MACHOP (2)	Yes		95	86 (2 y)
Cazals-Hatem, 1996 (6)	141	Intensive regimens	No	31	48	61 (3 y)
Lazzarino et al., 1997 (41)	106	Doxorubicin regimens	Yes	42	23	50 (3 y)
Martelli, 1998 (61)	37	F-MACHOP (10), MACOP-B (27)	No	90	10	70 (5 y)
Abou Ellela, 1999 (56)	43	CAP-BOB and variants	NR		63	39 (5 y)
Zinzani et al., 1999 (47)	50	MACOP-B	Yes		86	93 (8 y)
Bieri et al., 1999 (59)	27	Doxorubicin regimens	Yes	15	55	44 (10 y)
Nguyen et al., 2000 (60)	40	Doxorubicin regimens	Yes	41	41	67 (5 y)
Zinzani et al., 2001 (62)	89	MACOP-B	Yes	4	88	91 (9 y)
Zinzani et al., 2002 (65)	426	CHOP (105)	Yes	20	61	35
		MACOP-B/VACOP-B (277)		8	79	67
		HDS/ABMT (44)		13	75	78 (12 y)
Todeschini et al., 2004 (66)	138	CHOP (43)	Yes	7	51	39.5
		MACOP-B/VACOP-B (95)		10	80	75.7 (9 y)

ABMT, autologous bone marrow transplantation; CAP-BOP, Cyclophosphamide, Adriamycin (doxorubicin), procarbazine, bleomycin, Oncovin, and prednisone; CHOP-B, CHOP and bleomycin; C-MOPP, Cyclophosphamide, mechlorethamine, Oncovin (vincristine), procarbazine, and prednisone; FFS, failure-free survival; HDS, high-dose sequential; m-BACOD, moderate-dose methotrexate, bleomycin, Adriamycin (doxorubicin), Cyclophosphamide, Oncovin (vincristine), and dexamethasone; NR, not reported; PR, partial response; RT, radiation therapy.

Whereas the CHOP regimen has been used by American investigators, several European centers have suggested that the methotrexate, Adriamycin (doxorubicin), cyclophosphamide, Oncovin (vincristine), prednisone, and bleomycin (MACOP-B) regimen may be superior to CHOP (41,47,51,52,62). However, the debate is still open because it is difficult to compare the advantages of the different types of protocols, and it is also difficult to explain the rather different complete response and survival rates reported by different institutions using similar regimens in phase II studies potentially influenced by patient selection bias. Considering the published phase II data by centers that have used both first-generation chemotherapy regimens like CHOP and other more aggressive third-generation ones like MACOP-B, the results have clearly favored the latter. Todeschini et al. (52) used CHOP in six patients without achieving a single complete response; in the 15 patients treated with MACOP-B or 5-fluorouracil, methotrexate, cytosine arabinoside, cyclophosphamide, doxorubicin, Oncovin (vincristine), and prednisone (F-MACHOP) (64) regimens, 87% achieved a complete response. Lazzarino et al. (44) treated 30 patients; the complete response rate after CHOP was 36%, whereas that after MACOP-B or Vepesid (etoposide), Adriamycin (doxorubicin), cyclophosphamide, Oncovin (vincristine), prednisone, and bleomycin (VACOP-B) was 73%. In a multicenter study of 106 patients, the 3-year relapse-free survival was 38% in the 47 patients treated with CHOP, whereas it was 58% in the 62 patients treated with MACOP-B or VACOP-B (41). In two previous studies (47,62), we used the MACOP-B regimen in 50 patients (a two-center prospective trial), and in 89 patients (an Italian multicenter prospective trial), the complete response rates were 86% and 88%, respectively, whereas the 5-year relapse-free survival rates were 93% and 91%, respectively (Table 21.3).

Recently, two retrospective studies have reported data regarding the comparison between CHOP and CHOP-like regimens versus MACOP-B and MACOP-B-like regimens as induction chemotherapy in patients with PMBL (65,66). Our mulitinational retrospective study compared the outcomes of 426 patients with PMBL after first-generation (CHOP and CHOP-like regimens; 105 patients), third-generation (MACOP-B, VACOP-B, prednisone, methotrexate, doxorubicin, cyclophosphamide, and epipodophyllotoxin VP-16 Cytarabine, bleomycin, vincristine, methotrexate, and leucovorin; 277 patients), and high-dose chemotherapy schedules (high-dose sequential and autologous bone marrow transplantation; 44 patients) (65). In all these groups, the most patients underwent radiation therapy after chemotherapy. With chemotherapy, complete response rates were 49%, 51%, and 53%, with first-generation, third-generation, and high-dose chemotherapy strategies, respectively. The final complete response rates, after radiation therapy on the mediastinum, became 61% for CHOP and CHOP-like regimens, 79% for MACOP-B and other regimens, and 75% for high-dose strategies. Projected 10-year OS rates were 44%, 71%, and 77%, respectively (Fig. 21.3); and projected 10-year progression-free survival rates were 35%, 67%, and 78%,

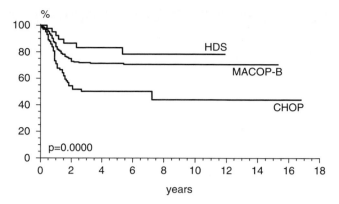

FIGURE 21.3 OS curves of the three main chemotherapy subgroups. (Reprinted with permission from Zinzani PL, Martelli M, Bertini M, et al. Induction chemotherapy strategies for primary mediastinal large B-cell lymphoma with sclerosis: a retrospective multinational study on 426 previously untreated patients. Haematologica 2002;87:1258–1264.)

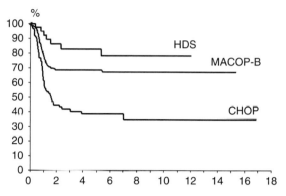

FIGURE 21.4 Progression-free survival curves of the three main chemotherapy subgroups. (Reprinted with permission from Zinzani PL, Martelli M, Bertini M, et al. Induction chemotherapy strategies for primary mediastinal large B-cell lymphoma with sclerosis: a retrospective multinational study on 426 previously untreated patients. Haematologica 2002;87:1258–1264.)

respectively (Fig. 21.4). In addition, after the radiation therapy, 81% of the patients who had already achieved a partial response obtained complete response status. Todeschini et al. (66) reported the long-term results from a retrospective multicenter Italian experience in 138 patients with PMBL treated with CHOP (43 patients) or MACOP-B/VACOP-B (95 patients). Complete response was 51% in the CHOP group and 80% in MACOP-B/VACOP-B. The addition of radiation therapy on mediastinum mass consolidation improved the outcome regardless of the type of chemotherapy. These two retrospective studies confirm the superiority of the third-generation chemotherapy strategies over first-generation ones. In addition, they highlight the role of radiation therapy for converting cases of partial response to complete response, and probably also of reinforcing existing complete responses.

The role of high-dose approaches, including autologous stem cell transplantation and high-dose sequential treatment, needs to be confirmed because the actual reported data do not prove the superiority of high-dose chemotherapy over conventional chemotherapy in phase II trials (67–69). The use of high-dose chemotherapy supported by stem cell transplantation to consolidate the initial response in high-risk patients is a matter of debate (67,70–72).

On the basis of the reported nonrandomized trials, the best results in terms of complete response and relapse-free survival rates seem to come from the combination of MACOP-B/VACOP-B regimens. Randomized prospective studies are needed to define the optimal first-line chemotherapy.

Radiation Therapy

The issue of adjuvant radiation therapy after chemotherapy also remains open, although it seems likely that it could play an important role in this locally aggressive disease, particularly in the presence of bulky disease. However, the excellent results obtained in the Groupe d'Etude des Lymphomes de l'Adulte study (6) without radiation therapy have called into question its necessity. The data from four recent publications (47,62,65,66) have indicated that the addition of radiation therapy after chemotherapy is of pivotal importance for the eradication of PMBL in terms of increasing the complete response rate or reinforcing existing complete responses after induction chemotherapy. In particular, in the first report (47), with the use of computed tomography scans, 70% of the patients had residual mediastinal tumor masses after chemotherapy (MACOP-B), and after radiation therapy, 44% of the patients had residual masses on computed tomography scan. Regarding gallium-67 scanning, 66% of the patients showed persistent abnormal uptake after MACOP-B, whereas after radiation therapy, 19% of the patients still had a positive gallium-67 scan. In the second study (62), after the chemotherapy regimen (MACOP-B), 26% of the patients achieved a complete response, and 66% obtained a partial response, giving an overall response rate of 92%. After radiation therapy, 93% of the patients who had already achieved a partial response obtained complete response status. Thus, after the combined modality treatment, 88% of the patients achieved a complete response.

Treatment of Recurrent Disease

Generally, patients with PMBL who obtain a complete response lasting >18 to 24 months after diagnosis are likely to be cured. In fact, most relapses occur within the first 12 months after the completion of the frontline treatment. A standard therapeutic option for patients with relapsed disease has not yet been identified. However, considering the young age of these patients and the pattern of relapse that spares the bone marrow, high-dose chemotherapy supported by autologous stem cell transplantation is suitable for individual clinical use (68,69). With this strategy, patients with relapsed mediastinal lymphoma seem to have a better prognosis than those with the other diffuse large cell lymphomas, with 5-year disease-free survival rates of 55% and 35%, respectively. In contrast, patients treated with conventional second-line chemotherapy or with radiation therapy to the mediastinum (for patients who did not undergo radiation therapy after the frontline chemotherapy regimen) have a median survival after relapse of a few months.

FUTURE DIRECTIONS

Further improvements in the management of PMBL depend on the design of prospective multicenter trials to assess the test chemotherapeutic regimen (first vs. third generation) to be combined with the radiation therapy, taking into account the pivotal role of the [18F]-2-fluoro-2-deoxyglucose-positron emission tomography in posttreatment imaging reevaluation. In addition, it will be important and interesting to add to the new therapeutic armamentarium of PMBL the anti-CD20 monoclonal antibody alone or conjugated to radionuclides (radioimmunoconjugates) in an effort to increase the complete response and survival rates.

Regarding the role of rituximab in PMBL treatment, so far there are only a few short reports (73,74) presented by two groups: the former (73) observed a statistically significant advantage for the combination of rituximab plus Dose Adjusted Etoposide, Prednisone, Vincristine, Cyclophosphamide, Doxorubicin; and the latter (74) reported a percent increase in terms of complete response, failure-free survival, and OS of the CHOP plus rituximab versus CHOP alone. Anyway, in this last study, the data obtained with the combined treatment were equivalent to the previously published MACOP-B/VACOP-B data without rituximab. In a retrospective study, Savage et al. (75) showed some patients treated with CHOP plus rituximab in comparison with patients treated with MACOP-B/VACOP-B who obtained the same results in terms of 5-year OS.

In the near future, probably the potential best treatment could be the sequential treatment of chemotherapy plus immunotherapy (as induction phase) and then radioimmunotherapy (as a consolidation phase) instead of local radiotherapy.

References

1. Lichtenstein AK, Levine A, Taylor CR, et al. Primary mediastinal lymphoma in adults. *Am J Med* 1980;68:509–514.
2. Levitt LJ, Aisenberg AC, Harris NL, et al. Primary non-Hodgkin's lymphoma of the mediastinum. *Cancer* 1982;50:2486–2492.
3. Harris NL, Jaffe ES, Stein H, et al. A revised European-American classification of lymphoid neoplasms: a proposal from the International Lymphoma Study Group. *Blood* 1994;84:1361–1392.
4. Jaffe ES, Harris NL, Stein H, et al. Pathology and genetics of tumors of hematopoietic and lymphoid tissues. In: Kleihues P, Sobin L, eds. *World Health Organization classification of tumours*, vol. 3. Lyon, France: IARC Press, 2001.
5. Swerdlow SH, Campo E, Harris NL, et al. WHO Classification of Tumours of Haematopoietic and Lymphoid Systems. 4th ed. Lyon: IARC; 2008.
6. Cazals-Hatem D, Lepage E, Brice P, et al. Primary mediastinal large B-cell lymphoma. A clinicopathologic study of 141 cases compared with 916 nonmediastinal large B-cell lymphomas, a GELA ("Groupe d'Elude des Lymphomes de l'Adulte") study. *Am J Surg Pathol* 1996;20:877–888.
7. A clinical evaluation of the International Lymphoma Study Group classification of non-Hodgkin's lymphoma. Non-Hodgkin's Lymphoma Classification Project. *Blood* 1997;89:3909–3918.
8. Armitage JO, Weisenburger DD. New approach to classifying non Hodgkin's lymphomas: clinical features of the major histologic subtypes. *J Clin Oncol* 1998;16:2780–2795.
9. Moller P, Lammler B, Eberlein-Gonska M, et al. Primary mediastinal clear cell lymphoma of B-cell type. *Virchows Arch A Pathol Anat Histopathol* 1986;409:79–92.
10. Hamlin PA, Portlock CS, Straus DJ, et al. Primary mediastinal large B-cell lymphoma: optimal therapy and prognostic factor analysis in 141 consecutive patients treated at Memorial Sloan Kettering from 1980 to 1999. *Br J Haematol.* 2005;130:691–699.
11. Paulli M, Sträter J, Gianelli U, et al. Mediastinal B-cell lymphoma: a study of its histomorphologic spectrum based on 109 cases. *Hum Pathol* 1999;30:178–187.
12. Barth TF, Leithauser F, Joos S, et al. Mediastinal (thymic) large B-cell lymphoma: where do we stand? *Lancet Oncol* 2002;3:229–234.
13. Pileri SA, Gaidano G, Zinzani PL, et al. Primary mediastinal B-cell lymphoma: high frequency of BCL-6 mutations and consistent expression of the transcription factors OCT-2, BOB.1, and PU.1 in the absence of immunoglobulins. *Am J Pathol* 2003;162:243–253.
14. Traverse-Glehen A, Pittaluga S, Gaulard P, et al. Mediastinal gray zone lymphoma: the missing link between classic Hodgkin's lymphoma and mediastinal large B-cell lymphoma. *Am J Surg Pathol* 2005;29:1411–1421.
15. Kanavaros P, Gaulard P, Charlotte F, et al. Discordant expression of immunoglobulin and its associated molecule mb-1/CD79a is frequently found in mediastinal large B cell lymphomas. *Am J Pathol* 1995;146:735–741.
16. Higgins JP, Warnke RA. CD30 expression is common in mediastinal large B-cell lymphoma. *Am J ClinPathol* 1999;112:241–247.
17. Möller P, Moldenhauer G, Momburg F, et al. Mediastinal lymphoma of clear cell type is a tumor corresponding to terminal steps of B cell differentiation. *Blood* 1987;69:1087–1095.
18. Copie-Bergman C, Gaulard P, Maouche-Chretien L, et al. The MAL gene is expressed in primary mediastinal large B-cell lymphoma. *Blood* 1999;94:3567–3575.
19. Copie-Bergman C, Plonquet A, Alonso M, et al. MAL expression in lymphoid cells: further evidence for MAL as a distinct molecular marker of primary mediastinal large B-cell lymphomas. *Mod Pathol* 2002;15:1172–1180.
20. de Leval L, Ferry JA, Falini B, et al. Expression of bcl-6 and CD10 in primary mediastinal large B-cell lymphoma: evidence for derivation from germinal center B cells? *Am J Surg Pathol* 2001;25:1277–1282.
21. Rodig SJ, Savage KJ, LaCasce AS, et al. Expression of TRAF1 and nuclear c-Rel distinguishes primary mediastinal large cell lymphoma from other types of diffuse large B-cell lymphoma. *Am J Surg Pathol* 2007;31:106–112.
22. Möller P, Herrmann B, Moldenhauer G, et al. Defective expression of MHC class I antigens is frequent in B-cell lymphomas of high-grade malignancy. *Int J Cancer* 1987;40:32–39.
23. Leithäuser F, Bäuerle M, Huynh MQ, et al. Isotype-switched immunoglobulin genes with a high load of somatic hypermutation and lack of ongoing mutational activity are prevalent in mediastinal B-cell lymphoma. *Blood* 2001;98:2762–2770.
24. Bentz M, Barth TF, Brüderlein S, et al. Gain of chromosome arm 9p is characteristic of primary mediastinal B-cell lymphoma (MBL): comprehensive moelcular cytogenetic analysis and presentation of a novel MBL cell line. *Genes Chromosomes Cancer* 2001;30:393–401.
25. Joos S, Otano-Joos MI, Ziegler S, et al. Primary mediastinal (thymic) B-cell lymphoma is characterized by gains of chromosomal material including 9p and amplification of the REL gene. *Blood* 1996;87:1571–1578.
26. Wessendorf S, Barth TFE, Viardot A, et al. Further delineation of chromosomal consensus regions in primary mediastinal B-cell lymphomas–an analysis of 37 tumor samples using high resolution genomic profiling (array-CGH). *Leukemia* 2007;21:2463–2469.
27. Weniger MA, Pulford K, Gesk S, et al. Gains of the proto-oncogene BCL11A and nuclear accumulation of BCL11AXL protein are frequent in primary mediastinal B-cell lymphoma. *Leukemia* 2006;20:1880–1882.
28. Weniger MA, Gesk S, Ehrlich S, et al. Gains of REL in primary mediastinal B-cell lymphoma coincide with nuclear accumulation of Rel protein. *Genes Chromosomes Cancer* 2007;46:406–415.
29. Melzner I, Bucur AJ, Brüderlein S, et al. Biallelic mutation of SOCS-1 impairs JAK2 degradation and sustains phosphor-JAK2 action in MedB-1 mediastinal lymphoma line. *Blood* 2005;105:2535–2542.
30. Rosenwald A, Wright G, Leroy K, et al. for the Lymphoma/Leukemia Molecular Profiling Project. Molecular diagnosis of primary mediastinal B cell lymphoma identifies a clinically favorable subgroup of diffuse large B cell lymphoma related to Hodgkin lymphoma. *J Exp Med* 2003;198:851–862.
31. Feuerhake F, Kutok JL, Monti S, et al. NFkappaB activity, function, and target-gene signatures in primary mediastinal large B-cell lymphoma and diffuse large B-cell lymphoma subtypes. *Blood* 2005;106:1392–1399.
32. Savage KJ, Monti S, Kutok JL, et al. The molecular signature of mediastinal large B-cell lymphoma differs from that of other diffuse large B-cell lymphomas and shares features with Hodgkin lymphoma. *Blood* 2003;102:3871–3879.
33. Guiter C, Dusanter-Fourt I, Copie-Bergman C, et al. Constitutive STAT6 activation in primary mediastinal large B-cell lymphoma. *Blood* 2004;104:543–549.
34. Weniger MA, Melzner I, Menz CK, et al. Mutations of the tumor suppressor gene SOCS-1 in classical Hodgkin lymphoma are frequent and associated with nuclear phospho-STAT5 accumulation. *Oncogene* 2006;25:2679–2684.
35. Tsang P, Cesarman E, Chadburn A, et al. Molecular characterization of primary mediastinal B cell lymphoma. *Am J Pathol* 1996;148:2017–2025.
36. Scarpa A, Moore PS, Rigaud G, et al. Molecular features of primary mediastinal B-cell lymphoma:involvement of p16INK4A, p53 and c-myc. *Br J Hematol* 1999;107:106–113.
37. Loddenkemper C, Anagnostopoulos I, Hummel M, et al. Differential Emu enhancer activity and expression of BOB.1/OBF.1, Oct2, PU.1, and immunoglobulin in reactive B-cell populations, B-cell non-Hodgkin lymphomas, and Hodgkin lymphomas. *J Pathol* 2004;202:60–69.
38. Ritz O, Leithäuser F, Hasel C, et al. Downregulation of internal enhancer activity contributes to abnormally low immunoglobulin expression in the MedB-1 mediastinal B-cell lymphoma cell line. *J Pathol* 2005;205:336–348.
39. Jacobson JO, Aisenberg AC, Lamane L, et al. Mediastinal large cell lymphoma: an uncommon subset of adult lymphoma curable with combined modality therapy. *Cancer* 1988;62:1893–1898.

40. Falini B, Venturi S, Martelli M, et al. Mediastinal large B-cell lymphoma: clinical and immunohistological findings in 18 patients treated with different third-generation regimens. *Br J Haematol* 1995;89:780–789.

41. Lazzarino M, Orlandi E, Paulli M, et al. Treatment outcome and prognostic factors for primary mediastinal (thymic) B-celllymphoma: a multicenter study of 106 patients. *J Clin Oncol* 1997;15:1646–1653.

42. Zinzani PL, Bendandi M, Frezza G, et al. Primary mediastinal B-cell lymphoma with sclerosis: clinical and therapeutic evaluation of 22 patients. *Leuk Lymphoma* 1996;21:311–316.

43. Haioun C, Gaulard P, Roudot-Thoraval F, et al. Mediastinal diffuse large B-cell lymphoma with sclerosis: a condition with a poor prognosis. *Am J Clin Oncol* 1989;12:425–429.

44. Lazzarino M, Orlandi E, Paulli M, et al. Primary mediastinal B-cell lymphoma with sclerosis: an aggressive tumor with distinctive clinical and pathological features. *J Clin Oncol* 1993;11:2306–2313.

45. Bishop P, Wilson W, Pearson D, et al. CNS involvement in primary mediastinal large B-cell lymphoma. *J Clin Oncol* 1999;17:2479–2485.

46. Abrahamsen AF, Lien HH, Aas M, et al. Magnetic resonance imaging and 67gallium scan in mediastinal malignant lymphoma: a prospective pilot study. *Ann Oncol* 1994;5:433–436.

47. Zinzani PL, Martelli M, Magagnoli M, et al. Treatment and clinical management of primary mediastinal large B-cell lymphoma with sclerosis: MACOP-B regimen and mediastinal radiotherapy monitored by (67) gallium scan in 50 patients. *Blood* 1999;94:3289–3293.

48. Carbone PP, Kaplan HS, Musshoff K, et al. Report of the Committee on Hodgkin's Disease Staging Classification. *Cancer Res* 1971;31:860–1861.

49. Lavabre-Bertrand T, Donadio D, Fegueux N, et al. A study of 15 cases of primary mediastinal lymphoma of B-cell type. *Cancer* 1992;69:2561–2566.

50. Rohatiner AZ, Whelan JS, Ganjoo RK, et al. Mediastinal large-cell lymphoma with sclerosis (MLCLS). *Br J Cancer* 1994;69:601–604.

51. Bertini M, Orsucci L, Vitolo D, et al. Stage II large B-cell lymphoma with sclerosis treated with MACOP-B. *Ann Oncol* 1991;2:733–737.

52. Todeschini G, Ambrosetti A, Meneghini V, et al. Mediastinal large-B cell-lymphoma with sclerosis: a clinical study of 21 patients. *J Clin Oncol* 1990;8:804–808.

53. Kim D, Mauch P, Shaffer K, et al. Large-cell and immunoblastic lymphoma of the mediastinum: prognostic and pathologic features in 57 patients. *J Clin Oncol* 1993;11:1336–1343.

54. Aisenberg AC. Primary large-celllymphoma of the mediastinum. *J Clin Oncol* 1993;11:2291–2298.

55. Rodriguez J, Pugh WC, Romaguera JE, et al. Primary mediastinal large cell lymphoma. *Hematol Oncol* 1994;12:175–184.

56. Abou-Elella AA, Weisenburger DD, Vose JM, et al. Primary mediastinal large B-cell lymphoma: a clinicopathologic study of 43 patients from the Nebraska Lymphoma Study Group. *J Clin Oncol* 1999;17:784–790.

57. Perrone T, Frizzera G, Rosai J. Mediastinal diffuse large-cell lymphoma with sclerosis. A clinicopathologic study of 60 cases. *Am J Clin Pathol* 1986;10:176–191.

58. AI-Sharabati M, Chittal S, Duga-Neulet I, et al. Primary anterior mediastinal B-celllymphoma: a clinicopathological and immunohistochemical study of 16 cases. *Cancer* 1991;67:2579–2583.

59. Bieri S, Roggero E, Zucca E, et al. Primary mediastinal large B-cell lymphoma (PMLCL): the need for prospective controlled clinical trials. *Leuk Lymphoma* 1999;35:139–146.

60. Nguyen LN, Ha CS, Hess M, et al. The outcome of combined-modality treatments for stage I and II primary large B-cell lymphoma of the mediastinum. *Int J Radiat Oncol Biol Phys* 2000;47:1281–1285.

61. Martelli MP, Martelli M, Pescarmona E, et al. MACOP-B and involved field radiation therapy is an effective therapy for primary mediastinal large B-cell lymphoma with sclerosis. *Ann Oncol* 1998;9:1027–1029.

62. Zinzani PL, Martelli M, De Renzo A, et al. Primary mediastinal large B-cell lymphoma with sclerosis: a clinical study of 89 patients treated with MACOP-B chemotherapy and radiation therapy. *Haematologica* 2001;86:187–191.

63. Fisher RI, Gaynor ER, Dahlberg S, et al. Comparison of a standard regimen (CHOP) with three intensive chemotherapy regimens for advanced non-Hodgkin's lymphoma. *N Engl J Med* 1993;329:1002–1006.

64. Guglielmi C, Amadori S, Anselmo AP, et al. Sequential combination chemotherapy of high-grade non-Hodgkin's lymphoma with 5-fluorouracil, methotrexate, cytosine arabinoside, cyclophosphamide, doxorubicin, vincristine and prednisone (F-MACHOP). *Cancer Invest* 1987;5:159–169.

65. Zinzani PL, Martelli M, Bestini M, et al. Induction chemotherapy strategies for primari mediastinal large B-cell lymphoma with sclerosis: a retrospective multinational study of 426 previously untreated patients. *Haematologica* 2002;87:1258–1264.

66. Todeschini G, Secchi S, Morra E, et al. Primary mediastinal large B-cell lymphoma (PMBL): long-term results from a retrospective multicentre Italian experience in 138 patients treated with CHOP or MACOP-B/VACOP-B. *Br J Cancer* 2004;90:372–376.

67. Nademanee A, Molina A, O'Donnell M, et al. Results of high-dose therapy and autologous bone marrow/stem cell transplantation during remission in poor-risk intermediate and high-grade lymphoma: international index high and high-intermediate risk group. *Blood* 1997;90:3844–3852.

68. Popat D, Przepiork D, Champlin R, et al. High-dose chemotherapy for relapsed and refractory diffuse large B-celllymphoma: mediastinal localization predicts for a favorable outcome. *J Clin Oncol* 1998;16:63–69.

69. Sehn LH, Antin JH, Shulman LN, et al. Primary diffuse large B-cell lymphoma of the mediastinum. Outcome after high-dose chemotherapy and autologous hematopoietic cell transplantation. *Blood* 1998;91:717–723.

70. Aisenberg AC. Primary large cell lymphoma of the mediastinum. *Semin Oncol* 1999;26:251–258.

71. Van Besien K, Kelta M, Bahaguna P. Primary mediastinal B-cell lymphoma: a review of pathology and management. *J Clin Oncol* 2001;19:1855–1864.

72. Rodriguez J, Conde E, Gutierrez A, et al. Primary mediastinal large cell lymphoma (PMBL): frontline treatment with autologous stem cell transplantation (ASCT). The GEL-TAMO experience. *Hematol Oncol* 2008;26:171–178.

73. Dunleavy K, Pittaluga S, Janik J, et al. Primary mediastinal large B-cell lymphoma (PMBL) outcome is significantly improved by the addition of rituximab to dose adjusted (DA)-EPOCH and overcomes the need for radiation. *Blood* 2005,106:929. (abstract)

74. Vassilakopoulos TP, Angelopoulou MK, Galani Z, et al. Excellent outcome with Rituximab-CHOP (R-CHOP) combined with radiotherapy (RT) in primary mediastinal large B-Cell lymphoma (PMBL). *Blood* 2005,106:935. (abstract)

75. Savage KJ, Al-Rajhi N, Voss N, et al. Favorable outcome of primary mediastinal large B-cell lymphoma in a single institution: the British Columbia experience. *Ann Oncol* 2006:17:123–130.

CHAPTER 22 ■ BURKITT LYMPHOMA

RANDY D. GASCOYNE, IAN T. MAGRATH, AND LAURIE SEHN

Burkitt lymphoma was one of the first tumors shown to be curable by chemotherapy alone, thus providing critical support to pioneer chemotherapists. It was the first tumor to be shown to be associated with a virus (Epstein-Barr virus [EBV]), an association that remains unexplained but that may eventually lead to highly specific targeted therapy. It was also one of the first tumors to be shown to be associated with a nonrandom chromosomal translocation, the first in which antigen receptor gene sequences were involved (now known to be a frequent occurrence in lymphoid neoplasia), and the first in which the consequences of the translocation are quite well understood, being the deregulation of an oncogene, *MYC*. It remains possible that this finding, too, may eventually be relevant to targeted therapeutic approaches; indeed, experiments with antisense directed against the c-myc gene have provided at least "proof of principle" in this context. For now, however, the tumor can be cured in a high fraction of cases with intensive conventional chemotherapy: approximately 90% in children and possibly a similar fraction in adults, although more information is needed in the latter, particularly in elderly patients.

The tumor occurs at any age, although its peak incidence is in the 1st decade of life. It is almost unknown in children younger than the age of 2 years, and although usually considered a tumor of childhood, given that there are more decades of life in adults, the numbers of cases of adults and children are approximately equal at least in affluent countries. The incidence of the tumor varies quite markedly throughout the world, ranging from some one to three per 1 million children in North America and Europe, to some five to ten per 1 million in equatorial Africa. The tumor is sometimes associated with a herpes-type virus, EBV (i.e., multiple viral genomes are present in the tumor cell nuclei), but the proportion of positive cases varies in different geographic regions and, doubtless, populations, to at least some degree in proportion to the incidence. Thus, in equatorial Africa, where the incidence is highest, quite probably because holoendemic malaria, which causes B-cell hyperplasia, is a cofactor, almost all cases are EBV associated (a few percentage are EBV negative). In affluent countries, only 10% to 20% are EBV positive. Burkitt lymphoma also occurs in the context of human immunodeficiency virus (HIV) infection, in which approximately 30% are EBV associated. In addition, the tumor, in this circumstance, is most often associated with a phase of HIV infection in which the immune system is relatively intact. In Africa, however, there does not appear to be an increased incidence of the disease in the context of HIV infection, at least in children. The reason for this remains unknown.

DISCOVERY OF THE TUMOR

Burkitt lymphoma was first recognized as a distinct clinicopathologic entity in Africa. The eponymous designation is probably well deserved, however, because Burkitt, a surgeon working in Kampala, Uganda, can certainly be said to have put the tumor "on the map," even though, as is so often the case, others, primarily pathologists, had made similar observations in Africa before Burkitt's classic 1958 paper (1). This tumor, which Burkitt referred to as a *sarcoma*, had a number of different clinical presentations, including jaw tumors and intra-abdominal tumor (2–6), and it was the frequent association of the two that led Burkitt to propose that many children with isolated abdominal tumors had the same disease as those who presented with isolated jaw tumors. Unknown to Burkitt, O'Conor and Davies (7), pathologists also working at Mulago Hospital in Kampala, were at the same time undertaking a survey of the departmental collection of malignant tumors in children and were able to confirm Davies' earlier observation (3) that approximately one-half of them were tumors of the "reticulo-endothelial system." Thus, it soon became clear that the tumor recognized clinically by Burkitt was a lymphoma. Burkitt went on to recognize that the "African lymphoma," as it became known, had a high frequency in a broad band across equatorial Africa and that its distribution in Africa was climatically determined (8,9). Haddow, working in the Entebbe Virus Research Institute also in Uganda, found the distribution to be very similar to that of several viral diseases vectored by mosquitoes. This observation prompted Epstein et al. (10), then working at the Middlesex Hospital in London, to search for virus particles in Burkitt lymphoma tumor cells and, thus, led directly to the discovery of EBV, although not in fresh tumor cells but in a tiny fraction of cells in cell lines derived from tumor samples. Subsequently, however, it has become clear, given the ubiquitous distribution of EBV, that the climatic distribution in Africa is not due to the virus association. Most of the evidence supports the hypothesis, originally proposed by Dalldorf et al. (11), that it is holoendemic malaria, which has a similar distribution to other insect-vectored diseases in equatorial Africa, that accounts for the geographic distribution on that continent. The distribution elsewhere has not been demonstrated to be climatically determined.

Subsequent to its discovery in Africa, pathologists who had worked there recognized that tumors with identical histology accounted for a fraction of the lymphomas occurring in children in other world regions (12–14). Initially, there was a general sense that patients with a leukemic presentation, almost unknown in Africa (although bone marrow involvement, in association with other disease sites, occurs in <10% of patients), had a different disease. However, through recognition that the molecular genetic abnormalities are identical to those with a more typical presentation and response to therapy is optimal with the same kinds of regimens, but not with regimens designed for acute lymphoblastic leukemia (ALL), it has become accepted that leukemic presentations (i.e., with bone marrow and peripheral blood involvement, and frequently with lymphadenopathy, hepatosplenomegaly, or both of Burkitt lymphoma [usually referred to as *acute B-cell leukemia* or *ALL-L3* by pediatric oncologists]) occur relatively frequently outside Africa. It has become conventional to refer to the disease as *acute B-cell leukemia* when the fraction of blast cells in the bone marrow is >25% (15–21).

Diagnosis

Burkitt lymphoma and Burkitt leukemia are considered part of the same disease spectrum and, thus, will be discussed together. They are distinguished by the primary site of presentation and more specifically, by the number of blast cells present in the bone marrow at diagnosis (15–18,20–24). Burkitt lymphoma occurs in three clinical settings, including endemic, sporadic, and immunodeficiency related variants.

Morphology

Classic Burkitt Lymphoma

Virtually all cases of endemic Burkitt lymphoma, the majority of sporadic Burkitt lymphoma, and many cases of acquired immunodeficiency syndrome (AIDS)-related Burkitt lymphoma have identical morphologic features, described as classic type (20,21,23–28). The architecture is diffuse with a distinct starry-sky pattern evident at low-power magnification (Fig. 22.1). The latter feature imparts a "moth-eaten" appearance and is due to the presence of many benign phagocytic histiocytes engulfing the nuclear debris that results from the apoptotic death of the lymphoma cells. Rare cases with a follicular pattern may be seen, but it is not possible to distinguish a true follicular growth pattern from colonization of residual benign lymphoid follicles in the majority of these cases (27). The cells are medium sized with a monotonous and somewhat uniform appearance (Fig. 22.2). The cell size approximates the nuclear size of the macrophages in the same section. A so-called "squaring-off" of the cytoplasm may be encountered because the cell borders appear to abut one another (Fig. 22.3) (29). This feature is particularly characteristic when using mercury based fixatives such as B5. The nuclear appearance is uniform with round to oval-shaped nuclei. The chromatin is clumped with relatively clear parachromatin and two to five centrally located small basophilic nucleoli. B5 fixation may enhance the tendency for the cells to have single, central prominent nucleoli. There is a small amount of deeply basophilic cytoplasm that frequently contains lipid vacuoles. The latter feature is best seen in imprint preparations of lymph nodes or bone marrow aspirates and although common, is not a universal finding (29). Multinucleated cells are uncommon.

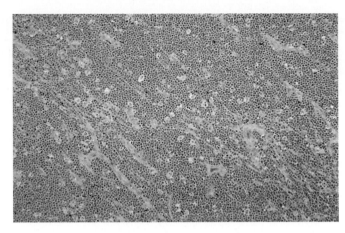

FIGURE 22.1 Low-power image of classic Burkitt lymphoma with prominent starry-sky appearance.

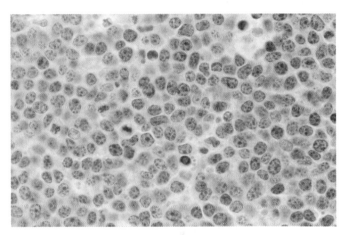

FIGURE 22.2 High magnification of classic Burkitt lymphoma showing the typical cytology of the neoplastic cells. Note the uniform appearance of the cells and the scattered mitotic figures.

Occasional cases of Burkitt lymphoma may show slight morphologic and/or immunophenotypic variation such as minimal heterogeneity of cell size and nuclear shape or weak expression of BCL2 protein. These cases are still considered Burkitt lymphoma, but definitive diagnosis often requires documentation of a *MYC* translocation using molecular genetic techniques such as fluorescence in situ hybridization (FISH). The terms atypical Burkitt lymphoma and Burkitt-like lymphoma are no longer used to describe these cases (24). The classic diagnostic features of Burkitt lymphoma are listed in Table 22.1 together with features that distinguish them from unclassifiable B-cell lymphomas with features intermediate between diffuse large B-cell lymphoma (DLBCL) and Burkitt lymphoma (see Table 22.1).

Variant Burkitt Lymphoma with Plasmacytoid Appearance

In the setting of HIV infection, a variant form of Burkitt lymphoma may be encountered that shares morphologic features with both classic Burkitt lymphoma and DLBCL (20,21,25,30–32). There is slight variation in cell size and shape imparting a

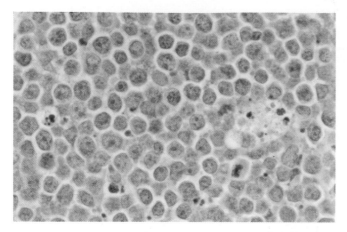

FIGURE 22.3 Classic Burkitt lymphoma at high magnification showing "squaring-off" of the cytoplasm. This feature is most easily seen in thin, formalin-fixed sections. Note the slight nuclear irregularity seen in classic Burkitt lymphoma at increased magnification.

minimal degree of heterogeneity to the sections. The nuclei may be slightly eccentric, and the nucleoli are more often single and central, resembling small plasmacytoid immunoblasts. This appearance of Burkitt lymphoma has been referred to as the "intermediate" form because it shares morphologic features intermediate between classic Burkitt lymphoma and DLBCL. Rarely, multinucleated cells may be present.

B-Cell Lymphoma, Unclassifiable, with Features Intermediate Between Diffuse Large B-Cell Lymphoma and Burkitt Lymphoma

In 2008, the World Health Organization (WHO) released the fourth edition of its classification of tumors of hematopoietic and lymphoid tissues (23). The classification introduced a new category of "B cell lymphoma, unclassifiable, with features intermediate between DLBCL and Burkitt lymphoma" (33). This new category almost certainly includes more than one entity but importantly recognizes that a proportion of de novo lymphomas and perhaps a greater frequency of transformed follicular lymphoma (FL) cases show features that are intermediate between typical DLBCL and classic Burkitt lymphoma. These "grey-zone" cases characteristically show morphologic features intermediate between DLBCL and Burkitt lymphoma, with some medium-sized cells reminiscent of Burkitt lymphoma and some larger cells admixed typical of DLBCL. These cases often have a starry-sky appearance and a high proliferative rate, and many have an immunophenotype consistent with Burkitt lymphoma (Fig. 22.4). However, a diagnosis of Burkitt lymphoma is not made because these cases show a variable combination of atypical morphology, immunophenotype, or genetic features that are not consistent with classic Burkitt lymphoma. Importantly, this new category of B-cell lymphoma should not be used in cases of otherwise typical DLBCL that happen to have a *MYC* rearrangement (approximately 5% to 8% of DLBCLs). Similarly, otherwise classic Burkitt lymphoma cases in which a *MYC* translocation cannot be

TABLE 22.1

DIAGNOSTIC FEATURES DISTINGUISHING CLASSIC BURKITT LYMPHOMA (BL) FROM UNCLASSIFIABLE B-CELL LYMPHOMAS, INTERMEDIATE BETWEEN BURKITT LYMPHOMA AND DLBCL

Feature	Classic BL	Unclassifiable BL/DLBCL
Architecture	Diffuse	Diffuse, rarely nodular
Starry-sky pattern	Usually present	May be absent
Mitoses	Many	Many
Cytology	Monomorphic	Pleomorphic with irregular nuclei
Nuclear shape	Round or oval	Usually irregular
Nuclear size	Medium-large	Medium size, some admixed larger cells
Nucleoli	Multiple (2–5), basophilic	May be single and more prominent
Cytoplasm	Basophilic and often vacuolated. Squared-off appearance present	Basophilic. Vacuoles may be absent and usually lack of squared-off appearance
CD10 expression	++	+/−
BCL6 expression	++	+/−
BCL2 expression	Negative/weak	++/−
Proliferation	> 95%	Variable 50–100%
Cytogenetics	t(8;14) or variant t(2;8) or t(8;22) Rare cases lack a *MYC* translocation	May lack *MYC* or have both *MYC* and *BCL2* in the same metaphase
Molecular	*MYC* rearrangement	+/− *MYC* +/− *BCL2* +/− *BCL6*
IG-MYC	Yes	Sometimes
Non-*IG-MYC*	No	Sometimes
Double-hit	No	Sometimes
Simple karyotype	Yes	No
Complex karyotype	No	Yes

Modified from Swerdlow SH, Campo E, Harris NL, et al. *WHO classification of tumours of hematopoietic and lymphoid tissues*, 4th ed. Lyon, France: International Agency for Research on Cancer, 2008.

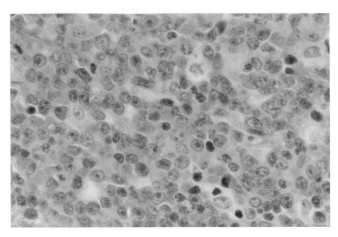

FIGURE 22.4 Unclassifiable B-cell lymphoma intermediate between Burkitt lymphoma/DLBCL case with prominent starry-sky pattern. The cells have more nuclear irregularity and single central nucleoli than is normally seen in classic Burkitt lymphoma.

demonstrated should still be classified as Burkitt lymphoma. Helpful features that allow distinction of Burkitt lymphoma from DLBCL and unclassifiable B-cell lymphomas with intermediate features are listed in Table 22.1.

A sizable proportion of these unclassifiable BL/DLBCL cases represent transformed low-grade lymphomas, most commonly FL harboring a t(14;18). These so-called dual translocation or double-hit cases occur in two clinical scenarios: 50% arise as a *de novo* presentation of an aggressive lymphoma in which the *MYC* translocation is thought to occur early in the genetic evolution of the malignant clone, and the other half is discovered following biopsy for relapse or progression in a patient with antecedent FL (34–44). In both settings, the neoplastic cells harbor both t(14;18) and a *MYC* translocation, and are typically very clinically aggressive lymphomas (45,46).

Is MYC Translocation Specific to Burkitt Lymphoma?

The role of dominant oncogenes can be either primary or secondary. A primary role in pathogenesis is exemplified by the function of *MYC* in Burkitt lymphoma. Secondary alterations are those that occur in the setting of clonal evolution and often herald a change to a more aggressive phenotype. A typical example would be the significant role that the *MYC* gene plays in the downstream events that characterize clonal evolution in multiple myeloma (47,48). Thus, it is worth remembering that a *MYC* translocation, although characteristic of classic Burkitt lymphoma, is by no means specific. The presence of a *MYC* translocation is well described in *de novo* DLBCL cases (49–58). They can be found in approximately 5% to 8% of *de novo* DLBCLs (49,58,59). Surrogate markers such as a proliferation rate in excess of 95% or a classic Burkitt lymphoma immunophenotype (CD10⁺, BCL6⁺, BCL2⁻) cannot be reliably used to recognize *MYC* translocation-positive DLBCL, although previous studies suggested some minor immunophenotypic changes, including a lower proliferation rate, expression of BCL2 protein, and less frequent CD10 expression, were more common in these cases (55,60–62).

Based on the gene expression profiling data described in the section on gene expression profiling novel immunohistochemical markers have recently been described, including TCL-1, CD38, and CD44, that may be of value in recognizing DLBCL with a *MYC* rearrangement (62). Burkitt lymphoma was shown to overexpress TCL-1 and CD38, with diminished expression of CD44 in contrast to *MYC*-negative cases (48). This phenotype (TCL1⁺, CD38⁺, CD44⁻) was shown to be a reliable marker of *MYC* translocation-positive cases, and was superior to the combination of CD10 and BCL2. These findings, however, require validation because very few typical DLBCL cases were included in these studies.

High-grade transformation of FL may involve the acquisition of a *MYC* translocation as a secondary cytogenetic alteration on a background of t(14;18) (44,63). The resultant morphology is highly variable, including DLBCL, Burkitt lymphoma, and terminal deoxynucleotidyl transferase (Tdt)-positive lymphoblastic lymphoma (36,44,63,64). The atypical morphology, immunophenotypic findings, and molecular alterations usually allow distinction from classic Burkitt lymphoma. The concomitant presence of the t(14;18) in such cases would preclude a diagnosis of classic Burkitt lymphoma in any setting. These tumors almost universally express BCL2 protein, and cytogenetic studies reveal complex karyotypes in most cases. Clinically they are usually very aggressive and have in the past been included under the rubric of Burkitt-like lymphomas. Use of this terminology is discouraged, such that in 2008 many of these cases would fall within the category of unclassifiable B-cell lymphoma, intermediate between Burkitt lymphoma and DLBCL (33). Rarely these cases may appear "blastoid" and show expression of nuclear Tdt (34–36,43,64,65). A *de novo* presentation with these features is best classified as lymphoblastic lymphoma, although the presence of both a *MYC* and a *BCL2* translocation should be included with the diagnosis. Cases that arise as a result of histologic transformation of FL are best classified as "high-grade transformation of FL, unclassifiable." Rarely such cases may present as acute leukemia, typically in adults (64,66–73). Importantly, half of the patients with dual translocations of *BCL2* and *MYC* may present *de novo*, presumably due to both the t(14;18) and t(8;14), or variant occurring in rapid succession or simultaneously, and, therefore, not associated with a clinically apparent FL (44). In this setting, classification of the tumor may be difficult as is recognition of the combination of these important molecular alterations. Typically, the morphology is not that of classic Burkitt lymphoma. The cells usually show a moderate to marked degree of nuclear irregularity, and admixed centroblasts are often present. A starry-sky pattern may be apparent. The immunophenotype is not typical of Burkitt lymphoma because the cells are usually strongly BCL2 positive, may fail to express CD10, and often display a lower proliferation rate (<95% Ki-67 or MIB-1 immunostains) (44,55). The cases would not harbor latent EBV. Molecular studies need to be carefully coordinated to search for the presence of both *BCL2* and *MYC* alterations. Moreover, standard cytogenetic or locus-specific FISH techniques may be required because fully half of these dual translocation cases have variant *MYC* translocations that would normally be missed by Southern blot or polymerase chain reaction (PCR) (74). *MYC* alterations occurring as secondary events have also been described in mantle cell lymphoma, splenic marginal zone lymphoma, and myeloma (48,75,76).

Immunophenotype

The tumor cells in classic Burkitt lymphoma and atypical Burkitt lymphoma variants are mature B cells, and, thus, express CD19, CD20, CD22, and CD79a. Usually the cells express membrane immunoglobulin (Ig) M with light chain restriction (19–21,29,77,78). The cells are frequently positive for both CD10 and BCL6, which helps to define Burkitt lymphoma as a germinal center cell lymphoma (Fig. 22.5) (79). Burkitt lymphoma cells are negative for CD5, CD23, cyclin D1, and Tdt. BCL2 is characteristically negative, although rare, weakly positive cases may be seen (80,81). CD21, which represents the receptor for both the C3d component of human complement and EBV, is commonly expressed on the cell surface of endemic Burkitt lymphoma. Sporadic Burkitt lymphoma is typically CD21 negative, a finding in keeping with the lower incidence of latent EBV infection in these cases. Cases of HIV-associated Burkitt lymphoma with the "intermediate" morphology may be shown to express monotypic intracytoplasmic Ig (32). Moreover, Burkitt lymphoma cases in the setting of AIDS are phenotypically distinct from both DLBCL and immunoblastic lymphomas in patients with HIV (82). Burkitt lymphoma cases are BCL6+, and lack expression of MUM1/IRF4 and CD138 (syndecan). Although they are uniformly latent membrane protein (LMP)-1 negative, they harbor latent EBV, as evidenced by in situ hybridization for Epstein-Barr-encoded ribonucleic acid in approximately 30% of cases (83).

When Burkitt lymphoma presents in leukemic form (L3 ALL), the blast cells have a mature immunophenotype and, thus, differ significantly from classic precursor B-cell ALL (Fig. 22.6) (16,17). The CD45 expression is brighter than typical ALL; the cells express monotypic Ig and lack expression of nuclear Tdt.

Endemic Burkitt lymphoma differs from both sporadic Burkitt lymphoma and AIDS-related regarding the frequency of latent EBV infection. Endemic Burkitt lymphoma demonstrates EBV with a latency type I pattern in >90% of cases (84). Sporadic Burkitt lymphoma on the hand is EBV positive in only 5% to 30% of cases (19). AIDS-associated Burkitt lymphoma reveals the presence of latent EBV in

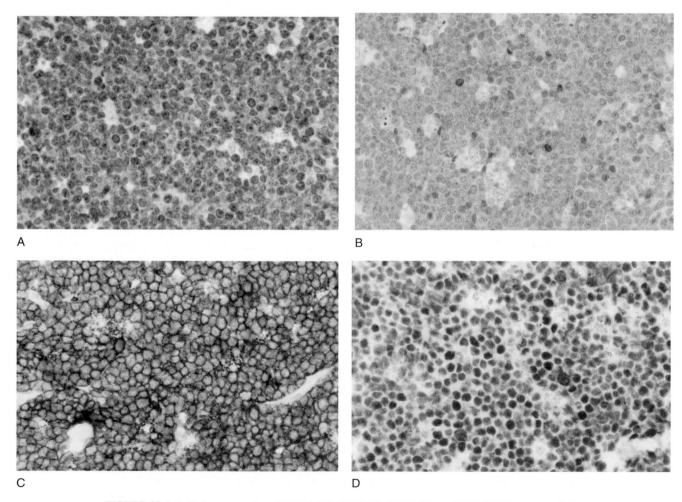

A B C D

FIGURE 22.5 A–D: Immunostains of MIB-1 (**A**), BCL2 (**B**), CD10 (**C**), and BCL6 (**D**) in a case of classic Burkitt lymphoma. Note that all cells are proliferating as defined by positive MIB-1 staining except the phagocytic histiocytes in the section. CD10 is strongly expressed by the malignant cells, and BCL2 is negative. Note several small, reactive lymphocytes in the section staining positively for BCL2 that serve as an internal control. **D:** BCL6 staining shows strong nuclear expression (see also Color Plate 37).

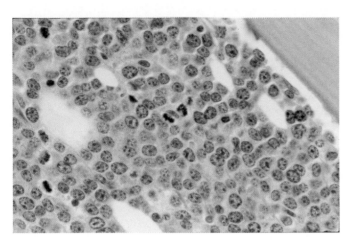

FIGURE 22.6 Bone marrow biopsy showing heavy infiltration with Burkitt lymphoma. The packed bone marrow led to a diagnosis of L3-ALL.

approximately 25% to 40% of cases (32). Virtually all cases of Burkitt lymphoma show a germinal center B-cell immunophenotype, with expression of CD10, BCL6, CD43, and lack of expression of BCL2 (60,85). Infrequent cases show aberrant expression of MUM1 and FOXP1, two genes not usually expressed by normal germinal center B cells (60,86). A characteristic feature in the majority of cases of Burkitt lymphoma is the lack of a host immune response, evidenced by few CD3+ T cells in most biopsies.

Genetics and Cytogenetics

The germinal center origin of Burkitt lymphoma cells is supported by the finding of somatic mutations within the variable-region *IGH* genes (77,87,88). Similarly, mutations in the 5' noncoding region of the *BCL6* gene serve as a molecular marker of transit through the germinal center. These are found in all clinical variants of Burkitt lymphoma, occurring in approximately 37% of cases (89–91).

In 1972, Manolov and Manolova (92) identified a marker chromosome 14, which was subsequently shown by Zech et al. (93) in 1976 to be a balanced reciprocal translocation between chromosomes 8q24 and 14q32. Thus, Burkitt lymphoma represents the first lymphoma for which a recurrent chromosomal aberration was described. Classic Burkitt lymphoma demonstrates translocation t(8;14)(q24;q32) in approximately 75% to 80% of the cases, or less frequently one of its variants t(8;22)(q24;q11) or t(2;8)(p12;q24) (94,95). Thus, the diagnosis of Burkitt lymphoma in a case having a clonal karyotype should reveal the presence of one of these *MYC* translocations; otherwise, an alternative diagnosis should be sought. The lack of a *MYC* translocation in an otherwise typical Burkitt lymphoma does not exclude the diagnosis because alternative mechanisms of *MYC* deregulation may rarely occur (96). It is likely that the standard commercially available *MYC* break-apart FISH assay does not identify all breakpoints that lead to *MYC* deregulation because distant 5' and 3' breakpoints and small insertions are not detected (97,98). However, the opposite is not true because *MYC* translocations or other alterations involving the *MYC* locus are seen in a number of different lymphomas, including FLs, transformed FL, mantle cell lymphomas, mul-

tiple myeloma, DLBCL, and others (described previously) (44,48,50,52,75,99,100). In these malignancies, the t(8;14) and variants frequently constitute secondary chromosomal changes, distinguishing them from classic Burkitt lymphoma in which *MYC* alterations are considered primary events. These cases typically show more complex karyotypes in contrast to classic Burkitt lymphoma, in which a low complexity of chromosomal abnormalities is characteristic (49,81). Those cases of classic Burkitt lymphoma that do show minimal karyotypic aberrations typically involve copy number gains of 1q, 7 and 12, and losses involving 6q, 13q32–34, and 17p. So-called double-hit or dual translocation cases refer to lymphomas in which both a *MYC* translocation and another typical translocation, such as t(14;18) or less commonly t(3;14), are present. The *MYC* translocation partners in these cases often involve non-Ig loci. When Ig genes are involved, the classic t(8;14) is less common because one chromosome 14 allele is already involved in the primary translocation, leaving the remaining IgH allele available for a functional variable (V) diversity (D) joining (J) rearrangement. These cases typically show complex karyotypes in contrast to classic Burkitt lymphoma.

At the molecular level, the t(8;14) and variants juxtapose the *MYC* gene located at chromosome region 8q24 next to one of the Ig gene loci, namely the Ig heavy chain (IGH) locus at chromosome region 14q32, the Ig κ locus in 2p12, or the Ig λ locus in 22q11. As a result of these translocations to the Ig loci, control of normal *MYC* expression is lost, leading to constitutive expression of the protein throughout the cell cycle. *MYC* encodes a transcription factor that can function both as transcriptional activator and transcriptional repressor capable of inducing apoptosis as well as proliferation (94,95,101).

The molecular breakpoints within the *MYC* locus at 8q24 depend on the translocation partners and show considerable interindividual variation (98,102,103). In the case of classic t(8;14), the breakpoints in 8q24 typically lie within the centromeric (5') part of the *MYC* locus. These have been classified according to the position of the chromosomal breakpoints relative to the *MYC* gene (Fig. 22.7). Translocations with breakpoints in the first (5') exon or intron of *MYC* have been designated as class I, those with breakpoints immediately upstream of the gene as class II, and those with distant breakpoints as class III. In sporadic and immunodeficiency associated Burkitt lymphoma, class I (and II) translocations are predominant, whereas in endemic Burkitt lymphoma (African) cases, class III translocations with breakpoints dispersed over about 300 kb upstream of the gene are most frequent (94,95,104). The t(8;14), thus, leads to activation of *MYC* on the der(14) chromosome containing the intact coding region of the gene. The breakpoints in the IGH locus at 14q32 usually occur 5' of the intron enhancer in a J or D segment in endemic Burkitt lymphoma, and 3' of the intron enhancer in the switch μ region in sporadic and HIV-associated Burkitt lymphoma, suggesting that these translocations occur during an aberrant VDJ- or class-switch recombination process, respectively (94,95,104). There is also evidence that Burkitt translocations might be the result of a misdirected somatic mutation (105). Somatic and in part ongoing V_H mutations have been observed in some cases of Burkitt lymphoma. Similarly, mutations of the *MYC* gene are very frequent, particularly in endemic Burkitt lymphoma carrying t(8;14), presumably owing to somatic

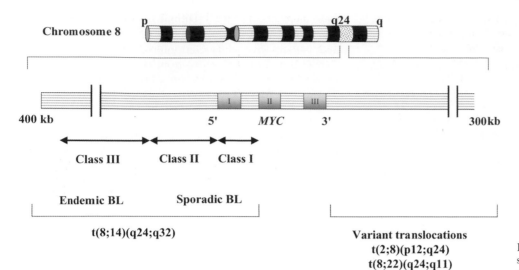

FIGURE 22.7 Schematic of chromosome 8q24 showing different breakpoints within the *MYC* oncogene. BL, Burkitt lymphoma.

hypermutation driven by the Ig sequences juxtaposed to the *MYC* locus on the derivative chromosome 14 (105,106). Such mutations can alter *MYC* transcription or influence phosphorylation, stability, and activity of the protein (107–109). They frequently cluster near the 3′ boundary of the first *MYC* exon. A surrogate marker for the presence of these mutations is the status of the hypermutable PvuII site in the first exon of the *MYC* gene (100,110).

In contrast to the classic Burkitt translocation t(8;14), both variant translocations t(2;8) and t(8;22) lead to deregulation of *MYC* on the derivative chromosome 8 caused by juxtaposition next to the Ig κ and Ig λ genes, respectively. The chromosome 8 breakpoints of these variants are located 3′ of *MYC* and can be dispersed over a region up to 300 kb telomeric of the *MYC* gene (103). The breaks on chromosomes 2 and 22 occur usually 5′ of the Ig κ and Ig λ gene constant region segments, respectively (94,95).

Ideally, to establish a confident diagnosis of a Burkitt lymphoma, the detection of a *MYC* translocation should be sought. Conventional cytogenetic analysis using chromosomal banding techniques is still the gold standard for the analysis of Burkitt lymphoma. In addition to the detection of the diagnostic translocations, cytogenetic analyses can identify variant *MYC* translocations involving non-Ig loci, as well as other characteristic primary chromosomal aberrations that may indicate an aggressive transformation of a variety of different underlying low-grade non-Hodgkin lymphomas (NHLs). Moreover, chromosomal banding analysis is the only technique providing a complete genomic overview of balanced and unbalanced secondary changes (111,112).

Molecular methods such as Southern blot or PCR-based approaches have been used for the diagnosis of Burkitt-associated *MYC* alterations but suffer because of the requirement for fresh or cryopreserved material as well as from the widely dispersed breakpoints over several hundred kilobases for both *MYC* and Ig loci. For example, alterations of *MYC* occurring as secondary events in FL often involve the light chain genes, which are more difficult to detect using Southern blot and/or PCR approaches (34,74). This molecular variability requires the application of multiple probes or sequence-specific primers that render Southern blot and PCR analysis time consuming and expensive. Nevertheless, long-distance PCR techniques using various sets of primers have been described to reliably detect *IG-MYC* junctions in classic and variant Burkitt translocations (113).

The most robust technique currently available for the routine detection of the Burkitt translocation is interphase FISH, which can be applied to virtually every type of tissue (114–119). In principle, two different types of FISH assays have been developed for the use in Burkitt lymphoma, including break-apart and colocalization assays. Break-apart assays are on the whole more robust and represent the new gold standard for the molecular analysis of most oncogene alterations.

Gene Expression Profiling

Two major gene expression profiling studies have been performed with the goal of defining the molecular profile of Burkitt lymphoma and its distinction from DLBCL (81). Hummel et al. (81) profiled 220 mature aggressive B-cell lymphomas that included classic Burkitt lymphoma, so-called atypical Burkitt lymphoma, and DLBCL. They used a small core group of eight cases, all of which showed characteristic Burkitt lymphoma morphology, immunophenotype, and had a *MYC* translocation to establish a molecular signature of 58 genes used to define molecular Burkitt lymphoma. In addition to FISH studies, array based comparative genomic hybridization was used to determine genetic gains and losses (chromosomal complexity) for all cases (81). Using a novel statistical approach coined *core group extension*, the gene expression profiles of the remaining cases were studied to determine their similarity to the core group of eight cases of molecular Burkitt lymphoma. This analysis revealed that 22% of the cases met the criteria of molecular Burkitt lymphoma, 20% were considered intermediate cases, and 58% were not molecular Burkitt lymphoma. The array based comparative genomic hybridization studies also revealed that chromosomal complexity increased as one went from molecular Burkitt lymphoma with its low cytogenetic complexity through the intermediate and nonmolecular Burkitt lymphoma categories that carried a higher load of chromosomal gains and losses. These authors made several other important observations including: (a) cases with clear-cut morphologic features of DLBCL showed a gene expression profile of molecular Burkitt lymphoma, thus extending the morphologic spectrum of the presumed biological entity; (b) a small number of the cases of molecular Burkitt lymphoma did not appear to have a *MYC* translocation, suggesting that alternative mechanisms may be capable of deregulating *MYC* expression; (c) infrequently, cases of molecular Burkitt lymphoma with classic Burkitt lymphoma morphology can express *BCL2* protein; (d) cases of nonmolecular Burkitt lymphoma with the morphology of DLBCL that harbor a *MYC* translocation show inferior overall survival as compared with DLBCL cases without a *MYC* translocation when treated with cyclophosphamide, hydroxydaunorubicin, Oncovin (vincristine), and prednisone or cyclophosphamide, hydroxydaunorubicin, Oncovin (vincristine), and prednisone-like regimens; and, finally, (e) non-Ig *MYC* translocations are more common in the intermediate and nonmolecular Burkitt lymphoma cases (49,81).

In an independent study conducted by the Lymphoma and Leukemia Molecular Profiling Project, 303 cases of diffuse aggressive B-cell lymphomas were studied using a custom oligonucleotide array (120). These authors used a different approach to identify the genes comprising a molecular signature of Burkitt lymphoma. First, a group of genes were defined as *MYC* target genes based on cell line experiments. The cases were then divided into two groups, those with a *MYC* target gene signature and those without. In a second step, cases with a *MYC* target gene signature were then compared with the expression profiles for germinal center B-cell DLBCL, activated B-cell subtype of DLBCL, and cases of primary mediastinal large B-cell lymphoma. Only those cases not classifiable as one of these predefined molecular subtypes were then considered molecular Burkitt lymphoma. This strategy explains the lack of an intermediate group similar to Hummel et al. (81) because any case with equivocal gene expression would default into one of the DLBCL categories. Moreover, the small number of cases with dual translocation lymphoma (e.g., both *MYC* and a *BCL2* translocation) fell within the molecular Burkitt lymphoma category, in contrast to the study by Hummel et al. (81), where similar cases were for the most part included in the intermediate and nonmolecular Burkitt lymphoma categories and associated with a higher chromosomal complexity score. Additional features of the molecular Burkitt lymphoma signature from the Lymphoma and Leukemia Molecular Profiling Project study included overexpression of a small subset of germinal center B-cell genes and low expression of both major histocompatibility complex class I genes and nuclear factor-κB target genes (120). Similar to the study by Hummel et al. (81), these authors also found that cases with a molecular profile of Burkitt lymphoma show improved survival if treated with intensive regimens better suited to Burkitt lymphoma.

A careful examination of the gene expression signatures of molecular Burkitt lymphoma between these two studies show almost no overlap of individual genes, yet both predictors work to identify cases of Burkitt lymphoma. Importantly, gene expression profiling outperforms even expert pathologists in identifying such cases (85). Moreover, a mod-

erate number of typical DLBCL cases were classified as molecular Burkitt lymphoma, raising the question of whether these cases might benefit from treatment strategies used to treat Burkitt lymphoma.

A recent molecular profiling study of pediatric mature B-cell lymphomas revealed several important findings (121). First, cases of pediatric and adult molecular Burkitt lymphoma are virtually identical with respect to expression of CD10, *BCL2*, *BCL6*, and Ki-67 detected using immunohistochemistry. Genomic imbalances detected using array based comparative genomic hybridization show very low cytogenetic complexity in both. Second, although nonmolecular Burkitt lymphoma cases exist within the category of DLBCL in children, a higher frequency of DLBCL cases with a molecular signature of Burkitt lymphoma exist, helping to explain the increased frequency of *MYC* translocations in this group. Finally, with current treatment regimens used in children, this distinction does not have clinical consequences as it does in adults.

A Practical Approach to the Diagnosis of Burkitt Lymphoma

Perhaps the most important diagnostic challenge facing hematopathologists today is the timely distinction between Burkitt lymphoma and its mimics, particularly in adults. In the pediatric setting, this distinction is not clinically relevant because treatment decisions are based more on clinical risk factors. That said, the molecular overlap between classic Burkitt lymphoma and DLBCL in children is much more significant as compared with adults, in part explaining the similar outcomes for these two histologies. Moreover, dual translocation cases do not occur. Pediatric cases with typical morphology and characteristic immunophenotype do not likely require FISH studies because virtually all will have an *IG-MYC* translocation and low-level cytogenetic complexity. These findings underscore the fact that pediatric Burkitt lymphoma is for the most part the prototype of "true" Burkitt lymphoma (Fig. 22.8).

In adults, the problem is much more complex, and an accurate distinction between Burkitt lymphoma and DLBCL does have major treatment implications (60,61,122–124). Even cases with classic morphology and prototypical immunophenotype (CD20$^+$, CD79a$^+$, CD10$^+$, BCL6$^+$, CD43$^+$, p53$^{+/-}$, and BCL2$^-$) should have FISH studies performed to document the presence of a *MYC* translocation. Typically, this would involve both *MYC* break-apart assays and a determination of the *MYC* partner because there is a suggestion that cases with Ig-*MYC* translocations have inferior survival in contrast with non-Ig *MYC* partners (R.D. Gascoyne, *unpublished observations*, 2009). In this scenario, BCL2 protein is negative, and, thus, the likelihood of a dual translocation is exceedingly small, precluding the need for *BCL2* FISH. Classic cytogenetic studies are also helpful because classic Burkitt lymphoma is characterized by infrequent additional secondary karyotypic aberrations. Atypical morphology or immunophenotype, particularly the strong expression of BCL2, makes it imperative that *BCL2* FISH studies also be performed. The presence of both translocations (*MYC* and *BCL2*) precludes a diagnosis of true Burkitt lymphoma, and, thus, dual translocation cases are best labeled as unclassifiable B-cell lymphomas with intermediate features of Burkitt lymphoma/DLBCL (33). How such cases are optimally treated is a matter of

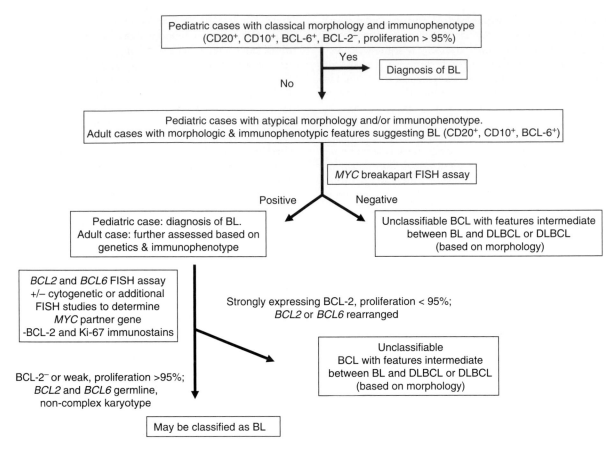

FIGURE 22.8 Diagnostic algorithm for Burkitt lymphoma (BL).

speculation, although retrospective data suggest that rituximab with cyclophosphamide, hydroxydaunorubicin, Oncovin (vincristine), and prednisone fails to cure the majority of these patients (63,85,122). Translocations of *MYC* can also be seen with *BCL6* translocation and are also considered as dual translocation lymphomas, but the clinical implications of this molecular finding are largely unknown (81). The most challenging group is those cases referred to as discrepant molecular Burkitt lymphoma, where the histology clearly favors DLBCL, but the molecular profile is Burkitt lymphoma. It is likely that these cases are more effectively treated with an intensified Burkitt lymphoma-like regimen, but this remains speculative until tested in prospective clinical trials.

Pathogenetic Mechanisms

The hallmark translocations involving *MYC* and Ig genes, coupled to experimental data indicating that c-*MYC* expression can be induced by juxtaposed enhancer elements from Ig loci (125,126), leave no doubt that the translocations are a central element of Burkitt lymphoma pathogenesis. However, because abnormal expression of c-*MYC* normally results in diversion of the cell to an apoptotic pathway, it appears that the translocations need to be associated with lesions that simultaneously inhibit apoptosis. Such lesions have been described in Burkitt lymphoma, in which the Fas pathway is frequently abrogated, and mutations in the proapoptotic protein bax have been described (127,128); although it must be

pointed out that abrogation of specific pathways does not prevent the induction of apoptosis via others (127), which may be relevant to treatment. In addition to lesions in EBV-associated apoptotic genes, however, another potential means whereby Burkitt lymphoma cells may avoid apoptosis is through the expression of viral genes. In this respect, recent reports that the EBV Epstein-Barr early region small molecular weight ribonucleic acid, highly expressed in EBV-associated Burkitt lymphoma, can protect against apoptosis are of considerable interest, although it also remains possible that this molecule may be relevant to pathogenesis in other ways (129–131). Although the pattern of EBV protein expression is restricted in Burkitt lymphoma, it is possible that before full malignant transformation, other viral proteins are expressed that inhibit apoptosis (either directly or via up-regulation of BCL2), as occurs when B cells are transformed by EBV when the full range of Epstein-Barr nuclear antigens and LMPs are expressed (a so-called latency III pattern). These proteins, with the exception of Epstein-Barr nuclear antigen 1, are highly immunogenic, and their expression in Burkitt lymphoma would lead to an immune reaction against the tumor cells. It is likely that they are expressed in vivo only in privileged sites, such as germinal centers where cytotoxic T cells are essentially absent. Recently, evidence supporting the possibility that Burkitt lymphoma evolves from EBV-transformed cells expressing a latency III pattern has been provided by the observation of Burkitt lymphomas in which Epstein-Barr nuclear antigen 2 has been deleted. Such cells also fail to express the LMPs that are regulated by Epstein-Barr nuclear antigen 2 (132). It is interesting to note that the expression of Epstein-Barr nuclear antigen 2, although necessary for the transformation of B cells, antagonizes c-myc and appears to have a negative impact on the growth of Burkitt lymphoma cells (133,134). This may be because Epstein-Barr nuclear antigen 2 inhibits *MYC* expression via its ability to inhibit the IG µ gene, which, by virtue of the t(8;14), regulates *MYC* in Burkitt lymphoma (135). But Burkitt lymphoma cells lack immunogenicity for other reasons; in particular, the peptide transporters are inactive, and there is reduced human leukocyte antigen class I protein expression such that there is an inability to present endogenously expressed EBV-latent proteins to cytotoxic T cells. Although Epstein-Barr nuclear antigen 1 is not immunogenic, a small number of additional proteins expressed in latency I are, such that this mechanism of reducing immunogenicity from virally derived proteins is critically important to the survival of Burkitt lymphoma cells. It is interesting to note that all of these characteristics can be produced in lymphoblastoid cell lines transformed by EBV simply by overexpressing c-*MYC* (136), suggesting that the oncogene does more than simply drive cell proliferation.

The mechanism whereby the latency switch (type III to type I), if indeed it does occur, is accomplished as cells undergo progressive transformation remains unknown. It is not due to overexpression of c-*MYC* (137) but could, instead, result from a mechanism operative when normal B cells infected by EBV leave the germinal center; peripheral memory cells that contain EBV express either no EBV proteins, or when they undergo cell division, a latency I pattern, suggesting the existence of such a mechanism. A latency switching mechanism may be critical to EBV's survival strategy in the host because cells expressing the highly immunogenic latency III pattern of viral proteins are immediately eliminated by EBV antigen-specific cytotoxic T cells; without this mechanism, EBV infection might always result, eventually, in massive B-cell proliferation and death of the host. Although c-*MYC* cannot induce a latency I pattern, it is able to replace the growth-stimulating effects of Epstein-Barr nuclear antigen 2 (138) such that the Burkitt lymphoma cells are independent of the need for expression of Epstein-Barr nuclear antigen 2 and the LMPs.

In the normal germinal center, the drive to proliferation is antigen. Recent gene expression profiling data suggest that the naive B cells become centroblasts through a proliferation program that does not include c-*MYC* expression (139). Such cells are primed to undergo apoptosis in the absence of antigen stimulation. Thus, if the transcriptional data reflect the protein data (which remain open to question) (140), even modest levels of c-myc expression induced by the *MYC* translocation are clearly abnormal for germinal center cells, and c-myc alone may not be sufficient to rescue them from apoptosis, in fact, its abnormal expression is more likely to drive the cell into an apoptotic pathway. EBV, through its ability to mimic antigen stimulation and CD40 binding (through the LMPs), is able to prevent apoptosis and presumably permit the cell to exit the germinal center and become a memory cell, thus ensuring its own survival in the host.

Together, these findings suggest that EBV⁺ Burkitt lymphoma arises from a B cell that has been transformed by EBV and that first expresses a latency III pattern, perhaps in the context of a germinal center. Because the latency III pattern is incompatible with the survival of Burkitt lymphoma cells in an immunologically normal host (such proteins often are expressed in EBV-containing lymphomas in immunodeficient hosts), the c-myc expression, brought about by the *MYC* chromosomal translocations, is necessary before exit from the germinal center, both to replace the normal transforming but immunogenic EBV proteins, thereby ensuring continued proliferation, and to reduce the immunogenicity of the tumor cells. A latency I pattern further contributes to the reduced immunogenicity and also avoids inhibition of expression of the translocated c-myc gene by Epstein-Barr nuclear antigen 2. The recent demonstration that c-*MYC* can enhance the expression of the potentially antiapoptotic Epstein-Barr early region ribonucleic acids (141) supports, if indirectly, the notion that Epstein-Barr early region expression is relevant to Burkitt lymphoma transformation.

Given the probable cooperation between EBV and the *MYC* translocation in the pathogenesis of Burkitt lymphoma, it seems likely that individuals carrying more EBV-transformed lymphocytes and perhaps releasing more virus capable of transforming other cells would be at greater risk for developing Burkitt lymphoma. This is entirely consistent with the observation of Geser et al. (142), that individuals with higher antiviral capsid antigen in Africa are at higher risk for the development of Burkitt lymphoma and with the finding that acute malaria is associated with an increased number of circulating EBV-containing cells (as is HIV infection) (143). Malaria may also increase the risk of the development of Burkitt lymphoma in Africa through its ability to cause B-cell hyperplasia and potentially, therefore, increase the likelihood that a chromosomal translocation will occur.

This hypothesis, constructed on the basis of available information, is also entirely consistent with the markedly increased incidence of Burkitt lymphoma in equatorial Africa, where EBV infection occurs at a very early age, and malaria is holoendemic. EBV-negative Burkitt lymphoma may well use similar pathways but is much less likely to occur because the role played by EBV must be subserved by, presumably, a series of genetic events. It is not known whether the differences in clinical behavior between endemic Burkitt lymphoma and Burkitt lymphoma in other world regions (see below) are a consequence of differences in the molecular abnormalities present in the tumor, differences in the host, or both.

CLINICAL FEATURES

The clinical features of Burkitt lymphoma overlap throughout the world, but regional variation in sites of involvement can be readily discerned. In particular, jaw tumors are present in 50% to 70% of patients in equatorial Africa, and are generally age associated. Almost all young children of 3 years of age present with a jaw or orbital tumor, or both, whereas only 25% of patients older than the age of 16 years present with jaw tumors. In the endemic region of Africa itself, the percentage of patients with jaw tumors appears to be inversely proportional to the incidence of the disease. In addition, the median age of patients tends to be higher in lower incidence areas, such as highlands or arid regions (144). Jaw involvement in sporadic Burkitt lymphoma, in contrast to endemic Burkitt lymphoma, occurs in a small percentage of patients at presentation (<10% in most series) and is not age related (145). Such patients frequently have involvement of other bony sites or of the bone marrow, suggesting that jaw

TABLE 22.2

CHARACTERISTIC GENETIC FEATURES OF BURKITT LYMPHOMA (BL)

Feature	Endemic BL	Sporadic BL	AIDS-associated BL
Usual class of *MYC* breakpoint	Class III	Class I and II	Class I
MYC breakpoint site	Centromeric (5′) of *MYC*	Within the first exon or intron of *MYC*, or centromeric of *MYC* (class II)	Within the first exon or intron of *MYC*
Predominant *IGH* breakpoint in t(8;14)(q24;q32)	VDJ region	Switch region	Switch region
Somatic *IGH* mutations	Yes	Yes	Yes
BCL6 mutations	Yes	Yes	Yes

involvement may be due to a different pathobiologic process than in African patients (146). A higher percentage of patients with jaw tumors than is seen in the United States and Europe has been reported in some Asian countries, South Africa (where both whites and nonwhites appear to have as high a frequency of jaw tumors as in the endemic form of the disease), Turkey, Japan, and equatorial Brazil (15,147–152).

Between 50% and 90% of patients with Burkitt lymphoma throughout the world present with abdominal involvement, which can give rise to abdominal pain or swelling, bowel intussusception, a change in bowel habits, nausea and vomiting, evidence of gastrointestinal bleeding, or rarely, intestinal perforation (15,152–157). Presentation with a right iliac fossa mass is quite frequent outside Africa, occurring in perhaps 25% of patients (158), and can be confused with an inflammatory appendiceal mass. Such presentations are uncommon, however, in the endemic form of disease. Frequently at surgery, multiple enlarged mesenteric lymph nodes and multiple peritoneal plaques may be observed. Involvement of retroperitoneal structures, including kidneys and pancreas, is second only to bowel and mesenteric involvement, whereas liver and particularly splenic involvement is seen somewhat less frequently. Ovarian involvement is frequent in females. Pleural effusions and ascites, which nearly always contain Burkitt lymphoma cells, and bone involvement are common. Pharyngeal or nasopharyngeal sites of disease, as well as paranasal sinus involvement, are all occasionally seen. Thyroid and salivary gland involvement is occasionally observed in patients with endemic disease but appears to be less common outside Africa. Adrenal gland involvement is occasionally seen. Isolated lymphadenopathy, tonsillar (or any form of pharyngeal tumor), splenic, and testicular involvement are all rare in African Burkitt lymphoma and somewhat more common in other world regions. Breast involvement, regardless of geography, occurs almost exclusively in pubertal girls or lactating women (159–162).

Bone marrow involvement is more common in sporadic Burkitt lymphoma, occurring in approximately 20% of patients (163). Interestingly, bone marrow involvement has been less frequently reported in several series from outside the United States or Europe, as is the case in equatorial Africa (164–166). Central nervous system disease, either cerebrospinal fluid pleocytosis or cranial nerve palsies, is more frequently observed in endemic Burkitt lymphoma than in the sporadic variety, occurring in approximately one third of patients at presentation in one Ugandan series. Any cranial nerve can be involved, but the ophthalmic nerves and the facial nerve are most often affected (150,167). Very rarely, cranial nerve involvement and cerebrospinal fluid pleocytosis have been the sole sites of disease (168), and peripheral neuropathy is occasionally seen (169). Also rare, the optic nerve may be infiltrated, giving rise to blindness. In Uganda, approximately 15% of patients present with isolated epidural lymphoma and paraplegia, requiring laminectomy for diagnosis (150,167). Intracerebral disease has been described but is usually seen only at recurrence (170). In patients with sporadic disease, intracranial disease may be extradural (171). When central nervous system disease occurs in patients with sporadic disease, it is usually associated with bone marrow involvement (approximately two-thirds of patients with marrow disease have central nervous system disease) or with multiple other bony sites of disease. It may consist of cerebrospinal fluid pleocytosis or cranial nerve palsies. Compression of the inferior alveolar nerve as it passes through the mandible with numbness of the lip and chin occurs quite frequently in patients with widespread bone marrow disease, and this, as with compression of cranial nerves by orbital tumor, is not a sign of central nervous system involvement, although such patients are at high risk for developing central nervous system disease(172).

A comparison of sites of disease at presentation in endemic (Ugandan) and sporadic (United States) Burkitt lymphoma is shown in Tables 22.2 and 22.3. In addition to the differences in jaw involvement, there are striking differences in the frequency of bone marrow involvement (higher in sporadic) and involvement of the central nervous system, including spinal epidural disease (higher in endemic).

STAGING

It is imperative that patients with Burkitt lymphoma undergo a rapid staging assessment so that treatment can be initiated in a timely fashion. Routine staging investigations should include computed tomography scans of the neck, chest, abdomen, and pelvis, bone marrow aspiration and biopsy, routine laboratory testing for blood counts, serum lactate dehydrogenase (LDH) level, liver and kidney function, and HIV status. LDH levels correlate well with stage (as do anti-EBV early antigen titers in equatorial African patients) (173). A lumbar puncture for cerebral spinal fluid evaluation should also be performed.

The most widely used staging system in children and young adults has been the St. Jude staging system, which is

TABLE 22.3

DISEASE SITES AT PRESENTATION IN ENDEMIC
AND SPORADIC BURKITT LYMPHOMA

	Patients with involvement (%)	
Site	Endemic	Sporadic
Abdomen	58	91
Pleural effusion	3	19
Bone marrow	7	20
Peripheral nodes	9	13
Bone	8	9
Central nervous system	19	14
Paraspinal	17	2
Testis	2	6
Pharynx	0	10
Jaw	58	7
Orbit	11	1

TABLE 22.4

ST. JUDE STAGING SYSTEM FOR CHILDHOOD NHL

Stage Definition

I   Single tumor (extranodal) or single nodal site, excluding mediastinum or abdomen

II   Single extranodal site with regional node involvement
Primary gastrointestinal tumor with or without involvement of associated mesenteric nodes only (if grossly completely resected then considered stage IIR)
On same side of diaphragm
a. Two or more nodal areas
b. Two extranodal sites with or without regional node involvement

III   On both sides of the diaphragm
a. Two single tumors (extranodal)
b. Two or more nodal areas
All primary intrathoracic tumors (mediastinal, pleural, thymic)
All extensive primary intra-abdominal disease
All primary paraspinal or epidural tumors regardless of other sites

IV[a] Any of the aforementioned with initial central nervous system or bone marrow involvement

[a] Patients with >25% of tumor cells in the bone marrow are generally referred to as having acute B-cell leukemia.

shown in Table 22.4. Although the Ann Arbor staging system is typically utilized for adult NHL, the St. Jude system has been largely employed in the pediatric Burkitt lymphoma literature, as well as in many adult studies and has formed the basis of many risk-adapted treatment strategies.

GENERAL PRINCIPLES OF CHEMOTHERAPY OF BURKITT LYMPHOMA

Progress in the treatment of Burkitt lymphoma in both children and adults has been dramatic, with long-term remission rates improving from approximately 25% to 80% to 90% (with the most effective protocols) since the 1960s. This success has been accomplished through a series of improvements in multiagent chemotherapy regimens used in children in which have been adopted in the adult setting (at least up to the age of 60 years). Independent, simultaneous efforts were made by Berlin-Frankfurt-Münster (BFM), Societé Française d'Oncologie Pediatrique (SFOP), the U.S. National Cancer Institute (NCI), and cooperative group investigators (22,174–190), who improved on the initial successes achieved in African patients in the 1960s (150,191–196). Clinical trials at the NCI in the last 3 decades have shown that it is possible to achieve the same degree of success in children and young adult patients with Burkitt lymphoma by using identical regimens (22,175,176). The NCI approach has also been employed by the United Kingdom Lymphoma Group, which achieved very good results in adults with Burkitt lymphoma using a similar protocol (60,197).

A review of the Burkitt lymphoma regimens developed in the last 30 years demonstrates that several strategies have played a crucial role in improving the long-term outlook for these patients: (a) dose intensity; (b) the addition of high-dose methotrexate and high-dose cytarabine, which are both active in central nervous system and systemic disease; (c) the inclusion of additional agents, such as etoposide and possibly ifosfamide; (d) central nervous system prophylactic therapy and central nervous system-directed therapy; (e) risk stratification and risk-adapted therapy; (f) exclusion of radiotherapy; (g) short-duration regimens; and (h) prompt initiation of successful treatment cycles as soon as the bone marrow has recovered (neutrophil count, 500 to 1,000 per mm^3, platelet count, $\geq$50,000 per mm^3).

Dose Intensity

Maintaining an appropriate dose intensity based on risk category is an important component of effective therapy. Most of the modern chemotherapy regimens are dose intensive and of short duration. Several studies have clearly shown that there is no benefit to long-duration treatment regimens (175,176,182,184–186). This remains true for patients with high-risk or extensive disease.

High-Dose Methotrexate and High-Dose Cytarabine

The BFM, SFOP, and NCI regimens have been very effective in Burkitt lymphoma, and all three regimens have given significant emphasis to high-dose methotrexate and high-dose cytarabine, which were first evaluated in patients with recurrent disease (198–200). In BFM trials, increasing the dose of methotrexate from 500 to 5,000 mg per m^2 for patients with stage III abdominal disease and LDH levels >500 resulted in an increase in event-free survival from 43% to 81%, whereas for patients with leukemic presentation, event-free survival improved from 50% to 78% (186). High-dose cytarabine is an important component of all these protocols for high-risk patients. At the NCI, addition of high-dose cytarabine along with etoposide and ifosfamide improved the survival rate in high-risk patients from <20% to approximately 80% (176).

Additional Agents

Good responses to ifosfamide and etoposide have been shown in relapsed and refractory settings, even in patients previously treated with high cumulative doses of cyclophosphamide (201,202). The incorporation of these two drugs, along with cytarabine, into early primary treatment at the NCI resulted in two major gains. First, there was a dramatic improvement in the survival of high-risk patients; second, the number of cycles of chemotherapy for these patients was reduced from 15 to four with an improved outcome (175,176). Alternating noncross-resistant regimens appeared to prevent the emergence of drug-resistant clones, which is crucial to a successful outcome. Although there is no direct information that can be brought to bear on the issue, it may also be critical to use these drugs early in treatment rather than later as consolidation therapy because resistant clones might, by then, have already emerged.

Central Nervous System Prophylaxis and Therapy

Central nervous system involvement in Burkitt lymphoma is a poor prognostic feature; survival for patients with central nervous system involvement in the United States and Europe was extremely poor when only intrathecal chemotherapy and radiation were used to treat central nervous system disease (181,182). The addition of high-dose methotrexate and cytarabine along with intrathecal chemotherapy has improved the results from approximately 20% to 75% to 80%. High-dose methotrexate and cytarabine, being active in both systemic and central nervous system disease, are likely to play a major role in improving the outcome of patients with central nervous system involvement or of patients who have a high risk for central nervous system relapse.

Risk Stratification and Risk-Adapted Therapy

The dramatically different survival rates of children with limited and advanced disease were most obvious when therapy was less intensive (22,158,177). Patients with limited disease continue to achieve high survival rates with less intensive therapy (178,179,185,190), whereas patients with more advanced disease have exhibited better outcomes as the intensity of therapy has been progressively increased in successive trials (176,182,184,185,187,188). Stratification by risk permits patients to be separated into different prognostic categories so that each group of patients can receive the appropriate dose and combination of drugs (175,181,186).

This strategy has been a very important part of all pediatric studies. BFM protocols have recognized four different risk categories, and the treatment is tailored to each of these risk groups so that treatment toxicity is minimized for low-risk patients, and more intensive therapy is used only in patients with higher risk disease. Appropriate risk stratification must take into consideration various prognostic features in addition to stage of disease. For example, in BFM protocols, patients with stage III abdominal disease have been divided

into two subgroups based on LDH levels of more than or <500. The BFM group has shown that these two groups of patients with stage III disease have a big difference in their outcome when treated with a low-dose methotrexate regimen (186). Risk stratification has not been used in many of the adult protocols, except for those in which a regimen developed in childhood Burkitt lymphoma has been used without modification (17,22,175). Risk stratification must clearly be a component of any effective modern chemotherapy regimen.

The risk stratification schemes and therapeutic strategies employed in NCI, SFOP, and BFM protocols are listed in Tables 22.5 through 22.10. These protocols have yielded excellent results demonstrating the principles of risk stratification, whereby patients with higher risk disease can achieve near comparable outcomes with more intensive therapy (Table 22.11). In particular, the German BFM-95 protocol included >500 patients with event-free survival rates ranging from 81% to 94% in the highest and lowest risk groups, respectively. Comparable results have been obtained by the NCI protocol 89-C-41, but the number of patients

TABLE 22.5

DEFINITIONS OF THERAPY ARMS FOR BURKITT LYMPHOMA AND LARGE B-CELL LYMPHOMA IN BFM PROTOCOL NHL-BFM 95

Risk group	Definition
1	Complete surgical resection
2	Incomplete surgical resection
	Stages I and II
	Stage III and LDH <500 U per L
3	Incomplete surgical resection
	Stage III and LDH 500–999 U per L
	Stage IV or B-cell leukemia and LDH <1,000 U per L; CNS negative
4	Incomplete surgical resection
	Stage III and LDH >999 U per L
	Stage IV or B-cell leukemia and LDH >999 U per ± CNS

CNS, central nervous system.

TABLE 22.6

DEFINITIONS OF THERAPY GROUPS IN FRENCH-AMERICAN-BRITISH PROTOCOL LMB 96 FOR B-CELL LYMPHOMAS

Therapy group	Definition
A	Complete surgical resection stage I or abdominal stage II
B	All patients not eligible for group A or C
C	Any central nervous system[a] involvement or bone marrow involvement ≥25% blasts

[a] Central nervous system involvement is defined as: any blasts in cerebrospinal fluid; cranial nerve palsies not explained by extracranial tumor; clinical spinal cord compression; isolated intracerebral mass; and parameningeal extension, cranial or spinal.

TABLE 22.7

DEFINITIONS OF THERAPY GROUPS IN NCI PROTOCOL 89-C-41 FOR B-CELL LYMPHOMAS

Therapy group	Definition
Low-risk patients	Stage I or II and LDH <150% of normal
High-risk patients	All other patients

TABLE 22.8

OUTLINE OF THERAPY IN PROTOCOL BFM-NHL 95 FOR B-CELL LYMPHOMAS

Risk group	Therapy[a]
1	Cycles A and B (no prephase and vincristine is omitted)
2	Prephase followed by 4 cycles: A-B-A-B
3	Prephase followed by 5 cycles: AA-BB-CC-AA-BB
4	Prephase followed by 6 cycles: AA-BB-CC-AA-BB-CC

A cycles consist of dexamethasone, VePesid, cytarabine, intermediate-dose methotrexate, ifosfamide, and triple intrathecal therapy. B cycles consist of dexamethasone, Adriamycin, intermediate-dose methotrexate, cyclophosphamide, and triple intrathecal therapy. In AA and BB cycles, high-dose methotrexate is given instead of intermediate-dose methotrexate, and vincristine is added to the regimen. CC cycles consist of dexamethasone, vindesine, high-dose cytarabine, VePesid, and triple intrathecal therapy.
[a] Trial included a randomization between methotrexate administration over 24 vs. 4 hours.

TABLE 22.9

OUTLINE OF THERAPY IN PROTOCOL FRENCH-AMERICAN-BRITISH LMB 96[a]

Therapy group	Therapy
A	Two cycles of COPAD
B[b]	COP
	COPADM 1
	COPADM 2
	COPADM 2 (reduced cyclophosphamide)
	CYM 1 and 2
	COPADM 3
C[c]	COP
	COPADM 1
	COPADM 2
	CYVE 1 and 2
	Mini-CYVE 1 and 2
	CYVE and intrathecal therapy and high-dose methotrexate
	Mini-CYVE and intrathecal therapy and high-dose methotrexate
	Maintenance 1
	Maintenance 2–4
	COPADM 3

AD, doxorubicin; C, cyclophosphamide; CY, cytarabine (cytarabine); M, methotrexate with leucovorin rescue; O, vincristine; P, prednis(ol)one; VE, etoposide.
[a] Intrathecal therapy is administered in all cycles except COPAD, CYVE, mini-CYVE, and maintenance courses 2–4, except when indicated.
[b] Early responding patients were randomized to receive standard doses vs. a reduced intensity approach (reduced cyclophosphamide in COPADM2 or omission of COPADM3)
[c] Patients with central nervous system disease receive additional high-dose methotrexate after CYVE 1 or mini-CYVE 1 and additional intrathecal drugs at the beginning of CYVE or mini-CYVE.

TABLE 22.10

OUTLINE OF THERAPY IN NCI PROTOCOL 89-C-41 FOR B-CELL LYMPHOMAS[a]

Therapy group	Therapy
Low-risk patients	Three A cycles
High-risk patients	Four cycles: A-B-A-B

[a] A cycles consist of cyclophosphamide, Adriamycin, vincristine, and high-dose methotrexate (given on day 10). B cycles consist of IVAC.

accrued is much smaller (175,176). In these modern protocols, the significance of prognostic factors has largely been lost. Even patients with stage IV disease (bone marrow disease, central nervous system disease, or both) do not have a significantly worse prognosis, although central nervous system disease in some studies may be associated with a worse outcome (180).

Exclusion of Local Radiotherapy

Although radiation has been used in the past for central nervous system prophylaxis, central nervous system therapy, consolidation treatment at sites of bulk disease, or in spinal cord compression, in the last 3 decades, it has become clear that radiation has essentially no role in the therapy of Burkitt lymphoma. Indeed, early studies in Africa with standard fractions of radiation demonstrated the poor response of irradiated tumors (203). A randomized clinical trial has shown that there is no benefit to adding radiation therapy in limited-stage disease (204), and although not formally studied, patients with central nervous system disease, bulky sites, and even testicular disease no longer receive radiation without detriment (176,180,186,205,206). On the other hand, combined modality therapy causes more acute and long-term complications, including acute and late neurologic toxicity from central nervous system radiation (in combination with

intrathecal therapy) and potentially second malignancies (207). Because more patients with Burkitt lymphoma are now being cured, particular attention must be paid to late complications.

Surgery, also once considered a useful therapeutic modality if almost all tumor could be removed (208), has become of limited value in the era of highly effective chemotherapy. At the present time, surgery is limited to obtaining a diagnostic sample (which may entail complete resection of a small abdominal mass) or to the management of complications such as an acute abdomen (209–211).

TABLE 22.11

RESULTS OF FRENCH (LMB 96), GERMAN-AUSTRIAN (BFM 95), AND NCI (89-C-41) PROTOCOLS IN THE TREATMENT OF B-CELL LYMPHOMAS

Protocol	No. of patients	Event-free survival (EFS) at 3 y (%)
LMB 96		
Group A	137	98
Group B	762	90 (4 y EFS)
Group C	235	79 (4 y EFS)
BFM 95		
Risk group 1	48	94
Risk group 2	233	94
Risk group 3	82	85
Risk group 4	142	81
NCI 89-C-41		
Low risk	18	100
High risk	66	85

Short-Duration, Dose-Intensive Therapy

The experience with Burkitt lymphoma in Africa during the 1960s and 1970s demonstrated that short-duration therapy of even one or a few doses of a single agent could cure Burkitt lymphoma; in fact a high fraction of patients with limited disease (perhaps 70% to 80%) were curable with a single agent (191–196). This experience has been recently repeated (212). In the 1970s, given the success of the treatment of ALL and the notion, at that time, that lymphomas were a variant form of leukemia and should be treated as such (213), the question of whether long-duration leukemia-like therapy (i.e., with multiple different treatment cycles, including induction, consolidation, and maintenance) is superior to short-duration regimens with repeated cycles of the same drug combinations was considered of primary importance. In 1977, the Children's Cancer Study Group initiated a study in which children with NHL were randomized to a regimen based on therapy for ALL, LSA$_2$-L$_2$, or to the cyclophosphamide, vincristine, methotrexate, and prednisone (COMP) regimen. The duration of therapy for both regimens was 18 months, and radiation was given to sites of bulk disease. The results were better with COMP for advanced-stage Burkitt lymphoma, whereas patients with lymphoblastic lymphoma had a better outcome with LSA$_2$-L$_2$ (177). In a subsequent study, the Children's Cancer Study Group compared 6 months of COMP with 18 months of COMP for patients with localized Burkitt lymphoma and showed that 6 months was as good as 18 months (178).

Protocol NCI 7704, a regimen consisting of cyclophosphamide, vincristine, doxorubicin (CODOX), and prednisone alternating with high-dose methotrexate (CODOX-M), was used to treat both adult and pediatric patients with Burkitt lymphoma and Burkitt-like lymphoma; patients with "high-risk" disease received 15 cycles of therapy. Overall, between 50% and 60% of patients achieved long-term survival (22).

A subsequent NCI regimen, 89-C-41, consisting of only four cycles of alternating CODOX-M therapy, with a combination of ifosfamide, etoposide, and high-dose cytarabine (IVAC) was shown to be effective in patients with recurrent disease after cyclophosphamide-containing regimens (175,176). Despite the drastic reduction in the number of cycles, this short-duration therapy resulted in a markedly superior outcome for both low-risk and high-risk patients. A study from the Pediatric Oncology Group in pediatric patients with limited-stage non-lymphoblastic lymphoma showed that 9 weeks of chemotherapy was as efficacious as 8 months of chemotherapy whether or not radiation was used (204). In another study, cure of a high fraction of patients with Burkitt lymphoma with an intensive regimen of only 45 days has been reported (214). These studies clearly support the concept that short-duration therapy with an effective regimen is sufficient to cure Burkitt lymphoma and that long-duration therapies appear to offer no advantage. In fact, long-duration regimens containing fewer drugs are clearly inferior in terms of their curative potential, especially in high-risk patients.

Prompt Initiation of Successive Cycles of Chemotherapy

Burkitt lymphoma has a very high proliferative index and very short tumor-doubling time. This is perhaps one of the reasons that these tumors are particularly responsive to chemotherapy, but it also has implications for the therapeutic strategy. Successful treatment regimens for Burkitt lymphoma allow as little delay between therapy cycles as possible; subsequent chemotherapy cycles are started as soon as there are signs of bone marrow recovery (usually based on the neutrophil count). Waiting for a fixed period of time between cycles, as may be reasonable for much more slowly growing solid tumors, may be detrimental; it is not unusual to see progressive growth before the next cycle of therapy when the tumor is resistant to chemotherapy. Because of the urgency of commencing the next cycle of therapy, it is considered inappropriate to wait for full marrow recovery.

The target neutrophil count required to initiate the next treatment cycle has varied among the different protocols. In BFM-95, a neutrophil count of 200 per mm^3 was required in early cycles and 500 per mm^3 in later cycles, with a platelet count of $\geq$50,000 per mm^3 (187). For NCI 89-C-41 (175), a neutrophil count of $\geq$1,000 per mm^3 and a platelet count of 50,000 per mm^3 were used, whereas in SFOP trials, a neutrophil count of $\geq$1,500 per mm^3 and platelet count of $\geq$100,000 per mm^3 have been required (181). Because all of these protocols appear equally successful, it appears that once marrow recovery has begun, it is safe to proceed with the next therapy cycle.

These general principles apply to both pediatric and adult patients with Burkitt lymphoma, although in adult patients with significant comorbidities and in patients who are very elderly, the application of these therapeutic principles may not be possible. In one multicenter study in which patients were treated with a slightly modified 89-C-41 protocol, only 43% of patients received the treatment as planned (197). In this group of patients, significant modifications in the doses may be required, and newer strategies may be necessary.

CHEMOTHERAPY REGIMENS AND RESULTS OF TREATMENT

Limited-Stage Disease

Patients with limited disease, i.e., localized or completely resected intra-abdominal disease (stages I and II, St. Jude), have an excellent prognosis with cure rates between 90% and 100%. The definition of limited-stage or low-risk patients varies among the different protocols. The NCI protocol has only two risk groups, SFOP protocols have three risk groups, and BFM has four risk groups (Tables 22.5, 22.6, and 22.7). Patients with limited disease can be treated with only two or three cycles of chemotherapy (without radiation), which is also less intensive than the therapy used for patients with extensive disease; yet published NCI, BFM, and SFOP trials have all reported 100% cure rates in these patients (175,180,185). A randomized study from the Pediatric Oncology Group has shown no benefit of combined chemoradiation when compared with chemotherapy alone in patients with limited disease (204).

The importance of not undertreating patients with a limited tumor burden must be emphasized. Occasional patients with stage I disease have quite an extensive tumor (e.g., a localized mass of >10 cm). Although there are insufficient published data from which to draw firm conclusions, it seems that such patients ought to be included in a higher risk category than would be the case if stage alone were the determinant of therapy. These patients may also be anticipated to have elevated serum LDH levels. If this were included as a marker of risk, they would receive more intensive therapy. Risk stratification should not, therefore, be based exclusively on clinical stage (not, at least, as determined by the existing staging systems).

Extensive-Stage Disease

Patients with Burkitt lymphoma had a very poor prognosis in the 1970s, especially patients with bone marrow involvement, central nervous system involvement, or both. The newer, more intensive short-duration regimens, which consist of seven to nine drugs instead of the four to five drug regimens used in the 1970s for 1 year to 18 months, have dramatically improved overall survival. These regimens have also demonstrated that chemotherapy alone is sufficient to treat sites of bulky disease, treat central nervous system disease (including paraplegia), prevent central nervous system disease, and even treat disease in so-called sanctuary sites, such as testicular disease, all of which were previously treated with radiation therapy.

Several regimens have been developed that result in cure rates in adults in the range of 60% to 90% for patients with more advanced-stage disease (17,175,215,216) These regimens have largely been extrapolated from advances made within the pediatric literature. For patients with extensive disease, the basic cyclophosphamide, vincristine, and methotrexate (with or without prednisone) has been supplemented with higher dose methotrexate (5 to 8 g per m^2) and frequently high-dose cytarabine, in addition to other drugs, such as etoposide and sometimes ifosfamide (176,181,185,217), shown to be active in patients with recurrent disease (17,198–202).

Of considerable significance is the observation that despite the shorter number of cycles, the survival rate for patients with marrow or central nervous system involvement improved from 20% to 80%. High-dose cytarabine and etoposide are used in NCI, BFM, and SFOP regimens for high-risk patients. In the NCI and BFM regimens, ifosfamide replaces cyclophosphamide in every other cycle. Although designed independently, it is clear that these three regimens (NCI, BFM, and SFOP) have more similarities than differences.

Although adult patients with Burkitt lymphoma comprise <2% of lymphomas, they have had major survival benefit (from approximately 25% to 30% cure rates to 60% to 90% cure rates) from these newer regimens (17,197,218–221). Because these protocols have not been directly compared and outcomes reported are greatly influenced by the clinical characteristics of the patients treated, it is difficult to identify the optimal regimen. The most commonly used regimen in North America has been CODOX-M/IVAC, which alternates seven chemotherapeutic agents, including the use of high-dose methotrexate and cytarabine, and intrathecal therapy for treatment of the central nervous system (175). Although demonstrating notable efficacy, tolerability of the original regimen developed by Magrath et al. (175) was challenged by significant neurologic toxicity, myelosuppression, and mucositis. Additional studies have confirmed the efficacy of this protocol and have attempted to minimize toxicity with dose modifications (197,222). In a recent publication by Mead et al. (60), a dose-modified CODOX-M/IVAC regimen was evaluated in patients with highly proliferative aggressive B-cell lymphoma, including patients with Burkitt lymphoma and DLBCL. Methotrexate was dosed at 3 g per m^2 (compared with the original dose of 6.72 g per m^2) and further reduced to 1 g per m^2 in patients >65 years of age. Two-year progression-free survival was 64% for patients with Burkitt lymphoma. Overall outcome appeared comparable to a historical group of patients treated with the unmodified protocol (197) with an apparent reduction in toxicity.

Variations in individual and cumulative drug dosages, timing, and total treatment duration exist among the several protocols in use. Emphasis in recent and ongoing trials is on "fine tuning" existing regimens (i.e., refining drug dosage and administration and reducing toxicity). Although the evidence suggests that more than four or five active drugs are necessary to achieve excellent results, it is difficult to determine the relative value of each drug in any given regimen. In this respect, it is of interest that corticosteroids are not included in one effective protocol (175,176). Data from the recent BFM-95 study demonstrated that a 4-hour methotrexate infusion was less toxic and effective for patients with limited disease. However, the 24-hour methotrexate infusion seemed to provide more benefit for higher risk patients (risk categories three and four) (187). In the recent LMB-96 trial, patients in the intermediate risk group were randomized to a less intensive treatment (either lower doses of cyclophosphamide or omission of a maintenance cycle) if they were early responders (>20% tumor response at day 7) (189). There was no significant difference in outcome between patients receiving standard doses and those receiving the less intensive approach in this response-based strategy. A major focus of future studies should be to better tailor therapy according to patient clinical characteristics, response to therapy, and, in particular, biologic features of the tumor.

Newer Therapeutic Strategies

Other intensive combination chemotherapy approaches have also been investigated but require validation in larger numbers of patients (223,224). More enticing strategies would be to incorporate newer targeted agents, such as monoclonal antibodies, which may improve efficacy while limiting toxicity. There is good evidence from in vitro experiments in Burkitt lymphoma cell lines and animal studies using Burkitt lymphoma cell line xenografts that anti-CD20 antibody has antitumor activity by itself and also enhances the efficacy of chemotherapy or radiation (225). Studies in patients with DLBCL have demonstrated a superior outcome for the combination of chemotherapy plus the anti-CD20 antibody rituximab when compared with chemotherapy alone (226). However, the utility of immunochemotherapy in Burkitt lymphoma remains unproven. Given that the mechanism of action of rituximab may largely be mediated through overcoming resistance to BCL2, it may not offer the same advantage in Burkitt lymphoma that does not express BCL2, although a recent study of rituximab added to hyper-CODOX and dexamethasone alternating with methotrexate and cytarabine suggested an improved event-free survival and overall survival when compared with historical patients treated with hyper-CODOX and dexamethasone alternating with methotrexate and cytarabine alone (227). Similarly, the possibility of using radioimmunoconjugates, such as yttrium and ^{131}I tagged to CD20 antibody, which presumably act independently of any effect on BCL2, should be considered (228). Thus far, minimal information is available on the use of these agents in Burkitt lymphoma, and given the limited utility of radiation therapy in this entity, it is unknown whether these agents would provide benefit.

Given the high mitotic rate of tumor cells in Burkitt lymphoma, a different strategy that has been explored is the use of continuous infusional chemotherapy. A preliminary unpublished report of an infusional regimen, dose-adjusted etoposide, prednisone, vincristine, cyclophosphamide, doxorubicin, and rituximab has demonstrated encouraging results with a complete remission rate of 100% and a 2-year event-free survival of 92% in 17 patients (229). This approach offers several potential advantages, including: continuous exposure of rapidly dividing cells to cytotoxic agents, escalation of doses based on level of cytopenias seen, and less toxicity compared with standard Burkitt regimens. However, this approach will require further validation in a larger number of patients.

Treatment and Prevention of Central Nervous System Disease

Patients with central nervous system disease have long been considered to have a particularly poor prognosis. There are several possible explanations for this. Such patients could have biologically different disease, which is more resistant to the particular chemotherapy in use. Central nervous system disease may be associated with particularly extensive systemic disease, or the chemotherapy used may be less effective because of poor penetration into the central nervous system. Of interest in this context is the observation that African patients with Burkitt lymphoma and central nervous system disease do not appear to have a worse prognosis than other

patients. Indeed, even with the therapy delivered in the 1960s and 1970s, 50% of patients could be expected to achieve long-term survival (193,230). This is probably related to the fact that in endemic Burkitt lymphoma, central nervous system disease is frequently associated with rather small tumor burdens. In contrast, in sporadic Burkitt lymphoma, it is associated with extensive systemic disease, frequently including bone marrow involvement (205).

The use of high-dose S-phase agents [i.e., methotrexate and cytarabine, both of which are highly active in Burkitt lymphoma (198,200–202) and provide effective drug levels in the spinal fluid and central nervous system parenchyma] has dramatically improved the results of therapy in patients with central nervous system disease (182). Before this, intrathecal therapy and radiation were the only therapeutic modalities used specifically against the central nervous system. However, the potential role of better systemic therapy in improving the results in patients with central nervous system disease must also be considered. Both high-dose methotrexate and high-dose cytarabine are also effective against systemic disease. High-dose cytarabine and high-dose methotrexate are potential neurotoxins, and this must be taken into consideration in protocol design because neurotoxicity may be considerably increased if other potential neurotoxins are used (231). The risk of enhancing the neurotoxicity of these drugs with radiation is another reason to avoid central nervous system irradiation.

In adults as well as children with Burkitt lymphoma, prophylaxis against the spread of tumor to the central nervous system is an essential component of therapy for the majority of patients. At the present time, the only patient groups that do not routinely receive prophylaxis against central nervous system disease are those with minimal disease, such as patients with intra-abdominal disease that is completely resected or patients with stage I disease that is not in proximity to the central nervous system (i.e., not in the head and neck region or epidural area) in whom central nervous system spread is extremely rare. Intrathecal therapy with methotrexate alone or methotrexate and cytarabine has been the mainstay of central nervous system prophylactic therapy, but in patients with extensive disease, high-dose intravenous infusions of the S-phase–specific agents, methotrexate and cytarabine, are administered in most effective protocols and clearly play a role in preventing central nervous system spread or dealing with occult central nervous system involvement.

Radiation of the cranium or craniospinal axis is generally not considered to have an advantage over chemotherapeutic central nervous system prophylactic therapy in children with lymphoma, and in some studies in patients with B-cell lymphomas, it has been shown to be ineffective (232,233). Moreover, prophylactic cranial irradiation in ALL, in which there is considerably more experience with this approach, has been associated with significant toxicity, including impaired growth, intellectual impairment, and secondary brain tumors (234,235).

TREATMENT OF ELDERLY PATIENTS WITH BURKITT LYMPHOMA

Despite the fact that most modern Burkitt lymphoma regimens can cure 80% to 90% of pediatric and young adult patients, the treatment of elderly patients is a challenge. Most adults treated on intensive protocols designed for Burkitt lymphoma have been ≤60 years of age. Elderly patients (patients >65 or 70 years of age) have a high incidence of comorbid conditions that may include cardiac problems, renal insufficiency, pulmonary problems, neurologic problems, and poor performance status. These factors can make it impossible to treat these patients with unmodified short-duration, dose-intensive regimens, which, in elderly patients, have a high likelihood of being associated with increased morbidity and mortality from toxicity. Treatment regimens for the elderly may need to be individualized, depending on extent of disease, renal function, cardiac status, and overall health, with the aim to minimize toxicity while still maintaining reasonable efficacy. However, there is very limited published information available, largely because it is difficult to conduct clinical trials in this age group given the rarity of Burkitt lymphoma and the frequent presence of significant comorbidities.

Treatment of Elderly Patients with Limited Disease

Elderly patients with localized nonbulky disease or with completely resected intra-abdominal disease may tolerate therapy as well as younger patients because it is less intensive and shorter. If a regimen with methotrexate is preferred, then an intermediate dose of methotrexate, such as 500 to 1,000 mg per m^2, may be preferable. Based on the studies in elderly patients with DLBCL, it may be reasonable to use rituxan along with chemotherapy because this may increase the efficacy of treatment. Cure rates for elderly patients with limited disease are likely to be as good, or only slightly worse, as in younger patients. The need for intrathecal prophylaxis is presumably similar to younger patients, although there are no data in this regard.

Treatment of Elderly Patients with Extensive Disease

Treatment of this group of patients is extremely challenging because the risks and benefits of therapy have to be delicately weighed in the balance. Modifications in drug dosages may need to be made accordingly. Extreme care should be given to postchemotherapy supportive care because the treatment-related morbidity and mortality can be significant. Elderly patients (>70 years of age) may have particular problems in handling high-dose methotrexate; in patients >70 years of age and in patients with significant associated medical problems, it may be safer to limit the dose of methotrexate to 1 to 3 g per m^2 or less. In a recent study by Mead et al. (60), patients >65 years of age received a modified CODOX-M/IVAC regimen with only 1 g per m^2 of methotrexate with excellent tolerance and comparable outcomes to previously reported results. In some patients (especially those with renal insufficiency), it may not be possible to give any methotrexate.

If an NCI 89-C-41 regimen is used, then doses of CODOX may also have to be modified (based on patients' total disease burden and the ability to tolerate the toxicity of therapy). Patients who have a high disease burden (who are at particular risk for central nervous system involvement) and those who already have central nervous system involvement should receive the highest tolerated dose of methotrexate. Patients who are in good physical condition and who have normal renal function may tolerate full doses of methotrexate without serious complications (if extreme care is taken to facilitate elimination of methotrexate by hyperhydration and alkalinization). Cyclophosphamide and ifosfamide as well as cytarabine may need dose reduction, but Adriamycin and vincristine may not in the absence of cardiac or neurologic problems, respectively. Similarly, individualized dose and schedule modification of BFM or SFOP regimens may be required in patients >70 years of age. In making such modifications, it must be recognized that there is likely to be an associated reduction in the chance for a good outcome. The use of prophylactic antibiotics, antiviral and antifungal medication, growth factor support, and very close follow-up until complete recovery from the treatment toxicity are particularly important in the elderly. In the near future, with advances in biologic therapies and targeted therapies directed to specific molecular lesions, treatment may become less toxic and more efficacious, perhaps equally effective and minimally toxic in elderly patients too.

Role of Stem Cell Transplantation

In light of the efficacy of modern short-duration multidrug regimens, which although intensive do not require stem cell rescue, there appears to be no routine role for stem cell transplantation in Burkitt lymphoma. Although induction of remission followed by transplantation has been used by some in an attempt to improve survival rates, particularly in adults, there seems to be no advantage to this approach. Indeed, anecdotally such approaches have yielded worse results (17,236,237). In a recent trial, patients were treated with a short course of intensive therapy followed by consolidation with high-dose carmustine, etoposide, cytarabine, and melphalan, and autologous stem cell support (238). The median age of patients enrolled was 36 years, and the 5-year event-free survival was 73%, a result that is comparable to outcomes reported without transplant. In another trial, Song et al. (239) demonstrated that patients treated with an approach that included autologous stem cell transplantation only had a cure rate of 50%, with many patients having progression before transplantation. There has been limited information on the use of allogeneic transplantation in Burkitt lymphoma. In a review of European registry data, 71 patients with Burkitt lymphoma who underwent allogeneic transplantation had a median survival of only 4.7 months, with a high rate of treatment-related mortality (240). Currently, the role of transplantation in the management of Burkitt lymphoma is unclear, and may best be reserved for the management of relapsed disease.

Treatment of B-Cell Lymphoma, Unclassifiable, with Features Intermediate between Diffuse Large B-Cell Lymphoma and Burkitt Lymphoma

In clinical practice, cases of aggressive B-cell lymphoma are encountered that may meet some, but not all, diagnostic criteria for Burkitt lymphoma, displaying features intermediate between Burkitt lymphoma and DLBCL. The WHO has recognized morphologic variants, including "atypical Burkitt lymphoma" and "Burkitt-like lymphoma" to account for these cases (19). However, the classification of these variants has been associated with low interobserver and intraobserver reproducibility among pathologists that has raised questions regarding their clinical significance and implications for treatment. It is difficult from the historical literature to assess optimal treatment strategies for these patients because they have been variably defined, and have been included in cohorts of patients with both DLBCL and Burkitt lymphoma (44,46).

The recently updated WHO classification designates a new category called "B-cell lymphoma, unclassifiable, with features intermediate between DLBCL and Burkitt lymphoma" to account for these aberrant cases (23). It will be important for future studies to separately categorize these patients, so that treatment strategies can be better defined. It is clear that standard therapy for DLBCL has proven ineffective for Burkitt lymphoma, thus patients within this category who have biologic features in keeping with Burkitt lymphoma may be harmed by treatment aimed at DLBCL. As discussed previously, two recent gene expression profiling studies evaluating aggressive B-cell lymphomas (including classic Burkitt lymphoma, atypical Burkitt lymphoma, and DLBCL) have explored the molecular complexity of these entities (81,120). Most, but not all, cases of atypical Burkitt lymphoma had a Burkitt lymphoma signature, whereas 17% to 34% of cases morphologically in keeping with DLBCL also displayed a Burkitt lymphoma molecular signature. Whether gene expression profiling will allow for a more reproducible classification in the future that can be used to better tailor therapy remains to be investigated.

SUPPORTIVE CARE

The success of treatment in Burkitt lymphoma is equally dependent on: (a) the effectiveness of the regimen, and (b) the efficacy of supportive care. Because of the intensive nature of most of the effective regimens, patients require very intensive postchemotherapy supportive care. Effective and careful management of treatment-related toxicity and complications is very critical to a successful outcome. Important aspects of postchemotherapy care include: (a) prevention and management of tumor lysis syndrome; (b) before and after high-dose methotrexate hyperhydration and alkalinization to maintain a good urine output (>100 to 150 mL per hour) and an alkaline urine pH (pH >7.0); (c) growth factor support; (d) prophylactic antibiotics, antifungals, and antivirals; and (e) close follow-up care as an inpatient or outpatient (almost daily visits to the clinic or physician's office).

Prevention and Management of Uric Acid Nephropathy and Tumor Lysis Syndrome

In patients with a large tumor burden, pretreatment uricemia is likely to be present, perhaps associated with renal failure from uric acid nephropathy. This syndrome can be compounded by obstruction to the renal outflow tract, and such patients are at heightened risk for the development of a tumor lysis syndrome (241–243). Management includes the use of alkaline hyperhydration and allopurinol or, probably more effective, a urate oxidase. In extreme circumstances, or

in cases in which treatment must be begun urgently, management includes hemodialysis or filtration. In general, it is wise not to commence therapy until the serum uric acid level is normal or close to normal and the patient has an excellent urine output because such patients are at particular risk for developing a tumor lysis syndrome. In the first few days of therapy, continuation of the aforementioned measures, with the exception of alkalinization (because hyperphosphatemia occurs after therapy, and phosphates are less soluble in an alkaline urine), is essential, the most important component being hydration because all oxypurines can be dissolved in a sufficiently large volume of urine. Patients must be monitored carefully, particularly with respect to fluid intake and output, such that additional measures (diuretics, dialysis, filtration) may be taken if necessary. It is advisable to avoid intravenous potassium or calcium in these patients because potassium levels tend to rise rapidly within hours of therapy, whereas elevated phosphorus can lead to deposition of calcium in soft tissues. In general, because of the significant risks and close monitoring required, most patients at risk for a tumor lysis syndrome (i.e., with a significant tumor burden) should be cared for in an acute care facility.

Before and After High-Dose Methotrexate Hydration and Alkalinization

Most of the effective Burkitt lymphoma regimens include high-dose methotrexate as an important component of the regimen. Among all the other drugs used in these regimens, high-dose methotrexate administration demands utmost care. Despite the fact that high-dose methotrexate is potentially very toxic or even fatal if care is not taken to facilitate its timely elimination, it can be administered safely by following a number of simple principles. For patients <70 years of age, these include the following:

1. Premethotrexate hydration and alkalinization.
2. Monitoring urine pH.
3. Strict monitoring of serum methotrexate levels, and, of course, input and output, as well as renal and hepatic function.
4. Prompt initiation of leucovorin rescue. Carboxypeptidase, which cleaves methotrexate, can be used if levels remain high, particularly in the presence of renal failure.
5. Temporary discontinuation of all potentially nephrotoxic drugs and drugs that compete with methotrexate for renal excretion (including nonsteroidal antiinflammatory agents, aminoglycosides, and acyclovir) before, during, and until complete clearance of methotrexate. It is very important to make sure the patient's renal function is normal or adequate (creatinine clearance of 50 to 60) before high-dose methotrexate administration; if renal function is suboptimal secondary to lymphoma or tumor lysis, then methotrexate should be withheld until renal function is satisfactory to meet the guidelines.
6. Patients with localized fluid accumulation (e.g., pleural effusion, ascites) may accumulate methotrexate in the fluid with resultant delayed elimination and toxicity. In such cases, drainage of the fluid or very careful monitoring of methotrexate excretion may be necessary.

Growth Factor Support

Many of the serious complications related to intensive chemotherapy are secondary to severe pancytopenia. All of the effective regimens used in Burkitt lymphoma cause prolonged severe neutropenia, which invariably leads to neutropenic infections (in most, if not all, patients) without prophylactic antibiotics. Granulocyte colony-stimulating factor or granulocyte-macrophage colony-stimulating factor can reduce the number of days of neutropenia and shorten the time for neutrophil recovery. By reducing the number of days of severe neutropenia, the risks of infection are lessened. Neutrophil recovery also increases the likelihood of, and potentially speeds, recovery from an existing infection. The use of growth factors should result in patients being treated in a timely fashion and maintaining the dose intensity of these highly effective regimens. In practice, although the kinetics of neutrophil recovery can be clearly demonstrated (176), the impact on rate of infection and number of days in the hospital has not been clearly documented, and may depend on dose, patient age group, and many other factors.

Prophylactic Antibiotics, and Antifungal and Antiviral Medications

Because most patients develop neutropenic infections because of the depth and duration of neutropenia from these regimens, the use of antibiotics during periods of neutropenia may help to reduce infection (in protocol 89-C-41, e.g., 80% to 90% of cycles are associated with febrile neutropenia in the absence of prophylactic antibiotics, such that patients are at very high risk). Antifungal and antiviral prophylaxis may also be valuable when given before the onset of neutropenia until recovery from neutropenia. Antiviral prophylaxis should not be given during high-dose methotrexate administration.

Close Follow-Up

Effective but intensive Burkitt lymphoma regimens demand close physician follow-up for a successful outcome. Follow-up care should be similar to that for patients with transplant and acute myelogenous leukemia. If close, detailed follow-up care cannot be provided, these patients should be referred to an institution where such care is available. In most instances, patients need inpatient care, but in places where outpatient transplant and leukemia therapy is given, it is possible to treat at least some patients on an outpatient basis, usually seeing them every day.

TREATMENT OF RELAPSE

When the highly effective, short-duration, high-intensity therapies described previously are used in primary therapy, the patients who relapse tend to have highly resistant disease. It is also highly unlikely that these patients who relapse after intensive therapy will be salvaged by additional intensive therapy (e.g., accompanied by autologous stem cell rescue). In this situation, salvage therapy accompanied by allogeneic transplantation appears to be a reasonable approach, which at least has the theoretic benefit of a potential graft versus tumor effect (244). Combinations containing platinum compounds (e.g., ifosfamide, carboplatin, and etoposide) are frequently chosen, particularly in patients who have not already been treated with ifosfamide and etoposide.

FUTURE DIRECTIONS

During the last 2 decades, huge advances have occurred in the management of Burkitt lymphoma that have resulted in a significant improvement in outcomes. Ongoing challenges include: refinement of the diagnosis, possibly with the use of molecular tools that may clarify aberrant cases; improved risk stratification that may allow for the use of lower intensity regimens in good-risk patients and the use of alternate therapies in patients who are unlikely to respond; and the development of newer treatment modalities that selectively target the underlying biologic mechanisms at play in this highly aggressive lymphoma. Given the rarity of this entity in adults, both national and international collaboration will be essential to ensuring timely progress.

References

1. Burkitt D. A sarcoma involving the jaws in African children. *Br J Surg* 1958;46:218–223.
2. Smith EC, Elmes BGT. Malignant disease in natives of Nigeria. *Ann Trop Med Parasitol* 1934;28:461–512.
3. Davies JN. Pathology of Central African natives. *East Afr Med J* 1948;25:117–122.
4. Edington GM. Malignant disease in the Gold Coast. *Br J Cancer* 1956;10:41–54.
5. Thijs A. Malignant tumors of Belgium Congo and Ruanda-Urundi natives; 2,536 case reports [in French]. *Ann Soc Belg Med Trop (1920)* 1957;37:483–484 passim.
6. De Smet MP. Clinical observations on malignant tumors of reticuloendothelial and hemolymphopoietic tissues at the Belgian Congo [in French]. *Ann Soc Belg Med Trop (1920)* 1956;36:53–70.
7. O'Conor GT, Davies JN. Malignant tumors in African children. With special reference to malignant lymphoma. *J Pediatr* 1960;56:526–535.
8. Burkitt D. Determining the climatic limitations of a children's cancer common in Africa. *Br Med J* 1962;2:1019–1023.
9. Burkitt D. A children's cancer dependent on climatic factors. *Nature* 1962;194:232–234.
10. Epstein MA, Achong BG, Barr YM. Virus particles in cultured lymphoblasts from Burkitt's lymphoma. *Lancet* 1964;1:702–703.
11. Dalldorf G, Linsell CA, Barnhart FE, et al. An epidemiologic approach to the lymphomas of African children and Burkitt's sarcoma of the jaws. *Perspect Biol Med* 1964;7:435–449.
12. O'Conor GT, Rappaport H, Smith EB. Childhood lymphoma resembling "Burkitt Tumor" in the United States. *Cancer* 1965;18:411–417.
13. Dorfman RF. Childhood lymphosarcoma in St. Louis, Missouri, clinically and histologically resembling Burkitt's tumor. *Cancer* 1965;18:418–430.
14. Wright DH. Burkitt's tumour in England. A comparison with childhood lymphosarcoma. *Int J Cancer* 1966;1:503–514.
15. Magrath IT, Sariban E. Clinical features of Burkitt's lymphoma in the USA. *IARC Sci Publ* 1985:119–127.
16. Preudhomme C, Dervite I, Wattel E, et al. Clinical significance of p53 mutations in newly diagnosed Burkitt's lymphoma and acute lymphoblastic leukemia: a report of 48 cases. *J Clin Oncol* 1995;13:812–820.
17. Soussain C, Patte C, Ostronoff M, et al. Small noncleaved cell lymphoma and leukemia in adults. A retrospective study of 65 adults treated with the LMB pediatric protocols. *Blood* 1995;85:664–674.
18. van der Burg M, Barendregt BH, van Wering ER, et alJ. The presence of somatic mutations in immunoglobulin genes of B cell acute lymphoblastic leukemia (ALL-L3) supports assignment as Burkitt's leukemia-lymphoma rather than B-lineage ALL. *Leukemia* 2001;15:1141–1143.
19. Jaffe ES, Harris NL, Stein H, et al. *Pathology and genetics of tumours of haematopoietic and lymphoid tissues.* Lyon, France: IARC Press, 2001.
20. Harris NL, Jaffe ES, Stein H, et al. A revised European-American classification of lymphoid neoplasms: a proposal from the International Lymphoma Study Group. *Blood* 1994;84:1361–1392.

21. Harris NL, Jaffe ES, Diebold J, et al. World Health Organization classification of neoplastic diseases of the hematopoietic and lymphoid tissues: report of the Clinical Advisory Committee meeting-Airlie House, Virginia, November 1997. *J Clin Oncol* 1999;17:3835–3849.

22. Magrath IT, Janus C, Edwards BK, et al. An effective therapy for both undifferentiated (including Burkitt's) lymphomas and lymphoblastic lymphomas in children and young adults. *Blood* 1984;63:1102–1111.

23. Swerdlow SH, Campo E, Harris NL, et al. *WHO classification of tumours of hematopoietic and lymphoid tissues*, 4th ed. Lyon, France: International Agency for Research on Cancer, 2008.

24. Leoncini L, Raphael M, Stein H, et al. Burkitt lymphoma. In: Booman M, Jaffe ES, Lakhani SR, et al., editors. *WHO classification of tumours of haematopoietic and lymphoid tissues*, 4th ed. Lyon, France: International Agency for Research on Cancer, 2008:262–264.

25. Hui PK, Feller AC, Lennert K. High-grade non-Hodgkin's lymphoma of B-cell type. I. Histopathology. *Histopathology* 1988;12:127–143.

26. Histopathological definition of Burkitt's tumour. *Bull World Health Organ* 1969;40:601–607.

27. National Cancer Institute sponsored study of classifications of non-Hodgkin's lymphomas: summary and description of a working formulation for clinical usage. The Non-Hodgkin's Lymphoma Pathologic Classification Project. *Cancer* 1982;49:2112–2135.

28. Wright DH. What is Burkitt's lymphoma? *J Pathol* 1997;182:125–127.

29. Warnke RA, Weiss LM, Chan JDC, et al. *Tumors of the lymph nodes and spleen*, 3rd ed. Washington, DC: Armed Forces Institute of Pathology, 1994.

30. Carbone A, Gloghini A, Gaidano G, et al. AIDS-related Burkitt's lymphoma. Morphologic and immunophenotypic study of biopsy specimens. *Am J Clin Pathol* 1995;103:561–567.

31. Raphael M, Gentilhomme O, Tulliez M, et al. Histopathologic features of high-grade non-Hodgkin's lymphomas in acquired immunodeficiency syndrome. The French Study Group of Pathology for Human Immunodeficiency Virus-Associated Tumors. *Arch Pathol Lab Med* 1991;115:15–20.

32. Carbone A. AIDS-related non-Hodgkin's lymphomas: from pathology and molecular pathogenesis to treatment. *Hum Pathol* 2002;33:392–404.

33. Kluin PM, Harris NL, Stein H, et al. B-cell lymphoma, unclassifiable, with features intermediate between large B-cell lymphoma and Burkitt lymphoma. In: Swerdlow SH, Campo E, Harris NL, et al., eds. *WHO classification of tumours of haematopoietic and lymphoid tissues*, 4th ed. Lyon, France: International Agency for Research on Cancer, 2008:265–266.

34. Thangavelu M, Olopade O, Beckman E, et al. Clinical, morphologic, and cytogenetic characteristics of patients with lymphoid malignancies characterized by both t(14;18)(q32;q21) and t(8;14)(q24;q32) or t(8;22)(q24;q11). *Genes Chromosomes Cancer* 1990;2:147–158.

35. Kroft SH, Domiati-Saad R, Finn WG, et al. Precursor B-lymphoblastic transformation of grade I follicle center lymphoma. *Am J Clin Pathol* 2000;113:411–418.

36. De Jong D, Voetdijk BM, Beverstock GC, et al. Activation of the c-myc oncogene in a precursor-B-cell blast crisis of follicular lymphoma, presenting as composite lymphoma. *N Engl J Med* 1988;318:1373–1378.

37. Donti E, Falini B, Giuseppe Pelicci P, et al. Immunological and molecular studies in a case of follicular lymphoma with an extra chromosome 12 and t(2;8) translocation. *Leukemia* 1988;2:41–44.

38. Lee JT, Innes DJ Jr, Williams ME. Sequential BCL2 and c-myc oncogene rearrangements associated with the clinical transformation of non-Hodgkin's lymphoma. *J Clin Invest* 1989;84:1454–1459.

39. Wlodarska I, Mecucci C, De Wolf-Peeters C, et al. Two translocations: a follicular variant 2;18 and a Burkitt 8;14 in a small non cleaved non Hodgkin's lymphoma. *Leuk Lymphoma* 1991;5:65–69.

40. Aventin A, Mecucci C, Guanyabens C, et al. Variant t(2;18) translocation in a Burkitt conversion of follicular lymphoma. *Br J Haematol* 1990;74:367–369.

41. Carli MG, Cuneo A, Piva N, et al. Lymphoblastic lymphoma with primary splenic involvement and the classic 14;18 translocation. *Cancer Genet Cytogenet* 1991;57:47–51.

42. Gauwerky CE, Haluska FG, Tsujimoto Y, et al. Evolution of B-cell malignancy: pre-B-cell leukemia resulting from MYC activation in a B-cell neoplasm with a rearranged BCL2 gene. *Proc Natl Acad Sci U S A* 1988;85:8548–8552.

43. Gauwerky CE, Hoxie J, Nowell PC, et al. Pre-B-cell leukemia with a t(8;14) and a t(14; 18) translocation is preceded by follicular lymphoma. *Oncogene* 1988;2:431–435.

44. Macpherson N, Lesack D, Klasa R, et al. Small noncleaved, non-Burkitt's (Burkitt-like) lymphoma: cytogenetics predict outcome and reflect clinical presentation. *J Clin Oncol* 1999;17:1558–1567.

45. Kanungo A, Medeiros LJ, Abruzzo LV, et al. Lymphoid neoplasms associated with concurrent t(14;18) and 8q24/c-MYC translocation generally have a poor prognosis. *Mod Pathol* 2006;19:25–33.

46. Le Gouill S, Talmant P, Touzeau C, et al. The clinical presentation and prognosis of diffuse large B-cell lymphoma with t(14;18) and 8q24/c-MYC rearrangement. *Haematologica* 2007;92:1335–1342.

47. Shou Y, Martelli ML, Gabrea A, et al. Diverse karyotypic abnormalities of the c-myc locus associated with c-myc dysregulation and tumor progression in multiple myeloma. *Proc Natl Acad Sci U S A* 2000;97:228–233.

48. Avet-Loiseau H, Gerson F, Magrangeas F, et al. Rearrangements of the c-myc oncogene are present in 15% of primary human multiple myeloma tumors. *Blood* 2001;98:3082–3086.

49. Boerma EG, Siebert R, Kluin PM, et al. Translocations involving 8q24 in Burkitt lymphoma and other malignant lymphomas: a historical review of cytogenetics in the light of todays knowledge. *Leukemia* 2009;23:225–234.

50. Sigaux F, Berger R, Bernheim A, et al. Malignant lymphomas with band 8q24 chromosome abnormality: a morphologic continuum extending from Burkitt's to immunoblastic lymphoma. *Br J Haematol* 1984;57:393–405.

51. Vitolo U, Gaidano G, Botto B, et al. Rearrangements of BCL6, BCL2, c-myc and 6q deletion in B-diffuse large-cell lymphoma: clinical relevance in 71 patients. *Ann Oncol* 1998;9:55–61.

52. Ladanyi M, Offit K, Jhanwar SC, et al. MYC rearrangement and translocations involving band 8q24 in diffuse large cell lymphoma. *Blood* 1991;77:1057–1063.

53. Kramer MH, Hermans J, Wijburg E, et al. Clinical relevance of BCL2, BCL6, and MYC rearrangements in diffuse large B-cell lymphoma. *Blood* 1998;92:3152–3162.

54. Akasaka T, Akasaka H, Ueda C, et al. Molecular and clinical features of non-Burkitt's, diffuse large-cell lymphoma of B-cell type associated with the c-MYC/immunoglobulin heavy-chain fusion gene. *J Clin Oncol* 2000;18:510–518.

55. Nakamura N, Nakamine H, Tamaru J, et al. The distinction between Burkitt lymphoma and diffuse large B-cell lymphoma with c-myc rearrangement. *Mod Pathol* 2002;15:771–776.

56. Cigudosa JC, Parsa NZ, Louie DC, et al. Cytogenetic analysis of 363 consecutively ascertained diffuse large B-cell lymphomas. *Genes Chromosomes Cancer* 1999;25:123–133.

57. Niitsu N, Okamoto M, Miura I, et al. Clinical features and prognosis of de novo diffuse large B-cell lymphoma with t(14;18) and 8q24/c-MYC translocations. *Leukemia* 2009;23:777–783

58. Klapper W, Stoecklein H, Zeynalova S, et al. Structural aberrations affecting the MYC locus indicate a poor prognosis independent of clinical risk factors in diffuse large B-cell lymphomas treated within randomized trials of the German High-Grade Non-Hodgkin's Lymphoma Study Group (DSHNHL). *Leukemia* 2008;22:2226–2229.

59. Lima FP, Bousquet M, Gomez-Brouchet A, et al. Primary diffuse large B-cell lymphoma of bone displays preferential rearrangements of the c-MYC or BCL2 gene. *Am J Clin Pathol* 2008;129:723–726.

60. Mead GM, Barrans SL, Qian W, et al. A prospective clinicopathologic study of dose-modified CODOX-M/IVAC in patients with sporadic Burkitt lymphoma defined using cytogenetic and immunophenotypic criteria (MRC/NCRI LY10 trial). *Blood* 2008;112:2248–2260.

61. McClure RF, Remstein ED, Macon WR, et al. Adult B-cell lymphomas with Burkitt-like morphology are phenotypically and genotypically heterogeneous with aggressive clinical behavior. *Am J Surg Pathol* 2005;29:1652–1660.

62. Rodig SJ, Vergilio JA, Shahsafaei A, et al. Characteristic expression patterns of TCL1, CD38, and CD44 identify aggressive lymphomas harboring a MYC translocation. *Am J Surg Pathol* 2008;32:113–122.

63. Lin P, Medeiros LJ. High-grade B-cell lymphoma/leukemia associated with t(14;18) and 8q24/MYC rearrangement: a neoplasm of germinal center immunophenotype with poor prognosis. *Haematologica* 2007;92:1297–1301.

64. Fiedler W, Weh HJ, Zeller W, et al. Translocation (14; 18) and (8; 22) in three patients with acute leukemia/lymphoma following centrocytic/centroblastic non-Hodgkin's lymphoma. *Ann Hematol* 1991;63:282–287.

65. Young KH, Xie Q, Zhou G, et al. Transformation of follicular lymphoma to precursor B-cell lymphoblastic lymphoma with c-myc gene rearrangement as a critical event. *Am J Clin Pathol* 2008;129:157–166.

66. Hammami A, Chan WC, Michels SD, et al. Mature B-cell acute leukemia: a clinical, morphological, immunological, and cytogenetic study of nine cases. *Hematol Pathol* 1991;5:109–118.

67. Smith SR, Bown N, Wallis JP. Acute lymphoblastic leukemia of Burkitt type (L3) with a (14;18) and an atypical (8;22) translocation. *Cancer Genet Cytogenet* 1992;62:197–199.

68. Gluck WL, Bigner SH, Borowitz MJ, et al. Acute lymphoblastic leukemia of Burkitt's type (L3 ALL) with 8;22 and 14;18 translocations and absent surface immunoglobulins. *Am J Clin Pathol* 1986;85:636–640.

69. Kramer MH, Raghoebier S, Beverstock GC, et al. De novo acute B-cell leukemia with translocation t(14;18): an entity with a poor prognosis. *Leukemia* 1991;5:473–478.

70. Brito-Babapulle V, Crawford A, Khokhar T, et al. Translocations t(14;18) and t(8;14) with rearranged BCL2 and c-myc in a case presenting as B-ALL (L3). *Leukemia* 1991;5:83–87.

71. Marosi C, Bettelheim P, Chott A, et al. Simultaneous occurrence of t(14;18) and t(8;22) common acute lymphoblastic leukemia. *Ann Hematol* 1992;64:101–104.

72. Mufti GJ, Hamblin TJ, Oscier DG, et al. Common ALL with pre-B-cell features showing (8;14) and (14;18) chromosome translocations. *Blood* 1983;62:1142–1146.

73. Stamatoullas A, Buchonnet G, Lepretre S, et al. De novo acute B cell leukemia/lymphoma with t(14;18). *Leukemia* 2000;14:1960–1966.

74. Karsan A, Gascoyne RD, Coupland RW, et al. Combination of t(14;18) and a Burkitt's type translocation in B-cell malignancies. *Leuk Lymphoma* 1993;10:433–441.

75. Au WY, Horsman DE, Viswanatha DS, et al. 8q24 translocations in blastic transformation of mantle cell lymphoma. *Haematologica* 2000;85:1225–1227.

76. Batanian JR, Dunphy CH, Richart JM, et al. Simultaneous presence of t(2;8)(p12;q24) and t(14;18)(q32;q21) in a B-cell lymphoproliferative

disorder with features suggestive of an aggressive variant of splenic marginal-zone lymphoma. *Cancer Genet Cytogenet* 2000;120:136–140.

77. Klein U, Klein G, Ehlin-Henriksson B, et al. Burkitt's lymphoma is a malignancy of mature B cells expressing somatically mutated V region genes. *Mol Med* 1995;1:495–505.
78. Mann RB, Jaffe ES, Braylan RC, et al. Non-endemic Burkitt's lymphoma. A B-cell tumor related to germinal centers. *N Engl J Med* 1976;295:685–691.
79. Dogan A, Bagdi E, Munson P, et al. CD10 and BCL6 expression in paraffin sections of normal lymphoid tissue and B-cell lymphomas. *Am J Surg Pathol* 2000;24:846–852.
80. Lai R, Arber DA, Chang KL, et al. Frequency of BCL2 expression in non-Hodgkin's lymphoma: a study of 778 cases with comparison of marginal zone lymphoma and monocytoid B-cell hyperplasia. *Mod Pathol* 1998;11:864–869.
81. Hummel M, Bentink S, Berger H, et al. A biologic definition of Burkitt's lymphoma from transcriptional and genomic profiling. *N Engl J Med* 2006;354:2419–2430.
82. Carbone A, Gaidano G, Gloghini A, et al. Differential expression of BCL6, CD138/syndecan-1, and Epstein-Barr virus-encoded latent membrane protein-1 identifies distinct histogenetic subsets of acquired immunodeficiency syndrome-related non-Hodgkin's lymphomas. *Blood* 1998;91:747–755.
83. Carbone A, Gloghini A, Larocca LM, et al. Expression profile of MUM1/IRF4, BCL6, and CD138/syndecan-1 defines novel histogenetic subsets of human immunodeficiency virus-related lymphomas. *Blood* 2001;97:744–751.
84. Tao Q, Robertson KD, Manns A, et al. Epstein-Barr virus (EBV) in endemic Burkitt's lymphoma: molecular analysis of primary tumor tissue. *Blood* 1998;91:1373–1381.
85. Harris NL, Horning SJ. Burkitt's lymphoma—the message from microarrays. *N Engl J Med* 2006;354:2495–2498.
86. Gualco G, Queiroga EM, Weiss LM, et al. Frequent expression of multiple myeloma 1/interferon regulatory factor 4 in Burkitt lymphoma. *Hum Pathol* 2009;40:565–571.
87. Chapman CJ, Mockridge CI, Rowe M, et al. Analysis of VH genes used by neoplastic B cells in endemic Burkitt's lymphoma shows somatic hypermutation and intraclonal heterogeneity. *Blood* 1995;85:2176–2181.
88. Tamaru J, Hummel M, Marafioti T, et al. Burkitt's lymphomas express VH genes with a moderate number of antigen-selected somatic mutations. *Am J Pathol* 1995;147:1398–1407.
89. Capello D, Vitolo U, Pasqualucci L, et al. Distribution and pattern of BCL6 mutations throughout the spectrum of B-cell neoplasia. *Blood* 2000;95:651–659.
90. Gaidano G, Pastore C, Capello D, et al. Involvement of the BCL6 gene in AIDS-related lymphomas. *Ann Oncol* 1997;8(suppl 2):105–108.
91. Gaidano G, Carbone A, Pastore C, et al. Frequent mutation of the 5' noncoding region of the BCL6 gene in acquired immunodeficiency syndrome-related non-Hodgkin's lymphomas. *Blood* 1997;89:3755–3762.
92. Manolov G, Manolova Y. Marker band in one chromosome 14 from Burkitt lymphomas. *Nature* 1972;237:33–34.
93. Zech L, Haglund U, Nilsson K, et al. Characteristic chromosomal abnormalities in biopsies and lymphoid-cell lines from patients with Burkitt and non-Burkitt lymphomas. *Int J Cancer* 1976;17:47–56.
94. Hecht JL, Aster JC. Molecular biology of Burkitt's lymphoma. *J Clin Oncol* 2000;18:3707–3721.
95. Boxer LM, Dang CV. Translocations involving c-myc and c-myc function. *Oncogene* 2001;20:5595–5610.
96. Leucci E, Cocco M, Onnis A, et al. MYC translocation-negative classical Burkitt lymphoma cases: an alternative pathogenetic mechanism involving miRNA deregulation. *J Pathol* 2008;216:440–450.
97. Einerson RR, Law ME, Blair HE, et al. Novel FISH probes designed to detect IGK-MYC and IGL-MYC rearrangements in B-cell lineage malignancy identify a new breakpoint cluster region designated BVR2. *Leukemia* 2006;20:1790–1799.
98. Joos S, Haluska FG, Falk MH, et al. Mapping chromosomal breakpoints of Burkitt's t(8;14) translocations far upstream of c-myc. *Cancer Res* 1992;52:6547–6552.
99. Ladanyi M, Offit K, Parsa NZ, et al. Follicular lymphoma with t(8;14)(q24;q32): a distinct clinical and molecular subset of t(8;14)-bearing lymphomas. *Blood* 1992;79:2124–2130.
100. Yano T, Jaffe ES, Longo DL, et al. MYC rearrangements in histologically progressed follicular lymphomas. *Oncogene* 1992;80:758–767.
101. Willis TG, Dyer MJ. The role of immunoglobulin translocations in the pathogenesis of B-cell malignancies. *Blood* 2000;96:808–822.
102. Joos S, Falk MH, Lichter P, et al. Variable breakpoints in Burkitt lymphoma cells with chromosomal t(8;14) translocation separate c-myc and the IgH locus up to several hundred kb. *Hum Mol Genet* 1992;1:625–632.
103. Zeidler R, Joos S, Delecluse HJ, et al. Breakpoints of Burkitt's lymphoma t(8;22) translocations map within a distance of 300 kb downstream of MYC. *Genes Chromosomes Cancer* 1994;9:282–287.
104. Bower M. Acquired immunodeficiency syndrome-related systemic non-Hodgkin's lymphoma. *Br J Haematol* 2001;112:863–873.
105. Kuppers R, Dalla-Favera R. Mechanisms of chromosomal translocations in B cell lymphomas. *Oncogene* 2001;20:5580–5594.
106. Pasqualucci L, Neumeister P, Goossens T, et al. Hypermutation of multiple proto-oncogenes in B-cell diffuse large-cell lymphomas. *Nature* 2001;412:341–346.

107. Cesarman E, Dalla-Favera R, Bentley D, et al. Mutations in the first exon are associated with altered transcription of c-myc in Burkitt lymphoma. *Science* 1987;238:1272–1275.
108. Gu W, Bhatia K, Magrath IT, et al. Binding and suppression of the Myc transcriptional activation domain by p107. *Science* 1994;264:251–254.
109. Raffeld M, Yano T, Hoang AT, et al. Clustered mutations in the transcriptional activation domain of Myc in 8q24 translocated lymphomas and their functional consequences. *Curr Top Microbiol Immunol* 1995;194:265–272.
110. Pelicci PG, Knowles DM 2nd, Magrath I, et al. Chromosomal breakpoints and structural alterations of the c-myc locus differ in endemic and sporadic forms of Burkitt lymphoma. *Proc Natl Acad Sci U S A* 1986;83:2984–2988.
111. Schlegelberger B, Zwingers T, Harder L, et al. Clinicopathogenetic significance of chromosomal abnormalities in patients with blastic peripheral B-cell lymphoma. Kiel-Wien-Lymphoma Study Group. *Blood* 1999;94:3114–3120.
112. Johansson B, Mertens F, Mitelman F. Cytogenetic evolution patterns in non-Hodgkin's lymphoma. *Blood* 1995;86:3905–3914.
113. Akasaka T, Muramatsu M, Ohno H, et al. Application of long-distance polymerase chain reaction to detection of junctional sequences created by chromosomal translocation in mature B-cell neoplasms. *Blood* 1996;88:985–994.
114. Siebert R, Matthiesen P, Harder S, et al. Application of interphase fluorescence in situ Hybridization for the detection of the Burkitt translocation t(8;14)(q24;q32) in B-cell lymphomas. *Blood* 1998;91:984–990.
115. Taniwaki M, Matsuda F, Jauch A, et al. Detection of 14q32 translocations in B-cell malignancies by in situ hybridization with yeast artificial chromosome clones containing the human IgH gene locus. *Blood* 1994;83:2962–2969.
116. Veronese ML, Ohta M, Finan J, et al. Detection of myc translocations in lymphoma cells by fluorescence in situ hybridization with yeast artificial chromosomes. *Blood* 1995;85:2132–2138.
117. Rack KA, Delabesse E, Radford-Weiss I, et al. Simultaneous detection of MYC, BVR1, and PVT1 translocations in lymphoid malignancies by fluorescence in situ hybridization. *Genes Chromosomes Cancer* 1998;23:220–226.
118. Tamura A, Miura I, Iida S, et al. Interphase detection of immunoglobulin heavy chain gene translocations with specific oncogene loci in 173 patients with B-cell lymphoma. *Cancer Genet Cytogenet* 2001;129:1–9.
119. Martin-Subero JI, Harder L, Gesk S, et al. Interphase FISH assays for the detection of translocations with breakpoints in immunoglobulin light chain loci. *Int J Cancer* 2002;98:470–474.
120. Dave SS, Fu K, Wright GW, et al. Molecular diagnosis of Burkitt's lymphoma. *N Engl J Med* 2006;354:2431–2442.
121. Klapper W, Szczepanowski M, Burkhardt B, et al. Molecular profiling of pediatric mature B-cell lymphoma treated in population-based prospective clinical trials. *Blood* 2008;112:1374–1381.
122. Sevilla DW, Gong JZ, Goodman BK, et al. Clinicopathologic findings in high-grade B-cell lymphomas with typical Burkitt morphologic features but lacking the MYC translocation. *Am J Clin Pathol* 2007;128:981–991.
123. Nomura Y, Karube K, Suzuki R, et al. High-grade mature B-cell lymphoma with Burkitt-like morphology: results of a clinicopathological study of 72 Japanese patients. *Cancer Sci* 2008;99:246–252.
124. Cogliatti SB, Novak U, Henz S, et al. Diagnosis of Burkitt lymphoma in due time: a practical approach. *Br J Haematol* 2006;134:294–301.
125. Kanda K, Hu HM, Zhang L, et al. NF-kappa B activity is required for the deregulation of c-myc expression by the immunoglobulin heavy chain enhancer. *J Biol Chem* 2000;275:32338–32346.
126. Hu HM, Arcinas M, Boxer LM. A Myc-associated zinc finger protein-related factor binding site is required for the deregulation of c-myc expression by the immunoglobulin heavy chain gene enhancers in Burkitt's lymphoma. *J Biol Chem* 2002;277:9819–9824.
127. Hussain M, Doucet JP, Gutierrez M, et al. Tumor necrosis factor-related apoptosis-inducing ligand (TRAIL) and Fas apoptosis in Burkitt's lymphomas with loss of multiple pro-apoptotic proteins. *Haematologica* 2003;88:167–175.
128. Gutierrez MI, Cherney B, Hussain A, et al. Bax is frequently compromised in Burkitt's lymphomas with irreversible resistance to Fas-induced apoptosis. *Cancer Res* 1999;59:696–703.
129. Nanbo A, Takada K. The role of Epstein-Barr virus-encoded small RNAs (EBERs) in oncogenesis. *Rev Med Virol* 2002;12:321–326.
130. Nanbo A, Inoue K, Adachi-Takasawa K, et al. Epstein-Barr virus RNA confers resistance to interferon-alpha-induced apoptosis in Burkitt's lymphoma. *EMBO J* 2002;21:954–965.
131. Takada K, Nanbo A. The role of EBERs in oncogenesis. *Semin Cancer Biol* 2001;11:461–467.
132. Kelly G, Bell A, Rickinson A. Epstein-Barr virus-associated Burkitt lymphomagenesis selects for downregulation of the nuclear antigen EBNA2. *Nat Med* 2002;8:1098–1104.
133. Pajic A, Staege MS, Dudziak D, et al. Antagonistic effects of c-myc and Epstein-Barr virus latent genes on the phenotype of human B cells. *Int J Cancer* 2001;93:810–816.
134. Kempkes B, Zimber-Strobl U, Eissner G, et al. Epstein-Barr virus nuclear antigen 2 (EBNA2)-oestrogen receptor fusion proteins complement the EBNA2-deficient Epstein-Barr virus strain P3HR1 in transformation of primary B cells but suppress growth of human B cell lymphoma lines. *J Gen Virol* 1996;77(Pt 2):227–237.

135. Jochner N, Eick D, Zimber-Strobl U, et al. Epstein-Barr virus nuclear antigen 2 is a transcriptional suppressor of the immunoglobulin mu gene: implications for the expression of the translocated c-myc gene in Burkitt's lymphoma cells. *EMBO J* 1996;15:375–382.

136. Staege MS, Lee SP, Frisan T, et al. MYC overexpression imposes a non-immunogenic phenotype on Epstein-Barr virus-infected B cells. *Proc Natl Acad Sci U S A* 2002;99:4550–4555.

137. Pajic A, Polack A, Staege MS, et al. Elevated expression of c-myc in lymphoblastoid cells does not support an Epstein-Barr virus latency III-to-I switch. *J Gen Virol* 2001;82(Pt 12):3051–3055.

138. Polack A, Hortnagel K, Pajic A, et al. c-myc activation renders proliferation of Epstein-Barr virus (EBV)-transformed cells independent of EBV nuclear antigen 2 and latent membrane protein 1. *Proc Natl Acad Sci U S A* 1996;93:10411–10416.

139. Klein U, Tu Y, Stolovitzky GA, et al. Transcriptional analysis of the B cell germinal center reaction. *Proc Natl Acad Sci U S A* 2003;100:2639–2644.

140. Cutrona G, Dono M, Pastorino S, et al. The propensity to apoptosis of centrocytes and centroblasts correlates with elevated levels of intracellular myc protein. *Eur J Immunol* 1997;27:234–238.

141. Niller HH, Salamon D, Ilg K, et al. The in vivo binding site for oncoprotein c-Myc in the promoter for Epstein-Barr virus (EBV) encoding RNA (EBER) 1 suggests a specific role for EBV in lymphomagenesis. *Med Sci Monit* 2003;9:HY1–HY9.

142. Geser A, de Thé G, Lenoir G, et al. Final case reporting from the Ugandan prospective study of the relationship between EBV and Burkitt's lymphoma. *Int J Cancer* 1982;29:397–400.

143. Whittle HC, Brown J, Marsh K, et al. T-cell control of Epstein-Barr virus-infected B cells is lost during P. falciparum malaria. *Nature* 1984;312:449–450.

144. Kitinya JN, Lauren PA. Burkitt's lymphoma on Mount Kilimanjaro and in the inland regions of Northern Tanzania. *East Afr Med J* 1982;59:256–260.

145. Sariban E, Donahue A, Magrath IT. Jaw involvement in American Burkitt's lymphoma. *Cancer* 1984;53:1777–1782.

146. Haddy TB, Keenan AM, Jaffe ES, et al. Bone involvement in young patients with non-Hodgkin's lymphoma: efficacy of chemotherapy without local radiotherapy. *Blood* 1988;72:1141–1147.

147. Sabbah RS, Ali MA, Lewall DB, et al. Burkitt's lymphoma in Saudi Arabia: clinical, pathological, and epidemiological analyses of 16 cases. *King Faisal Spec Hosp Med J* 1982;2:77–83.

148. Suvatte V, Mahasandana C, Tanphaichitr VS, et al. Burkitt's lymphoma in Thai children: an analysis of 25 cases. *Southeast Asian J Trop Med Public Health* 1983;14:385–393.

149. Wood RE, Nortje CJ, Hesseling P, et al. Involvement of the maxillofacial region in African Burkitt's lymphoma in the Cape Province and Namibia. *Dentomaxillofac Radiol* 1988;17:57–60.

150. Magrath IT. African Burkitt's lymphoma. History, biology, clinical features, and treatment. *Am J Pediatr Hematol Oncol* 1991;13:222–246.

151. Cavdar AO, Yavuz G, Babacan E, et al. Burkitt's lymphoma in Turkish children: clinical, viral [EBV] and molecular studies. *Leuk Lymphoma* 1994;14:323–330.

152. Ertem U, Duru F, Pamir A, et al. Burkitt's lymphoma in 63 Turkish children diagnosed over a 10 year period. *Pediatr Hematol Oncol* 1996;13:123–134.

153. Sandlund JT, Fonseca T, Leimig T, et al. Predominance and characteristics of Burkitt lymphoma among children with non-Hodgkin lymphoma in northeastern Brazil. *Leukemia* 1997;11:743–746.

154. Madanat FF, Amr SS, Tarawneh MS, et al. Burkitt's lymphoma in Jordanian children: epidemiological and clinical study. *J Trop Med Hyg* 1986;89:189–191.

155. Amr SS, Tarawneh MS, Jitawi SA, et al. Malignant neoplasms in Jordanian children. *Ann Trop Paediatr* 1986;6:161–166.

156. Hathirat P, Isarangkura P, Nitiyanant P, et al. Lymphoma in children: study of 100 cases. *Southeast Asian J Trop Med Public Health* 1986;17:135–137.

157. Thomas OA, Abdelaal MA, Ayoub DA. Childhood lymphoma in Saudi Arabia: experience at the King Khalid National Guard Hospital. *East Afr Med J* 1996;73:343–345.

158. Janus C, Edwards BK, Sariban E, et al. Surgical resection and limited chemotherapy for abdominal undifferentiated lymphomas. *Cancer Treat Rep* 1984;68:599–605.

159. Shepherd JJ, Wright DH. Burkitt's tumour presenting as bilateral swelling of the breast in women of child-bearing age. *Br J Surg* 1967;54:776–780.

160. Durodola JI. Burkitt's lymphoma presenting during lactation. *Int J Gynaecol Obstet* 1976;14:225–231.

161. Plantaz D, Bachelot C, Dyon JF, et al. Massive breast involvement in Burkitt's lymphoma [in French]. *Arch Fr Pediatr* 1987;44:199–200.

162. Hugh JC, Jackson FI, Hanson J, et al. Primary breast lymphoma. An immunohistologic study of 20 new cases. *Cancer* 1990;66:2602–2611.

163. Magrath IT, Ziegler JL. Bone marrow involvement in Burkitt's lymphoma and its relationship to acute B-cell leukemia. *Leuk Res* 1980;4:33–59.

164. Advani S, Pai S, Adde M, et al. Preliminary report of an intensified, short duration chemotherapy protocol for the treatment of pediatric non-Hodgkin's lymphoma in India. *Ann Oncol* 1997;8:893–897.

165. Chantada GL, Felice MS, Zubizarreta PA, et al. Results of a BFM-based protocol for the treatment of childhood B-non-Hodgkin's lymphoma and B-acute lymphoblastic leukemia in Argentina. *Med Pediatr Oncol* 1997;28:333–341.

166. Gad-el-Mawla N, Hamza MR, Abdel-Hadi S, et al. Prolonged disease-free survival in pediatric non-Hodgkin's lymphoma using ifosfamide-containing combination chemotherapy. *Hematol Oncol* 1991;9:281–286.

167. Ziegler JL, Magrath IT. Burkitt's lymphoma. In: Ioachim HL, ed. *Pathobiology annual.* New York, NY: Appleton Century Croft, 1974:129–142.

168. Osuntokun BO, Osuntokun O, Adeloye A, et al. Primary neuro-ophthalmological presentation of Burkitt's lymphoma. *Afr J Med Sci* 1973;4:111–117.

169. Nkrumah FK, Perkins IV. Neurological manifestations of Burkitt's lymphoma in Ghana. *Afr J Med Sci* 1973;4:209–214.

170. Magrath IT, Mugerwa J, Bailey I, et al. Intracerebral Burkitt's lymphoma: pathology, clinical features and treatment. *Q J Med* 1974;43:489–508.

171. Sanchez Pina C, Pascual-Castroviejo I, Martinez Fernandez V, et al. Burkitt's lymphoma presenting as Tolosa-Hunt syndrome. *Pediatr Neurol* 1993;9:157–158.

172. Landesberg R, Yee H, Datikashvili M, et al. Unilateral mandibular lip anesthesia as the sole presenting symptom of Burkitt's lymphoma: case report and review of literature. *J Oral Maxillofac Surg* 2001;59:322–326.

173. Magrath I, Lee YJ, Anderson T, et al. Prognostic factors in Burkitt's lymphoma: importance of total tumor burden. *Cancer* 1980;45:1507–1515.

174. Ziegler JL. Treatment results of 54 American patients with Burkitt's lymphoma are similar to the African experience. *N Engl J Med* 1977;297:75–80.

175. Magrath I, Adde M, Shad A, et al. Adults and children with small non-cleaved-cell lymphoma have a similar excellent outcome when treated with the same chemotherapy regimen. *J Clin Oncol* 1996;14:925–934.

176. Adde M, Shad A, Venzon D, et al. Additional chemotherapy agents improve treatment outcome for children and adults with advanced B-cell lymphomas. *Semin Oncol* 1998;2(suppl 4):33–39.

177. Anderson JR, Jenkin RD, Wilson JF, et al. Long-term follow-up of patients treated with COMP or LSA2L2 therapy for childhood non-Hodgkin's lymphoma: a report of CCG-551 from the Childrens Cancer Group. *J Clin Oncol* 1993;11:1024–1032.

178. Meadows AT, Sposto R, Jenkin RD, et al. Similar efficacy of 6 and 18 months of therapy with four drugs (COMP) for localized non-Hodgkin's lymphoma of children: a report from the Childrens Cancer Study Group. *J Clin Oncol* 1989;7:92–99.

179. Link MP, Shuster JJ, Donaldson SS, et al. Treatment of children and young adults with early-stage non-Hodgkin's lymphoma. *N Engl J Med* 1997;337:1259–1266.

180. Patte C, Auperin A, Michon J, et al. The Societe Francaise d'Oncologie Pediatrique LMB89 protocol: highly effective multiagent chemotherapy tailored to the tumor burden and initial response in 561 unselected children with B-cell lymphomas and L3 leukemia. *Blood* 2001;97:3370–3379.

181. Patte C, Michon J, Frappaz D, et al. Therapy of Burkitt and other B-cell acute lymphoblastic leukaemia and lymphoma: experience with the LMB protocols of the SFOP (French Paediatric Oncology Society) in children and adults. *Baillieres Clin Haematol* 1994;7:339–348.

182. Patte C, Philip T, Rodary C, et al. High survival rate in advanced-stage B-cell lymphomas and leukemias without CNS involvement with a short intensive polychemotherapy: results from the French Pediatric Oncology Society of a randomized trial of 216 children. *J Clin Oncol* 1991;9:123–132.

183. Patte C. Treatment of mature B-ALL and high grade B-NHL in children. *Best Pract Res Clin Haematol* 2002;15:695–711.

184. Reiter A, Schrappe M, Ludwig WD, et al. Favorable outcome of B-cell acute lymphoblastic leukemia in childhood: a report of three consecutive studies of the BFM group. *Blood* 1992;80:2471–2478.

185. Reiter A, Schrappe M, Parwaresch R, et al. Non-Hodgkin's lymphomas of childhood and adolescence: results of a treatment stratified for biologic subtypes and stage—a report of the Berlin-Frankfurt-Munster Group. *J Clin Oncol* 1995;13:359–372.

186. Reiter A, Schrappe M, Tiemann M, et al. Improved treatment results in childhood B-cell neoplasms with tailored intensification of therapy: a report of the Berlin-Frankfurt-Munster Group Trial NHL-BFM 90. *Blood* 1999;94:3294–3306.

187. Woessmann W, Seidemann K, Mann G, et al. The impact of the methotrexate administration schedule and dose in the treatment of children and adolescents with B-cell neoplasms: a report of the BFM Group Study NHL-BFM95. *Blood* 2005;105:948–958.

188. Cairo MS, Gerrard M, Sposto R, et al. Results of a randomized international study of high-risk central nervous system B non-Hodgkin lymphoma and B acute lymphoblastic leukemia in children and adolescents. *Blood* 2007;109:2736–2743.

189. Patte C, Auperin A, Gerrard M, et al. Results of the randomized international FAB/LMB96 trial for intermediate risk B-cell non-Hodgkin lymphoma in children and adolescents: it is possible to reduce treatment for the early responding patients. *Blood* 2007;109:2773–2780.

190. Gerrard M, Cairo MS, Weston C, et al. Results of the FAB international study in children and adolescents (C+A) with localized, resected B cell lymphoma (large Cell [LCL], Burkitt [BL] and Burkitt-like [BLL]). *Proc Amer Soc Clin Oncol* 2003;22:795.

191. Burkitt D. Long-term remissions following one and two-dose chemotherapy for African lymphoma. *Cancer* 1967;20:756–759.

192. Clifford P, Singh S, Stjernsward J, et al. Long-term survival of patients with Burkitt's lymphoma: an assessment of treatment and other factors which may relate to survival. *Cancer Res* 1967;27:2578–2615.

193. Ziegler JL, Magrath IT, Olweny CL. Cure of Burkitt's lymphoma. Ten-year follow-up of 157 Ugandan patients. *Lancet* 1979;2:936–938.
194. Ziegler JL, Morrow RH Jr, Fass L, et al. Treatment of Burkitt's tumor with cyclophosphamide. *Cancer* 1970;26:474–484.
195. Olweny CL, Katongole-Mbidde E, Kaddu-Mukasa A, et al. Treatment of Burkitt's lymphoma: randomized clinical trial of single-agent versus combination chemotherapy. *Int J Cancer* 1976;17:436–440.
196. Olweny CL, Katongole-Mbidde E, Otim D, et al. Long-term experience with Burkitt's lymphoma in Uganda. *Int J Cancer* 1980;26:261–266.
197. Mead GM, Sydes MR, Walewski J, et al. An international evaluation of CODOX-M and CODOX-M alternating with IVAC in adult Burkitt's lymphoma: results of United Kingdom Lymphoma Group LY06 study. *Ann Oncol* 2002;13:1264–1274.
198. Djerassi I, Kim JS. Methotrexate and citrovorum factor rescue in the management of childhood lymphosarcoma and reticulum cell sarcoma (non-Hodgkin's lymphomas): prolonged unmaintained remissions. *Cancer* 1976;38:1043–1051.
199. Jones GR, Ettinger LJ. Continuous infusion of high-dose cytosine arabinoside for treatment of childhood acute leukemia and non-Hodgkin's lymphoma in relapse. *Semin Oncol* 1985;12(suppl 3):150–154.
200. Patte C, Bernard A, Hartmann O, et al. High-dose methotrexate and continuous infusion Ara-C in children's non-Hodgkin's lymphoma: phase II studies and their use in further protocols. *Pediatr Hematol Oncol* 1986;3:11–18.
201. Gentet JC, Patte C, Quintana E, et al. Phase II study of cytarabine and etoposide in children with refractory or relapsed non-Hodgkin's lymphoma: a study of the French Society of Pediatric Oncology. *J Clin Oncol* 1990;8:661–665.
202. Magrath I, Adde M, Sandlund J, et al. Ifosfamide in the treatment of high-grade recurrent non-Hodgkin's lymphomas. *Hematol Oncol* 1991;9:267–274.
203. Norin T, Clifford P, Einhorn J, et al. Conventional and superfractionated radiation therapy in Burkitt's lymphoma. *Acta Radiol Ther Phys Biol* 1971;10:545–557.
204. Link MP, Donaldson SS, Berard CW, et al. Results of treatment of childhood localized non-Hodgkin's lymphoma with combination chemotherapy with or without radiotherapy. *N Engl J Med* 1990;322:1169–1174.
205. Magrath IT, Haddy TB, Adde MA. Treatment of patients with high grade non-Hodgkin's lymphomas and central nervous system involvement: is radiation an essential component of therapy? *Leuk Lymphoma* 1996;21:99–105.
206. Kellie SJ, Pui CH, Murphy SB. Childhood non-Hodgkin's lymphoma involving the testis: clinical features and treatment outcome. *J Clin Oncol* 1989;7:1066–1070.
207. Haddy TB, Adde MA, McCalla J, et al. Late effects in long-term survivors of high-grade non-Hodgkin's lymphomas. *J Clin Oncol* 1998;16:2070–2079.
208. Magrath IT, Lwanga S, Carswell W, et al. Surgical reduction of tumour bulk in management of abdominal Burkitt's lymphoma. *Br Med J* 1974;2:308–312.
209. Attarbaschi A, Mann G, Dworzak M, et al. The role of surgery in the treatment of pediatric B-cell non-Hodgkin's lymphoma. *J Pediatr Surg* 2002;37:1470–1475.
210. LaQuaglia MP, Stolar CJ, Krailo M, et al. The role of surgery in abdominal non-Hodgkin's lymphoma: experience from the Childrens Cancer Study Group. *J Pediatr Surg* 1992;27:230–235.
211. Reiter A, Zimmermann W, Zimmermann M, et al. The role of initial laparotomy and second-look surgery in the treatment of abdominal B-cell non-Hodgkin's lymphoma of childhood. A report of the BFM Group. *Eur J Pediatr Surg* 1994;4:74–81.
212. Kazembe P, Hesseling PB, Griffin BE, et al. Long term survival of children with Burkitt lymphoma in Malawi after cyclophosphamide monotherapy. *Med Pediatr Oncol* 2003;40:23–25.
213. Arseneau JC, Canellos GP, Banks PM, et al. American Burkitt's lymphoma: a clinicopathologic study of 30 cases. I. Clinical factors relating to prolonged survival. *Am J Med* 1975;58:314–321.
214. Spreafico F, Massimino M, Luksch R, et al. Intensive, very short-term chemotherapy for advanced Burkitt's lymphoma in children. *J Clin Oncol* 2002;20:2783–2788.
215. Bernstein JI, Coleman CN, Strickler JG, et al. Combined modality therapy for adults with small noncleaved cell lymphoma (Burkitt's and non-Burkitt's types). *J Clin Oncol* 1986;4:847–858.
216. Hoelzer D, Ludwig WD, Thiel E, et al. Improved outcome in adult B-cell acute lymphoblastic leukemia. *Blood* 1996;87:495–508.
217. Brecher ML, Schwenn MR, Coppes MJ, et al. Fractionated cyclophosphamide and back to back high dose methotrexate and cytosine arabinoside improves outcome in patients with stage III high grade small noncleaved cell lymphomas (SNCCL): a randomized trial of the Pediatric Oncology Group. *Med Pediatr Oncol* 1997;29:526–533.
218. Holte H, Smeland S, Blystad AK, et al. Intensive chemotherapy in Burkitt's lymphoma and aggressive non-Hodgkin's lymphoma [in Norwegian]. *Tidsskr Nor Laegeforen* 2002;122:364–369.
219. Pees HW, Radtke H, Schwamborn J, et al. The BFM-protocol for HIV-negative Burkitt's lymphomas and L3 ALL in adult patients: a high chance for cure [abstract]. *Ann Hematol* 1992;65:201–205. Abstract.
220. Todeschini G, Tecchio C, Degani D, et al. Eighty-one percent event-free survival in advanced Burkitt's lymphoma/leukemia: no differences in outcome between pediatric and adult patients treated with the same intensive pediatric protocol. *Ann Oncol* 1997;(suppl 1):77–81.
221. Evens AM, Gordon LI. Burkitt's and Burkitt-like lymphoma. *Curr Treat Options Oncol* 2002;3:291–305.
222. Lacasce A, Howard O, Lib S, et al. Modified Magrath regimens for adults with Burkitt and Burkitt-like lymphomas: preserved efficacy with decreased toxicity. *Leuk Lymphoma* 2004;45:761–767.
223. Thomas DA, Cortes J, O'Brien S, et al. Hyper-CVAD program in Burkitt's-type adult acute lymphoblastic leukemia. *J Clin Oncol* 1999;17:2461–2470.
224. Rizzieri DA, Johnson JL, Niedzwiecki D, et al. Intensive chemotherapy with and without cranial radiation for Burkitt leukemia and lymphoma: final results of Cancer and Leukemia Group B Study 9251. *Cancer* 2004;100:1438–1448.
225. Chow KU, Sommerlad WD, Boehrer S, et al. Anti-CD20 antibody (IDEC-C2B8, rituximab) enhances efficacy of cytotoxic drugs on neoplastic lymphocytes in vitro: role of cytokines, complement, and caspases. *Haematologica* 2002;87:33–43.
226. Coiffier B. Rituximab in combination with CHOP improves survival in elderly patients with aggressive non-Hodgkin's lymphoma. *Semin Oncol* 2002;29(suppl 6):18–22.
227. Thomas DA, Faderl S, O'Brien S, et al. Chemoimmunotherapy with hyper-CVAD plus rituximab for the treatment of adult Burkitt and Burkitt-type lymphoma or acute lymphoblastic leukemia. *Cancer* 2006;106:1569–1580.
228. Pagel JM, Hedin N, Subbiah K, et al. Comparison of anti-CD20 and anti-CD45 antibodies for conventional and pretargeted radioimmunotherapy of B-cell lymphomas. *Blood* 2003;101:2340–2348.
229. Dunleavy K, Pittaluga S, Janik J, et al. Novel treatment of Burkitt lymphoma with dose-adjusted EPOCH-Rituximab: preliminary results showing excellent outcome. *Blood* 2006;108:774a.
230. Ziegler JL, Bluming AZ, Morrow RH, et al. Central nervous system involvement in Burkitt's lymphoma. *Blood* 1970;36:718–728.
231. Macdonald DR. Neurologic complications of chemotherapy. *Neurol Clin* 1991;9:955–967.
232. Olweny CL, Atine I, Kaddu-Mukasa A, et al. Cerebrospinal irradiation of Burkitt's lymphoma. Failure in preventing central nervous system relapse. *Acta Radiol Ther Phys Biol* 1977;16:225–231.
233. Gasparini M, Lombardi F, Bellani FF, et al. Childhood non-Hodgkin's lymphoma: long-term results of an intensive chemotherapy regimen. *Cancer* 1981;48:1508–1512.
234. Smibert E, Anderson V, Godber T, et al. Risk factors for intellectual and educational sequelae of cranial irradiation in childhood acute lymphoblastic leukaemia. *Br J Cancer* 1996;73:825–830.
235. Walter AW, Hancock ML, Pui CH, et al. Secondary brain tumors in children treated for acute lymphoblastic leukemia at St Jude Children's Research Hospital. *J Clin Oncol* 1998;16:3761–3767.
236. Jost LM, Jacky E, Dommann-Scherrer C, et al. Short-term weekly chemotherapy followed by high-dose therapy with autologous bone marrow transplantation for lymphoblastic and Burkitt's lymphomas in adult patients. *Ann Oncol* 1995;6:445–451.
237. Sweetenham JW, Pearce R, Taghipour G, et al. Adult Burkitt's and Burkitt-like non-Hodgkin's lymphoma—outcome for patients treated with high-dose therapy and autologous stem-cell transplantation in first remission or at relapse: results from the European Group for Blood and Marrow Transplantation. *J Clin Oncol* 1996;14:2465–2472.
238. van Imhoff GW, van der Holt B, MacKenzie MA, et al. Short intensive sequential therapy followed by autologous stem cell transplantation in adult Burkitt, Burkitt-like and lymphoblastic lymphoma. *Leukemia* 2005;19:945–952.
239. Song KW, Barnett MJ, Gascoyne RD, et al. Haematopoietic stem cell transplantation as primary therapy of sporadic adult Burkitt lymphoma. *Br J Haematol* 2006;133:634–637.
240. Peniket AJ, Ruiz de Elvira MC, Taghipour G, et al. An EBMT registry matched study of allogeneic stem cell transplants for lymphoma: allogeneic transplantation is associated with a lower relapse rate but a higher procedure-related mortality rate than autologous transplantation. *Bone Marrow Transplant* 2003;31:667–678.
241. Cohen LF, Balow JE, Magrath IT, et al. Acute tumor lysis syndrome. A review of 37 patients with Burkitt's lymphoma. *Am J Med* 1980;68:486–491.
242. Cabanillas F. Metabolic abnormalities in lymphoma. *Clin Lymphoma* 2002;3(suppl 1):S32–S36.
243. Cairo MS. Prevention and treatment of hyperuricemia in hematological malignancies. *Clin Lymphoma* 2002;(suppl 1):S26–S31.
244. Grigg AP, Seymour JF. Graft versus Burkitt's lymphoma effect after allogeneic marrow transplantation. *Leuk Lymphoma* 2002;43:889–892.

CHAPTER 23 ■ PLASMA CELL NEOPLASMS: MULTIPLE MYELOMA AND PLASMACYTOMA

JEAN-LUC HAROUSSEAU, HERVE AVET-LOISEAU, AND PHILIPPE MOREAU

Plasma cell neoplasms are a group of related disorders associated with the accumulation and proliferation of monoclonal immunoglobulin (Ig)-secreting plasma cells. They are characterized by the secretion of electrophoretically and immunologically homogeneous (monoclonal) proteins. Therefore, another frequently used word to describe these diseases is monoclonal gammopathies. In terms of incidence and severity, the most important is multiple myeloma (MM).

In MM, malignant plasma cells accumulate in the bone marrow and produce an entire monoclonal Ig (usually IgG or IgA) or only light chains (κ or λ). Common complications of symptomatic MM include osteolytic bone lesions, anemia, renal insufficiency, and recurrent infections. The incidence of MM is four to six per 100,000 per year, and it is primarily a disease of the elderly with a median age at diagnosis between 65 and 70 years. Plasmacytomas are rare plasma cell tumors that can arise in bone (solitary plasmacytoma of bone) or outside the bone marrow (extramedullary plasmacytomas).

DIAGNOSIS OF PLASMA CELL NEOPLASMS

In contrast to many other hematologic malignancies, the diagnosis of MM is not that easy. It is based on three types of evaluation: detection of the monoclonal protein (M component), detection of bone marrow plasma cell infiltration, and detection of related organ or tissue impairment (ROTI) (1). Using these three parameters, the International Myeloma Working Group has reviewed the criteria for the diagnosis of three different entities that correspond to different prognosis and patient management: monoclonal gammopathy of unknown significance (MGUS), asymptomatic or smoldering MM, and symptomatic MM (Table 23.1).

MGUSs are defined as plasma cell disorders characterized by a M component in the serum at a low level, that is, <30 g per L, and a bone marrow plasmacytosis <10%, the absence of any sign or symptom related to B-cell malignancies, and the absence of ROTI.

Asymptomatic MM is defined by the same exclusion criteria, but bone marrow plasmacytosis may be >10%.

The diagnosis of symptomatic MM, a malignancy that requires specific treatment, is based on the evidence of a plasma cell expansion, associated with specific organ damages. The recently reviewed diagnostic criteria require three major positive criteria:

1. Evidence for a M component in the serum or the urine (without minimal levels),

2. An excess of plasma cells in the bone marrow (>5%), or a histologically proven plasmacytoma,

3. Evidence for ROTI criteria. These criteria are: hypercalcemia (calcium level >2.75 mmol per L); renal insufficiency (creatinine level >173 mmol per L), anemia (hemoglobin level <100g per L); or bone lesions (calcemia, renal insufficiency, anemia, and bone lesions).

The first required parameter is the M component. This monoclonal component is IgG in 60% to 65% of the patients, IgA in 20% to 25%, and rarely IgD, IgM, or IgE (<3%). In these cases, the monoclonal component is present in the serum, and is detected on the serum protein electrophoresis (SPEP) and characterized by the immunofixation (IFX), which types heavy and light chains. In 15% to 20% of the cases, no M component is detected in the serum, but the urines present a high level of monoclonal proteins, the so-called "Bence-Jones proteinuria." In these latter cases, malignant plasma cells excrete only light chains that are rapidly eliminated in the urines. To detect, characterize, and quantify this M component, a urine protein electrophoresis (UPEP) and IFX on the 24-hour urines are required. A

TABLE 23.1

CLASSIFICATION OF MONOCLONAL GAMMOPATHIES ACCORDING THE INTERNATIONAL WORKING GROUP

Monoclonal gammopathy of undetermined significance (MGUS)

M-protein in serum <30 g/l
Bone marrow clonal plasma cells <10% and low level of plasma cell infiltration in a trephine biopsy (if done)
No evidence of other B-cell proliferative disorders
*No related organ or tissue impairment (no end organ damage, including bone lesions)

Smoldering (or asymptomatic) MM (AMM)

M-protein in serum ≥30 g/l <u>and/or</u>
Bone marrow clonal plasma <u>cells</u> ≥10%
No related organ or tissue impairment (no end organ damage, including bone lesions) or symptoms

Symptomatic MM
M-protein in serum and/or urine
Bone marrow (clonal) plasma cells* or plasmacytoma
Related organ or tissue impairment (end organ damage, including bone lesions)

quantitative evaluation of serum IgG, IgA, and IgM enables evaluation of "immunoparesis," that is the quantitative repression of nonmonoclonal Ig.

The second required parameter is the presence of malignant plasma cells. The malignant plasma cells are usually located within the bone marrow, and are evidenced by the analysis of bone marrow smears or trephine biopsies. A simple bone marrow smear is usually sufficient to detect and quantify the plasma cells. When negative, the bone marrow evaluation must be completed by a guided biopsy of a suspected plasmacytoma (see below Special Issues Solitary plasmacytomas). The third parameter is the demonstration of ROTI.

The most prominent is related to the bone disease. In the absence of specific symptoms such as pain or fractures, a radiologic skeletal bone survey, including skull, spine, pelvis, humerus, and femurs, should be performed. Typically, the bone lesions are osteolytic, with fractures, although osteocondensation might be rarely encountered. Magnetic resonance imaging (MRI) may be useful to evaluate specific risks, especially at the spine level. A complete blood count is necessary to measure hemoglobin level, which is <100 g per L in about half of the patients. It can also assess possible thrombocytopenia and, more rarely, circulating plasma cells. Finally, a chemistry screen, including calcium and creatinine, is mandatory to assess hypercalcemia (observed in 10% to 15% of the patients) and renal insufficiency (present in up to 20% of the patients at diagnosis).

Special Issues

These parameters enable MM diagnosis in the very large majority of patients. However, in some cases, diagnosis is more difficult.

"Non-secretory" myeloma is characterized by the presence of monoclonal malignant plasma cells in the bone marrow, but the absence of the M component, both in the serum and urine. In these cases, detection and quantification of serum free light chains are very useful (Freelite test, The Binding Site, Birmingham, UK). In fact, the term "non-secretory" is not well chosen. Malignant plasma cells do actually secrete light chains, but not enough to be adequately measured in the urines. A related entity is the so-called "low-secreting" myeloma, which is defined as a plasma cell clone secreting low amounts of M component. These diseases are defined by a monoclonal component lower than the "measurable disease" (serum M component >10 g per L, or urine M component >0.2 g per 24 hours). In these patients with non or low-secreting myeloma, response evaluation is more difficult, and serum free light chain measurement may be useful to assess response to treatment.

Solitary plasmacytomas of bone are rather uncommon (<3% of plasma cell neoplasms), and are characterized by an apparently unique (when standard x-rays are used) plasma cell bone tumor, usually involving the spine, without bone marrow involvement, and usually with low amounts of M component in the serum and/or urines. MRI or positron emission tomography may be useful to detect other bone lesions that are not detected on standard x-rays (multifocal plasmacytomas). Usually, the treatment is based on local control by high-dose radiotherapy. The prognosis is relatively favorable with longer survival than in MM. However, virtually all patients will develop systemic disease if followed for sufficient periods. The risk is higher in patients with multifocal plasmacytomas on MRI or if the M component does not disappear after local treatment. Solitary plasmacytomas may also occur outside of the bone marrow (extramedullary plasmacytoma). The less rare forms involve the upper respiratory tract, but virtually every organ may be involved. Treatment is also local, and disease-free survival is usually longer than in plasmacytomas of the bone.

Finally, a very rare presentation is the plasma cell leukemia (PCL). As usual, the definition is arbitrary: >2.0 g per L of circulating plasma cells, or >20% plasma cells in the peripheral blood differential white cell count. PCLs are classified as "primary" and "secondary," the latter corresponding to leukemic transformations of previous classic MM phases. Even when "primary," PCLs are associated with a very poor outcome.

Prognostic Factors

Although MM remains a fatal disease, with exceptional cases of possible cure, it is characterized by an extraordinary heterogeneity in outcome, with life expectancy from a few weeks up to ≥10 years. Several prognostic factors have been described, some associated with the tumor mass, others associated with the intrinsic biology of the malignant plasma cell. More recent prognostic models have included genetics, similarly to other hematologic malignancies.

Classic "Old" Parameters

Many prognostic parameters have been identified in MM (2). Age and performance status are among the most powerful. For many years, the most widely used staging system has been the Durie-Salmon classification, which was based on the tumor mass evaluation (M-component quantification, presence of anemia, and number of bone lesions on standard x-rays) and on renal function. β2-microglobulin (β2m) level has also been identified as a very strong prognostic factor, higher levels being associated with shorter survival. β2m levels are correlated as well to the tumor mass, and to the renal function. Other factors such as anemia, or lactate dehydrogenase and C-reactive protein levels, are also inversely correlated with survival. The plasma cell proliferation, as measured by labeling index, is also an important prognosis factor, although rarely used in clinical practice.

The International Staging System

In 2005, on behalf of the International Myeloma Foundation, a simple prognostic model has been reported, known as the "International Staging System (ISS)" (2). To build this model, authors gathered biologic data from >10,000 patients treated in 17 institutions or groups. They built a two-variable prognostic model, based on the β2-m and albumin levels. The model identifies three groups of patients, with an increasing risk of early death. Stage I is defined by a β2m level <3.5 mg per L and an albumin level >35 g per L. Stage 3 is defined by a β2m ≥5.5 mg per L. Stage 2 is defined by patients who do not meet criteria for stages 1 or 3. The median survival for patients with stages 1, 2, and 3 disease was 62, 44, and 29 months, respectively. This model is now widely used in clinical trials.

Cytogenetics

More recently, investigators have used cytogenetics and, more specifically, fluorescence in situ hybridization to assess the prognostic in myeloma. They did identify several prognostic parameters, including del (13), t(4;14), del (17p), and t(14;16), all predicting poor outcome (3–5). The strongest prognostic chromosomal abnormalities are the t(4;14) and the del (17p). The role of del (13) is more subject to debate; its prognostic power could be related to the t(4;14) and del (17p), frequently associated. These parameters are now widely used in clinical trials, at least for the stratification of the patients. For instance, the survival of patients with t(4;14) or del (17p) and especially if combined with a high β2m level, is in the 18 to 24-month range, even with tandem intensive strategies (6).

Gene Expression Profiling and Copy Number Changes

With the development of high throughput genetic tools, it becomes possible to interrogate several thousands of markers at the same time, enabling to get a more powerful system for prognostication. The first models have used gene expression profiling to find genes whose deregulation is associated with a good or poor prognostic. Actually, because the follow-up of the cohorts is usually short, most models have been focused on predicting short survival. Two models have been published, one based on 17 genes (7), and the second on 15 genes (8). Although no common gene is present in each model, it is both equally effective on control cohorts of patients. More recently, data have been reported using deoxyribonucleic acid microarrays to analyze the gains and losses of genetic material throughout the whole genome (9). These techniques, known as comparative genomic hybridization array or single nucleotide polymorphism array, are currently used to identify a small set of copy number changes that could be analyzed by fluorescence in situ hybridization. There is no doubt that these techniques will be used in the future in a clinical setting.

But also, we have to keep in mind that most of these prognostic models have been built in the era of "old conventional drugs." Some data are suggesting that the novel drug may overcome these prognostic parameters. This would mean that all these models should be revisited for patients treated with the novel therapies.

What is the clinical assessment at diagnosis. When MM is suspected, the clinical assessment should be:

- Physical examination
- Complete blood count
- Chemistry, including calcium and creatinine
- SPEP and IFX
- Quantitation of IgG, IgA, and IgM
- UPEP and IFX, on 24-hour urine collection
- Radiologic skeletal bone survey, ± MRI
- Bone marrow aspirate for smear analysis and fluorescence in situ hybridization
- β2m, C reactive protein, and lactate dehydrogenase for prognostic assessment
- Freelite in low-secreting myeloma

The evaluation of the M component must be performed on the SPEP and UPEP, not on the Freelite. During follow-up, the response evaluation must be performed using the same tests, and in the same laboratory, to avoid any differences related to technical reasons. When the SPEP and UPEP become negative (if ever), complete remission (CR) must be confirmed by serum and urine IFX. Bone marrow evaluation must be performed only if CR on serum and urine tests, or in case of suspicion of relapse.

TREATMENT OF MULTIPLE MYELOMA

MGUS should not be treated because the M-component level may remain constant over many years. The risk of transformation into an overt MM is estimated at 1% per year, and because there is currently no simple method to evaluate the risk of transformation in a given patient, it is recommended to follow these patients (watch and wait).

In the absence of curative treatment, smoldering MM should not be treated, and treatment is indicated only for symptomatic MM.

MM is not a chemosensitive malignancy. Alkylating agents and glucocorticoids are the most effective drugs against MM. During three decades, the combination of oral melphalan and prednisone (MP) has been the standard treatment (10). Combinations with other cytotoxic agents (Vinca alkaloids, anthracyclines, nitrosoureas) have not significantly improved the outcome. With these treatments, CRs were very rare, all patients ultimately relapsed, and the prognosis was invariably fatal, with a median overall survival (OS) of 3 years. Therefore, the first advance was the introduction almost 25 years ago of high-dose therapy (11), which was shown as much safer with a support by autologous hematopoietic stem cell transplantation (ASCT) (12,13). This approach has rapidly been considered the standard of care for younger patients, and MM has become the first indication of ASCT worldwide (14).

More recently, three novel agents have been successively introduced in the treatment of relapsed MM. These agents are thalidomide, the proteasome-inhibitor bortezomib (Velcade), and lenalidomide (Revlimid), which is a thalidomide analog with a different efficacy-toxicity ratio. They are different from cytotoxic agents because they act not only on the myeloma clone itself but also on the microenvironment and the cytokine circuit that are necessary for plasma cell proliferation and survival, and on the immune system. Their use in relapse treatment has already increased OS by offering new possibilities that can be given sequentially. Moreover, their introduction in frontline treatment is dramatically changing the scenario both in patients who are eligible for ASCT and in elderly or more frail patients.

Autologous Stem Cell Transplantation

Autologous Stem Cell Transplantation versus Conventional Chemotherapy

The Intergroupe Francophone du Myelome (IFM) was the first to conduct a randomized trial showing the superiority of high-dose therapy with ASCT compared with conventional chemotherapy as frontline therapy in 200 patients < 65 years of age (15). In this trial, high-dose therapy significantly improved response rate, including CR rate, event-free

TABLE 23.2

CONVENTIONAL CHEMOTHERAPY VS. HIGH-DOSE THERAPY: RESULTS OF RANDOMIZED STUDIES

Group/trial (reference)	No. of patients	Age (y)	Median follow-up	CR rate (%) or CR/VGPR rate		Median EFS (mo)		Median OS (mo)	
				CC	HDT	CC	HDT	CC	HDT
IFM 90 (15)	200	<65	7 y	5[a]	22[a]	18[a]	28[a]	44[a]	57[a]
MRC7 (16)	407	<65	42 mo	8[a]	44[a]	19[a]	31[a]	42[a]	54[a]
MAG91 (17)	190	55–65	56 mo	5[a]	19[a]	19[a]	24[a]	50	55
Italian MMSG (18)	195	<70	39 mo	6[a]	25[a]	15.6[a]	28[a]	42[a]	58+[a]
Pethema (19)	164	<65	44 mo	11[a]	30[a]	33	42	66	61
MAG95 (20)	190	55–65	10 y	20[a]	48[a]	19[a]	25[a]	48	48
US S9321 (21)	516	≤70	76 mo	15	17	7 y 14%	7 y 17%	7 y 38%	7 y 38%

[a] Significant.

survival (EFS), and OS. Similar results were published 7 years later by the British Medical Research Council (16), which, retrospectively, fully justified the use of ASCT as part of frontline treatment at least in patients up to 65 years of age without renal dysfunction. However, five other randomized studies have been published in the past 10 years, and not all were that positive (17–21). The results of all studies comparing ASCT and conventional chemotherapy are in Table 23.2.

In all but one study, the CR rate was superior in the ASCT arm, and in five of these six studies, this better tumor reduction translated into a significantly longer EFS. In the two studies that failed to show a significantly improved EFS, randomization was performed only after induction treatment, and patients with progressive disease were excluded from the comparison, whereas it has been shown that ASCT is a useful salvage treatment in primary refractory MM (14). Therefore, patients who do not respond to their induction therapy should receive ASCT as well.

- In only three of seven studies, OS was significantly improved, and a metaanalysis of 2,411 patients included into randomized trials confirms that ASCT improves progression-free survival (PFS) without significant benefit on survival (22). This is partly explained by the impact of ASCT at relapse in patients initially treated with conventional chemotherapy, and in one of these studies, there was no difference in OS between early and late (at progression) ASCT (17). However, the use of ASCT either initially or at relapse did improve OS (median OS 50 to 57 months).
- There is a strong relationship between quality of response and the final outcome. Although the prognostic impact of CR achievement could not be demonstrated with conventional chemotherapy because CR was such a rare event, in studies on high-dose therapy, CR or CR plus very good partial remission (VGPR) (>90 % reduction of the M component) is significantly associated with a better long-term outcome (15,23). As a consequence, response criteria in MM have been redefined to introduce the concept of CR and VGPR (24,25) (Table 23.3). In the U.S. Intergroup study, which failed to show any advantage of ASCT, the results of ASCT were not inferior to those achieved in other studies, but the results of conventional chemotherapy were better, especially the CR rate, which

was identical to that achieved with ASCT (21). Therefore, if results of conventional chemotherapy could be improved, for instance with novel agents, the superiority of ASCT might be no longer significant.

- Almost all studies have been performed in patients aged ≤65 years and without renal dysfunction. There have been encouraging pilot studies, but no randomized study in patients with renal failure (14). In older patients, there are conflicting results regarding the interest of two courses of intermediate-dose melphalan supported by ASCT (18,26). Currently, ASCT should not be proposed to elderly patients or to patients with renal failure out of a clinical trial.

THE CURRENT AUTOLOGOUS STEM CELL TRANSPLANTATION PROCEDURE

Studies performed since the early 1980s have clearly defined the standard of care for stem cell collection and conditioning regimen

Stem Cell Collection

Peripheral blood progenitor cells have completely replaced bone marrow as the source of stem cells because of easier accessibility and availability, faster hematopoietic recovery, and, possibly, lower tumor cell contamination (27). There is a significant correlation between the number of CD34+ cells infused and the speed of engraftment, especially of platelet recovery. The minimal dose of CD34+ cells necessary for safe engraftment is 2×10^6 per kg (28). Two methods are currently used for mobilizing stem cells into the peripheral blood, either high-dose cyclophosphamide plus granulocyte colony-stimulating factor or higher doses of granulocyte colony-stimulating factor alone. When stem cells are collected early in the course of the disease and without prior exposure to alkylating agents, the proportion of poor mobilizers is very low (<5%). Therefore, stem cells are usually collected after two to four courses of a dexamethasone-based induction regimen like vincristine, Adriamycin, and dexamethasone (VAD). Attempts to reduce contamination of the graft by tumor cells have not been convincing so far.

TABLE 23.3

CRITERIA FOR DEFINITION OF RESPONSE

	EBMT criteria[a] Blade et al. (24)	IMWG uniform criteria[b] Durie et al. (25)
sCR	ND	CR plus normal FLC ratio Absence of clonal plasma cells by immunochemistry or fluorescence
CR	- Absence of M protein in serum and urine by IFX - <5% bone marrow plasma cells - No increase of lytic bone lesions - Disappearance of soft tissue - Plasmacytomas	Same definition
VGPR	ND	Serum and urine M protein detectable by IFX but not on electrophoresis or 90% or greater reduction in serum M protein plus urine M-protein <100 mg per 24 h
PR	- ≥50% reduction of serum M protein - and reduction in 24-h urinary M protein by 90% or <200 mg - for nonsecretory MM ≥50% reduction in bone marrow plasma cells - ≥50% reduction in the size of soft tissue plasmacytomas	Same definition plus for nonsecretory MM, ≥50% decrease in the difference between involved and uninvolved FLC
MR	- 25-49% reduction of serum M protein - 50-89% reduction in 24-h urinary M protein - for nonsecretory MM 25-49% reduction in bone marrow plasma cells - 25-49% reduction in the size of soft tissue plasmacytomas	ND
NC or SD	Not meeting criteria for MR or PD	Not meeting criteria for PR or PD
PD	- >25% increase in serum M protein - >25% increase in 24-h urinary M protein - >25% increase in bone marrow plasma cells - >25% increase in the size of soft tissue plasmacytomas or new bone lesions	Same definition plus - absolute increase in serum M protein ≥0.5 g per dL - absolute increase in urine M protein ≥200 mg per 24 h - for nonsecretory MM, increase in the difference between involved and uninvolved FLC >10 mg per dL

FLC, free light chain; MR, minimal response; NC, no change; ND, not defined; PD, progressive disease; PR, partial remission; sCR, stringent CR; SD, stable disease.
[a] Maintained at least 6 weeks.
[b] Two consecutive assessments before any new therapy.

Conditioning Regimen

The standard conditioning regimen is melphalan 200 mg per m^2, which has replaced the combination of melphalan 140 mg per m^2 plus total body irradiation due to a better efficacy-toxicity ratio (29). Until now no randomized study has shown the superiority of any other regimen compared with melphalan 200 mg per m^2.

Single versus Double Autologous Stem Cell Transplantation

The concept of double-intensive therapy was introduced in the late 1980s with the objective of further increasing the CR rate (30). The Arkansas group has developed a series of intensive programs named Total Therapy based on the use of double ASCT in newly diagnosed patients (31,32). The IFM was again the first to conduct a randomized trial comparing single and double ASCT, and showed that the more aggressive

strategy was significantly superior in terms of EFS and OS (33). Two other randomized studies confirmed that double ASCT prolonged EFS but failed to show an OS benefit (34,35) (Table 23.4). Although the feasibility and safety of this tandem ASCT approach have been confirmed, many investigators considered that the benefit for the patients was marginal, and were concerned by cost and morbidity issues. Therefore, defining which patients benefit from double ASCT is crucial. Until now, the only parameter predicting for the interest of the second is the result of the first because the outcome was not better after the second transplantation in patients achieving CR or VGPR after the first (33,34).

Allogeneic Stem Cell Transplantation

Allogeneic stem cell transplantation (allo-SCT) was introduced in the treatment of MM in the early 1980s but still remains a controversial issue (36). When given in newly diagnosed patients, allo-SCT may induce molecular remissions (37), and one-third of patients obtain long-term disease-free

TABLE 23.4

SINGLE VS. DOUBLE ASCT: RESULTS OF PUBLISHED RANDOMIZED TRIALS

	Number of patients	EFS	OS
IFM 94 (33)	399	7 y = 10% vs. 20% (p <0.03)	7 y 21% vs. 42% (p <0.01)
Bologna 96 (34)	321	Median 23 vs. 35 mo (p< 0.001)	7 y 46% vs. 43% (p = 0.90)
Hovon 24 (35)	304	Median 22 vs. 21 mo	Median 50 vs. 55 mo (p = 0.51)
		6 y 15% vs. 7% (p = 0.013)	

survival (38). Therefore, allo-SCT appears to be the only available therapy with a potential for cure at least in some patients. However, toxicity is extremely high, with a transplant-related mortality up to 50%, related to graft versus host disease and infections (39,40). Moreover, allo-SCT could only be proposed to patients <55 years of age, and only a small minority of patients with a human leukocyte antigen identical donor were eligible. Although toxicity is lower when allo-SCT is performed early (41), two prospective studies on allo-SCT as primary therapy yielded very poor results (21,42), and classic allo-SCT with myelo-ablative conditioning regimen has been almost completely abandoned.

More recently, reduced intensity conditioning (RIC) regimens were proposed to reduce transplant-related toxicity while harnessing the immunologic effect of donor lymphoid cells. Large retrospective surveys have confirmed that this approach is feasible, even with unrelated donors and in patients up to the age of 65 (43,44). Although graft versus host disease is still a concern, toxicity is reduced, compared with myelo-ablative regimens. However, relapse risk is higher, especially in patients with relapsed or progressive disease. Currently, RIC allo-SCT is mostly used after tumor reduction with high-dose melphalan plus ASCT (45,46). Prospective studies comparing ASCT/RIC allo-SCT and double ASCT in newly diagnosed patients yield controversial results.

An Italian study showed the superiority of RIC allo-SCT, due to a higher CR rate and a lower relapse risk (47). However, two other studies did not fully confirm this result because there was no benefit from RIC allo-SCT in terms of EFS or OS (48,49) (Table 23.5).

This difference in the outcome could be explained by differences in the conditioning regimen and in the selection of patients. But more importantly, 1-year transplant-related mortality remains as high as 10% to 15%, and reduction of the relapse risk is partly related to the occurrence of chronic graft versus host disease, which may significantly impact quality of life and induce life-threatening delayed complications. Considering that the prognosis in younger patients has already been improved by ASCT, with much less morbidity and mortality, and that it might be further improved with the addition of novel agents, the risk of RIC allo-SCT does not appear to be justified in newly diagnosed patients without poor risk characteristics.

Novel Agents in Relapsed Multiple Myeloma

Results of large studies with novel agents in relapsed MM are shown in Table 23.6.

TABLE 23.5

PROSPECTIVE STUDIES COMPARING TANDEM AUTOLOGOUS/REDUCED INTENSITY ALLO-SCT AND TANDEM ASCT

	Bruno et al. (47)		Garban et al. (48)		Rosinol et al. (49)	
	Auto/Ric Allo	Double Auto	Auto/Ric Allo	Double Auto	Auto/Ric Allo	Double Auto
Number of patients	58	46	46	166	25	85
Selection criteria	No		Poor-risk MM (high β2m plus deletion 13)		Patients failing to achieve at least n-CR after first ASCT	
Conditioning regimen	Low-dose TBI (200 cGy)		Busulfan ATG Fludarabine		Fludarabine/melphalan	
CR rate (%)	55%	26%	62%	51%	40%	11%
TRM	10%	2%	11%		16%	5%
AGVH $\geq$2	43%	–	24%	–	32%	–
cGVH	32%	–	36%	–	66%	–
Median OS	NR at 46 mo	46 mo	35	47	NR 62% at 5 y	58 mo 61% at 5 y
Median EFS	43 mo	33 mo	32	35	19.6 mo	26 mo

aGVH, acute graft-versus-host disease; Allo, allogeneic stem cell transplantation; Auto, autologous stem cell transplantation; cGVH, chronic graft versus host disease; nCR, near-complete response; NR, not reached; Ric, reduced-intensity conditioning; TBI, total body irradiation; TRM, transplant-related mortality.

TABLE 23.6

NOVEL AGENTS IN RELAPSED/REFRACTORY MM

	Thalidomide (54)	Bortezomib (61,68)	Bortezomib + PLD (68)	Lenalidomide + Dex (71, 72)
Response rate	28%	43–44%	52%	59%
CR rate	2%	16%	17%	13–15%
PFS	35% at 1 y	med 6 mo	med 9 mo	med 11–15 mo

med, median; PLD, pegylated liposomal doxorubicin.

Thalidomide

The Arkansas group was the first to report on the efficacy of thalidomide as a single agent at a dose range of 200 to −800 mg per day, with an overall response rate of 25% in heavily pretreated patients (50). The rationale for using thalidomide was based on its antiangiogenic properties because in MM, increased microvessel density has been correlated to survival (51). However, thalidomide has multiple modes of action, including immunomodulatory effects (52,53). This initial experience generated a great enthusiasm, and a large number of phase II trials were rapidly conducted. A systematic review of 42 such trials on >1,600 patients confirms that the response rate is 28% with an estimated 1-year OS of 60% (54). The well-known teratogenicity of thalidomide is not a major concern in patients with MM but justifies careful information of patients and programs to avoid drug exposure in women of childbearing potential. The major toxicities of thalidomide are fatigue, somnolence, constipation, and mostly peripheral neuropathy, which is related to the daily dosage and to treatment duration (52,55). The overall incidence of peripheral neuropathy is 30% but may be higher if treatment is prolonged for >1 year. Because this complication may be disabling and sometimes irreversible, patients should decrease the dose or stop treatment if significant paresthesia or numbness occurs.

Thalidomide has been rapidly combined with dexamethasone or cytotoxic agents with the objective of increasing efficacy and of reducing toxicity by decreasing the daily dosage. The combination of lower doses of thalidomide (100 to 200 mg per day) with dexamethasone does apparently increase the response rate to 45% (52) and is superior to conventional chemotherapy in first relapse in a historical comparison (56). Combination with cytotoxic agents (alkylating agents like melphalan or cyclophosphamide, or anthracyclines) may be even more active (60% to 65% response rate) (52,55). However, until now no randomized study has been conducted to confirm the superiority of combinations versus single agent. Moreover, combinations have increased infections, and generated a new and unexpected adverse event, i.e., deep vein thrombosis/pulmonary embolism. The incidence of this complication is up to 15% with dexamethasone and up to 30% in anthracycline-containing regimens. The risk is higher in patients with a high tumor burden, and prophylaxis with low-molecular weight heparin or oral anticoagulants should be considered in high-risk patients (52,55).

Bortezomib

Bortezomib (Velcade) is the first agent of a new class, proteasome inhibitors, that has demonstrated significant in vitro and in vivo activity on myeloma cell lines and in murine model (57,58). These studies led to the rapid development of this drug in relapsed MM. Two phase II studies (SUMMIT Study of Uncontrolled Multiple Myeloma Managed with Proteasome Inhibition Therapy and CREST Clinical Response and Efficacy Study of bortezomib in the Treatment of relapsing myeloma trials) have shown that in heavily pretreated patients, response rate with bortezomib alone is 25% to 30% and can be increased to 45% to 50% with the addition of dexamethasone (59,60). Following these studies, the drug has been rapidly approved in the United States and Europe. It is administered intravenously at a dose of 1.3 mg per m^2 on days 1, 4, 8, and 11 of 28-day cycles. The large randomized phase III trial, Assessment of Proteasome Inhibition for Extending Remissions (APEX), has demonstrated that bortezomib is superior to dexamethasone in patients with relapsed disease, in terms of response rate, time to progression, and OS (61). This superiority was confirmed in a subanalysis focusing on patients having received only one line of treatment (first relapse) (62). Based on these phase II–III trials, the toxicity profile of the drug is well defined. The most frequent side effects are gastrointestinal symptoms, which are usually mild. Bortezomib is not myelotoxic but induces rapidly reversible thrombocytopenia (40% to 60% decrease in the platelet count) (63). Peripheral neuropathy is observed in 30% to 40% of cases (grade 3 or 4 in 10% to 15%). Signs and symptoms are reversible in two of three of cases after dose reduction or drug discontinuation (64). Bortezomib appears to be as effective in older patients (65) and can be prescribed safely in patients with renal failure (66), even in patients on dialysis (67).

Bortezomib has been rapidly combined with dexamethasone or cytotoxic agents as well. A large randomized phase III trial has shown the superiority of bortezomib plus pegylated liposomal doxorubicin compared with bortezomib alone in terms of time to progression (68).

Lenalidomide

Lenalidomide (Revlimid) is a thalidomide analog with comparable modes of action but with a more potent in vitro efficacy. This agent is also active in myelodysplastic syndromes associated with chromosome 5 long arm deletion and is currently evaluated in a number of hematologic malignancies. Clinical development has been rapid as well. After the phase I study, it became apparent that the toxicity profile of lenalidomide was completely different (69). Constipation, somnolence, fatigue, and peripheral neuropathy that are frequent with thalidomide were rarely observed. The most frequent side effect was myelosuppression, mostly after 28 days. In phase II trials, the drug was administered orally for 21 consecutive days (70). In heavily pretreated patients, response rate was 25% and was further increased by the addition of dexamethasone. Therefore, for subsequent clinical development, lenalidomide (at a dose of 25 mg per day for 21 days in 28-day cycles) was combined with dexamethasone. Two large randomized trials with a similar design were conducted in the United States and Europe (71,72). They both showed the superiority of this combination compared with dexamethasone plus placebo, in terms of response rate, time to progression, and OS. Based on these results, lenalidomide was approved for the treatment of relapsed MM both in the United States and Europe. However, like with thalidomide, this combination increases the risk of deep vein thrombosis and justifies prophylaxis at least with low-dose aspirin. This drug should be used with caution in patients with renal dysfunction (73). Because it is mostly eliminated by the kidney, myelotoxicity (especially thrombocytopenia) is higher in patients with <50 ml per minute creatinine clearance

Combinations with cytotoxic agents are currently being evaluated in patients with relapsed disease.

Combination of Novel Agents

Because the toxicity profile of these agents is different, it appeared logical to combine them with the objective of increasing efficacy without increasing toxicity. Moreover, combination of an immunomodulatory drug (thalidomide or lenalidomide) with bortezomib was attractive due to a possible synergy of agents having different modes of action. Thalidomide and bortezomib have been combined with either dexamethasone or melphalan-prednisone, with promising results and an acceptable toxicity (74,75). However, because both agents may induce neurologic toxicity, the combination of lenalidomide and bortezomib could be even more attractive (76).

Novel Agents for Frontline Therapy in Older Patients

Older patients (>65 years) did not benefit from the improvement related to high-dose therapy plus ASCT, whereas they represent >50% of patients with MM. The standard of care for patients with de novo MM older than 65 years remained the classic MP regimen and no significant improvement had occurred in the past 40 years. The introduction of novel agents is dramatically changing the prognosis.

Melphalan-Based Combinations

Thalidomide

The IFM and the Italian group have published randomized studies comparing the addition of thalidomide with the MP protocol (MPT) to MP alone (26,77). In both studies, the response rate and PFS were significantly superior in the MPT arm. However, whereas in the French study, OS was also better with thalidomide (Fig. 23.1), in the Italian study, there was no significant difference between the two arms, due to a better salvage (including salvage with thalidomide) after relapse in the no-thalidomide arm (78). The consequence of these two studies is that at last MP should not be considered any longer the standard and should be replaced by MPT. In April 2008, the European Medicines Agency granted approval of MPT as frontline therapy in elderly patients. In another IFM randomized study, only patients >75 years were included, and again MPT (with lower doses of melphalan and thalidomide) was superior to MP in terms of response rate, PFS, and OS, meaning that this treatment could be proposed to very old patients (79). Two other randomized studies have been reported in meetings (80,81). Results of all five studies are in Table 23.7. Overall, in all five studies, response rates (including CR/VGPR rates) were superior in the MPT arm, which translated into a significantly longer PFS in four out of five studies. However, OS was significantly better with MPT only in the two IFM studies. Remaining questions are the optimal doses and duration of treatment because toxicity was a significant concern. In the Nordic group trial, the doses of melphalan and thalidomide might have been too high for those patients over the age of 75 or in poor general condition, which probably explains the absence of PFS benefit in the MPT arm (80).

Bortezomib

The Spanish group has published a phase I/II pilot study evaluating the efficacy and toxicity of bortezomib combined with MP in elderly patients (82). The unprecedented 35% CR rate was the rationale for the randomized trial, Velcade* as Initial STAndard therapy (VISTA) in multiple myeloma, which has been recently completed in >650 patients who were not eligible for ASCT (83). This trial fully confirms the efficacy of bortezomib combined with MP with an overall response of 82%, including a 35% CR defined by a negative IFX. This impressive result translated into a significantly better time-to-progression (TTP) and OS compared with MP. Results were equally good in older patients and in patients with renal dysfunction. The major toxicity associated with bortezomib was peripheral neuropathy, but the duration of treatment was not shorter in the MPT arm. Therefore, bortezomib combined with MP should also be considered as a new standard of care in older patients, and bortezomib was approved by the U.S. Food and Drug Administration in June 2008 for frontline treatment of MM.

Lenalidomide

The Italian group has published encouraging results with the combination of MP plus lenalidomide (84), which are the basis of an ongoing randomized trial comparing MP and MP plus lenalidomide.

Dexamethasone-Based Combinations

Pilot studies with thalidomide plus dexamethasone in newly diagnosed patients showed response rates of 65% to 70% (85,86). In a recently reported randomized study, this combination did increase the response rate compared with MP, but the final outcome did not appear to be superior due to a higher toxicity (87).

The combination of lenalidomide plus dexamethasone (RD) in frontline therapy for elderly patients appears to be more attractive. Preliminary results of a randomized trial show that the combination is clearly superior to dexamethasone alone in patients ineligible for ASCT (88). An Eastern Cooperative Oncology Group randomized trial has compared lenalidomide with either high-dose dexamethasone (RD) (three 4-day blocks per month) or low-dose dexamethasone (Rd) (once weekly)

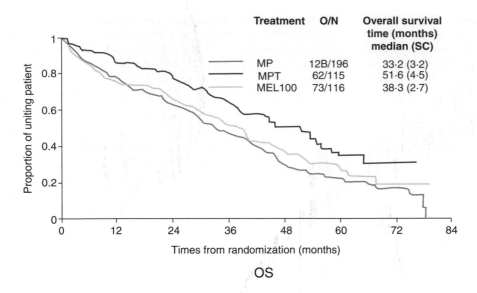

OS

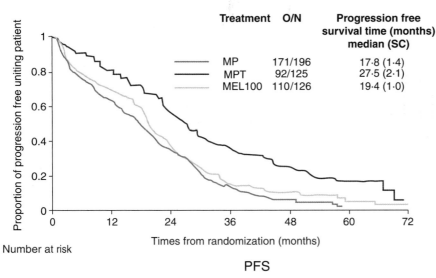

Number at risk

PFS

FIGURE 23.1 Comparison of MP, intermediate-dose melphalan plus ASCT, and MPT. **A:** OS. **B:** PFS. O/N, Number of Observed Events/total Number of Patients; SE, standard error. (Adapted from Facon T, Mary JY, Hulin C, et al. Melphalan and prednisone plus thalidomide versus melphalan and prednisone or reduced-intensity autologous stem cell transplantation in elderly patients with multiple myeloma (IFM 99-06): a randomized trial. *Lancet* 2007;370:1209–1218.)

TABLE 23.7

MPT VS. MP IN ELDERLY PATIENTS. RESULTS OF RANDOMIZED STUDIES

	GIMEMA (77)		IFM 99.06 (26)		IFM 01.01 (79)		NMSG (80)		HOVON (81)	
No. of patients	331 (67)		447 (126)		232 (13)		362 (182)		301 (152)	
Age (median)	60–85 (72)		65–75 (69)		76–91 (78.5)		49–92 (74.5)		(72)	
WHO ≥3 (%)	5		8		7		30		4	
MPT regimen										
No. of cycles	6		12		12		Until plateau		Until plateau	
Daily dosage of thalidomide (mg)	100		Up to 400		100		Up to 400		200	
Maintenance	+		−		−		+		+	
Comparison MPT vs. MP	MPT	MP	MPT	MP	MPT	MP	MPT	MP	MPT	MP
Response rate (%)	69	48	76	35	61	31	57	40	63	48
CR + VGPR (%)	29	11	47	7	23	8	23	7	29	9
Median PFS (mo)	22	14.5	27.5	18	24	19	16	14	$p < 0.001$	$p < 0.001$
Median OS (mo)	45	47	51.5	33	45	27.5	29	33	$p =$ NS	$p =$ NS

NS, not significant; WHO, World Health Organization.

(89). Although RD induced more responses, 2-year OS was superior in the Rd arm in patients over the age of 65. Although the follow-up time is still short, the very high OS rates indicate that Rd could be another standard of care in elderly patients. A randomized trial comparing MPT and RD in elderly patients is just starting.

NOVEL AGENTS FOR FRONTLINE THERAPY IN YOUNGER PATIENTS

Currently, ASCT is the standard of care for frontline therapy in younger patients. Although long-term PFS was achieved in patients with initial good risk characteristics, the majority of patients had relapse, and median PFS is in the range of 24 months with single ASCT and of 30 to 36 months with double ASCT. Consolidation chemotherapy may further improve the outcome, especially in patients without cytogenetic abnormalities (32), but dose intensification is limited by toxicity and is not useful in patients with poor risk cytogenetics (14). Therefore, the introduction of novel agents in the ASCT paradigm represents a new hope. Novel agents can be used before and/or after ASCT.

Novel Agents After Autologous Stem Cell Transplantation

Because almost all patients ultimately have relapse after ASCT, maintenance therapy is a logical approach to prolong remission duration.

Three randomized studies have evaluated the impact of thalidomide given as maintenance treatment after ASCT (90–92). Results are in Table 23.8. All three studies showed a significant benefit in terms of CR/VGPR rates, PFS, and OS, and as a consequence, thalidomide could be proposed as maintenance therapy after ASCT. However, two questions remain:

1. Should maintenance therapy with thalidomide be given to all patients? In the IFM study, post-ASCT thalidomide was useful only in patients who did not achieve at least VGPR after ASCT (90), which was not confirmed by the Australian study (92).

2. What are the optimal dose and duration of treatment? Peripheral neuropathy was the limiting factor for prolonged treatment and was less frequent in the Tunisian study in which patients received only 6 months of treatment (91).

Randomized trials are currently testing bortezomib and lenalidomide in this setting.

Novel Agents Before Autologous Stem Cell Transplantation

In the ASCT setting, there is a correlation between CR/VGPR achievement and the final outcome. One way to increase the CR/VGPR rate is to improve the initial treatment before ASCT (induction treatment).

Standard induction treatments (dexamethasone alone or VAD) yield <10% CR before ASCT and 25% to 40% CR after ASCT. The objective of using novel agents as induction treatments was, therefore, to increase the CR (or CR/VGPR) rate both before and after ASCT.

Thalidomide-Based Regimens

Thalidomide combined with dexamethasone was the first novel agent to be tested in this setting, and was compared with standard induction treatment in one historical control and two randomized studies (Table 23.9) (93–95). In all three studies, Thalidomide plus Dexamethasone (TD) induced more responses before ASCT, but there was no significant increase of the CR rate both before and after ASCT. Therefore, the addition of a third agent (cyclophosphamide or Adriamycin) looks more attractive with a significant increase of the CR/VGPR after ASCT (Table 23.9) (96,97).

Bortezomib-Based Regimens

Phase II studies of bortezomib plus dexamethasone (VD) regimens showed very high response rates (66% to 88%), and an apparent increase of CR/VGPR rates both before (22% to 31%) and after (approximately 55%) ASCT (98–100). In a small pilot study, the addition of Adriamycin appeared to further increase CR/VGPR rates up to 60% before and 80% after ASCT (101). The randomized IFM 2005-01 trial has confirmed that VD is superior to VAD in terms of CR/VGPR

TABLE 23.8

THALIDOMIDE AS MAINTENANCE THERAPY AFTER ASCT. RESULTS OF RANDOMIZED STUDIES.

Author	Number of patients	Dose and duration of treatment	CR rate (%)	PFS/EFS	OS	Peripheral neuropathy grade 3/4 (%)	Thalidomide discontinuation (%)
Attal et al. (90)	597	Median dose 300 mg per d. After ASCT and until progression or adverse event.	67 vs. 55 vs. 57[a]	3-y EFS 52% vs. 36% vs. 37%	4-y OS 87% vs. 77% vs. 74%	7	39
Abdelkefi et al. (91)	195	100 mg per d 6 mo after ASCT	68 vs. 54[a]	3-y PFS 85% vs. 57%	3-y OS 85% vs. 65%	4	9
Spencer et al. (92)	243	200 mg d 12 mo after ASCT	61 vs. 38[a]	3-y PFS 41% vs. 24%	3-y OS 86% vs. 75%	10	31

[a] CR + VGPR within 2 y.

TABLE 23.9

THALIDOMIDE-BASED INDUCTION REGIMENS BEFORE ASCT. RESULTS OF COMPARATIVE STUDIES

	TD vs. VAD	TD vs. VAD	TD vs. D	TAD vs. VAD	TLD vs. CVAD
Author	Cavo et al. (93)	Rajkumar et al. (94)	Macro et al. (95)	Lokhorst et al. (96)	Morgan et al. (97)
Number of patients	200	201	204	406	251
RR after induction	RR = 76% vs. 52% CR = NS	RR = 69% vs. 51% CR = NS	≥ VGPR 35% vs. 17%	≥ VGPR 33% vs. 15%	≥ VGPR 38% vs. 26%
RR after ASCT	NA	NA	≥ VGPR 44% vs. 42%	≥ VGPR 49% vs. 32%	≥ VGPR 67% vs. 43%
DVT	15% vs. 2%	17% vs. 3%	23% vs. 7.5%	8% vs. 4%[a]	NA

DVT, deep-vein thrombosis; NA, not applicable; NS, not significant; RR, response rate.
[a] Prophylaxis with low-molecular weight heparin.

TABLE 23.10

BORTEZOMIB-BASED INDUCTION REGIMENS BEFORE ASCT. RESULTS OF RANDOMIZED STUDIES

	VAD vs. VD (4 cycles) Harousseau et al. (102)	TD vs. VTD (3 cycles) Cavo et al. (103)
Number of patients	482	256
Before ASCT		
CR (%)	8 vs. 19	0 vs. 36
CR + VGPR (%)	19 vs. 47	27 vs. 60
After ASCT		
CR (%)	23 vs. 35	28 vs. 57
CR + VGPR (%)	45 vs. 63	54 vs. 77
Peripheral neuropathy		
Grade 3 (%)	1 vs. 6	2 vs. 7

VTD, thalidomide, bortezomib, and dexamethasone.

rates before and after ASCT (102). With VD, stem cell collection was adequate in 96% of patients, and the most important toxicity was peripheral neuropathy (grade 2 in 18% and grade 3 in 7% of patients) (Table 23.10).

Ongoing randomized trials are testing the addition of a third agent (Adriamycin or thalidomide) to VD. Preliminary results of a randomized Italian trial suggest that the addition of thalidomide to VD is superior to TD and might yield CR/VGPR rates superior to 70% (103).

However, it is too early to know whether the better tumor burden reduction achieved with VD regimens will translate into better PFS and OS. If this was the case, VD-based regimens might be considered the new standard induction treatments before ASCT.

Lenalidomide-Based Regimens

Experience with lenalidomide in induction treatment before ASCT is more limited.

Phase II and III studies with RD as primary therapy are difficult to evaluate because only a subgroup of patients was actually candidates to ASCT, but preliminary results are very encouraging with high 2-year PFS, up to 85%, for patients undergoing ASCT (89,104,105). However, there are some concerns regarding the hematopoietic quality of stem cell collection with granulocyte colony-stimulating factor alone (106,107). Therefore, more studies are needed to assess the efficacy-toxicity ratio of this promising combination as induction treatment before ASCT. More recently, the combination of RD and bortezomib has shown an impressive response rate of 98% in newly diagnosed patients (108) and could also be a new induction treatment before ASCT.

Novel Agents Before and After Autologous Stem Cell Transplantation

The first trial using novel agents before and after ASCT was the so-called Total Therapy 2, developed by the Arkansas group (109). This protocol consisted of four consecutive phases: induction chemotherapy, double ASCT, consolidation with chemotherapy, and maintenance with dexamethasone plus interferon. Patients were randomly assigned to receive thalidomide from treatment initiation to progression or undue toxicity, or no thalidomide. With a median follow-up of 5 years, the median EFS and OS for the 668 patients enrolled in this trial were respectively 4.8 and 8 years, whereas in the previous study from the same group, with a less intensive strategy and without thalidomide, the median EFS and OS were only 2.6 and 5.7 years (110). Although the comparison between Total Therapy 1 and Total Therapy 2 was not randomized, adjusting for prognostic variables in multivariate and pair-mates analyses supports the superiority of Total Therapy 2. This outstanding result appears to be related both to a more aggressive treatment and to thalidomide.

In Total Therapy 3, the same group has incorporated bortezomib up-front in a tandem-ASCT regimen derived from Total Therapy 2 (111). In this complex protocol, bortezomib was added to thalidomide and chemotherapy both during induction and consolidation, and maintenance was administered during 1 year with bortezomib, thalidomide, and dexamethasone, and during one additional year with thalidomide plus dexamethasone. Preliminary results with a median follow-up of 2 years are impressive with 90% 2-year CR rate and an estimated 2-year EFS of 89%.

Novel Agents with or without Up-Front Autologous Stem Cell Transplantation?

Combinations of MP with novel agents as primary therapy in older patients have obtained impressive results with CR rates and PFS that are comparable to those achieved in younger patients with one course of intensive therapy plus ASCT. One can speculate that these results could be at least similar if not better in younger patients. Combinations of lenalidomide plus dexamethasone yield very high CR/VGPR rates if treatment is prolonged or if bortezomib is added (105,108), and although follow-up is too short to be sure that these unexpectedly high tumor burden reductions will translate into sustained disease control, some investigators consider that ASCT should be abandoned as primary treatment for younger patients and could be saved for salvage treatment. Randomized studies comparing these two approaches will start soon.

Treatment of Special Entities

Solitary Plasmacytoma

For both solitary plasmacytoma of bone and extramedullary plasmacytoma, the treatment of choice is local radiotherapy at a total dose of at least 4,000 to 4,500 cGy (112). Currently, there is no role for systemic treatment that should be deferred until there is evidence of disease progression.

Approximately 30% of patients with solitary plasmacytoma remain long-term disease-free. Patients with the best prognosis are those in whom the M component disappears after radiotherapy.

The prognosis of solitary extramedullary plasmacytoma is even better because 70% remain disease free 10 years after radiotherapy.

Radiation therapy can also provide excellent palliation for pain, signs of cord or nerve root compression, and significant bone destruction to help reduce a risk of fracture. Doses of 30 Gy in 300-cGy fractions or 40 to 44 Gy in 200-cGy fractions provide excellent long-term control of disease.

Plasma Cell Leukemia

PCL is a severe form of plasma cell disorder, with a median survival of only 8 to 12 months, due to an aggressive behavior and a high incidence of poor risk features (113, 114). Treatment with conventional chemotherapy is ineffective. There have been some anecdotal reports of prolonged survival with ASCT (115,116). The role of novel agents in this disease is not yet known, although preliminary reports with bortezomib look promising (117,118).

CONCLUSION

Although there has been no significant change in the prognosis of MM during the last 30 years, the treatment and outcome have dramatically changed in the past 15 years.

In the 1990s, the introduction of high-dose therapy plus ASCT was the first improvement. By increasing the quality of response, ASCT prolonged PFS and OS, but only for younger patients without comorbidities. Although the great majority of patients undergoing ASCT ultimately have

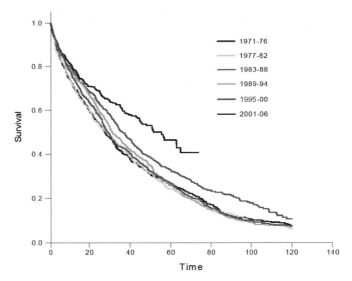

FIGURE 23.2 Improvement of OS related to the introduction of novel therapies. (Adapted from Kumar S, Rajkumar SV, Dispenzieri A, et al. Improved survival in multiple myeloma and the impact of novel therapies. *Blood* 2008;111:2516–2520.)

relapse, long-term PFS can be obtained in patients with good prognostic characteristics (119).

More recently, the introduction of thalidomide, bortezomib, and lenalidomide has already markedly improved the outcome of patients of all ages. Their successive use for relapsed MM has induced a 50% improvement of OS according to the Mayo Clinic experience (120) (Fig. 23.2). The addition of novel agents to frontline therapy (MP or dexamethasone) is becoming the new standard of care for elderly patients, more than 40 years after the introduction of MP.

Finally, novel agents are also improving the results of ASCT. When given after ASCT, they increase the CR/VGPR rate and prolong PFS.

When given before ASCT, they yield very high CR/VGPR rates that will hopefully translate into longer PFS. Preliminary results of studies in which they are given both before and after ASCT induce impressive short-term results. Even without ASCT, novel agents as primary therapy obtain 2-year PFS and OS that are quite comparable to those achieved with high-dose therapy.

In the near future, results of ongoing randomized studies will help to assess the role of novel agents in combination with ASCT, to understand the optimal duration of treatment with these agents, and to clarify the respective role of ASCT and novel agents in younger patients.

References

1. The International Myeloma Working Group. Criteria for the classification of monoclonal gammopathies, multiple myeloma and related disorders: a report of the International Myeloma Working Group. *Br J Haematol* 2003;121:749–757.
2. Greipp RR, San Miguel J, Durie BG, et al. International staging system for multiple myeloma. *J Clin Oncol.* 2005;23:3412–3420.
3. Moreau P, Facon T, Leleu X, et al. Recurrent 14q32 translocations determine the prognosis of multiple myeloma, especially in patients receiving intensive chemotherapy. *Blood* 2002;100:1579–1583.
4. Fonseca R, Blood E, Rue M, et al. Clinical and biologic implications of recurrent genomic aberrations in myeloma. *Blood* 2003;101:4569–4575.
5. Chang H, Qi C, Yi QL, et al. P53 gene deletion detected by fluorescence in situ hybridization is an adverse prognostic factor for patients with

multiple myeloma following autologous stem cell transplantation. *Blood* 2005;105:358–360.

6. Avet-Loiseau H, Attal M, Moreau P, et al. Genetic abnormalities and survival in multiple myeloma : the experience of the Intergroupe Francophone du Myélome. *Blood* 2007;109:3489–3495.

7. Shaughnessy JD Jr, Zhan F, Burington B, et al. A validated gene expression model of high-risk multiple myeloma is defined by deregulated expression of genes mapping to chromosome 1. *Blood* 2007;109: 2276–2284.

8. Decaux O, Lodé L, Magrangeas F, et al. Prediction of survival in multiple myeloma based on gene expression profiles reveals cell cycle and chromosomal instability signatures in high-risk patients and hyperdiploid signatures in low-risk patients: a study of the Intergroupe Francophone du Myélome. *J Clin Oncol* 2008;26:4798–4805.

9. Carrasco DR, Tonon G, Huang Y, et al. The differentiation and stress response factor XBP-1 drives multiple myeloma pathogenesis. *Cancer Cell* 2007;11:349–360.

10. Bataille R, Harousseau JL. Multiple myeloma. *N Engl J Med* 1997;23: 1657–1664.

11. McElwain TJ, Powles RL. High-dose intravenous melphalan for plasma-cell leukaemia and myeloma. *Lancet* 1983;16:822–824.

12. Barlogie B, Hall R, Zander A, et al. High-dose melphalan with autologous bone marrow transplantation for multiple myeloma. *Blood* 1986; 67:1298–1301.

13. Barlogie B, Alexanian R, Dicke KA, et al. High-dose chemoradiotherapy and autologous bone marrow transplantation for resistant multiple myeloma. *Blood* 1987;70:869–872.

14. Harousseau JL. Role of stem cell transplantation. *Hematol Oncol Clin North Am* 2007;21:1157–1174.

15. Attal M, Harousseau JL, Stoppa AM, et al. A prospective randomized trial of autologous bone marrow transplantation and chemotherapy in multiple myeloma. *N Engl J Med* 1996;335:91–97.

16. Child JA, Morgan GJ, Davies FE, et al. High-dose chemotherapy with hematopoietic stem-cell rescue for multiple myeloma. *N Engl J Med* 2003;348:1875–1883.

17. Fermand JP, Ravaud P, Chevret S, et al. High-dose therapy and autologous peripheral blood stem cell transplantation in multiple myeloma: upfront or rescue treatment? Results of a multicenter sequential randomized trial. *Blood* 1998;92:3131–3136.

18. Palumbo A, Bringhen S, Petrucci MT, et al. Intermediate-dose melphalan improves survival of myeloma patients aged 50-70: results of a randomized controlled trial. *Blood* 2004;104:3052–3057.

19. Blade J, Rosinol L, Sureda A, et al. High-dose therapy intensification compared with continued standard chemotherapy in multiple myeloma patients responding to the initial chemotherapy: long-term results from a prospective randomized trial from the Spanish Cooperative Group PETHEMA. *Blood* 2005;106:3755–3759.

20. Fermand JP, Katsahian S, Divine M, et al. High-dose therapy and autologous blood stem-cell transplantation compared with conventional treatment in myeloma patients aged 55 to 65 years: long-term results of a randomized control trial from the Group Myelome-Autogreffe. *J Clin Oncol* 2005;23:9227–9233.

21. Barlogie B, Kyle RA, Anderson KC, et al. Standard chemotherapy compared with high-dose chemoradiotherapy for multiple myeloma: final results of Phase III US Intergroup trial S9321. *J Clin Oncol* 2006;24; 929–936.

22. Koreth J, Cutler CS, Djulbegovic B, et al. High-dose therapy with single autologous transplantation versus chemotherapy for newly diagnosed multiple myeloma: a systematic review and meta-analysis of randomized controlled trials. *Biol Blood Marrow Transplant* 2007;13:183–196.

23. van de Velde HJK, Liu X, Chen G, et al. Complete response correlates with long-term survival and progression-free survival in high-dose therapy in multiple myeloma. *Haematologica* 2007;92:1399–1406.

24. Blade J, Samson D, Reece D, et al. Criteria for evaluating disease response and progression in patients treated with high-dose therapy and haematopoietic stem cell transplantation. *Br J Haematol* 1998;102: 1115–1123.

25. Durie BG, Harousseau JL, San Miguel JS, et al. International uniform response criteria for multiple myeloma. *Leukemia* 2006;20:1467–1473.

26. Facon T, Mary JY, Hulin C, et al. Melphalan and prednisone plus thalidomide versus melphalan and prednisone or reduced-intensity autologous stem cell transplantation in elderly patients with multiple myeloma (IFM 99-06): a randomized trial. *Lancet* 2007;370:1209–1218.

27. Harousseau JL. Optimizing peripheral blood progenitor cell autologous transplantation in multiple myeloma. *Haematologica* 1999;84:548–553.

28. Tricot G, Jagannath S, Vesole D, et al. Peripheral blood stem cell transplants for multiple myeloma: identification of favourable variables for rapid engraftment in 225 patients. *Blood* 1996;85:588–596.

29. Moreau P, Facon T, Attal M, et al. Comparison of 200mg/m2 melphalan and 8Gy total body irradiation plus 140 mg/m² melphalan as conditioning regimen for peripheral blood stem cell transplantation in patients with newly diagnosed multiple myeloma: final analysis of the Intergroupe Francophone du Myelome 9502 trial. *Blood* 2002; 99:731–735.

30. Harousseau JL, Milpied N, Laporte JP, et al. Double intensive therapy in high-risk multiple myeloma. *Blood* 1992;79:2827–2833.

31. Barlogie B, Jagannath S, Desikan KR, et al. Total therapy with tandem autotransplants for newly diagnosed multiple myeloma. *Blood* 1999;93:55–65.

32. Barlogie B, van Rhee F, Shaughnessy Jr JD, et al. Making progress in treating multiple myeloma with total therapies: issue of complete remission and more. *Leukemia* 2008;22:1633–1636.

33. Attal M, Harousseau JL, Facon T, et al. Intergroupe Francophone du Myelome: single versus double autologous stem cell transplantation for multiple myeloma. *N Engl J Med* 2003;349:2495–2502.

34. Cavo M, Tosi P, Zamagni E, et al. Prospective randomized study of single compared with double autologous stem cell transplantation for multiple myeloma: Bologna 96 clinical study *J Clin Oncol* 2007;25:2434–2441.

35. Sonneveld P, van der Holt B, Segeren CM, et al. Intermediate-dose melphalan compared with myeloablative treatment in multiple myeloma: long-term results of the Dutch Cooperative group HOVON 24 trial. *Haematologica* 2007;92:928–935.

36. Harousseau JL. The allogeneic dilemma. *Bone Marrow Transplant* 2007;40:1123–1128.

37. Corradini P, Voena C, Tarella C, et al. Molecular and clinical remissions in multiple myeloma: role of autologous and allogeneic transplantation of hematopoietic cells. *J Clin Oncol* 1999;17:208–215.

38. Gahrton G, Tura S, Ljungman P, et al. Prognostic factors in allogeneic bone marrow transplantation for multiple myeloma. *J Clin Oncol* 1995;13:1312–1322.

39. Bensinger WI, Buckner CD, Anasetti C, et al. Allogeneic marrow transplantation for multiple myeloma: an analysis of risk factors on outcome. *Blood* 1996;88:2787–2793.

40. Mehta J. Allogeneic hematopoietic stem cell transplantation in myeloma. In: Mehta J, Singhal S, eds. *Myeloma.* London, UK: Martin Dunitz London, 2002:349–365.

41. Gahrton G, Svensson H, Cavo M, et al. Progress in allogeneic bone marrow and peripheral blood stem cell transplantation for multiple myeloma: a comparison between transplants performed 1983–93 and 1994–98 at European Group for Blood and Marrow Transplantation Centres. *Br J Haematol* 2001;113:209–216.

42. Lokhorst HM, Segeren CM, Verdonck LF, et al. Partially T-cell depleted allogeneic stem-cell transplantation for first-line treatment of multiple myeloma: a prospective evaluation of patients treated in the phase III study Hovon 24 MM. *J Clin Oncol* 2003;21:1728–1733.

43. Crawley C, Lalancette M, Szydlo R, et al. Outcomes of reduced-intensity allogeneic transplantation for multiple myeloma: an analysis of prognostic factors from the Chronic Leukemia Working Party of the EBMT. *Blood* 2005;105:4532–4539.

44. Crawley C, Iacobelli S, Björkstrand B, et al. Reduced-intensity conditioning for myeloma: lower nonrelapse mortality but higher relapse rates compared with myeloablative conditioning. *Blood* 2007;109:3588–3594.

45. Kroger N, Schwerdtfeger R, Kiehl M, et al. Autologous stem cell transplantation followed by a dose-reduced allograft induced high complete remission rate in multiple myeloma. *Blood* 2002;100:755–760.

46. Maloney D, Molina A, Sahebi F, et al. Allografting with nonmyeloablative conditioning following cytoreductive autografts for the treatment of patients with multiple myeloma. *Blood* 2003;101:3447–3454.

47. Bruno B, Rotta M, Patriarca F, et al. A comparison of allografting with autografting for newly diagnosed myeloma. *N Engl J Med* 2007;356:1110–1120.

48. Garban F, Attal M, Michallet M, et al. Prospective comparison of autologous stem cell transplantation followed by dose-reduced allograft (IFM 99-03 trial) with tandem autologous stem cell transplantation (IFM 99-04 trial) in high-risk de novo multiple myeloma. *Blood* 2006;107:3474–3480.

49. Rosinol L, Perez-Simon JA, Sureda A, et al. A prospective Pethema study of tandem autologous transplant versus autograft followed by reduced-intensity conditioning allogeneic transplant in newly diagnosed multiple myeloma. *Blood* 2008;112:3591–3593.

50. Singhal S, Mehta J, Desikan R, et al. Antitumor activity of thalidomide in refractory multiple myeloma. *N Engl J Med* 1999;341:1565–1571.

51. Vacca A, Ribatti D, Ron Cali L, et al. Bone marrow angiogenesis and progression in multiple myeloma. *Br J Haematol* 1994;87:503–508.

52. Harousseau JL. Thalidomide in multiple myeloma: past, present and future. *Future Oncol* 2006;2:577–589.

53. Dimopoulos MA, Anagnostopoulos A, Weber D. Treatment of plasma cell dyscrasia with thalidomide and its derivates. *J Clin Oncol* 2003;21:4444–4452.

54. Glasmacher A, Hahn C, Hoffman F, et al. A systematic review of phase-II trials of thalidomide monotherapy in patients with relapsed or refractory multiple myeloma. *Br J Haematol* 2006;132:584–593.

55. Palumbo A, Facon T, Sonneveld P, et al. Thalidomide for treatment of multiple myeloma: 10 years later. *Blood* 2008;111:3968–3977.

56. Palumbo A, Giaccone L, Bertola A, et al. Low-dose thalidomide plus dexamethasone is an effective salvage therapy for advanced myeloma. *Haematologica* 2001;86:399–403.

57. Hideshima T, Richardson P, Chauhan D, et al. The proteasome inhibitor PS-341 inhibits growth, induces apoptosis, and overcomes drug resistance in human multiple myeloma cells. *Cancer Res* 2001;61:3071–3076.

58. Le Blanc R, Catley LP, Hideshima T, et al. Proteasome inhibitor PS-341 inhibits human myeloma cell growth in vivo and prolongs survival in a murine model. *Cancer Res* 2002;62:4996–5000.

59. Richardson P, Barlogie B, Berenson J, et al. A phase 2 study of bortezomib in relapsed, refractory myeloma. *N Engl J Med* 2003;348:2609–2617.

60. Jagannath S, Barlogie B, Berenson J, et al. A phase 2 study of two doses of bortezomib in relapsed or refractory multiple myeloma. *Br J Haematol* 2004;127:165–171.

61. Richardson PG, Sonneveld P, Schuster MW, et al. Bortezomib or high-dose dexamethasone for relapsed multiple myeloma. *N Engl J Med* 2005;352:2487–2498.

62. Sonneveld P, Richardson PG, Schuster MW, et al. Bortezomib at first relapse is superior to high-dose dexamethasone and more effective that when given later in relapsed multiple myeloma. *Haematologica* 2005;90:146–147.

63. Lonial S, Waller FK, Richardson PG, et al. Risk factors and kinetics of thrombocytopenia associated with bortezomib for relapsed, refractory multiple myeloma. *Blood* 2005;106:3777–3784.

64. Richardson PG, Briemberg H, Jagannath S, et al. Frequency, characteristics and reversibility of peripheral neuropathy during treatment of advanced multiple myeloma with bortezomib. *J Clin Oncol* 2006;24:3113–3120.

65. Richardson PG, Sonneveld P, Schuster MW, et al. Safety and efficacy of bortezomib in high-risk elderly patients with relapsed multiple myeloma. *Br J Hematol* 2007;137:429–435.

66. San Miguel JF, Richardson PG, Sonneveld P, et al. Efficacy and safety of bortezomib in patients with renal impairment: results from the APEX phase 3 study. *Leukemia* 2008;22:842–849.

67. Chanan-Khan AA, Kaufman JL, Mehta J, et al. Activity and safety of bortezomib in multiple myeloma patients with advanced renal failure: a multicenter retrospective study. *Blood* 2007;109:2604–2606.

68. Orlowski RZ, Nagler A, Sonneveld P, et al. Randomized phase III study of pegylated liposomal doxorubicin plus bortezomib versus bortezomib alone in relapsed or refractory multiple myeloma: combination therapy improves time to progression. *J Clin Oncol* 2007,25.3892 3901.

69. Richardson PG, Schlossman RL, Weller E, et al. Immunomodulatory drug CC-5013 overcomes drug resistance and is well tolerated in patients with relapsed multiple myeloma. *Blood* 2002;100:3063–3067.

70. Richardson PG, Blood E, Mitsiades CS, et al. A randomized phase 2 study of lenalidomide therapy for patients with relapsed or relapsed refractory multiple myeloma. *Blood* 2006;108:3458–3464.

71. Weber DM, Chen C, Nievisky R, et al. Lenalidomide plus dexamethasone for relapsed multiple myeloma in North America. *N Engl J Med* 2007;357:2133–2142.

72. Dimopoulos M, Spencer A, Attal M, et al. Lenalidomide plus dexamethasone for relapsed or refractory multiple myeloma. *N Engl J Med* 2007;357:2123–2132.

73. Chen N, Lau H, Kong L, et al. Pharmacokinetics of lenalidomide in patients with various degrees of renal impairment and in subjects on hemodialysis. *J Clin Pharmacol* 2007.47:1466–1475.

74. Zangari M, Barlogie B, Burns MJ, et al. Velcade, thalidomide, dexamethasone for advanced and refractory multiple myeloma. Long-term follow-up of phase I-II trial UARK 2001-37: superior outcome in patients with normal cytogenetics and no prior therapy [abstract]. *Blood* 2005;106:717a. Abstract 2552.

75. Palumbo A, Ambrosini MT, Benevolo G, et al. Bortezomib, melphalan, prednisone and thalidomide for relapsed multiple myeloma. *Blood* 2007;109:2767–2772.

76. Richardson P, Jagannath S, Jakubowiak A, et al. Lenalidomide, bortezomib, and dexamethasone in patients with relapsed/refractory multiple myeloma: encouraging response rates and tolerability with correlation of outcome and adverse cytogenetics in a Phase II study. *Blood* 2008;112:614. Abstract 1742.

77. Palumbo A, Bringhen S, Caravita T, et al. Oral melphalan and prednisone chemotherapy plus thalidomide compared with melphalan alone in elderly patients with MM: randomized controlled trial. *Lancet* 2006;367:825–831.

78. Palumbo A, Bringhen S, Liberati AM, et al. Oral melphalan, prednisone, and thalidomide in elderly patients: updated results of a randomized, controlled trial. *Blood* 2008;112:3107–3114.

79. Hulin C, Facon T, Rodon P, et al. Melphalan-prednisone-thalidomide demonstrates a significant survival advantage in elderly patients ≥75 years with multiple myeloma compared with melphalan-prednisone in a randomized, double-blind, placebo-controlled trial, IFM 01/01 [abstract]. *Blood* 2007;110:31a. Abstract 75.

80. Waage A, Gimsing P, Juliusson G, et al. Melphalan-prednisone-thalidomide to newly diagnosed patients with multiple myeloma: a placebo-controlled randomized phase 3 trial [abstract]. *Blood* 2007;110:32a. Abstract 78.

81. Wijermans P, Schaafsma P, Van Norden Y, et al. Melphalan Prednisone versus Melphalan Prednisone Thalidomide in induction therapy for Multiple Myeloma in Elderly patients: First interim results of the Dutch cooperative group HOVON. *Blood* 2008;112:649a. Abstract 649.

82. Mateos MV, Hernandez JM, Hernandez MT, et al. Bortezomib plus melphalan and prednisone in elderly untreated patients with multiple myeloma: results of a multicenter phase 1/2 study. *Blood* 2006;108:2165–2171.

83. San Miguel J, Schlag R, Khuageva N, et al. MMY-3002: a phase 3 study comparing bortezomib-melphalan-prednisone with melphalan-prednisone in newly diagnosed multiple myeloma [abstract]. *Blood* 2007;111:76a. Abstract 76.

84. Palumbo A, Falco P, Corradini P, et al. Melphalan, prednisone and lenalidomide treatment for newly diagnosed myeloma: a report from the GIMEMA-Italian Multiple Myeloma Network. *J Clin Oncol* 2007;25:4459–4465.

85. Rajkumar SV, Hayman S, Gertez M, et al. Combination therapy with thalidomide plus dexamethasone for newly diagnosed myeloma. *J Clin Oncol* 2002;20:4319–4323.

86. Weber D, Rankin K, Gavino M, et al. Thalidomide alone or with dexamethasone for previously untreated multiple myeloma. *J Clin Oncol* 2003;21:16–19.

87. Ludwig H, Tothova E, Hajek R, et al. Thalidomide-dexamethasone vs melphalan-prednisone as first line treatment and thalidomide-interferon maintenance therapy in elderly patients with multiple myeloma [abstract]. *Blood* 2007;110:163a. Abstract.

88. Zonder JA, Crowley JJ, Hussein M, et al. Superiority of lenalidomide plus high-dose dexamethasone compared to high-dose dexamethasone alone as treatment of newly diagnosed multiple myeloma patients: results of the randomized, double-blind, placebo-controlled Southwest Oncology Group trial S0232. *Blood* 2007;110:32a. Abstract 77.

89. Rajkumar SV, Jacobus S, Callander N, et al. a randomized trial of lenalidomide plus high-dose dexamethasone versus lenalidomide plus low-dose dexamethasone in newly diagnosed multiple myeloma: a trial coordinated by the Eastern Cooperative Oncology Group *Blood* 2007;110:31a. Abstract 74.

90. Attal M, Harousseau JL, Leyvraz S, et al. Maintenance therapy with thalidomide improves survival in multiple myeloma patients. *Blood* 2006;15:3289–3294.

91. Abdelkefi A, Ladeb S, Torjman L, et al. Single autologous stem cell transplantation followed by maintenance therapy with thalidomide is superior to double autologous transplantation in multiple myeloma: results of a multicenter randomized clinical trial. *Blood* 2008;111:1805–1810.

92. Spencer A, Prince HM, Roberts AW, et al. Consolidation therapy with low-dose thalidomide and prednisolone prolongs the survival of multiple myeloma patients undergoing a single autologous stem-cell transplantation procedure. *J Clin Oncol* 2009;27:1788–1793.

93. Cavo M, Zamagni, Tosi P, et al. Superiority of thalidomide and dexamethasone over vincristine-doxorubicin-dexamethasone (VAD) as primary therapy in preparation for autologous transplantation for multiple myeloma. *Blood* 2005;106:35–39.

94. Rajkumar SV, Blood E, Vesole D, et al. Phase III clinical trial of thalidomide plus dexamethasone compared with dexamethasone alone in newly diagnosed multiple myeloma: a clinical trial coordinated by the Eastern Cooperative Oncology Group. *J Clin Oncol* 2006;24:431–436.

95. Macro M, Divine M, Uzunban Y, et al. Dexamethasone + thalidomide compared to VAD as pre-transplant treatment in newly diagnosed multiple myeloma: a randomized trial. *Blood* 2006;108:22a. Abstract 57.

96. Lokhorst HM, Schidt-Wolf I, Sonneveld P, et al. Thalidomide in induction treatment increases the very good partial remission rate before and after high-dose therapy in previously untreated multiple myeloma. *Haematologica* 2008;93:124–127.

97. Morgan GJ, Davies FE, Owen RG, et al. Thalidomide combinations improve response rates: results from the MRC IX study [abstract]. *Blood* 2007;110:1051a. Abstract 3593.

98. Jagannath S, Durie B, Wolf J, et al. Bortezomib therapy alone and in combination with dexamethasone for previously untreated symptomatic multiple myeloma. *Br J Haematol* 2005;129:776–783.

99. Harousseau JL, Attal M, Leleu X, et al. Bortezomib plus dexamethasone as induction treatment prior to autologous stem cell transplantation in patients with newly diagnosed multiple myeloma. *Haematologica* 2006;91:1498–1505.

100. Rosinol L, Oriol A, Mateos MV, et al. Phase II Pethema trial of alternating bortezomib and dexamethasone as induction regimen before autologous stem-cell transplantation in younger patients with multiple myeloma: efficacy and clinical implications of tumor response kinetics. *J Clin Oncol* 2007;25:4452–4458.

101. Popat R, Oakervee HE, Hallam S, et al. Bortezomib, doxorubicin and dexamethasone–PAD) front-line treatment of multiple myeloma: updated results after long-term follow-up *Br J Haematol* 2008;141:512–516.

102. Harousseau JL, Mathiot C, Attal M, et al. Bortezomib/dexamethasone versus VAD as induction prior to autologous stem-cell transplantation in previously untreated multiple myeloma. Updated results from IFM 2005/01 trial [abstract]. *J Clin Oncol* 2008;26:455s. Abstract.

103. Cavo M, Patriarca F, Tacchetti P, et al. Bortezomib-thalidomide-dexamethasone vs thalidomide-Dexamethasone in preparation for autologous stem-cell transplantation in newly diagnosed multiple myeloma [abstract]. *Blood* 2007;110:30a. Abstract 73.

104. Lacy MQ, Gertz M, Dispenzieri A, et al. Long-term results of response to therapy, time to progression, and survival with lenalidomide plus dexamethasone in newly diagnosed myeloma. *Mayo Clin Proc* 2007;82:1179–1184.

105. Niesvizky R, Jayabalan DS, Christos PJ, et al. BiRD (Biaxin/Revlimid/Dexamethasone) combination therapy results in high complete and overall response rates in treatment-naïve symptomatic multiple myeloma. *Blood* 2008;111:1101–1109.

106. Kumar S, Dispenzieri QA, Lacy MG, et al. Impact of lenalidomide on stem cell mobilization and engraftment post-peripheral blood stem cell transplantation in patients with newly diagnosed multiple myeloma. *Leukemia* 2007;21:2035–2042.

107. Mark T, Stern J, Furst JR, et al. Stem cell mobilization with cyclophosphamide overcomes the suppressive effect of lenalidomide therapy on stem cell collection in multiple myeloma. *Biol Blood Marrow Transplant* 2008;14:795–798.

108. Richardson PG, Lonial S, Jakubowiak S, et al. Safety and efficacy of lenalidomide, bortezomib and dexamethasone in patients with newly diagnosed multiple myeloma [abstract]. *J Clin Oncol* 2008;26:459s. Abstract.

109. Barlogie B, Tricot G, Anaissie E, et al. Thalidomide and hematopoietic stem cell transplantation for multiple myeloma. *N Engl J Med* 2006; 354:1021–1030.

110. Zangari M, van Rhee F, Anaissie E, et al. Eight-year survival in multiple myeloma after Total therapy 2: roles of thalidomide and consolidation chemotherapy in the context of Total therapy 1. *Br J Haematol* 2008; 141:433–444.

111. Pineda-Roman M, Zangari M, Haessler J, et al. Sustained complete remissions in multiple myeloma linked to bortezomib in total therapy 3: comparison with total therapy 2. *Br J Haematol* 2008;140:625–634.

112. Dimopoulos MA, Hamilos G. Solitary bone plasmocytoma and extramedullary plasmocytoma. *Curr Treat Options Oncol* 2002;3:255–259.

113. Garcia-Sanz R, Orfao A, Gonzalez M, et al. Primary plasma cell leukaemia: clinical, immunophenotypic, DNA ploidy and cytogenetic characteristics. *Blood* 1999;93:1032–1037.

114. Noel P, Kyle RA. Plasma cell leukaemia: an evaluation of response to therapy. *Am J Med* 1987;83:1062–1068.

115. Hovenga S, de Wolf JTh, Klip H, et al. Consolidation therapy with autologous stem cell transplantation in plasma cell leukemia after VAD, high-dose cyclophosphamide and EDAP courses: a report of three cases and a review of the literature. *Bone Marrow Transplant* 1997;20: 901–904.

116. Sica S, Chiusolo P, Salutari P, et al. Long-lasting complete remission in plasma cell leukemia after aggressive chemotherapy and CD34-selected autologous peripheral cell transplant: Molecular follow-up of minimal residual disease. *Bone Marrow Transplant* 1998;22:823–825.

117. Finnegan DP, Kettle P, Drake M, et al. Bortezomib is effective in primary plasma cell leukaemia. *Leuk Lymphoma* 2006;47:1670–1673.

118. Jaskiewicz AD, Herrington JD, Wong L. Tumour lysis syndrome after bortezomib therapy for plasma cell leukaemia. *Pharmacotherapy* 2005; 25:1820–1825.

119. Barlogie B, Tricot G, van Rhee F, et al. Long-term outcome results of the First tandem autotransplant trial for multiple myeloma. *Br J Haematol* 2006;135:158–164.

120. Kumar S, Rajkumar SV, Dispenzieri A, et al. Improved survival in multiple myeloma and the impact of novel therapies. *Blood* 2008;111:2516–2520.

CHAPTER 24 ■ PRIMARY CUTANEOUS B-CELL LYMPHOMA

CHRISTIANE QUERFELD, JOAN GUITART, AND STEVEN T. ROSEN

Primary cutaneous B-cell lymphomas (PCBCLs) are distinct clinicopathologic entities (1–4). They are defined as a B-cell lymphoma originating in the skin. There is no evidence of extracutaneous disease at presentation as assessed by adequate staging procedures. At present, PCBCLs constitute 20% to 25% of all cutaneous lymphomas. Three main different types are highlighted in the most recent World Health Organization and European Organization for Research and Treatment of Cancer (EORTC) consensus classification of cutaneous lymphomas, and include primary cutaneous marginal zone B-cell lymphoma (PCMZL), primary cutaneous follicle center lymphoma (PCFCL), and primary cutaneous diffuse large B-cell lymphoma, leg type (PCLBCL, large type [LT]). Each PCBCL has a unique epidemiology, pathology, clinical presentation, therapy, and prognosis.

INCIDENCE AND EPIDEMIOLOGY

PCBCLs are rare malignancies. The overall annual incidence is approximately 0.1 per 100,000 individuals. The most common entity is PCFCL, representing about 55% to 60% of PCBCL cases, PCMZL accounts for 20% to 25%, and PCLBCL, LT 15% to 20% (4,5). The origin and homing mechanisms of B cells to the skin are poorly understood. It has been proposed that chronic antigen stimulation may play a role. A number of viruses, including human T-lymphocyte virus-1, herpes simplex virus, Epstein-Barr virus, and hepatitis C virus, have been implicated in the etiology of PCBCL without definitive proof (6–8). An association of *Borrelia burgdorferi* with PCBCL has been reported by European investigators but not confirmed in the United States or Asia (9–12).

CLINICAL PRESENTATION

Primary Cutaneous Marginal Zone B-Cell Lymphoma

The median age of diagnosis is about 55 years, but ranges from 20s to 90s without gender predilection. PCMZL presents with indolent erythematous to violaceous papules, plaques, or nodules preferentially involving the upper extremities or trunk (Fig. 24.1) (4,5,13–17). Subcutaneous nodules may also occur. Multifocal lesions are typical, and ulceration is infrequent. Spontaneous involution of lesions may be seen. Dissemination to extracutaneous sites is exceedingly rare. Systemic autoimmune disease may be present in a subpopulation of patients.

Primary Cutaneous Follicle Center Lymphoma

PCFCL (Fig. 24.2) shows predilection for the head, neck, and trunk in elderly patients with a medium age of 60 and male predominance of approximately 1.5:1. The characteristic

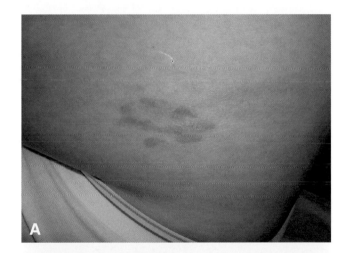

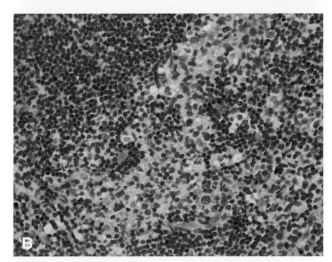

FIGURE 24.1 **A:** A patient diagnosed with primary cutaneous MZL presenting with an irregularly shaped, erythematous plaque on the left flank (see also Color Plate 38). **B:** Biopsy reveals a dense, pleomorphic infiltrate with atypical lymphocytes, plasma cells, and lymphoplasmacytoid cells (hematoxylin and eosin; original magnification ×200) (see also Color Plate 39). (Courtesy of Christiane Querfeld, MD.)

373

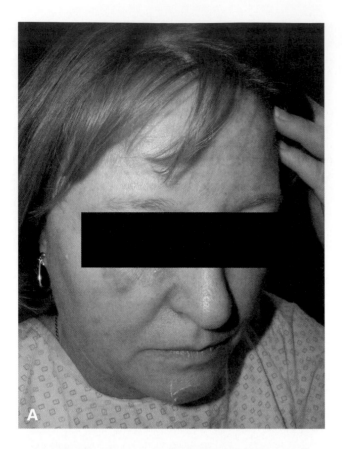

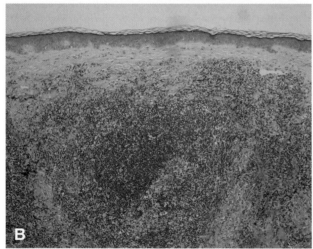

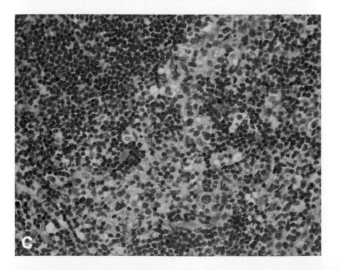

clinical presentation consists of solitary or grouped plaques, papules, and nodules. Arcuate plaques can occasionally be seen. Multifocal cutaneous lesions involving different anatomic regions are seen in a minority of patients. Extensive cutaneous lesions should alert the clinician for the possibility of a secondary lymphoma of primary systemic origin. Ulceration and pruritus are rarely associated with PCFCL lesions.

Primary Cutaneous Diffuse Large B-Cell Lymphoma, Leg Type

PCLBCL, large type (Fig. 24.3) is typically seen in elderly patients with a median age of 78 and female predominance of 2:1. Rapidly growing red or bluish-red tumors on one or both legs are common, but tumors may arise on other parts of the body as well. Marked edema of the legs is common, and the tumors tend to be large and bulky with common ulceration.

DIAGNOSIS

Persistent or recurrent erythematous or violaceous papules, plaques, or nodules should have an adequately large excisional or incisional (elliptical) biopsy rather than small punch or shave biopsy. It is important that the specimen be large enough to include subcutaneous fat, to facilitate optimal evaluation of architecture, depth of involvement, and cell morphology. The diagnosis of PCBCL or determining the subtype is often difficult to make based on histopathologic criteria alone. Immunophenotyping using flow cytometry or immunohistochemistry, and genotyping are critical to adequately characterize the tumor (1–3,18). For this reason, fresh tissue may be necessary with optimal preservation requiring freezing be performed within 2 to 3 hours of tissue acquisition.

PATHOLOGY AND BIOLOGIC PROPERTIES

Primary Cutaneous Marginal Zone B-Cell Lymphoma

PCMZL (Fig. 24.1B) has features of mucosa-associated lymphoid tissue lymphomas, and shows a nodular or diffuse dermal infiltrate often tracing adnexal structures and involving the deep reticular dermis and the subcutaneous tissue (19–29). The morphology is heterogeneous with collections of small to medium-sized marginal zone B lymphocytes with centrocyte-like or monocytoid configuration, lymphoplasmacytoid cells, plasma cells, admixed with small numbers of centroblast or immunoblast-like large cells. Reactive germinal centers are often present and colonized by neoplastic cells. The epidermis is not involved. Periodic acid-Schiff (PAS)-positive intranuclear or intracytoplasmic inclusions may be present when there is a predominance of lymphoplasmacytoid cells. Besides the sheets of small to

FIGURE 24.2 **A:** This patient presented with erythematous papules and nodules on the face (see also Color Plate 40). **B:** A skin biopsy shows a dense dermal infiltrate with a follicular growth pattern (hematoxylin and eosin; original magnification ×100). There is a grenz zone with uninvolved epidermis (see also Color Plate 41). **C:** Follicles are composed of centrocytes and centroblasts surrounded by small lymphocytes (hematoxylin and eosin; original magnification ×200) (see also Color Plate 42). (Courtesy of Christiane Querfeld, MD.)

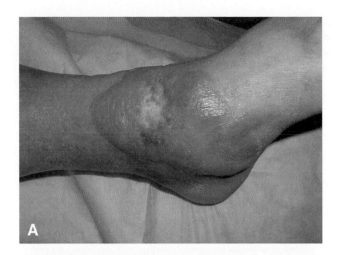

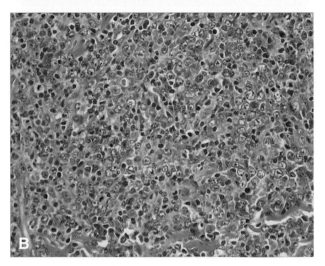

FIGURE 24.3 **A:** DLBCL, leg type presenting as a thick, indurated, erythematous, and ulcerated plaque on the lower leg (see also Color Plate 43). **B:** Histologic evaluation demonstrates a diffuse dermal infiltrate with predominately large lymphocytes with multilobulated nuclei, comprised of centroblasts and immunoblasts (hematoxylin and eosin; original magnification ×100) (see also Color Plate 44) (Courtesy of Christiane Querfeld, MD.)

medium-sized cells with irregular nuclei, inconspicuous nucleoli, and abundant pale cytoplasm (marginal zone B cells), a rich reactive T-cell infiltrate is commonly present giving a polytypic appearance that may pose diagnostic difficulties in some cases. Monotypic plasma cells may accumulate at the periphery of the infiltrates. Large transformed cells are present in some patients; however, transformation to diffuse large cell B-cell lymphoma is uncommon. This diagnosis includes cases previously designated as primary cutaneous immunocytoma and cutaneous follicular lymphoid hyperplasia with monotypic plasma cells. Cases reported as cutaneous plasmacytoma are probably also closely related to marginal zone lymphoma (MZL) and immunocytoma. The diagnosis of MZL continues to be a challenge for the pathologists due to the presence of various elements like many T cells, germinal centers, and mature plasma cells. Furthermore, some cases may also show scattered interstitial eosinophils.

The immunophenotype of PCMZL shows expression of CD20, CD79a, and bcl-2 on the marginal zone B cells, but absence of CD5, CD10, cyclin D1, and bcl-6 staining. The monocyte and T-cell marker CD43 is also often expressed

among the neoplastic cells. The reactive germinal centers will typically express both bcl-6 and CD10, but not bcl-2. Plasma cells are positive for CD138, CD79a, and MUM-1, and show monotypic cytoplasmic immunoglobulin (Ig) light chain expression without the presence of CD20. Some MZLs present with more immature features lacking obvious plasma cell differentiation. Clonality can be demonstrated in the majority of such cases with light chain in situ hybridization. However, rare cases of MZL may lack light chain restriction by in situ messenger ribonucleic acid or protein analysis. Molecular alterations in PCMZL include the clonal rearrangement of Ig heavy chain (IgH) genes. MZL may have extensive somatic hypermutations that could compromise clonal detection by routine polymerase chain reaction-based tests targeting the IgH. The most frequently reported chromosomal abnormality is the t(14;18)(q32;21) IgH/mucosa-associated lymphoid tissue-1 translocation. The t(14;18)(q32;q21)IgH/BCL2 translocation, t(3;14)(p14.1;q32) IGH/FOXP1, and trisomy 3 have also been found. The lack of a specific molecular signature suggests evolution through a variety of pathologic pathways. Translocations noted in gastric mucosa-associated lymphoid tissue lymphomas, such as t(11;18)(q21;q21) and t(1;14) (p22;q32), have not been seen in PCMZL.

Primary Cutaneous Follicle Center Lymphoma

PCFCL (Fig. 24.2, B and C) is defined as a proliferation of centrocytes (small to large cleaved cells) and centroblasts (large round cells with prominent nuclei) showing a nodular or diffuse infiltrate in the majority of cases, and rarely demonstrating a true follicular pattern (13,30–39). A follicular growth pattern is more commonly associated with scalp and small/early lesions. The dermal infiltrate spares the epidermis in almost all instances. Early lesions present with a nodular pattern and a predominance of small centrocytes, whereas more mature older lesions will have a diffuse pattern with an increased number of large cells. However, these patterns, which in nodal follicle center lymphoma correspond to low and high-grade tumors, have no prognostic significance in the skin. The course of PCFCL lesions may still behave in an indolent manner, regardless of architectural pattern and cytology. Usually a prominent stromal sclerotic component is present. Lesions may present with a peculiar spindle cell pattern resembling a sarcoma.

The immunophenotype of PCFCL is characterized by the expression of CD20 and CD79a on the neoplastic cells. Monotypic staining for surface Igs can be detected in frozen sections or fresh flow cytometry samples. However, light chain evaluation on paraffin sections is noncontributory. Furthermore, tumor lesions with a predominance of large follicle center cells may not have detectable surface Ig. The bcl-6 protein is consistently expressed. FoxP1 is present in a minority of cases. CD10 is usually observed in infiltrates composed of a follicular growth pattern. The antigens CD5, CD43, and MUM-1/IRF4 are absent. In most instances, the bcl-2 protein is not expressed or shows faint staining on a minority of neoplastic B cells. Strong bcl-2 expression is suspicious for a systemic follicular lymphoma with skin involvement.

Clonal rearrangement of the Ig genes is a characteristic feature to confirm the diagnosis. The follicle center cell origin of these lymphomas is supported by the evidence that somatic hypermutation of variable heavy and light chain genes is seen. In contrast to systemic follicular center lymphomas, primary cutaneous types do not carry the t(14;18) translocation. Some PCFCLs have the gene expression profile of germinal center-like large B-cell lymphomas. Inactivation of p15 and p16 tumor suppressor genes by promoter hypermethylation has been reported in a minority of cases.

Primary Cutaneous Diffuse Large B-Cell Lymphoma, Leg Type

PCLBCL, large type (Fig. 24.3B) shows a diffuse dermal infiltrate with predominance of a monotonous population of large round B cells with subtle multilobulated nuclei, comprised of centroblasts and immunoblasts (30,40–45). The cells are fragile, and nuclear debris and pyknotic cells or necrotic areas are commonly seen. The infiltrate often extends into the subcutaneous tissue.

The immunophenotype of PCLBCL, large type is characterized by the expression of monotypic surface Ig and/or cytoplasmic Ig by immunohistochemistry on frozen tissue sections or by flow cytometry. The classic B-cell markers CD20 and CD79a are uniformly expressed. Regardless of the tumor location (and in contrast to PCFCL), strong bcl-2 expression is seen. MUM-1/IRF4, FOXP1, and bcl-6 are typically positive. CD10 is generally negative.

Chromosomal imbalances have been demonstrated in up to 85% of PCLBCL, large type with gains in 18q and 7p and loss of 6q as the most common findings. Translocations involving myc, bcl-6, and IgH genes have been witnessed in a significant number of cases. Inactivation of p15 and p16 tumor suppressor genes by promoter hypermethylation has been noted. An activated B-cell profile is usually seen by gene expression profiling. Although strong bcl-2 staining is observed, the t(14;18) translocation is not seen. In some instances, amplification of the bcl-2 gene is present.

STAGING EVALUATION

After a diagnosis of PCBCL is established, complete clinical staging is appropriate (46,47). Recommendations for staging in cutaneous lymphomas other than mycosis fungoides/Sézary syndrome have recently been published by the International Society for Cutaneous Lymphoma and the EORTC. The tumor, node, metastases classification system advocated should improve the communication about the state of the disease, selection of appropriate management, standardization of enrollment/response criteria in clinical trials, and collection/analysis of prospective survival data (46). A complete history, review of systems (B symptoms, organ-specific signs), and a thorough physical examination should be performed. Photographs of select lesions may be of benefit (for later assessment of response). Laboratory evaluation should include a complete blood count with differential, a comprehensive chemistry panel, lactate dehydrogenase and serum protein electrophoresis to exclude a monoclonal gammopathy, and in selected instances, peripheral blood immunophenotyping by flow cytometry. In cases of PCMZL, serologic tests for *Borrelia*, *Helicobacter pylori*, and hepatitis as well as antinuclear and antigliadin

antibodies or other autoimmune panels may be helpful to distinguish primary cutaneous from secondary cutaneous involvement.

Adequate imaging studies of the chest, abdomen, and pelvis, and of the neck for patients with skin lesions on the head or neck should be obtained. Positron emission tomography scans have been employed by many investigators for patients with PCLBCL, large type and selected patients with PCFCL for both staging and response assessment. Bone marrow evaluation is indicated for patients with PCLBCL, LT and PCFCL. Due to the clinical and pathologic heterogeneity of PCBCL, the newly proposed tumor, node, metastases staging classification of cutaneous lymphomas other than mycosis fungoides/Sézary syndrome (Table 24.1) is purely an anatomic documentation of disease extent.

TABLE 24.1

INTERNATIONAL SOCIETY FOR CUTANEOUS LYMPHOMA/EORTC PROPOSAL ON TUMOR, NODE, METASTASES CLASSIFICATION OF CUTANEOUS LYMPHOMA OTHER THAN MF/SS45

Classification

T (skin)*	
T1	Solitary skin involvement
T1a	A solitary lesion <5 cm diameter
T1b	A solitary lesion >5 cm diameter
T2	Regional skin involvement: multiple lesions limited to 1 body region or 2 contiguous body regions
T2a	All-disease encompassing in a <15-cm diameter circular area
T2b	All-disease encompassing in a >15 and <30-cm diameter circular area
T2c	All-disease encompassing in a >30-cm diameter circular area
T3	Generalized skin involvement
T3a	Multiple lesions involving 2 noncontiguous body regions
T3b	Multiple lesions involving ≥3 body regions
N (nodes)**	
N0	No clinical or pathologic lymph node involvement
N1	Involvement of 1 peripheral lymph node region that drains an area of current or prior skin involvement
N2	Involvement of ≥2 peripheral lymph node regions or involvement of any lymph node region^a that does not drain an area of current or prior skin involvement
N3	Involvement of central lymph nodes
M (viscera)	
M0	No evidence of extracutaneous nonlymph node disease
M1	Extracutaneous nonlymph node disease present

*Designated body regions: head & neck, chest, abdomen & genital, upper back, lower back & buttocks, each upper arm, each lower arm & hand, each upper leg, each lower leg & foot..
**Designated lymph node regions according to the Ann Arbor classification. Peripheral: antecubital, cervical, supraclavicular, axillary, inguinal-femoral, popliteal. Central: mediastinal, pulmonary hilar, paraaortic, iliac.

PROGNOSIS AND PREDICTIVE FACTORS

The prognosis of PCMZL is excellent with exceedingly rare disease-related deaths at 5 and 10 years (1,4,17,47–54). Skin relapses are common. Large cell transformation and systemic involvement are seen in a minority of patients. The clinical course of PCFCL is usually indolent with 5-year disease-specific survival rates of approximately 95%. Similar to PCMZL, skin relapses are often witnessed during the course of the disease. Two multivariate analyses on PCFCL from the Dutch lymphoma group revealed that localization on the leg and expression of FOXP1 correlated with a poor prognosis. Growth pattern, expression of bcl-2 (though extensive bcl-2 expression suggests a systemic follicular lymphoma), or MUM-1 had no significant overall survival effect. Bone marrow involvement may be present in approximately 10% of patients at the time of diagnosis. Individuals with bone marrow involvement had a 5-year overall and disease-specific survival of 44% and 63%, respectively, compared with 84% and 95% for patients without marrow involvement.

The prognosis of PCLBCL, large type is the least favorable of all PCBCLs. The disease-specific survival is approximately 50%, and half of the patients develop clinically documented extracutaneous disease. In the previously noted report by Willemze et al. (1), by univariate analysis, only age and extent of skin lesions were associated with a worse outcome. The 5-year overall survival for patients with a solitary tumor was 70% compared with 27% and 0% for patients presenting with localized or multifocal disease, respectively. Gender, localization on the leg, expression of bcl-2, MUM-1, and FOXP1 did not affect prognosis. Of note, no difference in survival was seen in patients presenting with lesions on the leg versus other cutaneous sites.

TREATMENT

A recent publication from the International Society for Cutaneous Lymphoma/EORTC highlights consensus recommendations for the management of PCBCL (Table 24.2). This was a collaborative effort by an international team of dermatologists, pathologists, and medical oncologists with significant expertise in the field. In a separate report addressing prognostic factors in PCBCL by Zinzani et al. (5), it was noted that for PCMZL and PCFCL, a plateau in disease-free survival did not occur until 15 years, and for PCLBCL, LT not until 10 years from diagnosis and treatment (6).

Primary Cutaneous Marginal Zone B-Cell Lymphoma

Patients presenting with solitary or few scattered skin lesions should be treated with local radiotherapy (20 to 36 Gy) or surgical excision (4,5,47,49,55–73). Almost all treated patients achieve a complete remission; however, a cutaneous relapse will occur in about one half of these individuals. In patients with extensive skin lesions, a spectrum of approaches is considered acceptable, including oral chlorambucil, interferon α, rituximab, and other agents utilized for indolent low-grade systemic lymphomas. Observation is an acceptable alternative in patients with multifocal lesions who are not bothered by the cosmetic consequences of their disease. PCMZL associated with *B. burgdorferi* infection should receive a trial of antibiotics, but limited efficacy data are available. Patients who transform with a large cell phenotype and extracutaneous manifestations should be treated as having diffuse large B-cell lymphoma (DLBCL).

TABLE 24.2

RECOMMENDATIONS FOR INITIAL MANAGEMENT OF THE THREE MAIN DIFFERENT TYPES OF PCBL4

	Extent	First-line therapy	Alternative therapies
PCMZL	Solitary/localized	■ Local radiotherapy ■ Excision ■ Antibiotics[a]	■ IFN-α i.l. ■ Rituximab i.l. ■ Steroids i.l.
	Multifocal	■ Observation ■ Local radiotherapy ■ Chlorambucil[b] ■ Rituximab i.v. ■ Antibiotics[a]	■ IFN-α i.l. ■ Rituximab i.l. ■ Topical or i.l. steroids
PCFCL	Solitary/localized	■ Local radiotherapy ■ Excision	■ IFN-α i.l. ■ Rituximab i.l.
	Multifocal	■ Wait and see ■ Local radiotherapy ■ Rituximab i.v.	■ R-CVP/CHOP[c]
PCLBCL, LT	Solitary/localized	■ R-CHOP ± RT	■ Local radiotherapy ■ Rituximab i.v.
	Multifocal	■ R-CHOP	■ Rituximab i.v.

IFN, interferon; i.l., intralesional; i.v., intravenous; RT, local radiotherapy.
[a] In case of *B. burgdorferi* infection.
[b] *Single* or combination regimens appropriate for low-grade B-cell lymphomas.
[c] In selected cases or for patients developing extracutaneous disease.

Primary Cutaneous Follicle Center Lymphoma

Patients presenting with solitary or localized skin lesions should receive spot radiation treatment with a dose of at least 30 Gy and a margin of clinically uninvolved skin of at least 1 to 1.5 cm (4,5,47,74–96). Similar to PCMZL, almost all patients will enter a complete remission; however, a cutaneous relapse will be witnessed in one half of the individuals. Solitary lesions that are small and well demarcated can be treated with surgical excision. For patients presenting with generalized skin lesions, observation is an acceptable alternative. Patients requesting intervention should be treated with single-agent rituximab or rituximab combined with systemic chemotherapy; single-agent or combination drug regimens have been used. Interferon α also has activity against PCFCL. Patients who transform with a large cell phenotype and extracutaneous manifestations should be treated as having an intermediate-grade lymphoma.

Primary Cutaneous Diffuse Large B-Cell Lymphoma, Leg Type

The consensus is that PCLBCL, large type has morphologic, phenotypic, molecular genetic features and a clinical behavior similar to that of a systemic DLBCL, and should be treated in a comparable manner (4,5,47,97–110). There is much debate among experts on whether patients with solitary small lesions should receive radiation therapy alone. Reported relapse rates are around 60%, and a substantial number of patients have recurrence with systemic involvement. The value of rituximab combined with multiagent chemotherapy such as cyclophosphamide, doxorubicin, vincristine, and prednisolone (R-CHOP) or etoposide, prednisolone, vincristine, cyclophosphamide, and doxorubicin (R-EPOCH) with or without involved-field consolidation radiation treatment remains to be proven (though appealing based on results with DLBCL). Positron emission tomography scanning may provide insight into which patients benefit from combining chemoimmunotherapy with subsequent radiation treatment. For younger patients with relapsed disease, the issues of autologous or allogeneic stem cell transplantation are similar to patients with DLBCL.

References

1. Willemze R, Jaffe ES, Burg G, et al. WHO-EORTC classification for cutaneous lymphomas. *Blood* 2005;105:3768–3785.
2. Querfeld C, Kuzel TM, Guitart J, et al. Primary cutaneous B-cell lymphomas: clinico-pathologic aspects and current status of treatment. *Contemp Oncol* 2003;2:1–8.
3. Pandolfino TL, Siegel RS, Kuzel TM, et al. Primary cutaneous B-cell lymphoma: review and current concepts. *J Clin Oncol* 2000;18:2152–2168.
4. Senff NJ, Hoefnagel JJ, Jansen PM, et al. Reclassification of 300 primary cutaneous B-Cell lymphomas according to the new WHO-EORTC classification for cutaneous lymphomas: comparison with previous classifications and identification of prognostic markers. *J Clin Oncol* 2007;25:1581–1587.
5. Zinzani PL, Quaglino P, Pimpinelli N, et al. Prognostic factors in primary cutaneous B-cell lymphoma: the Italian Study Group for Cutaneous Lymphomas. *J Clin Oncol* 2006;24:1376–1382.
6. Wagner M, Rose VA, Linder R, et al. Human pathogenic virus-associated pseudolymphomas and lymphomas with primary cutaneous manifestation in humans and animals. *Clin Infect Dis* 1998;27:1299–1308.
7. Wechsler J, Willemze R, van der Brule A, et al. Differences in Epstein-Barr virus expression between primary and secondary cutaneous angiocentric lymphomas. French Study Group of Cutaneous Lymphomas. *Arch Dermatol* 1998;134:479–484.
8. Viguier M, Rivet J, Agbalika F, et al. B-cell lymphomas involving the skin associated with hepatitis C virus infection. *Int J Dermatol* 2002;41:577–582.
9. Grange F, Wechsler J, Guillaume JC, et al. Borrelia burgdorferi-associated lymphocytoma cutis simulating a primary cutaneous large B-cell lymphoma. *J Am Acad Dermatol* 2002;47:530–534.
10. Cerroni L, Zochling N, Putz B, et al. Infection by Borrelia burgdorferi and cutaneous B-cell lymphoma. *J Cutan Pathol* 1997;24:457–461.
11. de la Fouchardiere A, Vandenesch F, Berger F. Borrelia-associated primary cutaneous MALT lymphoma in a nonendemic region. *Am J Surg Pathol* 2003;27:702–703.
12. Wood GS, Kamath NV, Guitart J, et al. Absence of Borrelia burgdorferi DNA in cutaneous b-cell lymphomas from the United States. *J Cutan Pathol* 2001;28:502–507.
13. Pimpinelli N, Santucci M, Bosi A, et al. Primary cutaneous follicular centre-cell lymphoma—a lymphoproliferative disease with favourable prognosis. *Clin Exp Dermatol* 1989;14:12–19.
14. Long JC, Mihm MC, Qazi R. Malignant lymphoma of the skin: a clinicopathologic study of lymphoma other than mycosis fungoides. *Cancer* 1976;38:1282–1296.
15. Burke JS, Hoppe RT, Cibull ML, et al. Cutaneous malignant lymphoma: a pathologic study of 50 cases with clinical analysis of 37. *Cancer* 1981;47:300–310.
16. Santucci M, Pimpinelli N, Arganini L. Primary cutaneous B-cell lymphoma: a unique type of low-grade lymphoma. Clinicopathologic and immunologic study of 83 cases. *Cancer* 1991;67:2311–2326.
17. Gerami P, Wickless SC, Rosen S, et al. Applying the new TNM classification system for primary cutaneous lymphomas other than mycosis fungoides and Sézary syndrome in primary cutaneous marginal zone lymphoma. *J Am Acad Dermatol* 2008;59:245–254.
18. Lukowsky A, Marchwat M, Sterry W, et al. Evaluation of B-cell clonality in archival skin biopsy samples of cutaneous B-cell lymphoma by immunoglobulin heavy chain gene polymerase chain reaction. *Leuk Lymphoma* 2006;47:487–493.
19. LeBoit PE, McNutt NS, Reed JA, et al. Primary cutaneous immunocytoma. A B-cell lymphoma that can easily be mistaken for cutaneous lymphoid hyperplasia. *Am J Surg Pathol* 1994;18:969–978.
20. Cerroni L, Signoretti S, Hofler G, et al. Primary cutaneous marginal zone B-cell lymphoma: a recently described entity of low-grade malignant cutaneous B-cell lymphoma. *Am J Surg Pathol* 1997;21:1307–1315.
21. Tomaszewski MM, Abbondanzo SL, Lupton GP. Extranodal marginal zone B-cell lymphoma of the skin: a morphologic and immunophenotypic study of 11 cases. *Am J Dermatopathol* 2000;22:205–211.
22. de Leval L, Harris NL, Longtine J, et al. Cutaneous b-cell lymphomas of follicular and marginal zone types: use of Bcl-6, CD10, Bcl-2, and CD21 in differential diagnosis and classification. *Am J Surg Pathol* 2001;25:732–741.
23. Servitje O, Gallardo F, Estrach T, et al. Primary cutaneous marginal zone B-cell lymphoma: a clinical, histopathological, immunophenotypic and molecular genetic study of 22 cases. *Br J Dermatol* 2002;147:1147–1158.
24. Li C, Inagaki H, Kuo TT, et al. Primary cutaneous marginal zone B-cell lymphoma: a molecular and clinicopathologic study of 24 Asian cases. *Am J Surg Pathol* 2003;27:1061–1069.
25. Schreuder MI, Hoefnagel JJ, Jansen PM, et al. FISH analysis of MALT lymphoma-specific translocations and aneuploidy in primary cutaneous marginal zone lymphoma. *J Pathol* 2005;205:302–310.
26. de la Fouchardiere A, Gazzo S, Balme B, et al. Cytogenetic and molecular analysis of 12 cases of primary cutaneous marginal zone lymphomas. *Am J Dermatopathol* 2006;28:287–292.
27. Gallardo F, Bellosillo B, Espinet B, et al. Aberrant nuclear BCL10 expression and lack of t(11;18)(q21;q21) in primary cutaneous marginal zone B-cell lymphoma. *Hum Pathol* 2006;37:867–873.
28. Palmedo G, Hantschke M, Rutten A, et al. Primary cutaneous marginal zone B-cell lymphoma may exhibit both the t(14;18)(q32;q21) IGH/BCL2 and the t(14;18)(q32;q21) IGH/MALT1 translocation: an indicator for clonal transformation towards higher-grade B-cell lymphoma? *Am J Dermatopathol* 2007;29:231–236.
29. Cerroni L, Gatter K, Kerl H. *An illustrated guide to skin lymphoma*, 2nd ed. Malden, Mass: Blackwell Publishing, 2004.
30. Geelen FA, Vermeer MH, Meijer CJ, et al. bcl-2 protein expression in primary cutaneous large B-cell lymphoma is site-related. *J Clin Oncol* 1998;16:2080–2085.
31. Dogan A, Bagdi E, Munson P, et al. CD10 and BCL-6 expression in paraffin sections of normal lymphoid tissue and B-cell lymphomas. *Am J Surg Pathol* 2000;24:846–852.
32. Cerroni L, Arzberger E, Putz B, et al. Primary cutaneous follicle center cell lymphoma with follicular growth pattern. *Blood* 2000;95:3922–3928.
33. Bergman R, Kurtin PJ, Gibson LE, et al. Clinicopathologic, immunophenotypic, and molecular characterization of primary cutaneous follicular B-cell lymphoma. *Arch Dermatol* 2001;137:432–439.

34. Franco R, Fernandez-Vazquez A, Rodriguez-Peralto JL, et al. Cutaneous follicular B-cell lymphoma: description of a series of 18 cases. *Am J Surg Pathol* 2001;25:875–883.

35. Mirza I, Macpherson N, Paproski S, et al. Primary cutaneous follicular lymphoma: an assessment of clinical, histopathologic, immunophenotypic, and molecular features. *J Clin Oncol* 2002;20:647–655.

36. Fung MA, Murphy MJ, Hoss DM, et al. Practical evaluation and management of cutaneous lymphoma. *J Am Acad Dermatol* 2002;46:325–357.

37. Goodlad JR, Krajewski AS, Batstone PJ, et al. Primary cutaneous follicular lymphoma: a clinicopathologic and molecular study of 16 cases in support of a distinct entity. *Am J Surg Pathol* 2002;26:733–741.

38. Child FJ, Scarisbrick JJ, Calonje E, et al. Inactivation of tumor suppressor genes p15(INK4b) and p16(INK4a) in primary cutaneous B cell lymphoma. *J Invest Dermatol* 2002;118:941–948.

39. Hoefnagel JJ, Vermeer MH, Jansen PM, et al. Bcl-2, Bcl-6 and CD10 expression in cutaneous B-cell lymphoma: further support for a follicle centre cell origin and differential diagnostic significance. *Br J Dermatol* 2003;149:1183–1191.

40. Vermeer MH, Geelen FA, van Haselen CW, et al. Primary cutaneous large B-cell lymphomas of the legs. A distinct type of cutaneous B-cell lymphoma with an intermediate prognosis. Dutch Cutaneous Lymphoma Working Group. *Arch Dermatol* 1996;132:1304–1308.

41. Fernandez-Vazquez A, Rodriguez-Peralto JL, Martinez MA, et al. Primary cutaneous large B-cell lymphoma: the relation between morphology, clinical presentation, immunohistochemical markers, and survival. *Am J Surg Pathol* 2001;25:307–315.

42. Hembury TA, Lee B, Gascoyne RD, et al. Primary cutaneous diffuse large B-cell lymphoma: a clinicopathologic study of 15 cases. *Am J Clin Pathol* 2002;117:574–580.

43. Narimatsu H, Morishita Y, Shimada K, et al. Primary cutaneous diffuse large B cell lymphoma: a clinically aggressive case. *Intern Med* 2003;42:354–357.

44. Grange F, Petrella T, Beylot-Barry M, et al. Bcl-2 protein expression is the strongest independent prognostic factor of survival in primary cutaneous large B-cell lymphomas. *Blood* 2004;103:3662–3668.

45. Hoefnagel JJ, Dijkman R, Basso K, et al. Distinct types of primary cutaneous large B-cell lymphoma identified by gene expression profiling. *Blood* 2005;105:3671–3678.

46. Kim YH, Willemze R, Pimpinelli N, et al. TNM classification system for primary cutaneous lymphomas other than mycosis fungoides and Sézary syndrome: a proposal of the International Society for Cutaneous Lymphomas (ISCL) and the Cutaneous Lymphoma Task Force of the European Organization of Research and Treatment of Cancer (EORTC). *Blood* 2007;110:479–484.

47. Senff NJ, Noordijk EM, Kim YH, et al. European Organization for Research and Treatment of Cancer and International Society for Cutaneous Lymphoma consensus recommendations for the management of cutaneous B-cell lymphomas. *Blood* 2008;112:1600–1609.

48. de la Fouchardiere A, Balme B, Chouvet B, et al. Pathological and clinical correlations in primary cutaneous B-cell lymphomas: a series of 44 cases [in French]. *Ann Pathol* 2005;25:8–17.

49. Hoefnagel JJ, Vermeer MH, Jansen PM, et al. Primary cutaneous marginal zone B-cell lymphoma: clinical and therapeutic features in 50 cases. *Arch Dermatol* 2005;141:1139–1145.

50. Aguilera NS, Tomaszewski MM, Moad JC, et al. Cutaneous follicle center lymphoma: a clinicopathologic study of 19 cases. *Mod Pathol* 2001;14:828–835.

51. Goodlad JR, Krajewski AS, Batstone PJ, et al. Primary cutaneous diffuse large B-cell lymphoma: prognostic significance of clinicopathological subtypes. *Am J Surg Pathol* 2003;27:1538–1545.

52. Grange F, Beylot-Barry M, Courville P, et al. Primary cutaneous diffuse large B-cell lymphoma, leg type: clinicopathologic features and prognostic analysis in 60 cases. *Arch Dermatol* 2007;143:1144–1150.

53. Barrans SL, Fenton JA, Banham A, et al. Strong expression of FOXP1 identifies a distinct subset of diffuse large B-cell lymphoma (DLBCL) patients with poor outcome. *Blood* 2004;104:2933–2935.

54. Senff NJ, Willemze R. The applicability and prognostic value of the new TNM classification system for primary cutaneous lymphomas other than mycosis fungoides and Sézary syndrome: results on a large cohort of primary cutaneous B-cell lymphomas and comparison with the system used by the Dutch Cutaneous Lymphoma Group. *Br J Dermatol* 2007;157:1205–1211.

55. Bailey EM, Ferry JA, Harris NL, et al. Marginal zone lymphoma (low-grade B-cell lymphoma of mucosa-associated lymphoid tissue type) of skin and subcutaneous tissue: a study of 15 patients. *Am J Surg Pathol* 1996;20:1011–1023.

56. Eich HT, Eich D, Micke O, et al. Long-term efficacy, curative potential, and prognostic factors of radiotherapy in primary cutaneous B-cell lymphoma. *Int J Radiat Oncol Biol Phys* 2003;55:899–906.

57. Gronbaek K, Moller PH, Nedergaard T, et al. Primary cutaneous B-cell lymphoma: a clinical, histological, phenotypic and genotypic study of 21 cases. *Br J Dermatol* 2000;142:913–923.

58. Kiyohara T, Kumakiri M, Kobayashi H, et al. Cutaneous marginal zone B-cell lymphoma: a case accompanied by massive plasmacytoid cells. *J Am Acad Dermatol* 2003;48:S82–S85.

59. Sah A, Barrans SL, Parapia LA, et al. Cutaneous B-cell lymphoma: pathological spectrum and clinical outcome in 51 consecutive patients. *Am J Hematol* 2004;75:195–199.

60. Senff NJ, Hoefnagel JJ, Neelis KJ, et al. Results of radiotherapy in 153 primary cutaneous B-Cell lymphomas classified according to the WHO-EORTC classification. *Arch Dermatol* 2007;143:1520–1526.

61. Smith BD, Glusac EJ, McNiff JM, et al. Primary cutaneous B-cell lymphoma treated with radiotherapy: a comparison of the European Organization for Research and Treatment of Cancer and the WHO classification systems. *J Clin Oncol* 2004;22:634–639.

62. Yap LM, Blum R, Foley P, et al. Clinical study of primary cutaneous B-cell lymphoma using both the European Organization for Research and Treatment of Cancer and World Health Organization classifications. *Australas J Dermatol* 2003;44:110–115.

63. Bachmeyer C, Khosrotehrani K, Moguelet P, et al. Primary cutaneous follicular B-cell lymphoma arising at the site of radiotherapy for breast cancer. *Br J Dermatol* 2007;156:198–199.

64. Bachmeyer C, Orlandini V, Aractingi S. Topical mechlorethamine and clobetasol in multifocal primary cutaneous marginal zone-B cell lymphoma. *Br J Dermatol* 2006;154:1207–1209.

65. Cozzio A, Kempf W, Schmid-Meyer R, et al. Intra-lesional low-dose interferon alpha2a therapy for primary cutaneous marginal zone B-cell lymphoma. *Leuk Lymphoma* 2006;47:865–869.

66. Fink-Puches R, Wolf IH, Zalaudek I, et al. Treatment of primary cutaneous B-cell lymphoma with rituximab. *J Am Acad Dermatol* 2005;52:847–853.

67. Gellrich S, Muche JM, Wilks A, et al. Systemic eight-cycle anti-CD20 monoclonal antibody (rituximab) therapy in primary cutaneous B-cell lymphomas–an applicational observation. *Br J Dermatol* 2005;153:167–173.

68. Kerl K, Prins C, Saurat JH, et al. Intralesional and intravenous treatment of cutaneous B-cell lymphomas with the monoclonal anti-CD20 antibody rituximab: report and follow-up of eight cases. *Br J Dermatol* 2006;155:1197–1200.

69. Kyrtsonis MC, Siakantaris MP, Kalpadakis C, et al. Favorable outcome of primary cutaneous marginal zone lymphoma treated with intralesional rituximab. *Eur J Haematol* 2006;77:300–303.

70. Soda R, Costanzo A, Cantonetti M, et al. Systemic therapy of primary cutaneous B-cell lymphoma, marginal zone type, with rituximab, a chimeric anti-CD20 monoclonal antibody. *Acta Derm Venereol* 2001;81:207–208.

71. Stanway A, Rademaker M, Kennedy I, et al. Cutaneous B-cell lymphoma of nails, pinna and nose treated with chlorambucil. *Australas J Dermatol* 2004;45:110–113.

72. Kutting B, Bonsmann G, Metze D, et al. Borrelia burgdorferi-associated primary cutaneous B cell lymphoma: complete clearing of skin lesions after antibiotic pulse therapy or intralesional injection of interferon alfa-2a. *J Am Acad Dermatol* 1997;36:311–314.

73. Wollina U, Hahnfeld S, Kosmehl H. Primary cutaneous marginal center lymphoma—complete remission induced by interferon alpha2a. *J Cancer Res Clin Oncol* 1999;125:305–308.

74. Piccinno R, Caccialanza M, Berti E. Dermatologic radiotherapy of primary cutaneous follicle center cell lymphoma. *Eur J Dermatol* 2003;13:49–52.

75. Ulutin HC, Ozturk B, Onguru O, et al. Treatment of primary cutaneous B-cell lymphoma with radiotherapy. *Radiat Med* 2005;23:292–295.

76. Wong KC, Weller PA. Primary cutaneous B cell lymphoma: outcomes and treatment. *Australas J Dermatol* 1998;39:261–264.

77. Zemtsov A, Camisa C. Treatment of primary cutaneous B cell lymphoma with local radiotherapy. *Cutis* 1990;45:435–438.

78. Rubegni P, De Aloe G, Pianigiani E, et al. Primary cutaneous B-cell lymphoma: treatment with low dose intralesional recombinant interferon-alpha 2A. *J Eur Acad Dermatol Venereol* 1999;12:70–71.

79. Zenone T, Catimel G, Barbet N, et al. Complete remission of a primary cutaneous B cell lymphoma treated with intralesional recombinant interferon alpha-2a. *Eur J Cancer* 1994;30A:246–247.

80. Heinzerling L, Dummer R, Kempf W, et al. Intralesional therapy with anti-CD20 monoclonal antibody rituximab in primary cutaneous B-cell lymphoma. *Arch Dermatol* 2000;136:374–378.

81. Paul T, Radny P, Krober SM, et al. Intralesional rituximab for cutaneous B-cell lymphoma. *Br J Dermatol* 2001;144:1239–1243.

82. Roguedas AM, Watier H, Paintaud G, et al. Intralesional therapy with anti-CD20 monoclonal antibody rituximab: local and systemic efficacy in primary cutaneous B-cell lymphoma. *Br J Dermatol* 2005;152:541–544.

83. Errante D, Bernardi D, Bianco A, et al. Rituximab-related urticarial reaction in a patient treated for primary cutaneous B-cell lymphoma. *Ann Oncol* 2006;17:1720–1721.

84. Gitelson E, Al-Saleem T, Millenson M, et al. Cutaneous B-cell lymphoma responds to rituximab: a report of five cases and a review of the literature. *Leuk Lymphoma* 2006;47:1902–1907.

85. Kennedy GA, Blum R, McCormack C, et al. Treatment of primary cutaneous follicular centre lymphoma with rituximab: a report of two cases. *Australas J Dermatol* 2004;45:34–37.

86. Lami MC, Vabres P, Dreyfus B, et al. Primary cutaneous B-cell lymphoma mimicking pyoderma gangrenosum: first-line treatment with rituximab. *Br J Dermatol* 2004;151:250–252.

87. Massengale WT, McBurney E, Gurtler J. CD20-negative relapse of cutaneous B-cell lymphoma after anti-CD20 monoclonal antibody therapy. *J Am Acad Dermatol* 2002;46:441–443.

88. Nagasaka A, Matsue H, Kawamura T, et al. Complete remission of a primary cutaneous follicle-center cell lymphoma (EORTC criteria)/diffuse large B-cell lymphoma (WHO criteria) by single first-line therapy with rituximab. *J Dermatol* 2006;33:377–379.

89. Schneider LA. Cutaneous B-cell lymphoma treated with rituximab infusions. *Acta Derm Venereol* 2006;86:550–551.

90. Heinzerling LM, Urbanek M, Funk JO, et al. Reduction of tumor burden and stabilization of disease by systemic therapy with anti-CD20 antibody (rituximab) in patients with primary cutaneous B-cell lymphoma. *Cancer* 2000;89:1835–1844.

91. Lacouture ME, Baron JM, Jani AB, et al. Treatment of radiation-relapsing primary cutaneous B-cell lymphoma with an anti-CD20 monoclonal antibody. *Clin Exp Dermatol* 2005;30:46–48.

92. Fierro MT, Savoia P, Quaglino P, et al. Systemic therapy with cyclophosphamide and anti-CD20 antibody (rituximab) in relapsed primary cutaneous B-cell lymphoma: a report of 7 cases. *J Am Acad Dermatol* 2003;49:281–287.

93. Fierro MT, Quaglino P, Savoia P, et al. Systemic polychemotherapy in the treatment of primary cutaneous lymphomas: a clinical follow-up study of 81 patients treated with COP or CHOP. *Leuk Lymphoma* 1998;31:583–588.

94. Sarris AH, Braunschweig I, Medeiros LJ, et al. Primary cutaneous non-Hodgkin's lymphoma of Ann Arbor stage I: preferential cutaneous relapses but high cure rate with doxorubicin-based therapy. *J Clin Oncol* 2001;19:398–405.

95. Rijlaarsdam JU, Toonstra J, Meijer OW, et al. Treatment of primary cutaneous B-cell lymphomas of follicle center cell origin: a clinical follow-up study of 55 patients treated with radiotherapy or polychemotherapy. *J Clin Oncol* 1996;14:549–555.

96. Imai Y, Isoda K, Ito E, et al. Primary cutaneous follicle center cell lymphoma of the scalp successfully treated with anti CD20 monoclonal antibody and CHOP combination therapy with no subsequent permanent loss of hair. *J Dermatol* 2003;30:683–688.

97. Bonnekoh B, Schulz M, Franke I, et al. Complete remission of a primary cutaneous B-cell lymphoma of the lower leg by first-line monotherapy with the CD20-antibody rituximab. *J Cancer Res Clin Oncol* 2002; 128:161–166.

98. Di Bella NJ, Khan MM, Dakhil SR, et al. Pegylated liposomal doxorubicin as single-agent treatment of low-grade non-Hodgkin's lymphoma: a phase II multicenter study. *Clin Lymphoma* 2003;3:235–240.

99. Dummer R, Hassel JC, Fellenberg F, et al. Adenovirus-mediated intralesional interferon-gamma gene transfer induces tumor regressions in cutaneous lymphomas. *Blood* 2004;104:1631–1638.

100. Urosevic M. Drug evaluation: TG-1042, an adenovirus-mediated IFN-gamma gene delivery for the intratumoral therapy of primary cutaneous lymphomas. *Curr Opin Investig Drugs* 2007;8:493–498.

101. Urosevic M, Fujii K, Calmels B, et al. Type I IFN innate immune response to adenovirus-mediated IFN-gamma gene transfer contributes to the regression of cutaneous lymphomas. *J Clin Invest* 2007;117:2834–2846.

102. Conill C, Navalpotro B, Lopez I, et al. Results of radiotherapy in primary cutaneous lymphoma. *Clin Transl Oncol* 2006; 8: 430–434.

103. De Sanctis V, Osti MF, Berardi F, et al. Primary cutaneous lymphoma: local control and survival in patients treated with radiotherapy. *Anticancer Res* 2007;27:601–605.

104. El-Helw L, Goodwin S, Slater D, et al. Primary B-cell lymphoma of the skin: the Sheffield Lymphoma Group Experience (1984-2003). *Int J Oncol* 2004;25:1453–1458.

105. Kirova YM, Piedbois Y, Le Bourgeois JP. Radiotherapy in the management of cutaneous B-cell lymphoma. Our experience in 25 cases. *Radiother Oncol* 1999;52:15–18.

106. Piccinno R, Caccialanza M, Berti E, et al. Radiotherapy of cutaneous B cell lymphomas: our experience in 31 cases. *Int J Radiat Oncol Biol Phys* 1993;27:385–389.

107. Brice P, Cazals D, Mounier N, et al. Primary cutaneous large-cell lymphoma: analysis of 49 patients included in the LNH87 prospective trial of polychemotherapy for high-grade lymphomas. Groupe d'Etude des Lymphomes de l'Adulte. *Leukemia* 1998;12:213–219.

108. Wollina U, Mentzel T, Graefe T. Large B-cell lymphoma of the leg–complete remission with perilesional interferon alpha. *Dermatology* 2001;203:165–167.

109. Wollina U. Complete response of a primary cutaneous T-cell-rich B cell lymphoma treated with interferon alpha2a. *J Cancer Res Clin Oncol* 1998;124:127–129.

110. Hofbauer GF, Kessler B, Kempf W, et al. Multilesional primary cutaneous diffuse large B-cell lymphoma responsive to antibiotic treatment. *Dermatology* 2001;203:168–170.

CHAPTER 25 ■ MYCOSIS FUNGOIDES AND SÉZARY SYNDROME

YOUN H. KIM, RANJANA ADVANI, JEFF D. HARVELL, AND RICHARD T. HOPPE

Mycosis fungoides is a cutaneous lymphoma of mature, predominately CD4$^+$ T cells. It is the most common type of cutaneous T-cell lymphoma, and is distinguished from other cutaneous T-cell lymphomas by its unique clinical and histologic features. It is important to note that not all cutaneous T-cell lymphomas are mycosis fungoides. This term was introduced at a time when the immunoperoxidase characteristics of the entire spectrum of cutaneous lymphomas had not been defined, and only mycosis fungoides/Sézary syndrome was identified as being of T-cell origin. We now appreciate that other cutaneous T-cell lymphomas exist, including many cases of CD30$^+$ anaplastic large cell lymphoma, cytotoxic T-cell lymphomas, and peripheral T-cell lymphoma, not otherwise specified. Therefore, the terms *mycosis fungoides* and *cutaneous T-cell lymphoma* are not synonymous.

EPIDEMIOLOGY

The estimated annual incidence rate of mycosis fungoides and Sézary syndrome in the United States has increased gradually since 1973 at a rate of 0.29 per 100,000 per decade to 0.64 per 100,000 at the end of study period in 2002 (1). It accounts for 4% of all non-Hodgkin lymphoma. It commonly affects older adults (median age 55 to 65 years), and there is a 2:1 male predominance without an established racial predilection.

The etiologies of mycosis fungoides and Sézary syndrome are unknown. Some retrospective studies have suggested a role for chemical exposure as a source of either chronic antigenic stimulation or toxic exposure. However, recent case-controlled studies refute this hypothesis (2,3). A viral etiology for mycosis fungoides was once proposed based on the isolation of human T-cell leukemia virus type 1 from the peripheral blood lymphocytes of a patient with a cutaneous lymphoma that resembled mycosis fungoides (4). However, it was later demonstrated that this patient actually had human T-cell leukemia virus type 1-associated T-cell lymphoma, a specific type of lymphoma that has now been described more precisely and is quite different from mycosis fungoides.

PATHOLOGY

Morphology

In patch lesions of mycosis fungoides, there is typically mild epidermal hyperplasia or atrophy associated with a perivascular or band-like infiltrate of small- to medium-sized atypical lymphocytes with hyperchromatic and convoluted (cerebriform) nuclei. The atypical cells exhibit epidermotropism, with individual lymphocytes arranged along the dermal-epidermal junction in a single-file pattern or scattered throughout all layers of the epidermis in the absence of spongiosis (Color Plate 45). Small intraepidermal collections of neoplastic lymphocytes are known as *Pautrier microabscesses* (Color Plate 46). Although such collections are virtually pathognomonic of mycosis fungoides, in early patch-stage lesions, Pautrier microabscesses may not be present. As lesions evolve from patches to plaques, the density of neoplastic cells within the dermis increases, and the degree of epidermotropism becomes more exaggerated. In tumorous lesions, the dermal infiltrate is very dense, involving the full breadth of the dermis, often extending into the subcutaneous fat, and epidermotropism tends to diminish.

Biopsies of patients with erythroderma show very similar histology to that of patch mycosis fungoides, but the infiltrate is typically more sparse, and the diagnosis is more difficult to establish. By definition, in the Sézary syndrome, Sézary cells with cerebriform nuclei are seen within the peripheral blood (Color Plate 47). For a definitive diagnosis, they should number at least 1,000 per mm^3 (5). Additional ancillary tests, which help to refine the diagnosis, include an expanded peripheral blood CD4$^+$ population with increased ratio of CD4 to CD8 T lymphocytes (>10:1), expanded populations of abnormal T cells with CD4$^+$/CD7$^-$ or CD4$^+$/CD26$^-$ phenotype, and molecular evidence of a relevant T-cell receptor gene rearrangement in the peripheral blood (5–7). Involved lymph nodes in mycosis fungoides or Sézary syndrome show a range of histologic features (Table 25.1). The disease may cause regional nodes to develop the changes of dermatopathic lymphadenitis, with or without scattered individual atypical cerebriform lymphocytes (category I). Category II lymph nodes demonstrate dermatopathic lymphadenitis with clusters of more than ten cytologically atypical lymphocytes confined to the paracortex. Category III is reserved for lymph nodes that demonstrate partial or total effacement of lymph node architecture by atypical lymphocytes (8–10). Because reactive lymph nodes can sometimes exhibit nonneoplastic lymphocytes with cerebriform nuclei, and because the diagnosis of early lymph node involvement by mycosis fungoides (i.e., category I) can be very difficult on histologic grounds alone, molecular methods for demonstrating T-cell clonality are gaining wide acceptance. Recent studies even suggest that patients with lymph nodes exhibiting rearranged T-cell receptor genes by molecular methods have a worse prognosis, regardless of the histologic grade (6,11).

TABLE 25.1

LYMPH NODE GRADING SYSTEM FOR MYCOSIS FUNGOIDES

Category I (LN0–LN2)	Dermatopathic lymphadenopathy without atypical lymphocytes (LN0). Scattered atypical cerebriform lymphocytes (not in clusters), with or without dermatopathic lymphadenopathy (LN1). Atypical lymphocytes forming small clusters, not more than six cells per cluster, with or without dermatopathic lymphadenopathy (LN2).
Category II (LN3)	Clusters of ten or more cytologically atypical lymphocytes confined to the paracortex, with or without dermatopathic lymphadenopathy (LN3).
Category III (LN4)	Partial or complete effacement of lymph node architecture by cytologically atypical lymphocytes (LN4).

From Clendenning WE, Rappaport H. Report of the Committee on Pathology of Cutaneous T Cell Lymphomas. *Cancer Treat Rep* 1979;63:719–724, with permission.

Immunophenotype

Most cases of conventional mycosis fungoides exhibit the following immunophenotype: CD2$^+$, CD3$^+$, CD4$^+$, CD8$^-$, CD5$^+$, CD7$^-$, CD25$^{-/+}$, CD30$^-$, and T-cell receptor α/β^+. Some cases exhibit a CD8$^+$/CD4$^-$ immunophenotype, and rare ones exhibit surface T-cell receptor γ/δ rather than T-cell receptor α/β. Mycosis fungoides-associated follicular mucinosis and granulomatous slack skin generally exhibit the same immunophenotype as conventional mycosis fungoides (12,13). The immunophenotype in pagetoid reticulosis is variable: CD4$^+$/CD8$^-$, CD4$^-$/CD8$^+$, or CD4$^-$/CD8$^-$. As in conventional mycosis fungoides, CD7 is absent. The Ki-67 proliferation fraction in pagetoid reticulosis is higher than in conventional mycosis fungoides, usually >30%, and unlike conventional mycosis fungoides, CD30 expression is common (14).

Molecular Diagnosis

Both Southern blot and polymerase chain reaction analyses are capable of detecting clonally rearranged T-cell receptor gene sequences in clinical material from patients with mycosis fungoides. In normal and neoplastic T-cell ontogeny, the γ region of the T-cell receptor gene is rearranged early on, such that most T-cell malignancies have detectable T-cell–receptor γ chain rearrangements, despite the fact that the α/β heterodimer is more often expressed at the cell surface. For various practical reasons, polymerase chain reaction analysis of the γ-chain region of the T-cell receptor (T cell receptor γ) has proved more useful than Southern blot analysis in the evaluation of T-cell lymphoproliferative disorders. Polymerase chain reaction of T-cell receptor γ represents a very useful adjunct to the histopathologic diagnosis of various cutaneous T-cell malignancies, especially early patch-stage

mycosis fungoides, and, at present, the sensitivity of the assay is approximately 70%. It is well established that nonneoplastic inflammatory dermatoses can exhibit detectable T-cell receptor gene rearrangements. The false-positive rate reported in the literature is quite variable, but the overall specificity is probably approximately 80% to 90% (15). Recently reported data suggest that the false-positive rate becomes lower when tissue samples from two anatomically different sites or different time points demonstrate the presence of identical clones (16).

PATHOGENESIS

Immunopathogenesis

Cytokines have been implicated in the pathophysiology of mycosis fungoides and Sézary syndrome (17–19). However, whether cytokine abnormalities are primarily involved or are secondary processes in the pathogenesis is unclear. Studies have reported that soluble interleukin (IL)-2 receptor values in Sézary syndrome were significantly higher than for other malignant or inflammatory T-cell diseases, and that the serum levels correlated with clinical course and Sézary cell count. The highest soluble IL-2 receptor levels were found in patients with advanced disease (19). Other investigators have shown that peripheral blood mononuclear cells from patients with the Sézary syndrome expressed higher levels of IL-4 and lower levels of IL-2 and interferon (IFN)-γ after phytohemagglutinin stimulation compared with normal controls (17).

A number of studies have suggested that the malignant T cells in Sézary syndrome account for aberrant cytokine production, with increased production of T-helper type 2 cytokines (e.g., IL-4, IL-5, IL-10) and decreased production of T-helper type 1 cytokines (e.g., IL-2 and IFN-γ) (20,21). Moreover, this aberrant cytokine production may be the cause for the immune abnormalities seen occasionally in Sézary syndrome. These immune abnormalities may include: decreased T-cell responses to antigens and mitogens; impaired cell-mediated cytotoxicity, including natural killer-cell and lymphokine-activated killer-cell activities; increased levels of serum immunoglobulin E and immunoglobulin A; and peripheral eosinophilia.

Molecular Biology

Genetic aberrations that contribute to the development and progression of mycosis fungoides or Sézary syndrome are becoming better elucidated. Cytogenetic studies have yet to disclose a consistent chromosomal change in all patients with mycosis fungoides, but alterations to 10q, including loss of heterozygosity and microsatellite instability, are reported (14). These may result in the loss of function of a tumor suppressor gene (or genes) found in this region, such as PTEN. Other studies have found evidence that p16(INK4a), a tumor suppressor gene located on 9p, may be selectively inactivated with progression of mycosis fungoides from patch to tumor stage (22). Recurrent chromosomal or genetic abnormalities have been reported in Sézary syndrome. In particular, utilizing high-resolution array based comparative genomic hybridization, the Sézary syndrome genome was characterized by gross chromosomal instability with highly recurrent gains and losses. Prominent among deregulated genes are those encoding c-myc, c-myc-regulating proteins, mediators of myc-induced apoptosis, and IL-2 signaling pathway components.(23). Preliminary data from transcriptional analysis with oligonucleotide microarrays in mycosis fungoides revealed promising clinically relevant gene signatures predictive of survival, disease progression, and response to therapy (24). However, further prospective long-term studies are needed to validate these early findings.

Postulated Cell of Origin

In most cases of mycosis fungoides and Sézary syndrome, the cell of origin is a clonal CD4$^+$ T lymphocyte with skin-homing (epidermotropic) properties.

Biology of Transformation

Histologically, transformation to large cell lymphoma is defined on the basis of either an infiltrate of large atypical lymphocytes that comprise >25% of the dermal infiltrate, or nodular expansile aggregates of atypical large lymphocytes (Color Plate 48) (25,26). This large cell transformation is associated with worse clinical outcome (27). In the majority of cases, increased mitotic activity is readily observed, and the Ki-67 proliferation rate by immunohistochemistry is >25% (25). Immunophenotypically, the transformed large lymphocytes can exhibit variable loss of one or more T-cell–associated antigens such as CD3, CD5, CD4, CD8, CD45RO, or CD43 (25,26). Also, the large cells may express lymphocyte activation markers such as CD30 and CD25 (25). In some cases, there are intermixed aggregates of small, medium, or large-sized B lymphocytes, which are presumably reactive and should not be erroneously interpreted as a secondary B-cell lymphoproliferative disorder. When CD30 expression is prominent among the transformed large lymphocytes, CD30$^+$ lymphoproliferative disorders (especially CD30$^+$ anaplastic large cell lymphoma) must be considered in the differential diagnosis. Histologic findings that favor a diagnosis of transformed mycosis fungoides include an accompanying infiltrate of smaller-sized lymphocytes that exhibit epidermotropism (as seen in earlier-stage mycosis fungoides lesions), epidermotropism by CD30$^+$ lymphocytes (which is usually not a feature of anaplastic large cell lymphoma), and a relatively low percentage of CD30$^+$ lymphocytes (as compared with cases of anaplastic large cell lymphoma, in which CD30$^+$ large lymphocytes are >75%). In some cases, correlation with the clinical findings is essential for a definitive diagnosis.

CLINICAL PRESENTATION

Mycosis fungoides often has a long natural history, and the median duration from the onset of skin symptoms to a diagnosis of mycosis fungoides may be ≥5 years (5). In many patients, the disease presents initially in a premycotic phase with nonspecific, slightly scaling skin lesions that wax and wane over a period of years. Biopsies are generally nondiagnostic during this phase of disease, and patients may respond to treatment with topical corticosteroids. Some of these patients will experience an evolution of their disease and develop more typical patches or infiltrated plaques, from which a definitive diagnostic biopsy may be obtained. Repeated biopsies must be obtained from patients suspected of having mycosis fungoides, even when an initial biopsy is negative.

The most common initial cutaneous presentation is patch and plaque disease; however, some patients may present with tumors or generalized erythroderma. There may be prominent poikiloderma (skin atrophy with telangiectasia), or associated alopecia or follicular mucinosis. Approximately 30% of patients present with limited patch and plaque disease (<10% of the skin surface involved [T1]), 35% to 40% with generalized patch and plaque (≥10% of the skin surface involved [T2]), 15% to 20% with tumorous (T3), and 15% with erythroderma (T4).

The typical patches of mycosis fungoides are slightly scaling and mildly erythematous (Color Plate 49). More infiltrated lesions evolve into palpable plaques (Color Plate 50). These plaques are erythematous and slightly scaling, with well-defined borders. The shape and distribution of lesions are variable. Many patients present with involvement in the "bathing trunk" distribution, although lesions may be present on any part of the body. Pruritus is the most common symptom even in the early phases of the disease and is often the problem that prompts a visit to the dermatologist.

Infiltrated plaques may evolve into ulcerating or fungating tumors (Color Plate 51). Tumors often become infected, and sepsis secondary to infection is often the cause of death in individuals so affected. Generalized dermal thickening from infiltrative disease may cause the classic but very unusual leonine facies of mycosis fungoides.

Another manifestation of skin involvement in mycosis fungoides is generalized erythroderma (Color Plate 52). The erythema may be accompanied by either atrophic or lichenified skin, and plaques or tumors may also be present. These patients are almost always intensely symptomatic from pruritus and scaling, and often have lymphadenopathy due to diffuse and severe skin involvement. Cells may be present in the peripheral blood that have the same microscopic appearance and immunophenotypic and genotypic characteristics as the cells that infiltrate the epidermis. Patients with this complex of findings, generalized erythroderma, lymphadenopathy, and significant numbers of atypical T cells (Sézary cells) in the peripheral blood have Sézary syndrome (28). Patients with Sézary syndrome have a worse prognosis than patients with erythroderma with mycosis fungoides who do not have the other findings of the Sézary syndrome.

Mycosis fungoides may be associated with follicular involvement with or without mucin deposit. In these cases, involvement of the hair follicles is clinically prominent, and biopsy shows a heavy infiltration of the hair follicle epithelium by atypical cerebriform lymphocytes. Often, the interfollicular epidermis is spared. In typical cases, there is expansion of the hair follicle epithelium by connective tissue mucin, sometimes resulting in small pools of follicular mucin. However, mucin deposition can be variable, and because of this variability, there has been a recent recommendation that cases of mycosis fungoides associated with folliculotropism be designated *folliculotropic mycosis fungoides* (12,28).

Pagetoid reticulosis, also known as Woringer-Kolopp disease, is a verrucous variant of mycosis fungoides that typically affects acral sites, such as the hands and feet, and features extensive epidermotropism by atypical lymphocytes (29). The degree of epidermotropism is greatly exaggerated as compared with conventional mycosis fungoides, to the point that atypical lymphocytes are almost exclusively confined to a markedly acanthotic epidermis.

Granulomatous slack skin is a variant of mycosis fungoides that results in pendulous folds of slack or lax skin. The laxity is due to macrophage-mediated destruction of the normal elastic fiber network of the dermis. Histologically, there is a diffuse granulomatous and lymphocytic infiltrate with well-formed granulomas containing multinucleated giant cells. Another distinctive feature is the finding of elastic fibers within the cytoplasm of multinucleated giant cells, a pathologic process known as *elastophagocytosis*. It is the histologic correlate of ongoing elastic fiber destruction, which in late stages of the disease results in near-complete obliteration of dermal elastic tissue. Superimposed on the granulomatous infiltrate is an infiltrate of small cerebriform lymphocytes that displays the typical epidermotropic changes encountered in conventional mycosis fungoides (30).

Multiple other clinical and histologic variants of mycosis fungoides have been reported. Of these variants, hypopigmented or depigmented mycosis fungoides is most commonly seen in children (31) and darker skinned ethnic groups (32).

Many patients with mycosis fungoides have evidence of cutaneous disease only throughout the course of their disease. Only 15% to 20% of patients with mycosis fungoides develop clinical problems related to extracutaneous disease. The most commonly identified site of extracutaneous disease is the regional lymphatics, usually in areas that drain significant sites of skin involvement. Visceral disease may be identified subsequently. The most common visceral sites of involvement identified are the lungs, oral cavity/pharynx, and the central nervous system, but virtually any organ may be involved at autopsy in patients who have died of the disease.

STAGING

Along with a revised clinical staging system for patients with mycosis fungoides and Sézary syndrome, a consensus recommendation for staging evaluation has been established (6,7). Conventional staging for patients with mycosis fungoides includes a comprehensive physical examination with careful examination of the skin (including the scalp, palms, soles, and perineum) and lymph nodes, a complete blood count with Sézary cell studies, screening chemistries (including lactate dehydrogenase), and chest x-ray. Additional imaging studies for patients with T1 or T2 skin involvement are not recommended unless the patient has very extensive skin disease, lymphadenopathy, or parameters associated with worse clinical outcome, such as folliculotropic disease or blood involvement. However, patients with T3 or T4 disease are at increased risk for extracutaneous involvement, and further imaging, such as a contrast-enhanced chest/abdomen/pelvis computed tomography scan or whole body 18-fluoro-deoxy-glucose-positron emission tomography /computed tomography, is appropriate. The usefulness of added functional information with 18-fluoro-deoxyglucose-positron emission tomography has been demonstrated in mycosis fungoides and Sézary syndrome (33). Lymph node biopsies should be obtained if lymphadenopathy is present. Suspected sites of visceral involvement should be confirmed by appropriate biopsy. Bone marrow involvement may often be detected in patients who meet the clinical criteria for Sézary syndrome (34) but is extremely uncommon in classic mycosis fungoides. Therefore, a bone marrow biopsy is not routinely used as part of the initial staging.

A tumor-node-metastasis-blood (TNMB) staging system that has proved useful for mycosis fungoides was proposed at the Workshop on Mycosis Fungoides held at the National Cancer Institute in 1978 (35). This original staging system has been revised to reflect the updated prognostic information, and be more consistent with current practice and management (6). Tables 25.2 and 25.3 summarize the revised TNMB categories and staging classification, respectively.

The T classification reflects the extent and type of skin involvement. The N category indicates the presence or absence of lymph node involvement. The M category indicates visceral disease. In the B (blood) category, the absence or presence of a significant proportion of abnormal, cerebriform (Sézary) cells should be noted. Clinically insignificant, low levels of Sézary-like cells can be detected in the peripheral blood of patients with benign skin conditions.

PROGNOSTIC AND PREDICTIVE FACTORS

The T classification and presence of extracutaneous disease are the most important predictors of survival in patients with mycosis fungoides (36,37). Among patients with T4 disease (erythroderma), age >60 years, peripheral blood involvement, and extracutaneous disease are independent adverse

TABLE 25.2

TNMB CLASSIFICATION

T (skin)	
T1	Limited patch/plaque (<10% of total skin surface)
T2	Generalized patch/plaque (≥10% of total skin surface)
T3	Tumors
T4	Generalized erythroderma
N (nodes)	
N0	Lymph nodes clinically uninvolved
N1	Lymph nodes enlarged, histologically uninvolved (includes "reactive" and "dermatopathic" nodes)
N2	Lymph nodes clinically uninvolved, histologically involved
N3	Lymph nodes enlarged and histologically involved
M (viscera)	
M0	No visceral involvement
M1	Visceral involvement
B (blood)	
B0	No circulating atypical (Sézary) cells (<5% of total lymphocytes)
B1	Circulating atypical (Sézary) cells (≥5% of total lymphocytes)

TABLE 25.3

TNMB CLINICAL STAGING SYSTEM FOR MYCOSIS FUNGOIDES

Clinical stages	Tumor-Node-Metastasis classification[a]		
IA	T1	N0	M0
IB	T2	N0	M0
IIA	T1–2	N1	M0
IIB	T3	N0–1	M0
IIIA	T4	N0	M0
IIIB	T4	N1	M0
IVA	T1–4	N2–3	M0
IVB	T1–4	N0–3	M1

[a] The B classification does not alter clinical stage.

predictive factors for survival (38). Other worse prognostic factors include folliculotropic (12) or large cell-transformed disease (27).

TREATMENT

The nonspecific, symptomatic treatment of mycosis fungoides and Sézary syndrome is an integral component of the overall therapeutic regimen. Pruritus and xerosis, either as a result of the disease or therapy, may be severe. Thus, supportive measures, such as aggressive emolliation, topical steroids, and oral antipruritics, should be used as necessary.

There are multiple therapeutic options for mycosis fungoides and the Sézary syndrome. Selection of treatment is based primarily on the clinical stage of the disease (16,39). However, other factors, such as access to special treatment approaches, the patient's age, and other social and medical problems, as well as the cost to benefit ratio, should be taken into consideration. Also, patients with folliculotropic, any blood involvement, or transformed disease may receive more intensive therapy. For patients with patch or plaque skin involvement (T1 and T2) without extracutaneous disease, the treatment plan may be limited to skin-directed therapeutic measures, whereas patients with any extracutaneous disease should receive systemic (biologic or cytoxic) therapy as part of their management. It has been demonstrated in a prospective randomized clinical trial that there is no advantage to early aggressive combined modality therapy compared with conservative sequential therapies in the management of limited or advanced disease (40).

Topical Chemotherapy

Topical nitrogen mustard (mechlorethamine) is an effective topical therapy for mycosis fungoides (41–43). The mechanism of action when nitrogen mustard is applied topically is not well defined and may not be related simply to its alkylating-agent properties. Its activity may be mediated by immune mechanisms or by interaction with the epidermal cell-Langerhans cell-T cell axis.

Topical nitrogen mustard may be prepared as an aqueous solution or mixed in an ointment. Both preparations are

generally applied at a concentration of 10 to 20 mg per 100 cc. The aqueous and ointment preparations have similar efficacy. The choice is often dependent on convenience, patient preference, or cost. The ointment preparation uses less nitrogen mustard for similar response. Also, the aqueous preparation is associated with a much higher incidence (>30%) of hypersensitivity reaction compared with the low rate (<5%) reported with the ointment preparation.

Nitrogen mustard may be applied locally or to the entire skin. It is applied at least once daily during the clearing phase. Other areas of disease activity may become evident secondary to the inflammatory reaction provoked by the nitrogen mustard. After a period of several weeks, treatment may be limited to the affected region. Alternatively, if the disease is initially limited in distribution, the nitrogen mustard may be applied only to the affected anatomic region or regions, with careful follow-up to detect any new areas of involvement. Treatment is continued on a daily basis until skin clearance is complete. This may require ≥6 months and is then followed by a variable duration of maintenance therapy (3 to 6 months). If response is particularly slow, the concentration of the topical nitrogen mustard may be increased, or the frequency of application may be increased. The complete response rate for topical nitrogen mustard for limited patch or plaque (T1) disease is 70% to 80%. The median time to skin clearance is 6 to 8 months. When treatment is discontinued, more than one-half of patients will have relapse in the skin, but most will respond to a resumption of therapy. The proportion of patients treated with topical nitrogen mustard who have a durable complete response (>10 years) is 20% to 25%. In patients with a discrete number of refractory lesions, treatment may be supplemented with local irradiation.

The primary acute complication of topical nitrogen mustard is a cutaneous hypersensitivity reaction. Desensitization may be achieved by a variety of topical or systemic desensitization programs. There is no systemic absorption of topical nitrogen mustard, thus systemic complications such as bone marrow suppression or sterility are not an issue. Occasional patients treated with topical nitrogen mustard develop secondary squamoproliferative lesions of the skin. This risk is the greatest among patients who have had long-term sequential therapy with multiple topical modalities.

Another topical chemotherapeutic agent that has been used for patients with limited disease is carmustine (BCNU) (44). The efficacy of topical BCNU is similar to topical nitrogen mustard; however, because of the systemic absorption of BCNU, the potential hematologic complications are greater, and the maximum duration of treatment is limited. In addition, patients treated with BCNU tend to develop significant telangiectasias in areas where the drug is applied.

Phototherapy

Phototherapy involves using ultraviolet (UV) radiation in the form of UVA or UVB wavelengths, which can be used alone, together, or with psoralen, a photosensitizing agent, as psoralen plus UVA, or PUVA. The long-wave UVA has the advantage over UVB in its greater depth of penetration into the dermal infiltrates of mycosis fungoides. For early limited disease, UVB alone (45) or home UV phototherapy (UVA plus UVB) (46) has been shown to be effective.

More recently, narrow-band UVB (311 nm) phototherapy has been shown to be more effective than the traditional broad-band UVB. Narrow-band UVB is considered to have less associated toxicities than broadband UVB or PUVA. Several published studies using narrow-band UVB in mycosis fungoides have shown clinical efficacy that is superior than the broadband UVB (47); however, not more effective than PUVA (48).

PUVA therapy was first used in the treatment of psoriasis but also has been shown to be effective for patients with mycosis fungoides (49). In the presence of UVA, the psoralen drug intercalates with deoxyribonucleic acid (DNA), forming both monofunctional and bifunctional adducts. This process results in direct cytotoxic and antiproliferative effects, as well as possibly immunomodulatory effects, through either a direct effect on T cells or an indirect effect by modulating cytokine production.

During the clearing phase, which may require up to 6 months, patients are treated two to three times weekly. After this phase is completed, patients continue on a maintenance program with decreased frequency of treatment. If the disease begins to recur during the maintenance phase, then the frequency of treatment is increased in an effort to achieve better control.

With PUVA treatment, the complete clearance rate is 50% to 90% among patients with patch or plaque disease, and the likelihood of clearance is dependent on the initial extent of skin involvement. Long-term durable responses have been reported in patients treated with PUVA (50). The response is less impressive among patients with erythrodermic or tumor disease.

The primary acute complications of PUVA therapy include nausea and phototoxic reactions such as erythroderma and blistering, as well as skin dryness. Patients should shield their skin and eyes from the sun for at least 24 hours after psoralen ingestion. The potential long-term complications of PUVA therapy include cataract formation (requiring the use of UVA-opaque goggles during therapy) and secondary cutaneous malignancies. Among patients treated for mycosis fungoides, this risk is greatest for patients who have undergone long-term treatment with multiple topical therapies (50,51).

Topical Retinoids

Bexarotene (Targretin) 1% gel is the most commonly used topical retinoid for treating mycosis fungoides. The reported overall response rate (ORR) is 63%, with a complete response rate of 21% (40). Due to the irritant effect of the retinoids, it is only feasible to use this agent when there are a discrete number of patches or plaques. It is not intended for generalized application. Bexarotene gel is applied with a thin application to the patches or plaques and is most effective when used twice daily. The most common toxicity is irritation at sites of gel application, which occurs in the majority of patients with variable intensity. Because of the erythema from the irritant reaction, it may be necessary to withhold therapy for a few weeks to assess for residual active disease.

Radiation Therapy

Mycosis fungoides is an exquisitely radiosensitive neoplasm, and irradiation may be exploited in several ways for its man-

agement (52). Individual plaques or tumors of mycosis fungoides may be treated to total doses of 15 to 25 Gy in 1 to 3 weeks, with a high likelihood of achieving long-term local control. For the unusual patient with unilesional or localized mycosis fungoides, local electron beam therapy achieves the most efficient and complete clearance of the disease.

Local disease may be treated with low-energy x-rays or electrons. Electrons have an intrinsic advantage over x-rays because the depth of penetration of electrons can be controlled by the appropriate selection of electron energy. The relative dose contribution to the subcutaneous and deeper tissues is greater with even low-energy photons, compared with electrons. Peripheral margins of up to 2 cm are recommended but may be dependent on location and proximity to sensitive tissues.

Several centers have developed expertise in the use of total skin electron beam therapy (52–54). ORRs are nearly 100%, with complete response rates ranging from 40% to 98%, depending on the extent of skin involvement. As many as 50% of patients with limited plaque disease and 25% of patients with generalized plaque disease may remain free of disease for >5 years after completion of a single course of electron beam therapy. Although the curative potential of this treatment remains disputed, there is no doubt that it provides an important palliative benefit, especially for patients with extensive disease. Often, when disease recurs, it is in a more limited distribution and may be controlled more readily with localized topical therapies.

The widespread use of total skin electron beam therapy was facilitated by the development of the modern medical linear accelerator; the first adaptation of that device for total skin treatment with electrons was at Stanford University (55). The basic concept used in the "Stanford technique" was to replace the target at the end of the linear accelerator with an electron-scattering foil to generate a diffuse electron beam. The patient stood approximately 10 ft from the end of the accelerator, and his or her entire surface could be treated with the broad electron beam. By using multiple field techniques, it was possible to irradiate the entire cutaneous surface.

Patients are treated with a six-field technique that includes anterior, posterior, and four opposed oblique fields (55). A full "cycle" of treatment is administered over a 2-day period. On the first day, the anterior and two posterior oblique fields are treated at each of the two accelerator angles. On the second day, the posterior and two anterior oblique fields are treated at each of the two accelerator angles. The dose administered with each cycle is 1.5 to 2.0 Gy. Most patients will tolerate 2.0 Gy per cycle, but lower doses are used for patients with erythroderma, atrophic skin, or a previous course of electron beam therapy. The prescribed total dose is 30 to 36 Gy administered over a 9- to 10-week period. A 1-week split may be used after a dose of 18 to 20 Gy has been delivered to provide some relief from the generalized skin erythema that usually accompanies treatment.

With this technique, certain portions of the body surface are "shadowed" and receive relatively lower total doses of irradiation. These areas include the top of the scalp, the perineum, and the soles of the feet. Other areas may be problematic in individual patients because of body habitus, such as underneath the breasts of some women and under the panniculus of obese individuals. To compensate for this effect, we routinely treat the perineum and soles of the feet. Supplemental treatment is provided to the vertex of the scalp only if there is scalp involvement because permanent alopecia may result. Additional treatment also is administered underneath the breasts and panniculus of individual patients, as indicated. Also, some patients with a discrete number of tumorous lesions will receive boost treatment to these tumors at the outset of electron beam therapy to reduce their thickness and permit better penetration by the electrons.

The essentials of the Stanford technique have been adopted widely for the management of patients with mycosis fungoides. In addition, individual modifications have been introduced to suit local needs, such as treatment with a nonangulated electron beam (56), the use of a rotational patient platform (57), electron-arc therapy using a reclined patient position (58), and electron beams of varying energies (59).

Total skin electron beam therapy should be considered as initial therapy for patients with generalized very thickened plaque or tumorous disease because the effective depth of treatment of electron beam therapy is more substantial than either topical nitrogen mustard or phototherapy. It is also appropriate for patients with a recent history of rapid progression of disease and for those patients for whom topical nitrogen mustard, bexarotene gel, or phototherapy was not effective. Generally, after completion of total skin electron beam therapy, adjuvant treatment with topical nitrogen mustard with or without systemic adjuvant (e.g., oral bexarotene, photopheresis) is indicated and may be continued for up to 6 to 12 months.

In patients who have lymph node involvement or in some situations of localized visceral disease, megavoltage (4 to 15 MeV) photon irradiation may be helpful in providing important additional palliation. Doses of 30 to 36 Gy in 3 to 4 weeks are often sufficient to achieve local control of lymph nodes or other extracutaneous sites of disease. This is often combined with systemic chemotherapy or biologic therapy (IFN-α or bexarotene), depending on the extent of the extracutaneous involvement.

The most common acute complications of total skin electron beam therapy are erythema and dry desquamation (55,60). Intermediate-term complications include alopecia, which is incomplete and only temporary if the scalp dose is limited to 25 Gy (60). Most patients also experience temporary loss of fingernails and toenails 2 to 4 months after completion of therapy. Most patients report the inability to sweat properly for 6 to 12 months after therapy (61) and chronically dry skin thereafter, which requires the regular use of emolliation. In long-term follow-up, evidence for chronic radiation dermatitis is uncommon (62). Although secondary malignancies, such as squamous cell and basal cell cancers of the skin, are increased after the use of total skin electron beam therapy, the only patients in whom these have become problematic are those who have received repeated treatment with multiple therapies, including irradiation, topical nitrogen mustard, and PUVA (51).

Extracorporeal Photopheresis

Photopheresis (extracorporeal photopheresis [ECP] or systemic photochemotherapy) is a method of delivering PUVA systemically by using an extracorporeal technique (63). The patient's white blood cells are collected (leukapheresis), exposed to a photoactivating drug, and then irradiated with UVA. The irradiated cells then are returned to the patient. The mechanism of action of ECP remains unclear. It is

hypothesized that there may be a dual effect: a direct cytotoxic or antiproliferative effect on the neoplastic cells and an immune-enhancing effect on the competent lymphocytes against the neoplastic cells. Photopheresis is usually administered every 4 weeks, but in patients with severe disease, the frequency can be as often as every 2 weeks. Once complete clearance is achieved, the frequency can be gradually reduced and then discontinued.

In refractory disease with ECP monotherapy or in Sézary syndrome with high peripheral blood Sézary burden, ECP can be used successfully in combination with other systemic biologic agents such as IFNs or retinoids (e.g., bexarotene) (64). In addition, skin-directed therapies such as topical steroid, topical nitrogen mustard, phototherapy, or total skin electron beam therapy can be combined with ECP if additional skin-directed treatment is needed (39,65).

Compared with other systemic therapies, ECP has minimal adverse effects (63). Some patients may experience nausea, mostly due to the ingested psoralen, and some have a transient low-grade fever or slight malaise after treatment. There are no reports of organ injury or bone marrow or immune suppression.

Interferon-α

IFN-α is indicated primarily for the palliative management of refractory or advanced disease. It may be used alone or, more often, combined with topical or other systemic therapies. The dosage of IFN-α for mycosis fungoides is usually initiated at 3 to 5 million units daily or three times per week and is gradually increased, depending on the clinical response and the severity of adverse effects. Reported ORRs when used as monotherapy are 53% to 74%, with complete response rates of 21% to 35% (66,67).

PUVA can be given in combination with IFN-α. In one of the largest studies of this combination, a complete response rate of 33% and partial response rate of 50% were observed in patients with stage IIB disease (68). Studies using PUVA alone for patients with erythroderma (stage III) have reported complete response rates of 33% to 70% (49,69,70). Despite these good response rates, the majority of the patients have relapses during maintenance therapy. In another study, the complete response and partial response rates for a combination regimen of PUVA plus IFN-α in stage III disease were 62% and 25%, respectively (68). It is thought that the combined regimen may improve clinical response or response duration beyond that observed with PUVA or IFN-α alone. However, there is no clear evidence that prolongation of response duration leads to improvement in the overall survival.

Retinoids

Systemic therapy with retinoids, most commonly bexarotene, has been shown to be beneficial in the management of mycosis fungoides and Sézary syndrome (71). The reported response rate is approximately 45% to 55%, with a 10% to 20% complete response rate, depending on the dose of bexarotene and the severity of disease (71,72). Oral retinoids can be used successfully in combination with other skin-directed or systemic therapies, including PUVA, IFN-α, or total skin electron beam therapy (73–75). Combinations of systemic biologic therapies have been used successfully and with potential synergistic effects when individual therapies fail to attain adequate responses (64,76).

Bexarotene is administered orally. The initial dose is 200 to 300 mg per m² per day depending on the patient's toxicity risk and severity of disease, which can be adjusted according to clinical response and the severity of adverse effects. The most common adverse effects include photosensitivity, xerosis, myalgia, arthralgia, headaches, and impaired night vision. The well-known teratogenic effects of retinoids must be carefully addressed in female patients. Because of its potential hepatotoxic and hyperlipidemic effects, liver function and serum lipid levels should be monitored in each patient during treatment. In addition, central hypothyroidism is often induced, so patients are routinely started on levothyroxine (Synthroid) immediately before or simultaneously with bexarotene.

Recombinant Fusion Proteins

Recombinant fusion protein therapy, such as the IL-2–diphtheria toxin fusion protein (Ontak, denileukin diftitox), involves the use of growth factor-diphtheria toxin fusion proteins designed specifically to kill defined neoplastic cell populations. Ontak has undergone a multicenter phase III trial in patients with IL-2 receptor (CD25⁺)-expressing mycosis fungoides (77). Patients with intermediate or advanced stages of disease were included in the phase III trial. The ORR was 30%, with complete response and partial response rates of 10% and 20%, respectively. The main complication is related to a "capillary leak" syndrome that may be ameliorated by pretreatment with corticosteroids.

Histone Deacetylase Inhibitors

Histone deacetylase inhibitors are a novel class of agents that can induce tumor cell growth arrest, differentiation, or apoptosis by affecting gene expression and protein function. Vorinostat (suberoylanilide hydroxamic acid) is an orally available pan-histone deacetylase inhibitor that has been shown to have activity in patients with mycosis fungoides and Sézary syndrome. The clinical efficacy and safety were studied in a multicenter trial followed by U. S. Food and Drug Administration approval for the treatment of cutaneous manifestations of cutaneous T-cell lymphoma in patients with refractory disease (78). The ORR was 30% ($n = 74$), with only one patient achieving complete response. Vorinostat is available as 100-mg capsules, and the recommended starting dose is 400 mg daily.

The most common vorinostat-related toxicities were fatigue, diarrhea, nausea, anorexia, dysgeusia, and thrombocytopenia. Other hematologic abnormalities were less common and mild. The heart-rate corrected QT interval (QTc) interval prolongation has been observed, but none was considered clinically significant or associated with new cardiac symptoms.

Systemic Chemotherapy

Systemic chemotherapy is appropriate for patients with extracutaneous disease, advanced or refractory disease, or when biologic therapies have failed. Most chemotherapy regimens result in only temporary palliative responses. Recently, the National Comprehensive Cancer Network has published guidelines that recommend stage-based therapy, and only a minority of patients with mycosis fungoides (10% to 20%) require systemic management (39). With combination chemotherapy regimens, overall complete response or partial response rates can reach 80% to 100%; however, in most cases, the median duration of response is <1 year, and in many patients, shorter than several months (79,80). Virtually all drugs that have proved useful in the management of patients with non-Hodgkin lymphomas have been tested in patients with mycosis fungoides and Sézary syndrome. Chemotherapy may be used alone or in combination with topical therapy (e.g., radiation) or biologic response modifiers (e.g., retinoids, IFN-α). However, a randomized trial that compared electron beam radiation plus chemotherapy with sequential topical therapies in the initial treatment of mycosis fungoides did not demonstrate an improved survival with the more aggressive management approach (40).

Methotrexate, pegylated liposomal doxorubicin, gemcitabine, etoposide, chlorambucil, or purine analogs (fludarabine, 2′-deoxycoformycin) are the most commonly used single-agent chemotherapy regimens in mycosis fungoides and Sézary syndrome (39,79,80). The greatest experience with single agents has been with methotrexate. More commonly, lower doses of methotrexate (≤100 mg per week) are used in mycosis fungoides and Sézary syndrome. With low-dose methotrexate, the ORR ranges from 33% to 58%, and the time to treatment failure is 15 to 32 months, depending upon the extent of prior therapy (81). Another common single agent has been chlorambucil administered daily or intermittently with corticosteroids titrating the dose according to hematologic toxicity (82). The purine analogs showed promise in early clinical trials, but complications related to immunosuppression are significant. Fludarabine, which causes profound decreases in peripheral T-cell counts, has demonstrated clinical activity against mycosis fungoides, chronic lymphocytic leukemia, and the low-grade lymphomas (83). Another drug that may be useful is 2′-deoxycoformycin, which inhibits adenosine deaminase, an enzyme with a high level of activity in T cells, and leads to inhibition of DNA synthesis. The response rate may be as high as 70% (84,85).

Single-agent gemcitabine has been reported to achieve complete and partial response rates of 12% and 59%, respectively, with median durations of 15 and 10 months (86). More recent studies confirmed efficacy of gemcitabine in patients with advanced mycosis fungoides and Sézary syndrome, however, the complete remission rate was low (87). Pegylated liposomes are stable, long-circulating carriers useful for delivering doxorubicin to tumor sites with a lower toxicity than the free drug. In a study of patients who had refractory or relapsed mycosis fungoides or Sézary syndrome, pegylated doxorubicin (Doxil) was given as 20 mg per m² every month, with response rates of up to 80% (88). The most frequent side effects were mild anemia, lymphopenia, and palmoplantar erythrodysesthesia. An ORR of 33% has also been reported in patients with refractory stage IVB disease (89). Recently, another pegylated agent (Caelyx) has been evaluated prospectively in patients with refractory or relapsed mycosis fungoides or Sézary syndrome at higher doses of 40 mg per m² administered intravenously once every

4 weeks with a response rate of 56% and progression free survival of 5 months (90). In this prospective study, the response rate was lower than those reported by prior retrospective reports. This may be due to the inclusion of a larger number of patients with transformed disease or prior chemotherapy exposure.

Another new cytotoxic agent is temozolomide, which showed encouraging activity in mycosis fungoides and needs prospective further testing. Its mechanism of action is similar to other alkylating agents. It induces DNA damage by crosslinking, and resistance has been associated with high levels of the scavenger protein O 6-alkylguanine DNA alkyltransferase in tumor cells. Response rates from 26% to 33% have been reported in patients with relapsed stage IB to IVA disease (91). Proteosome inhibition with bortezomib has been shown to be an emerging effective strategy in non-Hodgkin lymphoma and multiple myeloma. Recently, it has been suggested that nuclear factor-κB may play a key role in mycosis fungoides/Sézary syndrome resistance to apoptosis (92). This observation supports a potential therapeutic role for bortezomib in the treatment of patients with cutaneous T-cell lymphoma. This agent has shown encouraging activity with a response rate of 67%, and was well tolerated in patients with mycosis fungoides and skin-limited peripheral T-cell lymphoma (93).

In contrast to other non-Hodgkin lymphomas, autologous bone marrow transplantation has not been actively investigated in mycosis fungoides and Sézary syndrome, and anecdotal experience in its use is limited (94,95). The ablative regimens used in these cases were combinations of total skin electron beam therapy, total body irradiation, and various combinations of cyclophosphamide, etoposide, BCNU, and cisplatin.

The concept of allogenic hematopoietic cell transplantation is provocative because even in the absence of a complete response, an allogenic graft versus tumor effect may provide an immune mechanism to control the malignant T-cell process. The published experience of allogenic hematopoietic stem cell transplantation (HSCT) is also limited with 21 patients reported and has been reviewed recently (96). Eligibility and preparatory regimens have varied across studies. Molina et al. (97) reported a complete response in all six patients transplanted for refractory disease. Five patients remained in complete response at a median follow-up of 17 months (range 3 to 65). Mild acute and chronic graft versus host disease developed in all patients, and chronic graft versus host disease was ongoing in patients with sustained remissions, suggesting a possible graft versus lymphoma effect. It appears that compared with autologous HSCT, allogenic HSCT may result in durable long-term remissions. Thus, allogeneic HSCT should be considered for patients with advanced mycosis fungoides or Sézary syndrome who have failed several systemic agents with short-lived responses or show refractory disease (7,39).

OUTCOME

Stage IA (Limited Patch or Plaque [T1]) Disease

The primary therapy for patients with stage IA (T1) disease is skin-directed (topical) treatments (7,39). This may include topical steroid, topical chemotherapy (usually nitrogen mustard), phototherapy (UVB or PUVA), bexarotene gel, or localized radiation therapy. The complete response rate to nitrogen mustard is 60% to 70% (43) and to total skin electron beam therapy is 85% to 95% (52). However, there is no evidence that any one approach is superior to the others with respect to long-term disease control or survival. Treatment selection is often based on convenience and cost.

Patients with limited patch or plaque (T1, overall stage IA) disease who are treated with conventional therapies have an excellent prognosis, with an overall long-term life expectancy that is similar to an age-, gender-, and race-matched control population. In a retrospective study of 122 patients with stage IA disease at Stanford, the median survival was not reached at 33 years (98). Nearly all patients with stage IA disease who die will die of causes other than mycosis fungoides. Furthermore, only 9% of treated patients at this stage ever have progression to a more advanced stage of disease. Early aggressive therapy with combination chemotherapy does not result in a more favorable survival outcome compared with patients managed more conservatively with sequential topical regimens (40).

Stage IB/IIA (Generalized Patch or Plaque [T2]) Disease

Topical nitrogen mustard, phototherapy (UVB or PUVA), and total skin electron beam therapy are commonly used for patients with T2 disease. Complete response rates using topical nitrogen mustard are 50% to 70%, whereas the complete response rate for total skin electron beam therapy is 80% to 90% (43,99). However, patients treated with total skin electron beam therapy do not have an improved long-term survival compared with those who received topical nitrogen mustard as initial therapy, despite the superior complete response rate (99). In patients treated with PUVA, the complete response rate ranges from 50% to 80% (49,50).

Patients who do not respond to one skin-directed therapy or who have progression after an initial response may be treated with an alternative skin-directed choice as demonstrated in the algorithmic display in the National Comprehensive Cancer Network practice guidelines (7). There is no evidence that development of resistance to one modality affects subsequent response to an alternative topical therapy (98,99). Combination skin-directed or skin-directed plus systemic therapies may also be used as initial therapy for patients with T2 disease. This may provide for better long-term control of disease, but the ultimate outcome is not usually affected (69,100,101). Patients who have generalized patch or plaque disease without evidence of extracutaneous involvement and who are treated with these modalities have a median survival >11 years, but 25% of deaths in this group are attributable to mycosis fungoides (99).

Stage IIB (Tumorous) Disease

Patients who have a limited number of cutaneous tumors in the setting of generalized patch or plaque disease may be treated with local radiation to the tumors plus one of the skin-directed therapies noted previously. However, those who have generalized tumorous disease will be treated most effectively with total skin electron beam therapy followed by maintenance therapy with nitrogen mustard (101) or combination with IFN-α (69) or oral bexarotene.

Alternatively, patients with generalized tumors can be treated up front with systemic therapies either alone or in combination (7,39). In patients with extensive tumors with large cell transformation, single-agent chemotherapy such as liposomal doxorubicin or gemcitabine may be very effective. These patients with advanced disease (stage IIB or greater) should be considered for investigative therapies whenever appropriate. Allogeneic HSCT maybe considered for those patients whose disease fails to respond to primary therapy options or who do not experience durable responses with any primary or salvage therapies. Patients with cutaneous tumors have a median survival of 3.5 to 4.0 years, and the majority of these patients die of mycosis fungoides.

Stage III (Erythrodermic [T4]) Disease

Patients with erythrodermic (T4) mycosis fungoides usually have very inflamed and itchy skin that may be irritated by topical therapies. Common treatments for these patients include ECP, PUVA, oral bexarotene, IFN-α, vorinostat, and single-agent methotrexate. With standard total skin electron beam therapy techniques, these patients may experience severe desquamation with relatively low total doses. Therefore, total skin electron beam therapy is generally not considered appropriate as the initial treatment. Treatment intent in these patients is almost always palliative, and most have progression through several therapies or combinations of therapy during the course of their disease.

The long-term outcome for these patients is quite variable, and is dependent on patient age at presentation (<65 vs. >65 years), overall stage (III vs. IV), and peripheral blood involvement (38). The median survival varies widely, depending on the number of independent adverse prognostic factors present.

Three distinct prognostic subgroups may be identified (favorable, intermediate, and unfavorable), with median survivals of 10.2, 3.7, and 1.5 years for patients with zero, one, or more than one unfavorable prognostic factor, respectively.

Stage IV (Extracutaneous Including Sézary Syndrome) Disease

Patients with extracutaneous disease have a poor prognosis. Appropriate management for these patients includes topical therapy suitable to the extent of skin involvement and, in addition, systemic therapy that may include biologics as well as chemotherapy depending on the primary site of extracutaneous disease. Patients with Sézary syndrome (stage IVA in the revised staging system) are managed as in patients with erythroderma with mycosis fungoides except that the systemic therapy regimens are used up front and often intensified by utilizing combination biologic regimens (e.g., ECP plus IFN or ECP plus oral bexarotene) (7,39). Given the poor prognosis and lack of any truly effective treatment, these patients are also candidates for investigational therapies, such as monoclonal antibodies, new histone deacetylase inhibitors, and new cytotoxic chemotherapy agents. Again, patients with stage IV disease are candidates for allogeneic HSCT. Patients who have localized nodal disease as the only evidence of stage IV disease may benefit from treatment with involved-field irradiation (30 to 36 Gy) in addition to systemic management.

In a retrospective study of a Stanford cohort, 77 patients either presented with or later developed extracutaneous (stage IV) disease (56 with stage IVA and 21 with stage IVB disease). The median survival of the 77 patients was only 13 months and was similar regardless of the extent of skin involvement (T2 vs. T3 vs. T4; $p = 0.69$ to 0.88) or the site of extracutaneous disease (IVA vs. IVB) (28).

The outcome of 525 patients treated for mycosis fungoides at Stanford over a period of nearly 40 years is displayed in Figure 25.1.

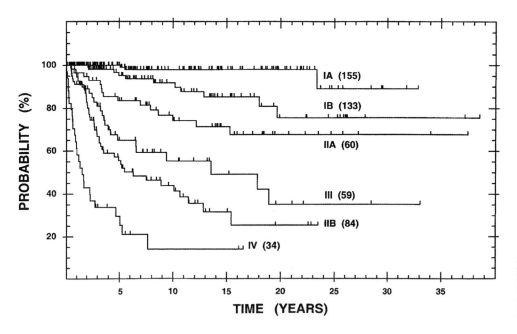

FIGURE 25.1 Disease-specific survival by initial disease stage for 525 patients with mycosis fungoides treated at Stanford University. (Adapted from *Arch Dermatol* 2003; 139:857–8.)

References

1. Criscione VD, Weinstock MA. Incidence of cutaneous T-cell lymphoma in the United States, 1973-2002. *Arch Dermatol* 2007;143:854–859.
2. Whittemore AS, Holly EA, Lee IM, et al. Mycosis fungoides in relation to environmental exposures and immune response: a case-control study. *J Natl Cancer Inst* 1989;81:1560–1567.
3. Tuyp E, Burgoyne A, Aitchison T, et al. A case-control study of possible causative factors in mycosis fungoides. *Arch Dermatol* 1987;123:196–200.
4. Poiesz BJ, Ruscetti FW, Gazdar AF, et al. Detection and isolation of type C retrovirus particles from fresh and cultured lymphocytes of a patient with cutaneous T-cell lymphoma. *Proc Natl Acad Sci U S A* 1980;77:7415–7419.
5. Kim YH, Hoppe RT. Mycosis fungoides and the Sézary syndrome. *Semin Oncol* 1999;26:276–289.
6. Olsen E, Vonderheid E, Pimpinelli N, et al. Revisions to the staging and classification of mycosis fungoides and Sézary syndrome: a proposal of the International Society for Cutaneous Lymphomas (ISCL) and the cutaneous lymphoma task force of the European Organization of Research and Treatment of Cancer (EORTC). *Blood* 2007;110:1713–1722.
7. Zelenetz A, Advani R, Byrd J, et al. Non-Hodgkin's lymphoma. In: NCCN *Clinical Practice Guidelines in Oncology.* v.2.2009 Available at: www.nccn.org.
7a. Clendenning WE, Rappaport H. Report of the Committee on Pathology of Cutaneous T Cell Lymphomas. *Cancer Treat Rep* 1979;63:719–724.
8. Colby TV, Burke JS, Hoppe RT. Lymph node biopsy in mycosis fungoides. *Cancer* 1981;47:351–359.
9. Scheffer E, Meijer CJ, Van Vloten WA. Dermatopathic lymphadenopathy and lymph node involvement in mycosis fungoides. *Cancer* 1980;45:137–148.
10. Ralfkiaer E. Mycosis fungoides and Sézary syndrome. In: Jaffe ES, World Health Organization, eds. *Pathology and genetics of tumours of haematopoietic and lymphoid tissues.* Lyon, France: IARC Press, 2001:216–220.
11. Kern DE, Kidd PG, Moe R, et al. Analysis of T-cell receptor gene rearrangement in lymph nodes of patients with mycosis fungoides. Prognostic implications. *Arch Dermatol* 1998;134:158–164.
12. van Doorn R, Scheffer E, Willemze R. Follicular mycosis fungoides, a distinct disease entity with or without associated follicular mucinosis: a clinicopathologic and follow-up study of 51 patients. *Arch Dermatol* 2002;138:191–198.
13. Haghighi B, Smoller BR, LeBoit PE. Pagetoid reticulosis (Woringer-Kolopp disease): an immunophenotypic, molecular, and clinicopathologic study. *Mod Pathol* 2000;13:502–510.
14. Scarisbrick JJ, Woolford AJ, Russell-Jones R, et al. Loss of heterozygosity on 10q and microsatellite instability in advanced stages of primary cutaneous T-cell lymphoma and possible association with homozygous deletion of PTEN. *Blood* 2000;95:2937–2942.
15. Kohler S, Jones CD, Warnke RA, et al. PCR-heteroduplex analysis of T-cell receptor gamma gene rearrangement in paraffin-embedded skin biopsies. *Am J Dermatopathol* 2000;22:321–327.
16. Thurber SE, Zhang B, Kim YH, et al. T-cell clonality analysis in biopsy specimens from two different skin sites shows high specificity in the diagnosis of patients with suggested mycosis fungoides. *J Am Acad Dermatol* 2007;57:782–790.
17. Vowels BR, Cassin M, Vonderheid EC, et al. Aberrant cytokine production by Sézary syndrome patients: cytokine secretion pattern resembles murine Th2 cells. *J Invest Dermatol* 1992;99:90–94.
18. Bernengo MG, Fierro MT, Novelli M, et al. Soluble interleukin-2 receptor in Sézary syndrome: its origin and clinical application. *Br J Dermatol* 1993;128:124–129.
19. Wasik MA, Vonderheid EC, Bigler RD, et al. Increased serum concentration of the soluble interleukin-2 receptor in cutaneous T-cell lymphoma. Clinical and prognostic implications. *Arch Dermatol* 1996;132:42–47.
20. Kim EJ, Hess S, Richardson SK, et al. Immunopathogenesis and therapy of cutaneous T cell lymphoma. *J Clin Invest* 2005;115:798–812.
21. Yoo EK, Cassin M, Lessin SR, et al. Complete molecular remission during biologic response modifier therapy for Sézary syndrome is associated with enhanced helper T type 1 cytokine production and natural killer cell activity. *J Am Acad Dermatol* 2001;45:208–216.
22. Navas IC, Algara P, Mateo M, et al. p16(INK4a) is selectively silenced in the tumoral progression of mycosis fungoides. *Lab Invest* 2002;82:123–132.
23. Vermeer MH, van Doorn R, Dijkman R, et al. Novel and highly recurrent chromosomal alterations in Sézary syndrome. *Cancer Res* 2008;68:2689–2698.
24. Shin J, Monti S, Aires DJ, et al. Lesional gene expression profiling in cutaneous T-cell lymphoma reveals natural clusters associated with disease outcome. *Blood* 2007;110:3015–3027.
25. Cerroni L, Rieger E, Hodl S, et al. Clinicopathologic and immunologic features associated with transformation of mycosis fungoides to large-cell lymphoma. *Am J Surg Pathol* 1992;16:543–552.
26. Salhany KE, Cousar JB, Greer JP, et al. Transformation of cutaneous T cell lymphoma to large cell lymphoma. A clinicopathologic and immunologic study. *Am J Pathol* 1988;132:265–277.
27. Vergier B, de Muret A, Beylot-Barry M, et al. Transformation of mycosis fungoides: clinicopathological and prognostic features of 45 cases. French Study Group of Cutaneous Lymphomas. *Blood* 2000;95:2212–2218.
28. Willemze R, Jaffe ES, Burg G, et al. WHO-EORTC classification for cutaneous lymphomas. *Blood* 2005;105:3768–3785.
29. Lee J, Viakhireva N, Cesca C, et al. Clinicopathologic features and treatment outcomes in Woringer-Kolopp disease. *J Am Acad Dermatol* 2008;59:706–712.
30. LeBoit PE. Granulomatous slack skin. *Dermatol Clin* 1994;12:375–389.
31. Wain EM, Orchard GE, Whittaker SJ, et al. Outcome in 34 patients with juvenile-onset mycosis fungoides: a clinical, immunophenotypic, and molecular study. *Cancer* 2003;98:2282–2290.
32. Lambroza E, Cohen SR, Phelps R, et al. Hypopigmented variant of mycosis fungoides: demography, histopathology, and treatment of seven cases. *J Am Acad Dermatol* 1995;32:987–993.
33. Tsai EY, Taur A, Espinosa L, et al. Staging accuracy in mycosis fungoides and Sézary syndrome using integrated positron emission tomography and computed tomography. *Arch Dermatol* 2006;142:577–584.
34. Salhany KE, Greer JP, Cousar JB, et al. Marrow involvement in cutaneous T-cell lymphoma. A clinicopathologic study of 60 cases. *Am J Clin Pathol* 1989;92:747–754.
35. Bunn PA Jr, Lamberg SI. Report of the Committee on Staging and Classification of Cutaneous T-Cell Lymphomas. *Cancer Treat Rep* 1979;63:725–728.
36. Sausville EA, Eddy JL, Makuch RW, et al. Histopathologic staging at initial diagnosis of mycosis fungoides and the Sézary syndrome. Definition of three distinctive prognostic groups. *Ann Intern Med* 1988;109:372–382.
37. Kim YH, Lieu HL, Mraz-Gernhard S, et al. Long-term outcome of 525 patients with mycosis fungoides and Sézary syndrome at Stanford: clinical prognostic factors and risks of disease progression and second cancer. *Arch Dermatol* 2003;139:857–866.
38. Kim YH, Bishop K, Varghese A, et al. Prognostic factors in erythrodermic mycosis fungoides and the Sézary syndrome. *Arch Dermatol* 1995;131:1003–1008.
39. Horwitz SM, Olsen EA, Duvic M, et al. Review of the treatment of mycosis fungoides and Sézary syndrome: a stage-based approach. *J Natl Compr Canc Netw* 2008;6:436–442.
40. Kaye FJ, Bunn PA Jr, Steinberg SM, et al. A randomized trial comparing combination electron-beam radiation and chemotherapy with topical therapy in the initial treatment of mycosis fungoides. *N Engl J Med* 1989;321:1784–1790.
41. Ramsay DL, Halperin PS, Zeleniuch-Jacquotte A. Topical mechlorethamine therapy for early stage mycosis fungoides. *J Am Acad Dermatol* 1988;19:684–691.
42. Vonderheid EC, Tan ET, Kantor AF, et al. Long-term efficacy, curative potential, and carcinogenicity of topical mechlorethamine chemotherapy in cutaneous T cell lymphoma. *J Am Acad Dermatol* 1989;20:416–428.
43. Kim YH, Martinez G, Varghese A, et al. Topical nitrogen mustard in the management of mycosis fungoides: update of the Stanford experience. *Arch Dermatol* 2003;139:165–173.
44. Zackheim HS, Epstein EH Jr, Crain WR. Topical carmustine (BCNU) for cutaneous T cell lymphoma: a 15-year experience in 143 patients. *J Am Acad Dermatol* 1990;22(pt 1):802–810.
45. Ramsay DL, Lish KM, Yalowitz CB, et al. Ultraviolet-B phototherapy for early-stage cutaneous T-cell lymphoma. *Arch Dermatol* 1992;128:931–933.
46. Resnik KS, Vonderheid EC. Home UV phototherapy of early mycosis fungoides: long-term follow-up observations in thirty-one patients. *J Am Acad Dermatol* 1993;29:73–77.
47. Boztepe G, Sahin S, Ayhan M, et al. Narrowband ultraviolet B phototherapy to clear and maintain clearance in patients with mycosis fungoides. *J Am Acad Dermatol* 2005;53:242–246.
48. Diederen PV, van Weelden H, Sanders CJ, et al. Narrowband UVB and psoralen-UVA in the treatment of early-stage mycosis fungoides: a retrospective study. *J Am Acad Dermatol* 2003;48:215–219.
49. Herrmann JJ, Roenigk HH Jr, Hurria A, et al. Treatment of mycosis fungoides with photochemotherapy (PUVA): long-term follow-up. *J Am Acad Dermatol* 1995;33(pt 1):234–242.
50. Querfeld C, Rosen ST, Kuzel TM, et al. Long-term follow-up of patients with early-stage cutaneous T-cell lymphoma who achieved complete remission with psoralen plus UV-A monotherapy. *Arch Dermatol* 2005;141:305–311.
51. Abel EA, Sendagorta E, Hoppe RT. Cutaneous malignancies and metastatic squamous cell carcinoma following topical therapies for mycosis fungoides. *J Am Acad Dermatol* 1986;14:1029–1038.
52. Jones GW, Hoppe RT, Glatstein E. Electron beam treatment for cutaneous T-cell lymphoma. *Hematol Oncol Clin North Am* 1995;9:1057–1076.
53. Hoppe RT. Total skin electron beam therapy in the management of mycosis fungoides. *Front Radiat Ther Oncol* 1991;25:80–89.

54. Jones GW, Tadros A, Hodson DI, et al. Prognosis with newly diagnosed mycosis fungoides after total skin electron radiation of 30 or 35 GY. *Int J Radiat Oncol Biol Phys* 1994;28:839–845.

55. Hoppe RT, Fuks Z, Bagshaw MA. Radiation therapy in the management of cutaneous T-cell lymphomas. *Cancer Treat Rep* 1979;63:625–632.

56. Tetenes PJ, Goodwin PN. Comparative study of superficial whole-body radiotherapeutic techniques using a 4-MeV nonangulated electron beam. *Radiology* 1977;122:219–226.

57. Podgorsak EB, Pla C, Pla M, et al. Physical aspects of a rotational total skin electron irradiation. *Med Phys* 1983;10:159–168.

58. Gerbi BJ, Khan FM, Deibel FC, et al. Total skin electron arc irradiation using a reclined patient position. *Int J Radiat Oncol Biol Phys* 1989;17:397–404.

59. Cox RS, Heck RJ, Fessenden P, et al. Development of total-skin electron therapy at two energies. *Int J Radiat Oncol Biol Phys* 1990;18:659–669.

60. Desai KR, Pezner RD, Lipsett JA, et al. Total skin electron irradiation for mycosis fungoides: relationship between acute toxicities and measured dose at different anatomic sites. *Int J Radiat Oncol Biol Phys* 1988;15:641–645.

61. Price NM. Electron beam therapy. Its effect on eccrine gland function in mycosis fungoides patients. *Arch Dermatol* 1979;115:1068–1070.

62. Price NM. Radiation dermatitis following electron beam therapy. An evaluation of patients ten years after total skin irradiation for mycosis fungoides. *Arch Dermatol* 1978;114:63–66.

63. Knobler R, Jantschitsch C. Extracorporeal photochemoimmunotherapy in cutaneous T-cell lymphoma. *Transfus Apher Sci* 2003;28:81–89.

64. Richardson SK, Lin JH, Vittorio CC, et al. High clinical response rate with multimodality immunomodulatory therapy for Sézary syndrome. *Clin Lymphoma Myeloma* 2006;7:226–232.

65. Wilson LD, Jones GW, Kim D, et al. Experience with total skin electron beam therapy in combination with extracorporeal photopheresis in the management of patients with erythrodermic (T4) mycosis fungoides. *J Am Acad Dermatol* 2000;43(pt 1):54–60.

66. Olsen EA, Rosen ST, Vollmer RT, et al. Interferon alfa-2a in the treatment of cutaneous T cell lymphoma. *J Am Acad Dermatol* 1989;20:395–407.

67. Vegna ML, Papa G, Defazio D, et al. Interferon alpha-2a in cutaneous T-cell lymphoma. *Eur J Haematol Suppl* 1990;52:32–35.

68. Kuzel TM, Roenigk HH Jr, Samuelson E, et al. Effectiveness of interferon alfa-2a combined with phototherapy for mycosis fungoides and the Sézary syndrome. *J Clin Oncol* 1995;13:257–263.

69. Roenigk HH Jr, Kuzel TM, Skoutelis AP, et al. Photochemotherapy alone or combined with interferon alpha-2a in the treatment of cutaneous T-cell lymphoma. *J Invest Dermatol* 1990;95(suppl):198S–205S.

70. Herrmann JJ, Roenigk HH Jr, Honigsmann H. Ultraviolet radiation for treatment of cutaneous T-cell lymphoma. *Hematol Oncol Clin North Am* 1995;9:1077–1088.

71. Duvic M, Hymes K, Heald P, et al. Bexarotene is effective and safe for treatment of refractory advanced-stage cutaneous T-cell lymphoma: multinational phase II-III trial results. *J Clin Oncol* 2001;19:2456–2471.

72. Duvic M, Martin AG, Kim Y, et al. Phase 2 and 3 clinical trial of oral bexarotene (Targretin capsules) for the treatment of refractory or persistent early-stage cutaneous T-cell lymphoma. *Arch Dermatol* 2001;137:581–593.

73. Duvic M, Lemak NA, Redman JR, et al. Combined modality therapy for cutaneous T-cell lymphoma. *J Am Acad Dermatol* 1996;34:1022–1029.

74. Knobler RM, Trautinger F, Radaszkiewicz T, et al. Treatment of cutaneous T cell lymphoma with a combination of low-dose interferon alfa-2b and retinoids. *J Am Acad Dermatol* 1991;24(pt 1):247–252.

75. Jones G, McLean J, Rosenthal D, et al. Combined treatment with oral etretinate and electron beam therapy in patients with cutaneous T-cell lymphoma (mycosis fungoides and Sézary syndrome). *J Am Acad Dermatol* 1992;26:960–967.

76. McGinnis KS, Junkins-Hopkins JM, Crawford G, et al. Low-dose oral bexarotene in combination with low-dose interferon alfa in the treatment of cutaneous T-cell lymphoma: clinical synergism and possible immunologic mechanisms. *J Am Acad Dermatol* 2004;50:375–379.

77. Olsen EA, Duvic M, Martin A, et al. Pivotal phase III trial of two dose levels of DAB389IL-2 (Ontak) for the treatment of cutaneous T-cell lymphoma (CTCL). *J Clin Oncol* 2001;19:376–388.

78. Olsen EA, Kim YH, Kuzel TM, et al. Phase IIb multicenter trial of vorinostat in patients with persistent, progressive, or treatment refractory cutaneous T-cell lymphoma. *J Clin Oncol* 2007;25:3109–3115.

79. Bunn PA Jr, Hoffman SJ, Norris D, et al. Systemic therapy of cutaneous T-cell lymphomas (mycosis fungoides and the Sézary syndrome). *Ann Intern Med* 1994;121:592–602.

80. Rosen ST, Foss FM. Chemotherapy for mycosis fungoides and the Sézary syndrome. *Hematol Oncol Clin North Am* 1995;9:1109–1116.

81. Zackheim HS, Kashani-Sabet M, McMillan A. Low-dose methotrexate to treat mycosis fungoides: a retrospective study in 69 patients. *J Am Acad Dermatol* 2003;49:873–878.

82. Coors EA, von den Driesch P. Treatment of erythrodermic cutaneous T-cell lymphoma with intermittent chlorambucil and fluocortolone therapy. *Br J Dermatol* 2000;143:127–131.

83. Von Hoff DD, Dahlberg S, Hartstock RJ, et al. Activity of fludarabine monophosphate in patients with advanced mycosis fungoides: a Southwest Oncology Group study. *J Natl Cancer Inst* 1990;82:1353–1355.

84. Greiner D, Olsen EA, Petroni G. Pentostatin (2'-deoxycoformycin) in the treatment of cutaneous T-cell lymphoma. *J Am Acad Dermatol* 1997;36(pt 1):950–955.

85. Tsimberidou AM, Giles F, Duvic M, et al. Phase II study of pentostatin in advanced T-cell lymphoid malignancies: update of an M.D. Anderson Cancer Center series. *Cancer* 2004;100:342–349.

86. Zinzani PL, Baliva G, Magagnoli M, et al. Gemcitabine treatment in pretreated cutaneous T-cell lymphoma: experience in 44 patients. *J Clin Oncol* 2000;18:2603–2606.

87. Duvic M, Talpur R, Wen S, et al. Phase II evaluation of gemcitabine monotherapy for cutaneous T-cell lymphoma. *Clin Lymphoma Myeloma* 2006;7:51–58.

88. Wollina U, Dummer R, Brockmeyer NH, et al. Multicenter study of pegylated liposomal doxorubicin in patients with cutaneous T-cell lymphoma. *Cancer* 2003;98:993–1001.

89. Di Lorenzo G, Di Trolio R, Delfino M, et al. Pegylated liposomal doxorubicin in stage IVB mycosis fungoides. *Br J Dermatol* 2005;153:183–185.

90. Quereux G, Marques S, Nguyen JM, et al. Prospective multicenter study of pegylated liposomal doxorubicin treatment in patients with advanced or refractory mycosis fungoides or Sézary syndrome. *Arch Dermatol* 2008;144:727–733.

91. Tani M, Fina M, Alinari L, et al. Phase II trial of temozolomide in patients with pretreated cutaneous T-cell lymphoma. *Haematologica* 2005;90:1283–1284.

92. Sors A, Jean-Louis F, Pellet C, et al. Down-regulating constitutive activation of the NF-kappaB canonical pathway overcomes the resistance of cutaneous T-cell lymphoma to apoptosis. *Blood* 2006;107:2354–2363.

93. Zinzani PL, Musuraca G, Tani M, et al. Phase II trial of proteasome inhibitor bortezomib in patients with relapsed or refractory cutaneous T-cell lymphoma. *J Clin Oncol* 2007;25:4293–4297.

94. Bigler RD, Crilley P, Micaily B, et al. Autologous bone marrow transplantation for advanced stage mycosis fungoides. *Bone Marrow Transplant* 1991;7:133–137.

95. Olavarria E, Child F, Woolford A, et al. T-cell depletion and autologous stem cell transplantation in the management of tumour stage mycosis fungoides with peripheral blood involvement. *Br J Haematol* 2001;114:624–631.

96. Duarte RF, Schmitz N, Servitje O, et al. Haematopoietic stem cell transplantation for patients with primary cutaneous T-cell lymphoma. *Bone Marrow Transplant* 2008;41(7):597–604.

97. Molina A, Zain J, Arber DA, et al. Durable clinical, cytogenetic, and molecular remissions after allogeneic hematopoietic cell transplantation for refractory Sézary syndrome and mycosis fungoides. *J Clin Oncol* 2005;23:6163–6171.

98. Kim YH, Jensen RA, Watanabe GL, et al. Clinical stage IA (limited patch and plaque) mycosis fungoides. A long-term outcome analysis. *Arch Dermatol* 1996;132:1309–1313.

99. Kim YH, Chow S, Varghese A, et al. Clinical characteristics and long-term outcome of patients with generalized patch and/or plaque (T2) mycosis fungoides. *Arch Dermatol* 1999;135:26–32.

100. Quiros PA, Jones GW, Kacinski BM, et al. Total skin electron beam therapy followed by adjuvant psoralen/ultraviolet-A light in the management of patients with T1 and T2 cutaneous T-cell lymphoma (mycosis fungoides). *Int J Radiat Oncol Biol Phys* 1997;38:1027–1035.

101. Chinn DM, Chow S, Kim YH, et al. Total skin electron beam therapy with or without adjuvant topical nitrogen mustard or nitrogen mustard alone as initial treatment of T2 and T3 mycosis fungoides. *Int J Radiat Oncol Biol Phys* 1999;43:951–958.

CHAPTER 26 ■ T-CELL CHRONIC LYMPHOCYTIC LEUKEMIA

KATHRYN FOUCAR, NNENNA OSUJI, ESTELLA MATUTES, CLAIRE DEARDEN, AND DANIEL CATOVSKY

T-CELL LARGE GRANULAR LYMPHOCYTIC LEUKEMIA

Definition

T-cell large granular lymphocytic leukemia is a clonal disorder of mature T cells with characteristic morphologic appearance. This condition has been referred to in the past as T-γ lymphoproliferative disorder, chronic T-cell lymphocytosis, and T-cell chronic lymphocytic leukemia, before the current descriptive term, *large granular lymphocytic leukemia*, proposed by Loughran et al. (1), was widely adopted. Cells show large size, pale cytoplasm, mature nuclear chromatin, and azurophilic granules of variable size. Such large granular lymphocytes, which represent 10% to 15% of circulating lymphocytes, may have a T cell or, rarely, a natural killer-cell phenotype. The World Health Organization (WHO) classification considers the cases derived from T cells, T-cell large granular lymphocytic leukemia (2), separately from those derived from natural killer cells, which are classified within the spectrum of natural killer-cell leukemias

Etiology and Epidemiology

The etiology of T-cell large granular lymphocytic leukemia is unknown. Recent evidence supports a role of chronic antigenic stimulation by autoantigen or infective antigen as an initial event leading to expansion of large granular lymphocytes (3). This is supported by the finding of nonrandom clonotypes on sequencing of the variable β-chain complementarity determining region 3 (4) of malignant T-cell large granular lymphocyte populations. To date, no single infective agent has been reliably identified, and early suggestions implicating Epstein-Barr virus or human T-cell leukemia (TCL) viruses in its pathogenesis have not been confirmed. Another explanation is that T-cell large granular lymphocytic leukemia is an autoimmune disorder (4,5) where an initial polyclonal expansion is followed by the expansion of a single clone of CD8+ cytotoxic cells. This is supported by the association of T-cell granular lymphocytic leukemia with a number of autoimmune conditions, including rheumatoid arthritis, systemic lupus erythematosus, Hashimoto thyroiditis (6,7), immune-mediated cytopenias, and bone marrow failure syndromes such as myelodysplastic syndrome and paroxysmal nocturnal hemoglobinuria (8). A history of rheumatoid arthritis is common and documented in 25% of patients (9). It has been shown that patients with T-cell large granular lymphocytic leukemia, like those with rheumatoid arthritis and/or Felty syndrome, express the human leukocyte antigen DR4 haplotype with a significantly higher frequency than the normal population. This suggests a similar immunogenetic basis for these two conditions (5). Dysregulation of several intracellular signaling pathways, including Fas/Fas ligand (10), phosphatidylinositol-3-kinase (11), and mitogen-activated protein kinase/extracellular signal-regulated kinase/Ras (12), are also described and may account, in part, for the inherent resistance to apoptosis in large granular T-lymphocytic cells. T-cell large granular lymphocytic leukemia preferentially affects adult patients with an equal male to female ratio and median age of 60 years. It is more common in the eastern hemisphere. The disease has rarely been documented in childhood.

Diagnosis

Although T-cell large granular lymphocytic leukemia is often suspected in patients with a sustained increase in cells with large granular lymphocyte morphology, its diagnosis requires a multiparameter approach integrating morphology, immunophenotyping, and T-cell receptor-gene rearrangement studies. Normally, the absolute large granular lymphocyte count ranges from 0.2 to 0.4×10^9 per L. Transient increases in circulating large granular lymphocytes are encountered in nonneoplastic conditions, especially viral infections, in which these cells are admixed with activated lymphocytes exhibiting heterogeneous morphology (6,13). A sustained large granular lymphocytosis is generally required for diagnosis. Most patients show increases $\geq 2 \times 10^9$ per L in absolute large granular lymphocyte counts. However, some patients with confirmed clonal disease have substantially fewer circulating cells (2,13). Monoclonal and oligoclonal populations of T-cell large granular lymphocytic leukemia are also detected with increasing age, viral infections (14), and autoimmune conditions. Evidence of clonal populations of T-cell large granular lymphocytes is, thus, in itself not sufficient to confirm diagnosis of this disorder. Four criteria have been suggested for diagnosis: a sustained expansion of T-cell large granular lymphocytes in the peripheral blood, demonstration of a characteristic immunophenotype, confirmation of a clonal T-cell population, and all in the context of characteristic clinical features (15). Bone marrow evaluation is becoming increasingly useful in diagnosing T-cell large granular lymphocytic leukemia, particularly in asymptomatic patients, when only a small clonal T-cell population is present, or for otherwise unexplained cytopenias (15,16).

By morphologic review of blood films, T-cell large granular lymphocytes have round nuclei with condensed chromatin,

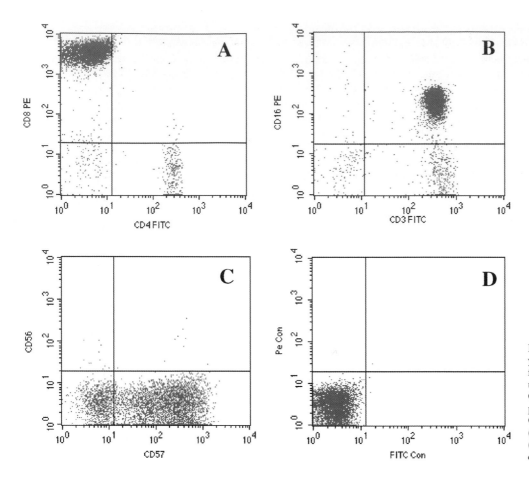

FIGURE 26.1 Flow cytometry analysis of a peripheral blood sample from a patient with T-cell large granular lymphocytic leukemia: CD8+, CD4–, CD57+, CD56–, and coexpression of CD16+ and CD3+. **A:** CD4 (–)FITC/CD8 (+)PE. **B:** CD3 (+)FITC/CD16 (+)PE. **C:** CD57 (+)FITC/CD56 (–)PE. **D:** Isotypic controls (–).

inconspicuous nucleoli, and abundant pale-blue cytoplasm containing sparse, coarse eosinophilic granules (Color Plate 53).

Membrane marker studies by flow cytometry show in most cases a CD2+, CD3+, and CD8+ phenotype with coexpression of natural killer-associated markers, usually CD57 and/or CD16, but only rarely CD56 (13). T-cell antigens are often aberrantly down-regulated (17) with CD5 and CD7 weakly expressed in 50% of cases, and may help to differentiate malignant T-cell large granular lymphocytes from normal T-lymphocytes, particularly when these are present as a homogenous population (Fig. 26.1). Less commonly found are CD4+CD8- (18), CD4+, CD8+, and CD4–CD8- variants. Some authors postulate that the CD4+CD8+ variant is a distinct clinical entity with restricted variable β13.1 usage seen in 44% of cases and possible association with concomitant B-cell disorders (18). Most T-cell large granular lymphocytic leukemia cases represent expansions of T cells bearing the T-cell receptor $\alpha\beta$, and a minority of cases is derived from T-cell receptor $\gamma\delta$-positive cells. Recent reviews suggest that CD56+ T-cell large granular lymphocytic leukemia and $\gamma\delta$ variants may have distinct clinical associations. CD56 expression is thought to define a subgroup of T-cell large granular lymphocytic leukemias with younger age of onset, more aggressive disease evolution, and shorter survival (19), whereas $\gamma\delta$ T-cell large granular lymphocytic leukemia shows more frequent neutropenia and double negativity for CD4 and CD8 (20). Expression of the more recently discovered killer immunoglobulin-like receptors (KIRs) and the C-type lectin receptors (CD94, CD161) has been investigated in T-cell large granular lymphocytic leukemia. CD94, like CD57,

is ubiquitously expressed (21), whereas KIR expression may show a clonal pattern (17,21). Both absence and overexpression of KIRs are considered pathologic and, therefore, potentially diagnostic. CD52 was reported to be strongly expressed in all of eight T-cell large granular lymphocytic samples tested (22).

Bone marrow involvement by T-cell large granular lymphocytic leukemia may be inconspicuous, consisting of poorly delineated interstitial or patchy infiltrates; these infiltrates may be particularly subtle in hypocellular specimens (Color Plate 54) (2,23). Immunohistochemical staining for CD3, CD8, and T-cell–restricted intracellular antigen (TIA)-1 is useful in highlighting these subtle infiltrates and for estimating the extent of infiltration by lymphocytes, which is generally more pronounced than suspected on hematoxylin-eosin-stained sections (Color Plate 55, 56) (24). In addition, because some cases exhibit reticulin fibrosis, large granular lymphocytes may not be well recognized on bone marrow aspirates (23). Many reports have focused on the malignant interstitial T-cell infiltrate. In general, substantially increased numbers of CD3+, CD8+, CD57+, and TIA-1+ T cells are evident diffusely or in at least eight cell clusters; intravascular/intrasinusoidal infiltrates may also be highlighted by immunohistochemical studies (Color Plates 55, 56) (16,24). B-cell aggregates are also present with sufficient frequency to represent a potential diagnostic epiphenomenon and are composed of polyclonal B cells surrounded by a corona of reactive CD4+ T cells (16). The successful diagnosis of T-cell large granular lymphocytic leukemia hinges on the recognition of increased numbers of clonal large granular lymphocytes in the blood and a high index of suspicion prompting immunohistochemical assessment of core biopsy specimens. Other bone marrow/blood findings that should prompt immunohistochemical assessment for occult T-cell large granular lymphocytic leukemia include acquired pure red cell aplasia, neutropenia, and the rare cases of adult-onset cyclic neutropenia.

In the spleen there is infiltration of the red pulp and preservation of the white pulp (25). Malignant infiltrates comprise medium-sized mature lymphocytes expressing TIA-1 and perforin. These cells show a CD5-, CD45RO- phenotype in contrast to the CD5+, CD45RO+ pattern of normal splenic red pulp tissue. The splenic white pulp displays germinal center hyperplasia with marked mantle zone expansion (25).

The diagnosis of T-cell large granular lymphocytic leukemia can be confirmed by documenting clonal T-cell receptor gene rearrangement of β or γ chains, or both by either Southern blot or polymerase chain reaction techniques.

Pathogenesis

Cytogenetic studies on T-cell large granular lymphocytic leukemias are limited, and clonal cytogenetics aberrations are infrequent, with no distinct genetic "markers" yet identified (1,2). Reported cytogenetic abnormalities include those involving the T-cell receptor gene loci at 7p14-p15 and 14q11, inversion of 12p and 14q, deletion of 5q, and trisomy of 3, 8, and 14 (6,26). Although large granular lymphocytes constitutively express both Fas (CD95) and Fas ligand, they are resistant to Fas-induced apoptosis due to a defective Fas apoptotic pathway (27).

The underlying mechanisms of the anemia may be multiple, including decrease or lack of erythroid precursors, Coombs-positive hemolytic anemia, or inhibition of the burst-forming and erythroid colony forming units by the leukemia (28). The mechanism responsible for the neutropenia is not well established, but it seems to be unrelated to hypersplenism or bone marrow infiltration. Although the presence of antineutrophil antibodies has been demonstrated in some cases, their pathogenic significance is uncertain because these patients often have circulating immunocomplexes. The postulated cell of origin of T-cell large granular lymphocytic leukemia is a postthymic immunocompetent (antigen-activated) cytotoxic T cell, including both memory and effector subsets (29).

Clinical and Laboratory Features

Approximately one-third of patients are asymptomatic at diagnosis, and the disease is discovered on a routine blood count that shows lymphocytosis, persistent neutropenia, or both (6). The most frequent symptoms are fever due to recurrent bacterial infections (usually mucocutaneous) or mouth ulcers; both are often related to neutropenia. Other presenting features are arthralgias and tiredness or fatigue, the latter unrelated to the degree of anemia, and, less often, thrombocytopenia, abdominal distension, maculopapular rash, and severe anemia (15). Eighty percent of patients with T-cell large granular lymphocytic leukemia are neutropenic, with severe neutropenia ($<0.5 \times 10^9$ per L) seen in almost half. Anemia, seen in 48% of patients, is transfusion dependent in 20% of cases. Pure red cell aplasia is commonly associated

(6), whereas autoimmune hemolytic anemia is uncommon, and thrombocytopenia is infrequent.

Physical examination shows moderate splenomegaly in 20% to 50% of patients, skin lesions in 20%, and hepatomegaly in a minority. Peripheral or intra-abdominal lymphadenopathy is rare (<10% patients). In some cases, the spleen is noted to be enlarged only by ultrasound or computed tomography.

Laboratory investigations show a normal or mildly raised white blood cell count ranging from 5 to 20×10^9 per L. Even if the absolute lymphocyte count is normal, the majority of circulating cells are large granular lymphocytes; a few patients are lymphopenic, but many develop lymphocytosis after splenectomy.

Liver biochemistry may show raised transaminases and alkaline phosphatase. Autoimmune screen may show a variety of immune abnormalities, such as the presence of rheumatoid factor, antinuclear antibodies, circulating immunocomplexes, and polyclonal hypergammaglobulinemia; rare patients may have severe hypogammaglobulinemia that relates to the suppressor activity of the large granular lymphocytes on the normal B lymphocytes.

Prognosis and Survival

The clinical course of the disease is chronic in the majority of patients. Overall, a mortality of 10% to 28% by 4 years is seen, with a median survival of >10 years (30). Up to one-quarter of patients, whether treated or not, survive beyond 20 years. Most deaths are due to bacterial sepsis and are more likely to occur in the presence of severe neutropenia. Rarely, death may occur due to disease progression. Although the vast majority of cases exhibit stable morphologic and immunophenotypic features, transformation to large cell lymphoma has been reported (31).

Therapy

At least a third of patients may never require treatment and have tolerable or minimal cytopenias. In these patients, a watch and wait strategy is appropriate (6). Indications for treatment include severe neutropenia (the most common indication) with or without life-threatening infections, symptomatic anemia or thrombocytopenia, progressive disease with B symptoms, organomegaly, and abnormal liver function tests (this is uncommon but may be seen in late stages). The main aim of treatment is to correct the neutropenia, which can be achieved without significant cytoreduction by using immunomodulatory agents such as weekly methotrexate (10 mg per m^2), cyclosporin A (5 to 10 mg per kg per day), or low-dose cyclophosphamide (50 to 100 mg per day) (6,30). Information relevant to treatment decisions is largely based on small case series with no randomized controlled trials to date. Although these agents are effective in ameliorating cytopenias in 50% to 80% of patients, the malignant clone has proven refractory. Symptoms of fatigue may improve before any improvement in blood count is observed.

Loughran et al. (32) reported good responses (correction of neutropenia, normalization of blood counts, and disappearance of circulating large granular lymphocytes) in five of ten patients treated with 10 mg per m^2 per week of oral methotrexate; one further patient had a partial response. In three of the five responders, the peripheral blood clone was no longer detectable, although relatively insensitive methods of detection were used. There is no information on bone marrow changes, but it is likely that infiltration persisted because the neutropenia, which improves in 1 to 4 months, tends to recur on discontinuation of therapy. In five of the ten patients, prednisolone was used initially with methotrexate and gradually tapered over several weeks. These results are echoed in other small series and more recently with responses in 85% of seven evaluable patients (30) (Table 26.1). Notably, methotrexate was able to induce a partial response in one of our patients who failed eight previous lines of therapy, including an autograft (33).

Cyclosporin A has similarly been shown to be effective in a number of cases (34). Optimum dosing of this agent is not established. Although initial therapeutic levels of 200 ng per L have been quoted, we found no direct correlation between cyclosporin A level and response among 23 treated patients (30), and doses may need to be titrated to response in the absence of toxicity. Reduction of cyclosporin maintenance to lowest effective doses, once neutrophil counts have normalized, should be enforced to avoid toxicities associated with long-term therapies, particularly among older patients (15). Cyclosporin A, like methotrexate, requires continuous long-term maintenance treatment due to the persistence of T-cell large granular lymphocytes, despite clinical improvement (34). Surprisingly, infrequent reports of continuing response off treatment, all seen in women, do exist (30). Adverse events with methotrexate and cyclosporin A are not severe and are more commonly seen with cyclosporin A, though they rarely prevent further treatment. Second malignancies were infrequently observed, and although it is not possible to attribute causality, these should prompt increased clinical vigilance, particularly in cases where intensive or prolonged immunosuppression is used.

The purine analogs remain relevant in any treatment algorithm for T-cell large granular lymphocytic leukemia. With response rates of 40% to 67% for single-agent pentostatin (35), fludarabine alone (36) or in combination (37), and cladribine, these agents are also distinguished by their independence from maintenance-type regimens and may, thus, represent particularly attractive options for younger patients. Like cyclophosphamide, the purine analogs are also moder-

ately myelosuppressive. This feature may account for the good remissions, including reduction of bone marrow infiltration, seen in some patients. Responses to cyclophosphamide are seen in one-third of patients when used with or without initial prednisolone therapy (30). In one of our patients, the response was sustained off therapy for >7 years, with a complete response in the bone marrow.

Newer agents, including the monoclonal antibodies (anti-CD52, anti-CD122, and anti-CD2) and the farnesyl transferase inhibitor tipifarnib (Zarnestra), may offer distinct more targeted therapeutic approaches. Anecdotal reports of successful treatment with the anti-CD52 antibody alemtuzumab in refractory disease (33) may be explained by the expression of this antigen on malignant cells. Similarly, in light of the dysregulation of the mitogen-activated protein kinase/Ras pathway, application of the farnesyl transferase inhibitor tipifarnib may offer therapeutic utility. Ongoing clinical trials for this disorder include the phase II Eastern Cooperative Oncology Group study of methotrexate 10 mg per m^2 weekly, with or without a 30 mg per day tapering dose of steroid, crossing over to low-dose cyclophosphamide 100 mg daily for nonresponders, a phase II study of tipifarnib, and a phase I study of the anti-CD2 antibody siplizumab.

Splenectomy is no longer considered as first-line treatment, but it may still offer some utility in the presence of immune thrombocytopenia (38) or symptomatic hypersplenism, and may offer diagnostic information in cases where T-cell large granular lymphocytic leukemia had not been previously suspected. Corticosteroids may be useful as part of the initial treatment with methotrexate and cyclophosphamide, to accelerate response. Growth factors are often useful because they may act synergistically with a number of immunosuppressive therapies.

Based on our experience, summarized in Table 26.1, the approach to treatment in T-cell large granular lymphocytic leukemia is to start with an agent such as methotrexate or cyclosporin A, with or without prednisolone or growth factors. Side effects appear less frequent with methotrexate, particularly for elderly patients whose renal function may be precarious. Monitoring of drug levels is also not needed with methotrexate. Attempts to induce remissions with pentostatin (which is mildly myelotoxic) or with cyclophosphamide, with or without prednisolone, may induce durable remissions. There is emerging information on the effect of alemtuzumab

TABLE 26.1

SUMMARY OF RESPONSES OF T-CELL LARGE GRANULAR LYMPHOCYTIC LEUKEMIA TO VARIOUS AGENTS FROM A RETROSPECTIVE CASE SERIES

Treatment	Number of patients	Median time to treatment (mo)	Duration of treatment (range)	Median follow-up (range)	CHR	PR	ORR (%)
MTX	8	1.0	22.2 mo (3–31.8)	22.8 mo (9.23–32.9)	1	5	85.7
CSA	23	1.0	23.1 mo (4–98.7)	31.8 mo (0–149.6)	7	11	78.2
DCF	4	0.75	3.25 mo (1–10)	55.5 mo	2	1	67
CTX	4	0.75	1.625 mo (1.25–10)	93 mo	1	0	33

CHR, complete hematological response; CSA, cyclosporin A; CTX, cyclophosphamide; DCF, 2-deoxycoformycin (pentostatin); MTX, methotrexate; ORR, overall response rate; PR, partial response.
Adapted from Osuji N, Matutes E, Tjonnfjord G, et al. T-cell large granular lymphocyte leukemia: a report on the treatment of 29 patients and a review of the literature. *Cancer* 2006;107:570–578, with permission.

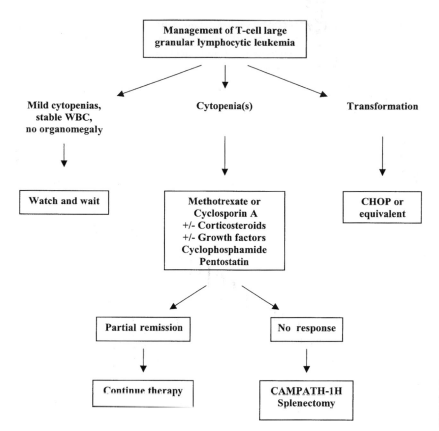

FIGURE 26.2 Flow chart summarizing the approach to treatment for T-cell large granular lymphocytic leukemia. CHOP, cyclophosphamide, hydroxydaunorubicin, Oncovin (vincristine), and prednisone; WBC, white blood cell count.

and other monoclonal antibodies. A flow chart summarizing our approach to management is shown in Figure 26.2.

T-CELL PROLYMPHOCYTIC LEUKEMIA

Definition

T-cell prolymphocytic leukemia is an aggressive disorder characterized by the proliferation of small to medium-sized lymphocytes with a mature T-cell phenotype. The disease was first recognized in 1973 in a patient whose circulating prolymphocytes were shown to be T cells by the formation of rosettes with sheep erythrocytes. The morphologic features, the recognition of a small cell variant, and the cytogenetics were subsequently reported in the 1980s (39), and in the early 1990s, the clinical and laboratory features were documented, enabling researchers to establish T-cell prolymphocytic leukemia as a distinct entity (40). T-cell prolymphocytic leukemia is now recognized as a disease entity in the WHO classification of lymphoid and hemopoietic tumors (41). Other designations used in the past to describe this condition are *"knobby-type" TCL* and *T-cell chronic lymphocytic leukemia.*

Epidemiology, Frequency, and Etiology

Epidemiologic information on the disease is scanty. T-cell prolymphocytic leukemia has been described in Western and Eastern countries, including Japan and China (Hong Kong), the Caribbean, and South America. Although this form of leukemia is more common than B-cell prolymphocytic leukemia, both diseases are rare and account for 2% of leukemias of mature lymphocytes. There is no evidence that environmental factors play a role in its development, and a familial clustering has not been described. However, there is a higher prevalence of T-cell prolymphocytic leukemia in patients with ataxia telangiectasia, in whom the disease has been described at a lower age of onset (42). Abnormalities of the ataxia telangiectasia mutated (ATM) gene localized at 11q23 have been documented by molecular analysis in the sporadic form of T-cell prolymphocytic leukemia (43,44). This suggests that the ATM gene plays a role in disease initiation; however, an increased risk for developing T-cell prolymphocytic leukemia in those heterozygous for the ATM gene has not been demonstrated.

Diagnosis

The diagnosis of T-cell prolymphocytic leukemia is best achieved by the integration of morphology, immunophenotype, and genetic features, with the greatest specificity provided by genotypic findings. However, the initial consideration of a diagnosis generally begins with the morphologic review of a blood film. Typical features include moderate to striking leukocytosis with variable anemia and thrombocytopenia (40,41). Although a spectrum of morphologic features has been described, most cases are characterized by small to intermediate-sized lymphocytes exhibiting regular or irregular nuclear outline, clumped chromatin, and generally distinct nucleoli (Color Plates 57, 58). Cytoplasm is scant to moderate, agranular, and basophilic; blebbing/cytoplasmic protrusions are common (40,41,45). A minority of cases demonstrates morphologic features that overlap with B-cell prolymphocytic leukemia, chronic lymphocytic leukemia, Sézary syndrome, or even adult TCL/lymphoma (46,47). The pattern of bone marrow infiltrates is diffuse (Color Plate 59) and often shows increased reticulin fibers, whereas lymph node sections show paracortical expansion by T-prolymphocytes with positivity for CD3 (Color Plate 60). Spleen histology shows a marked red pulp infiltration by prolymphocytes, and, unlike T-cell large granular lymphocytic leukemia, the picture here is more invasive, infiltrating the spleen capsule and the white pulp areas (25). The skin histology shows lymphoid infiltrates confined to the dermis, preferentially around the appendages with or without extending to the subcutaneous fat; epidermotropism is not seen in T-cell prolymphocytic leukemia.

Flow cytometry immunophenotyping provides critical diagnostic information by confirming the mature T-cell nature of this disorder. The leukemic cells express pan T-cell antigens such as CD2, CD5, CD7, and CD3; membrane expression of CD3 may be weak or rarely negative (40,41). Immature markers such as CD34, TdT, and CD1a are negative, and most patients are also CD25 and human leukocyte antigen-DR negative (40,45,46). Experience with 150 patients tested by our group shows that T-cell prolymphocytic leukemia typically exhibits a CD4$^+$/CD8$^-$ T-cell phenotype in 63% of patients. Twenty-three percent demonstrate CD4, CD8 coexpression, which is a distinctive feature of the disease, 13% of patients are CD4$^-$, CD8$^+$, and 1% are negative for CD4 and CD8. Natural killer-associated markers are, as a rule, negative except for CD161, which may be expressed in some cases and, in particular, in those whose cells are CD8+.

Two morphologic variants of T-cell prolymphocytic leukemia have been recognized: the small cell variant (approximately 20% of patients), in which the nucleoli may not be readily visible by light microscopy (39); and the cerebriform variant (5% of patients), in which the cells exhibit a morphology resembling Sézary cells (47).

Pathogenesis

T-cell prolymphocytic leukemia has distinct chromosome abnormalities. Studies in a large series show that 90% of patients have inv(14)(q11q32), and other translocations such as t(14;14)(q11;q32) are occasionally present (40,41,47–50). Abnormalities of chromosome 8 are also very common (80% of cases), and include idic(8)p11, tri(8)q, and t(8;8)(p11-12;q12) (50). In addition, del(12)p13 is also commonly found by fluorescent in situ hybridization studies (51). Likewise, recent studies also describe del(13)q14.3 in some cases of T-cell prolymphocytic leukemia (52). As predicted by the phenotype, a clonal T-cell receptor gene rearrangement is documented by standard molecular techniques.

Either translocation or inversion involving the TCL1 locus at chromosome 14q32.1 results in activation of TCL1 due to rearrangements with the regulatory elements of T-cell receptor genes at 14q11, and this is the likely causal event in the pathogenesis of T-cell prolymphocytic leukemia (53,54). Four genes are present at the TCL1 locus, including TCL1,

TCL1b, TNG1, and TNG2. Other less frequent translocations in T-cell prolymphocytic leukemia involve Xq28, the mature T-cell proliferation (MTCP) 1 locus (50). Activation of either TCL1 or MTCP1 results in overexpression of either p14^{TCL1} or p13^{MTCP1}, respectively, which share structural homology (53). Transgenic mice experiments with TCL1 and MTCP1 result in a TCL after 15 months of incubation but with a CD8$^+$ CD4$^-$ phenotype (55,56).

In addition, other molecular genetic events likely to play a role in the pathogenesis and progression of T-cell prolymphocytic leukemia include the inactivation of the tumor suppressor gene ATM at 11q22–23. Indeed, patients with ataxia telangiectasia often develop a variably indolent T-cell prolymphocytic leukemia-like picture (42,49), and knockout mice with an ataxia telangiectasia phenotype develop T-cell malignancies (57). T-cell prolymphocytic leukemia is in fact the first sporadic cancer in which missense mutations in the ATM gene have been demonstrated (43,44). Other candidate tumor suppressor genes at 13q14.3 may also play a role in the pathogenesis of this disorder (53).

Information on gene expression profile in T-cell prolymphocytic leukemia is scanty. A recent study combining single nucleotide polymorphism-based genomic mapping and global gene expression profiling on five cases with inv14 or t(14;14) points to a deregulation (up and down) of a variety of genes involved in lymphomagenesis, cell cycle, apoptosis, and deoxyribonucleic acid repair. The up-regulated genes were mainly clustered on chromosomes 6p and 8q, whereas the down-regulated were on 6q, 8p, 10p, 11q, and 18p. Although the number of cases is small, this study suggests novel genes involved in the pathogenesis of T-cell prolymphocytic leukemia (58). Combined single nucleotide polymorphism-based genomic mapping and global gene expression profiling identifies novel chromosomal imbalances, mechanisms, and candidate genes important in the pathogenesis of T-cell prolymphocytic leukemia with inv(14)(q11q32).

The postulated cell of origin in T-cell prolymphocytic leukemia is a mature (post-thymic) T lymphocyte. The distinctive CD4, CD8 coexpression in conjunction with weak CD3 membrane expression suggests an intermediate stage of differentiation between the cortical thymocyte stage and a circulating mature T lymphocyte.

Clinical and Laboratory Features

T-cell prolymphocytic leukemia affects adults in their mid-60s and is slightly more frequent in males. In the series investigated at the Royal Marsden Hospital, the median age was 63 years, and the male to female ratio was 3:1. Most patients are symptomatic at diagnosis and present with widespread disease. The main symptoms are abdominal distension, often resulting from splenomegaly, bulky nodes, skin rash, and, less often, anemia or bleeding; initial manifestations such as blurred vision due to infiltration of the retina by prolymphocytes are unusual, but we have seen this in two patients. A small number of patients, approximately 10%, are asymptomatic, and the diagnosis is made on a routine checkup that shows a low level of lymphocytosis. This group might be considered as having a form of smoldering T-cell prolymphocytic leukemia (45), but, almost invariably, the disease progresses in terms of months or, more rarely, years.

Physical examination shows splenomegaly in more than two-thirds of patients, hepatomegaly and lymphadenopathy in approximately half, and skin lesions in close to one-third. The skin lesions are manifested as a localized or generalized maculopapular rash, nodules, and, more rarely, erythroderma similar to that seen in Sézary syndrome (59). Other less common signs at diagnosis are pleural or pericardial effusions and ascites, but these features are common in the relapse phase or during disease progression. Central nervous system involvement manifested by meningeal disease with the presence of prolymphocytes in the central spinal fluid or brain deposits is rare but may be seen at diagnosis or relapse.

Peripheral blood counts show an elevated white blood cell count with values ranging between 10 and $1,000 \times 10^9$ per L, and >50% of patients have presenting counts >100 $\times$ 10^9 per L. A normochromic normocytic anemia or thrombocytopenia is present in 25% and 45% of patients, respectively. Cytopenias usually result from a combination of bone marrow infiltration and a degree of hypersplenism. Renal and liver biochemistry may be normal or show a mild impairment, and the serum urate and lactate dehydrogenase levels are often raised. Serum immunoglobulins are, as a rule, normal. Serology for the human TCL/lymphoma viruses types I and II is consistently negative, including patients of Japanese or Afro-Caribbean descent (40).

Prognostic Factors

Information is scanty regarding the variables that may have an influence on survival or the response to therapy. Hepatomegaly seemed to be a strong predictor for survival in our original series (40) and a predictor for response to therapy with Campath-1H (alemtuzumab) (60), whereas immunophenotype or molecular genetics does not appear to influence survival or response to therapy. In addition, response to therapy with either pentostatin or Campath-1H is a predictor for disease-free and overall survival (60). Thus, the median survival of the complete remitters with Campath-1H is close to 2 years, whereas in the partial responders, it is 9 months (61). A recent report showed a 5-year survival of 21% (62). Poorer outcome was associated with high white blood count, short lymphocyte doubling time, older age, high expression of TCL-1 protein as measured by flow cytometry and immunohistochemistry, and high levels of the serine-threonine kinase AKT (63).

Treatment

In the series of 78 cases reported in 1991 (40), the majority of patients were treated with alkylating agents, cyclophosphamide, hydroxydaunorubicin, Oncovin (vincristine), and prednisone, and/or with the adenosine deaminase inhibitor pentostatin, but results were disappointing. Most patients did not respond to alkylating agents, and one-third experienced short-lived responses to cyclophosphamide, hydroxydaunorubicin, Oncovin (vincristine), and prednisone. Pentostatin resulted in a higher response rate (45%), with few patients achieving a complete remission (40). The efficacy of pentostatin was further confirmed in a subsequent study that included 55 patients. These responses, however, were short lived. There is little information on the effect of other nucleoside analogs, such as cladribine and fludarabine, in T-cell prolymphocytic leukemia, but we have seen occasional responses with the former.

Currently, the best treatment is the humanized monoclonal antibody Campath-1H, directed against the CD52 antigen, which is widely expressed on normal and neoplastic lymphocytes. The standard regimen is to start with 5 mg intravenously and increase daily to reach 30 mg within 3 days, and subsequently this dose is given three times a week for 6 to 8 weeks, or longer if required, to clear the blood, bone marrow, and other tissues. The main side effects of Campath-1H are "first dose" infusion reactions, which can be readily controlled with premedication, mild transient myelosuppression, and, most importantly, profound immune suppression. The latter results in increased risk of opportunistic infections, including reactivation of latent viruses such as herpes and cytomegalovirus. Careful infection prophylaxis and weekly monitoring are recommended.

A recent update of our early results (60) shows that the complete remission rate with Campath-1H is 63% in 44 patients, the highest with any single agent in this disease (61). Patients with liver or central nervous system involvement, or with serous effusions, were more resistant to therapy. The majority of patients treated with Campath-1H had received prior therapy and were resistant to or had had relapse after first-line treatment with pentostatin or other agents. A retrospective analysis of 76 patients with T-cell prolymphocytic leukemia treated in a compassionate program reported a 51% overall response rate with 39% complete remissions. Median duration of responses was 8.7 months (14 months for responders) with a median time to progression of 4.5 months (62). The excellent results in T-cell prolymphocytic leukemia, better than in chronic lymphocytic leukemia and any other condition in which this agent has been used, may relate to the high density of CD52 expression in the T prolymphocytes (64). A strong case has been made for the use of Campath as first-line treatment (60–62): all five patients in our initial series treated with this antibody as first-line treatment all achieved a complete response with 6 to 8 weeks of therapy (61). We have subsequently treated a further 11 patients with first-line intravenous Campath, achieving an overall response rate of 94% with 88% complete remissions, confirming the efficacy of single-agent Campath in this disease. A recent pilot study evaluating subcutaneous Campath has indicated that this route of administration is not as effective as intravenous, with only three out of nine patients achieving complete remission.

Combination chemoimmunotherapy approaches have also been explored. The German Chronic Lymphocytic Leukemia Study Group (65) recently reported results of a prospective phase II trial of fludarabine, mitoxantrone, and cyclophosphamide followed by alemtuzumab consolidation in 18 patients. The overall response rate following this combination was 66%, increasing to 86% after alemtuzumab consolidation, with a median progression-free survival of 10.6 months and overall survival of 19.2 months.

Prognosis and Median Survival and Transformation

T-cell prolymphocytic leukemia has a poor prognosis. The median survival for patients treated with conventional therapy was 7 months (40). In 10% of patients with T-cell prolympho-cytic leukemia, the disease course may be initially stable or slowly progressive, but all patients finally show frank progression. The higher response rate with Campath-1H has resulted in a survival benefit as shown in the updated survival of 62 patients treated with this antibody, showing a median overall survival of 2 years for patients achieving a complete remission; nonresponders still have a poor outcome, with a median survival of only 4 months. It is unlikely, however, that Campath-1H treatment alone will result in a cure for patients with T-cell prolymphocytic leukemia. Transformation into a large cell lymphoma has not been reported. However, we have observed a patient who, after a 4-year remission with Campath-1H, had relapse with circulating blastoid cells and a rapid downward course suggestive of transformation. This was associated with immunophenotypic changes and down-regulation of CD52. The blast cells were shown by cytogenetic analysis to correspond to the same clone as the original prolymphocytes (66). Another patient whose cells became CD52 negative after Campath-1H therapy did not respond any longer to the antibody (66). The down-regulation of CD52 appears to be increasingly recognized as a mechanism of resistance to Campath-1H (67). It is, therefore, advisable to retest the cells for the expression of CD52 at the relapse phase, before embarking again with Campath-1H treatment.

Future Directions

Despite the high complete remission rate to Campath-1H, ultimately all patients relapse, and, thus, new strategies are needed to consolidate responses, with the aim of improving disease-free and overall survival. The fact that it is possible to clear the bone marrow and produce remissions undetected by flow cytometry or polymerase chain reaction for the T-cell receptor suggests that the next step is to use this good complete remission as a first step for attempts at high-dose therapy with stem cell rescue. Because stem cells do not express CD52, it is possible to collect adequate numbers of CD34 cells after remission with Campath-1H. In a recent study of 22 patients with T-cell prolymphocytic leukemia, who were in first or second complete remission, or had achieved a partial response following Campath-1H therapy, 13 were consolidated with an autologous, and nine with an allogeneic, stem cell transplant (five siblings, four unrelated donors) (68). In the patients who had autografts, 38% remain alive, with a median disease-free survival of 20 months (range 8 to 78 months). Of the nine patients who had an allograft, four had full-intensity conditioning and five reduced-intensity conditioning. Fifty-six percent remain alive, including one in continued complete remission 7 years after the transplant. Two patients died of transplant-related mortality, and both had received full-intensity conditioning. These results demonstrate that autologous stem cell transplants can increase disease-free survival, but one third of patients still have relapse. Although allogeneic stem cell transplant is an attractive option, patients should be selected carefully in view of the older age group of patients with this disease. Transplant-related mortality with full-intensity conditioning is high, and in older patients reduced-intensity conditioning should be explored, although it remains to be seen whether a graft versus leukemic effect is sufficient to hold this aggressive disease at bay.

NATURAL KILLER-CELL LEUKEMIA, INCLUDING CHRONIC LYMPHOPROLIFERATIVE DISORDERS OF NATURAL KILLER CELLS AND AGGRESSIVE NATURAL KILLER-CELL LEUKEMIA/LYMPHOMA

Definition

The natural killer-cell leukemias encompass a variety of neoplasms that arise from cells committed to the natural killer-cell lineage. They are considered in the WHO classification under the designations of *chronic lymphoproliferative disorders of natural killer cells* and *aggressive natural killer-cell leukemia/lymphoma* (69,70). The rare group of large granular lymphocytic leukemias with a natural killer phenotype has been designated chronic lymphoproliferative disorders of natural killer –cells, and these indolent disorders are distinct from aggressive natural killer-cell leukemias/lymphomas. Other neoplasms arising from natural killer cells are considered in the WHO classification within distinct subgroups of lymphomas, such as extranodal natural killer/T-cell lymphoma, nasal type. Indeed, it has been suggested that aggressive natural killer-cell leukemia may be the leukemic counterpart of the extranodal natural killer/T-cell lymphoma, nasal type. In this chapter we discuss both the chronic lymphoproliferative disorders of natural killer cells and the aggressive natural killer-cell leukemias, as per the WHO proposal.

CHRONIC LYMPHOPROLIFERATIVE DISORDERS OF NATURAL KILLER CELLS

Frequency, Epidemiology, and Etiology

Chronic lymphoproliferative disorders of natural killer cells are rare (71,72) and account for only a small proportion of large granular lymphocytic leukemias, which are usually derived from CD3+ CD8+ T –cells, as described earlier in this chapter. Chronic lymphoproliferative disorders of natural killer cells affect predominantly adults; many of these patients are asymptomatic. Transient increases in circulating natural killer cells can also be seen in patients with solid tumors, as well as viral infections, neurologic disorders, and autoimmune disorders (72,73). Unlike other more aggressive natural killer disorders, an association with Epstein-Barr virus is not typically identified in these indolent disorders. However, natural killer-cell activation from an, as yet, unknown cause may play a role in their pathogenesis (72,74–76).

Diagnosis

Although diagnostic criteria are not standardized, documentation of a sustained absolute increase in the number of circulating natural killer cells is required for diagnosis. Current recommendations are that a large granular lymphocyte count of at least 2×10^9 per L be sustained for at least 6 months for a diagnosis of a chronic lymphoproliferative disorder of natural killer cells (69). By morphologic review, these natural killer cells exhibit the classic morphology of large granular lymphocytes, which are characterized by mature, round nuclei, and moderate amounts of pale-blue–gray cytoplasm, which contains multiple variably distinct azurophilic granules. Flow cytometric immunophenotyping is essential to distinguish true natural killer cells (CD3 negative, CD16 positive, CD56 positive) from cytotoxic suppressor T cells (CD3 positive, CD8 positive, CD57 positive) (17,72,73,77). Patterns of aberrant antigen expression have been noted in these indolent natural killer disorders that may support a neoplastic rather than reactive etiology in a given patient (78,79). Expression patterns of the KIR family of natural killer-cell receptors may also be skewed, supporting a clonal process (17,73,80–82).

Pathogenesis

Because conventional karyotyping is usually normal and T-cell receptor gene rearrangements are not detected, the documentation of clonality is challenging in chronic lymphoproliferative disorders of natural killer cells. Either a skewed ratio of X-chromosome inactivation (Humara assay) or restricted KIR isoform genotype expression patterns may be useful, although neither test is used routinely in clinical practice (83–85). Recent studies show that by gene expression profiling, leukemic natural killer cells can be distinguished from reactive natural killer cells (86). However, because of the difficulties in confirming clonality in chronic natural killer-cell proliferations, it is likely that both neoplastic and nonneoplastic disorders are included in published series.

Clinical Features

Although most patients are asymptomatic, a minority manifest with fever, cytopenias, and, rarely, with lymphadenopathy and/or hepatosplenomegaly (72,77,87). Associations with solid tumors, viral infections, immune disorders, and neurologic disorders have been described, although the natural killer proliferations in these disorders may be secondary.

Therapy

Due to the typically prolonged, stable clinical course, therapy may not be necessary. Rare cases of spontaneous remission have been described (72,76,87). A more aggressive disease course has been linked to progressive symptomatology, progressive cytopenias, clonal cytogenetic aberrations, and transformation (88–90).

AGGRESSIVE NATURAL KILLER-CELL LEUKEMIA/LYMPHOMA

Definition

Aggressive natural killer-cell leukemia/lymphoma is a systemic disorder that is characterized by a clonal proliferation of natural killer cells often manifesting as widespread disease with frequent leukemic manifestation (70,91,92).

Frequency, Epidemiology, and Etiology

Aggressive natural killer-cell leukemia/lymphoma is a rare disorder with a relative greater frequency in Asian and selected Native American populations. Patients are typically younger (median age <40). An association with Epstein-Barr virus has been documented in the majority of cases, and this virus is considered to play a role in the pathogenesis of this disease (70,91,92).

Diagnosis

The diagnosis is based upon the morphologic and immunophenotypic features of the leukemia cells present in blood, bone marrow, or extramedullary sites. Although a spectrum of morphologic features has been described, in many cases the neoplastic cells have enlarged nuclei with variably prominent nucleoli and variably blastic chromatin, as well as moderate amounts of cytoplasm containing variably conspicuous azurophilic granules (92,93). In some cases the circulating cells are indistinguishable from acute leukemia (Color Plate 61). Immunophenotypic assessment is required to distinguish these leukemia cells from other neoplasms. The antigenic profile reflects natural killer derivation, CD3 negative, CD16 variably positive, CD56 positive, CD57 negative (92,93). In addition, nuclear Epstein-Barr virus ribonucleic acid can be demonstrated by Epstein-Barr encoded-ribonucleic acid in situ hybridization, a key diagnostic feature in cases in which the disease is Epstein-Barr virus driven (Color Plate 62). Additional features by immunohistochemical assessment include both cytoplasmic CD3 (εchain) and TIA-1/granzyme positivity; occasional cases express CD30 (Color Plates 63, 64). Detection of CD3 ε is likely to be due to cross-reactivity with the θ chain of the T-cell receptor, present in natural killer cells. T-cell receptor genes are germline (unrearranged). Florid, cytokine-mediated hemophagocytosis by admixed benign histiocytes may be a significant finding in some cases, with a potential to mask the underlying neoplastic aggressive natural killer-cell leukemia/lymphoma infiltrate (Color Plate 65).

Pathogenesis

By comparative genomic hybridization, recurrent regions of chromosomal gains and losses have been identified, suggesting a multistep neoplastic process. Recent reports of del(6q) in aggressive natural killer-cell leukemia/lymphoma and extranodal natural killer/T-cell lymphoma nasal type suggest a biologic link between these two Epstein-Barr virus-related disorders (92). In addition, the pathogenic role of Epstein-Barr virus is strongly suggested by the consistent Epstein-Barr virus-encoded small ribonucleic acid positivity in the leukemia cells. Various genes have been noted in the extranodal natural killer, nasal type Epstein-Barr virus-mediated neoplasms that may contribute to tumorigenesis, but the role of these genes in aggressive natural killer-cell leukemia/lymphoma has not been delineated (92).

Clinical Features

Systemic symptoms, such as fever and weight loss, in conjunction with multiorgan failure and marked organomegaly, are common features at presentation. Skin lesions may be present in one-third to one-half of the patients, and, in some patients, these lesions may precede the systemic manifestations (91–93). A few cases manifest with or develop extranodal involvement, such as pleural effusion, and in others the disease evolves with a hemophagocytic syndrome and profound pancytopenia (94,95). The latter may present diagnostic problems with a viral infection. Fever is a common symptom at presentation. Physical examination shows marked hepatosplenomegaly in the majority of cases, and in approximately half, lymphadenopathy. Anemia and thrombocytopenia and the presence of variable numbers of abnormal circulating cells are frequent findings. Biochemistry shows abnormal liver function tests and elevated urate and lactate dehydrogenase levels in the majority of patients. Liver dysfunction is possibly linked to the induction of hepatocyte apoptosis by Fas ligand-bearing natural killer cells (92). Hemophagocytic syndrome is commonly noted in bone marrow; up-regulation of tumor necrosis factor-α and other cytokines by tumor cells is a likely cause of this phenomenon (92,93). A few patients may have a coagulopathy, particularly those with a rapid downhill course (93).

Therapy/Survival

Most patients with aggressive natural killer-cell leukemia/lymphoma pursue a highly aggressive disease course with median survival times of only several months. This disease is typically refractory to therapy. There are case reports of successful allogeneic stem cell transplantation (92).

References

1. Loughran TP Jr, Kadin ME, Starkebaum G, et al. Leukemia of large granular lymphocytes: association with clonal chromosomal abnormalities and autoimmune neutropenia, thrombocytopenia, and hemolytic anemia. *Ann Intern Med* 1985;102:169–175.
2. Chan WC, Foucar K, Morice WG, et al. T-cell large granular lymphocytic leukaemia. In: Swerdlow SH, Campo E, Harris NL, et al, eds. *WHO classification of tumours of the haematopoietic and lymphoid tissues*, 4th ed. Lyon, France: International Agency for Research on Cancer, 2008; 272–273.
3. Epling-Burnette PK, Loughran TP Jr. Survival signals in leukemic large granular lymphocytes. *Semin Hematol* 2003;40:213–220.
4. Wlodarski MW, O'Keefe C, Howe EC, et al. Pathologic clonal cytotoxic T-cell responses: nonrandom nature of the T-cell-receptor restriction in large granular lymphocyte leukemia. *Blood* 2005;106:2769–2780.
5. O'Keefe CL, Plasilova M, Wlodarski M, et al. Molecular analysis of TCR clonotypes in LGL: a clonal model for polyclonal responses. *J Immunol* 2004;172:1960–1969.
6. Loughran TP Jr. Clonal diseases of large granular lymphocytes. *Blood* 1993;82:1–14.
7. Starkebaum G. Chronic neutropenia associated with autoimmune disease. *Semin Hematol* 2002;39:121–127.
8. Risitano AM, Maciejewski JP, Muranski P, et al. Large granular lymphocyte (LGL)-like clonal expansions in paroxysmal nocturnal hemoglobinuria (PNH) patients. *Leukemia* 2005;19:217–222.
9. Loughran TP Jr, Starkebaum G, Kidd P, et al. Clonal proliferation of large granular lymphocytes in rheumatoid arthritis. *Arthritis Rheum* 1988;31:31–36.
10. Lamy T, Liu JH, Landowski TH, et al. Dysregulation of CD95/CD95 ligand-apoptotic pathway in CD3(+) large granular lymphocyte leukemia. *Blood* 1998;92:4771–4777.
11. Schade AE, Powers JJ, Wlodarski MW, et al. Phosphatidylinositol-3-phosphate kinase pathway activation protects leukemic large granular lymphocytes from undergoing homeostatic apoptosis. *Blood* 2006;107:4834–4840.
12. Epling-Burnette PK, Bai F, Wei S, et al. ERK couples chronic survival of natural killer cells to constitutively activated Ras in lymphoproliferative disease of granular lymphocytes (LDGL). *Oncogene* 2004;23:9220–9229.
13. Semenzato G, Zambello R, Starkebaum G, et al. The lymphoproliferative disease of granular lymphocytes: updated criteria for diagnosis. *Blood* 1997;89:256–260.
14. Hodges E, Krishna MT, Pickard C, et al. Diagnostic role of tests for T cell receptor (TCR) genes. *J Clin Pathol* 2003;56:1–11.
15. Sokol L, Loughran TP Jr. Large granular lymphocyte leukemia. *Oncologist* 2006;11:263–273.
16. Osuji N, Beiske K, Randen U, et al. Characteristic appearances of the bone marrow in T-cell large granular lymphocyte leukemia. *Histopathology* 2007;50:547–554.
17. Morice WG, Kurtin PJ, Leibson PJ, et al. Demonstration of aberrant T-cell and natural killer-cell antigen expression in all cases of granular lymphocytic leukaemia. *Br J Haematol* 2003;120:1026–1036.
18. Lima M, Almeida J, Dos Anjos Teixeira M, et al. TCRalphabeta+/CD4+ large granular lymphocytosis: a new clonal T-cell lymphoproliferative disorder. *Am J Pathol* 2003;163:763–771.
19. Alekshun TJ, Tao J, Sokol L. Aggressive T-cell large granular lymphocyte leukemia: a case report and review of the literature. *Am J Hematol* 2007;82:481–485.
20. Bourgault-Rouxel AS, Loughran TP Jr, Zambello R, et al. Clinical spectrum of gammadelta+ T cell LGL leukemia: analysis of 20 cases. *Leuk Res* 2008;32:45–48.
21. Fischer L, Hummel M, Burmeister T, et al. Skewed expression of natural-killer (NK)-associated antigens on lymphoproliferations of large granular lymphocytes (LGL). *Hematol Oncol* 2006;24:78–85.
22. Osuji N, Del Giudice I, Matutes E, et al. CD52 expression in T-cell large granular lymphocyte leukemia–implications for treatment with alemtuzumab. *Leuk Lymphoma* 2005;46:723–727.
23. Foucar K. Chronic lymphoproliferative disorders. In: *Bone marrow pathology*, 2nd ed. Chicago, IL: ASCP Press, 2001:366–405.
24. Morice WG, Kurtin PJ, Tefferi A, et al. Distinct bone marrow findings in T-cell granular lymphocytic leukemia revealed by paraffin section immunoperoxidase stains for CD8, TIA-1, and granzyme B. *Blood* 2002;99:268–274.
25. Osuji N, Matutes E, Catovsky D, et al. Histopathology of the spleen in T-cell large granular lymphocyte leukemia and T-cell prolymphocytic leukemia: a comparative review. *Am J Surg Pathol* 2005;29:935–941.
26. Wong KF, Chan JC, Liu HS, et al. Chromosomal abnormalities in T-cell large granular lymphocyte leukemia: report of two cases and review of the literature. *Br J Haematol* 2002;116:598–600.
27. Perzova R, Loughran TP Jr. Constitutive expression of Fas ligand in large granular lymphocyte leukemia. *Br J Haematol* 1997;97:123–126.
28. Handgretinger R, Geiselhart A, Moris A, et al. Pure red-cell aplasia associated with clonal expansion of granular lymphocytes expressing killer-cell inhibitory receptors. *N Engl J Med* 1999;340:278–284.
29. Melenhorst JJ, Sorbara L, Kirby M, et al. Large granular lymphocyte leukemia is characterized by a clonal T-cell receptor rearrangement in both memory and effector CD8(+) lymphocyte populations. *Br J Haematol* 2001;112:189–194.
30. Osuji N, Matutes E, Tjonnfjord G, et al. T-cell large granular lymphocyte leukemia: a report on the treatment of 29 patients and a review of the literature. *Cancer* 2006;107:570–578.
31. Matutes E, Wotherspoon AC, Parker NE, et al. Transformation of T-cell granular lymphocyte leukemia into a high-grade large T-cell lymphoma. *Br J Haematol* 2001;115:801–806.
32. Loughran TP Jr, Kidd PG, Starkebaum G. Treatment of large granular lymphocyte leukemia with oral low-dose methotrexate. *Blood* 1994;84:2164–2170.
33. Osuji N, Matutes E, Wotherspoon A, et al. Lessons from a case of T-cell large granular lymphocytic leukemia suggesting that immunomodulatory therapy is more effective than intensive treatment. *Leuk Res* 2005;29:225–228.
34. Brinkman K, van Dongen JJ, van Lom K, et al. Induction of clinical remission in T-large granular lymphocyte leukemia with cyclosporin A, monitored by use of immunophenotyping with Vbeta antibodies. *Leukemia* 1998;12:150–154.
35. Tsirigotis P, Venetis E, Kapsimali V, et al. 2-deoxycoformycin in the treatment of T-large granular lymphocyte leukemia. *Leuk Res* 2003;27:865–867.
36. Sternberg A, Eagleton H, Pillai N, et al. Neutropenia and anaemia associated with T-cell large granular lymphocyte leukemia responds to fludarabine with minimal toxicity. *Br J Haematol* 2003;120:699–701.
37. Tse E, Chan JC, Pang A, et al. Fludarabine, mitoxantrone and dexamethasone as first-line treatment for T-cell large granular lymphocyte leukemia. *Leukemia* 2007;21:2225–2256.
38. Loughran TP Jr, Starkebaum G, Clark E, et al. Evaluation of splenectomy in large granular lymphocyte leukemia. *Br J Haematol* 1987;67:135–140.
39. Matutes E, Garcia-Talavera J, O'Brien M, et al. The morphological spectrum of T-prolymphocytic leukemia. *Br J Haematol* 1986;64:111–124.
40. Matutes E, Brito-Babapulle V, Swansbury J, et al. Clinical and laboratory features of 78 cases of T-prolymphocytic leukemia. *Blood* 1991;78:3269–3274.

41. Catovsky D, Müller-Hermelink HK, Ralfkiaer E. T-cell prolymphocytic leukaemia. In: Swerdlow SH, Campo E, Harris NL, et al., eds. *WHO classification of tumours of the haematopoietic and lymphoid tissues*, 4th ed. Lyon, France: International Agency for Research on Cancer, 2008; 270–271.

42. Taylor AMR, Metcalfe JA, Thick J, et al. Leukemia and lymphoma in ataxia telangiectasia. *Blood* 1996;87:423–438.

43. Vorechovsky I, Luo L, Dyer MJS, et al. Clustering of missense mutations in the ataxia-telangiectasia gene in a sporadic T-cell leukemia. *Nat Genet* 1997;17:96–99.

44. Stilgenbauer S, Schaffner C, Litterst A, et al. Biallelic mutations in the ATM gene in T-prolymphocytic leukemia. *Nat Med* 1997;3:1155–1159.

45. Garand R, Goasguen J, Brizard A, et al. Indolent course as a relatively frequent presentation in T-prolymphocytic leukemia. *Br J Haematol* 1998;103:488–494.

46. Hoyer JD, Ross CW, Li CY, et al. True T-cell chronic lymphocytic leukemia: a morphologic and immunophenotypic study of 25 cases. *Blood* 1995;86:1163–1169.

47. Brito-Babapulle V, Maljaie SH, Matutes E, et al. Relationship of T leukemias with cerebriform nuclei to T-prolymphocytic leukemia: a cytogenetic analysis with in situ hybridization. *Br J Haematol* 1997;96:724–732.

48. Brito-Babapulle V, Pomfret M, Matutes E, et al. Cytogenetic studies on prolymphocytic leukemia. II. T-cell prolymphocytic leukemia. *Blood* 1987;70:926–931.

49. Brito-Babapulle V, Catovsky D. Inversions and tandem translocations involving chromosome 14q11 and 14q32 in T-prolymphocytic leukemia and T-cell leukemias in patients with ataxia telangiectasia. *Cancer Genet Cytogenet* 1991;55:1–9.

50. Maljaic SH, Brito-Babapulle V, Hiorns LR, et al. Abnormalities of chromosomes 8, 11, 14 and X in T-prolymphocytic leukemia studied by fluorescence in situ hybridization. *Cancer Genet Cytogenet* 1998;103:110–116.

51. Salomon-Nguyen F, Brizard F, Le Coniat M, et al. Abnormalities of the short arm of chromosome 12 in T cell prolymphocytic leukemia. *Leukemia* 1998;12:972–975.

52. Brito-Babapulle V, Baou M, Matutes E, et al. Deletions of D13S25, D13S319 and RB-1 mapping to 13q14.3 in T-cell prolymphocytic leukemia. *Br J Haematol* 2001;114:327–332.

53. Pekarsky U, Hallas C, Croce CM. Molecular basis of mature T-cell leukemia. *JAMA* 2001;286:2308–2314.

54. Pekarsky Y, Hallas C, Isobe M, et al. Abnormalities at 14q32.1 in T cell malignancies involve two oncogenes. *Proc Natl Acad Sci U S A* 1999;96:2949–2951.

55. Virgilio L, Lazzeri C, Bichi R, et al. Deregulated expression of TCL1 causes T cell leukemia in mice. *Proc Natl Acad Sci U S A* 1998;95:3885–3889.

56. Gritti C, Dastot H, Soulier J, et al. Transgenic mice for MTCP1 develop T-cell prolymphocytic leukemia. *Blood* 1998;92:368–373.

57. Stoppa-Lyonnet D, Soulier J, Lauge A, et al. Inactivation of the ATM gene in T-cell prolymphocytic leukemias. *Blood* 1998;91:3920–3926.

58. Durig J, Bug S, Klein-Hitpass L, et al. Combined single nucleotide polymorphism-based genomic mapping and global gene expression profiling identifies novel chromosomal imbalances, mechanisms and candidate genes important in the pathogenesis of T-cell prolymphocytic leukemia with inv(14)(q11q32). *Leukemia* 2007;21:2153–2163.

59. Mallett RB, Matutes E, Catovsky D, et al. Cutaneous infiltration in T-cell prolymphocytic leukemia. *Br J Dermatol* 1995;132:263–266.

60. Dearden CE, Matutes E, Cazin B, et al. High remission rate in T-cell prolymphocytic leukemia with CAMPATH-1H. *Blood* 2001;98:1721–1726.

61. Dearden CE, Matutes E, Cazin B, et al. Longer follow up of T-prolymphocytic leukemia patients treated with Alemtuzumab (CAMPATH-1H) shows improved survival and higher response rates in previously untreated patients. *Blood* 2002;100:364a.

62. Keating MJ, Cazin B, Coutre S, et al. Campath-1H treatment of T-cell prolymphocytic leukemia in patients for whom at least one prior chemotherapy regimen has failed. *J Clin Oncol* 2002;20:205–213.

63. Herling M, Patel KA, Teitell MA, et al. High TCL1 expression and intact T-cell receptor signaling define a hyperproliferative subset of T-cell prolymphocytic leukemia. *Blood* 2008;111:328–337.

64. Ginaldi L, De Martinis M, Matutes E, et al. Levels of expression of CD52 in normal and leukemic B and T cells: correlation with in vivo therapeutic responses to CAMPATH-1H. *Leuk Res* 1998;22:185–191.

65. Hopfinger G, Busch R, Eichhorst B, et al. TPLL-1 protocol of the German CLL Study Group (GCLLSG)—a prospective phase II trial of fludarabine phosphate, mitoxantrone and cyclophosphamide (FMC) followed by alemtuzumab consolidation in T-PLL. *Blood* 2007;110:2039.

66. Tuset E, Matutes E, Brito-Babapulle V, et al. Immunophenotype changes and loss of CD52 expression in two patients with relapsed T-cell prolymphocytic leukemia. *Leuk Lymphoma* 2001;42:1379–1383.

67. Birhiray R, Shaw G, Guldan S, et al. Phenotypic transformation of CD52(+) to CD52(-) leukemic T-cells as a mechanism for resistance to CAMPATH-1H. *Leukemia* 2002;16:861–864.

68. Krishnan B, Cazin B, Ireland R, et al. Improved survival for patients with T-cell prolymphocytic leukaemia receiving alemtuzumab therapy followed by stem cell transplantation. *Leuk Lymphoma* 2007;48:S180.

69. Villamor N, Morice WG, Chan WC, et al. Chronic lymphoproliferative disorders of NK cells. In: Swerdlow SH, Campo E, Harris NL, et al., eds. *WHO classification of tumours of the haematopoietic and lymphoid tissues*, 4th ed. Lyon, France: International Agency for Research on Cancer, 2008;274–275.

70. Chan JKC, Jaffe ES, Ralfkiaer E, et al. Aggressive natural killer-cell leukemia/lymphoma. In: Swerdlow SH, Campo E, Harris NL, et al., eds. *WHO classification of tumours of the haematopoietic and lymphoid tissues*, 4th ed. Lyon, France: International Agency for Research on Cancer, 2008; 276–277.

71. Tefferi A, Li CY, Witzig T, et al. Chronic natural killer cell lymphocytosis: a descriptive clinical study. *Blood* 1994;84:2721–2725.

72. Lima M, Almeida J, Montero AG, et al. Clinicobiological, immunophenotypic, and molecular characteristics of monoclonal CD56-/+dim chronic natural killer cell large granular lymphocytosis. *Am J Pathol* 2004;165:1117–1127.

73. Pascal V, Schleintz N, Brunet C, et al. Comparative analysis of NK cell subset distribution in normal and lymphoproliferative disease of granular lymphocyte conditions. *Eur J Immunol* 2004;34:2930–2940.

74. Loughran TP Jr, Zambello R, Ashley R, et al. Failure to detect Epstein-Barr virus DNA in peripheral blood mononuclear cells of most patients with large granular lymphocyte leukemia. *Blood* 1993;81:2723–2727.

75. Zambello R, Loughran TP Jr, Trentin L, et al. Serologic and molecular evidence for a possible pathogenetic role of viral infection in CD3-negative natural killer-type lymphoproliferative disease of granular lymphocytes. *Leukemia* 1995;9:1207–1211.

76. Rabbani GR, Phyliky RL, Tefferi A. A long-term study of patients with chronic natural killer cell lymphocytosis. *Br J Haematol* 1999;106:960–966.

77. Lamy T, Loughran TP Jr. Clinical features of large granular lymphocyte leukemia. *Semin Hematol* 2003;40:185–195.

78. Morice W, Jevremovic D, Hanson C. The expression of the novel cytotoxic protein granzyme M by large granular lymphocytic leukemias of both T-cell and NK-cell lineage: an unexpected finding with implications regarding the pathobiology of these disorders. *B J Haemeatol* 2007;137:237–239.

79. Morice W The immunophenotypic attributes of NK cells and NK-cell lineage lymphoproliferative disorders. *Am J Clin Pathol* 2007;127:881–886.

80. Kelly A, Richards SJ, Sivakumaran M, et al. Clonality of CD3 negative large granular lymphocyte proliferations determined by PCR based X-inactivation studies. *J Clin Pathol* 1994;47:399–404.

81. Hoffmann T, De Libero G, Colonna M, et al. Natural killer-type receptors for HLA class I antigens are clonally expressed in lymphoproliferative disorders of natural killer and T-cell type. *Br J Haematol* 2000;110:525–536.

82. Warren HS, Christiansen FT, Witt CS. Functional inhibitory human leucocyte antigen class I receptors on natural killer (NK) cells in patients with chronic NK lymphocytosis. *Br J Haematol* 2003;121:793–804.

83. Zambello R, Falco M, Chiesa M, et al. Expression and function of KIR and natural cytotoxicity receptors in NK-type lymphoproliferative diseases of granular lymphocytes. *Blood* 2003;102:1797–1805.

84. Scquizzato E, Teramo A, Miorin M, et al. Genotypic evaluation of killer immunoglobulin-like receptors in NK-type lymphoproliferative disease of granular lymphocytes. *Leukemia* 2007;21:1060–1069.

85. Epling-Burnette PK, Painter JS, Chaurasia P, et al. Dysregulated NK receptor expression in patients with lymphoproliferative disease of granular lymphocytes. *Blood* 2004;103:3431–3439.

86. Choi YL, Makishima H, Ohashi J, et al. DNA microarray analysis of natural killer cell-type granular lymphocytes disease of granular lymphocytes with purified CD3-CD56+ fractions. *Leukemia* 2004;18:556–565.

87. Oshimi K, Yamada O, Kaneko T, et al. Laboratory findings and clinical courses of 33 patients with granular lymphocyte-proliferative disorders. *Leukemia* 1993;7:782–788.

88. Ohno Y, Amakawa R, Fukuhara S, et al. Acute transformation of chronic large granular lymphocyte leukemia associated with additional chromosome abnormality. *Cancer* 1989;64:63–67.

89. Huang Q, Chang K, Gaal K, et al. An aggressive extranodal NK-cell lymphoma arising from indolent NK-cell lymphoproliferative disorder. *Am J Surg Pathol* 2005;29:1540–1543.

90. Roullet M, Cornfield D. Large natural killer cell lymphoma arising from an indolent natural killer cell large granular lymphocyte proliferation. *Arch Pathol Lab Med* 2006;130:1712–1714.

91. Suzuki R, Suzumiya J, Nakamura S, et al. Aggressive natural killer-cell leukemia revisited: large granular lymphocyte leukemia of cytotoxic NK cells. *Leukemia* 2004;18:763–770.

92. Oshimi K. Progress in understanding and managing natural killer-cell malignancies. *Br J Haematol* 2007;139:532–544.

93. Cheung M, Chan J, Wonk KF. Natural killer cell neoplasms: a distinctive group of highly aggressive lymphomas/leukemias. *Semin Hematol* 2003;40:221–232.

94. Imamura N, Kusunoki Y, Kawa-Ha K, et al. Aggressive natural killer cell leukemia/lymphoma: report of four cases and review of the literature. Possible existence of a new clinical entity originating from the third lineage of lymphoid cells. *Br J Haematol* 1990;75:49–59.

95. Chan JKC, Sin VC, Wong KF, et al. Nonnasal lymphoma expressing the natural killer cell marker CD56: a clinicopathologic study of 49 cases of an uncommon aggressive neoplasm. *Blood* 1997;89:4501–4513.

CHAPTER 27 ■ HUMAN T-CELL LEUKEMIA VIRUS TYPE I-ASSOCIATED ADULT T-CELL LEUKEMIA LYMPHOMA

KENSEI TOBINAI, TOSHIKI WATANABE, AND ELAINE S. JAFFE

DEFINITION OF THE DISEASE

Adult T-cell leukemia lymphoma (ATL) was first recognized in Japan by Uchiyama et al. in 1977 (1). It is defined as a histologically or cytologically confirmed peripheral T-cell malignancy associated with a novel retrovirus, human T-cell lymphotropic virus type I (HTLV-1).

Retroviruses are unique among animal viruses in having a ribonucleic acid genome that replicates through a deoxyribonucleic acid (DNA) intermediate. The virally encoded reverse transcriptase converts the single-stranded ribonucleic acid genome into a double-stranded DNA copy, which is irreversibly integrated into a host chromosome where it resides as a provirus. HTLV-1 is the first retrovirus that was found to be associated with human malignant neoplasm.

FREQUENCY AND EPIDEMIOLOGY

Southwestern Japan is the district with the highest prevalence of HTLV-1 infection and the highest incidence of patients with ATL in the world. A high prevalence of HTLV-1 infection is also found in the Caribbean islands, tropical Africa, South America, and northern Oceania. Many patients who have been diagnosed as having ATL in Western countries are immigrants from the West Indies or tropical Africa.

A nationwide survey of HTLV-1 seroprevalence in adult populations in Japan showed the characteristic geographic variations from 0.2% in low endemic to 13% in high-endemic areas. It is estimated that approximately 1.2 million individuals infected with HTLV-1 reside in Japan, and the annual incidence of ATL is estimated to be approximately 700 in Japan. The annual rate of ATL development among HTLV-1 carriers >40 years is estimated at 1.5 per 1,000 in males and 0.5 per 1,000 in females. The cumulative risk of the development of ATL among the HTLV-1 carriers is estimated to be 2.5' during a 70-year lifespan (2).

In a national survey in Japan, the mean age of patients with ATL was 57.6 years, and this age appears to have increased with time. It was reported that the age of patients in areas outside Japan is somewhat lower, with an overall mean age in the mid 40s. There is a marked increase in HTLV-1 prevalence with age until age 70 years and an increased prevalence in females compared with males. In addition to transmission by sexual and blood-borne routes, a major reason for the increase in seroprevalence with age appears to be the decreasing prevalence of HTLV-1 in the population with time. This decrease in HTLV-1 carriers among younger blood donors may be explained by the improvement in sanitation and changes in lifestyle in recent years in Japan.

POTENTIAL STRATEGIES TO ELIMINATE ADULT T-CELL LEUKEMIA LYMPHOMA

It has been shown that HTLV-1 is transmitted via at least three routes: (a) mother-to-child transmission, mainly by HTLV-1–positive lymphocytes in breast milk; (b) sexual transmission, more commonly from males to females; and (c) blood-borne transmission, including blood transfusions and sharing needles by intravenous drug abusers. The overall infection rate of HTLV-1 in children by seropositive mothers has been estimated to be 10% to 30%. However, HTLV-1 infection has also been reported in children who had not been breast-fed, suggesting the possibility of intrauterine or transvaginal infection.

Several kinds of intervention trials have been conducted in some HTLV-1–endemic areas in Japan. Hino (3) investigated the influence of breast-feeding on HTLV-1 transmission in an intervention study in Nagasaki, Japan, during a 12-year period. More than 100,000 pregnant women in the third trimester were screened for anti-HTLV-1 antibody since 1987. The seropositive mothers were advised to refrain from breast-feeding. Without any intervention, the prevalence of seropositive women decreased significantly, from 8% for those born in 1945 to <2% for those born in 1975. Among the children born to carrier mothers, 18% of those breast-fed long term were infected with HTLV-1, in contrast to 3% of those bottle-fed (p <0.001). Considering the trend toward a decrease in maternal prevalence, the prevalence in the pregnant women born in 1987 is estimated to be 1%. The results confirm that breast-feeding plays the major role in the mother-to-child transmission of HTLV-1. It was also suggested that the intervention program has prevented approximately 800 new infections during the 12-year study period and is expected to prevent the development of 40 cases of ATL in the future.

To prevent HTLV-1 transmission through blood transfusions, serologic screening for HTLV-1 in all blood donors has been conducted in Japan since 1986. Since then, no episodes of seroconversion in transfusion recipients have been recognized.

DIAGNOSIS

Pathology

The cytologic spectrum of ATL is extremely diverse. Nevertheless, certain cytologic features are highly characteristic and may suggest the diagnosis, even if studies for HTLV-1 are not provided (4). These features are best appreciated in the peripheral blood. Most patients are leukemic at some point in the clinical course, although peripheral blood involvement may not be evident at presentation. The incidence of a leukemic blood picture is less in patients from the Western hemisphere than it is in patients from Japan.

The neoplastic cells in the peripheral blood are markedly polylobated and have been termed flower cells based on the petal-like appearance of the nuclear lobes, as shown in Color Plate 66 (5,6). The chromatin is condensed and usually hyperchromatic, although the flower cells usually do not manifest prominent nucleoli. The cytoplasm is basophilic, and cytoplasmic vacuoles may be seen. The basophilia of the cytoplasm and hyperchromasia are useful features in the differential diagnosis with Sézary syndrome (7). In addition, the nuclear irregularities in Sézary cells are much subtler, imparting the typical cerebriform appearance without separation into nuclear lobes.

These cytologic features are most evident in the acute type of ATL. In the chronic and smoldering forms of the disease, atypical cells are relatively sparse in the peripheral blood, and cytologic atypia are less evident (8,9). In addition, there are epidemiologic differences in the frequency of peripheral blood involvement. For example, a leukemic phase is less common in the Caribbean basin than in Japan (10,11).

Lymph node involvement is present in most patients. Lymph nodes typically show diffuse architectural effacement. In keeping with a leukemic pattern of involvement, in some instances the sinuses may be preserved or may contain neoplastic cells similar to those of the blood.

The cytologic composition of the neoplastic infiltrate is very diverse (7). Small pleomorphic lymphoid cells equivalent to the flower cells of the peripheral blood may predominate or may be admixed with larger cells. The larger cells have vesicular nuclei and usually multiple eosinophilic or basophilic nucleoli. In some instances, the large transformed cells comprise the major population, and the process may mimic a diffuse large B-cell lymphoma. Alternatively, the transformed cells may have more pleomorphic nuclear features. Giant cells with convoluted or cerebriform nuclear contours may be present. Although it is important for the pathologist to be aware of the diverse cytology that can be encountered in ATL, the cytologic composition does not impact the clinical course (7).

Some patients with the early or smoldering type may exhibit a Hodgkin-lymphoma–like histology in the lymph nodes (12,13). This pattern is recognized in the World Health Organization classification as a morphologic variant (14). Involved lymph nodes show expanded paracortical areas with diffuse infiltrates of small to medium-sized lymphocytes with mild nuclear irregularities, indistinct nucleoli, and scant cytoplasm. There are interspersed Reed-Sternberg–like cells and giant cells with lobulated or convoluted nuclei. These cells are Epstein-Barr virus-positive B lymphocytes that express CD30 and CD15. This variant of incipient disease usually progresses to overt disease within months. The expansion of Epstein-Barr virus-positive B cells is felt to be secondary to the underlying immunodeficiency seen in patients with ATL. Similar Reed-Sternberg–like cells have been described in other forms of peripheral T-cell lymphoma, most commonly angioimmunoblastic T-cell lymphoma (15).

Skin involvement is seen in >50% of patients with the disease. The dermis usually contains a superficial atypical lymphoid infiltrate, often with epidermotropism (16). Pautrier-like abscesses are common (7). However, in contrast to Sézary syndrome/mycosis fungoides, the neoplastic infiltrate is usually monomorphic, without numerous histiocytes or eosinophils. The smaller neoplastic cells predominate in the skin, and blastic forms are uncommon. In the smoldering and chronic types, cytologic atypia may be minimal. Hyperparakeratosis is variably present in the overlying epidermis. The skin lesions are clinically and histologically diverse, and may mimic inflammatory disorders (17,18).

Bone marrow involvement is typically not prominent. The marrow may contain patchy atypical lymphoid infiltrates. However, the degree of bone marrow infiltration is less than that expected, given the very marked lymphocytosis that may be present. Correlating with the clinical finding of hypercalcemia, one often sees evidence of bone resorption and osteoclastic activity (19). Bone trabeculae may show evidence of remodeling, and in some patients, lytic bone lesions can be present, even in the absence of tumoral bone infiltration (7,20).

Other frequent sites of involvement include lung and cerebrospinal fluid. Correlating with a leukemic phase, the pulmonary infiltrates are generally patchy and interstitial, without formation of tumor nodules. Cardiac involvement has been reported rarely, and is always associated with concomitant pulmonary involvement (21).

Involvement of the central nervous system is usually manifested as meningeal infiltration without nodular parenchymal lesions. However, rare cases with parenchymal tumor masses have been reported (22). Central nervous system involvement is nearly always associated with widespread systemic disease, but rare cases with isolated central nervous system involvement have been reported (23).

Immunophenotype

The neoplastic cells, regardless of cytologic subtype, are CD4+ T cells that strongly express the interleukin (IL)-2 receptor (IL-2R), CD25 (4). High levels of soluble IL-2R can also be found in the serum and correlate with disease activity (24). CD7 is nearly always absent, but CD3 and other mature T-cell antigens (CD2, CD5) are usually expressed. CD30 can be expressed in the larger blastic cells. Because many peripheral T-cell lymphomas have a CD3+, CD4+, CD7– immunophenotype, the most specific feature is the presence of strong CD25 positivity. With enhanced antigen-retrieval techniques, CD25 expression can be detected in formalin-fixed paraffin-embedded tissue sections (25). Recent studies have suggested that the cells of ATL may be the equivalent of regulatory T cells (26). In one study 68% of the cases tested were positive for FoxP3 in at least some of the neoplastic cells. No other T-cell lymphoma subtype was seen to express this transcription factor, which is a hallmark of regulatory T cells, in conjunction with CD25 and CD4. This finding helps to explain the immunodeficiency associated with ATL.

Mechanisms of Pathogenesis

The onset of ATL is preceded by a long period of latency, frequently lasting >4 decades. In addition, only about 5% of all infected individuals with HTLV-1 develop ATL. HTLV-1 has no classic viral oncogene. The insertional mutagenesis by HTLV-1 provirus was rejected as the leukemogenic mechanism because of random integration sites of the provirus depending on the patient (27). The age-specific occurrence of ATL suggested a multistep carcinogenesis model with five independent genetic events (28). Initial steps depend on viral gene products, among which a viral regulatory protein, Tax, plays pivotal roles. Tax was shown to be the major viral protein with oncogenic potential (29). Roles of Tax in the multistep leukemogenesis are shown in Figure 27.1.

Tax also exerts its pleiotropic functions through direct interaction with numerous cellular proteins (30), resulting in a unique phenotype of the infected cells. Effects of Tax on the host cells are summarized as follows: (a) transcriptional deregulation of cellular genes (30,31); (b) activation of signal transduction (32,33); (c) deregulation of cell cycle control (33); and (d) induction of genetic instability and chromosomal abnormality (34,35). Tax not only activates expression of viral genes via the viral long terminal repeat but also regulates the expression of a number of cellular genes by serving as a transcriptional cofactor for the adenosine 3c,5c-cyclic monophosphate responsive elements-binding protein, nuclear factor-κB (NF-κB), and the serum responsive factor pathways (30,31,36–39). Among the cellular genes that are the targets of Tax, those with growth-promoting capacities are found among those transactivated, such as IL-6 and lymphokine receptors such as IL-2R-α, and oncogenes such as c-fos. However, those with growth-retarding functions are included among those transrepressed, such as p18INK4c and Lck. Thus, transcriptional deregulation by Tax leads to efficient proliferation of infected cells (30,31,40).

Tax interacts with and activates specific components of growth factor signal-transduction pathways, such as IκB kinase-IκB-NF-κB, Ras/mitogen-activated protein kinase, and protein kinases A and C. Interaction with IκB kinase γ, a component of IκB kinase complex, results in constitutive activation of this kinase complex. Tax also participates in another NF-κB activation pathway involving p100 (32,33,41). Constitutive activation of the Janus kinas-signal transduction and activator of transcription pathway in HTLV-1–transformed cells was also reported (42). Thus, HTLV-1 infection results in aberrant activation of growth-promoting signaling pathways.

Tax also induces cell cycle progression by inhibiting negative cell cycle regulators, such as p53, p16, and INK4A, and stimulates positive cell cycle regulators, such as cdk4/6, D-type cyclins, and E2F, resulting in constant cell cycle progression of the infected cells (43).

Viral gene expression is absent in ATL cells in vivo (42,44). Integrated proviruses are frequently silenced by deletion (45) or mutations in the Tax coding region, or both, or are methylated in the 5′ region and 5′ long terminal repeat (46,47). Thus, in addition to direct growth promotion, Tax should endow the infected T cells with capacities that help to progress to transformed phenotypes in the absence of Tax. In this context, induction of a mutator phenotype (48) by Tax in the infected cells appears to be important. Tax impairs the cell's ability to repair DNA damage such as base excision repair and nucleotide excision repair, as well as homologous recombination pathway (49–53). Functional inactivation of p53 by Tax (54,55) allows HTLV-1–infected cells to survive and proliferate in the presence of unrepaired genomic damage.

One of the mitotic spindle assembly checkpoint proteins, MAD1, is inactivated by Tax by direct binding, which also causes chromosomal abnormalities (56). Tax directly binds and activates CDC20-associated anaphase promoting complex (Cdc20), resulting in a delay of S/G2/M-phase transition; in turn, this causes chromosomal instability (57). Thus, Tax not only stimulates proliferation of cells but also induces DNA damage and chromosomal abnormalities in HTLV-1–infected cells, which may constitute a basis for multistep leukemogenesis.

Recently, antisense transcripts of the HTLV-1 provirus have been reported (58). The transcript can encode a novel basic leucine zipper protein, named HBZ, which interacts with adenosine 3c,5c-cyclic monophosphate responsive elements-binding protein 2 and c-Jun, and suppresses the activity of Tax and activator protein-1, respectively. Several isoforms of HBZ transcripts were reported to be steadily expressed in

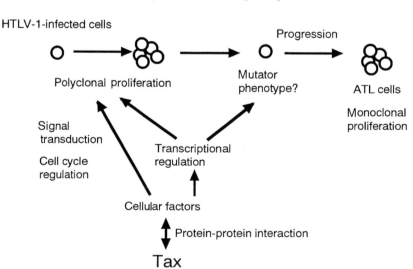

FIGURE 27.1 Roles of HTLV-1 transactivating viral factor (Tax) in the multistep leukemogenesis of ATL. Tax mainly exerts its biologic effects through protein-protein interaction, resulting in deregulation of transcription, cell cycle control, and signal transduction. It also impairs the cell's ability to repair DNA damage, which may lead to the mutator phenotype of the infected cells.

HTLV-1-infected cells and ATL cells. The functions of these transcripts and putative protein in the context of cellular transformation are now under investigation (59,60).

Presentation, Unique Aspects of Staging, and Unusual Syndromes

Based on the nationwide survey of 854 patients with ATL who were newly diagnosed between 1983 and 1987 in Japan, the diagnostic criteria of the four clinical subtypes were proposed (5). The leukemic subtypes include the *acute type*, with a rapidly progressive clinical course and most of the characteristic features of ATL: generalized lymphadenopathy, hepatomegaly, splenomegaly, skin involvement, hypercalcemia, and organ infiltration. The symptoms and signs include abdominal pain, diarrhea, ascites, pleural effusion, cough, sputum, and chest x-ray abnormalities. The *smoldering type* shows an indolent clinical course and only a small percentage of leukemic cells but may also include skin involvement. The *chronic type*, with a high percentage of leukemic cells, is occasionally associated with skin involvement, lymphadenopathy, and hepatosplenomegaly, and also shows an indolent clinical course. The *lymphoma type* is comprised of patients who present with the manifestations of lymphoma without circulating malignant cells in the peripheral blood. When patients with ATL are staged according to the Ann Arbor staging classification, most patients are categorized as having stage IV disease because leukemic cells are recognized even in clinically indolent forms. Therefore, in ATL, the clinical subtype is more important than the Ann Arbor stage for predicting prognosis and deciding treatment in each patient.

ATL, particularly the aggressive forms (acute and lymphoma types), has been found to infiltrate the stomach in 29% and the intestine in 25% of patients at autopsy (61). Patients with ATL experience a variety of abdominal symptoms, such as nausea, vomiting, abdominal fullness, and diarrhea, which may be attributable to the infiltration by neoplastic cells, but because of the associated immunodeficiency, various opportunistic infections, such as strongyloidiasis, may complicate the course.

Hepatic involvement of neoplastic cells may be found in up to one-fourth of patients with the acute or the lymphoma type, and is not infrequently manifested by jaundice and hepatic enzyme elevations. One hundred one patients with the acute type or the lymphoma type were analyzed for hepatic involvement and compared with 106 patients with non-Hodgkin lymphoma (NHL) other than ATL (62). There was more frequent palpable hepatomegaly, and higher total bilirubin, hepatic transaminase, lactate dehydrogenase, and alkaline phosphatase values than among other patients with NHL (p <0.0001). Autopsy liver samples disclosed that the portal area was most frequently infiltrated with ATL cells.

Pulmonary complications are due to leukemic infiltration in one-half of the patients, and to infections with a variety of bacterial and opportunistic organisms in the other half (63). Twenty-six percent of 854 Japanese patients with ATL had active infections at diagnosis (5). The incidence was highest in the chronic and smoldering types (36%), and lower in the acute (27%) and lymphoma types (11%). The encountered infections were bacterial (pneumonias, sepsis, and tuberculosis) in 43%, fungal in 31%, protozoal in 18%, and viral in 8% of patients. The immunodeficiency at presentation in ATL can be exacerbated by neutropenia produced by cytotoxic chemotherapy, leading to a high risk of infection throughout therapy. Infections are responsible for the patient's death in approximately half of the cases.

Central nervous system involvement, mostly leptomeningeal involvement, occurs in approximately 10% of patients with ATL (64). The initial symptoms include muscle weakness, altered mental status, paresthesia, headache, and urinary incontinence. Signs include nuchal rigidity and cranial nerve palsies. Hyponatremia secondary to the syndrome of inappropriate secretion of antidiuretic hormone is observed in some patients.

Laboratory Findings

Laboratory findings also depend on the clinical subtype (5). Leukocytosis is found in patients with the acute or the chronic type at presentation, exhibiting characteristic atypical lymphoid cells with marked polymorphic nuclei, so-called flower cells. Most patients with the acute or the lymphoma type have elevated serum lactate dehydrogenase levels.

The most striking laboratory finding in patients with ATL is hypercalcemia, which was found in 32% (5). Lytic bone lesions have been described in some patients; however, examinations of bone obtained at autopsy or from bone marrow biopsies usually reveal activated osteoclasts with increased bone resorption; infiltrating neoplastic T cells are rarely found. Patients with ATL have low phosphates, hypercalciuria, high levels of nephrogenous cyclic adenosine monophosphate, and low levels of 1,25-dihydroxyvitamin D. The following factors have been suggested to have roles in the hypercalcemia: parathyroid hormone-related peptide; osteoclast-activating factor; tumor necrosis factors-α and -β, IL-1α, IL-1β; and overexpression of the receptor activator of the NF-κB ligand gene.

Prognostic Factors

In all cases of ATL, age ($\geq$40 years), poor performance status (greater than or equal to two), high lactate dehydrogenase, hypercalcemia, and four or more involved lesions are unfavorable prognostic factors (65,66). For patients with the chronic type, the major prognostic factors are the serum values of lactate dehydrogenase, albumin, and blood urea nitrogen. Patients with the chronic type and normal values for the three factors have a prognosis as good as those with the smoldering type and account for 30% of the patients with the chronic type. In contrast, patients with the unfavorable chronic type, having an abnormal value in at least one of the three factors, would be targets for cytotoxic chemotherapy.

TREATMENT

Patients with the favorable chronic or smoldering type should be carefully monitored for the development of infectious complications and for signs of disease progression to the acute or lymphoma type.

Most previously untreated patients with aggressive forms (acute or lymphoma type) die within weeks or months of the

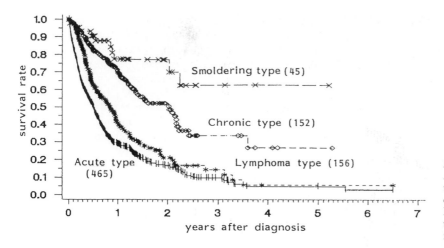

FIGURE 27.2 Survival curves of 818 patients with ATL, according to four clinical subtypes defined by the diagnostic criteria. Numbers in parentheses indicate the number of patients. (From Shimoyama M. Diagnostic criteria and classification of clinical subtypes of adult T-cell leukaemia-lymphoma. A report from the Lymphoma Study Group (1984–87). *Br J Haematol* 1991;79:428–437, with permission.)

diagnosis without treatment. Figure 27.2 shows the survival curves of 818 patients with ATL in Japan according to the four clinical subtypes (5). Most of the patients with the smoldering type lived well without chemotherapy for a long time. Approximately two-thirds of the patients with chronic type died within approximately 2.5 years from diagnosis. Patients with the lymphoma type had poor prognoses, with a median survival time of 10.2 months. The most aggressive type of ATL was acute type, with a median survival time of 6.2 months. The projected 4-year survival rates of patients with the lymphoma and acute types were only 5%. The clinical subtype clearly determines the prognosis of each patient with ATL.

Clinical Trials by the Japan Clinical Oncology Group

Seven chemotherapy trials have been consecutively conducted by the Lymphoma Study Group (LSG) of the Japan Clinical Oncology Group (JCOG) since 1978 (67–72) (Table 27.1). Between 1981 and 1983, JCOG conducted a phase III trial (JCOG8101), LSG1-VEPA, which consisted of vincristine, cyclophosphamide, prednisone, and Adriamycin (doxorubicin), versus LSG2-VEPA plus methotrexate, for patients with advanced NHL, including ATL (67,68). The complete response rate of LSG2-VEPA plus methotrexate for ATL (37%) was higher than that of LSG1-VEPA (17%) ($p = 0.09$). In the JCOG8101 trial, however, the complete response rate was significantly lower for ATL than for B-cell lymphoma and peripheral T-cell lymphoma other than ATL ($p < 0.001$). The median survival time of the 54 patients with ATL treated with LSG1/LSG2 was 6 months, and the estimated 4-year survival rate was only 8%.

In 1987, against advanced aggressive NHL, including ATL, JCOG initiated a phase II study (JCOG8701) of a multiagent combination chemotherapy called *LSG4*, consisting of three different regimens: (a) VEPA and bleomycin; (b) methotrexate, vindesine, cyclophosphamide, prednisone, and doxorubicin; and (c) vincristine, etoposide, procarbazine, prednisone, and bleomycin (69). The complete response rate (72%) of JCOG8701 trial in aggressive NHL was higher than that of the JCOG8101 trial (57%). The complete response rate for ATL was improved from 28% (JCOG8101) to 43% (JCOG8701). However, the complete response rate was significantly lower in ATL than in B-cell

lymphoma and peripheral T-cell lymphoma other than ATL ($p < 0.01$). The patients with ATL still showed a poor prognosis, with a median survival time of 8 months and a 4-year survival rate of 12%. A multivariate analysis of the 267 eligible patients with advanced aggressive NHL demonstrated that the clinical diagnosis of ATL was the most significant unfavorable prognostic factor (relative risk 3.185; $p = 0.0001$).

The disappointing results in patients with ATL treated with conventional chemotherapies have led to the search for new active agents. Deoxycoformycin (pentostatin), which is an inhibitor of adenosine deaminase, has been shown to be effective in a number of lymphoid malignancies. Based on the promising results of some single-institution studies, multicenter phase I and II studies of deoxycoformycin were conducted against ATL in Japan (66,73). The phase II study revealed a response rate of 32% (ten of 31) in relapsed or refractory ATL using the weekly intravenous administration of 5 mg per m². These encouraging results prompted us to conduct a deoxycoformycin-containing combination phase II trial (JCOG9109; LSG11) as the initial chemotherapy for ATL (70). In this trial, previously untreated patients with the acute, lymphoma, and unfavorable chronic types were eligible. Between 1991 and 1993, 62 patients with ATL (34 acute, 21 lymphoma, and seven chronic types) were enrolled. Vincristine (1 mg per m² intravenous on days 1 and 8), doxorubicin (40 mg per m² intravenous on day 1), etoposide (100 mg per m² intravenous on days 1 to 3), prednisone (40 mg per m² orally on days 1 and 2), and deoxycoformycin (5 mg per m² intravenous on days 8, 15, and 22) were administered every 28 days for ten cycles unless disease progression occurred. Among the 61 patients evaluable for toxicity, four patients (7%) died of infections. In the 60 eligible patients, there were 17 complete responses (28%) and 14 partial responses (overall response rate, 52%). The median survival time was 7.4 months, and the estimated 2-year survival was 17%, findings that were identical to those of the 43 patients with ATL who were treated with the previous JCOG8701. The prognosis of the patients with ATL remained poor, even though they were treated with a deoxycoformycin-containing combination chemotherapy.

In 1994, JCOG initiated a multiagent combination phase II trial (JCOG9303; LSG15), an eight-drug regimen consisting of vincristine, cyclophosphamide, doxorubicin, prednisone,

TABLE 27.1

RESULTS OF IMPORTANT CLINICAL TRIALS OF UNTREATED PATIENTS WITH ATL

Protocol	Drugs/regimen	No. of eligible patients	Complete response rate (%)	Median survival time (mo)	Survival rate	Reference
JCOG8101		54	28 (15/54)	7.5	8.3% (4 y)	(67,68)
LSG1-VEPA	VCR, CPA, PSL, DOX	24	17 (4/24)	NA	NA	
LSG2-VEPAM	VCR, CPA, PSL, DOX, MTX	30	37 (11/30)	NA	NA	
JCOG8701 (LSG4)	VCR, CPA, PSL, DOX, BLM, MTX, VDS, ETP, PCZ	43	42 (18/43)	8.0	11.6% (4 y)	(69)
JCOG9109 (LSG11)	VCR, DOX, ETP, PSL, DCF	60	28 (17/60)	7.4	15.5% (2 y)	(70)
JCOG9303 (LSG15)	VCR, CPA, PSL, DOX, MCNU, VDS, ETP, CBDCA	93	35 (33/93)	13	31% (2 y)	(71)
JCOG9801		118	32 (38/118)	NA	NA	(72)
LSG15	VCR, CPA, PSL, DOX, MCNU, VDS, ETP, CBDCA, MTX	57	40 (23/57)	12.7	24% (3 y)	
Biweekly CHOP	VCR, CPA, PSL, DOX, MTX	61	25 (15/61)	10.9	13% (3 y)	
Gill et al.	IFN-α, AZT	12	25 (3/12)	4.8	NA	(74)

AZT, zidovudine; BLM, bleomycin; CBDCA, carboplatin; CPA, cyclophosphamide; DCF, 2'-deoxycoformycin; DOX, doxorubicin; ETP, etoposide; IFN, interferon; MCNU, ranimustine; MTX, methotrexate; NA, not applicable; PCZ, procarbazine; PSL, prednisone; VCR, vincristine; VDS, vindesine.

ranimustine, vindesine, etoposide, and carboplatin for untreated patients with ATL (71). In this trial, the elevation of relative dose intensity was attempted with the prophylactic use of granulocyte colony-stimulating factor. In addition, non-cross-resistant agents, such as ranimustine and carboplatin, were incorporated. Ninety-six previously untreated patients with aggressive ATL were enrolled: 58 with acute, 28 with lymphoma, and ten with unfavorable chronic type. Eighty-one percent of the 93 eligible patients responded (75 of 93), with 33 patients obtaining a complete response (35%). Patients with the lymphoma type showed a better complete response rate (67%, 18 of 27) than patients with the acute type (20%, 11 of 56) and unfavorable chronic type (40%, four of ten). The overall survival of 93 eligible patients at 2 years was estimated to be 31%. The median survival time was 13 months, and the median follow-up duration of the 20 surviving patients was 4.2 years. A trend toward better survival for patients with lymphoma type (median survival time, 20 months) compared with patients with acute type (median survival time, 11 months) was recognized (hazard ratio, 1.65). Grade 4 hematologic toxicities of neutropenia and thrombocytopenia were observed in 65% and 53% of the patients, respectively, whereas grade 4 nonhematologic toxicity was observed in only one patient. It was concluded that the LSG15 protocol is feasible with mild nonhematologic toxicity and improved the clinical outcome of patients with ATL.

To confirm whether the LSG15 is a new standard for the treatment of patients with aggressive ATL, JCOG conducted a phase III trial comparing the LSG15 with biweekly (cyclophosphamide, doxorubicin, Oncovin [vincristine], and prednisone) (CHOP) (72). Previously untreated patients with aggressive ATL were assigned to receive either six courses of the LSG15 every 4 weeks or eight courses of biweekly

CHOP. Both treatments were supported with granulocyte colony-stimulating factor and intrathecal prophylaxis. A total of 118 patients were enrolled. The complete response rate was higher in the LSG15 arm than in the biweekly CHOP arm (40% vs. 25%, respectively; $p = 0.020$). Overall survival at 3 years was 24% in the LSG15 arm and 13% in the biweekly CHOP arm ($p = 0.085$, two-sided $p = 0.169$) (Fig. 27.3A). Progression-free survival rate at 1 year was 28% in the LSG15 arm compared with 16% in the biweekly CHOP arm ($p = 0.100$, two-sided $p = 0.200$) (Fig. 27.3B). For LSG15 versus biweekly CHOP, grade 4 neutropenia, grade 4 thrombocytopenia, and grade 3 or 4 infection rates were 98% versus 83%, 74% versus 17%, and 32% versus 15%, respectively. There were three toxic deaths in the LSG15 arm. The longer survival at 3 years and higher complete response rate with the LSG15 compared with biweekly CHOP suggest that LSG15 might be a more effective regimen at the expense of higher toxicities, providing the basis for future investigations in the treatment of ATL (72).

New Agent Development for Adult T-Cell Leukemia Lymphoma

Irinotecan hydrochloride (CPT-11) is a semisynthetic analog of camptothecin with inhibitory activity against topoisomerase I. CPT-11 has definitive activity against various kinds of solid tumors. Multicenter phase II studies of CPT-11 were conducted against relapsed or refractory NHL in Japan (75,76). The study revealed nine complete responses and 17 partial responses (response rate 38% [26 of 69]) using weekly intravenous administration of 40 mg per m^2 per day for three consecutive days. Among them, five (38%) of 13 patients

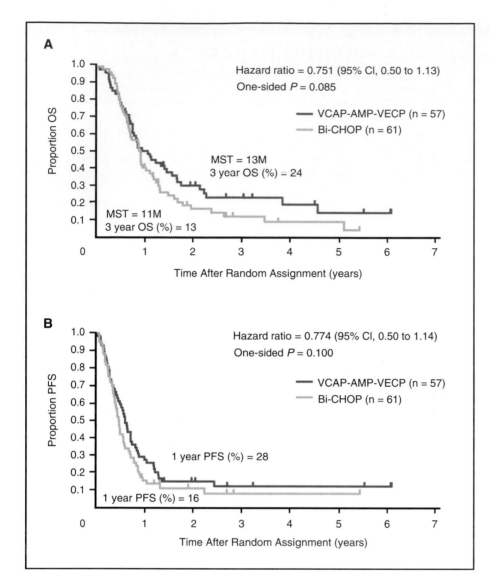

FIGURE 27.3 A: Kaplan-Meier estimate of overall survival (OS) for all randomly assigned patients. **B:** Kaplan-Meier estimate of progression-free survival (PFS) for all randomly assigned patients. AMP, doxorubicin, ranimustine, and prednisone; Bi-CHOP, biweekly CHOP; CI, confidence interval; VCAP, vincristine, cyclophosphamide, doxorubicin, and prednisone; VECP, vindesine, etoposide, carboplatin, and prednisone. (From Tsukasaki K, Utsunomiya A, Fukuda H, et al. VCAP-AMP-VECP compared with biweekly CHOP for adult T-cell leukemia-lymphoma: Japan Clinical Oncology Group Study JCOG9801. *J Clin Oncol* 2007;25:5458–5564, with permission.)

with ATL responded to CPT-11. The major toxicities of CPT-11 were leukopenia, diarrhea, and nausea and vomiting. To develop a new effective chemotherapy regimen against NHL and ATL, we conducted two kinds of phase I/II studies of CPT-11 in combination with carboplatin or etoposide for relapsed or refractory NHL. However, in both studies, dose escalation was halted because of the excessive toxicities.

Based on the preliminary documentation of the efficacy of interferon-α against ATL, two kinds of phase II trials of high-dose interferon-α (intravenous administration and subcutaneous administration) were conducted; however, the results were not promising. In 1995, Gill et al. (74) in the United States reported that 11 of 19 patients with acute or lymphomatous ATL achieved major responses (five complete responses and six partial responses) by the combination therapy of interferon-α and zidovudine. The therapeutic efficacy of this combination was also observed in a French study; major objective responses were obtained in all five patients with ATL (77). However, the median survival of previously untreated patients with ATL in the U.S. study was rather short (4.8 months) compared with those in the JCOG studies (7 to 13 months)

(74,78). Furthermore, the complete response rate in previously untreated patients (25%, three of 12) was not superior to the complete response rates in those treated with the JCOG8701, JCOG9109, and JCOG9303 (28% to 42%).

Recently, the results of a worldwide metaanalysis on the use of interferon-α and zidovudine for ATL were reported (79). One hundred patients received interferon-α and zidovudine as initial treatments. The overall response rate was 66%, including 43% of patients achieving complete response. In this retrospective subgroup analysis, the median survival time was 24 months, and the 5-year survival rate was 50% for first-line interferon-α and zidovudine, versus 7 months and 20% for 84 patients who received first-line chemotherapy. The median survival times of patients with acute-type ATL treated as first-line with interferon-α and zidovudine and chemotherapy were 12 and 9 months, respectively. Patients with lymphoma-type ATL did not benefit from interferon-α and zidovudine therapy; the median survival times of those treated as first-line with interferon-α and zidovudine and chemotherapy were 12 and 15 months, respectively. In addition, first-line interferon-α and zidovudine therapy in chronic- and smoldering-type ATL resulted in a 100% survival rate at a median follow-up of 5 years. Although the results for interferon-α and zidovudine in indolent ATL appear to be promising, the possibility of selection bias cannot be ruled out.

Cladribine (2-chlorodeoxyadenosine) is a chlorinated purine analog that is resistant to degradation by adenosine deaminase. Cladribine has been found to be effective against hairy cell leukemia, B-chronic lymphocytic leukemia, indolent B-cell NHL, and cutaneous T-cell lymphoma. In a Japanese phase I study of cladribine, one patient with relapse with ATL achieved a partial response (80). A multicenter phase II study of cladribine against ATL was conducted in Japan (81). Cladribine was administered as 0.09 mg per kg per day by 7-day continuous intravenous infusion every 28 days up to three courses. However, because the interim analysis revealed that only one of the 15 eligible patients showed a partial response (overall response rate, 7%; 90% confidence interval, 0% to 28%), the phase II study was discontinued.

Because most ATL cells express the α-chain of IL-2R (CD25), Waldmann (82) have treated patients with ATL using monoclonal antibodies to CD25. Six (32%) of 19 patients who were treated with anti-Tac showed objective responses lasting from 9 weeks to >3 years. One of the impediments to this approach is that a quantity of soluble IL-2R is shed by the tumor cells into the circulation. The soluble IL-2R can bind to anti-Tac and inhibit binding to the tumor cell.

Another strategy using the IL-2R as a target for the treatment of ATL is conjugation with an immunotoxin (*Pseudomonas* exotoxin) or radioisotope (yttrium-90). Anti-Tac coupled with *Pseudomonas* exotoxin, which inhibits protein synthesis, has been administered to patients with ATL, and tumor regressions were observed in some patients. The action of immunotoxins depends on the expression of the target antigen on all malignant cells and on the cell's ability to internalize the antigen-antibody complex containing the toxin. To circumvent findings that not all malignant cells express the target antigen and not all cells internalize bound substances, radiolabeled monoclonal antibodies were developed. Waldmann et al. (83) developed a stable conjugate of anti-Tac with yttrium-90. Among the 16 patients with ATL who received 5- to 15-mCi doses, nine (56%) showed objective responses. The response duration was longer than the previous results with unconjugated anti-Tac antibody. Grade 3 or greater toxicities were largely limited to hematologic toxicities. They concluded that radioimmunotherapy with yttrium-90–labeled anti-Tac may provide a useful approach for the treatment of ATL.

Monoclonal antibodies against molecules other than CD25 expressed on ATL cells, such as CD2, CD52, and chemokine receptor 4 (CCR4), appear to be promising in the recent clinical trials. Ishida et al. (84) conducted immunostaining analysis for CCR4 expression in 103 patients with ATL, and the overall survival of the patients with and without CCR4was compared. Ninety-one (88%) of the 103 cases were positive for CCR4 staining. Multivariate analysis revealed that CCR4 expression was a significant prognostic factor ($p < 0.05$) (84). A novel humanized anti-CCR4 monoclonal antibody has been developed, the Fc region of which is defucosylated to enhance antibody dependent cell-mediated cytotoxicity by increasing its binding affinity to Fc receptor on effector cells. A phase I study of this anti-CCR4 antibody in patients with CCR4-positive T-cell malignancy, including ATL, is being conducted in Japan (85).

Several new agents against ATL are now under investigation. One of the promising targeted therapies for ATL is the combination of arsenic trioxide and interferon-α, which targets both Tax and the NF-κB pathway. This combination exhibits clinical efficacy in patients with relapsed/refractory ATL (86) and is currently being evaluated in untreated patients.

Histone deacetylase inhibitors such as vorinostat (suberoylanilide hydroxamic acid), romidepsin, and panobinostat (LBH589) are also promising in preclinical and/or clinical studies. Pralatrexate, a novel antifolate, and forodesine, a purine nucleotide phosphorylase inhibitor, are potential new agents with potent preclinical activity in T-cell malignancies, including ATL (87). Other potential therapies for ATL under investigation include a proteasome inhibitor, bortezomib (88,89).

Allogeneic Stem Cell Transplantation

The results of allogeneic stem cell transplantation for ATL were reported by Japanese investigators (90,91). In the former series (90), ten patients tolerated well the conditioning regimens, including total body irradiation. The median disease-free survival after allogeneic stem cell transplantation was 17.5+ months (range 3.7 to 34.4+). Four patients died of acute graft versus host disease (grade IV), pneumonitis, gastrointestinal bleeding, or renal insufficiency. Two of ten patients with no symptoms of graft versus host disease had relapse. In the latter series (91), they analyzed 40 allogeneic stem cell transplantation for acute and lymphoma types of ATL between 1997 and 2002. All evaluable patients achieved complete response after allogeneic stem cell transplantation, and the median survival time was 9.6 months. The estimated 3-year overall and disease-free survivals were 45% and 34%, respectively. Among ten patients with relapsed ATL after allogeneic stem cell transplantation, five patients achieved complete response again: three by the reduction or cessation of immunosuppressive agents, which suggested a graft versus ATL effect. These results suggested that allogeneic stem cell transplantation was effective for some patients with aggressive ATL. In addition, Okamura et al. (92) reported the results of a multicenter feasibility study of reduced intensity allogeneic stem cell transplantation (RIST) against ATL. Sixteen patients all >50 years of age underwent allogeneic stem cell transplantation from HLA-matched sibling donors after a reduced intensity conditioning regimen consisting of fludarabine (180 mg per m^2), busulfan (8 mg per kg), and rabbit antithymocyte globulin (5 mg per kg). The observed regimen-related toxicities and nonhematologic toxicities were acceptable. Disease relapse was the main cause of treatment failure. Three patients who had a relapse subsequently responded to a rapid discontinuation of the immunosuppressive agent and thereafter achieved another remission. After RIST, the HTLV-1 proviral load became undetectable in eight patients. RIST is thus considered to be a feasible treatment for ATL. Subsequent multicenter trials of RIST are being conducted in Japan.

FUTURE DIRECTIONS

Despite the consecutive clinical trials by the JCOG to develop more effective chemotherapy regimens, most patients with ATL remain incurable with current chemotherapies. Further

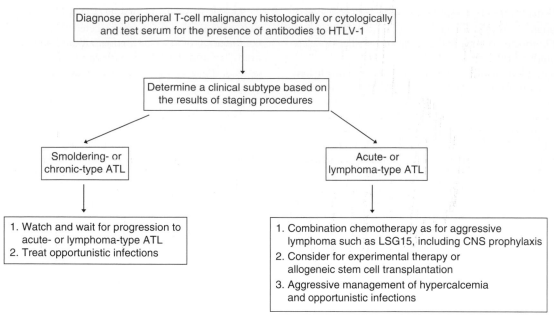

FIGURE 27.4 Approach to the patient with ATL. CNS, central nervous system.

efforts to incorporate new innovative treatment modalities are needed, such as new anticancer agents, monoclonal antibody therapy, and allogeneic hematopoietic stem cell transplantation, including nonmyeloablative, allogeneic hematopoietic stem cell transplantation.

Management Approach for Patients with Adult T-Cell Leukemia Lymphoma

An algorithm summarizing management approaches for patients with ATL is shown in Figure 27.4. When oncologists diagnose patients suspected of lymphoid malignancy, it is important to consider the possibility of ATL at any time. A routine check for serum HTLV-1 antibody is recommended at initial diagnosis. The following three points are essential for the diagnosis of ATL: (a) cytologically or histologically proven lymphoid malignancy; (b) mature T-cell phenotype, mostly CD4+, determined by flow cytometry or immunohistochemistry; and (c) testing positive for anti-HTLV-1 antibody. When a patient is diagnosed as having ATL, it is important to make an accurate diagnosis of clinical subtype for the treatment decisions. For patients with the smoldering or chronic type, close observation is recommended. Careful monitoring for opportunistic infections, including bacterial infection, fungal infection, or *Pneumocystis jiroveci* infection, is also needed. For patients with the acute or lymphoma type, the serum calcium level should be checked immediately. For those complicated with hypercalcemia, prompt management, including fluid therapy, bisphosphonate, and chemotherapy, is needed. For patients with the acute or lymphoma type requiring therapy, enrollment in a clinical trial is recommended. When there is no active trial or the patient is ineligible for the trial, chemotherapy used for aggressive NHL should be considered. For such patients, we recommend the LSG15 regimen based on the recent phase III study (72). Because most patients with ATL are not curable with current

chemotherapy regimens, it is reasonable to consider the applicability of allogeneic stem cell transplantation in patients who show responses to chemotherapy. For patients with relapsed or refractory disease, the possibility of enrollment in a new agent trial should be considered in addition to allogeneic stem cell transplantation.

References

1. Uchiyama T, Yodoi J, Sagawa K, et al. Adult T-cell leukemia: clinical and hematologic features of 16 cases. *Blood* 1977;50:481–492.
2. Tajima K. The 4th nation-wide study of adult T-cell leukemia/lymphoma (ATL) in Japan: estimates of risk of ATL and its geographical and clinical features. The T- and B-cell Malignancy Study Group. *Int J Cancer* 1990;45:237–243.
3. Hino S. Updated results of an intervention study against the mother-to-child transmission of human T-cell leukemia virus type-I. *Proceedings of the 15th International Symposium of Foundation for Promotion of Cancer Research*, January 15–17, 2002, Tokyo, Japan. Tokyo, Japan: Foundation for Promotion of Cancer Research 2002;15:43–44.
4. Levine PH, Cleghorn F, Manns A, et al. Adult T-cell leukemia/lymphoma: a working point-score classification for epidemiological studies. *Int J Cancer* 1994;59:491–493.
5. Shimoyama M. Diagnostic criteria and classification of clinical subtypes of adult T-cell leukaemia-lymphoma. A report from the Lymphoma Study Group (1984–87). *Br J Haematol* 1991;79:428–437.
6. Hanaoka M, Sasaki M, Matsumoto H, et al. Adult T cell leukemia. Histological classification and characteristics. *Acta Pathol Jpn* 1979;29:723–738.
7. Jaffe ES, Blattner WA, Blayney DW, et al. The pathologic spectrum of adult T-cell leukemia/lymphoma in the United States. *Am J Surg Pathol* 1984;8:263–275.
8. Kawano F, Yamaguchi K, Nishimura H, et al. Variation in the clinical courses of adult T-cell leukemia. *Cancer* 1985;55:851–856.
9. Yamaguchi K, Nishimura H, Kohrogi H, et al. A proposal for smoldering adult T-cell leukemia: a clinicopathologic study of five cases. *Blood* 1983;62:758–766.
10. Levine PH, Manns A, Jaffe ES, et al. The effect of ethnic differences on the pattern of HTLV-I-associated T-cell leukemia/lymphoma (HATL) in the United States. *Int J Cancer* 1994;56:177–181.
11. Pombo De Oliveira MS, Loureiro P, Bittencourt A, et al. Geographic diversity of adult T-cell leukemia/lymphoma in Brazil. *Int J Cancer* 1999;83:291–298.
12. Ohshima K, Suzumiya J, Kato A, et al. Clonal HTLV-I-infected CD4+ T-lymphocytes and non-clonal non-HTLV-I-infected giant cells in incipient ATLL with Hodgkin-like histologic features. *Int J Cancer* 1997;72:592–598.
13. Duggan D, Ehrlich G, Davey F, et al. HTLV-I induced lymphoma mimicking Hodgkin's disease. Diagnosis by polymerase chain reaction amplification of specific HTLV-I sequences in tumor DNA. *Blood* 1988;71:1027–1032.

14. Jaffe ES, Harris NL, Stein II, et al. *Pathology and genetics of tumours of haematopoietic and lymphoid tissues.* Lyon, France: IARC Press, 2001.

15. Quintanilla-Martinez L, Fend F, Moguel LR, et al. Peripheral T-cell lymphoma with Reed-Sternberg-like cells of B-cell phenotype and genotype associated with Epstein-Barr virus infection. *Am J Surg Pathol* 1999;23:1233–1240.

16. Mukai K, Sato Y, Watanabe S, et al. Non-Hodgkin lymphoma of the skin excluding mycosis fungoides and cutaneous involvement of adult T-cell leukemia/lymphoma. *J Cutan Pathol* 1988;15:193–200.

17. Ohtani T, Deguchi M, Aiba S. Erythema multiforme-like lesions associated with lesional infiltration of tumor cells occurring in adult T-cell lymphoma/leukemia. *Int J Dermatol* 2008;47:390–392.

18. Pezeshkpoor F, Yazdanpanah MJ, Shirdel A. Specific cutaneous manifestations in adult T-cell leukemia/lymphoma. *Int J Dermatol* 2008;47:359–362.

19. Yamaguchi K. Human T-lymphotropic virus type I in Japan. *Lancet* 1994;343:213–216.

20. Bunn PA Jr, Schechter GP, Jaffe E, et al. Clinical course of retrovirus-associated adult T-cell lymphoma in the United States. *N Engl J Med* 1983;309:257–264.

21. O'Mahony D, Debnath I, Janik J, et al. Cardiac involvement with human T-cell lymphotrophic virus type-1-associated adult T-cell leukemia/lymphoma: the NIH experience. *Leuk Lymphoma* 2008;49:439–446.

22. Kawasaki C, Ikeda H, Fukumoto T. Cerebral mass lesions associated with adult T-cell leukemia/lymphoma. *Int J Hematol* 1995;61:97–102.

23. Dungerwalla M, Osuji N, Waldman AD, et al. Isolated central nervous system involvement in adult T-cell lymphoma/leukaemia. *Br J Haematol* 2005;130:511–515.

24. Marcon L, Rubin LA, Kurman CC, et al. Elevated serum levels of soluble Tac peptide in adult T-cell leukemia: correlation with clinical status during chemotherapy. *Ann Intern Med* 1988;109:274–279.

25. Janik JE, Morris JC, Pittaluga S, et al. Elevated serum-soluble interleukin-2 receptor levels in patients with anaplastic large cell lymphoma. *Blood* 2004;104:3355–3357.

26. Roncador G, Garcia JF, Garcia JF, et al. FOXP3, a selective marker for a subset of adult T-cell leukaemia/lymphoma. *Leukemia* 2005:19:2247–2253.

27. Seiki M, Eddy R, Shows TB, et al. Nonspecific integration of the HTLV provirus genome into adult T-cell leukaemia cells. *Nature* 1984;309:640–642.

28. Okamoto T, Ohno Y, Tsugane S, et al. Multi-step carcinogenesis model for adult T-cell leukemia. *Jpn J Cancer Res* 1989;80:191–195.

29. Grassmann R, Aboud M, Jeang KT. Molecular mechanisms of cellular transformation by HTLV-1 Tax. *Oncogene* 2005;24:5976–5985.

30. Yoshida M. Discovery of HTLV-1, the first human retrovirus, its unique regulatory mechanisms, and insights into pathogenesis. *Oncogene* 2005;24:5931–5937.

31. Kashanchi F, Brady JN. Transcriptional and post-transcriptional gene regulation of HTLV-1. *Oncogene* 2005;24:5938–5951.

32. Sun SC, Yamaoka S. Activation of NF-κB by HTLV-I and implications for cell transformation. *Oncogene* 2005;24:5952–5964.

33. Hall WW, Fujii M. Deregulation of cell-signaling pathways in HTLV-1 infection. *Oncogene* 2005;24:5965–5975.

34. Lemoine1 FJ, Marriott SJ. Genomic instability driven by the human T-cell leukemia virus type I (HTLV-I) oncoprotein, Tax. *Oncogene* 2002;21:7230–7234.

35. Marriott SJ, Semmes OJ. Impact of HTLV-I Tax on cell cycle progression and the cellular DNA damage repair response. *Oncogene* 2005;24:5986–5995.

36. Wagner S, Green MR. HTLV-I Tax protein stimulation of DNA binding of bZIP proteins by enhancing dimerization. *Science* 1993;262:395–399.

37. Zhao LJ, Giam CZ. Human T-cell lymphotropic virus type I (HTLV-I) transcriptional activator, Tax, enhances CREB binding to HTLV-I 21-base-pair repeats by protein-protein interaction. *Proc Natl Acad Sci U S A* 1992;89:7070–7074.

38. Suzuki T, Hirai H, Yoshida M. Tax protein of HTLV-1 interacts with the Rel homology domain of NF-kappa B p65 and c-Rel proteins bound to the NF-kappa B binding site and activates transcription. *Oncogene* 1994;9:3099–3105.

39. Fujii M, Tsuchiya H, Chuhjo T, et al. Interaction of HTLV-1 Tax1 with p67SRF causes the aberrant induction of cellular immediate early genes through CArG boxes. *Genes Dev* 1992;6:2066–2076.

40. Yoshida M. Multiple viral strategies of HTLV-1 for dysregulation of cell growth control. *Annu Rev Immunol* 2001;19:475–496.

41. Xiao G, Cvijic ME, Fong A, et al. Retroviral oncoprotein Tax induces processing of NF-kappaB2=p100 in T cells: evidence for the involvement of IKKalpha. *EMBO J* 2001;20:6805–6815.

42. Migone TS, Lin JX, Cereseto A, et al. Constitutively activated Jak-STAT pathway in T cells transformed with HTLV-I. *Science* 1995;269:79–81.

43. Franchini G, Wong-Staal F, Gallo RC. Human T-cell leukemia virus (HTLV-I) transcripts in fresh and cultured cells of patients with adult T-cell leukemia. *Proc Natl Acad Sci U S A* 1984;81:6207–6211.

44. Kozuru M, Uike N, Takeichi N, et al. The possible mode of escape of adult T-cell leukaemia cells from antibody-dependent cellular cytotoxicity. *Br J Haematol* 1989;72:502–506.

45. Tamiya S, Matsuoka M, Etoh K, et al. Two types of defective human T-lymphotropic virus type I provirus in adult T-cell leukemia. *Blood* 1996;88:3065–3073.

46. Kitamura T, Takano M, Hoshino H, et al. Methylation pattern of human T-cell leukemia virus *in vivo* and *in vitro*: pX and LTR regions are hypomethylated *in vivo*. *Int J Cancer* 1985;35:629–635.

47. Koiwa T, Usami-Hamano A, Ishida T, et al. 5'-LTR-selective CpG methylation of latent HTLV-1 provirus *in vitro* and *in vivo*. *J Virol* 2002;76:9389–9397.

48. Loeb LA. A mutator phenotype in cancer. *Cancer Res* 2001;61:3230–3239.

49. Jeang KT, Widen SG, Semmes OJT, et al. HTLV-I trans-activator protein, tax, is a trans-repressor of the human beta-polymerase gene. *Science* 1990;247:1082–1084.

50. Philpott SM, Buehring GC. Defective DNA repair in cells with human T-cell leukemia/bovine leukemia viruses: role of tax gene. *J Natl Cancer Inst* 1999;91:933–942.

51. Kao SY, Marriott SJ. Disruption of nucleotide excision repair by the human T-cell leukemia virus type 1 Tax protein. *J Virol* 1999;73:4299–4304.

52. Nicot C, Mahieux R, Takemoto S, et al. Bcl-X(L) is up-regulated by HTLV-I and HTLV-II *in vitro* and in *ex vivo* ATLL samples. *Blood* 2000;96:275–281.

53. Saintigny Y, Dumay A, Lambert S, et al. A novel role for the Bcl-2 protein family: specific suppression of the RAD51 recombination pathway. *EMBO J* 2001;20:2596–2607.

54. Cereseto A, Diella F, Mulloy JC, et al. p53 functional impairment and high p21waf1/cip1 expression in human T-cell lymphotropic/leukemia virus type I-transformed T cells. *Blood* 1996;88:1551–1560.

55. Reid RL, Lindholm PF, Mireskandari A, et al. Stabilization of wild-type p53 in human T-lymphocytes transformed by HTLV-I. *Oncogene* 1993;8:3029–3036.

56. Jin DY, Spencer F, Jeang KT, et al. Human T cell leukemia virus type 1 oncoprotein Tax targets the human mitotic checkpoint protein MAD1. *Cell* 1998;93:81–91.

57. Liu B, Hong S, Tang Z, et al. HTLV-1 Tax directly bind the Cdc-20-associated anaphase-promoting complex and activates it ahead of schedule. *Proc Natl Acad Sci U S A* 2005;102:63–68.

58. Gaudray G, Gachon F, Basbous J, et al. The complementary strand of the human T-cell leukemia virus type 1 RNA genome encodes a bZip transcription factor that down-regulates viral transcription. *J Virol* 2002;76:12813–12822.

59. Satou Y, Yasunaga J, Yoshida M, et al. HTLV-I basic leucine zipper factor gene mRNA supports proliferation of adult T cell leukemia cells. *Proc Natl Acad Sci U S A* 2006;103:720–725.

60. Mesnard JM, Barbeau B, Devaux C. HBZ, a new important player in the mystery of adult T-cell leukemia. *Blood* 2006;108:3979–3982.

61. Utsunomiya A, Hanada S, Terada A, et al. Adult T-cell leukemia with leukemia cell infiltration into the gastrointestinal tract. *Cancer* 1988;61:824–828.

62. Yamada Y, Kamihira S, Murata K, et al. Frequent hepatic involvement in adult T-cell leukemia: comparison with non-Hodgkin's lymphoma. *Leuk Lymphoma* 1997;26:327–335.

63. Yoshioka R, Yamaguchi K, Yoshinaga T, et al. Pulmonary complications in patients with adult T-cell leukemia. *Cancer* 1985;55:2491–2494.

64. Teshima T, Akashi K, Shibuya T, et al. Central nervous system involvement in adult T-cell leukemia/lymphoma. *Cancer* 1990;65:327–332.

65. Lymphoma Study Group. Major prognostic factors of patients with adult T-cell leukemia-lymphoma: a cooperative study. *Leuk Res* 1991;15:81–90.

66. Shimoyama M. Chemotherapy of ATL. In: Takatsuki K, ed. *Adult T-cell leukaemia.* Oxford, UK: Oxford University Press, 1994:221–237.

67. Shimoyama M, Ota K, Kikuchi M, et al. Chemotherapeutic results and prognostic factors of patients with advanced non-Hodgkin's lymphoma treated with VEPA or VEPA-M. *J Clin Oncol* 1988;6:128–141.

68. Shimoyama M, Ota K, Kikuchi M, et al. Major prognostic factors of adult patients with advanced T-cell lymphoma/leukemia. *J Clin Oncol* 1988;6:1088–1097.

69. Tobinai K, Shimoyama M, Minato K, et al. Japan Clinical Oncology Group phase II trial of second-generation "LSG4 protocol" in aggressive T- and B-lymphoma: a new predictive model for T- and B-lymphoma [abstract]. *Proc Am Soc Clin Oncol* 1994;13:378. Abstract 1280.

70. Tsukasaki K, Tobinai K, Shimoyama M, et al. Deoxycoformycin-containing combination chemotherapy for adult T-cell leukemia-lymphoma: Japan Clinical Oncology Group study (JCOG9109). *Int J Hematol* 2003;77:164–170.

71. Yamada Y, Tomonaga M, Fukuda H, et al. A new G-CSF-supported combination chemotherapy, LSG15, for adult T-cell leukemia-lymphoma (ATL): Japan Clinical Oncology Group (JCOG) Study 9303. *Br J Haematol* 2001;113:375–382.

72. Tsukasaki K, Utsunomiya A, Fukuda H, et al. VCAP-AMP-VECP compared with biweekly CHOP for adult T-cell leukemia-lymphoma: Japan Clinical Oncology Group Study JCOG9801. *J Clin Oncol* 2007;25:5458–5564.

73. Tobinai K, Shimoyama M, Inoue S, et al. Phase I study of YK-176 (2'-deoxycoformycin) in patients with adult T-cell leukemia-lymphoma. *Jpn J Clin Oncol* 1992;22:164–171.

74. Gill PS, Harrington W, Kaplan MH, et al. Treatment of adult T-cell leukemia-lymphoma with a combination of interferon alfa and zidovudine. *N Engl J Med* 1995;332:1744–1748.

75. Ohno R, Okada K, Masaoka T, et al. An early phase II study of CPT-11: a new derivative of camptothecin, for the treatment of leukemia and lymphoma. *J Clin Oncol* 1990;8:1907–1912.

76. Tsuda H, Takatsuki K, Ohno R, et al. Treatment of adult T-cell leukemia-lymphoma with irinotecan hydrochloride. *Br J Cancer* 1994;70:771–774.

77. Hermine O, Blouscary D, Gessain A, et al. Treatment of adult T-cell leukemia-lymphoma with zidovudine and interferon alfa. *N Engl J Med* 1995;332:1749–1751.

78. Tobinai K, Kobayashi Y, Shimoyama M, et al. Interferon alfa and zidovudine in adult T-cell leukemia-lymphoma. *N Engl J Med* 1995;333:1285.

79. Bazarbachi A, Panelatti G, Ramos JC, et al. A worldwide meta-analysis on the use of zidovudine and interferon-alpha for the treatment of adult T-cell leukemia/lymphoma. American Society of Hematology, 2007 [abstract]. *Blood* 2007;110:610a–611a. Abstr 2049.

80. Tobinai K, Ogura M, Hotta T, et al. Phase I study of cladribine (2-chlorodeoxyadenosine) in lymphoid malignancies. *Jpn J Clin Oncol* 1997;27:146–153.

81. Tobinai K, Uike N, Saburi Y, et al. Phase II study of cladribine (2-chlorodeoxyadenosine) in relapsed or refractory adult T-cell leukemia-lymphoma. *Int J Hematol* 2003;77:512–517.

82. Waldmann TA. Multichain interleukin-2 receptor: a target for immunotherapy in lymphoma. *J Natl Cancer Inst* 1989;81:914–923.

83. Waldmann TA, White JD, Carrasquillo JA, et al. Radioimmunotherapy of interleukin-2Rα-expressing adult T-cell leukemia with yttrium-90-labeled anti-Tac. *Blood* 1995;86:4063–4075.

84. Ishida T, Utsunomiya A, Iida S, et al. Clinical significance of CCR4 expression in adult T-cell leukemia/lymphoma: its close association with skin involvement and unfavorable outcome. *Clin Cancer Res* 2003;9:3625–3634.

85. Ishida T, Ueda R. CCR4 as a novel molecular target for immunotherapy of cancer. *Cancer Sci* 2006;97:1139–1146.

86. Hermine O, Dombret H, Poupon J, et al. Phase II trial of arsenic trioxide (As2O3) and combination of alpha interferon (INF) and As2O3 in patients with relapsed/refractory adult T cell leukemia (ATL). *Hematol J* 2004;5:130–134.

87. O'Connor OA, Hamlin PA, Portlock C, et al. Pralatrexate, a novel class of antifol with high affinity for the reduced folate carrier-type 1, produces marked complete and durable remissions in a diversity of chemotherapy refractory cases of T-cell lymphoma. *Br J Haematol* 2007;139:425–428.

88. Tan C, Waldmann TA. Proteasome inhibitor PS-341, a potential therapeutic agent for adult T-cell leukemia. *Cancer Res* 2002;62:1083–1086.

89. Satou Y, Nosaka K, Koya Y, et al. Proteasome inhibitor, bortezomib, potently inhibits the growth of adult T-cell leukemia cells both in vivo and in vitro. *Leukemia* 2004;18:1357–1363.

90. Utsunomiya A, Miyazaki Y, Takatsuka Y, et al. Improved outcome of adult T cell leukemia/lymphoma with allogeneic hematopoietic stem cell transplantation. *Bone Marrow Transplant* 2001;27:15–20.

91. Fukushima T, Miyazaki Y, Honda S, et al. Allogeneic hematopoietic stem cell transplantation provides sustained long-term survival for patients with adult T-cell leukemia/lymphoma. *Leukemia* 2005;19:829–834.

92. Okamura J, Utsunomiya A, Tanosaki R, et al. Allogeneic stem-cell transplantation with reduced conditioning intensity as a novel immunotherapy and antiviral therapy for adult T-cell leukemia/lymphoma. *Blood* 2005;105:4143–4145.

CHAPTER 28 ■ ANAPLASTIC LARGE CELL LYMPHOMA

BRUNANGELO FALINI AND CHRISTIAN GISSELBRECHT

Anaplastic large cell lymphoma (ALCL) was first described by Stein et al. (1) in 1985. It was included, as a new entity, in the Revised European and American Lymphoma classification of lymphoid neoplasms (2) in 1994 and, subsequently, in the third edition of the World Health Organization (WHO) classification (3) of lympho-hemopoietic tissues in 2001. Characteristics of ALCL are the anaplastic appearance of tumor cells (Color Plate 73A–C), their propensity to grow cohesively and invade lymph node sinuses, and their consistent expression of the CD30 molecule (previously named Ki-1) (4), a 120-kDa transmembrane cytokine receptor of the tumor necrosis factor receptor family (5,6) (Color Plate 73D–E).

Further progress in the characterization of this lymphoma type had to wait for the observation by cytogeneticists that a proportion of ALCL cases, sometimes mimicking "malignant histiocytosis" (7,8), harbored a nonrandom t(2;5) (p23;q35) translocation (9–11). The next breakthrough was in 1994, when Morris et al. (12) at St. Jude Hospital demonstrated that the t(2;5) translocation caused the fusion of the NPM (nucleophosmin) gene with a previously unrecognized gene that was named ALK (anaplastic lymphoma kinase).

Several methods were subsequently developed to detect the t(2;5)-associated NPM-ALK fusion gene, including reverse transcriptase-polymerase chain reaction (PCR) (13–15), in situ hybridization (16), two-color fluorescence in situ hybridization (17), or detection of the encoded NPM-ALK chimeric protein by immunohistochemistry with anti-ALK specific antibodies (18,19) (Color Plate 73F). The latter technique, in particular, has greatly contributed to clarify controversies over ALCL morphologic and clinical heterogeneity, and to better define the borders between ALCL and other lymphoma entities, particularly Hodgkin lymphoma and peripheral T-cell lymphoma (PTCL).

Moreover, in the past 5 years, much information has accumulated on the role of ALK in the molecular pathogenesis of ALCL (20). Given these advances, the fourth edition of the WHO classification of lympho-hemopoietic tissues recognizes two types of systemic ALCL (21): a distinct disease entity showing unique molecular, pathologic, and clinical features that is called ALK-positive ALCL (ALCL, ALK+); and a provisional entity named ALK-negative ALCL (ALCL, ALK-). This chapter provides an overview of the progress in this field, and it will not be dealing with primary cutaneous ALCL that is extensively described in another section of the book (see Chapter 30).

ANAPLASTIC LARGE CELL LYMPHOMA, ANAPLASTIC LYMPHOMA KINASE POSITIVE

In the third edition of the WHO classification of lympho-hemopoietic tissues (3), ALCL, ALK+ and ALCL, ALK- were both covered under the broad term of "anaplastic large cell lymphoma." In the fourth WHO edition (2008) (21), ALCL, ALK+ is recognized as a new disease entity within the spectrum of mature T-cell neoplasms and as distinct from ALCL, ALK-.

ALK-positive ALCL most likely derives from an activated mature cytotoxic T cell. Neoplastic transformation is thought to be the consequence of constitutive expression and activation of oncogenic ALK fusion proteins, as a result of rearrangements of the ALK gene with the NPM gene (the majority of ALCL cases) or, less frequently, with gene partners other than NPM. However, close overlapping in the clinicopathologic features (22), gene expression profile (23), and molecular pathogenesis of ALCL carrying NPM-ALK versus other ALK variant fusion proteins justify their inclusion in the new WHO classification under the single term of ALCL, ALK+.

Morphology

Architectural features (propensity of lymphoma cells to grow cohesively and invade lymph node sinuses), the wide cytologic spectrum of tumor cells (ranging in size from small to large anaplastic), and the variable admixtures of reactive elements give rise to several morphologic patterns in ALCL, ALK+ (19,24–27).

The "common type" is the most frequent morphologic variant of ALCL, ALK+, occurring in about 60% of cases. The tumor cells are very large and have an abundant, often vacuolated, cytoplasm (1,2,26,28,29), and horseshoe or kidney-shaped nuclei containing multiple basophilic nucleoli (Color Plate 73A–C). Nuclear lobes sometimes surround the Golgi area, which appears as a clear, or more eosinophilic zone. Cells with these cytologic features have been referred to as "hallmark cells" (Color Plate 67A) (25) because they are detected in all cases of ALK-positive ALCLs, including the small cell and lymphohistiocytic morphologic variants. Recently, a relationship between anaplastic morphology and ALK activity has been suggested because the latter seems to control the cell shape and F-actin filament assembly of ALCL cells through Cdc42 activation (30).

In the "small cell variant" (5% to 10% of ALCL, ALK+), the predominant population consists of small- to medium-sized tumor cells with irregular, generally not cerebriform, nuclei (28,31) (Color Plate 67C). They are admixed with large anaplastic elements ("hallmark cells") that usually cluster around small vessels, as highlighted by immunostaining for CD30 (28) and ALK (19,25,32). Because the small cell component predominates, this variant may be misdiagnosed as PTCL not otherwise specified (PTCL-NOS) at conventional examination (21). Leukemic involvement appears to be more frequent in the "small cell variant" than in other ALCL, ALK+ morphologic variants, and is characterized by the presence of lymphoma cells with a flower-like appearance in the peripheral blood and/or bone marrow smears. Immunohistochemistry with anti-ALK antibodies is crucial for detecting marrow involvement in the "small cell variant" (29) because the small tumor cells are usually weakly positive or negative for CD30.

The "lymphohistiocytic variant" (33), which accounts for about 10% of ALK-positive ALCLs, is closely related to the "small cell variant" (34) because it often contains small neoplastic cells admixed with large anaplastic elements and many pale reactive histiocytes (CD68+) (Color Plate 67E), which sometimes show signs of erythrophagocytosis. The abundance of the histiocytic component may frequently mask the tumor cell population and lead to a misdiagnosis of atypical inflammatory lesions, hemophagocytic syndrome or malignant histiocytosis (28,33).

Morphologic features of the "Hodgkin-like pattern" (only 3% of ALCL, ALK+) usually mimic classic Hodgkin lymphoma, nodular sclerosis (35). Very rare morphologic patterns of ALCL, including cases with sarcomatoid (36,37), neutrophil-rich and hypocellular (39) appearance, have been reported, but no information was provided of whether these cases were ALK+ or ALK-. Recognition of these morphologic patterns is important because they can mimic either atypical inflammatory lesions or malignant tumors other than ALCL.

Patterns of Anaplastic Lymphoma Kinase Protein Expression in Anaplastic Large Cell Lymphoma, Anaplastic Lymphoma Kinase Positive

The ALK protein is not expressed in lymphoid tissues (18). Therefore, the immunohistochemical finding of ALK protein expression in lymphoma cells (16,19,26,27,40) reflects the presence of an ALK fusion product as a result of some kind of rearrangement of the *ALK* gene. Because of its specificity, simplicity, rapidity, and low cost, immunohistochemistry has largely supplanted molecular or fluorescence in situ hybridization assays for the diagnosis of ALCL, ALK+ (27). Additional advantages are that immunohistochemistry can be applied to archival paraffin-embedded material, and provides information on the identity of the labeled cells and their topographic distribution. Moreover, it is useful, as first screening, for identifying molecular variants

of ALCL, e.g., tumors expressing fusion proteins other than NPM-ALK.

Anaplastic Large Cell Lymphoma Expressing the Nucleophosmin -Anaplastic Lymphoma Kinase Fusion Protein

ALCL, ALK+ accounts for about 60% of all ALCLs. Approximately 85% of ALK-positive ALCLs bear an NPM-ALK fusion protein, i.e., the product of the t(2;5) translocation. Interestingly, the subcellular distribution of ALK moiety of the fusion protein tends to correlate with the size of neoplastic cells. In general, the large anaplastic tumor cells (which are the predominant population in the "common type") show ALK positivity not only in cytoplasm (the expected location site of wild-type ALK), but also in the nucleus (22,26,27,41) (Color Plates 67D,F and 70). This "ectopic" ALK nuclear expression is due to the fact that NPM, because of its nucleo-cytoplasmic shuttling properties, can transport the ALK fusion protein within the nucleus, through formation of NPM-ALK/wild-type NPM heterodimers (42). Notably, the small neoplastic cells, which constitute the predominant population in the "small cell" and "lympho-histiocytic" variants, exhibit a nuclear-restricted ALK protein expression (19) (Color Plate 67D,F).

In the "small cell variant" of ALCL with t(2;5), a few large anaplastic cells expressing ALK in cytoplasm and nucleus are found around vessels. ALK expression in both small and large tumor cells strongly supports the view that they belong to the same neoplastic clone and excludes the possibility that the large cells are subclones arising in a (2;5)-translocation-negative low-grade (small cell) lymphoma with the acquisition of the t(2;5) (43).

ALCL with t(2;5) shows a peculiar immunostaining pattern also when stained with antibodies that are specifically directed against the NPM N terminus (which is retained in NPM-ALK). In addition to the expected nuclear positivity, tumor cells also appear to express NPM aberrantly in the cytoplasm, which reflects the presence in this compartment of the NPM-ALK fusion protein (22,27,29,41). In contrast, in tissues devoid of NPM-ALK, NPM positivity is restricted to the nucleus (22,27,41). Interestingly, aberrant cytoplasmic expression of NPM caused by molecular events other than NPM-ALK rearrangement is also observed in acute myeloid leukemia carrying the NPM-MLF1 fusion protein (44) or mutations of the *NPM1* gene (45).

Anaplastic Large Cell Lymphoma Expressing Anaplastic Lymphoma Kinase Fusion Proteins Other than Nucleophosmin-Anaplastic Lymphoma Kinase

In about 15% of ALCL, ALK+ (18,19,25), the *ALK* gene fuses with a partner other than *NPM* to produce variant ALK fusion proteins (Color Plate 68). These cases can be clearly distinguished from the most common NPM-ALK positive ALCL by immunohistochemistry, Western blotting, cytogenetics/fluorescence in situ hybridization, and reverse transcriptase-PCR. Immunohistochemistry is the simplest first-line screening assay for identifying molecular variants of ALCL, ALK+ because they are characterized by cytoplasmic-restricted ALK positivity (18,19,22,25–27) (Color Plates 67B and 71) (Table 28.1). Moreover, unlike NPM-ALK+ ALCL,

TABLE 28.1

CHROMOSOMAL TRANSLOCATIONS AND ALK FUSION PROTEINS IN ALCL, ALK+

Chromosomal abnormality	ALK partner	ALK fusion protein (kDa)	ALK staining	NPM staining[a]	Frequency
t(2;5)(p23;q35)	NPM	80	Nuclear, diffuse cytoplasmic	Nuclear, diffuse cytoplasmic	~85%
t(1;2)(q25;p23)	TPM3	104	Diffuse cytoplasmic	Nuclear	~3%
Inv(2)(p23q35)	ATIC	96	Diffuse cytoplasmic	Nuclear	Rare
t(2;3)(p23;q21)	TFG XIong	113	Diffuse cytoplasmic	Nuclear	Rare
	TFG long	97	Diffuse cytoplasmic	Nuclear	Rare
	TFG short	85	Diffuse cytoplasmic	Nuclear	Rare
t(2;17)(p23;q23)	CLTC	250	Granular cytoplasmic	Nuclear	Rare
t(2;X)(p23;q11-12)	MSN	125	Diffuse cytoplasmic	Nuclear	Rare
t(2;19)(p23;p13.1)	TPM4	95	Diffuse cytoplasmic	Nuclear	Rare
t(2;22)(p23;q11.2)	MYH9	220	Diffuse cytoplasmic	Nuclear	Rare
t(2;17)(p23;q25)	ALO17	?	Diffuse cytoplasmic	Nuclear	Rare

ALO17, ALK lymphoma oligomerization partner on chromosome 17; MYH9, myosin heavy chain gene 9.
[a] Using monoclonal antibodies against the N-terminus portion of NPM.

cases harboring variant ALK fusion proteins show a nucleus-restricted expression for NPM (N terminus) (22) (not shown). Thus, the staining patterns of both ALK and NPM in ALCL carrying variant ALK-fusion proteins differ markedly from that observed in classic NPM-ALK positive ALCL (Color Plates 70–72). Western blotting provides further characterization of variant ALK fusion proteins because anti-ALK antibodies identify bands with molecular masses that are different to what is expected for NPM-ALK (46) (i.e., 80 kDa). Cytogenetic analysis of these cases has revealed a variety of genetic abnormalities leading to ALK rearrangements (47–49) (Table 28.1)

Other Immunohistochemical Markers

Although less specific than ALK expression, other immunohistochemical markers can assist in the diagnosis of ALCL, ALK+. Reproducibility of ALCL diagnosis on morphologic grounds alone is only 46%, but it is increased to up to 85% by immunostaining for CD30 (28,31). In the "common type variant," the totality of neoplastic cells appears to express the CD30 molecule, usually on the cell membrane and in the Golgi area (1,6,26) (Color Plate 73D–E). However, in the "small cell variant" of ALK-positive ALCL, only the large anaplastic cells, which are usually distributed around vessels, express the CD30 molecule; the small tumor cells are usually weakly positive or negative (28,31).

Although the majority of ALCL, ALK+ express one or more T-cell antigens (usually CD2, CD5, and CD4), some cases may show a "null phenotype" due to the loss of pan-T antigens (1,50). Despite this, the "null cell type" ALCL is thought to derive from T cells because tumor cells frequently express the cytotoxic molecules perforin, granzyme B, and T-cell–restricted intracellular antigen-1 (50,51), and harbor clonally rearranged T-cell receptor genes (51).

Epithelial membrane antigen positivity is often seen in ALCL, ALK+ (52,53), although in some cases, only a percentage of tumor cells appear positive. BCL2 expression was reported in ALK-negative but not ALK-positive ALCL (54). On the contrary, c-Myc nuclear expression was observed in pediatric ALK-positive but not ALK-negative ALCL (55). ALCL, ALK+ is consistently negative for Epstein-Barr virus markers (21,56).

Differential Diagnosis

Immunohistochemistry plays a pivotal role in the differential diagnosis between ALCL, ALK+ and other reactive or malignant conditions.

Anaplastic Large Cell Lymphoma, Anaplastic Lymphoma Kinase Positive versus Reactive Conditions

In the "lymphohistiocytic variant" of ALK-positive ALCL, the abundance of reactive histiocytes may mask the tumor cell population (Color Plate 67E), and lead to a misdiagnosis of atypical inflammatory lesions or hemophagocytic syndrome (28,33). Moreover, the neutrophil-rich (38) and hypocellular form of ALCL (39) can be confused with an inflammatory process in the lymph node (39) and skin (57,58). Immunostaining for CD30 and ALK usually provides a correct diagnosis.

Anaplastic Large Cell Lymphoma, Anaplastic Lymphoma Kinase Positive versus Extramedullary Tumors

ALCL, ALK+ growing within the sinuses or showing a "cohesive" growth pattern may mimic carcinoma. In this instance, the differential diagnosis is mainly based on detection of ALK protein (consistently negative in solid tumors) and cytokeratins (consistently negative in ALCL, ALK+). CD30 is a less reliable marker because it may be expressed in some carcinomas (6).

"Small Cell Variant" of Anaplastic Large Cell Lymphoma, Anaplastic Lymphoma Kinase-Positive versus Peripheral T-Cell Lymphoma-Not Otherwise Specified

The differential diagnosis is mainly based on detection of nuclear ALK positivity on the small atypical cells, which are usually CD30 negative (19,26) (Color Plate 67D). The distinction is clinically relevant because ALCL, ALK+ has a better prognosis than PTCL-NOS.

Anaplastic Large Cell Lymphoma, Anaplastic Lymphoma Kinase-Positive versus Classic Hodgkin Lymphoma

Differential diagnosis between ALCL, ALK+ and Hodgkin lymphoma, especially cases that are rich in neoplastic cells and show a nodular sclerosis pattern (59), is based mainly on study of the ALK protein because it is not detected by immunohistochemistry in classic Hodgkin lymphoma (35).

Anaplastic Large Cell Lymphoma, Anaplastic Lymphoma Kinase-Positive versus Anaplastic Lymphoma Kinase-Positive Large B-Cell Lymphoma

Both tumors strongly express the ALK protein, as a result of *ALK* gene rearrangements, but they can be easily differentiated by morphologic, immunophenotypic, and genetic criteria. In fact, unlike ALCL expressing the ALK protein, ALK-positive large B-cell lymphoma (60,61) is characterized by immunoblastic/plasmoblastic (rather than anaplastic) morphology, cytoplasmic expression of immunoglobulin A, and negativity or weak positivity for CD30 (61–63).

Anaplastic Large Cell Lymphoma, Anaplastic Lymphoma Kinase-Positive versus Anaplastic Lymphoma Kinase-Positive Histiocytosis

Chan et al. (64) recently reported three cases of infant histiocytosis characterized by ALK expression due, in at least one patient, to a *TPM3-ALK* rearrangement. Features that clearly distinguish ALK+ histiocytosis from ALCL, ALK+ are: (a) the histiocytic appearance of tumor cells and their positivity for the macrophage-restricted form of CD68 (65), and (b) negativity of tumor cells for the CD30 molecule.

Anaplastic Large Cell Lymphoma, Anaplastic Lymphoma Kinase-Positive verus Anaplastic Lymphoma Kinase-Positive Myofibroblastic Tumors

ALK protein expression due to a variety of *ALK* rearrangements has been reported in myofibroblastic tumors (66). The differential diagnosis between ALCL, ALK+ and ALK-positive inflammatory myofibroblastic tumors is mainly based on morphologic criteria and CD30 immunostaining (67). In fact, in ALK-positive inflammatory myofibroblastic tumors, the neoplastic cells are consistently CD30 negative.

Genetic Abnormalities of Anaplastic Large Cell Lymphoma, Anaplastic Lymphoma Kinase-Positive

In ALCL, the *ALK* gene fuses with *NPM* or other gene partners as a result of a variety of chromosomal translocations (26,27), which are listed in Table 28.1. Interestingly, expression of ALK fusion proteins can be also found in lymphomas other than ALCL and even in histiocytic proliferations (Fig. 28.1).

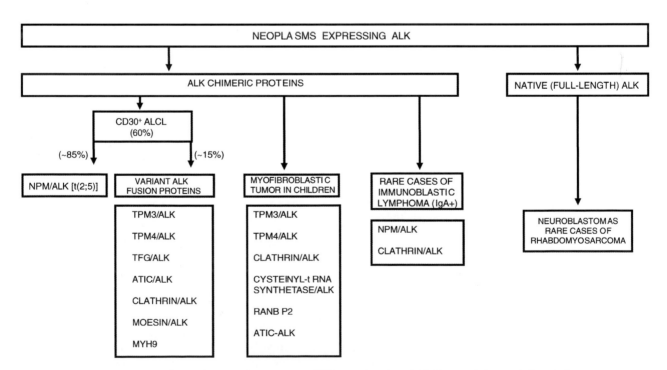

FIGURE 28.1 Hemopoietic neoplasm carrying ALK gene alterations. MYH9, myosin heavy chain gene 9.

The t(2;5) is the most frequent chromosomal translocation in ALCL, ALK+ (about 85% of cases) and generates the *NPM-ALK* fusion gene that encodes for a 80-kDa chimeric protein termed NPM-ALK (12) or p80 (68). In the NPM-ALK fusion protein, the NPM amino-terminal portion (amino acids 1 to 116) that contains the oligomerization domain fuses to the entire cytoplasmic region of ALK, that is, the last 563 amino acids that contain the tyrosine kinase domain (12) (Color Plate 68). *NPM* (69), the gene partner of *ALK* in the t(2;5), encodes for an ubiquitously expressed 38-kDa nucleolar (41) phosphoprotein that shuttles between the nucleus and cytoplasm (70). Thanks to its trafficking (70) and molecular chaperone (71,72) properties, NPM is involved in multiple functions (73), including regulation of ribosome biogenesis, control of centrosome duplication, and maintenance of integrity of the oncosuppressor p19Arf.

The second most frequent rearrangement in ALCL involves the *ALK* and *TPM3* (nonmuscle tropomyosin) genes, and is produced by the t(1;2)(q25;p23) translocation (49,74,75) (Table 28.1). The *TPM3-ALK* fusion gene encodes for a 104-kDa chimeric protein and also appears to be involved in the pathogenesis of a subset of myofibroblastic inflammatory tumors in children (76,77).

The *TFG* (tropomyosin receptor kinase [*TRK*]-fused gene)-*ALK* fusion gene (78) generates three different molecular mass chimeric proteins, i.e., 85 kDa (short TFG-ALK), 97 kDa (long TFG-ALK), and 113 kDa (extra-long TFG-ALK), corresponding to different breakpoints in the *TFG* gene (78,79). The TFG-ALK 97-kDa chimeric product is generated by the chromosomal translocation t(2;3)(p23;q21) (49) (Table 28.1).

The inv(2)(p23;q35) (48) leads to creation of a fusion gene named *ATIC-ALK*, which encodes for a chimeric protein composed of the entire cytoplasmic portion of ALK and the amino terminus of ATIC (5 Aminoimidazole-4-carboxamide-1-β-D-ribonucleotide transformylase/inosine monophosphate cyclohydrolase) (80–82) (Table 28.1). The latter is a bifunctional homodimeric enzyme that catalyzes the penultimate and ultimate steps of the de novo purine nucleotide biosynthesis (83).

Touriol et al. (84) reported ALCL, ALK+ cases in which *ALK* was fused with the *CLTCL* (*clathrin heavy polypeptide-like*) gene, which encodes for the main structural protein of coated vesicles. This chimeric *CLTCL-ALK* gene was generated by the t(2;17) (p23;q23) translocation (21) (Table 28.1), which interestingly, is predicted by immunohistochemistry with anti-ALK antibodies because CLTCL-ALK expression is associated with a characteristic cytoplasmic positivity of granular type (84) (Color Plate 72). This is due to the fact that the sequence responsible for clathrin heavy chain assemblage is retained in the CLTCL-ALK fusion protein, which can, therefore, participate in the formation of the clathrin coat on the surface of the vesicles.

Other rare ALK rearrangements in ALCL are shown in Table 28.1 and include: (a) fusion of *ALK* with the *TPM4* gene (85), as a result of t(2;19) (p23;p13.1); (b) fusion of *ALK* with the myosin heavy chain gene 9 gene, as a consequence of t(2;22) (p23;q11.2); (c) fusion of *ALK* with the ALK lymphoma oligomerization partner on chromosome 17 gene (21); and (d) fusion of *ALK* with the moesin (*MSN*) gene (86), as a result of t(2;X) (p23;q11-12) (21). The *ALK* breakpoint in this last translocation, unlike what has consistently been observed to date in other translocations involving the *ALK* gene, is localized within the exonic sequence coding for the *ALK* juxtamembrane portion (86). Notably, immunohistochemistry can predict the presence of the MSN-ALK fusion protein because ALK positivity appears to be restricted to the surface membrane, reflecting the physiologic association of MSN with this cell compartment (86) (Color Plate 72).

Anaplastic Lymphoma Kinase Rearrangements in Nonlympho-Hemopietic Tumors

Interestingly, the *ALK* gene may be involved also in the pathogenesis of some nonlympho-hemopietic neoplasms. ALK protein expression due to rearrangements involving the *ALK* gene and other partners such as *TPM3*, *TPM4* (66,76), or *cysteinyl-transfer ribonucleic acid (RNA)-synthetase* (87) has been reported in myofibroblastic tumors (66).

TPM4-ALK fusion protein has been detected by mass spectrometry in esophageal carcinoma (88,89), but the significance of this finding remains unknown. *Echinoderm microtubule-associated protein-like 4-ALK* rearrangements have been detected in nonsmall cell lung cancer (90). However, *echinoderm microtubule-associated protein-like 4-ALK* rearrangements in lung cancer are usually restricted to a small minority of tumor cells and do not result in expression of the ALK protein (at immunohistochemically detectable levels) (91). Therefore, the diagnostic and pathogenetic significance of *echinoderm microtubule-associated protein-like* 4-ALK in lung cancer remains controversial.

Recently, the *ALK* gene was found also to be a target of mutations (usually involving its kinase domain) in 6% to 8% of advanced neuroblastomas (92–94). The mutated kinases, in these cases, were autophosphorylated, and exhibited transforming activity both in vitro and in xenotransplanted nude mice (92).

Molecular Pathogenesis of Anaplastic Large Cell Lymphoma, Anaplastic Lymphoma Kinase Positive

NPM-ALK and the rarer "variant ALK fusion proteins" share several features that strongly suggest that they may contribute in similar ways to lymphomagenesis. In fact, in all ALCL-associated rearrangements so far identified (Table 28.1), ALK (which is silent in lymphoid tissues) is placed under the control of the strong promoter of a fusion partner gene, which is usually widely expressed in normal cells. This leads to the permanent and aberrant expression of the ALK chimeric RNA and corresponding fusion protein.

The second feature, which is common to all ALK fusion proteins, is that they carry at their N–terminus an oligomerization domain that is responsible for homodimer formation (26,29), through cross-linking with other ALK fusion proteins. Self-association of these chimeric molecules then leads to the constitutive activation of the ALK tyrosine kinase catalytic domain (74,78,86) that is a major contributor of transforming activity. A unique feature of NPM-ALK is its capability to form heterodimers with wild-type NPM, via the oligomerization domain.

Through this interaction, NPM-ALK is transported by wild-type NPM in the nucleolus. The ectopic (nuclear) expression of ALK is a useful immunohistochemical marker but is thought not to be pathogenetically relevant (42).

A number of experimental evidences support the view that ALK fusion proteins are the causative oncogenes in ALCL, ALK+. In vitro, NPM-ALK displayed strong transforming potential in hematopoietic and fibroblast cell lines (95). Transplantation of *NPM-ALK*-transduced bone marrow cells into irradiated recipient mice induced a lymphoma-like disease (96). Murine models available for defining the oncogenic role of NPM-ALK in lymphomas have been reviewed by Miething et al. (97).

NPM and other moieties (TPM3, ATIC, etc.) of the ALK fusion proteins would appear to play no other role in transformation beyond serving as an oligomerization domain for the chimera (98). On the other hand, the constitutive expression and activation of the ALK domain appear to be the most critical events for transformation. Thus, understanding the mechanism through which the ALK moiety in the fusion protein exerts its transforming activity implies knowledge of the wild-type ALK protein structure and function.

The wild-type ALK protein (now recognized by cluster designation as CD246) (99) is a large, 1,620 amino acid (210 kDa) single-chain transmembrane molecule that comprises a large extracellular ligand-binding region, a lipophilic transmembrane spanning segment, and a cytoplasmic tyrosine kinase domain (12,100,101). At present, the ALK protein is known to be activated physiologically by the endogenous ligands pleiotrophin (102) and midkine (103). When the ligand is missing, the wild-type ALK protein is inactive, and its expression increases apoptosis, whereas in the presence of the ligand, ALK becomes activated, and apoptosis is reduced (104). The wild-type ALK is normally detected only in the developing and mature central and peripheral nervous systems (18,101,105). In *ALK* knockout mice, Bilsland et al. (106) found no developmental, anatomic, or locomotor deficits but reported that they had an "antidepressant profile" with better learning and memory capabilities, which are closely associated with enhanced hippocampal progenitor proliferations. Although the function of ALK still remains elusive, these findings suggest that it may be involved in regulation of mood and cognitive processes. Interestingly, certain polymorphisms within the *ALK* gene locus were found to segregate with the development of schizophrenia (107).

In ALCL, ALK+, the self-association of ALK fusion protein via the N-terminus oligomerization domains leads to the constitutive expression and activation of the ALK domain. This event induces, in turn, phosphorylation and aberrant activation of multiple, potentially tumorigenic, downstream substrates and signaling cascades. At least two signaling cascades that are involved in control of proliferation and apoptosis appear to be activated by NPM-ALK in vitro (95). NPM-ALK was found to recruit phospholipase C-γ, which, in turn, enhanced inositol phosphate 3 production (108). The phospholipase C-γ/inositol phosphates 3 pathway seemed to be involved in NPM-ALK mediated mitogenicity (95). Moreover, NPM-ALK constitutively activated the antiapoptotic phosphatidylinositol-3 kinase/AKT pathway (109,110), resulting in phosphorylation and inactivation of the proapoptotic molecule BAD, which provides apoptosis protection in NPM-ALK bearing cells (95,109,110). NPM-ALK-mediated activation of

signal transduction and activator of transcription 3 (111,112) and signal transduction and activator of transcription 5 (113) could also play a role in lymphomagenesis. Over the past few years, an even more complex scenario has emerged (Color Plate 69) that has been described in recent reviews (20,114) to which the reader is referred. Elucidating the complex interactions of ALK protein with other molecules is of prime importance because it may lead to the design of new dugs for targeted therapy.

ANAPLASTIC LARGE CELL LYMPHOMA, ANAPLASTIC LYMPHOMA KINASE-NEGATIVE

In the third edition (2001) of the WHO classification of lympho-hemopoietic tissues (3), the broad entity "Anaplastic Large Cell Lymphoma" included ALCL, ALK+ together with ALK-negative ALCL. In the fourth WHO edition (2008), ALCL, ALK- is considered distinct from ALCL, ALK+ and PTCL-NOS, and is recognized as a new provisional entity within the spectrum of mature T-cell neoplasms (21). Thought to derive from an activated mature cytotoxic T cell, ALK-negative ALCL is defined as a CD30+ T-cell lymphoma that is morphologically indistinguishable from ALCL, ALK+, differing only in the lack of ALK protein expression.

Morphologic Features

Unfortunately, few detailed studies are available on the pathologic features of ALCL, ALK- (115). Although the morphologic spectra of ALCL, ALK- and ALCL, ALK+ are very similar, including the presence of the so-called "hallmark cells," ALK-negative ALCL cells tend to be larger, with a more pleomorphic appearance than the standard ALCL, ALK+ tumor cells (21). Rare cases may show a signet-ring appearance (116) (Color Plate 73B). Interestingly, ALCL, ALK- differs morphologically from ALCL, ALK+ because it does not have a "small cell morphological variant" (21).

Immunophenotype

By definition, ALCL, ALK- lacks expression of the ALK protein at immunohistochemistry (21). Strong CD30 expression by all neoplastic cells is its major immunophenotypic characteristic. This staining pattern clearly differs from that observed in PTCL-NOS, which is characterized by expression of CD30, at variable intensity, in only some tumor cells (21).

As in ALK-positive ALCL, T-cell markers are frequently lost. However, about 50% of ALCLs, ALK- express one or more T-cell molecules, usually CD2 and/or CD3. The CD4 antigen is also found in a significant percentage of cases. Most ALK-negative ALCLs express the cytotoxic-associated markers T-cell–restricted intracellular antigen 1, granzyme B, and/or perforin, but, unlike ALK-positive ALCL, epithelial membrane antigen expression is quite uncommon (21). ALK-negative ALCL is consistently negative for Epstein-Barr virus markers (i.e., Epstein-Barr-encoded RNA and latent membrane protein 1).

Differential Diagnosis

The main differential diagnoses of ALCL, ALK- are with PTCL-NOS and with classic Hodgkin lymphoma rich in tumor cells. ALCL, ALK- differs from PTCL-NOS because of the: (a) absence of small- to medium-sized neoplastic lymphocytes (frequently present in PTCL-NOS); (b) strong, homogeneous CD30 expression (variably expressed in PTCL-NOS); and (c) lack of T-cell receptor proteins (117) (usually retained in PTCL-NOS). However, because distinction between these two entities is not always straightforward, the WHO classification recommends diagnosing a case as ALCL, ALK- (rather than PTCL-NOS) only if the tumor cells closely resemble ALCL, ALK+ cells, despite the lack of ALK protein expression (21).

In distinguishing ALCL, ALK- from tumor cell rich forms of classic Hodgkin lymphoma, the major diagnostic criteria are: (a) nuclear negativity for the transcription factor PAX5 (118) (usually weakly expressed in Hodgkin lymphoma cells); (b) negativity for the Epstein-Barr virus markers Epstein-Barr-encoded RNA and latent membrane protein 1, which may be expressed in Hodgkin lymphoma; and (c) frequent evidence of clonal T-cell receptor rearrangements (usually absent in classic Hodgkin lymphoma). Thus, detailed immunophenotypic and genetic studies ensure ALK-negative ALCL and classic Hodgkin lymphoma to be distinguished in virtually all problematic cases.

It is also clinically important to distinguish between ALCL, ALK- and cutaneous ALCL because the latter pathologic condition has a more favorable prognosis. However, given the similar morphologic and immunophenotypic features between the two entities, their distinction mainly relies on correlation of clinical findings and staging procedures.

Finally, it should be pointed out that cases of ALCL, ALK- growing within the sinuses or showing a "cohesive" pattern may mimic carcinoma. In this instance, the differential diagnosis is mainly based on cytokeratin immunostaining (consistently negative in ALCL) because the CD30 molecule may be expressed in some carcinomas (6). Immunohistochemistry easily distinguishes between ALCL and malignant fibrous histiocytoma because the latter consistently lacks CD30 and other lymphoid markers (6,36).

Genetics and Molecular Pathogenesis

A T-cell receptor clonal rearrangement can be documented in most ALK-negative ALCL, regardless of T-cell marker expression status (51). Comparative genomic hybridization reveals different genetic aberrations in systemic ALK-negative versus ALK-positive ALCL (119), further supporting the view that they represent different entities. However, no recurrent genetic alteration (e.g., comparable to *ALK* rearrangement) has been identified to date in ALK-negative ALCL.

CLINICAL FEATURES: PRESENTATION, STAGING, AND UNUSUAL SYNDROMES

Overall, systemic ALCL accounts for 3% to 8% of all lymphomas and 10% to 15% of all childhood lymphomas.

Clinically, two distinct forms of primary ALCL are recognized: (a) primary cutaneous ALCL, which belongs to the spectrum of primary cutaneous CD30-positive T-cell lymphoproliferative disorders (120) and shows the phenotype ALK-, CLA+, epithelial membrane antigen/MUC1- (see Chapter 21 of the previous edition of this book); and (b) systemic ALCL, which comprises the two entities (ALK positive and ALK negative) recognized by new WHO classification (21).

The main clinical characteristics described in different series are reported in Table 28.2. Of particular interest are the comparisons within the same prospective study of treatment for ALCL and those with other types of lymphomas, including PTCLs (121,122). In one report (121), 146 patients with ALCL diagnosed based on morphology and CD30 expression were compared with 1,695 patients with diffuse non-ALCL. Both subtypes predominantly affected males <60 years of age. B symptoms were more frequent in patients with ALCL, and a majority of them had disseminated disease, with more skin and mediastinum lesions. Conversely, digestive tract involvement was less common in ALCL. According to that report, ALCL and non-ALCL cases had similar distributions in the different risk groups of the International Prognostic Index (IPI) (123), although a trend toward a lower risk category of the IPI presentation was found in the International Lymphoma Study Group (2). ALCL with T-cell phenotype (ALCL-T) had a higher rate of skin involvement, less disseminated disease, and lower lactate dehydrogenase (LDH) level when compared with B- and null cell ALCL. When compared with other non-ALCL T-cell lymphomas, the same trend was found. In addition, ALCL-T had less frequent bone marrow involvement or extranodal localizations, leading to an IPI score distribution with 39% having zero factors and 24% with only one factor (122).

Significant clinicopathologic differences have been found between ALK+ and ALK- ALCLs in most studies (22,124–127) (Table 28.2). ALCL, ALK+ mostly occurs in the first 3 decades of life, whereas ALCL, ALK- is much more frequent in older patients. B symptoms were observed in both groups, and patients with ALCL, ALK+ had significantly better performance status, and fewer had above normal LDH levels. Patients in both groups showed a nodal presentation, and >40% of children with disseminated disease had inguinal lymph node involvement. Mediastinal involvement was less common than in Hodgkin lymphoma. Skin, bone, and soft tissues were commonly affected extranodal sites. Pelvic muscle involvement is not infrequent and can be mistaken for a soft tissue sarcoma. Central nervous system involvement seems rare in adults and especially in children with ALK-positive ALCL. Bone marrow involvement is considered to be an uncommon event and can be difficult to detect on routine histologic examinations alone (32). In a series of 42 patients with ALCL, 17% had positive bone marrow with conventional examination. However, after immunohistochemical analysis, occult malignant cells were detected in 23% of the patients with negative bone marrow biopsies on routine histology (128). The only way to detect these cells is by immunocytochemical labeling with anti-CD30 and anti-ALK antibodies (128,129) or by reverse transcriptase-PCR for NPM-ALK (130). Using the latter method, bone marrow was positive in 47.5% of the 80 patients investigated. Results in bone marrow and peripheral blood strongly correlated. Positivity was correlated with clinical stage, mediastinal or

TABLE 28.2

ALCL: CLINICAL CHARACTERISTICS AND COMPARISON WITH NON-ALCL OR T-CELL LYMPHOMA

Reference	Histology subtype	No. of patients	Age (%)	M/F (%)	Stage I-II/III-IV (%)	PS >1 (%)	LDH >N (%)	B symptoms (%)	IPI 0-1 (%)	IPI ≥2 (%)	Skin involvement (%)	Bone involvement (%)	BM (%)	Med (%)
Tilly et al., 1997 (121)	ALCL CD30+	146	≤60 y (73)	64/36	40/60	27	47	53	62	33	15	8	14	38
Gisselbrecht et al., 1998 (122)	Non-ALCL B + T	1,695	≤60 y (58)	54/46	42/58	25	52	40	57	36	6	8	16	—
	Non-ALCL-T	228	≤60 y (76)	68/32	14/86	30	55	48	22	77	18	—	36	—
Suzuki et al., 2000 (126)	ALCL-T	60	≤60 y (75)	73/27	37/63	20	33	57	63	37	25	—	13	—
	ALK+	83	≤30 y (87)	63/37	34/66	19	41	54	78	22	21	12	11	6
	ALK−	60	≤30 y (21)	75/25	31/69	33	60	55	57	40	32	5	20	12
Falini et al., 1999 (32)	ALK+	53	≤35 y (88)	75/25	28/72	47	38	76	47	47	21	17	11	—
	ALK−	25	≤35 y (60)	48/52	56/44	28	40	60	68	28	4	4	0	—
Gascoyne et al., 1999 (124)	ALK+	36	≤60 y (51)	—	NA	28	36	—	—	—	—	—	—	—
	ALK−	34	≤60 y (52)	—	NA	41	50	—	—	—	—	—	—	—
Savage et al., 2008 (127)	ALCL	159	<60 y											
	ALK+	87	(86)	55/32	35/75	35	37	60	49	41	8	—	12	—
	ALK−	72	(58)	43/29	42/58	30	46	52	51	59	17	—	7	—
Seidemann et al., 2001 (136)	ALK+	35	≤17 y (100)	68/32	31/69	—	91	57	NA	—	11	17	—	26
Brugières et al., 1998 (135)	ALK−	8	≤17 y (100)	62/38	62/38	—	100	38	NA	NA	13	13	—	25
	ALK+ (93%)	82	≤17 y (100)	56/44	34/66	—	16	68	NA	NA	33	12	16	39
Brugières et al., 2009 (154)	ALCL	352	<16 y (94)	211/141	39/60	NA	NA	NA	47	53	19	19	12	47
	ALK+ 96%			41										
Le Deley et al., 2008 (193)	ALCL	225	≤17 y	140/85	25/75	NA	10 (>2 N)	54	NA	NA	26	14	8	36
	ALK+ (90%)		(100)											
Rosolen et al., 2005 (151)	ALCL	34	<15 y	18/16	29/70	NA	26	NA	NA	NA	12	24	6	47
	ALK+ (NA)													

BM, bone marrow; Med, mediastinum; M/F, male/female; N, normal; NA, not available; PS, performance status.
Adapted from Stein H, Mason DY, Gerdes J, et al. The expression of the Hodgkin's disease associated antigen Ki-1 in reactive and neoplastic lymphoid tissue: evidence that Reed-Sternberg cells and histiocytic malignancies are derived from activated lymphoid cells. *Blood* 1985;66:848–858.

visceral involvement. Moreover, positivity was associated with the cumulative incidence of relapse of 50% for the 38 patients with a positive PCR and 15% for the 42 with a negative one (130). Prominent leukemic involvement in ALCL is rare, it is usually observed in patients with the "small cell morphological variant," and carries a poor prognosis (131–134). The ALCL, ALK+ group was accorded lower IPI scores than was the ALCL, ALK- group. ALK expression is closely correlated with age and IPI. Clinical findings, such as those described for adult ALCL, ALK+ had been described in pediatric patients (135,136). In one report (135) on patients <17 years of age, 93% of patients with ALCL had ALK+ ALCL. Although not fully investigated in all series, ALK expression was high in young patients. Therefore, the entity, ALK+ ALCL, transcends the arbitrary boundaries of 15 or 20 years of age, so that there seems to be no good reason to divide this disease into pediatric and adult categories.

ALCL, ALK+ is rare in patients after transplant (137) and those infected with human immunodeficiency virus (138,139). In this setting, most ALCL cases appear to be related to the anaplastic variant of diffuse large cell B-cell lymphoma (138). Nevertheless, four of the eight cases of human immunodeficiency virus-associated ALCL reported in a New York series (140) had T-cell phenotype. Unfortunately, no information about ALK expression was available in these cases. Their prognosis was mainly determined by the immune status of the patient. An association between breast ALK-negative ALCL and silicone breast prostheses has recently been suggested (141), but these epidemiologic findings need to be confirmed in further studies.

Secondary ALCL may arise in the progression of other lymphomas, most commonly during the course of mycosis fungoides, PTCLs, Hodgkin lymphoma, or lymphomatoid papulosis (26), and is usually characterized by a poor prognosis (142).

Prognostic and Predictive Factors

The complete remission rate is generally higher for patients with ALCL than for those without ALCL (121). In patients with ALCL, survival is significantly longer than in those without ALCL. Multivariate analysis identified the anaplastic histology as an independent factor for survival. Moreover, patients with ALCL-T had significantly better survival than did those with non-ALCL large cell T-cell lymphoma (122,143) (Fig. 28.2). Event-free survival (EFS) and overall survival (OS) of the patients with ALCL with B-cell phenotype were reported to be similar to those of the ALCL T/null cases (121,124). The results obtained with large populations recognized low IPI as having positive prognostic value (32,121,126,127). The value of histology type remains an independent parameter according to multivariate analysis integrating histology along with the other parameters. Shiota et al. (125) reported a significant prognostic difference between ALK+ and ALK-ALCL, with the former having a far better 5-year survival rate (80%) than the latter (33%). This finding was subsequently confirmed by several other reports (32,124,126,127) (Fig. 28.3), except in children, because almost all of them have ALK+ ALCL.

Comparison of ALK-positive versus ALK-negative ALCL in adult patients identified risk groups described in the IPI

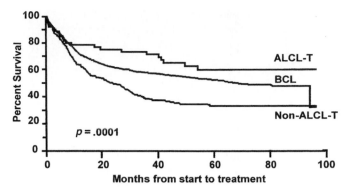

FIGURE 28.2 OS of 228 patients without ALCL-T and 60 with ALCL-T compared with 1,595 patients with diffuse BCL (B-cell lymphoma). (Adapted from Gisselbrecht C, Gaulard P, Lepage E, et al. Prognostic significance of T-cell phenotype in aggressive non-Hodgkin's lymphomas. Groupe d'Etudes des Lymphomes de l'Adulte (GELA). *Blood* 1998;92:76–82, with permission.)

with a significant difference in favor of patients with ALK+, although those with an IPI score of three were in the poor risk regardless of ALK status (127) (Fig. 28.4). The T cell prognostic index for T cell (PIT) (144) was predictive of OS and failure-free survival in both groups. These clinical findings further support the inclusion of ALCL, ALK+ as a distinct entity in the new WHO classification.

Interestingly, comparison of ALK+ and ALK- ALCL in patients >40 years of age revealed no difference in survival (127), suggesting that age is a prominent factor driving outcome difference. Suzuki et al. (126) found CD56 expression to be a prognostic factor independent of IPI and ALK expression in multivariate analysis. In fact, in both ALK+ and ALK- subgroups, CD56+ cases showed a poorer prognosis than did CD56- cases. In the large series of adults from the International Peripheral T-Cell Lymphoma Project (127), the biologic factors tested (CD8+ background and CD56 expression) did not reach statistical significance. Given the fact that survivin is a target of the signal transduction and activator of transcription 3 signaling pathway and is activated in ALCL, survivin expression was evaluated in 62 patients with ALCL: 30 with ALK+ and 32 with ALK- (145). Survivin was expressed in 34 patients and did not correlate with ALK expression. Survival was worse for patients with survivin for those with both ALK+ or ALK-. In multivariate analysis, this was an independent adverse prognostic factor. It is also possible that differences in expression of apoptosis-inhibiting proteins (146) might be responsible for the better prognosis of ALK+ as compared with ALK- ALCL.

Several series of childhood and adult ALCL have been reported, but they were often difficult to compare because of problems in defining entities, the heterogeneity of the treatments, or the lack of a common staging system (135,136,147–154). St. Jude's Hospital's classification has been used only for children, whereas the Ann Arbor staging system and the IPI scoring are used for adults.

Although ALK absence or presence in ALCL is useful, in association with the IPI score, for discriminating a patient's prognosis and to evaluate the impact of treatment in adult patients, it is not applicable for children because 90% of ALCLs at this age are ALK positive (135). The European Intergroup Study of ALCL (147) compared the results and prognoses of 225 children enrolled in trials designed to treat

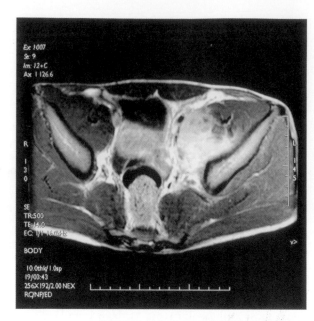
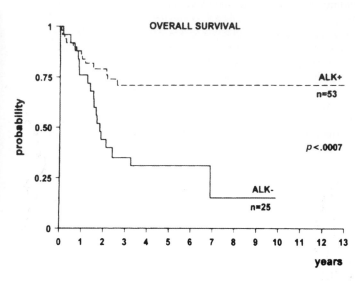

FIGURE 28.3 ALK+ ALCL: RNM image and survival curve. **Left:** Involvement of the left obturatory muscle in a 24-year-old patient with ALK+ ALCL (nuclear magnetic resonance). **Right:** ALK-positive ALCL shows better survival than ALK-negative ALCL. (Courtesy of Falini B, Pileri S, Zinzani PL, et al. ALK+ lymphoma: clinico-pathological findings and outcome. *Blood* 1999;93:2697–2706, with permission.)

childhood ALCL with short and intensive chemotherapy, similar to that used for B-cell lymphoma from the Berlin-Frankfurt-Munster group (88 patients), the French Society of Pediatric Oncology (82 patients), and the United Kingdom Childhood group (55 patients). Multivariate analysis adjusted for country has brought to light three prognostic factors: (a) mediastinal involvement; (b) visceral involvement defined as spleen, lung, or liver involvement; and (c) skin lesions. For the good prognosis group with no factors, the 5-year EFS was 89%; for the poor-risk group with at least two factors, the expected 5-year OS was 61% (147).

Treatment

In most European studies, ALCL is considered to be a separate entity, and is treated with either a short and intensive chemotherapy regimen, as for B-cell lymphoma (136,155), or with more prolonged chemotherapy derived from T-cell lymphoma protocols (156,157). However, North Americans treated all large cell lymphomas with the same chemotherapy regimen regardless of the histologic subgroup and immunophenotype (148,158). The opportunity to classify a case as either ALK-positive or ALK-negative ALCL according to the criteria of the new WHO classification, and to stratify patients into low- and high-risk categories, according to IPI score, is highly relevant for the design of optimal therapeutic strategies. This concept is particularly applicable to children, whose treatment has mainly been based on the highly aggressive regimens used for lymphoblastic leukemia and lymphoma. The low frequency (<5%) of central nervous system involvement by ALCL, ALK+ also calls into question the general policy of intrathecal prophylaxis, especially in children protocols.

Due to the relatively high frequency of ALCL in childhood, prospective nonrandomized studies have been per-

formed. Reports include generally successive protocols with stratification according to stage in Germany (Berlin-Frankfurt-Munster group) or the United States, whereas all patients received the same treatment regardless of stage in France (French Society of Pediatric Oncology). No randomized studies comparing different regimens have been reported so far. The main results obtained for children and adults are reported in Table 28.3. For the Berlin-Frankfurt-Munster group, after a cytoreductive prephase, treatment was stratified into three branches: nine patients in K1 (stage I and II resected) received three 5-day cycles (methotrexate [MTX] 0.5 g per m², dexamethasone, oxazaphorins, etoposide, cytarabine, doxorubicin, and intrathecal therapy); 65 patients in K2 (stage II nonresected and stage III) received six cycles without additional radiotherapy; and 14 patients in K3 (stage IV or multifocal bone disease) received six intensified cycles, including MTX 5 g per m² and high-dose cytarabine/etoposide. K1, K2, and K3 had similar 5-year EFS rates at 76%, 73%, and 79%, respectively (136). Therapy results of that study were similar to data previously obtained from 62 patients treated in earlier studies (155). Treatment lasted 2 months for localized resected stage I and II disease and 5 months for K3. In the French experience, after a cytoreductive prephase, children (135) received two cycles of MTX, cyclophosphamide, doxorubicin, vincristine, and prednisone, and 5 to 7 months of maintenance; radiotherapy was not used in localized stages. For all 82 children, the 3-year event-free survival rate was 66%, with a 3-year event-free survival rate of 47% for the 46 patients in the high-risk group, differing significantly from the 95% rate for the 29 children at low risk. The 18 children treated at St. Jude's Hospital (158) with six cycles of (cyclophosphamide, hydroxydaunorubicin, Oncovin [vincristine], and prednisone) (CHOP)-like regimens achieved a 5-year event-free survival rate of 75% for limited stages and 57% for extended stages. The results obtained in

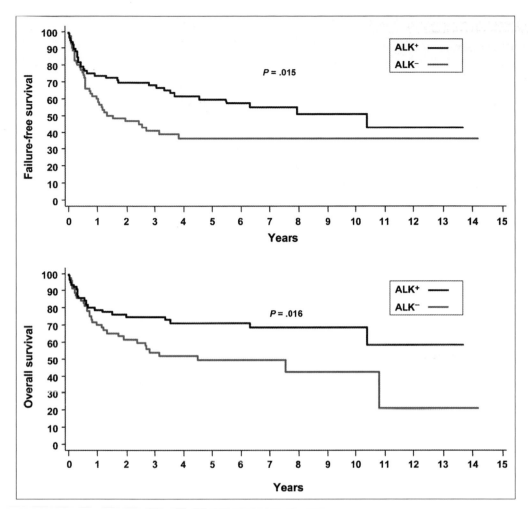

FIGURE 28.4 Survival systemic ALCL. **A:** Failure-free survival of ALK+ and ALK- ALCL. **B:** OS of ALK+ and ALK- ALCL. (Adapted from Savage KJ, Harris NL, Vose JM, et al. ALK- anaplastic large-cell lymphoma is clinically and immunophenotypically different from both ALK+ ALCL and peripheral T-cell lymphoma, not otherwise specified: report from the International Peripheral T-Cell Lymphoma Project. *Blood* 2008;111:5496–5504, with permission.)

86 pediatric ALCLs by the Pediatric Oncology Group, with protocols based on doxorubicin-prednisone-vincristine with intrathecal triple injections but without high-dose MTX, seem similar (153).

However, it must be kept in mind that those studies included variable and often small numbers of patients in each category, and no treatment was found superior to any other. Nevertheless, the impressive results obtained by the Berlin-Frankfurt-Munster group with low-cumulative doses of critical drugs, such as anthracyclines, were the basis of the largest international study completed on 352 pediatric and adolescent patients (154).

The overall complete remission rate was 88%, with a 2-year EFS of 74% and OS of 92% (Fig. 28.5). There was no significant difference in efficacy in terms of risk groups as defined by stage according to St. Jude and Ann Arbor or adverse factors for high risk group if they had at least one risk factor defined as the presence of skin, and/or mediastinal and/or visceral involvement (defined as lung, liver or spleen involvement) and standard risk if they had no risk factors.

No large comparative studies of adults have been published. Most investigators reported that the ALCL response rate to chemotherapy was good, ranging from 60% to 90%. Patients generally received the same treatment as that prescribed for diffuse large cell lymphoma, according to the policy of the institution or in prospective trials. Due to the retrospective nature of the data, the same debate on whether CHOP is the standard of treatment for lymphoma can be reproduced. In one study, 40 cases of Hodgkin-like ALCL were randomized to receive Hodgkin-type chemotherapy (Adriamycin [doxorubicin], bleomycin, vinblastine, and dacarbazine) or lymphoma treatment (MTX, Adriamycin [doxorubicin], cyclophosphamide, Oncovin [vincristine], prednisone, and bleomycin), and it was concluded that the two regimens were equivalent (159). Retrospectively, interpretation of these data is difficult because most cases that in the past were classified as "anaplastic large-cell lymphoma Hodgkin's like," are now thought to represent examples of classic Hodgkin lymphoma rich in tumor cells.

The OS of patients with localized stage without adverse IPI factors is known to exceed 90%. As in other adult studies, and in contrast to those in children, patients with more localized stages received radiotherapy. Patients with more advanced-stage disease frequently had relapse, and their

TABLE 28.3

ALCL: EVOLUTION AND TREATMENTS REPORTED

Authors	Histology subtype	No. of patients	Treatment	CR rate (%)	5-y survival (%)	ALK+/ALK- survival (%)	Risk factor (IPI): 5-y survival (%)			Prognostic factor (Cox model)
							0	1	2+	
Tilly et al., 1997 (121)	ALCL CD30+ T/B/Null	146	Dose-adjusted chemotherapy	75	66	Not done	82	78	50	IPI
	Non-ALCL B + T cells	1,695	CHOP/ACVB ASCT without RT	61	48	Not done	69	47	34	ALCL
Gisselbrecht et al., 1998 (122)	T-non-ALCL	228	idem	49	35	Not done	64	56	34	IPI
Zinzani et al., 1998 (159)	ALCL-HL	90	ABVD MACOP-B	73	60	Not available	—	—	—	Bulk/stage B symptoms
Suzuki et al., 2000 (126)	ALCL ALK+, ALK-	139	CHOP-like regimen	72	Not precise	Significantly different	—	—	—	ALK
Gascoyne et al., 1999 (124)	ALK+, ALK-	70	CHOP-like ± RT	NA	65	79/46	85	69	37	IPI/ALK
Falini et al., 1999 (32)	ALK+, ALK-	96	CHOP-like ±RT	72	—	71/15	94 (0–1)	—	41 (2+)	IPI/ALK
Savage et al., 2008 (127)	ALK+ ALK- Adult	87 / 72	Multiple Adult Regimen	88 ORR / 76 ORR	70 / 49	60 PFS / 36	80 (0–1) / 62 (0–1)		220 (3) / 116 (3)	Anemia IPI PIT
Seidemann et al., 2001 (136)	Pediatric	89	Dose duration	NA	76	NA	—	—	—	B symptoms
Brugieres et al., 1998 (135)	Pediatric ALK+ 93%	82	COPADM	95 (EFS)	66	NA	NA	NA	NA	Mediastinum, ENS, LDH[a]
Le Deley et al., 2007 (193)	Pediatric	225	BFM	88	81	NA	PFS 0 risk	89	OS 94	Mediastinal, skin, ENS
	ALK+ 90%		SFOP UK CCSG			PFS 71%	risk 1-3	61	OS 73	
Rosolen et al., 2005 (151)	Pediatric ALK+	34	LSA-L2 Modify	88	85	EFS 65%	NN A			No factor
Brugières et al., 2009 (154)	Pediatric ALK+ 96%	352	NHL BFM90 ALCL-R1	88	92 2 y	—		Similar	Non	No significant

ABVD, Adriamycin (doxorubicin), bleomycin, vincristine, and dacarbazine; ACVB, Adriamycin (doxorubicin), cyclophosphamide, vindesine, bleomycin, and prednisone; ASCT, autologous stem cell transplantation;COPADM, cyclophosphamide, prednisone, and MTX CR, complete remission; ENS, extranodal sites; HL, Hodgkin like; MACOP-B, MTX, Adriamycin (doxorubicin), cyclophosphamide, Oncovin (vincristine), prednisone, and bleomycin; NA, not available; ORR, overall response rate; RT, radiotherapy.

[a]IPI not used; replaced by prognostic factors mediastinum, extranodal sites, and LDH. Absent, low risk; 1 present, high risk (5-yr survival: 95% for low-risk and 47% for high-risk groups).

Adapted from Stein H, Mason DY, Gerdes J, et al. The expression of the Hodgkin's disease associated antigen Ki-1 in reactive and neoplastic lymphoid tissue: evidence that Reed-Sternberg cells and histiocytic malignancies are derived from activated lymphoid cells. Blood 1985;66:843–858.

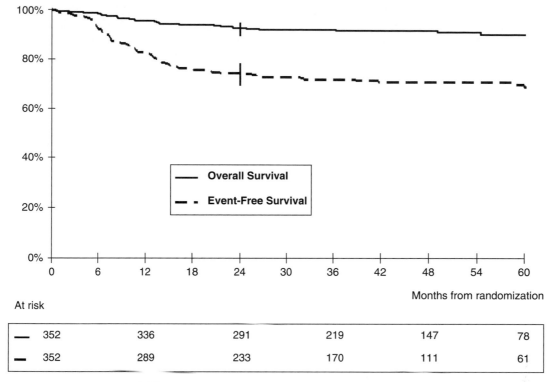

At risk

___ 352	336	291	219	147	78
▬ 352	289	233	170	111	61

FIGURE 28.5 EFS and OS of the whole study population and by treatment group. (Adapted from Brugières L, Le Deley MC, Rosolen A, et al. Impact of the methotrexate administration dose on the need for intrathecal treatment in children and adolescents with anaplastic large-cell lymphoma: results of a randomized trial of the EICNHL Group. *J Clin Oncol* 2009;27:897–903, with permission.)

prognosis, in comparison to that of patients with other large cell lymphomas, is controversial. Although a few studies have suggested that advanced-stage ALCL may have short disease-free survival and may require more intensive therapy (160,161), most investigators consider that ALCLs generally behave like high-grade lymphomas (133,162). However, several comparative studies on diffuse large cell lymphomas showed an association between CD30 expression and a favorable outcome (29,121,163–165) when patients were treated with chemotherapy regimens similar to those used for other types of lymphomas (e.g., CHOP). According to the Groupe d'Etude des Lymphomes de l'Adulte study (121), which included T/null- and B-cell ALCL, the 5-year OS rate for patients without adverse IPI factors was 82%, as compared with 78% for patients with one factor, 50% for the high-intermediate–risk group, and 25% for the high-risk group. Dose-intensive treatments have been used in this study according to initial stratification based on prognostic factors. However, in that investigation, stratification according to ALK positivity had not been done, and results may also reflect the different percentage of ALK+ lymphomas in adults. The age-adjusted IPI within the good prognosis group of ALK+ lymphomas showed that the 5-year OS rate was 94% for patients with no or one factor versus 41% for those with two or more factors (32). Although ALK positivity is considered a marker of better prognosis, patients with two or more IPI factors still have a poor prognosis (32), and new approaches are needed, and comparison with pediatric protocol should be made (154).

Systematic intensification of chemotherapy with the use of autologous stem cell support has been investigated in some institutions as part of a program designed for aggressive lymphoma (166–168). However, the good results observed in most series might be only reflecting the chemosensitivity of the disease, and consolidation has only a limited role if patients achieve complete remission. One study (166) described 16 consecutive ALCL cases, seven of which had an IPI score greater than or equal to two, autografted in first-line therapy with impressive 100% disease-free and OS rates at a median of 45 months. The other publication (167) on 15 patients, six with an IPI score greater than or equal to two and seven patients with ALK+ disease, reported a 5-year OS rate of 69%. In a retrospective study by the European Bone Marrow Transplantation group, the same authors reported on 64 patients with ALCL-T autografted during their treatment course, but the heterogeneity of patients and their therapeutic modalities prevented a clear appreciation of the role of autologous stem cell support (161).

In addition, the number of patients with severe adverse factors was too small to extrapolate from these favorable results a set of recommendations differing from those advocated by the Consensus Conference on Aggressive Lymphoma (169). Considering the response rate and the survival of patients with ALK-positive lymphoma, consolidation with autologous stem cell transplantation is not recommended if patients achieve a complete remission. For patients with ALK-negative lymphoma, the debate is still open for patients with at least two IPI adverse prognostic factors who can be considered for prospective study.

Guidelines for the treatment of ALCL in the absence of large prospective studies in adults are not easy. Two factors should be taken in consideration: ALK positivity and adverse prognostic factors. Dose and duration of treatment without radiotherapy have been adjusted in children; 90% have ALK-positive disease according to their aforementioned prognostic factors. The same recommendations can be made for adult patients with ALK+ lymphoma using the IPI as prognosis indicator, although the place of radiotherapy will remain controversial in localized stages (170,171). Comparison between CHOP and pediatric regimens could be of interest in the future.

Relapses occurred most frequently at the site of the primary tumor; however, involvement of new tumor sites distant from the initial manifestations was also observed frequently (135,136). Local recurrences of initial manifestations raise the question of additional local therapy with irradiation, as for other types of lymphomas. Questions not fully resolved by randomized studies include those of the potential late risks of radiotherapy and the fact that relapses may occur in new sites. As for other relapses, high-dose therapy with autologous stem cell support should be proposed to patients (161) chemosensitive to salvage chemotherapy. In the report from the Grupo Español de Linfomas/Trasplante Autólogo de Médula Osea on 115 PTCLs, 22% had ALCL, and the authors report that there was no difference in the outcome when compared with other T-cell subtypes (172,173). Generally, the ALK status is not fully reported in the different series, but data on limited numbers suggest that salvage with autologous stem cell transplantation is less efficient in patients with ALK-negative disease(174).

The role of allogeneic transplantation in patients with relapse is not extensively determined as in other aggressive lymphomas but might be easier to investigate in this young population and has been performed in children (175). Notably, allogeneic transplantation has emerged as a potentially useful treatment also for adult patients with relapsed or refractory ALK-positive ALCL (176–178). The major problem with interpretation of transplant data in ALCL is that studies have been mainly conducted in small cohorts of patients with T-cell lymphomas, including a few cases of ALCL, frequently not well characterized pathologically and in terms of ALK expression. For patients transplanted with a conventional myeloablative regimen, treatment-related mortality is high, reaching in registry data 42%. In the Japanese survey, in 233 patients there were 56 T-cell lymphomas allografted, including seven ALCLs. No difference was observed between the PTCL and non-PTCL (179).

In the French experience of 77 T-cell lymphomas treated with the myeloablative (74%) and nonmyeloablative regimen (26%), including 27 cases of ALCL (180), the 5-year OS was 55% and not different from the other histologic T subtypes. The transplant-related mortality was still high: 34% at 5 years. They observed a trend of longer OS and EFS for patients with ALCL, angioimmunoblastic T-cell lymphoma, or PTCL than for the so-called "other histopathologic subtypes" (180). Encouraging results have been reported with a reduction of transplant-related mortality down to 6% in the nonmyeloablative conditioning regimen (181), with a 3-year PFS of 64%.

Future Therapeutic Perspectives

It will also be important to look at the efficacy of innovative forms of therapy for ALK-positive ALCL with high IPI scores and for ALK-negative ALCL. Anti-CD30 monoclonal antibodies conjugated to toxins (116) or radioisotopes or vaccination strategies (182,183) may represent new tools. In the past years, multiple different antibodies to human CD30 have been generated. A fully human anti-CD30 immunoglobulin G1 antibody (MDX 060) that inhibits growth of CD30-expressing tumor cells in preclinical models was tested in 72 patients with relapsed or refractory CD30+ tumors, including seven cases of ALCL. Clinical responses were observed in six patients: four complete (including two ALCLs with predominantly skin disease) and two partial (in patients with Hodgkin lymphoma) (184). No information is provided by the authors of whether the responsive ALCL cases were ALK positive or negative. Using a chimeric monoclonal antibody SGN-30 (185) in a phase I study, including 24 patients with Hodgkin lymphoma and three with ALCL, a complete response was seen in one case of cutaneous ALCL. The use of drugs inhibiting NPM-ALK activity (186–189) or interfering with the downstream signaling pathways (190–192) may also be expected to play a future role in the therapy of ALK-positive ALCL.

References

1. Stein H, Mason DY, Gerdes J, et al. The expression of the Hodgkin's disease associated antigen Ki-1 in reactive and neoplastic lymphoid tissue: evidence that Reed-Sternberg cells and histiocytic malignancies are derived from activated lymphoid cells. *Blood* 1985;66:848–858.
2. Harris NL, Jaffe ES, Stein H, et al. A revised European-American classification of lymphoid neoplasms: a proposal from the International Lymphoma Study Group. *Blood* 1994;84:1361–1392.
3. Delsol G, Ralfkier E, Stein H, et al. Anaplastic large cell lymphoma. In: Jaffe ES, World Health Organization, eds. *Pathology and genetics of tumours of haematopoietic and lymphoid tissues.* Lyon, France: IARC Press, 2001:230–235.
4. Schwab U, Stein H, Gerdes J, et al. Production of a monoclonal antibody specific for Hodgkin and Sternberg- Reed cells of Hodgkin's disease and a subset of normal lymphoid cells. *Nature* 1982;299:65–67.
5. Durkop H, Latza U, Hummel M, et al. Molecular cloning and expression of a new member of the nerve growth factor receptor family that is characteristic for Hodgkin's disease. *Cell* 1992;68:421–427.
6. Falini B, Pileri S, Pizzolo G, et al. CD30 (Ki 1) molecule: a new cytokine receptor of the tumor necrosis factor receptor superfamily as a tool for diagnosis and immunotherapy. *Blood* 1995;85:1–14.
7. Benz-Lemoine E, Brizard A, Huret JL, et al. Malignant histiocytosis: a specific t(2;5)(p23;q35) translocation? Review of the literature. *Blood* 1988;72:1045–1047.
8. Kaneko Y, Frizzera G, Edamura S, et al. A novel translocation, t(2;5)(p23;q35), in childhood phagocytic large T-cell lymphoma mimicking malignant histiocytosis. *Blood* 1989;73:806–813.
9. Rimokh R, Magaud JP, Berger F, et al. A translocation involving a specific breakpoint (q35) on chromosome 5 is characteristic of anaplastic large cell lymphoma ('Ki-1 lymphoma'). *Br J Haematol* 1989;71:31–36.
10. Bitter MA, Franklin WA, Larson RA, et al. Morphology in Ki-1(CD30)-positive non-Hodgkin's lymphoma is correlated with clinical features and the presence of a unique chromosomal abnormality, t(2;5)(p23;q35). *Am J Surg Pathol* 1990;14:305–316.
11. Mason DY, Bastard C, Rimokh R, et al. CD30-positive large cell lymphomas ('Ki-1 lymphoma') are associated with a chromosomal translocation involving 5q35. *Br J Haematol* 1990;74:161–168.
12. Morris SW, Kirstein MN, Valentine MB, et al. Fusion of a kinase gene, ALK, to a nucleolar protein gene, NPM, in non-Hodgkin's lymphoma. *Science* 1994;263:1281–1284.
13. Downing JR, Shurtleff SA, Zielenska M, et al. Molecular detection of the (2;5) translocation of non-Hodgkin's lymphoma by reverse transcriptase-polymerase chain reaction. *Blood* 1995;85:3416–3422.
14. Lamant L, Meggetto F, al Saati T, et al. High incidence of the t(2;5)(p23;q35) translocation in anaplastic large cell lymphoma and its lack of detection in Hodgkin's disease. Comparison of cytogenetic analysis, reverse transcriptase-polymerase chain reaction, and P-80 immunostaining. *Blood* 1996;87:284–291.
15. Ladanyi M. The NPM/ALK gene fusion in the pathogenesis of anaplastic large cell lymphoma. *Cancer Surv* 1997;30:59–75.
16. Herbst H, Anagnostopoulos J, Heinze B, et al. ALK gene products in anaplastic large cell lymphomas and Hodgkin's disease. *Blood* 1995;86:1694–1700.

17. Mathew P, Sanger WG, Weisenburger DD, et al. Detection of the t(2;5)(p23;q35) and NPM-ALK fusion in non-Hodgkin's lymphoma by two-color fluorescence in situ hybridization. *Blood* 1997;89:1678–1685.
18. Pulford K, Lamant L, Morris SW, et al. Detection of anaplastic lymphoma kinase (ALK) and nucleolar protein nucleophosmin (NPM)-ALK proteins in normal and neoplastic cells with the monoclonal antibody ALK1. *Blood* 1997;89:1394–1404.
19. Falini B, Bigerna B, Fizzotti M, et al. ALK expression defines a distinct group of T/null lymphomas ("ALK lymphomas") with a wide morphological spectrum. *Am J Pathol* 1998;153:875–886.
20. Chiarle R, Voena C, Ambrogio C, et al. The anaplastic lymphoma kinase in the pathogenesis of cancer. *Nat Rev Cancer* 2008;8:11–23.
21. Delsol G, Falini B, Muller-Hermelink HK, et al. Anaplastic large cell lymphoma (ALCL), ALK-positive. In: Swerdlow SH, et al., eds. *WHO classification of tumours of haematopoietic and lymphoid tissues*, 4th ed. Lyon, France: International Agency for Research on Cancer, 2008:312–316.
22. Falini B, Pulford K, Pucciarini A, et al. Lymphomas expressing ALK fusion protein(s) other than NPM-ALK. *Blood* 1999;94:3509–3515.
23. Bohling SD, Jenson SD, Crockett DK, et al. Analysis of gene expression profile of TPM3-ALK positive anaplastic large cell lymphoma reveals overlapping and unique patterns with that of NPM-ALK positive anaplastic large cell lymphoma. *Leuk Res* 2008;32:383–393.
24. Pileri SA, Pulford K, Mori S, et al. Frequent expression of the NPM-ALK chimeric fusion protein in anaplastic large-cell lymphoma, lympho-histiocytic type. *Am J Pathol* 1997;150:1207–1211.
25. Benharroch D, Meguerian-Bedoyan Z, Lamant L, et al. ALK-positive lymphoma: a single disease with a broad spectrum of morphology. *Blood* 1998;91:2076–2084.
26. Stein H, Foss HD, Durkop H, et al. CD30(+) anaplastic large cell lymphoma: a review of its histopathologic, genetic, and clinical features. *Blood* 2000;96:3681–3695.
27. Falini B, Mason DY. Proteins encoded by genes involved in chromosomal alterations in lymphoma and leukemia: clinical value of their detection by immunocytochemistry. *Blood* 2002;99:409–426.
28. Kadin ME. Anaplastic large cell lymphoma and its morphological variants. *Cancer Surv* 1997;30:77–86.
29. Falini B. Anaplastic large cell lymphoma: pathological, molecular and clinical features. *Br J Haematol* 2001;114:741–760.
30. Ambrogio C, Voena C, Manazza AD, et al. The anaplastic lymphoma kinase controls cell shape and growth of anaplastic large cell lymphoma through Cdc42 activation. *Cancer Res* 2008;68:8899–8907.
31. Kinney MC, Collins RD, Greer JP, et al. A small-cell-predominant variant of primary Ki-1 (CD30)+ T-cell lymphoma. *Am J Surg Pathol* 1993;17:859–868.
32. Falini B, Pileri S, Zinzani PL, et al. ALK+ lymphoma: clinico-pathological findings and outcome. *Blood* 1999;93:2697–2706.
33. Pileri S, Falini B, Delsol G, et al. Lymphohistiocytic T-cell lymphoma (anaplastic large cell lymphoma CD30+/Ki-1+ with a high content of reactive histiocytes). *Histopathology* 1990;16:383–391.
34. Jaffe ES, Harris NL, Diebold J, et al. World Health Organization classification of lymphomas: a work in progress. *Ann Oncol* 1998;9:S25–S30.
35. Vassallo J, Lamant L, Brugieres L, et al. ALK-positive anaplastic large cell lymphoma mimicking nodular sclerosis Hodgkin's lymphoma: report of 10 cases. *Am J Surg Pathol* 2006;30:223–229.
36. Chan JK, Buchanan R, Fletcher CD. Sarcomatoid variant of anaplastic large-cell Ki-1 lymphoma. *Am J Surg Pathol* 1990;14:983–988.
37. Pereira EM, Maeda SA, Reis-Filho JS. Sarcomatoid variant of anaplastic large cell lymphoma mimicking a primary breast cancer: a challenging diagnosis. *Arch Pathol Lab Med* 2002;126:723–726.
38. Mann KP, Hall B, Kamino H, et al. Neutrophil-rich, Ki-1-positive anaplastic large-cell malignant lymphoma. *Am J Surg Pathol* 1995;19:407–416.
39. Cheuk W, Hill RW, Bacchi C, et al. Hypocellular anaplastic large cell lymphoma mimicking inflammatory lesions of lymph nodes. *Am J Surg Pathol* 2000;24:1537–1543.
40. Shiota M, Fujimoto J, Takenaga M, et al. Diagnosis of t(2;5)(p23;q35)-associated Ki-1 lymphoma with immunohistochemistry. *Blood* 1994;84:3648–3652.
41. Cordell JL, Pulford KA, Bigerna B, et al. Detection of normal and chimeric nucleophosmin in human cells. *Blood* 1999;93:632–642.
42. Mason DY, Pulford KA, Bischof D, et al. Nucleolar localization of the nucleophosmin-anaplastic lymphoma kinase is not required for malignant transformation. *Cancer Res* 1998;58:1057–1062.
43. Li G, Salhany KE, Rook AH, et al. The pathogenesis of large cell transformation in cutaneous T-cell lymphoma is not associated with t(2;5)(p23;q35) chromosomal translocation. *J Cutan Pathol* 1997;24:403–408.
44. Falini B, Bigerna B, Pucciarini A, et al. Aberrant subcellular expression of nucleophosmin and NPM-MLF1 fusion protein in acute myeloid leukaemia carrying t(3;5): a comparison with NPMc+ AML. *Leukemia* 2006;20:368–371.
45. Falini B, Mecucci C, Tiacci E, et al. Cytoplasmic nucleophosmin in acute myelogenous leukemia with a normal karyotype. *N Engl J Med* 2005;352:254–266.
46. Pulford K, Falini B, Cordell J, et al. Biochemical detection of novel anaplastic lymphoma kinase proteins in tissue sections of anaplastic large cell lymphoma. *Am J Pathol* 1999;154:1657–1663.
47. Pittaluga S, Wlodarska I, Pulford K, et al. The monoclonal antibody ALK1 identifies a distinct morphological subtype of anaplastic large cell lymphoma associated with 2p23/ALK rearrangements. *Am J Pathol* 1997;151:343–351.
48. Wlodarska I, De Wolf-Peeters C, Falini B, et al. The cryptic inv(2)(p23q35) defines a new molecular genetic subtype of ALK-positive anaplastic large-cell lymphoma. *Blood* 1998;92:2688–2695.
49. Rosenwald A, Ott G, Pulford K, et al. t(1;2)(q21;p23) and t(2;3)(p23;q21): two novel variant translocations of the t(2;5)(p23;q35) in anaplastic large cell lymphoma. *Blood* 1999;94:362–364.
50. Krenacs L, Wellmann A, Sorbara L, et al. Cytotoxic cell antigen expression in anaplastic large cell lymphomas of T- and null cell type and Hodgkin's disease: evidence for distinct cellular origin. *Blood* 1997;89:980–989.
51. Foss HD, Anagnostopoulos I, Araujo I, et al. Anaplastic large-cell lymphomas of T-cell and null-cell phenotype express cytotoxic molecules. *Blood* 1996;88:4005–4011.
52. Delsol G, Al Saati T, Gatter KC, et al. Coexpression of epithelial membrane antigen (EMA), Ki-1, and interleukin-2 receptor by anaplastic large cell lymphomas. Diagnostic value in so-called malignant histiocytosis. *Am J Pathol* 1988;130:59–70.
53. ten Berge RL, Snijdewint FG, von Mensdorff-Pouilly S, et al. MUC1 (EMA) is preferentially expressed by ALK positive anaplastic large cell lymphoma, in the normally glycosylated or only partly hypoglycosylated form. *J Clin Pathol* 2001;54:933–939.
54. Rassidakis GZ, Medeiros LJ, Herling M, et al. BCL-2 is expressed in ALK-negative but not ALK-positive anaplastic large cell lymphoma. *Blood* 2000;96.
55. Raetz EA, Perkins SL, Carlson MA, et al. The nucleophosmin-anaplastic lymphoma kinase fusion protein induces c-Myc expression in pediatric anaplastic large cell lymphomas. *Am J Pathol* 2002;161:875–883.
56. Tan BT, Seo K, Warnke RA, et al. The frequency of immunoglobulin heavy chain gene and T-cell receptor gamma-chain gene rearrangements and Epstein-Barr virus in ALK+ and ALK- anaplastic large cell lymphoma and other peripheral T-cell lymphomas. *J Mol Diagn* 2008;10.502–512.
57. Camisa C, Helm TN, Sexton C, et al. Ki-1-positive anaplastic large-cell lymphoma can mimic benign dermatoses. *J Am Acad Dermatol* 1993;29:696–700.
58. Simonart T, Kentos A, Renoirte C, et al. Cutaneous involvement by neutrophil-rich, CD30-positive anaplastic large cell lymphoma mimicking deep pustules. *Am J Surg Pathol* 1999;23:244–246.
59. Chittal SM, Delsol G. The interface of Hodgkin's disease and anaplastic large cell lymphoma. *Cancer Surv* 1997;30:87–105.
60. Delsol G, Campo E, Gascoyne R. ALK-positive large B-cell lymphoma. In: Swerdlow SH, et al., eds. *WHO classification of tumours of haematopoietic and lymphoid tissues*, 4th ed. Lyon, France: International Agency for Research on Cancer, 2008:254–255.
61. Momose S, Tamaru J, Kishi H, et al. Hyperactivated STAT3 in ALK-positive diffuse large B-cell lymphoma with clathrin-ALK fusion. *Hum Pathol* 2009;40:75–82.
62. Delsol G, Lamant L, Mariame B, et al. A new subtype of large B-cell lymphoma expressing the ALK kinase and lacking the 2; 5 translocation. *Blood* 1997;89:1483–1490.
63. Gascoyne RD, Lamant L, Martin-Subero JI, et al. ALK-positive diffuse large B-cell lymphoma is associated with Clathrin-ALK rearrangements: report of 6 cases. *Blood* 2003;102:2568–2573.
64. Chan JK, Lamant L, Algar E, et al. ALK+ histiocytosis: a novel type of systemic histiocytic proliferative disorder of early infancy. *Blood* 2008;112:2965–2968.
65. Falini B, Flenghi L, Pileri S, et al. PG-M1: a new monoclonal antibody directed against a fixative-resistant epitope on the macrophage-restricted form of the CD68 molecule. *Am J Pathol* 1993;142:1359–1372.
66. Griffin CA, Hawkins AL, Dvorak C, et al. Recurrent involvement of 2p23 in inflammatory myofibroblastic tumors. *Cancer Res* 1999;59:2776–2780.
67. Cessna MH, Zhou H, Sanger WG, et al. Expression of ALK1 and p80 in inflammatory myofibroblastic tumor and its mesenchymal mimics: a study of 135 cases. *Mod Pathol* 2002;15:931–938.
68. Fujimoto J, Shiota M, Iwahara T, et al. Characterization of the transforming activity of p80, a hyperphosphorylated protein in a Ki-1 lymphoma cell line with chromosomal translocation t(2;5). *Proc Natl Acad Sci U S A* 1996;93:4181–4186.
69. Chan PK, Chan FY, Morris SW, et al. Isolation and characterization of the human nucleophosmin/B23 (NPM) gene: identification of the YY1 binding site at the 5' enhancer region. *Nucleic Acids Res* 1997;25:1225–1232.
70. Borer RA, Lehner CF, Eppenberger HM, et al. Major nucleolar proteins shuttle between nucleus and cytoplasm. *Cell* 1989;56:379–390.
71. Okuwaki M, Matsumoto K, Tsujimoto M, et al. Function of nucleophosmin/B23, a nucleolar acidic protein, as a histone chaperone. *FEBS Lett* 2001;506:272–276.
72. Colombo E, Marine JC, Danovi D, et al. Nucleophosmin regulates the stability and transcriptional activity of p53. *Nat Cell Biol* 2002;4:529–533.
73. Grisendi S, Mecucci C, Falini B, et al. Nucleophosmin and cancer. *Nat Rev Cancer* 2006;6:493–505.

74. Lamant L, Dastugue N, Pulford K, et al. A new fusion gene TPM3-ALK in anaplastic large cell lymphoma created by a (1;2)(q25;p23) translocation. *Blood* 1999;93:3088–3095.

75. Siebert R, Gesk S, Harder L, et al. Complex variant translocation t(1;2) with TPM3-ALK fusion due to cryptic ALK gene rearrangement in anaplastic large-cell lymphoma. *Blood* 1999;94:3614–3617.

76. Lawrence B, Perez-Atayde A, Hibbard MK, et al. TPM3-ALK and TPM4-ALK oncogenes in inflammatory myofibroblastic tumors. *Am J Pathol* 2000;157:377–384.

77. Ladanyi M. Aberrant ALK tyrosine kinase signaling. Different cellular lineages, common oncogenic mechanisms. *Am J Pathol* 2000;157:341–345.

78. Hernandez L, Pinyol M, Hernandez S, et al. TRK-fused gene (TFG) is a new partner of ALK in anaplastic large cell lymphoma producing two structurally different TFG-ALK translocations. *Blood* 1999;94:3265–3268.

79. Hernandez L, Bea S, Bellosillo B, et al. Diversity of genomic breakpoints in TFG-ALK translocations in anaplastic large cell lymphomas: identification of a new TFG-ALK(XL) chimeric gene with transforming activity. *Am J Pathol* 2002;160:1487–1494.

80. Colleoni GW, Bridge JA, Garicochea B, et al. ATIC-ALK: a novel variant ALK gene fusion in anaplastic large cell lymphoma resulting from the recurrent cryptic chromosomal inversion, inv(2)(p23q35). *Am J Pathol* 2000;156:781–789.

81. Ma Z, Cools J, Marynen P, et al. Inv(2)(p23q35) in anaplastic large-cell lymphoma induces constitutive anaplastic lymphoma kinase (ALK) tyrosine kinase activation by fusion to ATIC, an enzyme involved in purine nucleotide biosynthesis. *Blood* 2000;95:2144–2149.

82. Trinei M, Lanfrancone L, Campo E, et al. A new variant anaplastic lymphoma kinase (ALK)-fusion protein (ATIC-ALK) in a case of ALK-positive anaplastic large cell lymphoma. *Cancer Res* 2000;60:793–798.

83. Beardsley GP, Rayl EA, Gunn K, et al. Structure and functional relationships in human pur H. *Adv Exp Med Biol* 1998;431:221–226.

84. Touriol C, Greenland C, Lamant L, et al. Further demonstration of the diversity of chromosomal changes involving 2p23 in ALK-positive lymphoma: 2 cases expressing ALK kinase fused to CLTCL (clathrin chain polypeptide-like). *Blood* 2000;95:3204–3207.

85. Meech S, Grump J, McGavran L, et al. Tropomyosin 4 (TPM4) is fused to ALK by a t(2:19)(p23;p13) in an unusual childhood ALCL with the immunophenotype and functional properties of a natural killer cell malignancy. *Blood* 2000;92.

86. Tort F, Pinyol M, Pulford K, et al. Molecular characterization of a new ALK translocation involving moesin (MSN-ALK) in anaplastic large cell lymphoma. *Lab Invest* 2001;81:419–426.

87. Cools J, Wlodarska I, Somers R, et al. Identification of novel fusion partners of ALK, the anaplastic lymphoma kinase, in anaplastic large-cell lymphoma and inflammatory myofibroblastic tumor. *Genes Chromosomes Cancer* 2002;34:354–362.

88. Jazii FR, Najafi Z, Malekzadeh R, et al. Identification of squamous cell carcinoma associated proteins by proteomics and loss of beta tropomyosin expression in esophageal cancer. *World J Gastroenterol* 2006;12:7104–7112.

89. Du XL, Hu H, Lin DC, et al. Proteomic profiling of proteins dysregulated in Chinese esophageal squamous cell carcinoma. *J Mol Med* 2007;85:863–875.

90. Soda M, Choi YL, Enomoto M, et al. Identification of the transforming EML4-ALK fusion gene in non-small-cell lung cancer. *Nature* 2007;448:561–566.

91. Martelli MP, Sozzi G, Hernandez L, et al. EML4-ALK rearrangement in non-small-cell lung cancer and non-tumor lung tissues. *Am J Pathol* 2009;174:661–670.

92. Chen Y, Takita J, Choi YL, et al. Oncogenic mutations of ALK kinase in neuroblastoma. *Nature* 2008;455:971–974.

93. Janoueix-Lerosey I, Lequin D, Brugieres L, et al. Somatic and germline activating mutations of the ALK kinase receptor in neuroblastoma. *Nature* 2008;455:967–970.

94. George RE, Sanda T, Hanna M, et al. Activating mutations in ALK provide a therapeutic target in neuroblastoma. *Nature* 2008;455:975–978.

95. Duyster J, Bai RY, Morris SW. Translocations involving anaplastic lymphoma kinase (ALK). *Oncogene* 2001;20:5623–5637.

96. Kuefer MU, Look AT, Pulford K, et al. Retrovirus-mediated gene transfer of NPM-ALK causes lymphoid malignancy in mice. *Blood* 1997;90:2901–2910.

97. Miething C, Peschel C, Duyster J. Targeting the oncogenic tyrosine kinase NPM-ALK in lymphoma: the role of murine models in defining pathogenesis and treatment options. *Curr Drug Targets* 2006;7:1329–1334.

98. Bischof D, Pulford K, Mason DY, et al. Role of the nucleophosmin (NPM) portion of the non-Hodgkin's lymphoma- associated NPM-anaplastic lymphoma kinase fusion protein in oncogenesis. *Mol Cell Biol* 1997;17:2312–2325.

99. Pulford K, Mason DY. CD246 antigen. In: Mason DY, International Workshop and Conference on Human Leucocyte Differentiation Antigens, eds. *Leucocyte typing VII: white cell differentiation antigens: proceedings of the Seventh International Workshop and Conference held in Harrogate, United Kingdom.* Oxford, UK: Oxford University Press, 2002.

100. Shiota M, Fujimoto J, Semba T, et al. Hyperphosphorylation of a novel 80 kDa protein-tyrosine kinase similar to Ltk in a human Ki-1 lymphoma cell line, AMS3. *Oncogene* 1994;9:1567–1574.

101. Morris SW, Naeve C, Mathew P, et al. ALK, the chromosome 2 gene locus altered by the t(2;5) in non-Hodgkin's lymphoma, encodes a novel neural receptor tyrosine kinase that is highly related to leukocyte tyrosine kinase (LTK). *Oncogene* 1997;14:2175–2188.

102. Powers C, Aigner A, Stoica GE, et al. Pleiotrophin signaling through anaplastic lymphoma kinase is rate- limiting for glioblastoma growth. *J Biol Chem* 2002;277:14153–14158.

103. Stoica GE, Kuo A, Powers C, et al. Midkine binds to anaplastic lymphoma kinase (ALK) and acts as a growth factor for different cell types. *J Biol Chem* 2002;277:35990–35998.

104. Allouche M. ALK is a novel dependence receptor: potential implications in development and cancer. *Cell Cycle* 2007;6:1533–1538.

105. Iwahara T, Fujimoto J, Wen D, et al. Molecular characterization of ALK, a receptor tyrosine kinase expressed specifically in the nervous system. *Oncogene* 1997;14:439–449.

106. Bilsland JG, Wheeldon A, Mead A, et al. Behavioral and neurochemical alterations in mice deficient in anaplastic lymphoma kinase suggest therapeutic potential for psychiatric indications. *Neuropsychopharmacology* 2008;33:685–700.

107. Kunugi H, Hashimoto R, Okada T, et al. Possible association between nonsynonymous polymorphisms of the anaplastic lymphoma kinase (ALK) gene and schizophrenia in a Japanese population. *J Neural Transm* 2006;113:1569–1573.

108. Bai RY, Dieter P, Peschel C, et al. Nucleophosmin-anaplastic lymphoma kinase of large-cell anaplastic lymphoma is a constitutively active tyrosine kinase that utilizes phospholipase C-gamma to mediate its mitogenicity. *Mol Cell Biol* 1998;18:6951–6961.

109. Slupianek A, Nieborowska-Skorska M, Hoser G, et al. Role of phosphatidylinositol 3-kinase-Akt pathway in nucleophosmin/anaplastic lymphoma kinase-mediated lymphomagenesis. *Cancer Res* 2001;61:2194–2199.

110. Bai RY, Ouyang T, Miething C, et al. Nucleophosmin-anaplastic lymphoma kinase associated with anaplastic large-cell lymphoma activates the phosphatidylinositol 3-kinase/Akt antiapoptotic signaling pathway. *Blood* 2000;96:4319–4327.

111. Zhang Q, Raghunath PN, Xue L, et al. Multilevel dysregulation of STAT3 activation in anaplastic lymphoma kinase-positive T/null-cell lymphoma. *J Immunol* 2002;168:466–474.

112. Zamo A, Chiarle R, Piva R, et al. Anaplastic lymphoma kinase (ALK) activates Stat3 and protects hematopoietic cells from cell death. *Oncogene* 2002;21:1038–1047.

113. Nieborowska-Skorska M, Slupianek A, Xue L, et al. Role of signal transducer and activator of transcription 5 in nucleophosmin/ anaplastic lymphoma kinase-mediated malignant transformation of lymphoid cells. *Cancer Res* 2001;61:6517–6523.

114. Amin HM, Lai R. Pathobiology of ALK+ anaplastic large-cell lymphoma. *Blood* 2007;110:2259–2267.

115. ten Berge RL, Oudejans JJ, Ossenkoppelc GJ, et al. ALK-negative systemic anaplastic large cell lymphoma: differential diagnostic and prognostic aspects—a review. *J Pathol* 2003;200:4–15.

116. Falini B, Liso A, Pasqualucci L, et al. CD30+ anaplastic large-cell lymphoma, null type, with signet-ring appearance. *Histopathology* 1997;30:90–92.

117. Bonzheim I, Geissinger E, Roth S, et al. Anaplastic large cell lymphomas lack the expression of T-cell receptor molecules or molecules of proximal T-cell receptor signaling. *Blood* 2004;104:3358–3360.

118. Foss HD, Reusch R, Demel G, et al. Frequent expression of the B-cell-specific activator protein in Reed- Sternberg cells of classical Hodgkin's disease provides further evidence for its B-cell origin. *Blood* 1999;94:3108–3113.

119. Salaverria I, Bea S, Lopez-Guillermo A, et al. Genomic profiling reveals different genetic aberrations in systemic ALK-positive and ALK-negative anaplastic large cell lymphomas. *Br J Haematol* 2008;140:516–526.

120. Ralfkier E, Willemze R, Paulli M, et al. Primary cutaneous CD30-positive T-cell lymphoproliferative disorders. In: Swerdlow SH, et al., eds. *WHO classification of tumours of haematopoietic and lymphoid tissues,* 4th ed. Lyon, France: International Agency for Research on Cancer, 2008:300–301.

121. Tilly H, Gaulard P, Lepage E, et al. Primary anaplastic large-cell lymphoma in adults: clinical presentation, immunophenotype, and outcome. *Blood* 1997;90:3727–3734.

122. Gisselbrecht C, Gaulard P, Lepage E, et al. Prognostic significance of T-cell phenotype in aggressive non-Hodgkin's lymphomas. Groupe d'Etudes des Lymphomes de l'Adulte (GELA). *Blood* 1998;92:76–82.

123. A predictive model for aggressive non-Hodgkin's lymphoma. The International Non-Hodgkin's Lymphoma Prognostic Factors Project. *N Engl J Med* 1993;329:987–994.

124. Gascoyne RD, Aoun P, Wu D, et al. Prognostic significance of anaplastic lymphoma kinase (ALK) protein expression in adults with anaplastic large cell lymphoma. *Blood* 1999;93:3913–3921.

125. Shiota M, Nakamura S, Ichinohasama R, et al. Anaplastic large cell lymphomas expressing the novel chimeric protein p80NPM/ALK: a distinct clinicopathologic entity. *Blood* 1995;86:1954–1960.

126. Suzuki R, Kagami Y, Takeuchi K, et al. Prognostic significance of CD56 expression for ALK-positive and ALK-negative anaplastic large-cell lymphoma of T/null cell phenotype. *Blood* 2000;96:2993–3000.

127. Savage KJ, Harris NL, Vose JM, et al. ALK- anaplastic large-cell lymphoma is clinically and immunophenotypically different from both ALK+ ALCL and peripheral T-cell lymphoma, not otherwise specified: report from the International Peripheral T-Cell Lymphoma Project. *Blood* 2008;111:5496–5504.

128. Fraga M, Brousset P, Schlaifer D, et al. Bone marrow involvement in anaplastic large cell lymphoma. Immunohistochemical detection of minimal disease and its prognostic significance. *Am J Clin Pathol* 1995;103:82–89.

129. Sadahira Y, Hata S, Sugihara T, et al. Bone marrow involvement in NPM-ALK-positive lymphoma: report of two cases. *Pathol Res Pract* 1999;195:657–661.

130. Damm-Welk C, Busch K, Burkhardt B, et al. Prognostic significance of circulating tumor cells in bone marrow or peripheral blood as detected by qualitative and quantitative PCR in pediatric NPM-ALK-positive anaplastic large-cell lymphoma. *Blood* 2007;110:670–677.

131. Bayle C, Charpentier A, Duchayne E, et al. Leukaemic presentation of small cell variant anaplastic large cell lymphoma: report of four cases. *Br J Haematol* 1999;104:680–688.

132. Chhanabhai M, Britten C, Klasa R, et al. t(2;5) positive lymphoma with peripheral blood involvement. *Leuk Lymphoma* 1998;28:415–422.

133. Greer JP, Kinney MC, Collins RD, et al. Clinical features of 31 patients with Ki-1 anaplastic large-cell lymphoma. *J Clin Oncol* 1991;9:539–547.

134. Takahashi D, Nagatoshi Y, Nagayama J, et al. Anaplastic large cell lymphoma in leukemic presentation: a case report and a review of the literature. *J Pediatr Hematol Oncol* 2008;30:696–700.

135. Brugieres L, Deley MC, Pacquement H, et al. CD30(+) anaplastic large-cell lymphoma in children: analysis of 82 patients enrolled in two consecutive studies of the French Society of Pediatric Oncology. *Blood* 1998;92:3591–3598.

136. Seidemann K, Tiemann M, Schrappe M, et al. Short-pulse B-non-Hodgkin lymphoma type chemotherapy is efficacious treatment for pediatric anaplastic large cell lymphoma: a report of the Berlin-Frankfurt-Munster Group Trial NHL-BFM 90. *Blood* 2001;97:3699–3706.

137. Costes-Martineau V, Delfour C, Obled S, et al. Anaplastic lymphoma kinase (ALK) protein expressing lymphoma after liver transplantation: case report and literature review. *J Clin Pathol* 2002;55:868–871.

138. Tirelli U, Vaccher E, Zagonel V, et al. CD30 (Ki-1)-positive anaplastic large-cell lymphomas in 13 patients with and 27 patients without human immunodeficiency virus infection: the first comparative clinicopathologic study from a single institution that also includes 80 patients with other human immunodeficiency virus-related systemic lymphomas. *J Clin Oncol* 1995;13:373–380.

139. Gabarre J, Raphael M, Lepage E, et al. Human immunodeficiency virus-related lymphoma: relation between clinical features and histologic subtypes. *Am J Med* 2001;111:704–711.

140. Chadburn A, Cesarman E, Jagirdar J, et al. CD30 (Ki-1) positive anaplastic large cell lymphomas in individuals infected with the human immunodeficiency virus. *Cancer* 1993;72:3078–3090.

141. de Jong D, Vasmel WL, de Boer JP, et al. Anaplastic large-cell lymphoma in women with breast implants. *JAMA* 2008;300:2030–2035.

142. Salhany KE, Cousar JB, Greer JP, et al. Transformation of cutaneous T cell lymphoma to large cell lymphoma. A clinicopathologic and immunologic study. *Am J Pathol* 1988;132:265–277.

143. Lopez-Guillermo A, Cid J, Salar A, et al. Peripheral T-cell lymphomas: initial features, natural history, and prognostic factors in a series of 174 patients diagnosed according to the R.E.A.L. Classification. *Ann Oncol* 1998;9:849–855.

144. Gallamini A, Stelitano C, Calvi R, et al. Peripheral T-cell lymphoma unspecified (PTCL-U): a new prognostic model from a retrospective multicentric clinical study. *Blood* 2004;103:2474–2479.

145. Schlette EJ, Medeiros LJ, Goy A, et al. Survivin expression predicts poorer prognosis in anaplastic large-cell lymphoma. *J Clin Oncol* 2004;22:1682–1688.

146. ten Berge RL, Meijer CJ, Dukers DF, et al. Expression levels of apoptosis-related proteins predict clinical outcome in anaplastic large cell lymphoma. *Blood* 2002;99:4540–4546.

147. Le Deley MC, Reiter A, Williams D, et al. Prognostic factors in childhood anaplastic large cell lymphoma: results of the European Intergroup Study. *Ann Oncol* 1999;10(suppl 3): abstract 81.

148. Anderson JR, Jenkin RD, Wilson JF, et al. Long-term follow-up of patients treated with COMP or LSA2L2 therapy for childhood non-Hodgkin's lymphoma: a report of CCG-551 from the Childrens Cancer Group. *J Clin Oncol* 1993;11:1024–1032.

149. Offit K, Ladanyi M, Gangi MD, et al. Ki-1 antigen expression defines a favorable clinical subset of non-B cell non-Hodgkin's lymphoma. *Leukemia* 1990;4:625–630.

150. Mori T, Kiyokawa N, Shimada H, et al. Anaplastic large cell lymphoma in Japanese children: retrospective analysis of 34 patients diagnosed at the National Research Institute for Child Health and Development. *Br J Haematol* 2003;121:94–96.

151. Rosolen A, Pillon M, Garaventa A, et al. Anaplastic large cell lymphoma treated with a leukemia-like therapy: report of the Italian Association of Pediatric Hematology and Oncology (AIEOP) LNH-92 protocol. *Cancer* 2005;104:2133–2140.

152. Williams DM, Hobson R, Imeson J, et al. Anaplastic large cell lymphoma in childhood: analysis of 72 patients treated on The United Kingdom Children's Cancer Study Group chemotherapy regimens. *Br J Haematol* 2002;117:812–820.

153. Laver JH, Kraveka JM, Hutchison RE, et al. Advanced-stage large-cell lymphoma in children and adolescents: results of a randomized trial incorporating intermediate-dose methotrexate and high-dose cytarabine in the maintenance phase of the APO regimen: a Pediatric Oncology Group phase III trial. *J Clin Oncol* 2005;23:541–547.

154. Brugières L, Le Deley MC, Rosolen A, et al. Impact of the methotrexate administration dose on the need for intrathecal treatment in children and adolescents with anaplastic large-cell lymphoma: results of a randomized trial of the EICNHL Group. *J Clin Oncol* 2009;27:897–903.

155. Reiter A, Schrappe M, Tiemann M, et al. Successful treatment strategy for Ki-1 anaplastic large-cell lymphoma of childhood: a prospective analysis of 62 patients enrolled in three consecutive Berlin-Frankfurt-Munster group studies. *J Clin Oncol* 1994;12:899–908.

156. Vecchi V, Burnelli R, Pileri S, et al. Anaplastic large cell lymphoma (Ki-1+/CD30+) in childhood. *Med Pediatr Oncol* 1993;21:402–410.

157. Massimino M, Gasparini M, Giardini R. Ki-1 (CD30) anaplastic large-cell lymphoma in children. *Ann Oncol* 1995;6:915–920.

158. Sandlund JT, Pui CH, Santana VM, et al. Clinical features and treatment outcome for children with CD30+ large-cell non-Hodgkin's lymphoma. *J Clin Oncol* 1994;12:895–898.

159. Zinzani PL, Martelli M, Magagnoli M, et al. Anaplastic large cell lymphoma Hodgkin's-like: a randomized trial of ABVD versus MACOP-B with and without radiation therapy. *Blood* 1998;92:790–794.

160. Shulman LN, Frisard B, Antin JH, et al. Primary Ki-1 anaplastic large-cell lymphoma in adults: clinical characteristics and therapeutic outcome. *J Clin Oncol* 1993;11:937–942.

161. Fanin R, Ruiz de Elvira MC, Sperotto A, et al. Autologous stem cell transplantation for T and null cell CD30-positive anaplastic large cell lymphoma: analysis of 64 adult and paediatric cases reported to the European Group for Blood and Marrow Transplantation (EBMT). *Bone Marrow Transplant* 1999;23:437–442.

162. Pileri S, Bocchia M, Baroni CD, et al. Anaplastic large cell lymphoma (CD30 +/Ki-1+): results of a prospective clinico-pathological study of 69 cases. *Br J Haematol* 1994;86:513–523.

163. A clinical evaluation of the International Lymphoma Study Group classification of non-Hodgkin's lymphoma. The Non-Hodgkin's Lymphoma Classification Project. *Blood* 1997;89:3909–3918.

164. Romaguera JE, Garcia-Foncillas J, Cabanillas F. 16-year experience at M. D. Anderson Cancer Center with primary Ki-1 (CD30) antigen expression and anaplastic morphology in adult patients with diffuse large cell lymphoma. *Leuk Lymphoma* 1995;20:97–102.

165. Zinzani PL, Bendandi M, Martelli M, et al. Anaplastic large-cell lymphoma: clinical and prognostic evaluation of 90 adult patients. *J Clin Oncol* 1996;14:955–962.

166. Fanin R, Silvestri F, Geromin A, et al. Primary systemic CD30 (Ki-1)-positive anaplastic large cell lymphoma of the adult: sequential intensive treatment with the F-MACHOP regimen (+/- radiotherapy) and autologous bone marrow transplantation. *Blood* 1996;87:1243–1248.

167. Deconinck E, Lamy T, Foussard C, et al. Autologous stem cell transplantation for anaplastic large-cell lymphomas: results of a prospective trial. *Br J Haematol* 2000;109:736–742.

168. Haioun C, Lepage E, Gisselbrecht C, et al. Survival benefit of high-dose therapy in poor-risk aggressive non-Hodgkin's lymphoma: final analysis of the prospective LNH87-2 protocol—a groupe d'Etude des lymphomes de l'Adulte study. *J Clin Oncol* 2000;18:3025–3030.

169. Shipp MA, Abeloff MD, Antman KH, et al. International Consensus Conference on high-dose therapy with hematopoietic stem cell transplantation in aggressive non-Hodgkin's lymphomas: report of the jury. *J Clin Oncol* 1999;17:423–429.

170. Miller TP, Dahlberg S, Cassady JR, et al. Chemotherapy alone compared with chemotherapy plus radiotherapy for localized intermediate- and high-grade non-Hodgkin's lymphoma. *N Engl J Med* 1998;339:21–26.

171. Reyes F, Lepage E, Ganem G, et al. Groupe d'Etude des Lymphomes de l'Adulte (GELA). ACVBP versus CHOP plus radiotherapy for localized aggressive lymphoma. *N Engl J Med* 2005;352:1197–205.

172. Rodriguez J, Caballero MD, Gutierrez A, et al. High-dose chemotherapy and autologous stem cell transplantation in peripheral T-cell lymphoma: the GEL-TAMO experience. *Ann Oncol* 2003;14:1768–1775.

173. Rodriguez J, Munsell M, Yazji S, et al. Impact of high-dose chemotherapy on peripheral T-cell lymphomas. *J Clin Oncol* 2001;19:3766–3770.

174. Zamkoff KW, Matulis MD, Mehta AC, et al. High-dose therapy and autologous stem cell transplant does not result in long-term disease-free survival in patients with recurrent chemotherapy-sensitive ALK-negative anaplastic large-cell lymphoma. *Bone Marrow Transplant* 2004;33:635–638.

175. Chakravarti V, Kamani NR, Bayever E, et al. Bone marrow transplantation for childhood Ki-1 lymphoma. *J Clin Oncol* 1990;8:657–660.
176. Liso A, Tiacci E, Binazzi R, et al. Haploidentical peripheral-blood stem-cell transplantation for ALK-positive anaplastic large-cell lymphoma. *Lancet Oncol* 2004;5:127–128.
177. Bordon V, De Paepe P, Dhooge C, et al. Successful treatment with allogeneic bone marrow transplantation of an early relapse of ALK-positive anaplastic large cell lymphoma. *Haematologica* 2005;90:ECR19.
178. Chen CH, Chen SW, Shen WL, et al. Successful allogeneic stem cell transplantation for an adult with refractory anaplastic lymphoma kinase-positive anaplastic large cell lymphoma. *Int J Hematol* 2007;85:105–107.
179. Kim SW, Tanimoto TE, Hirabayashi N, et al. Myeloablative allogeneic hematopoietic stem cell transplantation for non-Hodgkin lymphoma: a nationwide survey in Japan. *Blood* 2006;108:382–389.
180. Le Gouill S, Milpied N, Buzyn A, et al. Graft-versus-lymphoma effect for aggressive T-cell lymphomas in adults: a study by the Societe Francaise de Greffe de Moelle et de Therapie Cellulaire. *J Clin Oncol* 2008;26:2264–2271.
181. Corradini P, Dodero A, Zallio F, et al. Graft-versus-lymphoma effect in relapsed peripheral T-cell non-Hodgkin's lymphomas after reduced-intensity conditioning followed by allogeneic transplantation of hematopoietic cells. *J Clin Oncol* 2004;22:2172–2176.
182. Passoni L, Scardino A, Bertazzoli C, et al. ALK as a novel lymphoma-associated tumor antigen: identification of 2 HLA-A2.1-restricted CD8+ T-cell epitopes. *Blood* 2002;99:2100–2106.
183. Chiarle R, Martinengo C, Mastini C, et al. The anaplastic lymphoma kinase is an effective oncoantigen for lymphoma vaccination. *Nat Med* 2008;14:676–680.
184. Ansell SM, Horwitz SM, Engert A, et al. Phase I/II study of an anti-CD30 monoclonal antibody (MDX-060) in Hodgkin's lymphoma and anaplastic large-cell lymphoma. *J Clin Oncol* 2007;25:2764–2769.
185. Bartlett NL, Younes A, Carabasi MH, et al. A phase 1 multidose study of SGN-30 immunotherapy in patients with refractory or recurrent CD30+ hematologic malignancies. *Blood* 2008;111:1848–1854.
186. Turturro F, Arnold MD, Frist AY, et al. Model of inhibition of the NPM-ALK kinase activity by herbimycin A. *Clin Cancer Res* 2002;8:240–245.
187. Galkin AV, Melnick JS, Kim S, et al. Identification of NVP-TAE684, a potent, selective, and efficacious inhibitor of NPM-ALK. *Proc Natl Acad Sci U S A* 2007;104:270–275.
188. Li R, Morris SW. Development of anaplastic lymphoma kinase (ALK) small-molecule inhibitors for cancer therapy. *Med Res Rev* 2008;28:372–412.
189. McDermott U, Iafrate AJ, Gray NS, et al. Genomic alterations of anaplastic lymphoma kinase may sensitize tumors to anaplastic lymphoma kinase inhibitors. *Cancer Res* 2008;68:3389–3395.
190. Bonvini P, Gastaldi T, Falini B, et al. Nucleophosmin-anaplastic lymphoma kinase (NPM-ALK), a novel Hsp90- client tyrosine kinase: down-regulation of NPM-ALK expression and tyrosine phosphorylation in ALK(+) CD30(+) lymphoma cells by the Hsp90 antagonist 17-allylamino,17-demethoxygeldanamycin. *Cancer Res* 2002;62:1559–1566.
191. Gu L, Gao J, Li Q, et al. Rapamycin reverses NPM-ALK-induced glucocorticoid resistance in lymphoid tumor cells by inhibiting mTOR signaling pathway, enhancing G1 cell cycle arrest and apoptosis. *Leukemia* 2008;22:2091–2096.
192. Cho-Vega JH, Vega F, Medeiros LJ. An attractive therapeutic target, mTOR pathway, in ALK+ anaplastic large cell lymphoma. *Adv Anat Pathol* 2008;15:105–112.
193. Le Deley MC, Reiter A, Williams D, et al. Prognostic factors in childhood anaplastic large cell lymphoma: results of a large European intergroup study. *Blood* 2008;111:1560–1566.

CHAPTER 29 ■ MATURE NODAL AND EXTRANODAL T-CELL AND NATURAL KILLER-CELL LYMPHOMAS

JAMES O. ARMITAGE, ELAINE S. JAFFE, RAYMOND H. S. LIANG, JOHN W. SWEETENHAM, AND MARK RAFFELD

DEFINITION AND INTRODUCTION

Mature T-cell neoplasms are derived from mature or post-thymic T cells. Because natural killer (NK) cells are closely related, and share some immunophenotypic and functional properties with T cells, these two classes of neoplasms are considered together (1). In the broadest sense, any T-cell non-Hodgkin lymphoma (NHL) other than lymphoblastic lymphoma (i.e., the lymphoma that corresponds to T-cell acute lymphoblastic leukemia) is a peripheral T-cell lymphoma (PTCL). Some more common forms of PTCL, or those with distinctive clinical or epidemiologic features, are considered elsewhere in this text. These include anaplastic large cell lymphoma (ALCL), anaplastic lymphoma kinase (ALK) positive and ALK negative, mycosis fungoides, and adult T-cell leukemia/lymphoma (ATLL). This chapter will encompass a heterogeneous group of disorders that includes PTCL not otherwise specified (NOS) (i.e., those T-cell lymphomas not belonging to a defined entity) and several other less frequent disorders that represent distinctive clinical/pathologic syndromes. These include angioimmunoblastic T-cell lymphoma (AILT), subcutaneous panniculitis-like T-cell lymphoma, enteropathy associated T-cell lymphoma, extranodal NK/T lymphoma, and hepatosplenic lymphoma.

PTCLs are uncommon, accounting for <10% of all NHLs. Functionally, T-cell lymphomas are related to the two major arms of the immune system, the innate and adaptive immune systems. NK and T cells of the innate immune system recognize antigen in the absence of major histocompatibility complex (MHC) antigens, and are involved in mucosal immunity. The lymphomas derived from these cells often involve cutaneous and mucosal sites. The expression of cytotoxic molecules in these lymphomas may predispose to apoptosis by tumor cells and normal bystander cells. Hepatosplenic T-cell lymphoma (HSTCL) is a systemic disease derived from functionally immature innate effector cells, most often of $\gamma\delta$ T-cell origin. In contrast, most nodal T-cell lymphomas belong to the adaptive immune system. AILT is mostly likely derived from follicular helper T cells (T_{FH}), a finding that explains many of its pathologic and clinical features. Studies of these neoplasms may assist in further unraveling the functional diversity of their normal counterparts.

EPIDEMIOLOGY

Mature T-cell and NK-cell neoplasms are relatively uncommon, accounting for <10% of all NHLs on a worldwide basis (2,3). The most common subtypes of mature T-cell lymphomas are PTCL, unspecified (PTCL-NOS), AILT, and ALCL (Table 29.1). T-cell and NK-cell lymphomas show significant variations in incidence in different geographic regions and racial populations. For example, T/NK-cell lymphomas comprise a higher proportion of NHL in Asian populations. These differences result from both a true increased incidence, as well as a relative decrease in the frequency of many B-cell lymphomas, such as follicular lymphoma, seen commonly in North America and Europe. Human T-cell lymphotropic virus I accounts for an increase of ATLL risk in regions where it is endemic, including southwestern Japan and the Caribbean basin.

Another major factor affecting the incidence of T-cell and NK-cell lymphomas is racial predisposition. Extranodal NK-cell lymphomas, and nasal-type and aggressive NK-cell leukemia are much more common in Asians than they are in other

TABLE 29.1	
INTERNATIONAL T-CELL NHL STUDY: CONSENSUS DIAGNOSIS	
PTCL unspecified	23.0%
Angioimmunoblastic T cell	18.4%
ATLL	9.6%
Nasal NK/T cell	7.0%
Anaplastic large cell, ALK+	6.4%
Anaplastic large cell, ALK−	5.5%
Enteropathy type T cell	4.7%
Unclassifiable T cell	2.9%
NK/T-cell lymphoma, nasal type	2.7%
Primary cutaneous ALCL	1.7%
Hepatosplenic T cell	1.4%
Subcutaneous panniculitis	0.9%
Blastic NK-cell leukemia/lymphoma	0.2%
Peripheral γ-δ	0.1%
Other than mature T-cell NHL	11.1%

From Armitage J, Vose J, Weisenburger D. International peripheral T-cell and natural killer/T-cell lymphoma study: pathology findings and clinical outcomes. *J Clin Oncol* 2008;26:4124–4130, with permission.

races (4). Other groups at increased risk for these Epstein-Barr virus (EBV)-associated diseases are individuals of Native American descent in Central and South America, and Mexico (5). Other rare EBV-positive lymphomas derived from T cells showing a similar racial and geographic distribution include fulminant EBV-positive T-cell lymphoproliferative disorder (6), which has overlapping features with severe chronic active EBV infection (7), and hydroa vacciniforme-like lymphoma, a form of EBV-positive T-cell or NK-cell lymphoma seen mainly in children (8). Genetic factors linked to defective surveillance of EBV have been postulated to play a role in these epidemiologic differences. High viral load at the time of initial viral infection may be an additional risk factor.

$\gamma\delta$ PTCLs occur with increased frequency in the setting of immune suppression, especially following organ transplantation, a finding that is not well understood (9–11). Overall, the incidence of T-cell and NK-cell malignancies does not appear to be changing, although long-term epidemiologic data are not available because it is only recently with modern immunophenotypic and molecular tools that these neoplasms have been reliably distinguished from B-cell lymphomas.

Pathophysiology of T-Cell Subsets

T-cell lymphomas manifest the immunophenotypic features of post-thymic T lymphocytes, being derived from both $\alpha\beta$ T cells and $\gamma\delta$ T cells (12). This distinction is based on the structure of the T-cell receptor (TCR). γ-δ T cells, along with NK cells, are components of the innate immune system and do not require antigen sensitization to be active (13,14). The innate immune system is functional based only on genes encoded in the host genome. It is distinguished from the adaptive or antigen-specific immune system; most T cells in peripheral blood and peripheral lymphoid organs belong to the latter (Fig. 29.1).

$\gamma\delta$ T cells comprise <5% of all normal T cells, and show a restricted distribution, being found mainly in the splenic red pulp, intestinal epithelium, and other epithelial sites. It is notable that these sites are more commonly affected by $\gamma\delta$ T-cell lymphomas, which are rare in nodal sites (11,15). γ-δ T cells are not MHC restricted in their function, and represent a first line of defense against bacterial peptides, such as heat shock proteins (12). They are often involved in responses to mycobacterial infections, and both mucosal and cutaneous immunity.

Cells of the innate immune system represent a first line of defense, a more primitive type of immune response, and play a role in both mucosal and cutaneous immunity. It is interesting that many T-cell and NK-cell lymphomas observed commonly in the pediatric and young adult age group are derived from cells of the innate immune system (16). These include aggressive NK-cell leukemia, systemic EBV-positive T-cell lymphoproliferative disease of childhood, HSTCL, and $\gamma\delta$ T-cell lymphomas affecting mucocutaneous sites (13). ALCL is the most common pediatric T-cell lymphoma, and although it is of cytotoxic origin, it has a very aberrant phenotype and is difficult to relate to either the innate or adaptive immune system with certainty.

The T cells of the adaptive immune system are heterogeneous and functionally complex, and include naive, effector (regulatory and cytotoxic), and memory T cells. CD4-positive

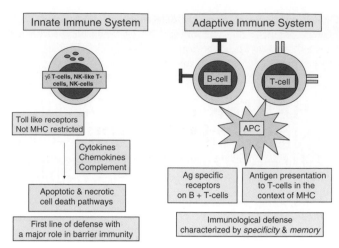

FIGURE 29.1 There are two main arms of the immune system: the innate immune system and the adaptive immune system. The diagram shows respective roles of lymphocyte subpopulations in the innate and adaptive immune responses. NK cells, NK-like T cells, and γ-δ T cells function with other cell types, including granulocytes and macrophages as a first line of defense. These cells have cytotoxic granules containing perforin and granzymes. The innate immune system lacks specificity and memory. In the adaptive immune system, B cells and T cells recognize antigens (Ag) through specific receptors, immunoglobulin and the TCR complex, respectively. Antigen presentation to T cells must take place via antigen-presenting cells (APC) in the context of the appropriate MHC class II antigens. T-cell lymphomas can be classified as to the origin from either the innate or adaptive immune system.

T cells are primarily regulatory, acting via cytokine production, whereas CD8-positive (and double negative) T cells are primarily cytotoxic. Recently, much has been learned about a unique T-cell subset found in the normal germinal center. These cells, termed T_{FH}, provide help to B cells in the context of the germinal center reaction. They have a unique phenotype, expressing the germinal center-associated markers BCL6 and CD10, normally found on B cells. T_{FH} express CD4, CD57, and produce the chemokines CXCR5 and CXCR13. CXCL13 causes induction and proliferation of follicular dendritic cells, and is involved in B-cell recruitment to the lymph node, by facilitating the adhesion of T cells to high endothelial venules (HEVs) and allowing them to transit the vessel wall.

Another T-cell malignancy, ATLL, has been linked to the T-regulatory cells based on expression of both CD25 and FoxP3 (17). T-regulatory cells are a specialized type of regulatory T cell that suppressed immune response, and, thus, this observation helps to explain the marked immunosuppression associated with ATLL. Additionally, the hypercalcemia associated with ATLL has been linked to secretion of factors with osteoclast-activating activity (18).

There have been relatively few studies correlating the subclassification of T-cell lymphomas with specific profiles of cytokine or chemokine expression (19). Nevertheless, data are now emerging that can relate the pathologic or clinical manifestations of T-cell lymphomas to cytokine or chemokine expression by the neoplastic cells, or accompanying accessory cells within the lymph node. The hemophagocytic syndrome seen in some T-cell and NK-cell malignancies has been associated with secretion of both cytokines and chemokines, in the setting of defective cytolytic function (20). More recently, the chemokine CXCL13 has been identified in AILTs, and its identification helps to elucidate many of the features of that T-cell subtype (21,22).

Classification of T-Cell and Natural Killer-Cell Lymphomas

PTCLs show great morphologic diversity, and a spectrum of histologic appearances can be seen within individual disease entities. The cellular composition can range from small cells with minimal atypia to large cells with anaplastic features. Such a spectrum is seen in ALCL, ATLL, and extranodal NK/T-cell lymphoma, as selected examples. However, cytologic atypia does not necessarily correlate with clinical behavior. For these reasons, it has been difficult to apply cytologic principles to the classification of PTCLs. In a similar vein, immunophenotypic markers have been less useful in classification T-cell lymphomas than B-cell lymphomas because often one marker is sharing by multiple disease entity. As an example, CD30, a hallmark of ALCL, is found in diverse lymphoid malignancies of T- and B-cell types. Finally, the molecular pathogenesis for most T-cell lymphomas is as yet undiscovered. For the aforementioned reasons, clinical features have played a major role in defining many of the specific entities included in the World Health Organization (WHO) classification (23) (Table 29.2).

TABLE 29.2

MATURE T-CELL AND NK-CELL NEOPLASMS

T-cell prolymphocytic leukemia
T-cell large granular lymphocytic leukemia
Chronic lymphoproliferative disorder of NK cells[a]
Aggressive NK-cell leukemia
Systemic EBV+ T-cell lymphoproliferative disease of
    childhood (associated with chronic active EBV infection)
Hydroa vacciniforme-like lymphoma
Adult T-cell Lymphomal/Leukemia (ATLL)
Extranodal NK/T-cell lymphoma, nasal type
Enteropathy associated T-cell lymphoma
Hepatosplenic T-cell lymphoma (HSTCL)
Subcutaneous panniculitis-like T-cell lymphoma
Mycosis fungoides
Sézary syndrome
Primary cutaneous ALCL
Primary cutaneous γ-δ T-cell lymphoma
*Primary cutaneous aggressive epidermotropic CD8-positive
    cytotoxic T-cell lymphoma[a]*
*Primary cutaneous small/medium CD4-positive T-cell
    lymphoma[a]*
PTCL, NOS
Angioimmunoblastic T-cell lymphoma (AILT)
Anaplastic large cell lymphoma (ALCL), ALK positive
ALCL, ALK negative[a]

[a] From Swerdlow SH. *WHO classification of tumours of haemato-poietic and lymphoid tissues*, 4th ed. Lyon, France: International Agency for Research on Cancer, 2008, with permission.

SPECIFIC DISEASE ENTITIES

Peripheral T-Cell Lymphoma Not Otherwise Specified

There is a rapid change in our understanding of PTCLs currently under way. From a heterogeneous group of disorders, specific clinical-pathologic syndromes are steadily being split away. Many of those are dealt with later in this chapter. Those PTCLs that do not fit into a recognized clinical-pathologic entity are lumped together in the category *PTCL NOS*. It is entirely possible that this category will decrease or disappear as new insights are gained by clinical observations, new histologic observations, or, more likely, by ongoing genetic studies. Initial studies using gene expression arrays suggest that this category is heterogenous (24).

Many of the papers describing the clinical characteristics and treatment outcome in PTCLs were published before any of the currently recognized specific clinical-pathologic entities were described. PTCLs are not geographically evenly distributed (25). PTCL or NK-cell lymphoma represented 2% of the cases studied in North America, 6% of the cases studied from Europe, 8% of the cases studied from southern Africa, and 18% of the cases studied from Hong Kong in one international study.

Pathology

PTCL, unspecified (PTCL-NOS) is the most common category of PTCL, and by definition is heterogeneous. PTCL-NOS is the "diffuse large B-cell" equivalent of PTCL. This subtype includes all cases not readily classified as one of the specific entities in the WHO classification. Two morphologic variants are delineated as T-zone lymphoma, and lymphoepithelioid cell lymphoma, but the evidence that these are distinct entities is lacking, and for that reason, the use of morphologic variants in diagnosis is optional. As a group, PTCLs-NOS are aggressive neoplasms, often present with advanced stage, and are seen mainly in older adults. They are most often nodal but can present with extranodal disease. They may contain a prominent background of inflammatory cells, be composed of a diverse population of pleomorphic tumor cells, or be monomorphic, resembling diffuse large B-cell lymphomas. For these reasons, the diagnosis of PTCL-NOS should always be based on confirmatory tests using immunophenotypic or genotypic methods.

In recent years, immunophenotypic, genomic, and genetic technologies have been utilized to better define clinical or prognostic groups in PTCL-NOS. For example, CD15 expression in PTCL-NOS appears to identify a subset with a very poor prognosis (26,27). A high proliferative rate, whether identified by Ki-67 expression (26) or by gene expression profiling (28), identifies a subset of cases with an especially poor prognosis. Overexpression of the SYK tyrosine kinase has been identified, but its clinical significance is unknown (29). Gene expression profiling has distinguished AILT from most other nodal PTCLs-NOS, but overlap exists in some cases (30).

Pathogenesis

PTCLs-NOS, comprise the largest group within the general category of PTCL. Nevertheless, our understanding of their pathogenesis is remarkably meager. The majority of cases show rearrangements of their TCR genes and are phenotypically

CD4-positive α/β cells (31). Occasional CD8-positive α/β-expressing nodal T-cell lymphomas have also been reported. Classic and array based comparative genomic hybridization (CGH) studies of this subset of T-cell lymphomas show gains on 1q, 3p, 5p, 7q, 8q, 11q, 17q, and 22q, and regions of loss on 5q, 6q, 9p, 10p, 10q, 12q, and 13q (32–34). These lymphomas do not appear to be a distinct clinicopathologic group but, rather, are likely to contain several entities, as is evidenced by their broad nonspecific phenotype, and nonrecurrent complex chromosomal abnormalities (35,36). One intriguing preliminary report suggests a pathogenetic role for a novel putative oncogene called human ralGDS-related (hrgr) (37). ralGDS-related (rgr) was originally identified as one of the subunits of the rabbit squamous cell carcinoma (rsc) oncogene isolated from a rsc. Truncated forms of rsc are able to transform NIH 3T3 cells (38). A preliminary screen of T and B-cell lymphomas has shown high levels of truncated transcript in the majority of PTCLs (nine of 11 cases), and in a small percentage of mycoses fungoides cases (two of seven) and ALCLs (two of five). Normal B and T cells and other forms of B and T-cell lymphomas did not express the aberrant transcripts (33,34,39,40).

There have been several recent gene expression profiling studies of PTCL, NOS, that confirm the heterogeneity of this group (28,41,42). In one such study, a proliferation signature was identified that correlated with patient survival and inversely with inflammatory response gene expression and the percentage of macrophages (28).

Translocations involving TCRs occur in about ≤2% cases (29). These include rare cases with t(14;19)(q11;q13) translocations involving the TRA/TRD locus on chromosome 14 and the poliovirus receptor-like 2 gene on chromosome 19 (43). This translocation results in overexpression the poliovirus receptor-like 2 gene as well as the nearby BCL3 gene, suggesting one or both of these genes may play a role in some cases of PTCL, NOS.

Rare translocations involving non-TCR loci have also been described. The most common of these is the t(5;9)(q33;q22) involving the ITK gene on chromosome 5 and the SYK gene on chromosome 9, which results in overexpression of a novel ITK/SYK fusion protein (44). Interestingly, this translocation seems to define a specific histologic subtype of PTCL, although it is currently categorized under PTCL, NOS (follicular variant). Histologically, these cases show infiltration of lymphoid follicles with medium to large atypical T cells that phenotypically resemble T_{FH} (CD3+, CD5+, CD4+, BCL6+, and CD10+). Despite what appears to be a common origin from T_{FH}, this translocation has not been reported in AILT. More recently, it has been reported that SYK is also overexpressed in the majority of t(5;9)(q33;q22)-negative T-cell lymphomas, suggesting that inappropriate SYK expression may be involved in the pathogenesis of many T-cell lymphomas (29).

Another candidate gene in PTCL pathogenesis is the hrgr gene (37). rgr was originally identified as the oncogenic portion of a fusion gene isolated from a rsc. Truncated forms of both rgr and hrgr are able to transform NIH 3T3 cells, and forced hrgr expression in thymocytes of transgenic mice leads to the development of thymic lymphomas (38,45). Although a preliminary screen of T- and B-cell lymphomas revealed high levels of truncated rgr transcripts in the majority of PTCLs studied (nine of 11 cases), the significance of this finding in PTCL lymphomagenesis is still not clear.

Clinical Features and Treatment Outcome

In a recent international study, 340 cases of PTCL-NOS were identified (46). The median age was 60 years, and 66% of the patients were male. Sixty-nine percent had stage III–IV disease, and 22% had positive bone marrows. The International Prognostic Index (IPI) scores were zero to one in 28% of patients and four to five in 15%. The 5-year overall survival was 32%, and the 5-year failure-free survival was 20%. Treatment outcome was predicted both by the IPI score and by the Prognostic Index developed especially for patients with T-cell lymphoma (47).

López-Guillermo et al. (48) described 184 patients with PTCL and subdivided them based on the WHO classification. Ninety-five patients had PTCL-NOS. Of these patients, 52% were >60 years of age, and 61% were male. Twenty-four percent had an Eastern Cooperative Oncology Group score of two or greater, and 57% of the patients had B symptoms. Some sign of extranodal disease was seen in 65% of the patients. Sixty-two percent had Ann Arbor stage IV disease, and 53% had a high lactate dehydrogenase level. A high β_2-microglobulin was seen in 62%. The IPI scores in these patients were zero to one for 28%, two for 26%, three for 22%, and four or five for 24%. The most frequent sites of extranodal involvement were the bone marrow (41%), skin (12%), and liver (13%).

Ansell et al. (49) reported 78 patients with PTCL seen at the Mayo Clinic. Forty-two percent of the patients were >60 years of age, and 62% were male. Eighty-two percent had Ann Arbor stage III/IV disease. Fifty-three percent of the patients had B symptoms, and 54% percent of the patients had an Eastern Cooperative Oncology Group score of two or greater. Extranodal involvement was frequently seen, with the most commonly involved organs being the gastrointestinal tract (29%), bone marrow (28%), and liver (21%). An elevated lactate dehydrogenase level was seen in 42% of the patients.

Many previous studies of treatment outcome included patients with PTCL-NOS and smaller numbers of other subtypes of PTCL. Liang et al. (50) found an 84% complete remission rate and a 60% overall survival at 18 months. In contrast, Greer et al. (51) found a 24% complete response rate in patients receiving combination chemotherapy regimens and only a 12% prolonged disease-free survival. Coiffier et al. (52) reported a 77% complete remission rate in 39 patients treated with Adriamycin (doxorubicin), cyclophosphamide, vindesine, bleomycin, and prednisone, with a 23% relapse rate. Armitage et al. (53) described 80 patients treated with chemotherapy regimens having curative potential in diffuse large B-cell lymphoma. Fifty percent of the patients achieved a complete remission, and the actuarial 4-year survival was 45%. Rudiger et al. (54) reported 69 patients treated with doxorubicin-containing combination chemotherapy regimens, with only a 20% 5-year failure-free survival. The Nebraska Lymphoma Study Group reported 19 patients with PTCL treated with cyclophosphamide, Adriamycin (doxorubicin), procarbazine, bleomycin, Oncovin (vincristine), and prednisone, with a 54% complete remission rate and 41% 3-year overall survival. The Group d'Etude des Lymphomes de l'Adulte reported a study of 108 patients treated with Adriamycin (doxorubicin), cyclophosphamide, vindesine, bleomycin, and prednisone that found a 72% complete remission rate and a 43% relapse rate.

TABLE 29.3

RESPONSE RATE AND OUTCOME OF T-CELL LYMPHOMAS

	No. of patients	CR (%)	CR/PR (%)	FFS (y)	OS (y)
PTCL-U	333	56	79	0.91	2.01
AILT	241	61	83	0.82	2.26
ATLL	126	34	69	0.57	0.79
Nasal NK/T	92	48	63	0.69	1.61
ETTL	61	46	63	0.55	0.88

CR, complete response; FFS, failure-free survival; OS, overall survival; Nasal NK/T, nasal NK/T-cell lymphoma; PR, partial response, PTCL-U, PTCL, unspecified.
From Armitage J, Vose J, Weisenburger D. International peripheral T-cell and natural killer/T-cell lymphoma study: pathology findings and clinical outcomes. *J Clin Oncol* 2008;26: 4124–4130, with permission.

In a series of 340 patients from multiple sites, the complete remission rate was 56% (55) (Table 29.3). The 5-year failure free and overall survivals were 20% and 32%, respectively (Fig. 29.2). There was no apparent advantage to receiving an anthracycline versus receiving a treatment regimen that did not contain an anthracycline.

A variety of new agents show activity in PTCL-NOS and might turn out to be important parts of future chemotherapy regimens. Pralatrexate is active and has a significant response rate in patients with refractory disease (56). Although only approximately 40% to 50% of patients with PTCL-NOS express C52 antigen (57), alemtuzumab appears to have clinical activity. An Italian Group reported the use of alemtuzumab added to cyclophosphamide, hydroxydaunorubicin, Oncovin (vincristine), and prednisone (CHOP) with a complete remission in 71% of patients (58). Gemcitabine is an active drug in PTCL and has been incorporated into combination regimens (59). CHOP has been combined with denileukin diftitox in a phase II trial (60).

Both autologous and allogeneic bone marrow transplantation have been utilized in patients with PTCL-NOS, although some series have probably contained patients with other subtypes of peripheral T-cell lymphoma. Vose et al. (61) reported no difference in disease-free and overall survival in 17 patients with T-cell lymphoma and 24 patients with diffuse aggressive lymphoma undergoing autologous transplantation. Rodriguez et al. reported 36 patients with aggressive B- or T-cell lymphoma, and found no difference between the outcome in B- and T-cell lymphomas with autologous transplantation. Blystad et al. (62) reported 27 patients with chemosensitive relapsed PTCL who underwent autologous transplantation, of whom 44% survived 4 years. Chen et al. (63) reported 53 patients with a variety of PTCLs who underwent autologous transplantation in first complete or partial remission, second or subsequent remission, or with refractory disease. Twenty-five percent of the patients had 5-year progression-free survival. Rodriguez et al. (64) reported 74 patients who received autotransplant in first complete remission with a 5-year progression-free survival of 63%. Feyler et al. (65) reported 64 patients who underwent autologous transplantation and found a 3-year progression-free survival of 33%.

Allogeneic transplantation appears to have activity in patients with PTCL, including those with PTCL-NOS. The French Bone Marrow and Cellular Therapy Group performed allogeneic bone marrow transplantation on 27 patients with PTCL-NOS. The 5-year overall survival was 63% (66). The Group interpreted this as supporting the existence of a graft versus lymphoma effect in PTCL. de Lavallade (67) and Corradini (68) et al. have reported the use of reduced intensity conditioning in PTCLs. Both groups reported sustained complete remissions, further supporting the existence of a graft versus lymphoma effect in PTCL.

Multiple salvage-chemotherapy regimens have been used in patients with PTCL for whom primary therapy was unsuccessful. These include platinum-based and fludarabine-based combination-chemotherapy regimens, pralatrexate (56), gallium nitrate (69), cyclosporine (70), pentostatin (71), cladribine (72), gemcitabine (73), retinoids (74), denileukin diftitox (75), interferon (76), darinaparsin (77), and immunotoxins

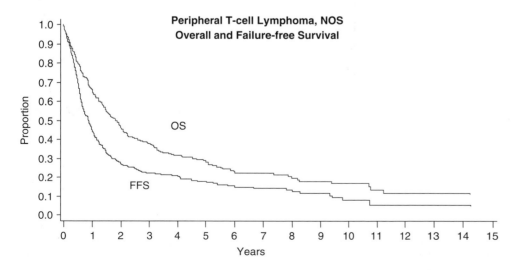

Peripheral T-cell Lymphoma, NOS Overall and Failure-free Survival

OS

FFS

FIGURE 29.2 The overall (OS) and failure-free (FFS) survival from a study of 333 patients with PTCL-NOS collected from multiple institutions as part of an international retrospective analysis. (Reprinted from Armitage J, Vose J, Weisenburger D. International peripheral T-cell and natural killer/T-cell lymphoma study: pathology findings and clinical outcomes. *J Clin Oncol* 2008;26:4124–4130, with permission.)

(78). All of these approaches have described some success. None has yet been advanced to frontline therapy.

Angioimmunoblastic T-Cell Lymphoma

Angioimmunoblastic lymphadenopathy with dysproteinemia was described by Frizzera et al. (79) in 1974. However, the same disorder had probably been reported by Flandrin et al. (80) in the French literature in 1972. The patients characteristically presented with generalized lymphadenopathy, hepatosplenomegaly, fever, hypergammaglobulinemia, and frequently a positive Coombs' test. A typical morphologic appearance involving proliferation of small arborizing vessels and a pleomorphic cellular infiltrate was described. Most patients had a short survival, although occasional patients seemed to have long-term benefit with prednisone therapy.

In 1987, Brice et al. (81) described five patients with PTCL that evolved from angioimmunoblastic lymphadenopathy. However, in 1979, Shimoyama et al. (82) had proposed an entity that they called *immunoblastic lymphadenopathy-like T-cell lymphoma*, which was probably the same entity. Today, the accepted name for this lymphoma is angioimmunoblastic T-cell lymphoma (AILT).

Pathology

AILT has emerged as a distinctive subtype of PTCL with unique pathobiological features. This disease is seen mainly in elderly adults with an equal male-female ratio. Originally thought to be a form of abnormal immune response, most patients present with generalized lymphadenopathy, hepatosplenomegaly, skin rash, and marked constitutional symptoms. Polyclonal hypergammaglobulinemia is an almost constant finding, and the lymph nodes usually contain polyclonal plasma cells, as well as frequent large B immunoblasts, despite the absence of well-formed follicles with germinal centers. The neoplastic T cells have clear cytoplasm and are distributed in a marked inflammatory background. Other features include prominent arborizing HEVs and expansion of dendritic meshworks outside the follicle, usually arising from the prominent HEVs. The neoplastic T cells are CD4-positive T cells that express CD10 and sometimes BCL6, features that suggested that the neoplastic cells might be derived from germinal center-based T cells (T_{FH}) (83).

Most recently, two groups have identified increased expression of CXCL13 in AILT, a finding that helps to link together many of these clinical and pathologic features (21,22). CXCL13 causes the induction and proliferation of follicular dendritic cells, and facilitates the entry of B cells into the lymph node through their attachment to the HEVs, thus helping to clarify the B-cell expansion characteristic of this disease. Gene expression profiling has confirmed a close association between AILT and the T_{FH} subset (30).

Another almost constant finding in AILT is the presence of EBV-positive B cells. It has been postulated that this finding is secondary to decreased immune surveillance and reactivation of EBV in the setting of a compromised immune system (84). However, EBV-positive B cells are found even very early in the course of the disease. In some cases this phenomenon progresses to an EBV-positive B-cell lymphoproliferative disorder, resembling posttransplant polymorphic

B-cell lymphoma. In other instances the EBV-positive B cells may resemble Reed-Sternberg cells, leading to an erroneous diagnosis of classic Hodgkin lymphoma (85).

Pathogenesis

AILTs comprise the second largest single group of PTCLs (PTCL, NOS being the largest), and are tumors of CD4+, α/β cells (86). TCR β-cell receptor β and γ chain gene rearrangements can be seen in up to 75% to 85% of cases (87–89). Cytogenetic studies have shown that virtually all cases have abnormal karyotypes, with frequent trisomy 3, 5, and +X, and structural abnormalities at 1p32-33 (40,90). Schlegelberger et al. (91) showed that the presence of multiple chromosomal abnormalities was associated with shortened survival. Up to 40% of AILTs show clonal immunoglobulin gene rearrangements (92–94). However, these have generally been attributed to clonal proliferations of EBV-infected B cells. EBV-infected B cells can be identified in up to 60% of cases and are believed to be a manifestation of the immune dysregulation associated with this disease (92). In up to 10% of cases, overt B-cell lymphoma may supervene (95,96).

The developmental pathogenesis of AILT remains controversial. Cytogenetic and spectral karyotyping studies have shown that virtually all cases have abnormal karyotypes, with frequent trisomy 3, 5, 21, and +X, structural abnormalities at 1p, frequent gains at 5q, and losses at 6q (34,40,90). Additional copy number changes have been reported using array based CGH, and include frequent gains of 22q, 19, and 11p11-q14 (11q13), and losses of 13q, 8p, and 9p (33). The combination of 5q losses and trisomy 21 is thought to be relatively specific to AILT as compared with other types of T-cell lymphomas. Although no specific chromosomal abnormality has been correlated with survival, the presence of multiple abnormalities is associated with a poor prognosis (34,91).

Much progress has been made in our understanding of the pathogenesis of this lymphoma. Initially, this disease was termed angioimmunoblastic lymphadenopathy with dysproteinemia, and was believed to be a systemic immunologic disease characterized by a variable clinical course, polyclonal gammopathy, a specific pattern of involvement of lymph nodes, and a predisposition for the development of T-cell lymphoma (97,98). With the development of improved methodologies to assess T-cell clonality and the identification of clonal T-cell populations in up to 75% to 95% of cases, the interpretation of this disease process has been shifting (92,99). The consensus opinion today is that this disease most likely represents a malignant T-cell lymphoma from its inception (therefore, the term AILT) and that the associated immunologic abnormalities are secondary to the lymphoma (100). However, there is a significant minority viewpoint that this disease represents a continuum from reactive polyclonal T-cell proliferations to highly malignant T-cell lymphomas. This viewpoint is supported by the 25% of cases without identifiable clonal T-cell populations, even using sophisticated microdissection technologies (89), in the existence of cases in oligoclonal T-cell populations (94,101), and from reports of cases with transient T-cell clones (93,102).

Approximately 10% of cases will show clonal immunoglobulin gene rearrangements (93,94). However, these have generally been attributed to clonal proliferations of EBV-infected B cells. EBV-infected B cells can be identified in a

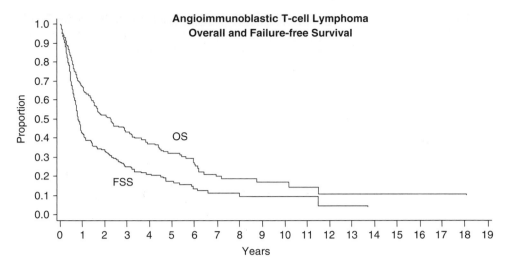

FIGURE 29.3 The overall (OS) and failure-free (FFS) survival from a study of 241 patients with AILT collected from multiple institutions as part of an international retrospective analysis. (Reprinted from Armitage J, Vose J, Weisenburger D. International peripheral T-cell and natural killer/T-cell lymphoma study: pathology findings and clinical outcomes. *J Clin Oncol* 2008;26:4124–4130, with permission.)

high proportion of AILTs and are believed to be a manifestation of the immune disturbance associated with this disease. In rare cases, overt B-cell lymphoma may supervene (95). In the past several years, evidence has accumulated that the tumor cells of AILT are derived from T_{FH}. Similar to T_{FH}, the atypical T cells in AILT express CD10, BCL6, CXCL13, SAP, and the cell death receptor PD1 (22,83,103–105). Furthermore, recent gene expression profiling studies have confirmed the relationship of these lymphomas to T_{FH} (30,42). Such studies have further identified a subset of PTCL, NOS that expresses a T_{FH} phenotype, suggesting that there is pathogenetic overlap between AILT and histologically defined PTCL, NOS.

Clinical Features and Treatment Outcome

Patients with AILT typically have generalized adenopathy, fever, weight loss, skin rash, polyclonal hypergammaglobulinemia, autoimmune manifestations that can include a positive Coombs' test, and frequent infections. A complicating factor in the care of patients in whom angioimmunoblastic-like T-cell lymphoma is considered can be whether or not the patient has a "benign" condition mimicking T-cell lymphoma that might respond to prednisone. In a German clinical trial that randomized patients to initial treatment with prednisone alone or an anthracycline-containing combination chemotherapy regimen, 28 patients were randomized to receive initial prednisone alone. The intent was to switch them to the combination chemotherapy regimen if prednisone failed. Eight patients (29%) achieved a complete remission with prednisone, and three patients were in continuous complete remission at the time of the report. It would appear that few, if any, patients diagnosed today with AILT have a "benign" condition, and all patients should receive initial chemotherapy for lymphoma.

Two large series of patients with AILT have recently been described. In an international cooperative study, 243 patients were reported (106). The median age of the patients was 65 years, and 56% were male. Generalized lymphadenopathy was noted at presentation in 76% of the patients, and 89% had stage III–IV disease. Hemolytic anemia and dysproteinemia were found in 13% and 50% of the patients, respec-

tively. Ninety-two percent of the patients were treated with an anthracycline-containing chemotherapy regimen. The 5-year overall survival was 33%, and the 5-year failure-free survival was 18% (Fig. 29.3 and Table 29.3).

The Groupe d'Etude des Lymphomes de l'Adulte reported 157 patients with AILT (107). The median age of the patients in this series was 62 years, and 60% were male. These were patients who were able to be included in Groupe d'Etude des Lymphomes de l'Adulte clinical trials. Eighty-one percent of the patients had stage III/IV disease, 72% had B symptoms, and 50% had hypergammaglobulinemia. The 7-year overall survival was 30%, and the 7-year failure-free survival was 23%.

The European Group for Blood and Marrow Transplantation reported 146 patients with AILT who underwent auto-transplant (108). The major determinant for treatment outcome was the disease status at the time of transplantation. Patients who were transplanted in first complete remission had a 56% 4-year progression-free survival in contrast to 30% failure-free survival for patients with chemotherapy sensitive relapse disease who were transplanted. Twenty-three percent of the patients who were transplanted for chemotherapy refractory disease survived 4 years progression free. Because some patients have long-term, disease-free survival with initial chemotherapy alone, and because patients were certainly selected for transplantation, it is still not clear that transplantation in initial remission improves the ultimate outcome. In one series of patients with PTCL undergoing allogeneic transplants, the best outcome was seen in AILT (66).

Other therapies have been noted to be active in patients with angioimmunoblastic T-cell lymphoma and might be incorporated into frontline regimens. Twelve patients treated with cyclosporine have been described in one series (109). Ten patients had prior therapy fail, and two elderly patients received cyclosporine as their initial treatment. Eight patients responded, and three had a continuing response at the time of the report. One patient who had several previous chemotherapy regimens fail was treated with bevacizumab and had a complete remission that lasted for 10 months (110). This is an interesting observation given the high density of blood vessels in these tumors.

Nasal and Extranasal Natural Killer/T-Cell Lymphoma

It is known that NK and T cells may have a common precursor. NK cells typically have abundant pale cytoplasm and azurophilic granules. Immunophenotypically, T-lineage-associated antigens such as CD2, CD7, and CD8 may be expressed. Surface CD3 antigen is usually negative but cytoplasmic CD3ε chain positive. CD56 surface antigen is consistently expressed. TCR and immunoglobulin gene rearrangements are uniformly absent. Functionally, NK cells are cytolytic cells targeting malignant or virally infected cells (111).

In the WHO classification for hematopoietic and lymphoid tumors, NK-cell malignancies are recognized as distinct clinicopathologic entities, and they include the extranodal NK/T-cell lymphoma, nasal type (ENKTL) (112). Many other terms, including *polymorphic reticulosis, lethal midline granuloma, progressive lethal granulomatous ulceration, malignant granuloma, nonhealing granuloma,* and *midline malignant reticulosis,* have all been used in the past to describe this clinically malignant lesion involving midline facial structures (113–121). Because this lymphoma may present in sites other than the upper airway and nose, the term *nasal type* was used originally in the WHO classification. Because the term "nasal type" has been recognized to be rather confusing and misleading, it has been suggested in the revised WHO classification that this type of lymphoma should be renamed as "Nasal or Extra-nasal NK/T-cell lymphoma."

Epidemiology

Nasal NK/T-cell lymphoma is an uncommon tumor, and it shows great variations in incidence in different racial populations and geographic locations (2,122,123). In Asia, the tumor is seen mainly in southern China, Japan, and Korea. In our International Lymphoma Study, nasal NK/T-cell lymphoma comprised 8% of all the NHL seen in Hong Kong. Nasal NK/T-cell lymphoma is also seen in patients of Native-American descent in Mexico and Central and South America, but it rarely affects whites. The tumor only accounts for <1% of all cases of NHL seen in Europe and North America. It has, however, been sporadically reported in patients with immunosuppression and posttransplantation.

Pathology

Extranodal NK/T-cell lymphoma is characterized by a broad cytologic spectrum (Table 29.4). The atypical cells may be small or medium in size. Large atypical and hyperchromatic cells may be admixed, or may predominate. If the small cells are in the majority, the disease may be difficult to distinguish from an inflammatory or infectious process. In early stages there may also be a prominent admixture of inflammatory cells, further causing difficulty in diagnosis (116,124). Most cases of nasal NK/T-cell lymphoma have extensive tissue necrosis, often with vascular infiltration and necrosis. This feature led to the earlier description of this lymphoma type as angiocentric lymphoma (120,125). More recent studies have implicated chemokines and cytokines, induced by EBV, as mediating the vascular damage (126,127).

Because virtually all cases of nasal NK/T-cell lymphoma are positive for EBV, in situ hybridization studies with probes to EBV–encoded small nuclear ribonucleic acid

---

TABLE 29.4

COMMON FEATURES OF EXTRANODAL T/NK-CELL LYMPHOMAS

Broad cytologic spectrum
Disease definition is heavily dependent upon clinical features, not morphology
Infrequent lymph node involvement, even with recurrences
Frequent spread to other extranodal sites
Cytotoxic T-cell or NK-cell phenotype
Frequent apoptosis and /or necrosis, with or without angioinvasion
Increased incidence of a hemophagocytic syndrome
Presence of EBV correlates with both anatomic site and geographic factors

---

(Epstein-Barr-encoded ribonucleic acid 1/2) may be very helpful in diagnosis and can detect even small numbers of neoplastic cells (128,129). Although the cells express some T-cell-associated antigens, most commonly CD2, other T-cell markers such as surface CD3, are usually absent (125). Cytoplasmic CD3ε can be found in paraffin sections. However, cytoplasmic CD3ε can be found in NK cells, and is not specific for a T-cell lineage. Studies for clonal T-cell gene rearrangement are generally negative. CD56 is expressed in nearly all cases, and is seen in nasal and extranasal sites (130). Expression of p53 has been reported in a variable proportion of cases (123) but appears not to have prognostic significance in this disease (130).

PATHOGENESIS

ENKTLs are generally tumors of NK cells lacking rearranged TCRs. The majority express T-cell-associated antigens CD2, CD43, cytoplasmic CD3ε, as well as the NK-cell-associated marker CD56 (13,131). By definition all cases express cytotoxic proteins and contain EBV. Rare cases comprised of CD8-positive tumor cells, possessing TCR rearrangements, that otherwise mimic cases with the NK phenotype have been described (130). ENKTLs show frequent overexpression of the p53 tumor suppressor gene (123,132–134). A subset of p53 overexpressing cases possess p53 mutations, and these are associated with large cell histology, advanced stage of disease, and poor prognosis (133,134).

There are few classic cytogenetic studies of these lymphomas, and among the reported abnormalities reported are trisomy 7, deletions of 6q, +X, trisomy 8, del (13q), and del (17p) (135). More recent studies using both chromosomal and array based CGH and loss of heterozygosity studies have confirmed the high incidence of chromosomal loss at 6q (up to 90% of cases) and 13q (approximately 70%, with percentage of cases), and the lower frequencies of loss of heterozygosity chromosomal loss observed at chromosomes 11q and 17p (in about 30% of cases) (136). Frequent chromosomal gains were identified including at 1p32-pter, 2q, 6p., 11q, 12q, 17q, 19p, 20q, and Xp. Recent studies using spectral karyotyping have identified the presence of cryptic translocations involving Xp21-pter and 8p23 (137). The genes involved are not known. These lymphomas show frequent overexpression of the p53 tumor suppressor gene (123). This finding combined with reports of 17p deletions suggest that inactivation of p53 may be a common occurrence in NK/T-cell lymphomas, however, there are a lack of confirmatory mutational studies. Other findings include chromosomal losses at 1p, 2p, 4q, 5p, 5q, 6q, and 11q (136,138). Detailed loss of heterozygosity studies has further refined the area of deletion on chromosome 6q to a 2.6-Mb region containing at least 18 known genes and an additional 25 hypothetical genes sequences (139). However, to date no candidate tumor suppressor loci genes have been studied or identified in the region. The presence of cryptic translocations involving Xp21-pter and 8p23 has been reported in rare cases through the use of spectral karyotyping, but the genes involved have also not been identified (137).

EBV is thought to play a prominent role in the pathogenesis of these tumors. EBV deoxyribonucleic acid sequences are found in 100% of tumors, and an EBV latency type II phenotype is usually seen (140). It is of interest that nearly all cases are infected with the EBV Epstein-Barr nuclear antigen (EBNA)-1 p-ala variant sequence. This virus subtype is virtually never found in other types of EBV-associated neoplasms, although it is one of the major viral subtypes found in reactive conditions (141). Remarkably, Gaal et al. (142) also identified ongoing mutations at a number of "hot spots" in the EBNA-1 sequence, although this finding is controversial. These observations raise interesting questions regarding the host-virus interaction and pathogenesis. Why are not the other viral EBNA-1 subtypes found in ENKTL, as they are in other EBV-associated cancers? Why is the p-ala EBNA-1 subtype selected specifically in NK cells? Are ongoing mutations an indication of genomic instability in these tumors?

Like their putative normal cellular progenitor, ENKTLs express several proteins capable of causing tissue destruction, including cytotoxic effectors such as perforin and granzyme B, and FAS ligand (FAS-L). Ng et al. (143) demonstrated a correlation between the percentage of perforin-positive cells and that the expression of both of these effectors is positively correlated with the degree of zonal necrosis and single cell apoptosis associated with the lesions (144). The expression of FAS-L is FAS-L, is capable of initiating apoptotic death through activation of the FAS death pathway. There was not found to be any obvious correlation between the expression of FAS-L and the degree of necrosis present (145).

Cytotoxic NK cells and lymphomas of NK cells appear to have evolved elaborate mechanisms to control their potentially lethal activities. NK cells express a family of regulatory receptors termed killer inhibitory receptors (KIRs), and they express the FAS receptor (145,146). The KIRs are MHC class 1-specific NK-cell receptors that primarily function to inhibit the NK-cytotoxic response. These receptors are comprised of two families the immunoglobulin superfamily receptors (CD158a, CD158b, and NKB1) and the lectin-like receptors (CD94/NKG2A). Studies of KIRs in NK/T-cell lymphomas indicate that these receptors continue to be expressed in lymphomas of NK cells, and it has been suggested that their presence may be important in modulating their potential antitumor activity (147,148). Although the specific KIR repertoire does not seem to correlate with clinical outcome, expression of the lectin-like receptor CD94 is associated with a significantly increased median survival (149).

It has been postulated that the expression of both FAS and FAS-L on are highly expressed in normal NK cells may also play a role in preventing uncontrolled NK-cell activity and proliferation. Although one may have predicted down-regulation of FAS on tumor cells, this is not the case. Interestingly, whereas NK-cell tumors continue to express FAS, as many as half of all ENKTLs show potentially inactivating FAS-coding region mutations, including point mutations and frameshifts (150,151). The majority of these mutations truncate the N-terminal death domain leaving the C-terminal ligand-binding domain intact. Furthermore, when these mutations were modeled, which in mice, they were shown to models confer resistance to FAS-mediated apoptosis. It has been suggested that these truncated FAS proteins may behave in a dominant negative manner in the cell, or alternatively result in a soluble ligand binding domain that can block FAS-L activity. Thus, the presence of these FAS mutations should inactivate, rendering the tumor cell resistant to FAS-mediated killing. In addition to the presence of FAS mutations, overexpression of cellular FLICE (caspase-8)-inhibitory protein has been reported in NK/T-cell lines that lack FAS mutations, and in a subset of primary NK/T-cell lymphomas (152). Cell lines overexpressing cellular FLICE (caspase-8)-inhibitory protein are resistant to FAS mediated apoptosis, suggesting that in addition to FAS mutation, cellular FLICE (caspase 8)-inhibitory protein overexpression may be another mechanism of inactivating this potent death-signaling pathway and provide the tumor with a survival advantage.

ENKTLs also express high levels of the serpin proteinase inhibitor 9 (PI9) (153). This is the only known protein able to inhibit the proteolytic activity of granzyme B. It has been suggested that this is yet another mechanism by which ENKTL tumor cells can protect themselves from autologous granzyme B, or enzyme directed from cytotoxic T cells, and escape from immune surveillance. However, a recent clinical study showed that the absence of PI9 expression was associated with poor survival (154). This is contrary to a prior study of ALCL in which a positive correlation between PI9 expression and clinical outcome was shown (155). The reason why PI9 expression confers a different clinical outcome in these two lymphomas is unclear.

Clinical Features

Nasal NK/T-cell lymphoma more commonly affects men, and the median age of the patients is approximately 50 years old (156–161). The tumor typically presents with nasal symptoms, including obstruction and bleeding, or a nasal mass. There may be local invasion into the orbit, nasal sinuses, nasopharynx, oropharynx, palate, and even larynx (Color Plate 74). Cranial nerves may also be involved, but meningeal involvement is not common (162,163). Systemic dissemination is often late but clinically very aggressive. Favorite metastatic sites include skin, gut, and testis, sites where CD56 is normally expressed. Patients may also present with a primary tumor in one of these sites. In a percentage of these patients, however, occult nasal disease may be present. Circulating lymphoma cells together with marrow involvement may be seen as a terminal event.

A high index of suspicion is essential for early diagnosis. Because of the anatomic location of the tumor, the size of the biopsy specimens from nasal endoscopy is often small. The presence of extensive necrosis, together with the marked

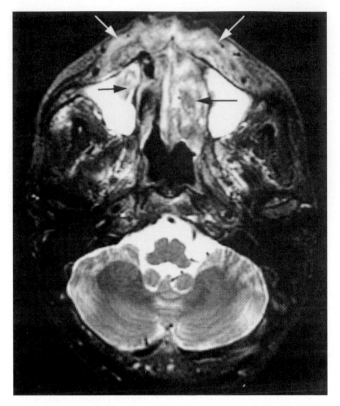

FIGURE 29.4 Nuclear magnetic resonance scan showing NK-cell lymphoma in the midline nasal cavity.

presence of inflammatory cellular infiltrates, makes this a big challenge for histopathologists. Multiple biopsies of adequate size are required before a definitive diagnosis can be made. For difficult cases, an opinion from an experienced histopathologist is beneficial, and the use of EBV markers may also provide additional clues (164).

A small subset of patients may have very aggressive disease at presentation. These patients have high fever, liver failure, and marrow failure. Features of hemophagocytosis may be observed. Studies have shown that this is usually associated with a high level of soluble FAS-L from the tumor (165). Other than the usual staging investigations for NHL, including computed tomographic scan of the thorax and abdomen and bone marrow biopsy, a computed tomographic scan or magnetic resonance imaging scan of the nasal region may give a better picture of the extent of local spread of the tumor (Fig. 29.4) (166,167). The role of positron emission tomography is uncertain.

Treatment and Monitoring

Local radiotherapy and chemotherapy are both effective treatments for primary nasal lymphoma (Table 29.3). However, with radiotherapy or chemotherapy alone, treatment failure is still common (162,168,169). Local recurrences are usually followed by systemic relapse. Better clinical outcome has been obtained with the combined use of chemotherapy and local radiotherapy. For patients with localized disease at presentation, local radiotherapy is an important treatment (170–172). Prolonged remission is achievable in approximately one half of cases. An adequate radiation dose together with an accurately planned radiation field is essential to minimize the chance of local failure. For patients with disseminated disease at presentation or at disease progression, the disease is almost invariably fatal. The relatively poor clinical outcome may be explained by the ischemic nature of the tumor as well as the primary cellular drug resistance. The results from an international series are presented in Figure 29.5.

There is no consensus on the optimal chemotherapeutic regimen for this tumor. Because of the relative rarity of this disease, prospective clinical studies are not available. An anthracycline-containing regimen, such as CHOP, is commonly used. It remains uncertain that other more complicated regimens, such as prednisone, methotrexate-leucovorin, Adriamycin (doxorubicin), cyclophosphamide, etoposide plus cytarabine, bleomycin, Oncovin (vincristine), and methotrexate, are more effective (163,173,174).

After therapy, it is essential to monitor the patient closely with nasal endoscopy and biopsy. Random blind biopsy is recommended even if the nasal mucosa appears normal on endoscopy because occult residual tumor cells may still persist. Interpretation of the biopsy specimens can be even more difficult at this stage. The use of EBV markers, such as

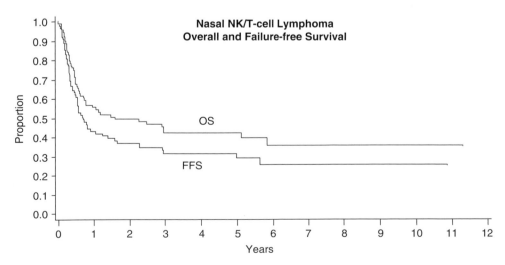

FIGURE 29.5 The overall (OS) and failure-free (FFS) survival from a study of 92 patients with nasal NK/T-cell lymphoma collected from multiple institutions as part of an international retrospective analysis. (Reprinted from Armitage J, Vose J, Weisenburger D. International peripheral T-cell and natural killer/T-cell lymphoma study: pathology findings and clinical outcomes. *J Clin Oncol* 2008;26:4124–4130, with permission.)

Epstein-Barr early region staining, may sometimes be helpful (175). Further studies are ongoing to see whether molecular markers, such as circulating EBV deoxyribonucleic acid, are even more useful (150,176,177).

The optimal timing of radiotherapy in relation to chemotherapy (i.e. which should be given first) is also uncertain, but it should not be delayed because of its effectiveness in local control of disease. The presence of residual tumor cells after 3 months of initial chemotherapy is usually indicative of inadequate response to therapy. A decision has to be made to give local radiotherapy early and to switch to an alternative chemotherapy regime. L-asparaginase has been shown to have good activity in the treatment of nasal NK/T-cell lymphoma, and further clinical studies are ongoing (178–182).

High-dose chemotherapy with autologous stem cell rescue may also have a role in the management of this tumor (183–185). The best result is seen when it is performed at the time of remission (186–188). There is very limited experience in the use of allogeneic transplants, including the nonmyeloablative approach, for this tumor (189).

Distant tumor dissemination appears to be the most important prognostic feature. It is well known that there is a wide variation in the cytologic appearance of the tumor. However, there is no evidence that the cytologic grade is useful in predicting prognosis. On the other hand, the IPI commonly used for B-cell tumors has been shown to be useful (190).

Hepatosplenic T-Cell Lymphoma

Hepatosplenic T-cell lymphoma (HSTCL) is an aggressive subtype of extranodal lymphoma accounting for <2% of all PTCLs in a recent international study (46). In 1990 a report of two patients with prominent infiltration of the spleen and liver led to a proposal that a new entity should be recognized based on the clinical presentation, the pattern of histologic involvement showing a sinusoidal tropism of neoplastic cells, and the $\gamma\delta$ TCR phenotype of the tumor cells (191).

Pathology

The great majority of cases are of $\gamma\delta$ T-cell origin (11,192), but an $\alpha\beta$ origin has been seen in a small subset of cases (193–195). The clinical presentation is very homogeneous, with most cases presenting in young males, 15 to 30 years of age. Many patients have a history of chronic antigenic stimulation in the setting of immunosuppression, with a number of reports occurring in patients with solid organ transplantation (11,196,197), or less commonly Crohn disease (9,198). Treatment with inhibitors of tumor necrosis factor appears to increase the risk of HSTCL (199,200), although interestingly antitumor necrosis factor therapy in rheumatoid arthritis is not associated with a similar risk. Crohn disease, with its defects in the intestinal barrier, may be susceptible because of the marked antigenic assault associated with the underlying disease.

The disease is disseminated at presentation by virtue of marked sinusoidal infiltration of liver, spleen, and bone marrow, despite the absence of lymph node involvement. Abnormal cells are usually present in the sinusoids of the bone marrow but may be difficult to identify without immunohistochemical stains. Peripheral blood involvement is usually not seen until late in the course. The neoplastic cells have a phenotype that resembles that of immature or resting $\gamma\delta$

T cells, often double negative for CD4 and CD8, and negative for CD5; CD56 is also positive (191,192). The cells express the cytotoxic granule-associated protein, T-cell intracellular antigen-1, but are generally negative for perforin and granzyme B. Isochromosome 7q is a consistent cytogenetic abnormality, usually in association with trisomy 8 (201–203).

Pathogenesis

HSTCLs are primarily tumors of nonactivated $\gamma\delta$–expressing T cells (191,192,204). These rare lymphomas express the cytotoxic granule-associated protein T-cell intracellular antigen-1 (205,206) but do not express the effector cytotoxic proteins, the granzymes and perforin (205). A few α/β–expressing cases have been reported (193,195). HSTCLs show rearrangements of their γ and β-TCR genes. The more common $\gamma\delta$–expressing lymphomas preferentially use the Vδ1 gene, reflecting the preferential use of this V-family gene in resident $\gamma\delta$ cells in the spleen (11,207). Regardless of which TCR gene is expressed, these lymphomas share identical nonrandom chromosomal abnormalities, specifically isochromosome 7q and trisomy 8 (11,201,203,207,208). However, neither of these abnormalities is a specific marker of HSTCL, and the presumed genes involved have not been identified. Gene expression profiling of a limited number of cases suggests that these lymphomas form a distinctive group, separate from other $\gamma\delta$–expressing T-cell lymphomas (209). HSTCLs express the NK-associated KIRs and CD94, which can be found on cytotoxic α/β or $\gamma\delta$– memory cells, suggesting a pathogenic relationship to this subset of normal cells (209,210).

Clinical Features and Treatment Outcome

The clinical entity $\gamma\delta$ HSTCL occurs primarily in young men, and typically presents with hepatosplenomegaly, no peripheral adenopathy, B symptoms, and cytopenias (11) (Table 29.3). In a recent international study (46), the median age was 34 years, and 68% of the patients were male. Ninety-five percent presented with stage III–IV disease, and 74% had positive bone marrow biopsies. An overt leukemic presentation was unusual, but careful examination of blood smears often identified a minor population of "atypical lymphoid cells." Patients occasionally presented with the hemophagocytic syndrome. This entity has been reported in patients with a known immune defect and in those receiving long-term immunosuppressive therapy (197,211,212). This entity can be diagnosed at autopsy if the clinicians do not consider the diagnosis in a patient whose presentation might suggest more of an infectious disease or another immune disorder. HSTCL has an extremely poor outcome, with no 5-year survivors in a series of 21 patients (11) and a 5-year survival of 7% in a recent large international study (46) (Fig. 29.6). Patients frequently respond to CHOP-like chemotherapy regimens but essentially all have relapse (11). Long-term survival has been reported with HyperCVAD (213) and with allogeneic bone marrow transplantation (214). Some newer agents appear to be active, and excellent responses have been reported with pentostatin, cladribine, and alemtuzumab (215,216).

Enteropathy Type T-Cell Lymphoma

Enteropathy type T-cell lymphoma (ETTL) is a rare type of NHL comprising <1% of all NHLs in the recent reports

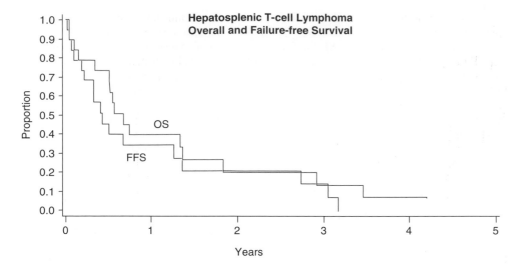

FIGURE 29.6 The overall (OS) and failure-free (FFS) survival from a study of 18 patients with HSTCL collected from multiple institutions as part of an international retrospective analysis. (Reprinted from Armitage J, Vose J, Weisenburger D. International peripheral T-cell and natural killer/T-cell lymphoma study: pathology findings and clinical outcomes. *J Clin Oncol* 2008;26:4124–4130, with permission.)

from the International Lymphoma Study Group (217). Before the development of the WHO classification of lymphoid tumors, ETTL was also known as *malignant histiocytosis of the intestine* (218) and *enteropathy associated T-cell lymphoma* (219). It is a tumor of intraepithelial T lymphocytes most commonly occurring in the jejunum or ileum and is closely associated with celiac disease. The prognosis is poor, with reported 5-year survival rates of <30%. Optimal treatment strategies for ETTL are unclear.

Epidemiology, Etiology, and Relationship to Celiac Disease

ETTL is a rare subtype of NHL that is most common in those areas with a high incidence of celiac disease (220–223). In a study of 175 cases of gastrointestinal lymphoma from the British National Lymphoma Investigation, only 16 cases (9%) were ETTL (224). In a more recent report of 199 patients with various subtypes of T-cell lymphoma from British Columbia, 5% were classified as having ETTL (225). The reported frequency of diagnosis corresponds with the overall frequency of celiac disease. In a series from the United Kingdom, where the incidence of celiac disease is higher than in North America, 34 of 120 patients with PTCL (28%) had ETTL (226). Patients with ETTL may have a history of celiac disease since childhood or a relatively brief history of adult-onset celiac disease before the development of lymphoma. It is thought that patients with adult-onset celiac disease may have occult clinical disease from early in life. In either case, a lack or loss of response of celiac disease to a gluten-free diet is often the first indication of the development of ETTL (227,228).

Most patients with ETTL have the human leukocyte antigen (HLA) DQA1*0501, DQB1*0201 genotype, which is also associated with an increased risk of celiac disease (229,230). However, additional HLA-DR/DQ-associated alleles that act independently may represent additional risk factors for ETTL but require further investigation (231). Recent data using whole genome analysis and HLA genotyping have suggested that two distinct subtypes of ETTL may exist, one of which may not be associated with celiac disease (232).

Pathology

ETTL occurs in adults, the majority of whom have a history of gluten–sensitive enteropathy. Patients usually present with abdominal symptoms such as pain, small bowel perforation, and associated peritonitis. The small bowel usually shows ulceration, frequently with perforation. A mass may or may not be present, and the intestinal involvement is often multifocal. The neoplastic cells infiltrate the overlying epithelium, mimicking normal intraepithelial lymphocytes (IELs). In refractory coeliac disease and ulcerative jejunitis, the IELs share clonal identity with the subsequent lymphomas developing in these patients (233,234). The clinical course is aggressive, with poor long-term survival.

The neoplastic cells in ETTL have a wide morphologic spectrum. The cells are generally medium to large in size, but in a subset they are markedly anaplastic and strongly CD30 positive (235). A marked tissue eosinophilia may partially mask the neoplastic population (236). The cells are $\alpha\beta$-cytotoxic T cells mimicking the phenotype of IEL. CD56 positivity is seen in a subset of cases, typically with more monomorphic cytology (237). Although some of the CD56-positive cases with monomorphic cytology are seen in patients with celiac disease, this form of intestinal lymphoma also occurs sporadically. The neoplastic cells are uniformly negative for EBV.

ETTL must be distinguished from other T-cell lymphomas presenting with intestinal disease, and not all *intestinal T-cell lymphomas* are ETTL. The intestinal tract is a common site of localization of extranodal NK/T-cell lymphoma, nasal type, which can be distinguished by its EBV positivity. Mucocutaneous $\gamma\delta$ T-cell lymphomas may also present with intestinal disease, and may appear similar both clinically and morphologically (14,238). They too are of cytotoxic T-cell derivation, and are associated with extensive apoptosis and necrosis.

Pathogenesis

ETTL is a clonal T-cell proliferation, presumably originating from cytotoxic IELs, in which the TCR βTRB and γ genes TRG are usually rearranged (239,240). Although the majority of these lymphomas express the α/β TCR, a minority express the γ/δ TCR (241). Although traditional cytogenetic studies that include cases of ETCL are rare. Recent studies using the application of molecular cytogenetic technologies have begun to provide some clues into the molecular genetics of these lymphomas. Classic chromosome-based CGH studies have demonstrated recurrent gains of chromosome 1q, 5q, 7q, and 9q (58% of cases), 7q (24%), 5q (18%), and 1q (16%), and chromosomal losses of 8p (24%), 9p, 13q (24%), and 9p (18%) (242). More recent high-resolution array CGH studies have further refined these major regions of losses and gains into several smaller regions, and have identified additional novel alterations, including regions of gain on chromosomes 5p, 7p, 20q, 21q, and 22q, and regions of loss at 17p, 10q, and 3p (232). Interestingly, the region of loss at chromosome 16q present in 23% of cases was narrowed to 2.5 Mb, and found to be mutually exclusive with the more prevalent 9q gains that occur in 70% of cases (232). Although the genes on chromosome 16q have not been identified, the region of gain on 9q (9q34) contains two potential oncogenes, ABL1 and NOTCH1, which are both amplified in most cases (243). Whether one or both of these genes play a role in the pathogenesis of this lymphoma has yet to be determined.

Like their nonneoplastic progenitors, ETCL cells express the homing and adhesion receptor CD103 (HML-1) (244,245). CD103 is a novel integrin composed of β 7 and α E subunits, implicated in homing and adhesion properties of the IELs (246). This receptor is expressed almost exclusively in ETCL, mycoses fungoides, and in hairy cell leukemia (242,247). The presence of this receptor may be responsible for the frequent intraepithelial spread of ETCL (240).

ETCLs often arise in patients with evidence of celiac disease and nearly all cases are associated with the HLA DQA1*0501, DQB1*0201 genotype that is characteristic of celiac disease (231). Patients who have progression and develop refractory sprue or ulcerative duodenitis frequently show intraepithelial lymphocytosis associated with clonal T-cell rearrangements (233,248). Furthermore, the IELs of noninvolved intestinal mucosa in patients with ETCL frequently display identical TCR gene rearrangements as those observed in their lymphoma (240). These observations suggest a stepwise progression from the polyclonal T-cell expansion seen in typical sprue, to an early monoclonal T-cell expansion/low-grade lymphoma seen in refractory sprue, and finally to a clinically evident overt T-cell lymphoma. Based on morphologic, immunophenotypic, cytogenetic, and HLA phenotypes, two distinct types of ETCLs have been recently recognized (232). Type 1 ETCL accounts for the majority of cases, is characterized by nonmonomorphic cytology, CD56 negativity, and chromosomal gains of 1q and 5q. This ETCL subtype appears to be linked pathogenetically to celiac disease, sharing genetic alterations and HLA-DQB1 genotype patterns. Type 2 ETL shows monomorphic small to medium-sized tumor cell morphology, CD56 positivity, *MYC* oncogene locus amplification, and generally lacks gains of chromosomes 1q and 5q. In contrast to type 1 ETCL, type 2 ETCL shows an HLA-DQB1 genotype pattern more closely resembling the normal white population, suggesting it arises independently of celiac disease.

Sites of Involvement

ETTL most commonly involves the jejunum or ileum, although involvement of other parts of the gastrointestinal tract, including the stomach, duodenum, and colon, has been reported. The typical macroscopic appearance is of circumferential ulceration of the bowel wall with marked edema of the adjacent small intestine (249). Enlargement of mesenteric lymph nodes in surgically resected specimens is observed in most cases, although only approximately 30% of these lymph nodes have evidence of infiltration by ETTL, with the remaining cases showing reactive changes only.

In addition to the histologic changes observed in the affected small bowel, most resected specimens show evidence of villous atrophy and crypt hyperplasia in the adjacent small bowel, with increased numbers of IELs with a CD3$^+$/CD8$^+$ phenotype. These changes reflect those associated with the underlying celiac disease.

Clinical Features

In view of the rarity of ETTL, there are very few reports that specifically describe this entity. In the largest published series, from the United Kingdom, the median age at onset of ETTL was 55 years (range 20 to 80 years); 74% of patients were male, and 26% female (249). Twelve of the patients in this series had a history of celiac disease, diagnosed between 3 months and 40 years before the diagnosis of ETTL. In a similar series from Ireland, where the prevalence of celiac disease is high, seven of 30 patients with ETTL had a previous diagnosis of celiac disease, from 12 to 252 months (median 44 months) earlier (250). Other series have reported the onset of ETTL between 3 and 5 years after the diagnosis of celiac disease in adults, suggesting that close monitoring of patients with adult-onset celiac disease, especially in the first few years after diagnosis, is essential (251). Previous studies have demonstrated that between 5% and 10% of patients with adult-onset celiac disease may be at risk for ETTL (252,253).

The role of adherence to a gluten-free diet in the development of enteropathy type intestinal T-cell lymphoma in patients with celiac disease is unclear, although Holmes et al. (254) have reported that treatment of celiac disease with a gluten-free diet for >5 years reduces the risk of lymphoma to that of the general population. Recent studies have investigated whether preemptive treatment of refractory celiac disease can prevent the emergence of ETTL. Cladribine, alemtuzumab, and the use of high-dose therapy with autologous stem cell transplantation have been investigated in this context in small series, but their impact on the subsequent development of ETTL is unclear despite evidence for an initial histologic response (255–257).

In the series from the United Kingdom (249), the most common presenting symptoms for ETTL were abdominal pain (84%), weight loss (81%), diarrhea (39%), and vomiting (29%). Small bowel perforation or small bowel obstruction was a presenting feature in 42%. In the series from Ireland, a similar proportion of patients without preceding celiac disease (60%) presented with intestinal obstruction or perforation (250). Night sweats and fevers are uncommon presenting symptoms in ETTL. Abdominal masses are uncommon (16%), and peripheral lymphadenopathy is very rare at presentation. Most patients present with high-intermediate or high-risk disease according to the IPI.

The diagnosis of ETTL is most commonly made at laparotomy (80%), although in some patients, endoscopic biopsies from the proximal small bowel are diagnostic. In reported series, approximately two thirds of patients have single-site disease in the small bowel, the remainder having multiple areas of involvement.

Most patients have clinical stage IE or IIE disease at presentation. Mesenteric lymph node involvement is relatively common, as is direct spread to the omentum or mesentery. Stage IV disease is uncommon, comprising only 20% of cases in the published series.

Techniques for the diagnosis and staging of ETTL have evolved in recent years. The advent of wireless capsule endoscopy (258) and double balloon endoscopy (259), which allow visualization of the entire small intestine, have enabled more accurate staging, and preliminary data suggest that fluorodeoxyglucose positron emission tomography may be superior to conventional imaging for this disease (260,261).

Treatment and Complications

The optimal treatment strategy for patients with ETTL is unclear. In previous series, a small proportion of patients with stage IE disease have been managed with surgical resection alone. However, in one published series, of six patients managed with surgery alone, five subsequently had relapse (249), and it is now widely accepted that all patients presenting with ETTL should receive combination chemotherapy. The most commonly used regimen for patients with ETTL is CHOP (3,262). However, the use of combination chemotherapy in these patients is complicated, and <50% of patients typically complete their planned course of chemotherapy (249). In part, this may reflect the impaired nutritional status of this group of patients. Approximately 30% require parenteral or enteral nutrition during chemotherapy (Table 29.3). Small bowel perforation is a well-documented complication of this treatment, most commonly after the first cycle of chemotherapy, when it is thought to be the result of tumor response in transmural disease. The risk of intestinal perforation in the UK series was four of 31 (13%). The risk of early treatment-related mortality in this group also appears to be high. In the same series, 21% of patients died of treatment-related complications (infection or gastrointestinal hemorrhage) after the first cycle of chemotherapy.

A small series of patients treated with cyclophosphamide, doxorubicin, etoposide, vincristine, and prednisone has been reported based on encouraging data for the use of this regimen in patients with diffuse large B-cell lymphoma (263). Of the ten patients included in this study, five had primary progressive disease, two had complete remissions, but only one was in continuing complete remission 10 months after completion of chemotherapy.

The use of high-dose therapy and autologous stem cell transplantation as consolidation of first complete response has also been reported in a number of case reports and small series (264–266). Long-term survival has been reported in some of these patients, although the reports are largely anecdotal, and the patient populations are likely to be highly selected. A formal prospective phase II evaluation of "early" autologous stem cell transplantation is currently in progress in Europe.

Response and Survival

Limited response data are available from previous reports, with complete response rates of 20% to 40% and overall response rates of 50% to 60%. Relapses typically occur at a median of 6 to 7 months from the completion of initial

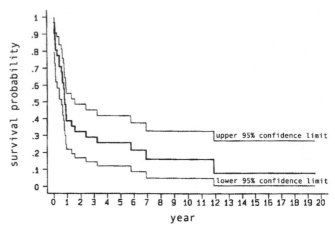

FIGURE 29.7 Overall survival for 31 patients with enteropathy type intestinal T-cell lymphoma. (Reprinted from Gale J, Simmonds PD, Mead GM, et al. Enteropathy-type intestinal T-cell lymphoma: clinical features and treatment of 31 patients in a single center. *J Clin Oncol* 2000;18:795–803, with permission.)

therapy, most commonly in the small intestine, although relapse at other sites, including the liver, spleen, and mesenteric lymph nodes, has been documented. Central nervous system relapse has also been documented.

Results of salvage therapy have been poor, with very few patients achieving long-term disease-free survival after conventional dose salvage. Although anecdotal reports of long-term survival after high-dose therapy and autologous stem cell transplantation exist, there is no proven role for this approach.

Overall survival data from the UK series are shown in Figure 29.7. Twenty-six of the 31 patients died of disease progression or treatment-related complications. The actuarial 1- and 5-year overall survival rates were 39% and 20%, respectively. In the Irish study, of 23 patients who received chemotherapy, nine were alive and disease free with a median follow-up of 74 months (range 10 to 196 months) (250). The latter series, however, included some patients in whom histologic review was not performed, and the outcome was not separately reported for the group that had undergone histologic review.

Novel treatment approaches are needed for ETTL, as for other PTCLs. The recent identification of amplification of the *NOTCH1* and *ABL1* genes in ETTL suggests that these may be potential future therapeutic targets (243). Other novel agents under evaluation in PTCL, summarized elsewhere in this chapter, may also have activity in ETTL.

Subcutaneous Panniculitis-Like T-Cell Lymphoma

The first report of this rare entity is often ascribed to Gonzalez et al. (267), who reported eight cases of T-cell lymphoma primarily involving subcutaneous adipose tissue and stressed the resemblance of these tumors to panniculitis. Ashworth et al. (268) had previously described similar cases, as had Tanaka et al. (269). Wang et al. (270), in 1996, described 23 patients seen at the Mayo Clinic. Many of the older cases were interpreted as an abnormal histiocytic proliferation, histiocytic cytophagic panniculitis. The diagnosis is only made when a

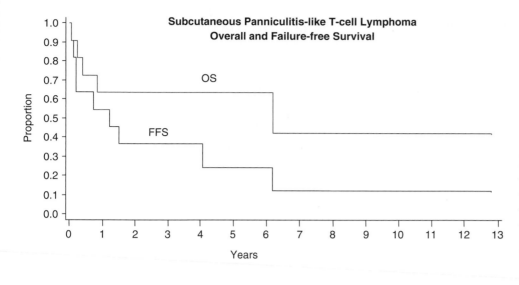

FIGURE 29.8 The overall (OS) and failure-free (FFS) survival from a study of 12 patients with subcutaneous panniculitis-like T-cell lymphoma collected from multiple institutions as part of an international retrospective analysis. (Reprinted from Armitage J, Vose J, Weisenburger D. International peripheral T-cell and natural killer/T-cell lymphoma study: pathology findings and clinical outcomes. *J Clin Oncol* 2008;26:4124–4130, with permission.)

hematopathologist or dermatopathologist who is familiar with the entity reviews a biopsy specimen.

Pathology

The cytologic composition of subcutaneous panniculitis-like T-cell lymphoma is extremely variable. The lesions may contain a predominance of small atypical lymphoid cells, often with clear cytoplasm, or larger atypical cells with hyperchromatic nuclei. Admixed reactive histiocytes are frequently present, particularly in areas of fat infiltration and destruction. The histiocytes are frequently vacuolated due to ingested lipid material. Vascular invasion may be seen in some cases, and necrosis and karyorrhexis are common.

The neoplastic cells invariably express a mature activated cytotoxic T-cell phenotype. Most cases are of $\alpha\beta$ T-cell origin, although in approximately 25% of cases, a $\gamma\delta$ T-cell phenotype can be seen. The $\gamma\delta$ T-cell cases are clinically more aggressive and display more varied histologic features. For example, both dermal and epidermal involvement are often seen, in contrast to most cases of panniculitis-like T-cell lymphoma, which are generally confined to subcutaneous tissue.

Pathogenesis

Subcutaneous panniculitis-like T-cell lymphomas are exceedingly rare lymphomas that show an activated cytotoxic phenotype, with most cases expressing cytotoxic granule protein T-cell intracellular antigen-1 and the cytotoxic effector granzymes and perforin. The necrosis often associated with these lymphomas is likely to be related, at least in part, to their expression of these cytotoxic proteins. Most cases are derived from CD8-positive α/β T cells, whereas a minority are CD4-CD8- and express the γ/δ TCR (271,272). All show clonal rearrangements of the TCR γ chain gene. The γ/δ cases exclusively utilize the Vδ2 gene, reflecting the predominant usage of this variable region gene in resident γ/δ cells of the skin (207). Cytogenetic and molecular classic cytogenetic studies of these lymphomas are virtually nonexistent, however, one recent comparative hybridization study revealed a large number of deoxyribonucleic acid copy number changes that included losses of chromosomes 1p, 2p, 2q, 5p, 7p, 9q, 10q, 11q, 12q, 17q, 16, 19, 20, and 22, and gains of chromo-

somes 2q, 4q, 5q, 6q, and 13q. Although most of these abnormalities have been reported in other cutaneous T-cell lymphomas, the gains of 5q and 13q were thought to be relatively unique to subcutaneous panniculitis-like T-cell lymphoma (273).

Clinical Features and Treatment Outcome

The clinical behavior of typical patients includes presentation with subcutaneous, sometimes painful, nodules that can resemble lipomas. The lesions are typically first seen on the extremities, and follow a several-year course of waxing and waning, but ultimately progressing. The nodules can sometimes ulcerate. Biopsies are frequently initially interpreted as showing panniculitis. When the diagnosis is made, it has been proposed that there is a distinction between those expressing $\alpha\beta$ TCRs and those expressing $\gamma\delta$ TCRs (274), with patients expressing $\gamma\delta$ TCRs being older, having a higher frequency of systemic symptoms, and having a shorter median survival (275). There is one case report of this lymphoma apparently being transmitted to the recipient of an allogeneic bone marrow transplant (276). The hemophagocytic syndrome is a well-described complication of subcutaneous panniculitis-like T-cell lymphoma (267,277) that is often fatal.

This lymphoma can follow a relatively indolent course. The survival from one international series is presented in Figure 29.8.

Patients with subcutaneous panniculitis-like T-cell lymphoma frequently respond to standard chemotherapy regimens, and complete remissions occur often in those with tumors expressing the $\alpha\beta$ TCRs but patients usually relapse (267,270,275,278–280). A variety of other drugs have been shown to be active in patients with subcutaneous panniculitis-like T-cell lymphoma, including platinum-based chemotherapy (280,281), 13 cis-retinoid acid (282), cyclosporine (282), α-interferon, zidovudine (270,283), and denileukin diftitox (284). Patients with tumors that express the $\gamma\delta$ TCRs and those who present with a hemophagocytic syndrome have a much poorer outlook (275). Occasional patients who have standard therapy fail might be salvaged with allogeneic hematopoietic stem cell transplantation.

FUTURE DIRECTIONS

PTCLs represent a wide variety of clinical/pathologic syndromes that are infrequent but, with the exception of anaplastic large T-cell lymphomas, share a poor prognosis. The explanation for a poor treatment outcome in patients with PTCL in contrast to patients with aggressive B-cell lymphomas remains uncertain. However, one possibility is that the rarity of these disorders has made them difficult to study, and the results for patients with PTCL in studies of the therapy of aggressive NHL are "lost" because these patients represent such a small proportion of those being studied. The one thing that can be said with certainty is that what we currently consider optimal treatments for diffuse large B-cell lymphoma is not equally efficacious for patients with PTCL.

Recognition of specific PTCLs as distinct entities should improve our ability to develop treatments for these disorders. A number of new agents, such as pralatrexate, denileukin diftitox, alemtuzumab, Ara-G, α-interferon, purine analogs, gemcitabine, dasatinib, and darinaparsin, are being studied in the treatment of patients with PTCL. An improved understanding of the biology of the various PTCLs will, in all likelihood, offer new targets for developing specific treatments. There is every reason to believe that currently available treatments are not being optimally used in the treatment of patients with these disorders, and that prognosis will improve with clinical trials focusing specifically on these varied disorders.

References

1. Spits H, Blom B, Jaleco AC, et al. Early stages in the development of human T, natural killer and thymic dendritic cells. *Immunol Rev* 1998;165:75–86.
2. A clinical evaluation of the International Lymphoma Study Group classification of non-Hodgkin's lymphoma. The Non-Hodgkin's Lymphoma Classification Project. *Blood* 1997;89:3909–918.
3. Savage KJ. Peripheral T-cell lymphomas. *Blood Rev* 2007;21:201–216.
4. Nava VE, Jaffe ES. The pathology of NK-cell lymphomas and leukemias. *Adv Anat Pathol* 2005;12:27–34.
5. Elenitoba-Johnson KS, Zarate-Osorno A, Meneses A, et al. Cytotoxic granular protein expression, Epstein-Barr virus strain type, and latent membrane protein-1 oncogene deletions in nasal T- lymphocyte/natural killer cell lymphomas from Mexico. *Mod Pathol* 1998;11:754–761.
6. Quintanilla-Martinez L, Kumar S, Fend F, et al. Fulminant EBV(+) T-cell lymphoproliferative disorder following acute/chronic EBV infection: a distinct clinicopathologic syndrome. *Blood* 2000;96:443–451.
7. Kimura H, Hoshino Y, Kanegane H, et al. Clinical and virologic characteristics of chronic active Epstein-Barr virus infection. *Blood* 2001;98:280–286.
8. Zhang Y, Nagata H, Ikeuchi T, et al. Common cytological and cytogenetic features of Epstein-Barr virus (EBV)-positive natural killer (NK) cells and cell lines derived from patients with nasal T/NK-cell lymphomas, chronic active EBV infection and hydroa vacciniforme-like eruptions. *Br J Haematol* 2003;121:805–814.
9. Navarro JT, Ribera JM, Mate JL, et al. Hepatosplenic T-gammadelta lymphoma in a patient with Crohn's disease treated with azathioprine. *Leuk Lymphoma* 2003;44:531–533.
10. Gardner RV, Velez MC, Ode DL, et al. Gamma/delta T-cell lymphoma as a recurrent complication after transplantation. *Leuk Lymphoma* 2004;45:2355–2359.
11. Belhadj K, Reyes F, Farcet JP, et al. Hepatosplenic gammadelta T-cell lymphoma is a rare clinicopathologic entity with poor outcome: report on a series of 21 patients. *Blood* 2003;102:4261–4269.
12. Delves PJ, Roitt IM. The immune system. First of two parts. *N Engl J Med* 2000;343:37–49.
13. Krenacs L, Smyth MJ, Bagdi E, et al. The serine protease granzyme M is preferentially expressed in NK-cell, gamma delta T-cell, and intestinal T-cell lymphomas: evidence of origin from lymphocytes involved in innate immunity. *Blood* 2003;101:3590–3593.
14. Jaffe ES, Krenacs L, Raffeld M. Classification of cytotoxic T-cell and natural killer cell lymphomas. *Semin Hematol* 2003;40:175–184.
15. Toro JR, Liewehr DJ, Pabby N, et al. Gamma-delta T-cell phenotype is associated with significantly decreased survival in cutaneous T-cell lymphoma. *Blood* 2003;101:3407–3412.
16. Jaffe ES. Mature T-cell and NK-cell lymphomas in the pediatric age group. *Am J Clin Pathol* 2004;122(suppl):S110–S121.
17. Roncador G, Garcia JF, Maestre L, et al. FOXP3, a selective marker for a subset of adult T-cell leukaemia/lymphoma. *Leukemia* 2005;19:2247–2253.
18. Nosaka K, Miyamoto T, Sakai T, et al. Mechanism of hypercalcemia in adult T-cell leukemia: overexpression of receptor activator of nuclear factor kappaB ligand on adult T-cell leukemia cells. *Blood* 2002;99:634–640.
19. Jones D, O'Hara C, Kraus MD, et al. Expression pattern of T-cell-associated chemokine receptors and their chemokines correlates with specific subtypes of T-cell non-Hodgkin lymphoma. *Blood* 2000;96:685–690.
20. Teruya-Feldstein J, Setsuda J, Yao X, et al. MIP-1alpha expression in tissues from patients with hemophagocytic syndrome. *Lab Invest* 1999;79:1583–1590.
21. Grogg KL, Attygalle AD, Macon WR, et al. Angioimmunoblastic T-cell lymphoma: a neoplasm of germinal-center T-helper cells? *Blood* 2005;106:1501–1502.
22. Dupuis J, Boye K, Martin N, et al. Expression of CXCL13 by neoplastic cells in angioimmunoblastic T-cell lymphoma (AITL): a new diagnostic marker providing evidence that AITL derives from follicular helper T cells. *Am J Surg Pathol* 2006;30:490–494.
23. Swerdlow SH. *WHO classification of tumours of haematopoietic and lymphoid tissues*, 4th ed. Lyon, France: International Agency for Research on Cancer, 2008.
24. Iqbal J, Weisenburger D, Greiner TC, et al. Molecular signatures to improve diagnosis, prognostication and identification of oncogenic pathways in peripheral T and NK cell lymphoma [abstract]. *Blood* 2008;112:1147. Abstract 3339.
25. Anderson JR, Armitage JO, Weisenburger DD. Epidemiology of the non-Hodgkin's lymphomas: distributions of the major subtypes differ by geographic locations. Non-Hodgkin's Lymphoma Classification Project. *Ann Oncol* 1998;9:717–720.
26. Went P, Agostinelli C, Gallamini A, et al. Marker expression in peripheral T-cell lymphoma: a proposed clinical-pathologic prognostic score. *J Clin Oncol* 2006;24:2472–2479.
27. Barry TS, Jaffe ES, Sorbara L, et al. Peripheral T-cell lymphomas expressing CD30 and CD15. *Am J Surg Pathol* 2003;27:1513–1522.
28. Cuadros M, Dave SS, Jaffe ES, et al. Identification of a proliferation signature related to survival in nodal peripheral T-cell lymphomas. *J Clin Oncol* 2007;25:3321–3329.
29. Feldman AL, Sun DX, Law ME, et al. Overexpression of Syk tyrosine kinase in peripheral T-cell lymphomas. *Leukemia* 2008;22:1139–1143.
30. de Leval L, Rickman DS, Thielen C, et al. The gene expression profile of nodal peripheral T-cell lymphoma demonstrates a molecular link between angioimmunoblastic T-cell lymphoma (AITL) and follicular helper T (TFH) cells. *Blood* 2007;109:4952–4963.
31. Takagi N, Nakamura S, Ueda R, et al. A phenotypic and genotypic study of three node-based, low-grade peripheral T-cell lymphomas: angioimmunoblastic lymphoma, T-zone lymphoma, and lymphoepithelioid lymphoma. *Cancer* 1992;69:2571–2582.
32. Zettl A, Rudiger T, Konrad MA, et al. Genomic profiling of peripheral T-cell lymphoma, unspecified, and anaplastic large T-cell lymphoma delineates novel recurrent chromosomal alterations. *Am J Pathol* 2004;164:1837–1848.
33. Thorns C, Bastian B, Pinkel D, et al. Chromosomal aberrations in angioimmunoblastic T-cell lymphoma and peripheral T-cell lymphoma unspecified: a matrix-based CGH approach. *Genes Chromosomes Cancer* 2007;46:37–44.
34. Nelson M, Horsman DE, Weisenburger DD, et al. Cytogenetic abnormalities and clinical correlations in peripheral T-cell lymphoma. *Br J Haematol* 2008;141:461–469.
35. Schlegelberger B, Himmler A, Godde E, et al. Cytogenetic findings in peripheral T-cell lymphomas as a basis for distinguishing low-grade and high-grade lymphomas. *Blood* 1994;83:505–511.
36. Lepretre S, Buchonnet G, Stamatoullas A, et al. Chromosome abnormalities in peripheral T-cell lymphoma. *Cancer Genet Cytogenet* 2000;117:71–79.
37. Leonardi P, Kassin E, Hernandez-Munoz I, et al. Human rgr: transforming activity and alteration in T-cell malignancies. *Oncogene* 2002;21:5108–5116.
38. D'Adamo DR, Novick S, Kahn JM, et al. rsc: a novel oncogene with structural and functional homology with the gene family of exchange factors for Ral. *Oncogene* 1997;14:1295–1305.
39. Hans CP, Weisenburger DD, Greiner TC, et al. Confirmation of the molecular classification of diffuse large B-cell lymphoma by immunohistochemistry using a tissue microarray. *Blood* 2004;103:275–282.
40. Schlegelberger B, Zhang Y, Weber-Matthiesen K, et al. Detection of aberrant clones in nearly all cases of angioimmunoblastic lymphadenopathy with dysproteinemia-type T-cell lymphoma by combined interphase and metaphase cytogenetics. *Blood* 1994;84:2640–2648.
41. Ballester B, Ramuz O, Gisselbrecht C, et al. Gene expression profiling identifies molecular subgroups among nodal peripheral T-cell lymphomas. *Oncogene* 2006;25:1560–1570.
42. Piccaluga PP, Agostinelli C, Califano A, et al. Gene expression analysis of peripheral T cell lymphoma, unspecified, reveals distinct profiles and new potential therapeutic targets. *J Clin Invest* 2007;117:823–834.

43. Almire C, Bertrand P, Ruminy P, et al. PVRL2 is translocated to the TRA@ locus in t(14;19)(q11;q13)-positive peripheral T-cell lymphomas. *Genes Chromosomes Cancer* 2007;46:1011–1018.

44. Streubel B, Vinatzer U, Willheim M, et al. Novel t(5;9)(q33;q22) fuses ITK to SYK in unspecified peripheral T-cell lymphoma. *Leukemia* 2006;20:313–318.

45. Jimenez M, Perez de Castro I, Benet M, et al. The Rgr oncogene induces tumorigenesis in transgenic mice. *Cancer Res* 2004;64:6041–6049.

46. Armitage J, Vose J, Weisenburger D. International peripheral T-cell and natural killer/T-cell lymphoma study: pathology findings and clinical outcomes. *J Clin Oncol* 2008;26:4124–4130.

47. Hayes RB, Yin SN, Dosemeci M, et al. Benzene and the dose-related incidence of hematologic neoplasms in China. Chinese Academy of Preventive Medicine–National Cancer Institute Benzene Study Group. *J Natl Cancer Inst* 1997;89:1065–1071.

48. López-Guillermo A, Cid J, Salar A, et al. Peripheral T-cell lymphomas: initial features, natural history, and prognostic factors in a series of 174 patients diagnosed according to the R.E.A.L. Classification. *Ann Oncol* 1998;9:849–855.

49. Ansell SM, Habermann TM, Kurtin PJ, et al. Predictive capacity of the International Prognostic Factor Index in patients with peripheral T-cell lymphoma. *J Clin Oncol* 1997;15:2296–2301.

50. Liang R, Todd D, Chan TK, et al. Peripheral T cell lymphoma. *J Clin Oncol* 1987;5:750–755.

51. Greer JP, York JC, Cousar JB, et al. Peripheral T-cell lymphoma: a clinicopathologic study of 42 cases. *J Clin Oncol* 1984;2:788–798.

52. Coiffier B, Berger F, Bryon PA, et al. T-cell lymphomas: immunologic, histologic, clinical, and therapeutic analysis of 63 cases. *J Clin Oncol* 1988;6:1584–1589.

53. Armitage JO, Greer JP, Levine AM, et al. Peripheral T-cell lymphoma. *Cancer* 1989;63:158–163.

54. Rudiger T, Weisenburger DD, Anderson JR, et al. Peripheral T-cell lymphoma (excluding anaplastic large-cell lymphoma): results from the Non-Hodgkin's Lymphoma Classification Project. *Ann Oncol* 2002;13:140–149.

55. Antman K, Chang Y. Kaposi's sarcoma. *N Engl J Med* 2000;342:1027–1038.

56. O'Connor OA, Hamlin PA, Portlock C, et al. Pralatrexate, a novel class of antifol with high affinity for the reduced folate carrier-type 1, produces marked complete and durable remissions in a diversity of chemotherapy refractory cases of T-cell lymphoma. *Br J Haematol* 2007;139:425–428.

57. Piccaluga PP, Agostinelli C, Righi S, et al. Expression of CD52 in peripheral T-cell lymphoma. *Haematologica* 2007;92:566–567.

58. Gallamini A, Zaja F, Patti C, et al. Alemtuzumab (Campath-1H) and CHOP chemotherapy as first-line treatment of peripheral T-cell lymphoma: results of a GITIL (Gruppo Italiano Terapie Innovative nei Linfomi) prospective multicenter trial. *Blood* 2007;110:2316–2323.

59. Arkenau HT, Chong G, Cunningham D, et al. Gemcitabine, cisplatin and methylprednisolone for the treatment of patients with peripheral T-cell lymphoma: the Royal Marsden Hospital experience. *Haematologica* 2007;92:271–272.

60. Foss F, Sjak-Shie N, Goy A, et al. Denileukin Diftitox (ONTAK) plus CHOP chemotherapy in patients with peripheral T-cell lymphomas (PTCL), the CONCEPT Trial [abstract]. *Blood* 2007;110:1011A. Abstract 3449.

61. Vose JM, Peterson C, Bierman PJ, et al. Comparison of high-dose therapy and autologous bone marrow transplantation for T-cell and B-cell non-Hodgkin's lymphomas. *Blood* 1990;76:424–431.

62. Blystad AK, Enblad G, Kvaloy S, et al. High-dose therapy with autologous stem cell transplantation in patients with peripheral T cell lymphomas. *Bone Marrow Transplant* 2001;27:711–716.

63. Chen AI, McMillan A, Negrin RS, et al. Long-term results of autologous hematopoietic cell transplantation for peripheral T cell lymphoma: the Stanford experience. *Biol Blood Marrow Transplant* 2008;14:741–747.

64. Rodriguez J, Conde E, Gutierrez A, et al. The results of consolidation with autologous stem-cell transplantation in patients with peripheral T-cell lymphoma (PTCL) in first complete remission: the Spanish Lymphoma and Autologous Transplantation Group experience. *Ann Oncol* 2007;18:652–657.

65. Feyler S, Prince HM, Pearce R, et al. The role of high-dose therapy and stem cell rescue in the management of T-cell malignant lymphomas: a BSBMT and ABMTRR study. *Bone Marrow Transplant* 2007;40:443–450.

66. Le Gouill S, Milpied N, Buzyn A, et al. Graft-versus-lymphoma effect for aggressive T-cell lymphomas in adults: a study by the Societe Francaise de Greffe de Moelle et de Therapie Cellulaire. *J Clin Oncol* 2008;26:2264–2271.

67. de Lavallade H, Cassier PA, Bouabdallah R, et al. Sustained response after reduced-intensity conditioning allogeneic stem cell transplantation for patients with relapsed peripheral T-cell non-Hodgkin lymphoma. *Br J Haematol* 2008;142:848–850.

68. Corradini P, Dodero A, Zallio F, et al. Graft-versus-lymphoma effect in relapsed peripheral T-cell non-Hodgkin's lymphomas after reduced-intensity conditioning followed by allogeneic transplantation of hematopoietic cells. *J Clin Oncol* 2004;22:2172–2176.

69. Huang Z, Higgins B, Foss F. Activity of gallium nitrate in refractory peripheral T-cell lymphoma. *Clin Lymphoma* 2005;6:43–45.

70. Cooper DL, Braverman IM, Sarris AH, et al. Cyclosporine treatment of refractory T-cell lymphomas. *Cancer* 1993;71:2335–2341.

71. Mercieca J, Matutes E, Dearden C, et al. The role of pentostatin in the treatment of T-cell malignancies: analysis of response rate in 145 patients according to disease subtype. *J Clin Oncol* 1994;12:2588–2593.

72. Saven A, Carrera CJ, Carson DA, et al. 2-Chlorodeoxyadenosine: an active agent in the treatment of cutaneous T- cell lymphoma. *Blood* 1992;80:587–592.

73. Zinzani PL, Baliva G, Magagnoli M, et al. Gemcitabine treatment in pretreated cutaneous T-cell lymphoma: experience in 44 patients. *J Clin Oncol* 2000;18:2603–2606.

74. Cheng AL, Su IJ, Chen CC, et al. Use of retinoic acids in the treatment of peripheral T-cell lymphoma: a pilot study. *J Clin Oncol* 1994;12:1185–1192.

75. Dang NH, Pro B, Hagemeister FB, et al. Phase II trial of denileukin diftitox for relapsed/refractory T-cell non-Hodgkin lymphoma. *Br J Haematol* 2007;136:439–447.

76. Armitage JO, Coiffier B. Activity of interferon-alpha in relapsed patients with diffuse large B-cell and peripheral T-cell non-Hodgkin's lymphoma. *Ann Oncol* 2000;11:1–3.

77. Craig M, Shah S, Tallman M, et al. A phase II trial of darinaparsin in advanced lymphomas: report on safety and activity [abstract]. *Blood* 2008;112:554. Abstract 1562.

78. Frankel AE, Laver JH, Willingham MC, et al. Therapy of patients with T-cell lymphomas and leukemias using an anti- CD7 monoclonal antibody-ricin A chain immunotoxin. *Leuk Lymphoma* 1997;26:287–298.

79. Frizzera G, Moran EM, Rappaport H. Angio-immunoblastic lymphadenopathy with dysproteinaemia. *Lancet* 1974;1:1070–1073.

80. Flandrin G, Daniel M, Yafi G, et al. Sarcomatoses ganglionnaires diffuses a differenciation plasmocytaire avec anemie hemolytique auto-immune. In: Bernard J, ed. *Actualites hematologiques*. Paris, France: Masson, 1972.

81. Brice P, Calvo F, d'Agay MF, et al. Peripheral T cell lymphoma following angioimmunoblastic lymphadenopathy. *Nouv Rev Fr Hematol* 1987;29:371–377.

82. Shimoyama M, Minato K, Saito H, et al. Immunoblastic lymphadenopathy (IBL)-like T-cell lymphoma. *Jpn J Clin Oncol* 1979;9:347.

83. Attygalle A, Al-Jehani R, Diss TC, et al. Neoplastic T cells in angioimmunoblastic T-cell lymphoma express CD10. *Blood* 2002;99:627–633.

84. Weiss LM, Jaffe ES, Liu XF, et al. Detection and localization of Epstein-Barr viral genomes in angioimmunoblastic lymphadenopathy and angioimmunoblastic lymphadenopathy-like lymphoma. *Blood* 1992;79:1789–1795.

85. Quintanilla-Martinez L, Fend F, Moguel LR, et al. Peripheral T-cell lymphoma with Reed-Sternberg-like cells of B-cell phenotype and genotype associated with Epstein-Barr virus infection. *Am J Surg Pathol* 1999;23:1233–1240.

86. Lee SS, Rudiger T, Odenwald T, et al. Angioimmunoblastic T cell lymphoma is derived from mature T-helper cells with varying expression and loss of detectable CD4. *Int J Cancer* 2003;103:12–20.

87. Weiss LM, Strickler JG, Dorfman RF, et al. Clonal T-cell populations in angioimmunoblastic lymphadenopathy and angioimmunoblastic lymphadenopathy-like lymphoma. *Am J Pathol* 1986;122:392–397.

88. Feller AC, Griesser H, Schilling CV, et al. Clonal gene rearrangement patterns correlate with immunophenotype and clinical parameters in patients with angioimmunoblastic lymphadenopathy. *Am J Pathol* 1988;133:549–556.

89. Willenbrock K, Roers A, Seidl C, et al. Analysis of T-cell subpopulations in T-cell non-Hodgkin's lymphoma of angioimmunoblastic lymphadenopathy with dysproteinemia type by single target gene amplification of T cell receptor- beta gene rearrangements. *Am J Pathol* 2001;158:1851–1857.

90. Schlegelberger B, Feller A, Godde E, et al. Stepwise development of chromosomal abnormalities in angioimmunoblastic lymphadenopathy. *Cancer Genet Cytogenet* 1990;50:15–29.

91. Schlegelberger B, Zwingers T, Hohenadel K, et al. Significance of cytogenetic findings for the clinical outcome in patients with T-cell lymphoma of angioimmunoblastic lymphadenopathy type. *J Clin Oncol* 1996;14:593–599.

92. Lachenal F, Berger F, Ghesquieres H, et al. Angioimmunoblastic T-cell lymphoma: clinical and laboratory features at diagnosis in 77 patients. *Medicine (Baltimore)* 2007;86:282–292.

93. Lipford EH, Smith HR, Pittaluga S, et al. Clonality of angioimmunoblastic lymphadenopathy and implications for its evolution to malignant lymphoma. *J Clin Invest* 1987;79:637–642.

94. Smith JL, Hodges E, Quin CT, et al. Frequent T and B cell oligoclones in histologically and immunophenotypically characterized angioimmunoblastic lymphadenopathy. *Am J Pathol* 2000;156:661–669.

95. Abruzzo LV, Schmidt K, Weiss LM, et al. B-cell lymphoma after angioimmunoblastic lymphadenopathy: a case with oligoclonal gene rearrangements associated with Epstein-Barr virus. *Blood* 1993;82:241–246.

96. Willenbrock K, Brauninger A, Hansmann ML. Frequent occurrence of B-cell lymphomas in angioimmunoblastic T-cell lymphoma and proliferation of Epstein-Barr virus-infected cells in early cases. *Br J Haematol* 2007;138:733–739.

97. Frizzera G, Moran EM, Rappaport H. Angio-immunoblastic lymphadenopathy. Diagnosis and clinical course. *Am J Med* 1975;59:803–818.

98. Pangalis GA, Moran EM, Nathwani BN, et al. Angioimmunoblastic lymphadenopathy. Long-term follow-up study. *Cancer* 1983;52:318–321.

99. Tan BT, Warnke RA, Arber DA. The frequency of B- and T-cell gene rearrangements and Epstein-Barr virus in T-cell lymphomas: a comparison between angioimmunoblastic T-cell lymphoma and peripheral T-cell lymphoma, unspecified with and without associated B-cell proliferations. *J Mol Diagn* 2006;8:466–475.

100. Jaffe E, Harris N, Vardiman J, et al. Pathology and genetics: neoplasms of the haematopoietic and lymphoid tissues. In: Kleihaus P, Sobin L, eds. *World Health Organization classification of tumours*. Lyon, France: IARC Press, 2001.

101. Hodges E, Quin CT, Wright DH, et al. Oligoclonal populations of T and B cells in a case of angioimmunoblastic T-cell lymphoma predominantly infiltrated by T cells of the VB5.1 family. *Mol Pathol* 1997;50:15–17.

102. Dogan A, et al. Angioimmunoblastic T-cell lymphoma. In: Swerdlow S, et al., eds. *WHO classification of tumours of haematopoietic and lymphoid tissues*, 4th ed. Lyon, France: International Agency for Research on Cancer, 2008:209–316.

103. Ree HJ, Kadin ME, Kikuchi M, et al. Bcl-6 expression in reactive follicular hyperplasia, follicular lymphoma, and angioimmunoblastic T-cell lymphoma with hyperplastic germinal centers: heterogeneity of intrafollicular T-cells and their altered distribution in the pathogenesis of angioimmunoblastic T-cell lymphoma. *Hum Pathol* 1999;30:403–411.

104. Dorfman DM, Brown JA, Shahsafaei A, et al. Programmed death-1 (PD-1) is a marker of germinal center-associated T cells and angioimmunoblastic T-cell lymphoma. *Am J Surg Pathol* 2006;30:802–810.

105. Roncador G, Garcia Verdes-Montenegro JF, Tedoldi S, t al. Expression of two markers of germinal center T cells (SAP and PD-1) in angioimmunoblastic T-cell lymphoma. *Haematologica* 2007;92:1059–1066.

106. Vose J, et al. Angioimmunoblastic T-cell lymphoma. Results from the International T-cell lymphoma project. Submitted.

107. Mourad N, Mounier N, Briere J, et al. Clinical, biologic, and pathologic features in 157 patients with angioimmunoblastic T-cell lymphoma treated within the Groupe d'Etude des Lymphomes de l'Adulte (GELA) trials. *Blood* 2008;111:4463–4470.

108. Kyriakou C, Canals C, Goldstone A, et al. High-dose therapy and autologous stem-cell transplantation in angioimmunoblastic lymphoma: complete remission at transplantation is the major determinant of Outcome Lymphoma Working Party of the European Group for Blood and Marrow Transplantation. *J Clin Oncol* 2008;26:218–224.

109. Advani R, Horwitz S, Zelenetz A, et al. Angioimmunoblastic T cell lymphoma: treatment experience with cyclosporine. *Leuk Lymphoma* 2007;48:521–525.

110. Aguiar Bujanda D. Complete response of relapsed angioimmunoblastic T-cell lymphoma following therapy with bevacizumab. *Ann Oncol* 2008;19:396–397.

111. Kwong YL, Chan AC, Liang RH. Natural killer cell lymphoma/leukemia: pathology and treatment. *Hematol Oncol* 1997;15:71–79.

112. Chan J, Jaffe E, Ralfkiaer. Extranodal NK/T cell lymphoma, nasal type. In: Jaffe E, Harris N, Stein H, et al., eds. *Pathology and genetics of tumours of haematopoietic and lymphoid tissues*. Lyon, France: IARC Press, 2001:204–207.

113. Jaffe ES, Krenacs L, Kumar S, et al. Extranodal peripheral T-cell and NK-cell neoplasms. *Am J Clin Pathol* 1999;111(suppl 1):S46–S55.

114. Harris NL, Jaffe ES, Diebold J, et al. World Health Organization classification of neoplastic diseases of the hematopoietic and lymphoid tissues: report of the Clinical Advisory Committee meeting-Airlie House, Virginia, November 1997. *J Clin Oncol* 1999;17:3835–3849.

115. Harris NL, Jaffe ES, Stein H, et al. A revised European-American classification of lymphoid neoplasms: a proposal from the International Lymphoma Study Group. *Blood* 1994;84:1361–1392.

116. Ho FC, Choy D, Loke SL, et al. Polymorphic reticulosis and conventional lymphomas of the nose and upper aerodigestive tract: a clinicopathologic study of 70 cases, and immunophenotypic studies of 16 cases. *Hum Pathol* 1990;21:1041–1050.

117. Vidal RW, Devaney K, Ferlito A, et al. Sinonasal malignant lymphomas: a distinct clinicopathological category. *Ann Otol Rhinol Laryngol* 1999;108:411–419.

118. Liang R, Ng RP, Todd D, et al. Management of stage I-II diffuse aggressive non-Hodgkin's lymphoma of the Waldeyer's ring: combined modality therapy versus radiotherapy alone. *Hematol Oncol* 1987;5:223–230.

119. National Cancer Institute sponsored study of classifications of non-Hodgkin's lymphomas: summary and description of a working formulation for clinical usage. The Non-Hodgkin's Lymphoma Pathologic Classification Project. *Cancer* 1982;49:2112–2135.

120. Chan JK. Natural killer cell neoplasms. *Anat Pathol* 1998;3:77–145.

121. Chan JK. Peripheral T-cell and NK-cell neoplasms: an integrated approach to diagnosis. *Mod Pathol* 1999;12:177–199.

122. Liang R, Loke SL, Ho FC, et al. Histologic subtypes and survival of Chinese patients with non-Hodgkin's lymphomas. *Cancer* 1990;66:1850–1855.

123. Quintanilla-Martinez L, Franklin JL, Guerrero I, et al. Histological and immunophenotypic profile of nasal NK/T cell lymphomas from Peru: high prevalence of p53 overexpression. *Hum Pathol* 1999;30:849–855.

124. Liang R. Diagnosis and management of primary nasal lymphoma of T-cell or NK-cell origin. *Clin Lymphoma* 2000;1:33–37.

125. Jaffe ES, Chan JK, Su IJ, et al. Report of the Workshop on Nasal and Related Extranodal Angiocentric T/Natural Killer Cell Lymphomas. Definitions, differential diagnosis, and epidemiology. *Am J Surg Pathol* 1996;20:103–111.

126. Teruya-Feldstein J, Jaffe ES, Burd PR, et al. The role of Mig, the monokine induced by interferon-gamma, and IP-10, the interferon-gamma-inducible protein-10, in tissue necrosis and vascular damage associated with Epstein-Barr virus-positive lymphoproliferative disease. *Blood* 1997;90:4099–4105.

127. Lay JD, Tsao CJ, Chen JY, et al. Upregulation of tumor necrosis factor-alpha gene by Epstein-Barr virus and activation of macrophages in Epstein-Barr virus-infected T cells in the pathogenesis of hemophagocytic syndrome. *J Clin Invest* 1997;100:1969–1979.

128. Dictor M, Cervin A, Kalm O, et al. Sinonasal T-cell lymphoma in the differential diagnosis of lethal midline granuloma using in situ hybridization for Epstein-Barr virus RNA. *Mod Pathol* 1996;9:7–14.

129. Tsang WY, Chan JK, Yip TT, et al. In situ localization of Epstein-Barr virus encoded RNA in non-nasal/nasopharyngeal CD56-positive and CD56-negative T-cell lymphomas. *Hum Pathol* 1994;25:758–765.

130. Ng SB, Lai KW, Murugaya S, et al. Nasal-type extranodal natural killer/T-cell lymphomas: a clinicopathologic and genotypic study of 42 cases in Singapore. *Mod Pathol* 2004;17:1097–1107.

131. Schwartz EJ, Molina-Kirsch H, Zhao S, et al. Immunohistochemical characterization of nasal-type extranodal NK/T-cell lymphoma using a tissue microarray: an analysis of 84 cases. *Am J Clin Pathol* 2008;130:343–351.

132. Li T, Hongyo T, Syaifudin M, et al. Mutations of the p53 gene in nasal NK/T-cell lymphoma. *Lab Invest* 2000;80:493–499.

133. Quintanilla-Martinez L, Kremer M, Keller G, et al. p53 Mutations in nasal natural killer/T-cell lymphoma from Mexico: association with large cell morphology and advanced disease. *Am J Pathol* 2001;159:2095–2105.

134. Takahara M, Kishibe K, Bandoh N, et al. P53, N- and K-Ras, and beta-catenin gene mutations and prognostic factors in nasal NK/T-cell lymphoma from Hokkaido, Japan. *Hum Pathol* 2004;35:86–95.

135. Wong KF, Zhang YM, Chan JK. Cytogenetic abnormalities in natural killer cell lymphoma/leukaemia—is there a consistent pattern? *Leuk Lymphoma* 1999;34:241–250.

136. Siu LL, Wong KF, Chan JK, et al. Comparative genomic hybridization analysis of natural killer cell lymphoma/leukemia. Recognition of consistent patterns of genetic alterations. *Am J Pathol* 1999;155:1419–1425.

137. Wong N, Wong KF, Chan JK, et al. Chromosomal translocations are common in natural killer-cell lymphoma/leukemia as shown by spectral karyotyping. *Hum Pathol* 2000;31:771–774.

138. Nakashima Y, Tagawa H, Suzuki R, et al. Genome-wide array-based comparative genomic hybridization of natural killer cell lymphoma/leukemia: different genomic alteration patterns of aggressive NK-cell leukemia and extranodal Nk/T-cell lymphoma, nasal type. *Genes Chromosomes Cancer* 2005;44:247–255.

139. Sun HS, Su IJ, Lin YC, et al. A 2.6 Mb interval on chromosome 6q25.2-q25.3 is commonly deleted in human nasal natural killer/T-cell lymphoma. *Br J Haematol* 2003;122:590–599.

140. Chiang AK, Tao Q, Srivastava G, et al. Nasal NK- and T-cell lymphomas share the same type of Epstein-Barr virus latency as nasopharyngeal carcinoma and Hodgkin's disease. *Int J Cancer* 1996;68:285–290.

141. Gutierrez MI, Spangler G, Kingma D, et al. Epstein-Barr virus in nasal lymphomas contains multiple ongoing mutations in the EBNA-1 gene. *Blood* 1998;92:600–606.

142. Gaal K, Weiss LM, Chen WG, et al. Epstein-Barr virus nuclear antigen (EBNA)-1 carboxy-terminal and EBNA-4 sequence polymorphisms in nasal natural killer/T-cell lymphoma in the United States. *Lab Invest* 2002;82:957–962.

143. Ng CS, Lo ST, Chan JK, et al. CD56+ putative natural killer cell lymphomas: production of cytolytic effectors and related proteins mediating tumor cell apoptosis? *Hum Pathol* 1997;28:1276–1282.

144. Ko YH, Park S, Jin H, et al. Granzyme B leakage-induced apoptosis is a crucial mechanism of cell death in nasal-type NK/T-cell lymphoma. *Lab Invest* 2007;87:241–250.

145. Ng CS, Lo ST, Chan JK. Peripheral T and putative natural killer cell lymphomas commonly coexpress CD95 and CD95 ligand. *Hum Pathol* 1999;30:48–53.

146. Binstadt BA, Brumbaugh KM, Leibson PJ. Signal transduction by human NK cell MHC-recognizing receptors. *Immunol Rev* 1997;155:197–203.

147. Haedicke W, Ho FC, Chott A, et al. Expression of CD94/NKG2A and killer immunoglobulin-like receptors in NK cells and a subset of extranodal cytotoxic T-cell lymphomas. *Blood* 2000;95:3628–3630.

148. Dukers DF, Vermeer MH, Jaspars LH, et al. Expression of killer cell inhibitory receptors is restricted to true NK cell lymphomas and a subset of intestinal enteropathy-type T cell lymphomas with a cytotoxic phenotype. *J Clin Pathol* 2001;54:224–228.

149. Lin CW, Chen YH, Chuang YC, et al. CD94 transcripts imply a better prognosis in nasal-type extranodal NK/T-cell lymphoma. *Blood* 2003;102:2623–2631.

150. Shen L, Liang AC, Lu L, et al. Frequent deletion of Fas gene sequences encoding death and transmembrane domains in nasal natural killer/T-cell lymphoma. *Am J Pathol* 2002;161:2123–2131.

151. Takakuwa T, Dong Z, Nakatsuka S, et al. Frequent mutations of Fas gene in nasal NK/T cell lymphoma. *Oncogene* 2002;21:4702–4705.

152. Jeon YK, Kim H, Park SO, et al. Resistance to Fas-mediated apoptosis is restored by cycloheximide through the downregulation of cellular FLIPL in NK/T-cell lymphoma. *Lab Invest* 2005;85:874–884.

153. Bladergroen BA, Meijer CJ, ten Berge RL, et al. Expression of the granzyme B inhibitor, protease inhibitor 9, by tumor cells in patients with non-Hodgkin and Hodgkin lymphoma: a novel protective mechanism for tumor cells to circumvent the immune system? *Blood* 2002;99:232–237.

154. Bossard C, Belhadj K, Reyes F, et al. Expression of the granzyme B inhibitor PI9 predicts outcome in nasal NK/T-cell lymphoma: results of a Western series of 48 patients treated with first-line polychemotherapy within the Groupe d'Etude des Lymphomes de l'Adulte (GELA) trials. *Blood* 2007;109:2183–2189.

155. ten Berge RL, Meijer CJ, Dukers DF, et al. Expression levels of apoptosis-related proteins predict clinical outcome in anaplastic large cell lymphoma. *Blood* 2002;99:4540–4546.

156. Chan JK, Sin VC, Wong KF, et al. Nonnasal lymphoma expressing the natural killer cell marker CD56: a clinicopathologic study of 49 cases of an uncommon aggressive neoplasm. *Blood* 1997;89:4501–4513.

157. Liang R, Todd D, Chan TK, et al. Nasal lymphoma. A retrospective analysis of 60 cases. *Cancer* 1990;66:2205–2209.

158. Yeh KH, Lien HC, Hsu SM, et al. Quiescent nasal T/NK cell lymphoma manifested as primary central nervous system lymphoma. *Am J Hematol* 1999;60:161–163.

159. Chim CS, Choy C, Liang R, et al. Isolated uterine relapse of nasal T/Nk cell lymphoma. *Leuk Lymphoma* 1999;34:629–632.

160. Kato N, Yasukawa K, Onozuka T, et al. Nasal and nasal-type T/NK-cell lymphoma with cutaneous involvement. *J Am Acad Dermatol* 1999;40(pt 2):850–856.

161. Au WY, Chan AC, Kwong YL. Scrotal skin ulcer in a patient with a previous tonsillectomy because of natural killer cell lymphoma. *Am J Dermatopathol* 1998;20:582–585.

162. Liang R, Todd D, Chan TK, et al. Treatment outcome and prognostic factors for primary nasal lymphoma. *J Clin Oncol* 1995;13:666–670.

163. Kwong YL, Chan AC, Liang R, et al. CD56+ NK lymphomas: clinicopathological features and prognosis. *Br J Haematol* 1997;97:821–829.

164. Chim CS, Ma ES, Loong F, et al. Diagnostic cues for natural killer cell lymphoma: primary nodal presentation and the role of in situ hybridisation for Epstein-Barr virus encoded early small RNA in detecting occult bone marrow involvement. *J Clin Pathol* 2005;58:443–445.

165. Han JY, Seo EJ, Kwon HJ, et al. Nasal angiocentric lymphoma with hemophagocytic syndrome. *Korean J Intern Med* 1999;14:41–46.

166. Ooi GC, Chim CS, Liang R, et al. Nasal T-cell/natural killer cell lymphoma: CT and MR imaging features of a new clinicopathologic entity. *AJR Am J Roentgenol* 2000;174:1141–1145.

167. Chim CS, Ooi GC, Shek TW, et al. Lethal midline granuloma revisited: nasal T/Natural-killer cell lymphoma. *J Clin Oncol* 1999;17:1322–1325.

168. Kim GE, Cho JH, Yang WI, et al. Angiocentric lymphoma of the head and neck: patterns of systemic failure after radiation treatment. *J Clin Oncol* 2000;18:54–63.

169. Cheung MM, Chan JK, Lau WH, et al. Primary non-Hodgkin's lymphoma of the nose and nasopharynx: clinical features, tumor immunophenotype, and treatment outcome in 113 patients. *J Clin Oncol* 1998;16:70–77.

170. Cheung MM, Chan JK, Lau WH, et al. Early stage nasal NK/T-cell lymphoma: clinical outcome, prognostic factors, and the effect of treatment modality. *Int J Radiat Oncol Biol Phys* 2002;54:182–190.

171. You JY, Chi KH, Yang MH, et al. Radiation therapy versus chemotherapy as initial treatment for localized nasal natural killer (NK)/T-cell lymphoma: a single institute survey in Taiwan. *Ann Oncol* 2004;15:618–625.

172. Koom WS, Chung EJ, Yang WI, et al. Angiocentric T-cell and NK/T-cell lymphomas: radiotherapeutic viewpoints. *Int J Radiat Oncol Biol Phys* 2004;59:1127–1137.

173. Au WY, Ma SY, Chim CS, et al. Clinicopathologic features and treatment outcome of mature T-cell and natural killer-cell lymphomas diagnosed according to the World Health Organization classification scheme: a single center experience of 10 years. *Ann Oncol* 2005;16:206–214.

174. Cheung MM, Chan JK, Wong KF. Natural killer cell neoplasms: a distinctive group of highly aggressive lymphomas/leukemias. *Semin Hematol* 2003;40:221–232.

175. Lei KI, Chan LY, Chan WY, et al. Quantitative analysis of circulating cell-free Epstein-Barr virus (EBV) DNA levels in patients with EBV-associated lymphoid malignancies. *Br J Haematol* 2000;111:239–246.

176. Au WY, Pang A, Choy C, et al. Quantification of circulating Epstein-Barr virus (EBV) DNA in the diagnosis and monitoring of natural killer cell and EBV-positive lymphomas in immunocompetent patients. *Blood* 2004;104:243–249.

177. Siu LL, Chan JK, Wong KF, et al. Aberrant promoter CpG methylation as a molecular marker for disease monitoring in natural killer cell lymphomas. *Br J Haematol* 2003;122:70–77.

178. Obama K, Tara M, Niina K. L-asparaginase-Based induction therapy for advanced extranodal NK/T-cell lymphoma. *Int J Hematol* 2003;78:248–250.

179. Yong W, Zheng W, Zhang Y, et al. L-asparaginase-based regimen in the treatment of refractory midline nasal/nasal-type T/NK-cell lymphoma. *Int J Hematol* 2003;78:163–167.

180. Matsumoto Y, Nomura K, Kanda-Akano Y, et al. Successful treatment with Erwinia L-asparaginase for recurrent natural killer/T cell lymphoma. *Leuk Lymphoma* 2003;44:879–882.

181. Ando M, Sugimoto K, Kitoh T, et al. Selective apoptosis of natural killer-cell tumours by l-asparaginase. *Br J Haematol* 2005;130:860–868.

182. Yamaguchi M, Suzuki R, Kwong YL, et al. Phase I study of dexamethasone, methotrexate, ifosfamide, L-asparaginase, and etoposide (SMILE) chemotherapy for advanced-stage, relapsed or refractory extranodal natural killer (NK)/T-cell lymphoma and leukemia. *Cancer Sci* 2008;99:1016–1020.

183. Liang R, Chen F, Lee CK, et al. Autologous bone marrow transplantation for primary nasal T/NK cell lymphoma. *Bone Marrow Transplant* 1997;19:91–93.

184. Nawa Y, Takenaka K, Shinagawa K, et al. Successful treatment of advanced natural killer cell lymphoma with high-dose chemotherapy and syngeneic peripheral blood stem cell transplantation. *Bone Marrow Transplant* 1999;23:1321–1322.

185. Mukai HY, Kojima H, Suzukawa K, et al. High-dose chemotherapy with peripheral blood stem cell rescue in blastoid natural killer cell lymphoma. *Leuk Lymphoma* 1999;32:583–588.

186. Au WY, Lie AK, Liang R, et al. Autologous stem cell transplantation for nasal NK/T-cell lymphoma: a progress report on its value. *Ann Oncol* 2003;14:1673–1676.

187. Suzuki R, Suzumiya J, Nakamura S, et al. Hematopoietic stem cell transplantation for natural killer-cell lineage neoplasms. *Bone Marrow Transplant* 2006;37:425–431.

188. Kim HJ, Bang SM, Lee J, et al. High-dose chemotherapy with autologous stem cell transplantation in extranodal NK/T-cell lymphoma: a retrospective comparison with non-transplantation cases. *Bone Marrow Transplant* 2006;37:819–824.

189. Murashige N, Kami M, Kishi Y, et al. Allogeneic haematopoietic stem cell transplantation as a promising treatment for natural killer-cell neoplasms. *Br J Haematol* 2005;130:561–567.

190. Chim CS, Ma SY, Au WY, et al. Primary nasal natural killer cell lymphoma: long-term treatment outcome and relationship with the International Prognostic Index. *Blood* 2004;103:216–221.

191. Farcet JP, Gaulard P, Marolleau JP, et al. Hepatosplenic T-cell lymphoma: sinusal/sinusoidal localization of malignant cells expressing the T-cell receptor gamma delta. *Blood* 1990;75:2213–2219.

192. Cooke CB, Krenacs L, Stetler-Stevenson M, t al. Hepatosplenic T-cell lymphoma: a distinct clinicopathologic entity of cytotoxic gamma delta T-cell origin. *Blood* 1996;88:4265–4274.

193. Macon WR, Levy NB, Kurtin PJ, et al. Hepatosplenic alphabeta T-cell lymphomas: a report of 14 cases and comparison with hepatosplenic gammadelta T-cell lymphomas. *Am J Surg Pathol* 2001;25:285–296.

194. Kumar S, Lawlor C, Jaffe ES. Hepatosplenic T-cell lymphoma of alphabeta lineage. *Am J Surg Pathol* 2001;25:970–971.

195. Suarez F, Wlodarska I, Rigal-Huguet F, et al. Hepatosplenic alphabeta T-cell lymphoma: an unusual case with clinical, histologic, and cytogenetic features of gammadelta hepatosplenic T-cell lymphoma. *Am J Surg Pathol* 2000;24:1027–1032.

196. Wu H, Wasik MA, Przybylski G, et al. Hepatosplenic gamma-delta T-cell lymphoma as a late-onset posttransplant lymphoproliferative disorder in renal transplant recipients. *Am J Clin Pathol* 2000;113:487–496.

197. Khan WA, Yu L, Eisenbrey AB, et al. Hepatosplenic gamma/delta T-cell lymphoma in immunocompromised patients. Report of two cases and review of literature. *Am J Clin Pathol* 2001;116:41–50.

198. Mittal S, Milner BJ, Johnston PW, et al. A case of hepatosplenic gammadelta T-cell lymphoma with a transient response to fludarabine and alemtuzumab. *Eur J Haematol* 2006;76:531–534.

199. Zeidan A, Sham R, Shapiro J, et al. Hepatosplenic T-cell lymphoma in a patient with Crohn's disease who received infliximab therapy. *Leuk Lymphoma* 2007;48:1410–1413.

200. Veres G, Baldassano RN, Mamula P. Infliximab therapy for pediatric Crohn's disease. *Expert Opin Biol Ther* 2007;7:1869–1880.

201. Wang CC, Tien HF, Lin MT, et al. Consistent presence of isochromosome 7q in hepatosplenic T gamma/delta lymphoma: a new cytogeneticclinicopathologic entity. *Genes Chromosomes Cancer* 1995;12:161–164.

202. Alonsozana EL, Stamberg J, Kumar D, et al. Isochromosome 7q: the primary cytogenetic abnormality in hepatosplenic gammadelta T cell lymphoma. *Leukemia* 1997;11:1367–1372.

203. Wlodarska I, Martin-Garcia N, Achten R, et al. Fluorescence in situ hybridization study of chromosome 7 aberrations in hepatosplenic T-cell lymphoma: isochromosome 7q as a common abnormality accumulating in forms with features of cytologic progression. *Genes Chromosomes Cancer* 2002;33:243–251.

204. Wong KF, Chan JK, Matutes E, et al. Hepatosplenic gamma delta T-cell lymphoma. A distinctive aggressive lymphoma type. *Am J Surg Pathol* 1995;19:718–726.

205. Boulland ML, Kanavaros P, Wechsler J, et al. Cytotoxic protein expression in natural killer cell lymphomas and in alpha beta and gamma delta peripheral T-cell lymphomas. *J Pathol* 1997;183:432–439.

206. Felgar RE, Macon WR, Kinney MC, et al. TIA-1 expression in lymphoid neoplasms. Identification of subsets with cytotoxic T lymphocyte or natural killer cell differentiation. *Am J Pathol* 1997;150:1893–1900.

207. Przybylski GK, Wu H, Macon WR, et al. Hepatosplenic and subcutaneous panniculitis-like gamma/delta T cell lymphomas are derived from different Vdelta subsets of gamma/delta T lymphocytes. *J Mol Diagn* 2000;2:11–19.

208. Jonveaux P, Daniel MT, Martel V, et al. Isochromosome 7q and trisomy 8 are consistent primary, non-random chromosomal abnormalities associated with hepatosplenic T gamma/delta lymphoma. *Leukemia* 1996;10:1453–1455.

209. Miyazaki K, Yamaguchi M, Imai H, et al. Gene expression profiling of peripheral T-cell lymphoma including gammadelta T-cell lymphoma. *Blood* 2009;113:1071–1074.

210. Morice WG, Macon WR, Dogan A, et al. NK-cell-associated receptor expression in hepatosplenic T-cell lymphoma, insights into pathogenesis. *Leukemia* 2006;20:883–886.

211. Francois A, Lesesve JF, Stamatoullas A, et al. Hepatosplenic gamma/delta T-cell lymphoma: a report of two cases in immunocompromised patients, associated with isochromosome 7q. *Am J Surg Pathol* 1997;21:781–790.

212. Ross CW, Schnitzer B, Sheldon S, et al. Gamma/delta T-cell posttransplantation lymphoproliferative disorder primarily in the spleen. *Am J Clin Pathol* 1994;102:310–315.

213. Tey SK, Marlton PV, Hawley CM, et al. Post-transplant hepatosplenic T-cell lymphoma successfully treated with HyperCVAD regimen. *Am J Hematol* 2008;83:330–333.

214. Machino T, Okoshi Y, Kaneko S, et al. Hepatosplenic alphabeta T-cell lymphoma successfully treated with allogeneic bone marrow transplantation. *Bone Marrow Transplant* 2007;39:513–514.

215. Grigg AP. 2'-Deoxycoformycin for hepatosplenic gammadelta T-cell lymphoma. *Leuk Lymphoma* 2001;42:797–799.

216. Jaeger G, Bauer F, Brezinschek R, et al. Hepatosplenic gammadelta T-cell lymphoma successfully treated with a combination of alemtuzumab and cladribine. *Ann Oncol* 2008;19:1025–1026.

217. Greiner TC, Raffeld M, Lutz C, et al. Analysis of T cell receptor-gamma gene rearrangements by denaturing gradient gel electrophoresis of GC-clamped polymerase chain reaction products. Correlation with tumor-specific sequences. *Am J Pathol* 1995;146:46–55.

218. Mead GM, Whitehouse JM, Thompson J, et al. Clinical features and management of malignant histiocytosis of the intestine. *Cancer* 1987;60:2791–2796.

219. O'Farrelly C, Feighery C, O'Briain DS, et al. Humoral response to wheat protein in patients with coeliac disease and enteropathy associated T cell lymphoma. *Br Med J (Clin Res Ed)* 1986;293:908–910.

220. Isaacson P, Wright DH. Intestinal lymphoma associated with malabsorption. *Lancet* 1978;1:67–70.

221. Isaacson P, Wright DH. Malignant histiocytosis of the intestine. Its relationship to malabsorption and ulcerative jejunitis. *Hum Pathol* 1978;9:661–677.

222. Whitehead R. Primary lymphadenopathy complicating idiopathic steatorrhoea. *Gut* 1968;9:569–575.

223. Gough K, Read A, Naish J. Intestinal reticulosis as a complication of idiopathic steatorrhoea. *Gut* 1962;3:232–239.

224. Morton JE, Leyland MJ, Vaughan et al. Primary gastrointestinal non-Hodgkin's lymphoma: a review of 175 British National Lymphoma Investigation cases. *Br J Cancer* 1993;67:776–782.

225. Savage KJ, Chhanabhai M, Gascoyne RD, et al. Characterization of peripheral T-cell lymphomas in a single North American institution by the WHO classification. *Ann Oncol* 2004;15:1467–1475.

226. Pellatt J, Sweetenham J, Pickering RM, et al. A single-centre study of treatment outcomes and survival in 120 patients with peripheral T-cell non-Hodgkin's lymphoma. *Ann Hematol* 2002;81:267–272.

227. Trier JS. Celiac sprue. *N Engl J Med* 1991;325:1709–1719.

228. Weinstein W. Intractable celiac sprue. In: *Difficult decisions in digestive diseases*, 2nd ed. St. Louis, Mo: Mosby, 1994:257–268.

229. Stokes PL, Asquith P, Holmes GK, et al. Inheritance and influence of histocompatibility (HL-A) antigens in adult coeliac disease. *Gut* 1973;14:627–630.

230. Hall M, Mazzilli M, Satz M, et al. *Celiac disease study.* Oxford, UK: Oxford University Press, 1992.

231. Howell WM, Leung ST, Jones DB, et al. HLA-DRB, -DQA, and -DQB polymorphism in celiac disease and enteropathy- associated T-cell lymphoma. Common features and additional risk factors for malignancy. *Hum Immunol* 1995;43:29–37.

232. Deleeuw RJ, Zettl A, Klinker E, et al. Whole-genome analysis and HLA genotyping of enteropathy-type T-cell lymphoma reveals 2 distinct lymphoma subtypes. *Gastroenterology* 2007;132:1902–1911.

233. Cellier C, Delabesse E, Helmer C, et al. Refractory sprue, coeliac disease, and enteropathy-associated T-cell lymphoma. French Coeliac Disease Study Group. *Lancet* 2000;356:203–208.

234. Bagdi E, Diss TC, Munson P, et al. Mucosal intra-epithelial lymphocytes in enteropathy-associated T-cell lymphoma, ulcerative jejunitis, and refractory celiac disease constitute a neoplastic population. *Blood* 1999;94:260–264.

235. Kluin PM, Feller A, Gaulard P, et al. Peripheral T/NK-cell lymphoma: a report of the IXth Workshop of the European Association for Haematopathology. *Histopathology* 2001;38:250–270.

236. Gallamini A, Carbone A, Lista P, et al. Intestinal T-cell lymphoma with massive tissue and blood eosinophilia mediated by IL-5. *Leuk Lymphoma* 1995;17:155–161.

237. Chott A, Haedicke W, Mosberger I, et al. Most CD56+ intestinal lymphomas are CD8+CD5-T-cell lymphomas of monomorphic small to medium size histology. *Am J Pathol* 1998;153:1483–1490.

238. Arnulf B, Copie-Bergman C, Delfau-Larue MH, et al. Nonhepatosplenic gammadelta T-cell lymphoma: a subset of cytotoxic lymphomas with mucosal or skin localization. *Blood* 1998;91:1723–1731.

239. Isaacson PG, O'Connor NT, Spencer J, et al. Malignant histiocytosis of the intestine: a T-cell lymphoma. *Lancet* 1985;2:688–691.

240. Murray A, Cuevas EC, Jones DB, et al. Study of the immunohistochemistry and T cell clonality of enteropathy-associated T cell lymphoma. *Am J Pathol* 1995;146:509–519.

241. Katoh A, Ohshima K, Kanda M, et al. Gastrointestinal T cell lymphoma: predominant cytotoxic phenotypes, including alpha/beta, gamma/delta T cell and natural killer cells. *Leuk Lymphoma* 2000;39:97–111.

242. Zettl A, Ott G, Makulik A, et al. Chromosomal gains at 9q characterize enteropathy-type T-cell lymphoma. *Am J Pathol* 2002;161:1635–1645.

243. Cejkova P, Zettl A, Baumgartner AK, et al. Amplification of NOTCH1 and ABL1 gene loci is a frequent aberration in enteropathy-type T-cell lymphoma. *Virchows Arch* 2005;446:416–420.

244. Stein H, Dienemann D, Sperling M, et al. Identification of a T cell lymphoma category derived from intestinal- mucosa-associated T cells. *Lancet* 1988;2:1053–1054.

245. Spencer J, Cerf-Bensussan N, Jarry A, et al. Enteropathy-associated T cell lymphoma (malignant histiocytosis of the intestine) is recognized by a monoclonal antibody (HML-1) that defines a membrane molecule on human mucosal lymphocytes. *Am J Pathol* 1988;132:1–5.

246. Micklem KJ, Dong Y, Willis A, et al. HML-1 antigen on mucosa-associated T cells, activated cells, and hairy leukemic cells is a new integrin containing the beta 7 subunit. *Am J Pathol* 1991;139:1297–1301.

247. Simonitsch I, Volc-Platzer B, Mosberger I, et al. Expression of monoclonal antibody HML-1-defined alpha E beta 7 integrin in cutaneous T cell lymphoma. *Am J Pathol* 1994;145:1148–1158.

248. Daum S, Weiss D, Hummel M, et al. Frequency of clonal intraepithelial T lymphocyte proliferations in enteropathy-type intestinal T cell lymphoma, cocliac disease, and refractory sprue. *Gut* 2001;49:804–812.

249. Gale J, Simmonds PD, Mead GM, et al. Enteropathy-type intestinal T-cell lymphoma: clinical features and treatment of 31 patients in a single center. *J Clin Oncol* 2000;18:795–803.

250. Egan LJ, Walsh SV, Stevens FM, et al. Celiac-associated lymphoma. A single institution experience of 30 cases in the combination chemotherapy era. *J Clin Gastroenterol* 1995;21:123–129.

251. Brandt L, Hagander B, Norden A, et al. Lymphoma of the small intestine in adult coeliac disease. *Acta Med Scand* 1978;204:467–470.

252. Cooper BT, Holmes GK, Cooke WT. Lymphoma risk in coeliac disease of later life. *Digestion* 1982;23:89–92.

253. Holmes GK, Stokes PL, McWalter R, et al. Proceedings: coeliac disease, malignancy, and gluten-frcc diet. *Gut* 1974;15:339.

254. Holmes GK, Prior P, Lane MR, et al. Malignancy in coeliac disease—effect of a gluten free diet. *Gut* 1989;30:333–338.

255. Al-Toma A, Goerres MS, Meijer JW, et al. Cladribine therapy in refractory celiac disease with aberrant T cells. *Clin Gastroenterol Hepatol* 2006;4:1322–13327.

256. Verbeek WH, Mulder CJ, Zweegman S. Alemtuzumab for refractory celiac disease. *N Engl J Med* 2006;355:1396–1397.

257. Al-toma A, Visser OJ, van Roessel HM, et al. Autologous hematopoietic stem cell transplantation in refractory celiac disease with aberrant T cells. *Blood* 2007;109:2243–2249.

258. Joyce AM, Burns DL, Marcello PW, et al. Capsule endoscopy findings in celiac disease associated enteropathy-type intestinal T-cell lymphoma. *Endoscopy* 2005;37:594–596.

259. Heine GD, Al-Toma A, Mulder CJ, et al. Milestone in gastrointestinal endoscopy: double-balloon enteroscopy of the small bowel. *Scand J Gastroenterol Suppl* 2006243:32–38.

260. Hoffmann M, Vogelsang H, Kletter K, et al. 18F-fluoro-deoxy-glucose positron emission tomography (18F-FDG-PET) for assessment of enteropathy-type T cell lymphoma. *Gut* 2003;52:347–351.

261. Hadithi M, Mallant M, Oudejans J, et al. 18F-FDG PET versus CT for the detection of enteropathy-associated T-cell lymphoma in refractory celiac disease. *J Nucl Med* 2006;47:1622–1627.

262. Armitage JO, Dick FR, Corder MP, et al. Predicting therapeutic outcome in patients with diffuse histiocytic lymphoma treated with cyclophosphamide, adriamycin, vincristine and prednisone (CHOP). *Cancer* 1982;50:1695–1702.

263. Wohrer S, Chott A, Drach J, et al. Chemotherapy with cyclophosphamide, doxorubicin, etoposide, vincristine and prednisone (CHOEP) is not effective in patients with enteropathy-type intestinal T-cell lymphoma. *Ann Oncol* 2004;15:1680–1683.

264. Jantunen E, Juvonen E, Wiklund T, et al. High-dose therapy supported by autologous stem cell transplantation in patients with enteropathy-associated T-cell lymphoma. *Leuk Lymphoma* 2003;44:2163–2164.

265. Bishton MJ, Haynes AP. Combination chemotherapy followed by autologous stem cell transplant for enteropathy-associated T cell lymphoma. *Br J Haematol* 2007;136:111–113.

266. Lennard A. Combination chemotherapy followed by autologous stem cell transplant for enteropathy-associated T-cell lymphoma. *Br J Haematol* 2007;137:170.

267. Gonzalez CL, Medeiros LJ, Braziel RM, et al. T-cell lymphoma involving subcutaneous tissue. A clinicopathologic entity commonly associated with hemophagocytic syndrome. *Am J Surg Pathol* 1991;15:17–27.

268. Ashworth J, Coady AT, Guy R, et al. Brawny cutaneous induration and granulomatous panniculitis in large cell non-Hodgkin's (T suppressor/cytotoxic cell) lymphoma. *Br J Dermatol* 1989;120:563–569.

269. Tanaka K, Hagari Y, Sano Y, et al. A case of T-cell lymphoma associated with panniculitis, progressive pancytopenia and hyperbilirubinaemia. *Br J Dermatol* 1990;123:649–652.

270. Wang CY, Su WP, Kurtin PJ. Subcutaneous panniculitic T-cell lymphoma. *Int J Dermatol* 1996;35:1–8.

271. Kumar S, Krenacs L, Medeiros J, et al. Subcutaneous panniculitic T-cell lymphoma is a tumor of cytotoxic T lymphocytes. *Hum Pathol* 1998;29:397–403.

272. Kong YY, Dai B, Kong JC, et al. Subcutaneous panniculitis-like T-cell lymphoma: a clinicopathologic, immunophenotypic, and molecular study of 22 Asian cases according to WHO-EORTC classification. *Am J Surg Pathol* 2008;32:1495–1502.

273. Hahtola S, Burghart E, Jeskanen L, et al. Clinicopathological characterization and genomic aberrations in subcutaneous panniculitis-like T-cell lymphoma. *J Invest Dermatol* 2008;128:2304–2309.

274. Wang H, Medeiros LJ, Jones D. Subcutaneous panniculitis-like T-cell lymphoma. *Clin Lymphoma* 2002;3:181–183.

275. Willemze R, Jansen PM, Cerroni L, et al. Subcutaneous panniculitis-like T-cell lymphoma: definition, classification, and prognostic factors: an EORTC Cutaneous Lymphoma Group Study of 83 cases. *Blood* 2008;111:838–845.

276. Berg KD, Brinster NK, Huhn KM, et al. Transmission of a T-cell lymphoma by allogeneic bone marrow transplantation. *N Engl J Med* 2001;345:1458–1463.

277. Parisi M, McNutt N. Subcutaneous panniculitis-like T-cell lymphoma associated with a hemophagocytic syndrome in a patients with polycythemia vera and interferon-alpha therapy. *J Cutan Pathol* 1998;25:580. Abstract.

278. Perniciaro C, Zalla MJ, White JW Jr, et al. Subcutaneous T-cell lymphoma. Report of two additional cases and further observations. *Arch Dermatol* 1993;129:1171–1176.

279. Matsue K, Itoh M, Tsukuda K, et al. Successful treatment of cytophagic histiocytic panniculitis with modified CHOP-E. Cyclophosphamide, adriamycin, vincristine, prednisone, and etoposide. *Am J Clin Oncol* 1994;17:470–474.

280. Weenig RH, Ng CS, Perniciaro C. Subcutaneous panniculitis-like T-cell lymphoma: an elusive case presenting as lipomembranous panniculitis and a review of 72 cases in the literature. *Am J Dermatopathol* 2001;23:206–215.

281. Abeloff M. *Clinical oncology*, 2nd ed. New York, NY: Churchill Livingstone, 2000.

282. Papenfuss JS, Aoun P, Bierman PJ, et al. Subcutaneous panniculitis-like T-cell lymphoma: presentation of 2 cases and observations. *Clin Lymphoma* 2002;3:175–180.

283. Salhany KE, Macon WR, Choi JK, et al. Subcutaneous panniculitis-like T-cell lymphoma: clinicopathologic, immunophenotypic, and genotypic analysis of alpha/beta and gamma/delta subtypes. *Am J Surg Pathol* 1998;22:881–893.

284. Hathaway T, Subtil A, Kuo P, et al. Efficacy of denileukin diftitox in subcutaneous panniculitis-like T-cell lymphoma. *Clin Lymphoma Myeloma* 2007;7:541–545.

CHAPTER 30 ■ PRIMARY CUTANEOUS CD30⁺ LYMPHOPROLIFERATIVE DISORDERS

CHRISTIANE QUERFELD, JOAN GUITART, AND STEVEN T. ROSEN

The primary cutaneous CD30-positive (CD30⁺) lymphoproliferative diseases (LPDs) represent the second most common types of cutaneous T-cell lymphomas (CTCLs), accounting for approximately 20% to 25% of all cutaneous lymphomas according to the World Health Organization and European Organization for Research and Treatment of Cancer (EORTC) consensus classification (1). The spectrum of CD30⁺ LPD includes lymphomatoid papulosis (LyP), cutaneous anaplastic large cell lymphoma (CALCL), and borderline cases that represent a range of disease with variable clinical behavior, morphology, and immunophenotype (1–4). The common hallmark of the tumor cells is CD30, a cell membrane receptor protein belonging to the tumor necrosis factor superfamily. This protein was initially described in Hodgkin lymphoma but also expressed in activated T and B cells. The protein leads to the activation of nuclear factor-κB and is a positive regulator of apoptosis.

CLINICAL MANIFESTATION AND DIFFERENTIAL DIAGNOSIS

Lymphomatoid Papulosis

LyP was first described in 1968 by Macaulay (5) to characterize a chronic self-healing disorder composed of erythematous papules and nodules on trunk and extremities that often occur in clusters or present as many disseminated lesions. They tend to ulcerate and regress spontaneously within weeks, leaving pox-like scars behind (Fig. 30.1). Unusual presentations include a large plaque variant composed of agminated and more persistent papules, follicular, vesicular, and pustular types, and involvement of oral mucosa has been rarely observed (6–8). The lesions wax and wane, and the process can eventually and permanently resolve or persist for decades. Therefore, the course is highly variable. Clinically, arthropod bites, pityriasis lichenoides, viral and parasitic infections, folliculitis, drug eruptions, and various cutaneous lymphomas may resemble LyP.

LyP was previously considered as a benign inflammatory process comprising a spectrum with pityriasis lichenoides (9). LyP is now regarded as an indolent cutaneous lymphoproliferative disorder but is associated with the development of a second malignant lymphoma in about 20% of cases, with mycosis fungoides (MF) as the most common one (1).

Histologic features depend largely on the stage of disease. Classic LyP shows a wedge-shaped pattern of dermal lymphoid infiltrates. Generally, three histologic types have been identified, characterized as types A, B, and C, which may present with overlapping features (Table 30.1). LyP, type A or histiocytic type and type C consist of large atypical lymphocytes resembling Reed-Sternberg cells. Type A cells are embedded in a dense inflammatory background with histiocytes, neutrophils, and eosinophils, and can resemble Hodgkin disease (HD), whereas type C cells are characterized by sheets of similar large atypical lymphocytes with prominent lavender nucleoli and open chromatin with fewer interspersed inflammatory cells (Fig. 30.2). Clinically, the main difference between type A and type C is that type A tends to preset as small papules, in contrast to the large, long-lasting, nodular lesions that are more typical of type C. Type B or lymphocytic type simulates classic MF, with epidermotropism and a dermal band-like infiltrate composed of small to medium-sized hyperconvoluted T cells. Differentiation

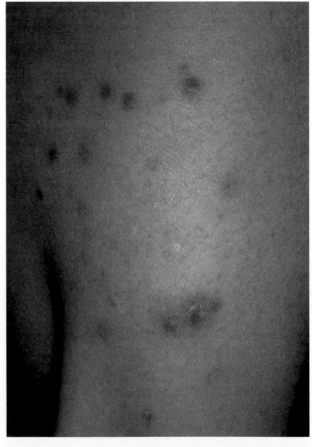

FIGURE 30.1 Patient diagnosed with LyP presenting with multiple erythematous papules on the upper arm (see also Color Plate 75).

TABLE 30.1			
KEY DIAGNOSTIC CRITERIA FOR LYP			
Criteria	Type A LyP (histiocytic type)	Type B LyP (lymphocytic type)	Type C LyP
Cutaneous infiltrate	➢ Scattered or small sheets of large anaplastic or pleomorphic lymphoid cells ➢ Numerous histiocytes, neutrophils, eosinophils ➢ Reed-Sternberg-like cells	➢ Band-like small to medium-sized lymphocytes with cerebriform nuclei ➢ Pautrier microabscesses	➢ Nodular infiltrate ➢ Cohesive sheets of large atypical lymphoid cells ➢ Few inflammatory cells
CD30 expression	➢ Positive	➢ Negative	➢ Positive
Epidermotropism	➢ Little	➢ Yes	➢ No
Differential diagnosis	➢ HD	➢ MF	➢ CD30⁺ ALCL

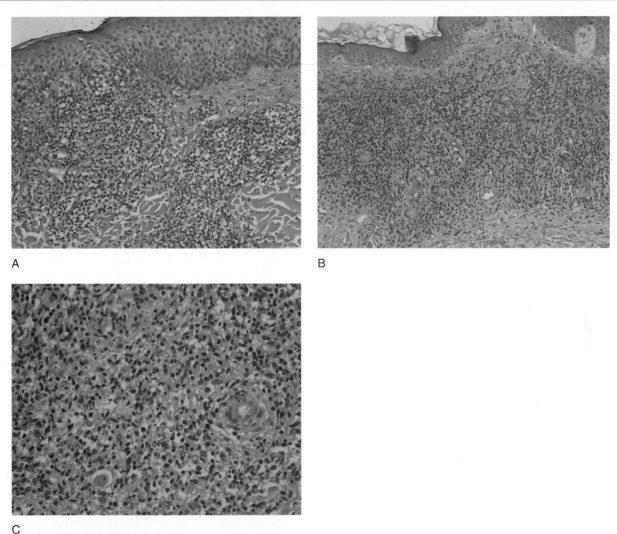

A

B

C

FIGURE 30.2 LyP type A with large atypical cells intermingled with histiocytes, eosinophils, and small lymphocytes (see also Color Plate 76) (**A**), and type B with band-like infiltrate of small to medium-sized lymphocytes and epidermotropism resembling histologic features of MF (hematoxylin and eosin; original magnification ×200) (**B**) (see also Color Plate 77). **C:** Type C reveals cohesive sheets of atypical lymphoid cells (hematoxylin and eosin; original magnification ×400) (see also Color Plate 78).

between LyP type B and MF cannot be made without immunophenotyping. Furthermore, incipient lesions of type A LyP may have a similar appearance as type B, and the coexistence of type A and type B lesions has been reported in the same patient.

The atypical lymphoid cells exhibit a CD4⁺ CD8⁻ CD30⁺ T-helper (Th) phenotype, and frequently express cytotoxic proteins such as T-cell–restricted intracellular antigen-1, and less commonly granzyme B and perforin (10). Occasionally LyP has a CD8⁺ or CD4⁻/CD8⁻ null phenotype. Pan-T-cell markers such as CD2, CD3, and CD5 are usually expressed, but CD7 is frequently absent (1,3). The expression of CD15, a marker for Hodgkin lymphoma and Reed-Sternberg cells, has been reported, but staining for CD15 is generally negative. The anaplastic lymphoma kinase (ALK) protein-1 is negative; coexpression of CD56 is observed in rare cases but does not appear to be associated with an unfavorable prognosis (11,12). Pseudocarcinomatous epidermal hyperplasia was found in cases of LyP and CD30⁺ CALCL, possibly associated with epidermal growth factor dysregulation (13). Recently published immunohistochemical data suggest that expression of fascin, survivin, Bcl-2, and TRAF in LyP may become a predictive marker for progression or development of a second lymphoid malignancy (14). Low or loss of CD134 expression may also predict disease progression (15).

PRIMARY CUTANEOUS ANAPLASTIC LARGE CELL LYMPHOMA

In 1985, Stein et al. (16) described a large cell lymphoma defined by cohesive sheets of large lymphoid cells expressing the Ki-1 (CD30) antigen. This has led to the further recognition of CD30 expression as a common phenotypic hallmark for LyP and CD30⁺ CALCL. CD30⁺ CALCL may present as primary or as secondary lymphoma arising from another lymphoma through transformation. Most cases of CD30⁺ CALCL present as solitary or regional nodules and/or tumors that often show ulceration (Fig. 30.3). The skin lesions may undergo spontaneous regression as in LyP, but often persist. Predilection sites are head and extremities. Generalized or multifocal lesions are seen in about 20% of the patients. Extracutaneous or regional lymph node involvement is seen in 10% of patients at presentation.

CD30⁺ CALCL shows histologic and immunophenotypic overlap with type C. LyP and may be difficult or impossible to distinguish at times. Therefore, clinical features are important in distinguishing CD30⁺ CALCL from LyP. A morphologic and immunophenotypic overlap with classic Hodgkin disease (HD) was also recognized. Histology shows a diffuse, dense,

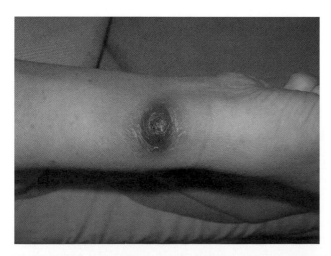

FIGURE 30.3 Patient diagnosed with CD30⁺ CALCL revealing a solitary violaceous tumor with central necrosis on the forearm. Courtesy of Christiane Querfeld, MD. (see also Color Plate 79).

nonepidermotropic infiltrate with cohesive proliferations of large CD30⁺ lymphocytes. In most cases, neoplastic cells show anaplastic features, less commonly a pleomorphic or immunoblastic appearance (Fig. 30.4). However, there is no difference in the prognosis and survival rate based on cytomorphology.

According to the World Health Organization-EORTC classification, CALCL is classified by the expression of CD30 in >75% of large atypical cells (1). However, it may show a wide morphologic spectrum, including neutrophil-rich tumors (17). The atypical cells generally show an activated CD4⁺ Th cell phenotype with variable loss of T-cell markers and frequent expression of cytotoxic proteins. Other activation markers such as CD25 (interleukin-2 receptor) and human leukocyte antigen-DR are also found. CD8⁺ T-cell phenotype, as well as a null CD4⁻CD8⁻ T-cell phenotype and coexpression of CD56 and CD30 have rarely been reported (17). Cytotoxic proteins such as granzyme B, T-cell–restricted intracellular antigen-1, and perforin may be found in about 50% of the cases (6). The overlying epidermis may show a variable degree of pseudoepitheliomatous hyperplasia mimicking squamous cell carcinoma, thereby leading to inappropriate diagnosis and treatment (Fig. 30.4) (13).

In contrast to systemic anaplastic large cell lymphoma (ALCL), primary CD30⁺ CALCLs do not carry the t(2;5) translocation and are ALCL kinase protein (ALK-1) negative (18,19). Clusterin is found in both CALCL and ALK+ ALCL (20). Epithelial membrane antigen and expression of c-kit receptor (CD117) are usually negative in CALCL and LyP (21).

BORDERLINE CASES

Borderline cases are characterized by differences between the clinical features and their histologic appearance. These include cases with the clinical presentation of a CD30⁺ CALCL with histologic features suggestive of LyP, and, conversely, cases with a recurrent, self-healing skin eruption that shows histologic features characteristic of a CD30⁺ CALCL (2). There are no current clinicopathologic criteria to allow a clear distinction. Borderline cases may exhibit features between LyP and CD30⁺ CALCL. LyP type C has been described as a borderline lesion of CD30⁺ CALCL. Thus, the clinical appearance and the clinical course over time are used as decisive criteria for the definite diagnosis and the choice of treatment. A recent study investigated the expression of multiple myeloma oncogene 1/IRF4 in CD30⁺ lymphoproliferative disorders of the skin. About 90% of the LyP biopsies were found to be multiple myeloma oncogene 1/IRF4 positive, whereas multiple myeloma oncogene 1/IRF4 was expressed only in 20% of CALCL biopsies and, thus, represents a new diagnostic marker that may allow for the distinction of LyP and ALCL (22).

EPIDEMIOLOGY

CD30⁺ LPDs represent the second most common CTCL after MF, comprising approximately 25% of all CTCL cases, with a male predominance of approximately 1.5 to 2.0:1. The prevalence rate of LyP is estimated at 1.2 to 1.9 cases per 1 million population in the United States and may occur less frequently in African-American patients (25). The prevalence

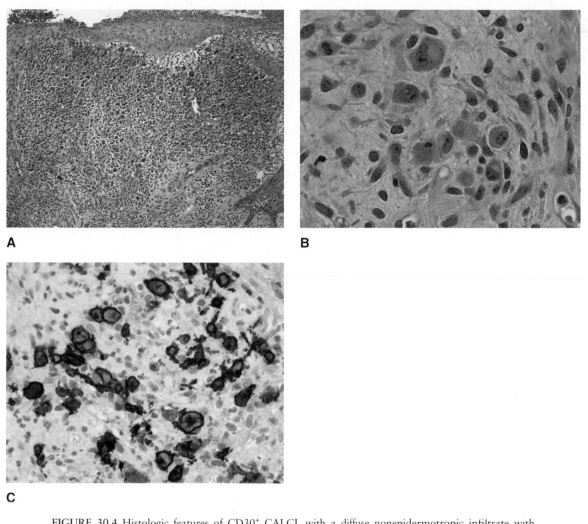

FIGURE 30.4 Histologic features of CD30⁺ CALCL with a diffuse nonepidermotropic infiltrate with cohesive sheets of large atypical lymphocytes. **A:** Numerous inflammatory cells (T cells, eosinophils, and neutrophils) are present (hematoxylin and eosin; original magnification ×200) (see also Color Plate 80). **B:** The tumor cells have the characteristic morphology of anaplastic cells, showing round, oval, or irregularly shaped nuclei with prominent (eosinophilic) nucleoli and abundant cytoplasm (hematoxylin and eosin; original magnification ×400) (see also Color Plate 81). **C:** Immunostaining for CD30 antigen produced a strong cytoplasmic membrane staining of the tumor cells (hematoxylin and eosin; original magnification ×400) C (see also Color Plate 82).

of CD30⁺ CALCL in the United States is not known. LyP generally occurs in adults between the 3rd and 4th decade, with a median age of 45 years at onset, although the disorder may affect any age. It has also been described in children (26). In addition, cases of regional LyP were more often found in children than adults. About 10% to 20% of the adult patients diagnosed with LyP coexist with, or develop, an associated lymphoid malignancy, in particular MF, CD30⁺ CALCL, and HD, but the prognosis for patients with LyP is otherwise excellent, showing a 100% 5-year survival (27). CD30⁺ CALCL may occur at any age but typically affects older patients in the 6th decade, with a median age of 61 years. Systemic therapy will often cure the associated lymphoid malignancy; however, the LyP will recur. Although rarely, CD30⁺ CALCL does appear in children, as confirmed by two retrospective studies with follow-up data for >20 years (26,28). A case-control study performed in patients with LyP found a significantly increased exposure to previous radiation therapy (24).

ETIOLOGY

CD30 expression in lymphocytes is up-regulated by select viruses such as Epstein-Barr virus, human herpesvirus, and human T-cell lymphotropic viruses 1 and 2, and has been implicated in the pathogenesis of CD30⁺ LPDs. Electron microscopy identified intranuclear and intracytoplasmic virus-like particles in cases of LyP, but further investigations have been negative to date (29–31). More recently, transcripts of human endogenous retroviral sequences in lesional tissue and cell lines of cutaneous CD30⁺ LPDs have been detected (32). Epstein-Barr virus has been found in rare cases of CD30⁺ CALCL and LyP as posttransplant lymphoproliferative disorders, after immunosuppressive therapy, or in human immunodeficiency virus infection (33–35). Reduced immunosurveillance, chronic antigenic stimulation due to the graft, a direct oncogenic effect of immunosuppressive drugs, and activation of oncogenic viruses have all been suggested as possible mechanisms, however, the exact pathologic process remains elusive (36,37).

BIOGLOIC PROPERTIES, MOLECULAR AND CYTOGENETIC ABNORMALITIES

The skin-homing mechanism of malignant T cells is not completely elucidated, although adhesion molecules and chemokines have been associated with the pathogenesis. Data have shown that expression of CLA and CCR3 with its ligand eotaxin/CCL11 plays a role in the homing of CD30[+] CTCL cells to the skin (38). More recent studies investigated the expression patterns of the chemokine receptors CXCR3, CCR4, and CCR3, and their ligands monokine-induced by interferon (IFN)-γ (CXCL9), thymus- and activation-regulated chemokine (CCL17), and RANTES (CCL5) in skin specimens of patients with CD30[+] cutaneous lymphoproliferative disorders (39). It appears that CCR3 and its ligand RANTES were coexpressed in CD30[+] CALCL (38,39), suggesting tumor cell growth via an autocrine mechanism. CXCR3 was detected in atypical lymphoid cells of LyP, especially in epidermotropic small to medium-sized lymphoid cells of type B LyP. The CXCR3 ligand monokine-induced by IFN-γ was expressed in lesional epidermal keratinocytes in LyP, thereby facilitating migration into the epidermis (39).

The preferential association of some chemokine receptors with human Th1 or Th2 cells has been reported (40). In vitro studies have proposed that human Th1 cells favor expression of CXCR3, whereas Th2 cells favor CCR3 and CCR4. Analysis of cytokine expression pattern of CCR3-bearing CD30[+] infiltrating CTCL cells showed a predominant Th2 profile with interleukin-4, but not IFN-γ protein expression, consistent with the hypothesis that CD30[+] CALCL might be characterized by a Th2-like cytokine profile and that LyP might be functionally of Th1 phenotype, in contrast to CD30[+] CALCL (38,39).

Little is known about apoptosis mechanisms that may underlie the clinical regression of skin lesions in CD30[+] LPDs. Apoptosis rates and expression of apoptosis-related proteins were analyzed in evolutional stages of LyP and CD30[+] CALCL, and CD30[+] lymphoma cell lines (41). A significantly higher apoptotic index was found in LyP than in CD30[+] CALCL (42). The proapoptotic protein Bax was expressed at high levels in evolutional stages of LyP and CD30[+] CALCL, and may play a crucial role in mediating apoptosis of tumor cells, however, no significant correlation was found between Bax expression and the tumor type and evolutional stage. Expression of bcl-2 appears to protect tumor cells from apoptosis in CD30[+] lymphoproliferative disorders. Stimulation of cell growth and apoptosis have been noted with activation of CD30, and, therefore, CD30 ligand-mediated cytotoxicity may participate in the pathophysiology of clinical regression (42,43). Interaction between Fas/APO-1 (CD95) and its ligand FasL have also been studied (44). CD95 expression appears to be expressed at high levels in all cutaneous CD30[+] lymphomas and suggests that CD95 activation may induce regression of CD30[+] skin lesions. FOXP3 expression in cutaneous and systemic CD30 LPD was also investigated. FoxP3 is expressed in tumor-infiltrating regulatory T cells. Significant higher numbers were recorded in ALK-negative systemic ALCL and LyP

biopsies than in primary CALCL, implicating the more favorable outcome of LyP (45). Increased expression of the Notch family member, Notch1, and its ligand Jagged1 was found in Lyp and primary cutaneous CD30[+] CALCL, but their mechanism of up-regulation and potential role in disease progression has not been established (46).

Molecular studies have found that nearly all primary cutaneous CD30[+] CALCLs are of clonal origin (47,48). Analyses of LyP cases for the presence of clonal T-cell receptor rearrangements have shown that only a proportion of patients with LyP have a monoclonal T-cell proliferation (49,50). However, identical clones have been found in LyP lesions and associated CTCL. Recent data demonstrated that the sensitivity of the polymerase chain reaction may be enhanced by microdissection of T cells in MF (51), but controversial data on clonality of neoplastic CD30[+] cells by microdissection and single-cell analysis in LyP have been reported (52–54). One group identified monoclonal patterns of T-cell receptor-γ chain rearrangements in the large CD30[+] T cells in nearly all cases (52), whereas a recent study showed that the small CD30[−] T cells represent the clonal population (53). The phenomenon of spontaneous regression and recurrence of skin lesions observed in patients with LyP and CALCL raised the question of persistence of a clonal T-cell population in the peripheral blood (55). Clonal T-cell receptor rearrangement in a high percentage of skin samples was demonstrated but differs from the T-cell clone in the blood in 35% and 86% of patients with LyP and ALCL, respectively.

The genetic background of CD30[+] LPDs is largely unknown. Microsatellite instability, consistent with deficits in deoxyribonucleic acid repair, has recently been identified in one patient with CD30[+] CALCL originating from LyP (56). Cytogenetic analysis revealed numeric and structural aberrations such as trisomy 7 in CD30[+] neoplastic cells with recurrent breakpoints observed at 1p36, 6p25, 8q24, and 10q24. Loss of genetic material occurred at 6q in one CD30[+] CALCL (57,58). Comparative genomic hybridization studies disclosed chromosomal imbalances in approximately 40% of the cases (59). The most frequent gains involved chromosome 1/1p and 5 (50% of the cases), 6, 7, 8/8p, and 19 (38%). Recurrent losses were detected at 6q21 and 18p11. Gains involving chromosome 9 and losses involving chromosome 6q and 18p were seen in patients with relapse (60).

Cellular insensitivity to growth inhibition by transforming growth factor(TGF)-β is a hallmark in the genesis and progression of human malignancies. Mutations in or loss of the TGF-β receptor genes I and II have been described in cell lines clonally derived from LyP in the progression to systemic lymphoma and have been linked directly to resistance to the growth inhibitory effects of TGF-β (61–63). JunB overexpression is a common finding in CD30[+] CALCL and LyP, and appears to be necessary for CD30 expression, but its potential pathogenetic role in these neoplasms has not been elucidated yet (64).

STAGING, SURVIVAL, AND PROGNOSIS

The tumor, node, metastases classification system has been used to stage patients with MF and Sézary syndrome, and has been in use for almost 30 years for prediction of survival and stratification of therapy (65). Recently, the International Society for Cutaneous Lymphomas and the cutaneous lymphoma task force of the EORTC have established a consensus proposal of a tumor, node, metastases classification system applicable for all primary cutaneous lymphomas other than MF and Sézary syndrome to improve the communication about the state of disease, selection of appropriate management, standardization of enrollment/response criteria in clinical trials, and collection/analysis of prospective survival data (66).

Routine evaluation should include complete physical examination, complete blood count with differential, chemistry panel with lactate dehydrogenase, skin biopsy for histology, immunophenotyping and gene rearrangement studies, and lymph node biopsies in cases with enlarged nodes at presentation to establish the diagnosis and staging. Immunostaining with anti-ALK monoclonal antibodies and/or reverse transcriptase-polymerase chain reaction can be performed to detect the t(2;5) translocation for diagnostic purposes. Imaging studies such as computed tomography and positron emission tomography scans should be reserved for patients with clinical and laboratory findings suggestive of systemic disease or prominent lymphadenopathy. Bone marrow biopsy is a consideration in patients with CD30⁺ CALCL. Histopathologic and molecular results should be correlated with clinical findings and patients classified according to the World Health Organization-EORTC consensus classification.

Many European studies have confirmed the excellent prognosis of CD30⁺ LPDs (67). This was confirmed by two recent reports from cutaneous lymphoma groups in Europe and United States, with 5- and 10-year disease-related survival rates exceeding 90% (28,68). However, a few cases of CD30⁺ CALCL with poor outcome have been observed. Patients presenting with multifocal skin lesions and/or limited regional lymph nodes have a similar prognosis to patients with only skin lesions. In contrast, the specific survival at 5 years was only 24% in patients presenting secondary cutaneous involvement during systemic lymphoma with large CD30⁺ cells (28). The occurrence of tumors with large CD30⁺ cell transformation of MF is also associated with poor prognosis (67). No difference in clinical presentation, clinical behavior, or prognosis is found between CD30⁺ CALCL cases with an anaplastic, pleomorphic, or immunoblastic morphology (1). Spontaneous regression and age <60 years are associated with a favorable prognosis (2). No patients with LyP died of disease. Patients diagnosed with LyP at a younger age tend to be at higher risk for malignant transformation (69). One investigation found that the cumulative risk for developing lymphoma over time begins after 5 years and approaches 80% after 15 years, but this has not been witnessed in our experience or by others investigators (69). A few cases have been reported showing that CD30/CD56 coexpression is associated with a disease progression, as well as increased fascin levels, but this was not confirmed by other investigators (14,70,71). In cases with progression, point mutations and deletions on TGF-β receptor genes I and II have been found, leading to the loss of its tumor suppressive properties (61,62).

TREATMENT OPTIONS

There is no curative treatment available. Historically, the most commonly reported treatment modalities in LyP are doxycycline, psoralens and ultraviolet (UV) light A, UVB, narrowband-UVB, low-dose methotrexate, IFN-α, topical steroid and bexarotene formulations, and radiation. However, none of these treatments alters the natural course of disease; therefore, the short-term benefits should be weighed against the potential harmful side effects. Observation in patients with few lesions is recommended, whereas in patients with more disseminated disease, low-dose methotrexate or UV light treatment might be effective in clearing disease (72,73). A few single case reports have found that topical carmustine, topical nitrogen mustard, topical methotrexate, intralesional IFN-α, low-dose cyclophosphamide, chlorambucil, medium-dose UVA₁ therapy, imiquimod, and dapsone may be effective (74–78). Data are scarce in children with LyP; reported treatment modalities include systemic antibiotics, low-dose methotrexate, topical steroids, psoralens and UV light A, and UVB (26,28).

Spot involved-field radiation therapy for solitary or localized lesions is the preferred treatment for CD30⁺ CALCL with systemic chemotherapy reserved for cases with large tumor burden and/or extracutaneous involvement. However, relapse occurs in approximately 40% of patients, despite treatment (28). Therapy regimens include cyclophosphamide, hydroxydaunorubicin, Oncovin [vincristine], and prednisone (CHOP) or cyclophosphamide, Oncovin [vincristine], and prednisone (CVP) chemotherapy, IFN-α, or oral bexarotene. The Dutch Cutaneous Lymphoma Group found that multiagent systemic chemotherapy, compared with single-agent therapy, did not result in a higher cure rate or prevent future relapses in their patients (28). More recently there has been reported efficacy of recombinant IFN-γ and combined treatment with bexarotene and IFN-α 2a (79,80). Patients with systemic progression following systemic combination chemotherapy are potential candidates for autologous or allogeneic stem cell transplantation, although there are limited data concerning this patient population. In our experience, pegylated doxorubicin is very effective as a single agent, presumably due to the increased efficacy of liposomal doxorubicin in the skin (81).

Experimental immunotherapies have targeted CD30⁺ cells in the setting of HD. SGN-30 is a chimeric anti-CD30 monoclonal antibody that demonstrated activity against HD and ALCL cell lines in vitro and in xenograft models (42,82). SGN-30 has been shown to cause objective tumor responses in patients with systemic ALCL. Moreover, preliminary results of a phase II trial in patients with cutaneous CD30⁺ lymphoproliferative disorders demonstrated promising results, with low toxicities reported (83). SGN-30 was given at a dose of 12 mg per kg every 2 to weeks, with six (35%) objective responses (complete and partial responses) observed.

References

1. Willemze R, Jaffe ES, Burg G, et al. WHO-EORTC classification for cutaneous lymphomas. *Blood* 2005;105:3768–3785.
2. Paulli M, Berti E, Rosso R, et al. CD30/Ki-1-positive lymphoproliferative disorders of the skin—clinicopathologic correlation and statistical analysis of 86 cases: a multicentric study from the European Organization for Research and Treatment of Cancer Cutaneous Lymphoma Project Group. *J Clin Oncol* 1995;13:1343–1354.
3. Burg G, Kempf W. *Cutaneous lymphomas*. London: Taylor and Francis 2005.
4. Querfeld C, Kuzel TM, Guitart J, et al. Primary cutaneous CD30+ lymphoproliferative disorders: new insights into biology and therapy. *Oncology (Williston Park)* 2007;21:689–696.

5. Macaulay WL. Lymphomatoid papulosis. A continuing self-healing eruption, clinically benign-histologically malignant. *Arch Dermatol* 1968;97:23–30.

6. Kempf W. CD30+ lymphoproliferative disorders: histopathology, differential diagnosis, new variants, and simulators. *J Cutan Pathol* 2006;33:(suppl 1):58–70.

7. Pujol RM, Muret MP, Bergua P, et al. Oral involvement in lymphomatoid papulosis. Report of two cases and review of the literature. *Dermatology* 2005;210:53–57.

8. Heald P, Subtil A, Breneman D, et al. Persistent agmination of lymphomatoid papulosis: an equivalent of limited plaque mycosis fungoides type of cutaneous T-cell lymphoma. *J Am Acad Dermatol* 2007;57:1005–1011.

9. Cerroni L. Lymphomatoid papulosis, pityriasis lichenoides et varioliformis acuta, and anaplastic large-cell (Ki-1+) lymphoma. *J Am Acad Dermatol* 1997;37:287.

10. Kummer JA, Vermeer MH, Dukers D, et al. Most primary cutaneous CD30-positive lymphoproliferative disorders have a CD4-positive cytotoxic T-cell phenotype. *J Invest Dermatol* 1997;109:636–640.

11. Harvell J, Vaseghi M, Natkunam Y, et al. Large atypical cells of lymphomatoid papulosis are CD56-negative: a study of 18 cases. *J Cutan Pathol* 2002;29:88–92.

12. Flann S, Orchard GE, Wain EM, et al. Three cases of lymphomatoid papulosis with a CD56+ immunophenotype. *J Am Acad Dermatol* 2006;55:903–906.

13. Scarisbrick JJ, Calonje E, Orchard G, et al. Pseudocarcinomatous change in lymphomatoid papulosis and primary cutaneous CD30+ lymphoma: a clinicopathologic and immunohistochemical study of 6 patients. *J Am Acad Dermatol* 2001;44:239–247.

14. Kempf W, Levi E, Kamarashev J, et al. Fascin expression in CD30-positive cutaneous lymphoproliferative disorders. *J Cutan Pathol* 2002;29:295–300.

15. Gniadecki R, Rossen K. Expression of T-cell activation marker CD134 (OX40) in lymphomatoid papulosis. *Br J Dermatol* 2003;148:885–891.

16. Stein H, Mason DY, Gerdes J, et al. The expression of the Hodgkin's disease associated antigen Ki-1 in reactive and neoplastic lymphoid tissue: evidence that Reed-Sternberg cells and histiocytic malignancies are derived from activated lymphoid cells. *Blood* 1985;66:848–858.

17. Boudova L, Kazakov DV, Jindra P, et al. Primary cutaneous histiocyte and neutrophil-rich CD30+ and CD56+ anaplastic large-cell lymphoma with prominent angioinvasion and nerve involvement in the forehead and scalp of an immunocompetent woman. *J Cutan Pathol* 2006;33:584–589.

18. Herbst H, Sander C, Tronnier M, et al. Absence of anaplastic lymphoma kinase (ALK) and Epstein-Barr virus gene products in primary cutaneous anaplastic large cell lymphoma and lymphomatoid papulosis. *Br J Dermatol* 1997;137:680–686.

19. Sasaki K, Sugaya M, Fujita H, et al. A case of primary cutaneous anaplastic large cell lymphoma with variant anaplastic lymphoma kinase translocation. *Br J Dermatol* 2004;150:1202–1207.

20. Lae ME, Ahmed I, Macon WR. Clusterin is widely expressed in systemic anaplastic large cell lymphoma but fails to differentiate primary from secondary cutaneous anaplastic large cell lymphoma. *Am J Clin Pathol* 2002;118:773–779.

21. Rassidakis GZ, Georgakis GV, Oyarzo M, et al. Lack of c-kit (CD117) expression in CD30+ lymphomas and lymphomatoid papulosis. *Mod Pathol* 2004;17:946–953.

22. Kempf W, Kutzner H, Cozzio A, et al. MUM1 expression in cutaneous CD30+ lymphoproliferative disorders: a valuable tool for the distinction between lymphomatoid papulosis and primary cutaneous anaplastic large-cell lymphoma. *Br J Dermatol* 2008;158:1280–1287.

23. Panhans A, Bodemer C, Macinthyre E, et al. Pityriasis lichenoides of childhood with atypical CD30-positive cells and clonal T-cell receptor gene rearrangements. *J Am Acad Dermatol* 1996;35:489–490.

24. Laube S, Shah F, Marsden J. Consequences of misdiagnosis of lymphomatoid papulosis. *Eur J Cancer Care (Engl)* 2006;15:194–198.

25. Wang HH, Lach L, Kadin ME Epidemiology of lymphomatoid papulosis. *Cancer* 1992;70:2951–2957.

26. Nijsten T, Curiel-Lewandrowski C, Kadin ME. Lymphomatoid papulosis in children: a retrospective cohort study of 35 cases. *Arch Dermatol* 2004;140:306–312.

27. Wang HH, Myers T, Lach LJ, et al. Increased risk of lymphoid and non-lymphoid malignancies in patients with lymphomatoid papulosis. *Cancer* 1999;86:1240–1245.

28. Bekkenk MW, Geelen FA, van Voorst Vader PC, et al. Primary and secondary cutaneous CD30(+) lymphoproliferative disorders: a report from the Dutch Cutaneous Lymphoma Group on the long-term follow-up data of 219 patients and guidelines for diagnosis and treatment. *Blood* 2000;95:3653–3661.

29. Sangueza OP, Galloway J, Eagan PA, et al. Absence of Epstein-Barr virus in lymphomatoid papulosis. An immunohistochemical and in situ hybridization study. *Arch Dermatol* 1996;132:279–282.

30. Jang KA, Choi JC, Choi JH. Expression of cutaneous lymphocyte-associated antigen and TIA-1 by lymphocytes in pityriasis lichenoides et varioliformis acuta and lymphomatoid papulosis: immunohistochemical study. *J Cutan Pathol* 2001;28:453–459.

31. Shamsuddin AK, Nedwich A, Toker C. Lymphomatoid papulosis. Ultrastructural study with demonstration of intranuclear and intracytoplasmic viruslike particles. *Dermatologica* 1980;161:238–242.

32. Kempf W, Kadin ME, Dvorak AM, et al. Endogenous retroviral elements, but not exogenous retroviruses, are detected in CD30-positive lymphoproliferative disorders of the skin. *Carcinogenesis* 2003;24:301–306.

33. Ravat FE, Spittle MF, Russell-Jones R. Primary cutaneous T-cell lymphoma occurring after organ transplantation. *J Am Acad Dermatol* 2006;54:668–675.

34. Wilkins K, Turner R, Dolev JC, et al. Cutaneous malignancy and human immunodeficiency virus disease. *J Am Acad Dermatol* 2006;54:189–206.

35. Dreno B, Milpied-Homsi B, Moreau P, et al. Cutaneous anaplastic T-cell lymphoma in a patient with human immunodeficiency virus infection: detection of Epstein-Barr virus DNA. *Br J Dermatol* 1993;129:77–81.

36. Lucioni M, Ippoliti G, Campana C, et al. EBV positive primary cutaneous CD30+ large T-cell lymphoma in a heart transplanted patient: case report. *Am J Transplant* 2004;4:1915–1920.

37. Salama S. Primary "cutaneous" T-cell anaplastic large cell lymphoma, CD30+, neutrophil-rich variant with subcutaneous panniculitic lesions, in a post-renal transplant patient: report of unusual case and literature review. *Am J Dermatopathol* 2005;27:217–223.

38. Kleinhans M, Tun-Kyi A, Gilliet M, et al. Functional expression of the eotaxin receptor CCR3 in CD30+ cutaneous T-cell lymphoma. *Blood* 2003;101:1487–1493.

39. Yamaguchi T, Ohshima K, Karube K, et al. Expression of chemokines and chemokine receptors in cutaneous CD30+ lymphoproliferative disorders. *Br J Dermatol* 2006;154:904–909.

40. Yamamoto J, Adachi Y, Onoue Y, et al. Differential expression of the chemokine receptors by the Th1- and Th2-type effector populations within circulating CD4+ T cells. *J Leukoc Biol* 2000;68:568–574.

41. Greisser J, Doebbeling U, Roos M, et al. Apoptosis in CD30-positive lymphoproliferative disorders of the skin. *Exp Dermatol* 2005;14:380–385.

42. Wahl AF, Klussman K, Thompson JD, et al. The anti-CD30 monoclonal antibody SGN-30 promotes growth arrest and DNA fragmentation in vitro and affects antitumor activity in models of Hodgkin's disease. *Cancer Res* 2002;62:3736–3742.

43. Mori M, Manuelli C, Pimpinelli N, et al. CD30-CD30 ligand interaction in primary cutaneous CD30(+) T-cell lymphomas: a clue to the pathophysiology of clinical regression. *Blood* 1999;94:3077–3083.

44. Paulli M, Berti E, Boveri E, et al. Cutaneous CD30+ lymphoproliferative disorders: expression of bcl-2 and proteins of the tumor necrosis factor receptor superfamily. *Hum Pathol* 1998;29:1223–1230.

45. Gjerdrum LM, Woetmann A, Odum N, et al. FOXP3 positive regulatory T-cells in cutaneous and systemic CD30 positive T-cell lymphoproliferations. *Eur J Haematol* 2008;80:483–489.

46. Kamstrup MR, Ralfkiaer E, Skovgaard GL, et al. Potential involvement of Notch1 signalling in the pathogenesis of primary cutaneous CD30-positive lymphoproliferative disorders. *Br J Dermatol* 2008;158:747–753.

47. Assaf C, Hummel M, Dippel E, et al. Common clonal T-cell origin in a patient with T-prolymphocytic leukaemia and associated cutaneous T-cell lymphomas. *Br J Haematol* 2003;120:488–491.

48. Kadin ME. Pathobiology of CD30+ cutaneous T-cell lymphomas. *J Cutan Pathol* 2006;33:(suppl 1):10–17.

49. Whittaker S, Smith N, Jones RR, et al. Analysis of beta, gamma, and delta T-cell receptor genes in lymphomatoid papulosis: cellular basis of two distinct histologic subsets. *J Invest Dermatol* 1991;96:786–791.

50. Wood GS, Crooks CF, Uluer AZ. Lymphomatoid papulosis and associated cutaneous lymphoproliferative disorders exhibit a common clonal origin. *J Invest Dermatol* 1995;105:51–55.

51. Dereure O, Levi E, Vonderheid EC, et al. Improved sensitivity of T-cell clonality detection in mycosis fungoides by hand microdissection and heteroduplex analysis. *Arch Dermatol* 2003;139:1571–1575.

52. Steinhoff M, Hummel M, Anagnostopoulos I, et al. Single-cell analysis of CD30+ cells in lymphomatoid papulosis demonstrates a common clonal T-cell origin. *Blood* 2002;100:578–584.

53. Gellrich S, Wernicke M, Wilks A, et al. The cell infiltrate in lymphomatoid papulosis comprises a mixture of polyclonal large atypical cells (CD30-positive) and smaller monoclonal T cells (CD30-negative). *J Invest Dermatol* 2004;122:859–861.

54. Greisser J, Palmedo G, Sander C, et al. Detection of clonal rearrangement of T-cell receptor genes in the diagnosis of primary cutaneous CD30 lymphoproliferative disorders. *J Cutan Pathol* 2006;33:711–715.

55. Humme D, Lukowsky A, Steinhoff M, et al. Dominance of nonmalignant T-cell clones and distortion of the TCR repertoire in the peripheral blood of patients with cutaneous CD30+ lymphoproliferative disorders. *J Invest Dermatol* 2009;129:89–98

56. Rubben A, Kempf W, Kadin ME, et al. Multilineage progression of genetically unstable tumor subclones in cutaneous T-cell lymphoma. *Exp Dermatol* 2004;13:472–483.

57. Peters K, Knoll JH, Kadin ME. Cytogenetic findings in regressing skin lesions of lymphomatoid papulosis. *Cancer Genet Cytogenet* 1995;80:13–16.

58. Ott G, Katzenberger T, Siebert R, et al. Chromosomal abnormalities in nodal and extranodal CD30+ anaplastic large cell lymphomas: infrequent detection of the t(2;5) in extranodal lymphomas. *Genes Chromosomes Cancer* 1998;22:114–121.

59. Mao X, Orchard G, Lillington DM, et al. Genetic alterations in primary cutaneous CD30+ anaplastic large cell lymphoma. *Genes Chromosomes Cancer* 2003;37:176–185.

60. Prochazkova M, Chevret E, Beylot-Barry M, et al. Chromosomal imbalances: a hallmark of tumour relapse in primary cutaneous CD30+ T-cell lymphoma. *J Pathol* 2003;201:421–429.

61. Schiemann WP, Pfeifer WM, Levi E, et al. A deletion in the gene for transforming growth factor beta type I receptor abolishes growth regulation by transforming growth factor beta in a cutaneous T-cell lymphoma. *Blood* 1999;94:2854–2861.

62. Kadin ME, Levi E, Kempf W. Progression of lymphomatoid papulosis to systemic lymphoma is associated with escape from growth inhibition by transforming growth factor-beta and CD30 ligand. *Ann N Y Acad Sci* 2001;941:59–68.

63. Knaus PI, Lindemann D, DeCoteau JF, et al. A dominant inhibitory mutant of the type II transforming growth factor beta receptor in the malignant progression of a cutaneous T-cell lymphoma. *Mol Cell Biol* 1996;16:3480–3489.

64. Rassidakis GZ, Thomaides A, Atwell C, et al. JunB expression is a common feature of CD30+ lymphomas and lymphomatoid papulosis. *Mod Pathol* 2005;18:1365–1370.

65. Bunn PA Jr, Lamberg SI. Report of the Committee on Staging and Classification of Cutaneous T-Cell Lymphomas. *Cancer Treat Rep* 1979;63:725–728.

66. Kim YH, Willemze R, Pimpinelli N, et al. TNM classification system for primary cutaneous lymphomas other than mycosis fungoides and Sezary syndrome: a proposal of the International Society for Cutaneous Lymphomas (ISCL) and the Cutaneous Lymphoma Task Force of the European Organization of Research and Treatment of Cancer (EORTC). *Blood* 2007;110:479–484.

67. Grange F, Bagot M. Prognosis of primary cutaneous lymphomas [in French]. *Ann Dermatol Venereol* 2002;129:30–40.

68. Liu HL, Hoppe RT, Kohler S, et al. CD30+ cutaneous lymphoproliferative disorders: the Stanford experience in lymphomatoid papulosis and primary cutaneous anaplastic large cell lymphoma. *J Am Acad Dermatol* 2003;49:1049–1058.

69. Cabanillas F, Armitage J, Pugh WC, et al. Lymphomatoid papulosis: a T-cell dyscrasia with a propensity to transform into malignant lymphoma. *Ann Intern Med* 1995;122:210–217.

70. Natkunam Y, Warnke RA, Haghighi B, et al. Co-expression of CD56 and CD30 in lymphomas with primary presentation in the skin: clinicopathologic, immunohistochemical and molecular analyses of seven cases. *J Cutan Pathol* 2000;27:392–399.

71. El Shabrawi-Caelen L, Kerl H, Cerroni L. Lymphomatoid papulosis: reappraisal of clinicopathologic presentation and classification into subtypes A, B, and C. *Arch Dermatol* 2004;140:441–447.

72. Vonderheid EC, Sajjadian A, Kadin ME. Methotrexate is effective therapy for lymphomatoid papulosis and other primary cutaneous CD30-positive lymphoproliferative disorders. *J Am Acad Dermatol* 1996;34:470–481.

73. Hughes PS. Treatment of lymphomatoid papulosis with imiquimod 5% cream. *J Am Acad Dermatol* 2006;54:546–547.

74. Esteve E, Bagot M, Joly P, et al. A prospective study of cutaneous intolerance to topical mechlorethamine therapy in patients with cutaneous T-cell lymphomas. French Study Group of Cutaneous Lymphomas. *Arch Dermatol* 1999;135:1349–1353.

75. Zackheim HS, Epstein EH Jr, Crain WR. Topical carmustine therapy for lymphomatoid papulosis. *Arch Dermatol* 1985;121:1410–1414.

76. Didona B, Benucci R, Amerio P, et al. Primary cutaneous CD30+ T-cell lymphoma responsive to topical imiquimod (Aldara). *Br J Dermatol* 2004;150:1198–1201.

77. Shehan JM, Kalaaji AN, Markovic SN, et al. Management of multifocal primary cutaneous CD30 anaplastic large cell lymphoma. *J Am Acad Dermatol* 2004;51:103–110.

78. Calzavara-Pinton P, Venturini M, Sala R. Medium-dose UVA1 therapy of lymphomatoid papulosis. *J Am Acad Dermatol* 2005;52:530–532.

79. Yagi H, Tokura Y, Furukawa F, et al. Th2 cytokine mRNA expression in primary cutaneous CD30-positive lymphoproliferative disorders: successful treatment with recombinant interferon-gamma. *J Invest Dermatol* 1996;107:827–832.

80. French LE, Shapiro M, Junkins-Hopkins JM, et al. Regression of multifocal, skin-restricted, CD30-positive large T-cell lymphoma with interferon alfa and bexarotene therapy. *J Am Acad Dermatol* 2001;45:914–918.

81. Wu JJ, Guitart J, Tucker RM, et al. Secondary cutaneous anaplastic large cell lymphoma treated with liposomal doxorubicin (Doxil) leading to complete remission. *Int J Dermatol* 2003;42:464–465.

82. Mir SS, Richter BW, Duckett CS. Differential effects of CD30 activation in anaplastic large cell lymphoma and Hodgkin disease cells. *Blood* 2000;96:4307–4312.

83. Duvic M, Kim Y, Reddy S, et al. Phase II preliminary results of SGN-30 (anti-CD30 mAb) in patients with CD30+ lymphoproliferative disorders. *Blood* 2006;108:773a. Abstract 2733.

SECTION V ■ LATE EFFECTS

CHAPTER 31 ■ SECOND TUMORS

ANDREA K. NG, FLORA VAN LEEUWEN, AND PETER M. MAUCH

The incidence of most histologic subtypes of non-Hodgkin lymphoma (NHL) has steadily increased in the last 3 decades, although in recent years, there is evidence of stabilization of the level of increase (1,2). Nevertheless, it is anticipated that the number of survivors of NHL will continue to rise as the cure rate of the disease improves. In a recent population-based study utilizing data from the Surveillance Epidemiology End Results (SEER) program, which collects information on incidence, survival, and prevalence from specific geographic areas representing 26% of the US populations, data on patients with NHL treated between 1990 and 2004 were reported (3). There was a significant improvement in prognosis over time, in part attributed to therapeutic advances, most notably the success of monoclonal antibodies (4,5), and the decrease in the human immunodeficiency virus-related NHL (6,7). The 10-year relative survival was found to increase from 39.4% to 56.3% between 1990 and 1992 and 2002 and 2004. Although there were improvements across all age groups, the improvement was especially notable among patients <45 years of age. The improvement in 10-year relative survival by age group and calendar year is shown in Figure 31.1.

With the increasing number of survivors of NHL, identifying late effects of treatment may have important implications in the long-term follow-up of these patients as well as in determining treatment strategies in newly diagnosed patients. Among the various late effects faced by survivors of cancer, second malignancy represents one of the most serious late events that can have a significant negative impact on their survival and quality of life. Although there are ample data documenting the risk of and risk factors for second malignancy after Hodgkin lymphoma (8–11), the data on second cancer risk after NHL are more limited. This may be related to the heterogeneity of the disease and its treatment, older age at diagnosis, and the less favorable survival rates. In addition, it is also important to recognize that although lymphoma therapy likely contributes to a significant proportion of the excess number of cases of second malignancy, other factors may also be responsible for the observed increased risk. These include shared etiologic factors such as compromised immune function, viral infections, genetic predisposition, and environmental exposures, including pesticides and organic solvents. As in other survivors of cancer, increased surveillance after initial diagnosis and treatment of the lymphoma may lead to an increased report of second cancers.

TYPES OF SECOND MALIGNANCY AFTER NON-HODGKIN LYMPHOMA

Some of the earlier studies on second malignancy after NHL have failed to detect a significantly elevated risk (12–14).

However, these studies mostly consisted of patients treated in an era before effective systemic therapy were available, and they may also be limited by insufficient power and underreporting of cases of second tumors. More recent data have shown an increased risk of various second cancers in patients treated for NHL (15–25). These include myelodysplasia/acute myelogenous leukemia, cancers of the bladder, lungs, and gastrointestinal tract, sarcoma, head and neck cancers, and mesothelioma. Although most of these cancers may be related to prior lymphoma therapy, other cancers frequently reported in survivors of NHL may be related to shared risk factors rather than treatment exposures, including other hematologic malignancies and skin cancers. The following sections summarize the data on the most widely reported types of second malignancy after NHL. It should be noted that the majority of studies that have systemically evaluated second malignancy after NHL are population-based studies using registry data. Although such data sources have the advantage of large patient number, detailed clinical information is often not available. In addition, although initial treatment data are provided, there is

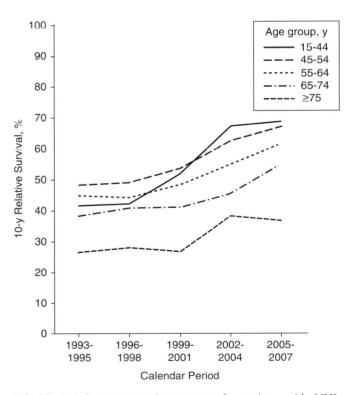

FIGURE 31.1 Improvement in outcomes for patients with NHL from 1993 to 2004. (Adapted from Pulte D, Gondos A, Brenner H. Ongoing improvement in outcomes for patients diagnosed as having non-Hodgkin lymphoma from the 1990s to the early 21st century. *Arch Intern Med* 2008;168:469–476, with permission.)

no information on subsequent therapy or salvage therapy. One major limitation of this type of study is, therefore, the inability to separate out second malignancy risk in patients who are in first remission after initial treatment, versus that in patients who have received additional salvage therapy. However, the second malignancy risk associated with high-dose therapy and stem cell transplantation will be separately discussed in a later section under second malignancy risk following high-dose therapy/bone marrow or stem cell rescue for lymphoma.

Acute Myelogenous Leukemia/Myelodysplasia

An increased risk of acute myelogenous leukemia after treatment for NHL was intially reported in the early 1980s. Greene et al. (26) was among the first to demonstrate a significant relationship between the risk of acute nonlymphocytic leukemia and the doses of radiation to active bone marrow and cyclophosphamide dose in patients treated for NHL, based on nine cases of acute nonlymphycytic leukemia that developed among 517 patients with NHL. It should be noted, however, that this study included patients treated between 1954 and 1975, with the routine use of large-field radiation therapy, including total body irradiation, hemibody irradiation, and total nodal irradiation, and higher cumulative doses of chemotherapy due to maintenance therapy. Another study that may be of historical relevance is a retrospective review of 61 patients with NHL who all received low-dose total body irradiation between 1965 and 1980 as part of primary treatment at the Harvard Joint Center for Radiation Therapy (27). Patients typically received 0.15 Gy twice weekly to a cumulative dose of 1.5 Gy. Three quarters of patients also received local radiation therapy. The estimated median cumulative dose to the active bone marrow, including doses from local radiation therapy, was 5.2 Gy. Forty-one patients (67%) subsequently received salvage alkylating chemotherapy. Five patients developed acute nonlymphocytic leukemia with a mean time from initial lymphoma treatment of 9 years. All five patients had received alkylating chemotherapy as salvage for relapsed lymphoma.

The risk of leukemia after NHL was later explored in a larger, international collaborative case-control study on 11,386 2-year survivors of NHL from three cancer registries treated between 1965 and 1989 (28). Thirty-five patients with NHL who developed acute nonlymphocytic leukemia were identified and matched to 140 control patients. The median time from NHL diagnosis to leukemia was 7.5 years. Detailed information on estimated radiation dose to the bone marrow and doses of individual chemotherapeutic agent were available. On multivariable analysis of the major alkylating agents, a significantly increased risk of acute nonlymphocytic leukemia was observed following treatment with chlorambucil (relative risk [RR] 2.4), prednimustine (RR 13.4), and combination regimens containing both (RR 12.6). In addition, a significant dose-response relationship was demonstrated for prednimustine and chlorambucil. The estimated median radiation dose to active bone marrow and the proportion of bone marrow receiving radiation, however, were not significantly associated with the leukemia risk.

Several more recent population-based studies that included patients with NHL treated in the modern era continued to find a significantly increased risk of leukemia after treatment (17,19,20). Table 31.1 summarizes studies based on registry data that included patients treated after 1990. All but one study showed a significantly elevated RR of acute leukemia, ranging from 1.7 to 8.8. The variation in the estimated risks may reflect differences in treatment from country to country, changes in treatment over time, and types of patients with NHL included in the studies. In the British Cohort Study by Mudie et al. (19), the authors found that the significantly increased RR of leukemia appeared to be limited to the first 10 years after treatment, a finding consistent with that observed in survivors of Hodgkin lymphoma. There was a significant trend of increasing RR of acute leukemia with younger age at treatment. The RR of leukemia among patient ages <45, 45 to 54, and 55 to 59 were 14.4, 8.6, and 6.5, respectively ($p < 0.001$). However, the absolute excess risks increased with increasing age, and were found to be 6.1, 9.0, and 10.8, respectively. With regard to treatment history, the significantly increased risk of leukemia was limited to patients who had received chemotherapy, whereas no leukemia cases were observed in patients who received radiation therapy alone. The RRs of leukemia after chemotherapy alone and after combined modality therapy were 10.5 (95% confidence interval [CI] 5.0 to 19.3) and 13 (95% CI 5.2 to 26.7), respectively. In the study based on SEER data by Tward et al. (20), it was found that the addition of radiation therapy did

---

TABLE 31.1

RECENT POPULATION-BASED STUDIES (INCLUDED PATIENTS TREATED AFTER 1990) REPORTING ON RRS OF LEUKEMIA AFTER NHL

Study	No. of pts with NHL	No. of person-years	Time period	RR of AML/MDS	(95% CI)
Australia (Brennan)	12,352	54,308	1972–1995	Myeloid leukemia: 0.78	(0.28–1.69)
				Other leukemia: 1.26	(0.26–3.67)
Sweden (Dong)	18,960	53,159	1958–1996	Lymphoid leukemia: 4.07	(3.05–5.33)
				Myeloid leukemia: 2.55	(1.65–3.77)
Britain (Mudie)	2,456	18,430	1973–2000	8.8	(5.1–14.1)
US/SEER (Curtis)	73,958	352,695	1973–2000	1.68 ($p < 0.05$)	–
US/SEER (Tward)	77,823	380,505	1973–2001	1.72	(1.51–1.95)

AML/MDS, acute myelogenous leukemia/myelodysplasia; pts, patients.

not further contribute to the subsequent leukemia risk. Among the 55,392 patients who did not receive radiation therapy, and among the 21,111 patients who received radiation therapy, the RRs of leukemia were 1.84 (95% CI 1.58 to 2.12) and 1.52 (95% CI 1.16 to 1.96), respectively.

Several studies have shown an association between treatment with fludarabine in patients with indolent lymphoma and the risk of myelodysplastic syndrome/acute myeloid leukemia. In a study by Tam et al. (29), among 137 patients treated with fludarabine combination regimens, ten patients developed myelodysplastic syndrome/acute myeloid leukemia at a median follow-up of 40 months, including one who had received no other therapy. The crude rate of myelodysplastic syndrome/acute myeloid leukemia was 2.5% for previously untreated patients and 9.3% for pretreated patients ($p = 0.28$). In another study from M. D. Anderson Cancer Center on 202 patients with stage IV indolent lymphoma (30), eight developed myelodysplasia between 1 and 5 years after therapy, including four who received only fludarabine, mitoxantrone, and dexamethasone for six to eight courses, with or without rituximab, followed by interferon α. Sacchi et al. (23) recently reported on the second malignancy risk after treatment for indolent NHL in 563 patients. At a median follow-up of 62 months, 39 patients (6.9%) developed a second malignancy, including 12 with myelodysplastic syndrome/acute myeloid leukemia and 27 with solid tumors. On multivariable analysis, older age at diagnosis, male gender, and fludarabine-containing therapy had a significant negative impact on time free of a second tumor.

There is a recent trend of using dose-escalated chemotherapy in the treatment of aggressive NHL in the hope of further increasing the cure rate of these patients (31–36). In light of the known dose-response relationship between specific types of alkylating agents and the subsequent development of leukemia, it is important to document the potential risks associated with these newer regimens. The Groupe d'Etude des Lymphomes de l'Adulte (GELA) (36) has developed the Adriamycin, cyclophosphamide, vindesine, bleomycin, and prednisone regimen, which consisted of four cycles of Adriamycin 75 mg m^2 day, cyclophosphamide 1,200 mg per m^2, vindesine 2 mg per m^2, and bleomycin 10 mg, followed by two cycles of methotrexate 3,000 mg per m^2, four cycles of ifosfamide 1,500 mg per m^2 and VP-16 300 mg per m^2, and two cycles of cytarabine 100 mg per m^2. Prophylactic intrathecal administration of 15 mg methotrexate was performed during the first four cycles. This regimen was initially designed for patients with advanced-stage disease and subsequently was also tested among patients with early stage disease. In a retrospective analysis of 2,837 patients who have received Adriamycin, cyclophosphamide, vindesine, bleomycin, and prednisone in three consecutive GELA trials, the late toxicities of the treatment, including second malignancy risk, were reported (18). Only 4% of the patient population also received radiation therapy. At a median follow-up of 74 months, 17 cases of acute myelogenous leukemia/myelodysplasia were found with a median time from NHL diagnosis to leukemia of 40 months. Compared with the normal population, the risk of leukemia was significantly increased among both male patients (RR 5.65; $p = 0.006$) and female patients (RR 19.9; $p < 0.001$). The median survival time from acute myelogenous leukemia/myelodysplasia diagnosis was 1 year. Other groups have also developed other dose-

dense and dose intense cyclophosphamide, doxorubicin, vincristine, and prednisone-like regimens for the treatment of aggressive lymphoma with reports of cases of leukemia, although a larger number of patients and longer follow-up time are needed to more clearly elucidate the risks.

In contrast to second malignancies after Hodgkin lymphoma in which solid tumors represent the majority of cases, in survivors of NHL, both leukemia and solid tumors appear to have a similar contribution to the overall risk.

In a British cohort study by Mudie et al. (19), the absolute excess risk of leukemia was 8.2 per 10,000 person-years, whereas that of solid tumor was 6.5 per 10,000 person-years. The types of solid tumors with the most data after NHL include cancers of the bladder, lungs, skin, and gastrointestinal tract. Similar to that observed in survivors of Hodgkin lymphoma, the risk of solid tumors after NHL appears to remain significantly elevated over time. In a population-based study by Travis et al. (37), the RRs of solid tumor at 2 to 4, 5 to 9, 10 to 14, and >15 years were 0.121, 1.28, 1.31, and 1.37, respectively, all of which were significantly elevated compared with the normal population ($p < 0.05$).

Bladder Cancer

The significantly increased risk of bladder cancer after NHL therapy was first reported by Pedersen-Bjergaard et al. (38). In this study, seven cases of bladder carcinomas occurred within a cohort of 471 patients treated for NHLs, with an estimated 8-year cumulative risk of 3.5%. Compared with the normal population, the RR was significantly increased at 6.8 (95% CI 3.2 to 14.2). In an international collaborative effort using registry data, a case-control study was conducted focusing on bladder and kidney cancers after NHL (21). A total of 33 cases of bladder cancer were identified among 6,171 patients with NHL treated between 1965 and 1980. Compared with patients without a history of exposure to cyclophosphamide, treatment with cyclophosphamide was associated with a 4.5-fold increased risk of bladder cancer (95% CI 1.5 to 13.6). In addition, the excess risk of bladder cancer was found to significantly increase with increasing cumulative doses of cyclophosphamide. Although the RR of bladder cancer was nonsignificant at 2.4 among patients who received cumulative doses of cyclophosphamide of <20 g, the RRs were significantly increased, ranging from 6 to 14.5, among patients who received >20 g of cyclophosphamide cumulatively ($p = 0.004$). It is notable that the high RRs of bladder cancer after NHL in both of these studies reflect the historical use of higher cumulative doses of cyclophosphamide, when maintenance therapy was routinely given to patients. In more recent studies, the RRs of bladder cancer continued to remain elevated but to a lesser extent, and some studies failed to detect a significantly increased risk (Table 31.2).

Data on the contribution of radiation therapy to the risk of bladder cancer in patients with NHL are conflicting. In the study by Travis et al. (21), radiation therapy given without cyclophosphamide was associated with a nonsignificant 2.8-fold risk of secondary bladder cancer compared with subjects whose treatment included neither radiation nor cyclophosphamide. A dose-response relationship between radiation and bladder cancer risk was also not apparent within this treatment group ($p = 0.42$). In the SEER study by Tward et al. (20), the patients with NHL were divided into no-radiotherapy

TABLE 31.2

STUDIES REPORTING ON RRS OF BLADDER CANCER AFTER NHL THERAPY

Study	No. of pts with NHL	No. of person-years	Time period	RR of bladder cancer*	(95% CI)
Australia (Brennan)	12,352	54,308	1972–1995	**1.64**	(1.19–2.21)
Sweden (Dong)	18,960	53,159	1958–1996	1.09	(0.85–1.37)
Sweden (Hemminki)	29,134	141,915	1961–2004	**1.43**	(1.2–1.60)
Britain (Mudie)	2,456	18,430	1973–2000	1.6	(0.7–3.2)
Multi-institutional (Travis)	6,171	n.r.	1965–1980	**1.77**	(1.26–2.42)
US/SEER (Travis)	29,153	90,979	1973–1987	**1.3**	(1.02–1.63)
US/SEER (Curtis)	73,958	352,695	1973–2000	**1.33** ($p < 0.05$)	–
US/SEER (Tward)	77,823	380,505	1973–2001	**1.32**	(1.19–1.46)

n.r., not reported; pts, patients.
* Bolded values indicate that they are statistically significantly elevated.

and radiotherapy groups. The RR of bladder cancer was significantly elevated in the no-radiotherapy group (RR 1.38; 95% CI 1.22 to 1.55), whereas a significantly increased risk was not seen in the radiotherapy group (RR 1.2; 95% CI 0.97 to 1.47). Similarly, in the National Cancer Institute monograph by Curtis et al. (22), the RR of bladder cancer was significantly increased in the 52,934 patients who did not receive initial radiotherapy (RR 1.38; $p < 0.05$), but the RR was not significantly increased among the 21,024 patients who received intial radiotherapy (RR 1.21). However, information was not available on the radiation treatment fields, doses, whether chemotherapy was received, and the types and doses of chemotherapy. In contrast, Mudie et al. (19) showed in the British Cohort study that whereas the RR of bladder cancer was not significantly increased among patients who received chemotherapy alone (RR 1.2; 95% CI 0.3 to 3.6), there was a significantly increased RR among patients who received radiation therapy alone (RR 4.5; 95% CI 1.5 to 10.4). However, it was noted that only two of the five patients who subsequently developed bladder cancer in the radiation therapy alone group had received treatment to below the diaphragm.

Age at treatment for NHL appears to affect the subsequent risk of bladder cancer. In the Swedish study by Hemminki et al. (39), the RRs of bladder cancers decreased with increasing age at treatment. The RRs of bladder cancer for patients who were diagnosed at ages 20 to 39, 40 to 49, and 50 to 59 years were significantly elevated at 4.22, 4.06, and 2.39, respectively. Significantly elevated excess risks were not observed in patients who were diagnosed at ages 60 to 69 and ≥70 years (RRs 0.96 and 0.83, respectively). Similarly, whereas the study by Tward et al. (20) showed that patients who received radiation therapy as a whole did not experience a significantly increased risk of bladder cancer, in the subgroup of patients aged 25 to 49 years who received radiation therapy, the RR of bladder cancer was significantly elevated at 2.38 ($p < 0.05$). Older patients in the radiation therapy group, however, did not have an increased risk of bladder cancer.

The risk of bladder cancer after NHL therapy appears to increase with increasing follow-up time. In the National Cancer Institute monograph (22), the RR of bladder cancer after NHL was signicantly increased only for patients who were ≥5 years after treatment. The RRs at <1, 1 to 4, 5 to 9, and ≥10 years out from treatment were 0.92, 1.02, 1.5, and 2.06, respectively.

Lung Cancer

Lung cancer is one of the most common second malignancies found in survivors of Hodgkin lymphoma, with significantly elevated RRs ranging from three to seven (8–10,40–42). In addition, the increased lung cancer risk is generally not observed in the first 5 years after treatment, but the risk remains significantly elevated for at least 20 years after treatment (8,42). For survivors of NHL, several studies have shown a modest increased risk of lung cancer, with most studies reporting a <2-fold increased risk compared witho the normal population (Table 31.3) (15–20,37,39). The variation in the lung cancer risk level may be due to differences in treatment exposures as well as prevalence of tobacco use among patients in the studies.

Chemotherapy has been shown to be a key contributor to the development of lung cancer after lymphoma therapy. For survivors of Hodgkin lymphoma, in an international collaborative study, lung cancer risk was strongly associated with prior exposures to mechlorethemine and procarbazine, and a significant trend of increasing RRs of lung cancer with increasing cumulative doses to either of the two agents was demonstrated (40). Similarly, lung cancer after NHL appears to be linked to not only radiation therapy, but also chemotherapy, specifically, alkylating agent chemotherapy. In the British Cohort study by Mudie et al. (19), approximately half of the study population received chemotherapy alone as initial treatment. Among the 1,274 patients who received chemotherapy alone, the RR of lung cancer was significantly increased at 1.9 (95% CI 1.1 to 3.1). Moreover, the RR of lung cancer was significantly elevated in the subcohort that received cyclophosphamide, doxorubicin, vincristine, and prednisone chemotherapy (RR 2.1; 95% CI 1.1 to 3.7), but not in patients who received chlorambucil (RR 1.1; 95% CI 0.4 to 2.4). Among the 328 patients who received radiation therapy alone, the RR of lung cancer was also significantly increased at 2.3 (95% CI 1.1 to 4.5). The comparable contribution of chemotherapy and radiation therapy to the risk of lung cancer after NHL was confirmed by the SEER study by Tward et al. (20). The risks of lung cancer were similarly significantly elevated among the 55,392 patients who did not receive radiation therapy and the 21,111 patients who received radiation therapy. The RRs were 1.32 (95% CI 1.23

TABLE 31.3

STUDIES REPORTING ON RRS OF LUNG CANCER AFTER NHL THERAPY

Study	No. of pts with NHL	No. of person-years	Time period	RR of lung cancer*	(95% CI)
Australia (Brennan)	12,352	54,308	1972–1995	1.01	(0.8–1.25)
Sweden (Dong)	18,960	53,159	1958–1996	1.08	(0.88–1.32)
GELA (Andre)	2837	n.r.	1984–2000	Male: 2.45	(1.48–3.83)
Sweden (Hemminki)	29,134	141,915	1961–2004	1.49	(1.29–1.72)
Britain (Mudie)	2,456	18,430	1973–2000	1.6	(1.1–2.3)
Multi-institutional (Travis)	6,171	n.r.	1965–1980	1.36	(1.07–1.69)
US/SEER (Travis)	29,153	90,979	1973–1987	1.57	(1.39–1.77)
US/SEER (Curtis)	73,958	352,695	1973–2000	1.32 ($p<0.05$)	–
US/SEER (Tward)	77,823	380,505	1973–2001	1.31	(1.23–1.39)

n.r., not reported; pts, patients.
* Bolded values indicate that they are statistically significantly elevated.

to 1.42) and 1.31 (95% CI 1.16 to 1.46), respectively. The risk of lung cancer after the Adriamycin, cyclophosphamide, vindesine, bleomycin, and prednisone regimen was addressed in the study by Andre et al. (18). In this study, only 4% of patients received radiation therapy. There was a total of 23 cases of lung cancer among the 2,837 patients, including nine cases of squamous cell cancer, eight small cell lung cancers, three adenocarcinomas, one large cell carcinoma, and two cases with unknown histology. The RR of lung cancer was found to be significantly increased among male patients (RR 2.45; 95% CI 1.48 to 3.83), but not among female patients.

The finding of an increased lung cancer risk limited to male survivors of NHL was also noted in the multi-institutional population-based study by Travis et al. (15). Although the overall RR of lung cancer was significantly elevated at 1.36 (95% CI 1.07 to 1.69), the increased risk was restricted to male survivors (RR 1.41; $p <0.05$). A likely explanation for the higher risk of lung cancer among male patients may be related to the higher prevalence of smoking in men. In the GELA study that was conducted between 1984 and 2000, the incidences of smoking in men and women during this period were estimated to be 30% to 47% and 19% to 27% (18), respectively. Another indirect support for an association between smoking and lung cancer risk after NHL therapy is the observed decrease in lung cancer RR in the two SEER studies that encompassed NHL treated from 1973 to 1987 and 1973 to 2001, respectively (20,37). The RR of lung cancer decreased from 1.57 in the earlier study to 1.31 in the more recent study. The authors hypothesized that one of the explanations may be related to the reduced prevalence of smoking in patients treated in the more modern era. The differences in lung cancer risk by gender have also been demonstrated among survivors of Hodgkin lymphoma (8,40).

It is noteworthy that although there is evidence of an association between increased risk of lung cancer after chemotherapy and radiation therapy for NHL, and the potential contribution of smoking to the risk, the dose-effect relationship and the interactive effect between treatment exposures and smoking remain unknown at this time. On the other hand, among survivors of Hodgkin lymphoma, it has been shown that smoking multiplies the RRs of lung cancer associated with exposures to alkylating chemotherapy and radiation therapy (40).

In addition to an increased risk of lung carcinoma, an increased risk of mesothelioma after NHL has also been demostrated. In the population-based studies by Tward (20) and Teta (43) et al., whereas patients who received initial radiation therapy for their NHL, the RR of mesothelioma was significantly increased at 2.26 (95% CI 1.03 to 4.28), although the risk was not increased among patients who did not receive initial radiation therapy. In a subsequent SEER study that included patients diagnosed with NHL through 2003 (43), a significantly elevated risk of mesothelioma limited to patients who received radiation therapy was again confirmed. The mean latency for mesothelioma among patients who received radiation therapy was 16 years. However, data on radiation fields and doses, chemotherapy, and other risks factors such as smoking and asbestos exposures were not available.

GASTROINTESTINAL CANCER

Several studies have demonstrated an elevated risk of specific subtypes of gastrointestinal cancers in survivors of NHL (17,20,39), although others have failed to show an increased risk of cancers of the gastrointestinal tract (16,18,19). Specifically, a significantly increased risk of cancers of the small intestine (17,39), stomach, anus, pancreas (39), and colon (20) has been reported. In most studies, the risk of individual types of gastrointestinal cancers was reported, and the power to detect significant differences from the background risk may have been limited after the subdivisions.

Unlike gastrointestinal cancer after Hodgkin lymphoma, which is likely related to the historical use of extended-field radiation therapy for the disease, the contribution of radiation therapy to the risk of gastrointestinal cancer after NHL is less clear. In the study by Mudie et al. (19), among the entire cohort of 2,456 patients with NHL, significant increases in the RRs for subsequent cancers of the esophagus, stomach, colon, rectum, and pancreas were not observed. However, when the risks were assessed based on treatment exposures, the RR of colorectal cancer was significantly increased among the 1,274 patients treated with chemotherapy alone (12 cases observed, RR 2.1; 95% CI 1.1 to 3.6), whereas the RRs were not significantly increased among the 856 patients who received combined modality therapy (five cases observed, RR 1.5; 95% CI 0.5 to 3.5) or the 328 patients treated with radiation therapy alone (RR 0). As in chemotherapy-related lung cancer from the same study, the increased risk of colorectal cancer after chemotherapy alone was limited to patients treated with cyclophosphamide, doxorubicin, vincristine, and prednisone (RR 2.4; 95% CI 1.1 to 4.3) and not observed among survivors treated with chlorambucil (RR 1.4; 95% CI 0.5 to 3.2). In the population-based study by Tward et al. (20), a significantly increased RR of colon cancer was found only among the 55,392 patients who did not receive radiation therapy (RR 1.14; 95% CI 1.04 to 1.25), but not among the 21,111 patients who received radiation therapy (RR 1.02; 95% CI 0.86 to 1.19). A potential explanation for this finding could be that patients who received radiation therapy may have received less chemotherapy. Also, one key limitation of population-based data is the lack of information on relapses and subsequent salvage therapy. The contribution of salvage therapy for relapses and cumulative treatment exposures to the risk is, therefore, unknown.

BREAST CANCER

In female survivors of Hodgkin lymphoma, a large amount of data is available on risk of breast cancer, which represents the most common second malignancy after Hodgkin lymphoma (8–11,42,44–48). Available data consistently showed that the risks become significantly increased only after at least 5 to 10 years from treatment. In addition, women irradiated at a young age to the chest area are at especially increased risk. In one study of survivors of pediatric Hodgkin lymphoma, the cumulative incidence of breast cancer was estimated to be 20% by the time a patient reaches age 45 (45). Increasing data are also available showing a significant radiation dose-effect, protective effect of treatment-induced ovarian failure, and the modifying effect of other traditional breast cancer risk factors (47,48).

In studies that reported on breast cancer risk after NHL, a significantly reduced risk compared with the general population was found in some of the studies, a finding of which is likely due to therapy related early menopause (16,17,20). In contrast to Hodgkin lymphoma, mediastinal irradiation is not routinely given as part of treatment for NHL. The main exception is in patients with localized mediastinal diffuse large–B-cell lymphoma, which has a tendency to affect young women (49). Although breast cancer risk after mediastinal irradiation for NHL has not been specifically assessed, there are data to suggest that there may be an association between young age at irradiation and breast cancer risk, as has been demonstrated in survivors of Hodgkin lymphoma and childhood malignancies. In the SEER study by Tward et al. (20) on 77,876 patients with NHL, the RR of breast cancer was significantly reduced only among patients who did not receive radiation therapy (RR 0.79; 95% CI 0.71 to 0.88), whereas the risk of breast cancer was no different than expected among women who received radiation therapy (RR 1; 95% CI 0.86 to 1.16). However, on subgroup analysis, women who were age <25 at diagnosis and who had

received radiation therapy, the RR of breast cancer was significantly increased at 5.05 (p <0.05). The RRs were no longer significantly increased in women who were over age 25 at the time of diagnosis and who had received radiation therapy. Presumably, the increased breast cancer risk in the young women was due to radiation therapy to the chest area, although this cannot be confirmed because sites of irradiation are not available in the SEER data. In the Swedish Cancer Registry study by Hemminki et al. (39) on 29,134 patients with NHL, when analyzing breast cancer risk according to age at NHL diagnosis, the RR of breast cancer was significantly increased only among women diagnosed between ages 20 and 39 years (RR 3.29; 95% CI 1.91 to 5.67), and not in older patients. However, data on treatment exposures were not provided. The contribution of radiation therapy to the increase of breast cancer in young women with NHL, therefore, cannot be directly confirmed.

SKIN CANCER

There is substantial evidence of an association between lymphoid malignancies and cutaneous malignancies (melanoma and nonmelanomatous cancer) (50–55). Potential explanations for the relationship include shared etiologies for both malignancies, including sun exposures, chronic immunosuppression, and genetic susceptibility. A case report study described three cases of activation of cutaneous squamous cell carcinoma during treatment with prolonged administration of rituximab (56). The observation of an increased risk of skin cancer in patients with NHL may also be due to increased awareness and heightened surveillance.

In a pooled analysis of published data on the association between melanoma and NHL (50), a total of 137,612 survivors of NHL and 109,532 survivors of melanoma were reviewed. A significantly increased risk of melanoma was found among patients with history of NHL (RR 1.42; 95% CI 1.26 to 1.58). Conversely, the RR of developing NHL among patients with melanoma was also significantly increased (RR 2.01; 95% CI 1.79 to 2.24). In three of the seven included studies, the RR of cutaneous melanoma was higher the first 3 years following the diagnosis of the NHL (17,51,52). When analyzed by gender, the increased risk was higher among males than females.

The increased risk of squamous cell carcinoma in patients with lymphoid malignancies appears to be even more pronounced. A multi-institutional population-based cohort study identified 34,641 patients with NHL treated between 1943 and 1989 from four cancer registries (54). The RR for developing squamous cell skin cancer was 5.5 (95% CI 4.6 to 6.6), and the risks remained elevated over <15 years of follow-up.

Given these findings of a significant association between lymphoma and skin cancers, the well-documented contributing role of ultraviolet radiation to both malignant melanoma and squamous cell skin cancer, as well as the potential systemic immunosuppression caused by ultraviolet radiation (57–59), it is important to encourage sun safety practice in patients with a history of NHL. In addition, regular screening skin examination in these patients should be considered, with low threshold to work up any suspicious skin lesions.

SECOND MALIGNANCY RISK FOLLOWING HIGH-DOSE THERAPY/BONE MARROW OR STEM CELL RESCUE FOR LYMPHOMA

High-dose therapy with bone marrow or stem cell rescue is increasingly used in the treatment of relapsed or refractory lymphoma, and in selected cases, as up-front treatment in high-risk patients. With the growing success of transplant programs and improvement in supportive treatment, the number of patients who survive bone marrow or stem cell transplantation is expected to rise. The risk of acute myeloid leukemia/myelodysplasia after transplant for lymphoma has been well documented, with an estimated risk at 10 years of approximately $\geq$10% (60–64).

Investigators from the University of Nebraska evaluated the cumulative risk of myelodysplasia among 511 patients with Hodgkin lymphoma and NHL who underwent autologous bone marrow or stem cell transplantation (65). A total of 12 cases of myelodysplasia were found. Among the 262 patients with NHL, there were six cases of subsequent myelodysplasia, after a median of 68 months from transplant. The estimated 7-year cumulative incidence was 8%. Risk factors significantly associated with the risk of developing myelodysplasia included age $\geq$40 at the time of transplant and the use of total body irradiation as part of the preparative regimen.

Stone et al. (64) retrospectively reviewed 262 patients who underwent autologous bone marrow transplantation for NHL at the Dana-Farber Cancer Institute. The 6-year actuarial risk of myelodysplasia or acute myeloid leukemia was 18%. Univariable analysis showed that the longer length of time from initial therapy to transplant, extent of prior chemotherapy, and history of pelvic irradiation were significantly associated with an increased risk. On multivariable analysis, independent predictors for development of myelodysplasia were age >38 years and platelet counts of <152,000 per μL at the time of transplant. In an expanded update from the same group (66), which included 552 patients who underwent autologous bone marrow transplantation for NHL, at a median follow-up of 75 months, the 10-year actuarial incidence was 19.8%. On multivariable analysis, a lower median number of cells infused per kilogram at the time of transplant, and history of prior radiation therapy were independent preidictive factors for the development of myelodysplasia. In the most recent update from the group (67), which included 605 patients, at a median follow-up of 9.5 years, the 10-year cumulative incidence was estimated at 11%. Age >44 years at transplant and prior radiation therapy were significantly associated with an increased risk. It is notable that in this update, a cumulative incidence model, which took into account competing events, was used. This may explain the substantially lower estimated risk in this most recent study than those from the two prior studies, which used Kaplan-Meier methods to estimate the actuarial risks, an approach that can lead to overestimation of risk levels.

In a retrospective review by Miller et al. (60), from the University of Minnesota, of 206 patients who underwent autologous bone marrow transplant for NHL or Hodgkin lymphoma, the 5-year cumulative incidence of myelodysplasia was 14.5%.

The use of peripheral blood stem cells was associated with a significantly higher incidence of myelodysplasia than if bone marrow cells were used (31% vs. 10.5%; $p = 0.0035$). However, patients who underwent peripheral stem cell collection may be at higher risk at the time of transplant. Whether stem cell source represents an independent predictor for the risk of development of myelodysplasia remains unclear.

In a study based on data from the European Bone Marrow Transplantation Lymphoma Registry (62), the risks of myelodysplasia/acute myeloid leukemia among 4,998 patients with NHL and Hodgkin lymphoma who underwent transplant between 1978 and 1996 were reviewed. Among the 3,205 patients with NHL, the incidence of myelodysplasia/acute myeloid leukemia at 2, 5, and 10 years was 0.7%, 3%, and 5.7%, respectively. On multivariable analysis, factors significantly associated with an increased risk of subsequent myelodysplasia/acute myeloid leukemia among the patients with NHL were older age at transplant, use of total body irradiation conditioning, higher number of prior transplant, and high-grade histology.

The City of Hope reported on its experience of therapy related leukemia and myelodysplasia following autologous transplantation for lymphoma (61). A total of 612 patients with NHL and Hodgkin lymphoma who underwent bone marrow or stem cell transplant between 1985 and 1998 were reviewed. Among the 394 patients with NHL, the 6-year estimated cumulative probability of developing leukemia or myelodysplasia was 9.1%. None of the following factors was significantly associated with an increased risk of subsequent leukemia or myelodysplasia: age at transplant, source of stem cell, or priming with VP-16 for peripheral stem cell collection. The authors also conducted a nested case-control study combining both patients with Hodgkin and NHL. It was found that VP-16 priming for stem cell mobilization was associated with a 12-fold increased risk of developing acute myeloid leukemia with 11q23/21q22 abnormalities ($p = 0.006$). In addition, among the cohort that had not received VP-16 priming, pretreatment radiation therapy was associated with a 3.2-fold risk of myelodysplasia/acute myeloid leukemia ($p = 0.05$).

Most studies showed that treatment-related myelodysplasia and acute myeloid leukemia are associated with a dismal prognosis, with a median survival of well <1 year. In a study from the Dana-Farber Cancer Institute (66), among the 41 patients who developed myelodysplasia after autologous bone marrow transplantation for NHL, it was found that the International Prognostic Scoring System for myelodysplastic syndrome failed to predict outcome in these patients. Thirteen patients underwent allogeneic bone marrow transplant as treatment for the myelodysplasia; 11 patients died of transplanted-related complications, and two died of relapsed disease, with a median survival of only 1.8 months.

Most of the data on second malignancy risk after high-dose therapy and transplant focused on myelodysplastic syndrome/acute leukemia. Limited data are available on the risk of solid tumor after transplant for NHL. Brown et al. (67), from the Dana-Farber Cancer Institute, reported on the incidence and outcome of solid tumors among 605 patients who underwent autologous bone marrow transplantation for B-cell NHL. All patients received cyclophosphamide and total body irradiation as conditioning. A total of 42 cases of solid tumors were observed at a median follow-up of

9.5 years. A higher than expected number of cases of cancers of the breast, prostate, lungs, gastrointestinal tract, bladder, ovaries, and thyroid, and melanoma and sarcoma were found. Overall, the 10-year cumulative incidence of second malignancy was 21%, and the 10-year cumulative incidence of tumors other than myelodysplasia/acute myeloid leukemia was 10%. The incidence of myelodysplasia/acute myeloid leukemia leveled off at 15 years, whereas all other tumors continued to increase with follow-up time. Older age at the time of transplant ($p \geq 44$ years) was the only significant predictor for the development of both solid tumors and myelodysplasia/acute myeloid leukemia.

CONCLUSIONS

With the increasing success of treatment for patients with NHL and the prolonged life expectancy of patients affected by the disease, there are emerging data on the risk of second malignancy in this population. As lymphoma therapy evolves over time, it is critical to continue efforts of describing the second malignancy risks, as well as to identify factors contributing to the risks. An improved recognition of therapy related second malignancies can allow tailored follow-up of survivors, as well as guide treatment modifications for newly diagnosed patients to minimize exposure to cytoxic agents. The role of early detection and screening for specific second malignancies in survivors of NHL is unknown at this time but should be considered in selected high-risk patients. Examples include routine screening skin examination by a dermatologist, mammography and breast magnetic resonance imaging screening in women who had received chest irradiation at a young age, and chest computed tomography screening for patients who have been exposed to alkylating chemotherapy, chest irradiation, and tobacco. In view of the potential contribution of other nontreatment-related factors to the risks of selected types of second malignancies, survivors of NHL may also benefit from preventative measures, including smoking cessation and avoidance of ultraviolet light exposures.

References

1. Groves FD, Linet MS, Travis LB, et al. Cancer surveillance series: non-Hodgkin's lymphoma incidence by histologic subtype in the United States from 1978 through 1995. *J Natl Cancer Inst* 2000;92:1240–1251.
2. Sandin S, Hjalgrim H, Glimelius B, et al. Incidence of non-Hodgkin's lymphoma in Sweden, Denmark, and Finland from 1960 through 2003: an epidemic that was. *Cancer Epidemiol Biomarkers Prev* 2006;15:1295–1300.
3. Pulte D, Gondos A, Brenner H. Ongoing improvement in outcomes for patients diagnosed as having non-Hodgkin lymphoma from the 1990s to the early 21st century. *Arch Intern Med* 2008;168:469–476.
4. Coiffier B, Lepage E, Briere J, et al. CHOP chemotherapy plus rituximab compared with CHOP alone in elderly patients with diffuse large-B-cell lymphoma. *N Engl J Med* 2002;346:235–242.
5. Pfreundschuh M, Trumper L, Osterborg A, et al. CHOP-like chemotherapy plus rituximab versus CHOP-like chemotherapy alone in young patients with good-prognosis diffuse large-B-cell lymphoma: a randomised controlled trial by the MabThera International Trial (MInT) Group. *Lancet Oncol* 2006;7:379–391.
6. Diamond C, Taylor TH, Im T, et al. Improved survival and chemotherapy response among patients with AIDS-related non-Hodgkin's lymphoma receiving highly active antiretroviral therapy. *Hematol Oncol* 2006;24:139–145.
7. Wolf T, Brodt HR, Fichtlscherer S, et al. Changing incidence and prognostic factors of survival in AIDS-related non-Hodgkin's lymphoma in the era of highly active antiretroviral therapy (HAART). *Leuk Lymphoma* 2005;46:207–215.

8. van Leeuwen FE, Klokman WJ, Veer MB, et al. Long-term risk of second malignancy in survivors of Hodgkin's disease treated during adolescence or young adulthood. *J Clin Oncol* 2000;18:487–497.
9. Swerdlow AJ, Barber JA, Hudson GV, et al. Risk of second malignancy after Hodgkin's disease in a collaborative British cohort: the relation to age at treatment. *J Clin Oncol* 2000;18:498–509.
10. Ng AK, Bernardo MV, Weller E, et al. Second malignancy after Hodgkin disease treated with radiation therapy with or without chemotherapy: long-term risks and risk factors. *Blood* 2002;100:1989–1996.
11. Hodgson DC, Gilbert ES, Dores GM, et al. Long-term solid cancer risk among 5-year survivors of Hodgkin's lymphoma. *J Clin Oncol* 2007;25:1489–1497.
12. MacDougall BK, Weinerman BH, Kemel S. Second malignancies in non-Hodgkin's lymphoma. *Cancer* 1981;48:1299–1301.
13. Zarrabi MH. Association of non-Hodgkin's lymphoma (NHL) and second neoplasms. *Semin Oncol* 1980;7:340–351.
14. Berg JW. The incidence of multiple primary cancers. I. Development of further cancers in patients with lymphomas, leukemias, and myeloma. *J Natl Cancer Inst* 1967;38:741–752.
15. Travis LB, Curtis RE, Boice JD Jr, et al. Second cancers following non-Hodgkin's lymphoma. *Cancer* 1991;67:2002–2009.
16. Brennan P, Coates M, Armstrong B, et al. Second primary neoplasms following non-Hodgkin's lymphoma in New South Wales, Australia. *Br J Cancer* 2000;82:1344–1347.
17. Dong C, Hemminki K. Second primary neoplasms among 53 159 haematolymphoproliferative malignancy patients in Sweden, 1958–1996: a search for common mechanisms. *Br J Cancer* 2001;85:997–1005.
18. Andre M, Mounier N, Leleu X, et al. Second cancers and late toxicities after treatment of aggressive non-Hodgkin lymphoma with the ACVBP regimen: a GELA cohort study on 2837 patients. *Blood* 2004;103:1222–1228.
19. Mudie NY, Swerdlow AJ, Higgins CD, et al. Risk of second malignancy after non-Hodgkin's lymphoma: a British Cohort Study. *J Clin Oncol* 2006;24:1568–1574.
20. Tward JD, Wendland MM, Shrieve DC, et al. The risk of secondary malignancies over 30 years after the treatment of non-Hodgkin lymphoma. *Cancer* 2006;107:108–115.
21. Travis LB, Curtis RE, Glimelius B, et al. Bladder and kidney cancer following cyclophosphamide therapy for non-Hodgkin's lymphoma. *J Natl Cancer Inst* 1995;87:524–530.
22. Curtis R, Freedman D, Ron E, et al. *New Malignancies Among Cancer Survivors: SEER Cancer Registries, 1973–2000.* Bethesda, MD: National Cancer Institute, 2006. NIH Publ. No. 05-5302.
23. Sacchi S, Marcheselli L, Bari A, et al. Secondary malignancies after treatment for indolent non-Hodgkin's lymphoma: a 16-year follow-up study. *Haematologica* 2008;93:398–404.
24. Bluhm EC, Ronckers C, Hayashi RJ, et al. Cause-specific mortality and second cancer incidence after non-Hodgkin lymphoma: a report from the Childhood Cancer Survivor Study. *Blood* 2008;111:4014–4021.
25. Huang KP, Weinstock MA, Clarke CA, et al. Second lymphomas and other malignant neoplasms in patients with mycosis fungoides and Sézary syndrome: evidence from population-based and clinical cohorts. *Arch Dermatol* 2007;143:45–50.
26. Greene MH, Young RC, Merrill JM, et al. Evidence of a treatment dose response in acute nonlymphocytic leukemias which occur after therapy of non-Hodgkin's lymphoma. *Cancer Res* 1983;43:1891–1898.
27. Travis LB, Weeks J, Curtis RE, et al. Leukemia following low-dose total body irradiation and chemotherapy for non-Hodgkin's lymphoma. *J Clin Oncol* 1996;14:565–571.
28. Travis LB, Curtis RE, Stovall M, et al. Risk of leukemia following treatment for non-Hodgkin's lymphoma. *J Natl Cancer Inst* 1994;86:1450–1457.
29. Tam CS, Seymour JF, Prince HM, et al. Treatment-related myelodysplasia following fludarabine combination chemotherapy. *Haematologica* 2006;91:1546–1550.
30. McLaughlin P, Estey E, Glassman A, et al. Myelodysplasia and acute myeloid leukemia following therapy for indolent lymphoma with fludarabine, mitoxantrone, and dexamethasone (FND) plus rituximab and interferon alpha. *Blood* 2005;105:4573–4575.
31. Trumper L, Zwick C, Ziepert M, et al. Dose-escalated CHOEP for the treatment of young patients with aggressive non-Hodgkin's lymphoma: I. A randomized dose escalation and feasibility study with bi- and tri-weekly regimens. *Ann Oncol* 2008;19:538–544.
32. Pfreundschuh M, Zwick C, Zeynalova S, et al. Dose-escalated CHOEP for the treatment of young patients with aggressive non-Hodgkin's lymphoma: II. Results of the randomized high-CHOEP trial of the German High-Grade Non-Hodgkin's Lymphoma Study Group (DSHNHL). *Ann Oncol* 2008;19:545–552.
33. Pfreundschuh M, Trumper L, Kloess M, et al. Two-weekly or 3-weekly CHOP chemotherapy with or without etoposide for the treatment of elderly patients with aggressive lymphomas: results of the NHL-B2 trial of the DSHNHL. *Blood* 2004;104:634–641.
34. Pfreundschuh M, Trumper L, Kloess M, et al. Two-weekly or 3-weekly CHOP chemotherapy with or without etoposide for the treatment of young patients with good-prognosis (normal LDH) aggressive lymphomas: results of the NHL-B1 trial of the DSHNHL. *Blood* 2004;104:626–633.

35. Reyes F, Lepage E, Ganem G, et al. ACVBP versus CHOP plus radiotherapy for localized aggressive lymphoma. *N Engl J Med* 2005;352:1197–1205.
36. Tilly H, Lepage E, Coiffier B, et al. Intensive conventional chemotherapy (ACVBP regimen) compared with standard CHOP for poor-prognosis aggressive non-Hodgkin lymphoma. *Blood* 2003;102:4284–4289.
37. Travis LB, Curtis RE, Glimelius B, et al. Second cancers among long-term survivors of non-Hodgkin's lymphoma. *J Natl Cancer Inst* 1993;85:1932–1937.
38. Pedersen-Bjergaard J, Ersboll J, Hansen VL, et al. Carcinoma of the urinary bladder after treatment with cyclophosphamide for non-Hodgkin's lymphoma. *N Engl J Med* 1988;318:1028–1032.
39. Hemminki K, Lenner P, Sundquist J, et al. Risk of subsequent solid tumors after non-Hodgkin's lymphoma: effect of diagnostic age and time since diagnosis. *J Clin Oncol* 2008;26:1850–1857.
40. Travis LB, Gospodarowicz M, Curtis RE, et al. Lung cancer following chemotherapy and radiotherapy for Hodgkin's disease. *J Natl Cancer Inst* 2002;94:182–192.
41. Swerdlow AJ, Schoemaker MJ, Allerton R, et al. Lung cancer after Hodgkin's disease: a nested case-control study of the relation to treatment. *J Clin Oncol* 2001;19:1610–1618.
42. Dores GM, Metayer C, Curtis RE, et al. Second malignant neoplasms among long-term survivors of Hodgkin's disease: a population-based evaluation over 25 years. *J Clin Oncol* 2002;20:3484–3494.
43. Teta MJ, Lau E, Sceurman BK, et al. Therapeutic radiation for lymphoma: risk of malignant mesothelioma. *Cancer* 2007;109:1432–1438.
44. Aisenberg AC, Finkelstein DM, Doppke KP, et al. High risk of breast carcinoma after irradiation of young women with Hodgkin's disease. *Cancer* 1997;79:1203–1210.
45. Bhatia S, Yasui Y, Robison LL, et al. High risk of subsequent neoplasms continues with extended follow-up of childhood Hodgkin's disease: report from the Late Effects Study Group. *J Clin Oncol* 2003;21:4386–4394.
46. Travis LB, Hill D, Dores GM, et al. Cumulative absolute breast cancer risk for young women treated for Hodgkin lymphoma. *J Natl Cancer Inst* 2005;97:1428–1437.
47. Travis LB, Hill DA, Dores GM, et al. Breast cancer following radiotherapy and chemotherapy among young women with Hodgkin disease. *JAMA* 2003;290:465–475.
48. van Leeuwen FE, Klokman WJ, Stovall M, et al. Roles of radiation dose, chemotherapy, and hormonal factors in breast cancer following Hodgkin's disease. *J Natl Cancer Inst* 2003;95:971–980.
49. van Besien K, Kelta M, Bahaguna P. Primary mediastinal B-cell lymphoma: a review of pathology and management. *J Clin Oncol* 2001;19:1855–1864.
50. Lens MB, Newton-Bishop JA. An association between cutaneous melanoma and non-Hodgkin's lymphoma: pooled analysis of published data with a review. *Ann Oncol* 2005;16:460–465.
51. Goggins WB, Finkelstein DM, Tsao H. Evidence for an association between cutaneous melanoma and non-Hodgkin lymphoma. *Cancer* 2001;91:874–880.
52. McKenna DB, Stockton D, Brewster DH, et al. Evidence for an association between cutaneous malignant melanoma and lymphoid malignancy: a population-based retrospective cohort study in Scotland. *Br J Cancer* 2003;88:74–78.
53. Hemminki K, Jiang Y, Steineck G. Skin cancer and non-Hodgkin's lymphoma as second malignancies. Markers of impaired immune function? *Eur J Cancer* 2003;39:223–229.
54. Adami J, Frisch M, Yuen J, et al. Evidence of an association between non-Hodgkin's lymphoma and skin cancer. *BMJ* 1995;310:1491–1495.
55. Levi F, Randimbison L, Te VC, et al. Non-Hodgkin's lymphomas, chronic lymphocytic leukaemias and skin cancers. *Br J Cancer* 1996;74:1847–1850.
56. Fogarty GB, Bayne M, Bedford P, et al. Three cases of activation of cutaneous squamous-cell carcinoma during treatment with prolonged administration of rituximab. *Clin Oncol (R Coll Radiol)* 2006;18:155–156.
57. Kripke ML. Effects of UV radiation on tumor immunity. *J Natl Cancer Inst* 1990;82:1392–1396.
58. Hersey P, Bradley M, Hasic E, et al. Immunological effects of solarium exposure. *Lancet* 1983;1:545–548.
59. Hersey P, Haran G, Hasic E, et al. Alteration of T cell subsets and induction of suppressor T cell activity in normal subjects after exposure to sunlight. *J Immunol* 1983;131:171–174.
60. Miller JS, Arthur DC, Litz CE, et al. Myelodysplastic syndrome after autologous bone marrow transplantation: an additional late complication of curative cancer therapy. *Blood* 1994;83:3780–3786.
61. Krishnan A, Bhatia S, Slovak ML, et al. Predictors of therapy-related leukemia and myelodysplasia following autologous transplantation for lymphoma: an assessment of risk factors. *Blood* 2000;95:1588–1593.
62. Milligan DW, Ruiz De Elvira MC, Kolb HJ, et al. Secondary leukaemia and myelodysplasia after autografting for lymphoma: results from the EBMT. EBMT Lymphoma and Late Effects Working Parties. European Group for Blood and Marrow Transplantation. *Br J Haematol* 1999;106:1020–1026.
63. Forrest DL, Nevill TJ, Naiman SC, et al. Second malignancy following high-dose therapy and autologous stem cell transplantation: incidence and risk factor analysis. *Bone Marrow Transplant* 2003;32:915–923.
64. Stone RM, Neuberg D, Soiffer R, et al. Myelodysplastic syndrome as a late complication following autologous bone marrow transplantation for non-Hodgkin's lymphoma. *J Clin Oncol* 1994;12:2535–2542.
65. Darrington DL, Vose JM, Anderson JR, et al. Incidence and characterization of secondary myelodysplastic syndrome and acute myelogenous leukemia following high-dose chemoradiotherapy and autologous stem-cell transplantation for lymphoid malignancies. *J Clin Oncol* 1994;12:2527–2534.
66. Friedberg JW, Neuberg D, Stone RM, et al. Outcome in patients with myelodysplastic syndrome after autologous bone marrow transplantation for non-Hodgkin's lymphoma. *J Clin Oncol* 1999;17:3128–3135.
67. Brown JR, Yeckes H, Friedberg JW, et al. Increasing incidence of late second malignancies after conditioning with cyclophosphamide and total-body irradiation and autologous bone marrow transplantation for non-Hodgkin's lymphoma. *J Clin Oncol* 2005;23:2208–2214.

CHAPTER 32 ■ LATE EFFECTS OF TREATMENT AFTER LYMPHOMA

MARC P. E. ANDRÉ

Because of the increasing incidence of non-Hodgkin lymphoma over the past 2 decades and improvements in curing this disease, long-term survivors should be observed for late toxicities. The relative contribution of the treatment modalities to the development of these toxicities may be approached in an attempt to improve the quality of life of long-term survivors. Second cancer is the most devastating toxicity of treatments and is reviewed in the previous chapter of this book. This chapter is dedicated to nonneoplastic toxicities. Whether these events can be addressed as complications of treatments in all cases remains unclear. Long-term follow-up of survivors of cancer and careful review of late effects are of major importance. Retrospective studies on this topic have described an incidence of late nonneoplastic toxicities ranging from 5% to 46% (1,2). Late effects reviewed in this section include toxicities that occurred after treatment was completed, as well as toxicities that occurred during therapy and continued after therapy was completed.

CARDIAC TOXICITY

For frequently used chemotherapy, such as anthracyclines, the risk of acute cardiovascular toxicity has been extensively evaluated and is well known (Table 32.1) (3). Data on long-term effects on survivors of childhood cancer treated with anthracycline-based chemotherapy regimens or of survivors of Hodgkin lymphoma treated with radiotherapy (4) have revealed that cardiovascular damage can manifest many years after the end of treatment (5). Today, the evaluation of long-term cardiovascular complications is of growing importance for adults and also for elderly patients who might expect cure with the currently available treatments. The study of long-term cardiac complications in the population between 40 and 60 years of age is more complicated because the risk of cardiovascular disease increases above the age of 50 years. Therefore, it is more difficult to establish whether the cardiovascular morbidity occurring during the follow-up period is the result of chemotherapy or the consequence of aging. Compared with the multitude of studies on long-term consequences of treatments in survivors of Hodgkin lymphoma, the literature on survivors of non-Hodgkin lymphoma is limited.

Radiation-Associated Cardiac Toxicity

Most of the data in the literature on radiotherapy late effects come from observation of survivors of Hodgkin lymphoma, most of whom received mediastinal irradiation. Pericarditis was an important complication in the 1960s and 1970s, but this complication has virtually vanished with new treatment approaches.

An association between coronary artery disease and irradiation was first reported in the late 1960s (6). The association between age at treatment and dose of radiotherapy in relation to risk remains uncertain, and conflicting results are reported in the literature (7,8) depending on treatment techniques, use of chemotherapy, and duration of observation.

So far, there is no evidence of a synergy between radiotherapy and chemotherapy; the combination increases neither the coronary risk associated with radiotherapy nor the chronic heart failure associated with chemotherapy. Although an additive risk of anthracyclines and radiotherapy on cardiac risk is suggested, the difference with radiotherapy alone did not reach statistical significance in several studies (9).

Chemotherapy Associated Cardiac Toxicity

For patients with advanced intermediate-grade or high-grade lymphoma, the cyclophosphamide, doxorubicin, vincristine, and prednisone (CHOP) regimen is considered the standard treatment and has been shown to improve the cure rate when combined with rituximab (10,11). However, various other standard or high-dose chemotherapy regimens are used after relapse or progression and might contain drugs with potential cardiac toxic effects, such as high-dose ifosfamide, paclitaxel, or vinca alkaloids.

Acute Cardiovascular Toxicity

Myocardial Toxicity. Although the initial anthracycline-induced damage to the myocyte occurs shortly after its administration, overt heart failure presents weeks, months, or years after chemotherapy. Acute cardiotoxic effects that can occur during or shortly (i.e., within hours) after administration of anthracyclines include electrocardiographic changes and rhythm disturbances (12). These changes appear to be of minor clinical relevance because they rarely happen with current treatment regimens and do not predict chronic cardiac toxicity (13). A long-term evaluation of cardiac function in children born from a mother who received anthracyclines during pregnancy did not show any clinically or echocardiogram evidence of late cardiac toxicity (14).

The other agent that can cause acute cardiotoxicity is cyclophosphamide, which is mainly cardiotoxic at higher doses, such as those used before stem cell transplantation. The reported

TABLE 32.1

CARDIAC TOXICITIES ASSOCIATED WITH THE TREATMENT OF LYMPHOMA

Type of treatment	Effects	References
Radiotherapy	Increases coronary risk	4
Chemotherapy	Acute	
	Myocardiotoxicity (anthracycline)	13–16,18,19
	Cardiovascular (vinca alkaloids)	20,21
	Other vascular effects (bleomycin)	22
	Late	
	Myocardiotoxicity	25–27
	Coronary vasculature	28,29
	Pulmonary vasculature	30
Interferon	Hypotension, arrhythmia, myocardial infarction, congestive cardiomyopathy	31–35
High-dose chemotherapy	Acute cardiomyopathy related to cyclophosphamide	36–37
	Late cardiomyopathy: infrequent	27

cardiotoxicity ranges from transient electrocardiographic changes to more severe cardiotoxicity, such as exudative pericardial effusion, ventricular hypertrophy, and fatal myocardial necrosis (15,16). The onset of the latter type of cardiac toxicity is acute, with death within 15 days. The cardiotoxic effect of cyclophosphamide may be potentiated by anthracycline administration (17). In 2000, Brockstein et al. (18) evaluated the risk factors in patients receiving high-dose cyclophosphamide before stem cell transplantation. In this series of 138 patients, a multivariate analysis showed that lymphoma (as opposed to breast cancer) and older age were the risk factors associated with cardiac toxicity. History of an abnormal ejection fraction and higher doses of anthracyclines before high-dose chemotherapy may also contribute to the cardiac toxicity (18). The authors concluded that patients who are seemingly poor cardiac risks may fare well with high-dose chemotherapy if carefully selected with the aid of a thorough cardiac evaluation. High-dose cyclophosphamide results in very acute cardiac toxicity characterized by cardiac dilatation in patients with non-Hodgkin lymphoma. This toxicity can be detected with elevated concentrations of natriuretic peptides, which are more sensitive than echocardiography or magnetic resonance imaging (19).

Another agent that can cause cardiac toxicity is high-dose ifosfamide. In one study, cardiac arrhythmias were observed (20). In another study by Quezado et al. (21) in 1993, high-dose ifosfamide was associated with severe but usually reversible myocardial depression and malignant arrhythmias. Given the close chemical resemblance between cyclophosphamide and ifosfamide, it is possible that they induce myocardial depression through a similar mechanism, even if no histopathologic evidence of hemorrhagic myocarditis, the hallmark of cyclophosphamide cardiomyopathy, could be found (22).

Although high-dose cyclophosphamide or ifosfamide is often used in the setting of autologous stem cell transplantation, cardiac toxicity is infrequent. Hertenstein et al. (23) reported an occurrence of <2%. Occurrence of cardiac toxicity was correlated with an echographic reduction in ejection fraction before bone marrow transplantation, but life-threatening cardiac toxicity could not be predicted in individual patients (23).

Other drugs, such as paclitaxel, may be associated with cardiac toxicity. One study of 60 patients treated with a 3-hour infusion of 200 mg per m^2 did not show any significant cardiac toxicity (24).

Cardiovascular Events. Although rare, patients have been described who developed acute myocardial infarction during or after chemotherapy for lymphomas (25,26). In these reports, the cause of these events was attributed to the administration of vinca alkaloids. The mechanism by which chemotherapy, specifically vinca alkaloids, could cause myocardial infarction remains speculative (26).

Other Vascular Events. There are at least two manifestations of acute vascular toxicity associated with chemotherapy for lymphomas. Bleomycin-containing regimens may induce pneumonitis, which is thought to be a result of damage to endothelium of the lung vasculature. Another manifestation of acute vascular toxicity may be the thromboembolic events that occur during chemotherapy. Clarke et al. (27) evaluated 85 patients with non-Hodgkin lymphoma and found thromboembolic events in four of 11 patients who received weekly chemotherapy; this was not the case in patients treated with a less-intensive schedule.

Late Cardiovascular Toxicity

Myocardial Toxicity. Of the agents used in the treatment for non-Hodgkin lymphoma, anthracyclines are the most important in causing direct injury to the heart. The exact mechanism of how anthracyclines affect the myocardium is not fully elucidated, but the formation of free radicals and calcium overload in the myocytes play an important role (28). These processes lead to patchy myocyte damage, leading to intramyocyte vacuolization and eventually myocyte death. As a consequence, cardiomyopathy develops, which can result in congestive heart failure (29). However, because the heart has considerable compensatory reserves, a long time elapses before heart failure manifests, if it does at all. The majority of chronic heart failure occurs within 1 year, and cardiotoxicity increases with the cumulative dose given; however, wide interindividual susceptibility exists. In survivors of childhood cancer, incidences of subclinical cardiotoxicity have been reported to increase with the extent of follow-up duration. These figures cannot be reliably extrapolated to adults, but they illustrate that the risk of chronic heart failure continues long after the completion of treatment. In a recent study on cardiac toxicity in elderly patients with diffuse B-cell non-Hodgkin lymphoma, Hershman et al. (30) showed that patients with prior heart disease were less likely than others to be treated with doxorubicin, and those who received doxorubicin were more likely than others to develop congestive heart failure (29% increase). Various cardiac risk factors increased congestive heart failure risk, but only hypertension was synergistic with doxorubicin, suggesting that some subgroups may benefit from efforts to reduce doxorubicin-related congestive heart failure risk (30). Hypertension, together with smoking and age >50, was also retrieved as a risk factor for cardiovascular disease in another study (1).

In the study by Miller et al. (31) in 1998, left ventricular dysfunction was found in seven of 201 patients treated with eight cycles of CHOP (cumulative dose of doxorubicin, 400 mg per m^2), whereas in the group treated with three cycles combined with radiotherapy, none of the 200 patients developed left ventricular dysfunction. Seven patients treated with eight cycles of CHOP and only two patients treated with three cycles of CHOP and radiotherapy subsequently died of heart disease. In the study by Haddy et al. (32) in 1998, 103 young long-term survivors were observed up to 20 years with a median time to cardiac evaluation of 9.9 years. Left ventricular dysfunction was detected in eight (14%) of 57 patients who had received cumulative doses of doxorubicin of 200 to 560 mg per m^2. Four were symptomatic, of whom two needed cardiac medication, and four were asymptomatic. Cardiac toxicity was the predominant major late effect observed in this series (32).

Although high-dose cyclophosphamide can cause acute cardiotoxicity, late toxicity in the 1st year after stem cell transplantation seems exceptional, as was recently described by Ghielmini et al. (33). However, longer follow-up is needed to exclude long-term cardiotoxicity with certainty.

Coronary Vasculature. Mediastinal irradiation is known to affect coronary arteries, but different large series were unable to find an association between chemotherapy and death from myocardial infarction, suggesting that chemotherapy alone was not directly affecting coronary artery disease (34,35). However, because cardiac death was not an end point in these trials, risk of coronary artery disease might be underestimated and, therefore, not detected.

Pulmonary Vasculature. Several cases of pulmonary venoocclusive disease have been described after chemotherapy for lymphoma. Although the number of cases is limited in the literature, this might be due to the failure to recognize this complication (36).

Interferon-Associated Cardiac Toxicity

In clinical trials, interferon has demonstrated activity in the treatment of several tumors, including follicular lymphoma (37). Adverse cardiovascular effects due to interferon have been reported infrequently, and consist mainly of transient hypotension and tachyarrhythmias that are commonly associated with the initial febrile reaction. More severe adverse cardiac events, including arrhythmia and myocardial infarction, have been reported (38,39). The etiologic role of interferon-α in the development of these adverse cardiac events, however,

cannot be firmly established due to the presence of preexisting heart disease or significant previous doxorubicin exposure. The development of congestive cardiomyopathy has also been infrequently described in patients receiving interferon-α (40,41). The cardiomyopathy occurred while receiving interferon and subsequently improved on discontinuation of interferon. The mechanism for the development of this cardiomyopathy remains unclear. In a randomized trial comparing an anthracycline-based chemotherapy with and without interferon, Solal-Celigny et al. (37) did not report any significant increase in cardiac toxicity among patients with follicular lymphoma.

High-Dose Chemotherapy Associated Cardiac Toxicity

Cardiac toxicity associated with high-dose chemotherapy and stem cell transplantation has been reported in different series (42–44). In two series, 12% of patients died of cardiac or pulmonary toxicities. Cardiac toxicity is clearly related to the high dose of cyclophosphamide as used in the carmustine (BCNU) (300 mg per m^2), VP16 (800 mg per m^2), cytarabine (800 mg per m^2), and cyclophosphamide (140 mg per kg) regimen, and has not been reported to be significant when cyclophosphamide is replaced by melphalan, such as in the BCNU (300 mg per m^2), VP16 (800 mg per m^2), cytarabine (800 mg per m^2), and melphalan (140 mg per m^2) regimen. In the series by Rapoport et al. (43) in 1993, toxicity appeared to be related to the bulk of disease at time of transplant, but for van Besien et al. (42) in 1995, cyclophosphamide-associated cardiac toxicity was unpredictable. It was not related to pretreatment left ventricular ejection fraction or any other pretreatment factors. Cardiac toxicity has been reported most frequently when cyclophosphamide was combined either with BCNU or cytarabine. BCNU can lead to intracellular glutathione depletion and, therefore, enhance cardiac toxicity (45). In addition, high-dose nitrosoureas can cause myocardial ischemia, hypotension, tachycardia, myocardial infarction, and even non-Q-wave infarction (46). It is also possible that high-dose cytarabine contributes to the cardiac toxicity of the BCNU (300 mg per m^2), VP16 (800 mg per m^2), cytarabine (800 mg per m^2), and cyclophosphamide (140 mg per kg) regimen, as suggested by the absence of cardiac toxicity in patients with Hodgkin lymphoma treated with cyclophosphamide, BCNU, and etoposide.

Association of High-Dose Chemotherapy and Radiotherapy

A study from Memorial Sloan-Kettering Cancer Center on 164 patients with relapsed/refractory diffuse large B-cell lymphoma treated with short-course, involved-field radiotherapy before high-dose chemotherapy and stem cell transplantation showed minimal treatment-related mortality and morbidity (47). In another study on 29 patients with relapsed B-cell lymphoma treated with iodine-131-labelled anti-CD20 antibody and autologous stem cell rescue, no significant late cardiopulmonary toxicities were observed (48).

Reducing the Risk

Studies evaluating the extent of cardiac toxicity have used various combinations of rest and exercise echocardiography and radionuclide scintigraphy scanning. However, it has become evident that chemotherapy induced left ventricular dysfunction often occurs without symptoms and that new tools to identify higher-risk patients needing close monitoring or cardiologic treatment are needed. In 2000, Cardinale et al. (49) reported a series of 204 patients treated with high-dose chemotherapy for various tumors, including 46 lymphomas. Cardiac troponin, a new specific marker of minor myocardial damage, was measured shortly after high-dose chemotherapy. In the troponin-negative group, left ventricular ejection fraction progressively decreased after the treatment, but this was transient and no longer detectable after later follow-up. In the troponin-positive group, left ventricular ejection depression was more marked and still evident at the end of follow-up. In this group, a close relationship between the short-term troponin increment and the greatest left ventricular ejection fraction reduction was found. All three patients developing symptoms of heart failure and needing treatment were in this group.

In general, efforts should be aimed at reducing all risk factors after treatments of patients with lymphoma to reduce potentially fatal cardiac complications. Cessation of cigarette smoking and optimal management of hypertension, lipids, and diabetes are absolutely mandatory.

PULMONARY TOXICITY

Development of pulmonary complications in patients with lymphoma is frequent and nonspecific (Table 32.2). Patients with lung damage frequently receive empirical antibiotics and frequently invasive diagnostic procedures to rule out infection before lung toxicity is suspected. In this context, cytomegalovirus pneumopathy should be carefully excluded because its incidence seems to be rising, possibly reflecting the use of more immunosuppressive agents such as fludarabine, rituximab, and alemtuzumab in the treatment of lymphoma (50).

Both radiotherapy, including total body irradiation used before autologous stem cell transplantation, and chemotherapeutic agents (mainly bleomycin, methotrexate, BCNU, and cyclophosphamide) may induce short- and long-term pulmonary toxicity. Because most patients receive combination chemotherapy, additional or synergistic effects may overlap and make the relative contribution of each different toxic effect difficult to evaluate. The toxic effects of both radiotherapy and mainly bleomycin have been the subject of many publications on Hodgkin lymphoma because of the use of the doxorubicin (Adriamycin), bleomycin, vinblastine, and dacarbazine (ABVD) regimen and long-term follow-up of many survivors (51–53). Although not demonstrated, it can be speculated that most of the information obtained in Hodgkin lymphoma might be translated to non-Hodgkin lymphoma.

Radiotherapy

Two successive phases of lung damage may occur after radiation therapy of the chest. The first phase is a radiation pneumonitis developing usually within the first 6 months of the radiotherapy and can cause radiographic changes. The second phase is the progressive development of fibrosis that occurs in the field of radiation therapy. Recent data suggest an activation of inflammatory reaction, mainly transforming growth factor-β and interleukin-1α, leading to the expression of a cytokine cascade and an overexpression of collagen genes (54). Actually, combination chemotherapy with or without radiotherapy is used because of reported inferior results with radiation alone in patients with clinically staged disease (55,56). In 1996, Lee and Levitt (57) reported a small series of patients with stage I large cell non-Hodgkin lymphoma treated exclusively with radiotherapy and did not report any significant lung toxicity. However, this treatment modality remains infrequently used, and most lung toxicity occurs after combination therapy, leading to difficulty in estimating the contribution of radiotherapy to this toxic effect.

Chemotherapy

It is quite well recognized that at a cumulative dose of approximately 400 to 450 mg of bleomycin, the incidence of pulmonary toxicity (e.g., interstitial chronic fibrosis) increases dramatically, reaching approximately 13%. However, the relationship between dose and toxicity is unclear, and severe interstitial pulmonary fibrosis (Fig. 32.1) has been shown to develop with cumulative doses of <50 mg in sensitive patients. Most patients with acute pulmonary damage associated with bleomycin respond favorably to steroids (58). There are recent

TABLE 32.2		
PULMONARY TOXICITIES ASSOCIATED WITH THE TREATMENT OF LYMPHOMA		
Type of treatment	Effects	References
Radiotherapy	Radiation pneumonitis	46–49
	Progressive fibrosis	
Chemotheraphy	Bleomycin toxicity	50
	Methotrexate toxicity	51–52
	Granulocyte colony-stimulating factor: poor evidence of association	53–59
High-dose chemotherapy	BCNU toxicity	63–64
	BCNU + cyclophosphamide toxicity	65–68

BCNU, carmusline.

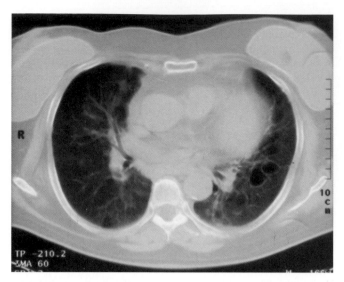

FIGURE 32.1 Bleomycin pulmonary toxicity in a 62-year-old patient treated with bleomycin-containing chemotherapy for lymphoma.

data showing the utility of 18-fluoro-deoxyglucose-positron emission tomography as a diagnostic tool and as an indicator of the resolution of bleomycin-induced lung toxicity, even in the presence of residual pulmonary scarring on computed tomography scan (59).

Methotrexate pneumonitis has been described in patients with hematologic and solid tumors. The pathogenesis of the pulmonary injury related to methotrexate is not identified, although some features, such as peripheral eosinophilia, suggest an immune-mediated hypersensitivity mechanism. It is interesting to note that methotrexate-leucovorin, doxorubicin, cyclophosphamide, vincristine, prednisone, and bleomycin (MACOP-B), which contains the same component drugs as methotrexate, bleomycin, doxorubicin, cyclophosphamide, vincristine, and dexamethasone (m-BACOD), has no reported pulmonary toxicity (60). These regimens differ in several ways, including the dosage and schedule of the component drugs and the use of steroids. High doses of steroids are administered throughout the MACOP-B treatment course, and the immunosuppressive and antiinflammatory properties of steroids may suppress methotrexate pneumonitis; short intermittent courses of steroids, such as in m-BACOD, may promote its development. Shapiro et al. (61) compared three different chemotherapy regimens (m-BACOD, methotrexate, calcium, leucovorin, doxorubicin, cyclophosphamide, vincristine, and dexamethasone, and CHOP) containing the same drugs but differing primarily in the addition of bleomycin and methotrexate. Pulmonary toxicity occurred in 24 of 134 (18%) of the patients treated with m-BACOD and in six of 43 (14%) of the patients treated with methotrexate, calcium, leucovorin, doxorubicin, cyclophosphamide, vincristine, and dexamethasone ($p = $ not significant). None of the patients treated with CHOP had pulmonary toxicity. This suggested that methotrexate may play an important role in the pathogenesis of pulmonary toxicity (61).

Some patients have developed pulmonary toxicity after receiving chemotherapy and granulocyte colony-stimulating factor (G-CSF) (62–65). The G-CSF increases the number and functional properties, such as superoxide production and expression of adhesion-related molecules, of neutrophils. Therefore, it might be speculated that G-CSF has a causal

association with the pulmonary toxicity. However, there is no full consensus that G-CSF is involved in the development of pulmonary toxicity (66,67). In one series, Yokose et al. (68) in 1998 retrospectively compared CHOP and CHOP with G-CSF. They reported six patients with pulmonary toxicity out of 52 patients (11.5%) in the G-CSF group and none in the CHOP-alone group. The mean peak leukocyte count with each therapy cycle was associated with the development of this toxicity. Because the toxicity was associated with a high mean peak leukocyte count and did not recur in readministration of G-CSF, an idiosyncratic reaction to G-CSF is unlikely to be the pathogenesis of this phenomenon. Early use of steroids and lowering the dose of G-CSF seem to be useful in the management of this toxicity. However, the probability of an increase of bleomycin-induced toxicity by G-CSF remains controversial and questionable. Two randomized Groupe d'Etude des Lymphomes de l'Adulte trials comparing placebo versus G-CSF after bleomycin-containing chemotherapy did not observe any increase in pulmonary toxicity in 278 patients (66).

Rituximab-Induced Interstitial Lung Disease

Recent publications have reported the occurrence of interstitial pneumonitis in patients receiving rituximab-containing chemotherapy, mostly rituximab with CHOP (R-CHOP). The pathogenesis is largely unknown. A potential explanation may include the induction and release of cytotoxic substances after the binding between CD20 and B cells (cytokines and complement activation). Therapy included corticosteroids, and the prognosis has been variable (69,70).

High-Dose Chemotherapy Associated Pulmonary Toxicity

The major risk factor for serious pulmonary toxicity is previous radiation therapy or prior treatment with bleomycin, as indicated by different studies (42,43,68,71–73). Mild delayed drug toxicity related to BCNU, cyclophosphamide, or previous radiotherapy might be responsive to treatment with steroids.

Drug-induced lung injury has been associated with the use of several alkylating agent-based high-dose chemotherapy regimens but is particularly problematic when high-dose BCNU is administered in combination with multiple alkylating agents. In the dose-finding series of Wheeler et al. (74) in 1990, it was reported that a BCNU dose escalation to 600 mg per m^2 was associated with a significant increase in the incidence of interstitial pneumonitis. In another study by Kalaycioglu et al. (75) in 1995, 30 of 59 patients required steroids for a decline in the diffusing capacity of the lung for carbon monoxide after high-dose chemotherapy combining BCNU at a dose of 600 mg per m^2 with etoposide and cyclophosphamide.

Pulmonary toxicity appears to be enhanced when BCNU is combined with high-dose cyclophosphamide (76,77). It has been suggested that cyclophosphamide and BCNU act synergistically by depleting reduced glutathione and impairing antioxidant defenses (78,79). Seiden et al. (77) in 1992 retrospectively evaluated the incidence of pulmonary toxicity after six high-dose chemotherapy cycles. Eighteen of 178 patients had fatal or life-threatening toxicity. A significant decrease in diffusing capacity of the lung for carbon monoxide and forced expiratory volume in 1-second values was observed in patients treated with a regimen containing cyclophosphamide and BCNU, respectively. In another study by Jones et al. (76) in 1993, 20 of 38 patients treated with high-dose cyclophosphamide, cisplatin, and BCNU at a dose of 600 mg per m^2 developed pulmonary toxicity. Thirteen of 20 patients were treated with steroids for shortness of breath, and the majority of patients were diagnosed 1 to 3 months after transplantation.

GONADAL TOXICITY

Because the annual incidence of lymphoma is increasing, especially among men <55 years (80), and the cure rate is increasing, the detrimental effect of treatment on fertility and its psychologic consequences are of growing interest to physicians.

Several reports have described severe gonadal toxicity in patients with Hodgkin lymphoma (ranging from 40% to 90%), particularly ovarian failure in women and infertility in men, after chemotherapy such as mechlorethamine, vincristine, procarbazine, and prednisone (81) or cyclophosphamide, vincristine, procarbazine, and prednisone (COPP)/ABVD (Table 32.3) (82). However, recent randomized trials have demonstrated that ABVD achieves comparable or better results than mechlorethamine, vincristine, procarbazine, and prednisone and alternating regimens (83). ABVD is now the standard systemic treatment for Hodgkin lymphoma. Because ABVD has been associated with 30% azoospermia but 100% recovery, and it seems that in patients receiving COPP/ABVD, the cyclophosphamide and procarbazine, as components of COPP, are mainly responsible for the occurrence of gonadal toxicity. The comparison of gonadal toxicity between patients with Hodgkin lymphoma and non-Hodgkin lymphoma is complicated by the differences in typical age at presentation and the fact that different drugs are used. However, patients with non-Hodgkin lymphoma have a lower incidence of long-term gonadal damage after therapy (84). In lymphoma, chemotherapy (mainly cyclophosphamide) and radiation, if directed to the pelvic/groin area, may contribute to gonadal damage. Fever, the general state of the patient, and psychologic factors have been suggested as other possible causes as well.

Ovary

Injury to the ovary can cause sterility and suppressed hormone production. The assessment of gonadal function after treatment of lymphoma in women is difficult because the ova and ovary are not easily accessible for study. Therefore, the surrogate markers of a woman's fertility are regular menses, estrogen levels >20 pmol per L, and the ability to become pregnant.

The dose of radiation that ablates ovarian function depends on whether the dose is fractionated and the age at the time of radiation. The ovary has a smaller number of cells that undergo meiotic activity than the testis and, therefore, is sensitive to radiation at a higher dosage than the testis. Subsequent to radiation, a woman may have months of amenorrhea followed by the return of normal menses because cessation of menses does not imply permanent sterility. However, in general, women >25 years who receive an ovarian dose >5 Gy tend to undergo ovarian castration (85). However, even after total body irradiation, pregnancies have been reported (86). If pelvic radiotherapy is planned in a patient who still desires pregnancy, oophoropexy may be performed. Shielding of the gonads is performed but is less successful in preserving the fertility of a woman than it is for a man. For chemotherapy, cyclophosphamide, age, dosage, and combination with pelvic radiation are risk factors for ovarian injury. The basic ovarian injuries after chemotherapy are fibrosis and follicle destruction (85). Protection of gonad function with hormonal manipulation has shown encouraging preliminary data but is still an area of investigation (87). Harvesting and cryopreservation of ovarian tissue must be considered, given the report of successful human pregnancies following reimplantation (88). Bokemeyer et al. (84) in 1994 reported on ten women with lymphoma treated with CHOP plus radiotherapy. One of the women showed an elevated level of serum gonadotropins and decreased estradiol as an indicator of gonadal toxicity, with abnormalities of the menstrual cycle. In a series of 36 patients <40 years old and treated with CHOP, all but two resumed menses, and 18 (50%) became naturally pregnant during first remission (89). In the series of Müller and Stahel (90) in 1993, one of seven women was found to have gonadal dysfunction after MACOP-B or doxorubicin, cyclophosphamide, etoposide, vincristine, prednisone, and bleomycin. After autologous transplantation, all patients became menopausal immediately after the procedure in the series by Schimmer et al. (91) in 1998. Twenty-nine percent recovered ovarian function, and younger age at transplantation predicted ovarian recovery, whereas use of total body irradiation had a borderline negative impact. Pregnancies have been reported, essentially for women <26 years of age. Brice et al. (92) found that a small number of normal pregnancies can be achieved in women treated with chemotherapy for non-Hodgkin lymphoma, regardless of whether high-dose therapy with autologous stem cell transplantation is included. The pregnancy rate did not

TABLE 32.3

GONADAL TOXICITIES ASSOCIATED WITH THE TREATMENT OF LYMPHOMA

Type of treatment	Effects	References
Radiotherapy	Women: ovarian castration if >5 Gy	74–75
	Men: sterility at 1–2 Gy	
Chemotherapy	Women: low effect	73,77,78
	Men: sterility with chlorambucil, cyclophosphamide, busulfan	75
High-dose chemotheraphy	Female: increased preterm labor and delivery, increase of low-birth-weight infants	77,82–85

seem to have been impaired in the group treated with high-dose chemotherapy. On the other hand, these pregnancies occurred in the youngest patients, and no pregnancy was observed in women >29 years at non-Hodgkin lymphoma diagnosis in this group (92). The question of pregnancy complications or birth defects after stem cell transplantation is difficult. Sanders et al. (86) reported in 1996 that women who received high doses of alkylating agents with total body irradiation were at increased risk for spontaneous abortion, and women who were treated with high-dose alkylating agents had an increased incidence of preterm labor and delivery, as well as an increased incidence of low birth weight infants (86).

Testes

Chemotherapy and radiotherapy affect gonadal function primarily by progressive, dose-related injury to the germinal epithelium of the seminiferous tubules. This damage can lead to oligospermia or aspermia that may be reversible. After therapy, the Leydig cells remain at normal values, whereas follicle-stimulating hormone increases secondary to the germinal aplasia. Drugs commonly associated with germinal aplasia include chlorambucil, cyclophosphamide, and busulfan. However, semen anomalies, which are reflected by low sperm count (<20 ∞ 10^6 per mL) and reduced sperm motility, are well documented in the range of 20% to 67% at diagnosis and before treatment (93,94). These anomalies were attributed to emotional stress, elevated body temperature, and immunologic influences (95). Spermatogonia are very sensitive to radiation therapy, and small doses can produce damage. Multiple small fractions of radiation are more toxic to spermatogenesis than are large, single fractions. Semen cryopreservation and testicular shielding are used to preserve gonadal function after treatment.

In a 2000 series of 33 patients with Hodgkin lymphoma and non-Hodgkin lymphoma, Tal et al. (96) found that patients with stage III and IV disease had a greater probability of long-lasting sperm anomalies after treatment, but that B symptoms had no predictive value. The overall incidence of long-term gonadal toxicity was 21% among men, but all of them received cyclophosphamide, vincristine, and prednisone maintenance therapy with cumulative doses of cyclophosphamide between 12 and 43 g. Similarly, in the series of Pryzant et al. (97) in 1993, cumulative cyclophosphamide doses >9.5 g per m^2 were associated with a high risk of permanent sterility in patients with lymphoma treated with the CHOP-bleomycin regimen; other drugs from this combination might increase the risk associated with cyclophosphamide alone. The fractions of patients whose sperm counts recovered were 83% and 47% for those who received <9.5 g per m^2 and >9.5 g per m^2, respectively. As expected, pelvic radiation therapy also had an increased risk of sterility, and all patients were azoospermic during treatment (97). Normal follicle-stimulating hormone values and spermatogenesis were found in 70% to 80% of the patients after treatments with COPP or the LNH-80 regimen (98,99). In the series of Müller and Stahel (90) in 1993, all patients had normal testosterone, luteinizing hormone, and follicle-stimulating hormone values after conventional treatment with MACOP-B or doxorubicin, cyclophosphamide, etoposide, vincristine, prednisone, and bleomycin. In contrast, three out of seven patients undergoing autologous stem cell transplantation showed abnormal values. Haddy et al. (32) showed that,

among 18 patients with lymphoma who elected to have a semen analysis performed after completion of radiotherapy, all showed azoospermia or oligospermia. Nine of the 18 patients later fathered children. Of the nine patients who did not father children, six were shown to have azoospermia or oligospermia 10 to 14 years later, and the others were not tested (31).

NEUROLOGIC TOXICITIES

Primary Central Nervous System Lymphoma

Late leukoencephalopathy is a common complication in patients treated with high-dose methotrexate and cranial radiation for primary central nervous system lymphoma (100,101). However, the exact incidence of this devastating neurologic dysfunction is not very well–known, and has been reported to be between 4% and 36% in different series (102,103). In the series of Blay et al. (104) in 1998, it was found to be 19% at 5 years, and correlated with the dose administered to the brain (>50 Gy) and with the use of postradiation chemotherapy. A hyperfractionated schedule might allow to reduce the dose without compromising progression free survival or overall survival; however, this regimen delayed but did not eliminate the severe neurotoxicity from a chemoradiation regimen (105). Haddy et al. (32) in 1998 reported a pediatric series of 103 young survivors. Two patients who received 3,000 cGy of cranial irradiation subsequently developed seizures and required continuous anticonvulsant therapy; both had leukomalacia shown by magnetic resonance imaging. One of them required a special education class at school. Two others who received 900 and 1,200 cGy of cranial irradiation did not develop neurologic deficits. Three patients who did not receive cranial irradiation developed seizures during or after chemotherapy. One of them required tutoring in school due to short-term memory loss. This late neurologic toxicity also contributes to the poor social outcome of patients with primary central nervous system lymphoma. In one series, only 6% of patients returned to work. In the study of Sandor et al. (100), the incidence of late neurologic effects (three out of 14, 21%) does not seem to be dramatically decreased by the use of chemotherapy alone, and case reports of fatal leukoencephalopathy after CHOP chemotherapy without radiotherapy have been reported (106).

The risk of significant neurotoxicity associated with cranial irradiation after high-dose methotrexate appears to be age related. The risk is significantly higher for patients who are age ≥60 years in the Memorial Sloan-Kettering Cancer Center experience (107). However, recent data from the same group suggested that lower doses of hyperfractionated radiation treatment after a complete response to chemotherapy may preserve neurocognitive function without compromise of disease control (108).

Vincristine

Vincristine, a common agent in treating lymphoma, is associated with peripheral, central, and autonomic neuropathies. In the series of Haim et al. (109) in 1994, mild to moderately severe neuropathy was seen in 92% of the patients with lymphoma exposed to the drug at full dose, without capping at a total of 2 mg. After discontinuation of vincristine, the median time to recovery was 3 months for paresthesia and motor weakness, and 5 months for muscle cramps. Residual minor abnormalities have, in some cases, persisted for years. Patients with relapsed or refractory disease may be treated with ifosfamide and cisplatin, both known to cause central and peripheral neurotoxicity. Fludarabine, used in indolent lymphomas, induces mild and reversible central nervous system toxicity in 15% of treated patients; however, delayed and severe encephalopathy has been reported (110).

Intrathecal Chemotherapy

Intrathecal chemotherapy is commonly provided as central nervous system prophylaxis in the treatment. Chemical meningitis is a common side effect of intrathecal methotrexate and cytarabine; the risk is estimated at about 10% Liposomal cytarabine is now approved for use in lymphomatous meningitis, and the use of concomitant corticosteroids has been shown to decrease the incidence of chemical meningitis with this drug. A less common side effect of intrathecal methotrexate and cytarabine is transverse myelopathy. Encephalopathy is rare with these agents (111)

Inadvertent intrathecal administration of vincristine has been reported and is uniformly fatal except in two of three cases treated with spinal fluid exchange (112).

ENDOCRINE TOXICITIES

The thyroid is likely to produce clinically significant abnormalities after external radiotherapy. Functional clinical changes after direct radiation exceeding 30 Gy are essentially related to hypothyroidism, which may be clinically overt or subclinical with normal serum free thyroxine levels and high thyrotropin concentrations (113). In the series by Hancock et al. (113) in 1991, 512 out of 1,677 irradiated patients with Hodgkin lymphoma presented with hypothyroidism, and 486 patients received thyroxine therapy; the 20-year actuarial risk among irradiated patients was 43%. The risk of hyperthyroidism (113), silent thyroiditis, and Hashimoto disease (114) is also increased after radiation therapy. Secondary hypothyroidism related to the irradiation of the hypothalamus and pituitary gland may arise with doses >40 to 50 Gy. After total body irradiation, subclinical thyroid dysfunction was seen in 39% of patients. No evidence of direct damage to the hypothalamic-pituitary axis was found in one series (115).

Thyroid dysfunction has been the most common late complication after myeloablative radioimmunotherapy with iodine-131–labeled anti-CD20 antibody. Seventeen of 29 patients developed abnormal elevations of thyroid-stimulating hormone during follow-up. The estimated cumulative probability of hypothyroidism is 62%. All patients who developed hypothyroidism have done so within the first year, and the median time to development of an elevated thyroid-stimulating hormone has been 6 months. No patient developed symptomatic hypothyroidism because thyroid replacement therapy was initiated as soon as monitoring showed elevated thyroid-stimulating hormone levels (48).

As the number of young patients surviving lymphoma increases, the growth impairment resulting from radiotherapy, especially from cranial radiation >24 Gy, or from aggressive chemotherapy has become a matter of concern. Growth hormone deficiency is of primary importance among the various potential alterations in hypothalamic and pituitary function associated with radiotherapy or chemotherapy, and the hypothalamus appears to be the main site of damage (116). Normal spontaneous growth hormone secretion during sleep but failure to show the normal growth hormone response to arginine, growth hormone-releasing factor, and glucagon-propanolol test suggest hypothalamic dysfunction and secondary pituitary atrophy, as demonstrated in patients with central nervous system relapse (117). Age at initial diagnosis and at central nervous system relapse seems to be the best predictive factor of the severity of the subsequent growth impairment. Children <2 years may be particularly sensitive to the radiation and systemic or intrathecal chemotherapy and, therefore, experience more severe growth impairment.

MISCELLANEOUS

Bone Damage

Ionizing radiation may induce an impairment of growing bone. This fact is of particular importance in children and represents the most important dose-limiting factor in the radiotherapeutic management of children with malignant disease. Scoliosis, epiphyseal slippage, avascular necrosis, and abnormalities of craniofacial growth may be observed after radiation. The child's age at the time of treatment, the location of irradiated bone, and irradiation characteristics may influence the radiation-related observed effects (118). There is no evidence that chemotherapy may affect bone growth in patients with lymphoma, as is suggested for medulloblastoma (119). In adults, pathologic analysis of mature bone after ionizing radiation exposure is rare, suggesting that it is difficult to draw a clear picture of the action of radiation on the bone. Osteoporosis, medullary fibrosis, and cytotoxicity on bone cells can lead to fracture or necrosis. Various factors can influence bone tolerance to radiation, such as bone involvement or infection, which is frequent in mandibular osteonecrosis. Technical improvements in radiation techniques have also decreased radiation-induced bone complication. The most common effect of chemotherapy is skeletal demineralization (osteoporosis) leading to fractures after use of corticosteroids.

Avascular necrosis of bone (AVNB) is a well-known but rare complication of chemotherapy for lymphoma, with a reported incidence ranging from 1% to 10%. Early diagnosis is essential for optimal therapeutic management. Using magnetic resonance imaging, the most sensitive means of detecting the earlier stages of AVNB, 100 patients treated with standard chemotherapy for lymphoma were assessed. Fifteen patients were found to have changes of AVNB, ten with early changes, but five with advanced segmental collapse of the femoral head. None of the patients with AVNB had more than the standard course of corticosteroids. Almost one fourth of the study group complained of joint pain during or after their treatment, one-third of whom were found to have

TABLE 32.4

RECOMMENDATIONS OF THE EUROPEAN BONE MARROW TRANSPLANTATION REGISTRY FOR VACCINATION AFTER STEM CELL TRANSPLANTATION

Vaccine	Allograft	Autograft	Delay after transplant
Tetanus	Recommended for all patients	Recommended for all patients	6–12 mo
Diphtheria	Recommended for all patients	Recommended for all patients	6–12 mo
Poliomyelitis (inactivated)	Recommended for all patients	Recommended for all patients	6–12 mo
Streptococcus pneumoniae (Pneumo 23)	Recommended for all patients (low efficacy)	Recommended for all patients (low efficacy)	6–12 mo
Haemophilus influenzae	Recommended for all patients	Recommended for children and patients with respiratory deficiency	4–5 mo
Flu	Recommended for all patients	Recommended for all patients	>6 mo and 1/yr for at least 2 yr
Hepatitis B	According to epidemiology	According to epidemiology	6–12 mo

AVNB, a strong indicator to screen all those with pain. However, 40% of those with AVNB were asymptomatic. The clinical significance of the "silent hip" has yet to be elucidated (120).

Muscle

There are few data regarding the adverse effects of chemotherapy or radiotherapy on skeletal muscle. This tissue is considered to be radioresistant, and the most common effect on muscle is hypoplasia, but the effects on strength are not pronounced. Therefore, the effect is more cosmetic than functional.

Skin

The skin response to ionizing radiation is characterized by an acute reaction during and after the treatment, and a chronic effect, subcutaneous fibrosis, resulting from a continuous and self-maintained local process, possibly sensitive to therapeutic intervention (121). At the present time, late skin effects should rarely be observed if appropriate dose, fractionation, and beam energy are used. Alopecia generally occurs in radiation field with doses of 25 to 40 Gy, and regrowth is generally seen within 3 months.

Cutaneous hyperpigmentation is observed after administration of doxorubicin and bleomycin, often at the sites of skin trauma. Nail changes, radiation recall reactions, and photosensitivity are also commonly observed.

Immune System

The different treatment modalities used in non-Hodgkin lymphoma may cause more or less pronounced immunodeficiency. Deficiencies in the humoral system, even using anti-CD20, an antigen present on every B cell, are generally not long lasting and not very clinically significant (11). In the trial comparing CHOP with R-CHOP, an update indicates a trend of increased occurrence of infections in all patients treated with R-CHOP after the end of treatment (12 in R-CHOP vs. six in the CHOP group) (122). However, T-cell reconstitution may be more affected by therapy. After autologous stem cell transplantation, T-cell CD3$^+$ repopulation typically occurs by 2 to 4 months. Low CD4$^+$/CD8$^+$ ratios may exist during the first 6 to 12 months, and T-cell function, as measured by mitogen studies, typically returns to baseline by 1 year (123). The introduction of the CD34$^+$ selection technique to reduce tumor contamination does not greatly influence long-term immunologic reconstitution. However, unusual viral infections, progressive multifocal leukoencephalopathy, and cytomegalovirus have recently been reported with concomitant use of CD34$^+$ selection and peritransplant rituximab (124). Recommendations for vaccination after stem cell transplantation have been proposed by the European Bone Marrow Transplantation Registry and U.S. Centers for Disease Control and Prevention (125) (Table 32.4).

References

1. Moser E, Noordijk E, Carde P, et al. Late non-neoplastic events in patients with aggressive non-Hodgkin's lymphoma in four randomized European Organisation for Research and Treatment of Cancer trials. *Clin Lymphoma Myeloma* 2005;6:122–130.
2. André M, Mounier N, Leleu X, et al. Second cancers and late toxicities after treatment of aggressive non-Hodgkin lymphoma with the ACVBP regimen: a GELA cohort study on 2837 patients. *Blood* 2004;103:1222–1228.
3. Singal PK, Iliskovic N. Doxorubicin-induced cardiomyopathy. *N Engl J Med* 1998;339:900–905.
4. Pohjola-Sintonen S, Totterman KJ, Salmo M, et al. Late cardiac effects of mediastinal radiotherapy in patients with Hodgkin's disease. *Cancer* 1987;60:31–37.
5. Lipshultz SE, Colan SD, Gelber RD, et al. Late cardiac effects of doxorubicin therapy for acute lymphoblastic leukemia in childhood. *N Engl J Med* 1991;324:808–815.
6. Cohn KE, Stewart JR, Fajardo LF, et al. Heart disease following radiation. *Medicine (Baltimore)* 1967;46:281–298.
7. Hancock SL, Tucker MA, Hoppe RT. Factors affecting late mortality from heart disease after treatment of Hodgkin's disease. *JAMA* 1993;270:1949–1955.
8. Boivin JF, Hutchison GB, Lubin JH, et al. Coronary artery disease mortality in patients treated for Hodgkin's disease. *Cancer* 1992;69:1241–1247.
9. Myrehaug S, Pintilie M, Tsang R, et al. Cardiac morbidity following modern treatment for Hodgkin lymphoma: supra-additive cardiotoxicity of doxorubicin and radiation therapy. *Leuk Lymphoma* 2008;49:1486–1493.
10. Fisher RI, Gaynor ER, Dahlberg S, et al. Comparison of a standard regimen (CHOP) with three intensive chemotherapy regimens for advanced non-Hodgkin's lymphoma. *N Engl J Med* 1993;328:1002–1006.
11. Coiffier B, Lepage E, Briere J, et al. CHOP chemotherapy plus rituximab compared with CHOP alone in elderly patients with diffuse large-B-cell lymphoma. *N Engl J Med* 2002;346:235–242.
12. Bristow MR, Billingham ME, Mason JW, et al. Clinical spectrum of anthracycline antibiotic cardiotoxicity. *Cancer Treat Rep* 1978;62:873–879.

13. Shan K, Lincoff AM, Young JB. Anthracycline-induced cardiotoxicity. *Ann Intern Med* 1996;125:47–58.

14. Aviles A, Neri N, Nambo MJ. Long-term evaluation of cardiac function in children who received anthracyclines during pregnancy. *Ann Oncol* 2006;17:286–288.

15. Laufman LR, Jones JJ, Morrice B, et al. Case report of a lethal cardiac toxic effect following high-dose cyclophosphamide. *J Natl Cancer Inst* 1995;87:539–540.

16. Tulleken JE, Kooiman CG, van der Werf TS, et al. Constrictive pericarditis after high-dose chemotherapy. *Lancet* 1997;350:1601.

17. Isberg B, Paul C, Jonsson L, et al. Myocardial toxicity of high-dose cyclophosphamide in rabbits treated with daunorubicin. *Cancer Chemother Pharmacol* 1991;28:171–180.

18. Brockstein BE, Smiley C, Al-Sadir J, et al. Cardiac and pulmonary toxicity in patients undergoing high-dose chemotherapy for lymphoma and breast cancer: prognostic factors. *Bone Marrow Transplant* 2000;25:885–894.

19. Kuittinen T, Husso-Saastamoinen M, Sipola P, et al. Very acute cardiac toxicity during BEAC chemotherapy in non-Hodgkin's lymphoma patients undergoing autologous stem cell transplantation. *Bone Marrow Transplant* 2005;36:1077–1082.

20. Kandylis K, Vassilomanolakis M, Tsoussis S, et al. Ifosfamide cardiotoxicity in humans. *Cancer Chemother Pharmacol* 1989;24:395–396.

21. Quezado ZM, Wilson WH, Cunnion RE, et al. High-dose ifosfamide is associated with severe, reversible cardiac dysfunction. *Ann Intern Med* 1993;118:31–36.

22. Gottdiener JS, Appelbaum FR, Ferrans VJ, et al. Cardiotoxicity associated with high-dose cyclophosphamide therapy. *Arch Intern Med* 1981;141:758–763.

23. Hertenstein B, Stefanic M, Schmeiser T, et al. Cardiac toxicity of bone marrow transplantation: predictive value of cardiologic evaluation before transplant. *J Clin Oncol* 1994;12:998–1004.

24. Younes A, Sarris A, Melnyk A, et al. Three-hour paclitaxel infusion in patients with refractory and relapsed non-Hodgkin's lymphoma. *J Clin Oncol* 1995;13:583–587.

25. House KW, Simon SR, Pugh RP. Chemotherapy-induced myocardial infarction in a young man with Hodgkin's disease. *Clin Cardiol* 1992;15:122–125.

26. Scholz KH, Herrmann C, Tebbe U, et al. Myocardial infarction in young patients with Hodgkin's disease—potential pathogenic role of radiotherapy, chemotherapy, and splenectomy. *Clin Investig* 1993;71:57–64.

27. Clarke CS, Otridge BW, Carney DN. Thromboembolism. A complication of weekly chemotherapy in the treatment of non-Hodgkin's lymphoma. *Cancer* 1990;66:2027–2030.

28. Klencke B, Kaplan L. Advances and future challenges in non-Hodgkin's lymphoma. *Curr Opin Oncol* 1998;10:422–427.

29. Shan K, Lincoff AM, Young JB. Anthracycline-induced cardiotoxicity. *Ann Intern Med* 1996;125:47–58.

30. Hershman DL, McBride RB, Eisenberg A, et al. Doxorubicin, cardiac risk and cardiac toxicity in elderly patients with diffuse B-cell non-Hodgkin's lymphoma. *J Clin Oncol* 2008;26:3159–65.

31. Miller TP, Dahlberg S, Cassady JR, et al. Chemotherapy alone compared with chemotherapy plus radiotherapy for localized intermediate- and high-grade non-Hodgkin's lymphoma. *N Engl J Med* 1998;339:21–26.

32. Haddy TB, Adde MA, McCalla J, et al. Late effects in long-term survivors of high-grade non-Hodgkin's lymphomas. *J Clin Oncol* 1998;16:2070–2079.

33. Ghielmini M, Zappa F, Menafoglio A, et al. The high-dose sequential (Milan) chemotherapy/PBSC transplantation regimen for patients with lymphoma is not cardiotoxic. *Ann Oncol* 1999;10:533–537.

34. Hancock SL, Tucker MA, Hoppe RT. Factors affecting late mortality from heart disease after treatment of Hodgkin's disease. *JAMA* 1993;270:1949–1955.

35. Henry-Amar M, Hayat M, Meerwaldt JH, et al. Causes of death after therapy for early stage Hodgkin's disease entered on EORTC protocols. EORTC Lymphoma Cooperative Group. *Int J Radiat Oncol Biol Phys* 1990;19:1155–1157.

36. Rose AG. Pulmonary veno-occlusive disease due to bleomycin therapy for lymphoma. Case reports. *S Afr Med J* 1983;64:636–638.

37. Solal-Celigny P, Lepage E, Brousse N, et al. Recombinant interferon alfa-2b combined with a regimen containing doxorubicin in patients with advanced follicular lymphoma. Groupe d'Etude des Lymphomes de l'Adulte. *N Engl J Med* 1993;329:1608–1614.

38. Dickson D. Deaths halt interferon trials in France. *Science* 1982;218:772.

39. Grunberg SM, Kempf RA, Itri LM, et al. Phase II study of recombinant alpha interferon in the treatment of advanced non-small cell lung carcinoma. *Cancer Treat Rep* 1985;69:1031–1032.

40. Deyton LR, Walker RE, Kovacs JA, et al. Reversible cardiac dysfunction associated with interferon alfa therapy in AIDS patients with Kaposi's sarcoma. *N Engl J Med* 1989;321:1246–1249.

41. Zimmerman S, Adkins D, Graham M, et al. Irreversible, severe congestive cardiomyopathy occurring in association with interferon alpha therapy. *Cancer Biother* 1994;9:291–299.

42. van Besien K, Tabocoff J, Rodriguez M, et al. High-dose chemotherapy with BEAC regimen and autologous bone marrow transplantation for intermediate grade and immunoblastic lymphoma: durable complete remissions, but a high rate of regimen-related toxicity. *Bone Marrow Transplant* 1995;15:549–555.

43. Rapoport AP, Rowe JM, Kouides PA, et al. One hundred autotransplants for relapsed or refractory Hodgkin's disease and lymphoma: value of pre-transplant disease status for predicting outcome. *J Clin Oncol* 1993;11:2351–2361.

44. Salloum E, Jillella AP, Nadkarni R, et al. Assessment of pulmonary and cardiac function after high dose chemotherapy with BEAM and peripheral blood progenitor cell transplantation. *Cancer* 1998;82:1506–1512.

45. Friedman HS, Colvin OM, Aisaka K, et al. Glutathione protects cardiac and skeletal muscle from cyclophosphamide-induced toxicity. *Cancer Res* 1990;50:2455–2462.

46. Kanj SS, Sharara AI, Shpall EJ, et al. Myocardial ischemia associated with high-dose carmustine infusion. *Cancer* 1991;68:1910–1912.

47. Hoppe BS, Moskovitz C, Filippa D, et al. Involved-field radiotherapy before high-dose therapy and autologous stem-cell rescue in diffuse large-cell lymphoma: long-term disease control and toxicity. *J Clin Oncol* 2008;26:1858–1864.

48. Liu SY, Eary JF, Petersdorf SH, et al. Follow-up of relapsed B-cell lymphoma patients treated with iodine-131-labeled anti-CD20 antibody and autologous stem-cell rescue. *J Clin Oncol* 1998;16:3270–3278.

49. Cardinale D, Sandri MT, Martinoni A, et al. Left ventricular dysfunction predicted by early troponin I release after high-dose chemotherapy. *J Am Coll Cardiol* 2000;36:517–522.

50. Chemaly R, Torres H, Hachem R, et al. Cytomegalovirus pneumonia in patients with lymphoma. *Cancer* 2005;104:1213–1220.

51. Villani F, De Maria P, Bonfante V, et al. Late pulmonary toxicity after treatment for Hodgkin's disease. *Anticancer Res* 1997;17:4739–4742.

52. Horning SJ, Adhikari A, Rizk N, et al. Effect of treatment for Hodgkin's disease on pulmonary function: results of a prospective study. *J Clin Oncol* 1994;12:297–305.

53. Hirsch A, Vander Els N, Straus DJ, et al. Effect of ABVD chemotherapy with and without mantle or mediastinal irradiation on pulmonary function and symptoms in early-stage Hodgkin's disease. *J Clin Oncol* 1996;14:1297–1305.

54. Rubin P, Johnston CJ, Williams JP, et al. A perpetual cascade of cytokines postirradiation leads to pulmonary fibrosis. *Int J Radiat Oncol Biol Phys* 1995;33:99–109.

55. Nissen NI, Ersboll J, Hansen HS, et al. A randomized study of radiotherapy versus radiotherapy plus chemotherapy in stage I-II non-Hodgkin's lymphomas. *Cancer* 1983;52:1–7.

56. Sutcliffe SB, Gospodarowicz MK, Bush RS, et al. Role of radiation therapy in localized non-Hodgkin's lymphoma. *Radiother Oncol* 1985;4:211–223.

57. Lee CK, Levitt SH. Long-term follow-up of pathologic stage I large cell non-Hodgkin's lymphoma patients after primary radiotherapy. *Am J Clin Oncol* 1996;19:93–98.

58. Kreisman H, Wolkove N. Pulmonary toxicity of antineoplastic therapy. *Semin Oncol* 1992;19:508–520.

59. Conerotte T, Lonneux M, De Meeus Y, et al. Use of 2-[18F]fluoro-2-deoxy-D-glucose positron emission tomography in the early diagnosis of asymptomatic bleomycin-induced pneumonitis. *Ann Haematol* 2008;87:943–945.

60. Klimo P, Connors JM. MACOP-B chemotherapy for the treatment of diffuse large-cell lymphoma. *Ann Intern Med* 1985;102:596–602.

61. Shapiro CL, Yeap BY, Godleski J, et al. Drug-related pulmonary toxicity in non-Hodgkin's lymphoma. Comparative results with three different treatment regimens. *Cancer* 1991;68:699–705.

62. Iki S, Yoshinaga K, Ohbayashi Y, et al. Cytotoxic drug-induced pneumonia and possible augmentation by G-CSF—clinical attention. *Ann Hematol* 1993;66:217–218.

63. Matthews JH. Pulmonary toxicity of ABVD chemotherapy and G-CSF in Hodgkin's disease: possible synergy. *Lancet* 1993;342:988.

64. Lei KI, Leung WT, Johnson PJ. Serious pulmonary complications in patients receiving recombinant granulocyte colony-stimulating factor during BACOP chemotherapy for aggressive non-Hodgkin's lymphoma. *Br J Cancer* 1994;70:1009–1013.

65. Couderc LJ, Stelianides S, Frachon I, et al. Pulmonary toxicity of chemotherapy and G/GM-CSF: a report of five cases. *Respir Med* 1999;93:65–68.

66. Bastion Y, Reyes F, Bosly A, et al. Possible toxicity with the association of G-CSF and bleomycin. *Lancet* 1994;343:1221–1222.

67. Bastion Y, Coiffier B. Pulmonary toxicity of bleomycin: is G-CSF a risk factor? *Lancet* 1994;344:474.

68. Yokose N, Ogata K, Tamura H, et al. Pulmonary toxicity after granulocyte colony-stimulating factor-combined chemotherapy for non-Hodgkin's lymphoma. *Br J Cancer* 1998;77:2286–2290.

69. Wagner S, Mehta A, Laber D. Rituximab-induced interstitial lung disease. *Am J Hematol* 2007;82:916–919.

70. Lui X, Hong X, Gu Y, et al. Interstitial pneumonitis during rituximab-containing chemotherapy for non-Hodgkin lymphoma. *Leuk Lymphoma* 2008;49:1778–1783.

71. Petersen FB, Appelbaum FR, Hill R, et al. Autologous marrow transplantation for malignant lymphoma: a report of 101 cases from Seattle. *J Clin Oncol* 1990;8:638–647.

72. Gingrich RD, Ginder GD, Burns LJ, et al. BVAC ablative chemotherapy followed by autologous bone marrow transplantation for patients with advanced lymphoma. *Blood* 1990;75:2276–2281.

73. Ghalie R, Szidon JP, Thompson L, et al. Evaluation of pulmonary complications after bone marrow transplantation: the role of pretransplant pulmonary function tests. *Bone Marrow Transplant* 1992;10:359–365.

74. Wheeler C, Antin JH, Churchill WH, et al. Cyclophosphamide, carmustine, and etoposide with autologous bone marrow transplantation in refractory Hodgkin's disease and non-Hodgkin's lymphoma: a dose-finding study. *J Clin Oncol* 1990;8:648–656.

75. Kalaycioglu M, Kavuru M, Tuason L, et al. Empiric prednisone therapy for pulmonary toxic reaction after high-dose chemotherapy containing carmustine (BCNU). *Chest* 1995;107:482–487.

76. Jones RB, Matthes S, Shpall EJ, et al. Acute lung injury following treatment with high-dose cyclophosphamide, cisplatin, and carmustine: pharmacodynamic evaluation of carmustine. *J Natl Cancer Inst* 1993; 85:640–647.

77. Seiden MV, Elias A, Ayash L, et al. Pulmonary toxicity associated with high dose chemotherapy in the treatment of solid tumors with autologous marrow transplant: an analysis of four chemotherapy regimens. *Bone Marrow Transplant* 1992;10:57–63.

78. Babson JR, Reed DJ. Inactivation of glutathione reductase by 2-chloroethyl nitrosourea-derived isocyanates. *Biochem Biophys Res Commun* 1978;82:754–762.

79. Friedman HS, Colvin OM, Aisaka K, et al. Glutathione protects cardiac and skeletal muscle from cyclophosphamide-induced toxicity. *Cancer Res* 1990;50:2455–2462.

80. Wingo PA, Ries LA, Rosenberg HM, et al. Cancer incidence and mortality, 1973-1995: a report card for the U.S. *Cancer* 1998;82:1197–1207.

81. Schilsky RL, Sherins RJ, Hubbard SM, et al. Long-term follow up of ovarian function in women treated with MOPP chemotherapy for Hodgkin's disease. *Am J Med* 1981;71:552–556.

82. Kreuser ED, Felsenberg D, Behles C, et al. Long-term gonadal dysfunction and its impact on bone mineralization in patients following COPP/ABVD chemotherapy for Hodgkin's disease. *Ann Oncol* 1992;3(suppl 4):105–110.

83. Canellos GP, Anderson JR, Propert KJ, et al. Chemotherapy of advanced Hodgkin's disease with MOPP, ABVD, or MOPP alternating with ABVD. *N Engl J Med* 1992;327:1478–1484.

84. Bokemeyer C, Schmoll HJ, van Rhee J, et al. Long-term gonadal toxicity after therapy for Hodgkin's and non-Hodgkin lymphoma. *Ann Hematol* 1994;68:105–110.

85. Chapman RM, Sutcliffe SB, Malpas JS. Cytotoxic-induced ovarian failure in women with Hodgkin's disease. I. Hormone function. *JAMA* 1979; 242:1877–1881.

86. Sanders JE, Hawley J, Levy W, et al. Pregnancies following high-dose cyclophosphamide with or without high-dose busulfan or total-body irradiation and bone marrow transplantation. *Blood* 1996;87:3045–3052.

87. Whitehead E, Shalet SM, Blackledge G, et al. The effect of combination chemotherapy on ovarian function in women treated for Hodgkin's disease. *Cancer* 1983;52:988–993.

88. Donnez J, Dolmans MM, Demylle D, et al. Livebirth after orthotopic transplantation of cryopreserved ovarian tissue. *Lancet* 2004;364:1405–1410.

89. Elis A, Tevet A, Yerushalmi R, et al. Fertility status among women treated for aggressive non-Hodgkin's lymphoma. *Leuk Lymphoma* 2006;47:623–627.

90. Müller U, Stahel RA. Gonadal function after MACOP-B or VACOP-B with or without dose intensification and ABMT in young patients with aggressive non-Hodgkin's lymphoma. *Ann Oncol* 1993;4:399–402.

91. Schimmer AD, Quatermain M, Imrie K, et al. Ovarian function after autologous bone marrow transplantation. *J Clin Oncol* 1998;16:2359–2363.

92. Brice P, Haioun C, André M, et al. Pregnancies after high-dose chemotherapy and autologous stem cell transplantation in aggressive lymphomas. *Blood* 2002;100:736.

93. Marmor D, Elefant E, Dauchez C, et al. Semen analysis in Hodgkin's disease before the onset of treatment. *Cancer* 1986;57:1986–1987.

94. Viviani S, Ragni G, Santoro A, et al. Testicular dysfunction in Hodgkin's disease before and after treatment. *Eur J Cancer* 1991;27:1389–1392.

95. Barr RD, Clark DA, Booth JD. Dyspermia in men with localized Hodgkin's disease. A potentially reversible, immune-mediated disorder. *Med Hypotheses* 1993;40:165–168.

96. Tal R, Botchan A, Hauser R, et al. Follow-up of sperm concentration and motility in patients with lymphoma. *Hum Reprod* 2000;15:1985–1988.

97. Pryzant RM, Meistrich ML, Wilson G, et al. Long-term reduction in sperm count after chemotherapy with and without radiation therapy for non-Hodgkin's lymphomas. *J Clin Oncol* 1993;11:239–247.

98. Dumontet C, Bastion Y, Felman P, et al. Long-term outcome and sequelae in aggressive lymphoma patients treated with the LNH-80 regimen. *Ann Oncol* 1992;3:639–644.

99. Roeser HP, Stocks AE, Smith AJ. Testicular damage due to cytotoxic drugs and recovery after cessation of therapy. *Aust N Z J Med* 1978;8:250–254.

100. Sandor V, Stark-Vancs V, Pearson D, et al. Phase II trial of chemotherapy alone for primary central nervous system and intraocular lymphoma. *J Clin Oncol* 1998;16:3000–3006.

101. Bessell EM, Graus F, Punt JA, et al. Primary non-Hodgkin's lymphoma of the CNS treated with BVAM or CHOD/BVAM chemotherapy before radiotherapy. *J Clin Oncol* 1996;14:945–954.

102. Glass J, Gruber ML, Cher L, et al. Preirradiation methotrexate chemotherapy of primary central nervous system lymphoma: long-term outcome. *J Neurosurg* 1994;81:188–195.

103. Abrey LE, DeAngelis LM, Yahalom J. Long-term survival in primary CNS lymphoma. *J Clin Oncol* 1998;16:859–863.

104. Blay JY, Conroy T, Chevreau C, et al. High-dose methotrexate for the treatment of primary cerebral lymphomas: analysis of survival and late neurologic toxicity in a retrospective series. *J Clin Oncol* 1998;16:864–871.

105. Fisher B, Seiferheld W, Schultz C, et al. Secondary analysis of Radiation Therapy Oncology Group study (RTOG) 9310: an intergroup phase II combined modality treatment of primary central nervous system lymphoma. *J Neurooncol* 2005;74:201–205.

106. Cain MS, Burton GV, Holcombe RF. Fatal leukoencephalopathy in a patient with non-Hodgkin's lymphoma treated with CHOP chemotherapy and high-dose steroids. *Am J Med Sci* 1998;315:202–207.

107. Gavrilovic IT, Hormigo A, Yahalom J, et al. Long-term follow-up of high-dose methotrexate-based therapy with and without whole brain irradiation for newly diagnosed primary CNS lymphoma. *J Clin Oncol* 2006;24:4570–4574.

108. Shah GD, Yahalom J, Correa DD, et al. Combined immunochemotherapy with reduced whole-brain radiotherapy for newly diagnosed primary CNS lymphoma. *J Clin Oncol* 2007;25:4730–4735.

109. Haim N, Epelbaum R, Ben-Shahar M, et al. Full dose vincristine (without 2-mg dose limit) in the treatment of lymphomas. *Cancer* 1994; 73:2515–2519.

110. Johnson PW, Fearnley J, Domizio P, et al. Neurological illness following treatment with fludarabine. *Br J Cancer* 1994;70:966–968.

111. Glass J. Neurologic complications of lymphoma and leukemia. *Semin Oncol* 2006;33:342–347.

112. Qweider M, Gilsbach JM, Rhode V. Inadvertent intrathecal vincristine administration: a neurosurgical emergency. Case report. *J Neurosurg Spine* 2007;6:280–283.

113. Hancock SL, Cox RS, McDougall IR. Thyroid diseases after treatment of Hodgkin's disease. *N Engl J Med* 1991;325:599–605.

114. Tamura K, Shimaoka K, Friedman M. Thyroid abnormalities associated with treatment of malignant lymphoma. *Cancer* 1981;47:2704–2711.

115. Littley MD, Shalet SM, Morgenstern GR, et al. Endocrine and reproductive dysfunction following fractionated total body irradiation in adults. *Q J Med* 1991;78:265–274.

116. Shalet SM, Clayton PE, Price DA. Growth and pituitary function in children treated for brain tumours or acute lymphoblastic leukaemia. *Horm Res* 1988;30:53–61.

117. Yamada S, Ishii E, Okabe Y, et al. Growth retardation in childhood leukemia and lymphoma. Special reference to patients with CNS relapse. *Am J Pediatr Hematol Oncol* 1992;14:236–240.

118. Willman KY, Cox RS, Donaldson SS. Radiation induced height impairment in pediatric Hodgkin's disease. *Int J Radiat Oncol Biol Phys* 1994;28:85–92.

119. Olshan JS, Gubernick J, Packer RJ, et al. The effects of adjuvant chemotherapy on growth in children with medulloblastoma. *Cancer* 1992; 70:2013–2017.

120. Ratcliffe MA, Gilbert FJ, Dawson AA, et al. Diagnosis of avascular necrosis of the femoral head in patients treated for lymphoma. *Hematol Oncol* 1995;13:131–137.

121. Lefaix JL, Delanian S, Leplat JJ, et al. Successful treatment of radiation-induced fibrosis using Cu/Zn-SOD and Mn-SOD: an experimental study. *Int J Radiat Oncol Biol Phys* 1996;35:305–312.

122. Feugier P, Van Hoof A, Sebban C, et al. Long-term results of the R-CHOP study in the treatment of elderly patients with diffuse large B-cell lymphoma: a study by the Groupe d'Etude des Lymphomes de l'Adulte. *J Clin Oncol* 2005;23:4117–4126.

123. Steingrimsdottir H, Gruber A, Bjorkholm M, et al. Immune reconstitution after autologous hematopoietic stem cell transplantation in relation to underlying disease, type of high-dose therapy and infectious complications. *Haematologica* 2000;85:832–838.

124. Goldberg SL, Pecora AL, Alter RS, et al. Unusual viral infections (progressive multifocal leukoencephalopathy and cytomegalovirus disease) after high-dose chemotherapy with autologous blood stem cell rescue and peritransplantation rituximab. *Blood* 2002;99:1486–1488.

125. Ljungman P. Immunization of transplant recipients. *Bone Marrow Transplant* 1999;23:635–636.

SECTION VI ■ SPECIAL CLINICAL SITUATIONS

CHAPTER 33 ■ LYMPHOMAS IN CHILDREN

JOHN T. SANDLUND, KAREN J. MARCUS, AND MIHAELA ONCIU

The malignant lymphomas, which include both Hodgkin lymphoma and non-Hodgkin lymphoma (NHL), are the third most common malignancy of childhood; only acute lymphoblastic leukemia (ALL) and brain tumors are more common (1–7). Among children <15 years of age, approximately 60% of cases are NHL; however, among children <18 years of age, there is a slight predominance of Hodgkin lymphoma (4,5).

There are significant differences between the NHLs that occur in children and in adults. The pediatric NHLs are primarily aggressive tumors, whereas in adults, indolent low-grade lymphomas are more common (8,9). Children with NHLs often present with diffuse extranodal disease, whereas adults more frequently present with primary nodal disease. These differences in histologic subtype are likely to reflect age-related differences in the immune system and associated susceptibility to malignant transformation (10,11).

There have been dramatic improvements in our understanding of these diseases with respect to pathogenesis, diagnosis, and treatment. As survival rates have improved, efforts to refine therapy have in part focused on reducing or eliminating the risk of treatment-related late effects such as cardiotoxicity, infertility, and second malignancy. This chapter will review these advances and discuss future directions.

EPIDEMIOLOGY

Approximately 500 new cases of pediatric NHL are diagnosed each year in the United States (5–7). The median age at the time of diagnosis is approximately 10 years (3). Although NHL can occur at any age, it is less common in children <3 years of age (3,12). Unlike Hodgkin lymphoma, which has a bimodal age distribution, NHL continues to increase in frequency with advancing age. For reasons that have yet to be elucidated, NHL is more common in the white than in the Black population and is two to three times more common in males than in females (3,10).

There are specific populations of children who are at increased risk for NHL (1–3). These groups include children with congenital immunodeficiency disorders such as common variable immunodeficiency, Wiskott-Aldrich syndrome, ataxia telangiectasia (13), and X-linked lymphoproliferative syndrome. It is important that these underlying conditions be recognized so that an appropriate management plan can be designed. For example, in children with ataxia telangiectasia, electron beam irradiation and use of radiomimetics such as bleomycin should be avoided, and judicious use of diagnostic x-rays is recommended. Additionally, patients with ataxia telangiectasia are at a much higher risk for late onset hemorrhagic cystitis when treated with cyclophosphamide or ifosfamide; thus, vigorous hydration and mesna uroprotection

should be implemented, even when low doses of these chemotherapeutic agents are used. Boys with X-linked lymphoproliferative syndrome are at increased risk for both fatal infectious mononucleosis and B-cell lymphoma. Because allogeneic bone marrow transplantation may be a treatment option for children with X-linked lymphoproliferative syndrome, the diagnosis should be considered in any male who presents with a B-cell lymphoma and whose brother has had either fatal infectious mononucleosis or B-cell lymphoma, or in any male who has two primary B-cell lymphomas. Children with acquired immunodeficiency conditions are also at increased risk for NHL (14–16). This group comprises children who are recipients of bone marrow or organ transplants and those who have the acquired immunodeficiency syndrome.

The incidence and distribution of histologic subtypes of NHL in children differ geographically (4,17–21). Although NHL is very rare in Japan, it is very common in equatorial Africa (20). The Burkitt subtype is the most common childhood malignancy in equatorial Africa, and is the most common histologic subtype of NHL in northeastern Brazil and areas of the Middle East (19). In contrast, the predominant histologic subtype in Southern India is lymphoblastic lymphoma (LBL).

CLINICAL FEATURES

The signs and symptoms seen of presentation in children with NHL are in large part determined by the sites of tumor involvement. There is a striking relationship between the primary site of disease at presentation and the LBL and Burkitt lymphoma (BL) histologic subtypes (3). Children with BL typically present with primary involvement of the abdomen or head and neck region, but not of the mediastinum, whereas children with LBL usually present with primary involvement of the head and neck area or mediastinum, but not of the abdomen. In contrast, children with large cell lymphoma may present with primary involvement at almost any location.

Children who have a mediastinal mass (e.g., those who have LBL, mediastinal large B-cell lymphoma [MLBCL], anaplastic large cell lymphoma [ALCL]) may present with a spectrum of respiratory symptoms ranging from slight cough to severe respiratory distress (10). An associated pleural effusion may contribute to worsening respiratory status. A mediastinal mass may also compromise venous return, resulting in a superior vena cava syndrome (10). This syndrome is characterized by prominent venous vasculature, and swelling in the shoulder and neck region: a condition that may favor the development of deep venous thrombosis. An abdominal mass with or without associated ascites is a common finding in children with advanced-stage BL. The tumor often arises from the terminal ileum, and may result in intussusception and/or nausea, vomiting, and abdominal pain. Extension of the mass into the pelvis may result in compression of the ureter and secondary hydronephrosis.

The extent of disease ranges from isolated peripheral node involvement with an otherwise normal physical examination to a leukemic picture with associated pallor and increased bruising. Involvement of the central nervous system may result in headache and vision changes or in the finding of cranial nerve palsy on physical examination. Bony invasion by tumor may result in local pain or limping. Skin lesions may be present in as many as 4% of children with NHL and are usually associated with CD30+ ALCL (22,23).

DIAGNOSIS

The diagnosis is best established by examination of tissue obtained by an open biopsy of the involved site. Sufficient tissue should be resected for histologic, flow cytometric, cytogenetic, and molecular pathologic studies. However, all patients should undergo bilateral iliac crest bone marrow aspiration and biopsy before open biopsy because the diagnosis may be established by studies of these specimens without the need for more invasive procedures. Some patients, such as those with a large mediastinal mass, may not be good candidates for general anesthesia. In those cases, the diagnosis may be established by examination of pleural fluid obtained by thoracentesis. If there is no pleural fluid, the diagnosis may be established in some cases by a parasternal core biopsy of the mass obtained under local anesthesia (24).

STAGING WORKUP

The treatment of children with NHL depends on both histologic subtype and disease stage. Therefore, after a diagnosis is established, an expeditious and comprehensive staging workup must be performed. Such a workup generally includes: computerized tomography of the neck, chest, abdomen, and pelvis; nuclear imaging (i.e., gallium scan and bone scan); bilateral iliac crest bone marrow aspiration and biopsy; and lumbar puncture for examination of cerebrospinal fluid (1,3). Positron emission tomography is commonly used in the staging workup of adults with malignant lymphoma, and is now routinely used in children at many centers (25). Studies are currently being designed to compare positron emission tomography with other nuclear imaging approaches in children. After completion of the staging workup, patients are generally classified according to the St. Jude staging system described by Murphy (9) (Table 33.1). A stage I or II classification is considered to denote limited-stage disease, whereas stage III or IV is considered to denote advanced-stage disease.

INITIAL MANAGEMENT

The NHLs of childhood are very rapidly growing malignancies; therefore, pathologic confirmation of the diagnosis, completion of staging workup, and initiation of chemotherapy should be expeditious. Before chemotherapy is started, various issues must be considered. A complete blood count and chemistry panel should be obtained. Children who are at high risk for tumor lysis syndrome, such as those who have advanced-stage BL and high-serum lactate dehydrogenase value, require excellent intravenous access, vigorous hydration, and management of hyperuricemia. Historically, hyperuricemia has been managed in the United States with hyperhydration, alkalinization, and administration of allopurinol. In France, the use of uricolytic agents such as uricozyme has proven to be very effective. More recently, the recombinant form of this drug (i.e., SR29142) has become available and has been studied in the United States (26). This agent directly cleaves uric acid, converting it to allantoin, which is readily excreted; uric acid is often undetectable in the serum within several hours of administration of the drug. In a recent study of recombinant uricozyme, renal function

---

TABLE 33.1

STAGES OF NHL

Stage I
A single tumor (extranodal) or involvement of a single anatomic area (nodal), with the exclusion of the mediastinum and abdomen.

Stage II
A single tumor (extranodal) with regional node involvement.
Two or more nodal areas on the same side of the diaphragm.
Two single (extranodal) tumors, with or without regional node involvement on the same side of the diaphragm.
A primary gastrointestinal tract tumor (usually in the ileocecal area), with or without involvement of associated mesenteric nodes, that is completely resectable.

Stage III
Two single tumors (extranodal) on opposite sides of the diaphragm.
Two or more nodal areas above and below the diaphragm.
Any primary intrathoracic tumor (mediastinal, pleural, or thymic).
Extensive primary intra-abdominal disease.
Any paraspinal or epidural tumor, whether or not other sites are involved.

Stage IV
Any of the aforementioned findings with initial involvement of the central nervous system, bone marrow, or both.

Based on the classification proposed by Murphy (9).

was preserved, and there were no significant problems with hyperphosphatemia or hyperkalemia (26). When SR29142 is administered, patients at risk for tumor lysis syndrome require hyperhydration but not alkalinization or administration of allopurinol.

SPECIFIC SUBTYPES OF PEDIATRIC LYMPHOMA

The major subtypes of NHL occurring in children include: Burkitt, B and T lymphoblastic, large B cell, and T/null anaplastic large cell. These groupings are recognized in the Revised European-American Lymphoma (REAL) classification (27) and the World Health Organization (WHO) classification of tumors of haematopoietic and lymphoid tissues (28). Table 33.2 summarizes the different classification terms used by these three schemes for the three major pediatric NHL subtypes. According to the National Cancer Institute (NCI) Working Formulation, which incorporates both morphologic features and clinical aggressiveness, the majority of pediatric NHLs are high-grade lesions. The more recent REAL and WHO systems incorporate clinical, histopathologic, and genetic features into distinct clinicopathologic entities. Table 33.3 summarizes the clinical and biologic features of each main subtype. For the classification of pediatric lymphoma, the REAL and WHO classifications are comparable, with both being a significant improvement over the older Working Formulation that did not recognize ALCL and MLBCL as distinct entities.

Burkitt Lymphoma

BL is a high-grade B-cell lymphoma of germinal center (GC) derivation, characterized by a mature B-cell phenotype, and overexpression of the c-myc gene. The latter is the result of its translocation that brings it under the control of the elements that regulate immunoglobulin (Ig) heavy chain or light chain expression. The chromosomal translocations that typically lead to these rearrangements include the t(8;14), t(8;22), and t(2;8). A proliferation index of >95% (as highlighted by immunohistochemical staining for Ki-67) is an acceptable surrogate when genetic studies for c-myc rearrangements are not available (28). Most of the BLs were classified as "small noncleaved cell lymphoma" in the Lukes-Collins classification and the NCI Working Formulation (8,29) (Table 33.2). Lukes and Collins (29) coined the term "small noncleaved cell lymphomas" because of the morphologic and biologic resemblance of the malignant lymphoid cells to similar cells in the normal lymph node GC. The intent of the authors of these systems was to separate this neoplastic process from large cell lymphomas with large noncleaved cells. The cells designated histologically as small noncleaved cells approximate the size of the adjacent macrophage nuclei (as large cells exceed this reference, and small cells are smaller than it). The updated REAL and new WHO classifications (27,28) include "small noncleaved cell lymphoma" under the BL category, which also includes the L3-ALL of the French-American-British classification of acute leukemia and some of the cases of small noncleaved Burkitt-like lymphoma from the previous classifications.

Histologically, BLs have a diffuse infiltrative growth pattern. A "starry-sky" appearance imparted by interspersed tingible-body macrophages is usually present. Frequent mitotic and apoptotic cells are present and reflect this lymphoma's high proliferative rate and apoptotic index, respectively. The classic variant (as designated in the WHO classification) is composed of uniform, medium-sized (small noncleaved) cells with moderate amounts of basophilic cytoplasm (27,28). The cells have round nuclei, clumped or condensed chromatin

---

TABLE 33.2

COMPARISON OF THE UPDATED REAL/WHO LYMPHOMA CLASSIFICATIONS WITH THE NCI WORKING FORMULATION FOR PEDIATRIC LYMPHOMAS

Updated REAL and WHO classifications	NCI working formulation
Common pediatric lymphomas	
B-cell lymphomas	
Precursor B-LBL/leukemia	Lymphoblastic
BL	Small noncleaved cell, Burkitt or non-Burkitt
DLBCL	Diffuse large cell/large cell immunoblastic
Mediastinal (thymic) large B-cell lymphoma	Diffuse large cell/large cell immunoblastic
T-cell lymphomas	
Precursor T-LBL/leukemia	Lymphoblastic
ALCL	Diffuse large cell, immunoblastic
Peripheral T-cell lymphoma	Diffuse, mixed small and large cell/large cell immunoblastic
Uncommon pediatric lymphomas	
FL (grade 1, 2, or 3)	Follicular, small cleaved, mixed small and large, or large cell
MZL (nodal or extranodal)	Small lymphocytic, lymphoplasmacytoid, diffuse small cleaved cell
Hepatosplenic T-cell lymphoma	not recognized (diffuse small cleaved cell)

From National Cancer Institute sponsored study of classifications of non-Hodgkin's lymphomas: summary and description of a working formulation for clinical usage. The Non-Hodgkin's Lymphoma Pathologic Classification Project. *Cancer* 1982;49:2112–2135, with permission. From Harris NL, et al. A revised European-American classification of lymphoid neoplasms: a proposal from the International Lymphoma Study Group. *Blood* 1994;84:1361–1392, with permission. From Jaffe ES, World Health Organization, et al. *Pathology and genetics of tumours of haematopoietic and lymphoid tissues*. Lyon, France: IARC Press, 2001, with permission.

TABLE 33.3

CLINICAL AND BIOLOGIC CHARACTERISTICS OF THE MOST COMMON SUBTYPES OF PEDIATRIC NHL

Subtype	Proportion of cases (%)[a]	Phenotype	Primary site	Translocation	Affected genes
Burkitt	39	Mature B cell	Abdomen or head and neck	t(8;14)(q24;q32) t(2;8)(p11;q24) t(8;22)(q24;q11)	IgH-cMYC Igκ-cMYC Igλ-cMYC
Lymphoblastic	28	Precursor T cell or B cell	Mediastinum (T) or head and neck (B)	t(1;14)(p32;q11)[b] t(11;14)(p13;q11)[b] t(11;14)(p15;q11)[b] t(10;14)(q24;q11)[b] t(7;19)(q35;p13)[b] t(8;14)(q24;q11)[b] t(1;7)(p34;q34)[b]	TCRαδ-TAL1[b] *TCRαδ-RHOMB2*[b] TCRαδ-RHOMB1[b] TCRαδ - HOX11[b] TCRβ - LYL1[b] TCRαδ- MYC[b] TCRβ-LCK[b]
Diffuse large B cell (including mediastinal)	~16	Mature B cell	Mediastinum, abdomen, head, and neck	t(14;18)(q14;q32)	IgH-BCL2
ALCL	~10	Peripheral T, null	Abdomen, head and neck, skin, lung, bone	t(2;5)(p23;q35)[b]	NPM-ALK

TCR, T-cell receptor.
[a] Proportion at St. Jude Children's Research Hospital; other histotypes account for approximately 7%.
[b] Applicable to T-LBL.

with clear parachromatin, and one to three small nucleoli. In Wright-Giemsa-stained cytologic preparations, the malignant cells characteristically have a deeply basophilic cytoplasm and multiple, clear cytoplasmic vacuoles that are highlighted by stains for lipid. The atypical variant of BL, as described by the WHO classification, encompassed lymphomas composed of larger, more pleomorphic cells, often with single, prominent, centrally located nuclei, which nevertheless have the immunophenotypic and genetic features that define this entity. Some of these cases would be designated as "small non-cleaved Burkitt-like" by the previous classifications. Finally, BL with plasmacytoid differentiation is composed of tumor cells with eccentric nuclei and a single central nucleolus (plasmacytoid cells) (27,28). This variant is uncommon in children and is frequently found in immunodeficiency related

BLs (30). No prognostic significance has been described for these morphologic variants in children.

BL and its variants have a characteristic immunophenotypic profile (Table 33.4): CD10+, CD19+, strong CD20+, CD22+, CD79α+, PAX-5; and Ki-67+ with moderately strong expression of surface IgM or, less commonly, IgA or IgG, with light chain κ or λ restriction (31). A small percentage of BLs have cytoplasmic Igμ with no detectable surface Ig, and a rare case may have neither (32,33). Nuclear BCL6 is present without evidence of BCL6 rearrangement (34). CD21, the receptor for complement fragment Cd3 and the Epstein-Barr virus (EBV), is often expressed and is more frequently detected in the endemic than sporadic form. Markers CD5 and BCL2 are invariably negative. The typical cases are also negative for the lymphoblastic markers CD34 and terminal

TABLE 33.4

IMMUNOPHENOTYPIC FEATURES OF PRECURSOR B AND T-BLS

Subtype	CD45	CD34	TdT	CD3[a]	CD5	CD7	CD19	CD20	CD22	CD79α[a]	CD10	Ig expression
Precursor-B	+[b]	+	+	−	−	−	+	±	+	+	+	cIgμ$^{+/-}$, sIgμ$^{-/+}$, κ−, λ−
Mature B[c]	+	±	±	−	−	−	+	±	+	+	+	cIgμ+, sIg μ+, κ ±, λ ±
T[d]	+	±	±	+	±	+	−	−	−	±	−	

cIgμ, cytoplasmic Igμ; sIgμ, surface Ig μ, κ, Ig light chain κ; λ, Ig light chain λ.
[a] Cytoplasmic antigen expression.
[b] Ten percent of cases may have very weak to no detectable CD45 antigen.
[c] Rare subtype not to be confused with BL.
[d] May be subclassified into early thymic stage (CD7+, cytoplasmic CD3+, CD5±, CD2±, CD1a−, CD4−, CD8−), midthymic stage (CD7+, CD5+, CD2+, cytoplasmic CD3+, surface CD3±, CD1a±, CD4±, CD8±), and late thymic stage (CD7+, CD5+, CD2+, surface CD3+, CD1a−, CD4+, or CD8+).

deoxynucleotidyl transferase (TdT), although exceptions may occur.

Translocations of c-myc on chromosome 8 at band q24 to the Ig heavy chain locus on chromosome band 14 q32, the λ Ig light chain loci on 2q11, or 22q11 are found in all cases of BL. The t(8;14)(q24;q32) occurs in approximately 80% of BLs (35). The breakpoint on chromosome 14 in endemic BL involves the heavy chain-joining region. Sporadic cases demonstrate a translocation of c-myc to the Ig switch region. As a result of these translocations, c-myc comes under the influence of the promoter region of the Ig genes, resulting in constitutive expression of c-myc (36). The deregulation of c-myc drives cells through the cell cycle and activates genes involved in apoptosis. As noted previously, c-myc translocations are not entirely specific for BL, having been reported in large B-cell lymphomas, follicular lymphomas (FLs), and precursor B-lymphoblastic transformation of FL. c-myc translocations are relatively easily detected by classic cytogenetic methods and more recently by fluorescence in situ hybridization of interphase nuclei (37). In addition, long-range polymerase chain reaction methodology can reliably identify the presence of the t(8;14) translocation.

The differential diagnosis of BL includes B-LBL and diffuse large B-cell lymphoma (DLBCL). There is morphologic overlap between DLBCL and the atypical variant of BL. In addition, c-myc translocations may also be present in some large B-cell lymphomas. Therefore, the distinction between these two entities may be very challenging. Typically, high-grade B-cell lymphomas showing a proliferation index of >95% (or nearly 100%) and lacking expression of BCL-2 are classified as BLs, whereas the reverse is true for DLBCLs. The differential diagnosis with precursor B-cell lymphoblastic leukemia/lymphoma becomes important (and sometimes equally challenging) in cases of so-called "precursor B-cell BL." These are neoplasms with often predominantly leukemic presentation that harbor BL-type chromosomal translocations, and show morphologic features intermediate between BL and LBL. Immunophenotypically, they show a mixture of mature and precursor B-cell markers, such as TdT and CD34 for the former, and strong surface CD20 and surface Ig with light chain restriction for the latter. These cases have been treated as BL (32,38).

Epidemiology

BL is of particular interest with respect to the geographic variation of clinical and biologic features (20). The endemic subtype, which occurs in equatorial Africa, is characterized clinically by younger age at diagnosis, and by frequent involvement of jaw, abdomen, orbit, and paraspinal area (19–21). In contrast, the sporadic subtype (which occurs in the United States and Western Europe) is characterized by an older median age at diagnosis, and frequent involvement of the abdomen, nasopharynx, and bone marrow. There are also geographic differences with respect to location of the c-myc breakpoint in BL cells. Among sporadic cases, the breakpoint tends to occur within the c-myc gene, whereas it tends to occur upstream of the c-myc gene in endemic cases (20).

The association of EBV with BL has also been shown to vary with geographic location (20,21). The overlap of the BL belt and the malaria belt in equatorial Africa first suggested the involvement of an infections agent in BL pathogenesis. This hypothesis led to the discovery that EBV is associated with the endemic (African) subtype. Although there is little direct evidence of its role in pathogenesis, the circumstantial evidence is provocative. EBV, a B-cell mitogen, is hypothesized to expand the target pool of cells susceptible to malignant transformation (20,21). This hypothesis is supported by studies demonstrating that expression of the recombination activating gene can be induced by EBV, theoretically increasing the chance of a chromosomal translocation during Ig gene rearrangement (39). The observation that lymphomas develop in transgenic mice expressing Epstein-Barr nuclear antigen-1 is also compelling (40). A more direct role of EBV in pathogenesis was suggested by the finding that the EBV-positive cell line Akata loses its malignant phenotype with spontaneous loss of EBV but regains the malignant phenotype upon reinfection with EBV (41). EBV is associated with approximately 85% of cases of endemic BL but with only 15% of sporadic cases (20). An intermediate degree of EBV association has been identified in other parts of the world (17).

Treatment

Two of the most successful early treatment regimens for the management of pediatric NHL were the cyclophosphamide-based cyclophosphamide, vincristine, methotrexate, and prednisone (COMP) regimen (42) and the multiagent anti-ALL regimen, LSA_2L_2 (42–44). The Children's Cancer Group performed a randomized trial of these two regimens (42). Children with limited-stage disease had excellent outcomes regardless of histologic subtype, whereas the outcomes of patients with advanced-stage disease depended on histologic subtype. Specifically, treatment with the COMP regimen was more effective for children with BL, whereas children with LBL had a superior outcome with the LSA_2L_2 regimen. Subsequent trials built on these observations (11,45–73).

For children with limited-stage disease, the primary focus of clinical trials has been to reduce treatment-related acute and late effects without compromising the excellent outcome (11,49). Therefore, trials investigated the reduction of the dose intensity and the duration of therapy. The Pediatric Oncology Group (POG) demonstrated in the first of two sequential trials that involved-field irradiation could be safely eliminated when three cycles of cyclophosphamide, doxorubicin, vincristine, and prednisone (CHOP) are followed by a 24-week maintenance phase of 6-mercaptopurine and methotrexate (49). The second trial demonstrated that the 24-week maintenance phase could be eliminated without compromising outcome, except in the case of lymphoblastic disease.

For children with advanced-stage disease, improvements in outcome have been achieved in part by refinement of a risk-adapted histology and an immunophenotype-directed approach. Treatment of BL was first improved by adding cytarabine and/or high-dose methotrexate to the cyclophosphamide-based COMP regimen (48,50,51,53,55,56). For example, the Total B regimen featured courses of fractionated cyclophosphamide, vincristine, and doxorubicin given in alternation with courses of high-dose methotrexate and cytarabine (48). The results were excellent for children with stage III disease (2-year event-free survival [EFS] estimate of 80%). However, patients who had bone marrow or central nervous system involvement had a 2-year EFS estimate of only approximately 20%. Over the last decade, further improvement in outcome has been achieved by dose intensification of

TABLE 33.5

TREATMENT OUTCOME FOR ADVANCED-STAGE SMALL NONCLEAVED-CELL NHL

Protocol	Stage	No. of patients	EFS rate	Reference
POG 8617	IV	34	4-y EFS = 79% ± 9%	(51)
	B-ALL	47	4-y EFS = 65% ± 8%	
LMB 89[a,b]	III	278	5-y EFS = 91% (95% CI 87%–94%)	(47)
	IV	62	5-y EFS = 87% (95% CI 77%–93%)	
	B-ALL	102	5-y EFS = 87% (95% CI 79%–92%)	
BFM 90[c]	III	169	6-y EFS = 86% ± 3%	(69)
	IV	24	6-y EFS = 73% ± 10%	
	B-ALL	56	6-y EFS = 74% ± 6%	

CI, confidence interval.
[a] Includes patients with B-cell large cell NHL.
[b] Excellent results confirmed in LMB-96 (75,76).
[c] Excellent results confirmed in BFM-95 (193).

cyclophosphamide, methotrexate, and cytarabine, and by the inclusion of new active agents such as etoposide (see Table 33.5) (47,53,66,69,72). One of the most successful regimens to date is the LMB-89 regimen designed by Patte et al. (47) (French Society of Pediatric Oncology). In this strategy, patients are grouped on the basis of disease extent and degree of resection. Group A comprises those with completely resected limited-stage disease. Group C comprises those with central nervous system involvement or >70% replacement of the bone marrow by lymphoma cells, and group B comprises the remainder of patients (i.e., those with incompletely resected limited-stage disease; stage III disease; or <70% replacement of the bone marrow). Eighty-five percent of children with advanced-stage disease are long-term event-free survivors with this regimen. This approach has also been very effective for adults with BL (74).

The largest and recently completed clinical trial for children with BL is the LMB-96 study, which was an international collaboration between institutions in France, the United States, and the United Kingdom (75,76). This randomized trial is designed to determine whether the duration and dose intensity of therapy of the highly successful French LMB-89 protocol can be reduced without compromising outcome (47). They found that the intensity of therapy could be safely reduced in group B patients without compromising outcome; however, for group C patients, treatment intensity could not be safely reduced. Immunotherapeutic approaches may ultimately permit additional reduction in the intensity of cytotoxic therapy (75,76). In this regard, the Children's Oncology Group (COG) has designed a pilot study that incorporates rituximab (i.e., anti-CD20) into the LMB-96 regimen. Preliminary results for group B patients suggest that this is feasible (77). If feasibility is confirmed, subsequent studies may focus on further reduction of cytotoxic dose intensity.

LYMPHOBLASTIC LYMPHOMA (PRECURSOR B- OR T-CELL LYMPHOBLASTIC LYMPHOMA/ LEUKEMIA)

LBLs and leukemias are neoplasms that resemble either T- or B-lineage lymphoid precursors (Tables 33.3 and 33.4). ALL and LBL have overlapping morphologic, immunophenotypic, and cytogenetic features, and, thus, the distinction between these two processes is considered by many to be largely arbitrary (78–80). The International Lymphoma Study Group and the WHO have designated these malignancies "precursor B- and T-lymphoblastic leukemia/lymphoma" in the updated REAL and WHO classifications (27,28). However, subtle immunophenotypic, molecular, and cytogenetic differences suggest that primary ALL and LBLs may be biologically different. Typically, the diagnosis of lymphoma is reserved for those patients presenting with predominantly extramedullary involvement, whereas the reverse is accepted for a diagnosis of leukemia. The cutoff for this distinction is largely arbitrary. Although the most widely accepted criteria define ALL by >25% lymphoblasts in the bone marrow, some require only 10% marrow lymphoblasts for this diagnosis (9,81).

Histologically, LBLs show a diffuse growth pattern and are composed of a uniform population of small to medium-sized blastic cells. The neoplastic cells are characterized by scanty cytoplasm, sometimes cleaved and convoluted nuclear outlines, finely and homogeneously dispersed nuclear chromatin, and small nucleoli.

Immunophenotypic studies have revealed only minor differences in antigen expression between B and T LBLs and their leukemic counterparts. However, as opposed to acute leukemia, approximately 90% of LBLs are of T lineage, and the remaining 10%, of B lineage (82–86). Rarely is LBL derived from a natural killer cell of origin (85,87,88). Precursor B-cell LBL typically expresses CD10, CD19, CD20 (may be very weak or absent), CD22, CD24, PAX-5, CD34, CD45 (weaker than normal lymphocytes), and human leukocyte antigen-DR. Cytoplasmic antigens include CD22, CD79a, and TdT, and in a subset of cases, μ Ig heavy chains (Igμ). Some of the cases that have cytoplasmic Igμ expression may also express weak surface Igμ (so called transitional pre-B ALL/LBL). Precursor B-cell lesions may be subclassified according to their pattern of Ig expression into several stages of maturation, without significant prognostic implications (Table 33.4). T-cell LBLs are more heterogeneous in their pattern of T-antigen expression. All T-cell LBLs express CD45 and cytoplasmic CD3, and many cases may show weak surface CD3 expression. Other T-cell antigens that are consistently expressed include CD2, CD5, and CD7. Very commonly, the blasts have a cortical thymic immunophenotype that also includes expression of CD1a, CD4, CD8, and CD21. Other antigens that may be expressed in these cases are CD10 and CD56. Notably, an occasional T-cell LBL may be negative for CD34, TdT, and human leukocyte antigen-DR. Careful exclusion of peripheral T-cell NHLs may be required in these cases. Aberrant expression of myeloid-associated antigen, a feature of some B- and T-lineage ALLs, can also occur in LBLs (83,89,90).

Reported cytogenetic studies of LBLs have been fewer than those for ALL and include small numbers of patients (91–93). Additionally, many reports describing molecular and cytogenetic findings of LBL include cases of ALL. Thus, an accurate summary of cytogenetic abnormalities in LBL devoid of the influence of ALL remains elusive. T LBL and T-cell ALL demonstrate similar chromosomal abnormalities for the most part. Chromosome abnormalities involving the T-cell receptor are relatively common, and include abnormalities at bands 7q34-36, 7p15, and 14q11 (92,93). The t(9;17) translocation appears more commonly in T LBL than in T-cell ALL (92,94). Patients with this translocation often present with a mediastinal mass and have an aggressive disease course. The t(8;13)(p11;q11-14) has been described in rare cases of T LBL that present with myeloid hyperplasia and eosinophilia (95–97). The t(10;11)(p13-14;q14-21) is an uncommon but recurring translocation associated with ALL, acute myelogenous leukemia, and LBL (98,99). Unlike the case in ALL, cytogenetic abnormalities have not been shown to be of prognostic significance in LBL. Gene expression profile (microarray) studies have demonstrated possible clinically relevant subgroups of T-cell ALL, but similar studies of LBL have yet to be reported (100,101).

Treatment

For children with LBL, various strategies have been implemented to further improve the treatment outcome achieved with LSA$_2$L$_2$ (see Table 33.6) (57,64,67,73). The French Society of Pediatric Oncology incorporated courses of high-dose methotrexate into an LSA$_2$L$_2$ backbone with excellent results (64). Other groups have also obtained successful outcomes with the inclusion of high-dose methotrexate (73). Of these, the German Berlin-Frankfurt-Münster (BFM) group has

reported results among the best (i.e., 5-year EFS of 90%) with a regimen (BFM-90) whose consolidation phase includes four courses of high-dose methotrexate (5 g per m^2 given every 2 weeks) (73). This improvement in outcome may be the result of higher intracellular levels of methotrexate polyglutamates achieved with a higher dose of methotrexate (102). A subsequent BFM trial demonstrated that prophylactic cranial irradiation (CRT) could be safely eliminated without compromising outcome (103). Other refinements in therapy that are thought to contribute to improved treatment outcome include the incorporation of a reinduction (i.e., reintensification) phase, as well as the incorporation of new active agents (57–59,73).

In the United States, the COG is currently performing a randomized trial to determine whether extended intrathecal administration methotrexate can be safely used as a substitute for high-dose methotrexate in the context of the very successful BFM regimen (73), which includes a consolidation phase featuring four doses of high-dose methotrexate at (5 g per m^2) given every other week. Data from a POG study suggested that high-dose methotrexate may not be necessary, in the context of a regimen based on anthracycline and L-asparaginase, for children with advanced-stage LBL (104), even though it was necessary for T-cell leukemia. The COG's current trial is also testing the benefit of an intensification phase of cyclophosphamide and an anthracycline. Early response, as measured by diagnostic imaging and minimal residual disease studies, will also be evaluated.

In the POG limited stage NHL trial, which featured three courses of CHOP followed by a 24-week maintenance phase of 6-mercaptopurine and methotrexate, one third of children with LBL experienced relapse even with the maintenance phase; however, the majority were successfully salvaged, and their overall survival did not differ from that of children with other histologic subtypes (49). Some groups, such as the French Society of Pediatric Oncology, take a more aggressive initial approach to avoid the need to retreat (64).

In an attempt to reduce the 30% rate of relapse observed with the POG approach (49) (three cycles of CHOP followed by a 24-week maintenance phase of 6-mercaptopurine and methotrexate) without exposing patients to the toxicity of therapy for high-risk T-cell ALL, the COG is currently studying a regimen similar in design to a treatment plan for standard-risk ALL.

TABLE 33.6

TREATMENT OUTCOME FOR ADVANCED-STAGE LYMPHOBLASTIC NHL

Protocol	Stage	No. of patients	EFS rate	Reference
LSA$_2$L$_2$ (modified) POG 7615	III	24	3-y EFS = 57%	(44)
LSA$_2$L$_2$ (modified) CCG-551	III/IV	124	5-y EFS = 64%	(194)
BFM 90[a]	III	82	5-y EFS = 90% ± 3%	(73)
	IV	19	5-y EFS = 95% ± 5%	
X-H SJCRH	III/IV	22	4-y DFS = 73%	(57)
APO (Dana-Farber)	III/IV	21	3-y DFS = 58% ± 23%	(58)
A-COP + (POG)	III	33	3-y DFS = 54% ± 9%	(59)

CCG, Children's Cancer Group; DFS, disease-free survival.
[a] Excellent results confirmed in BFM95 that featured elimination of prophylactic CRT (103).

TABLE 33.7

TISSUE MARKERS OF LARGE CELL LYMPHOMAS OF CHILDREN

	CD20	CD79	Ig	CD5	CD3	CD30	CD15	ALK	CA	BCL2	BCL6
ALCL[a]	–	–	–	–/+	–/+	+	–/+	+/–	+	–	–/+
PTL	–	–	–	+/–	+/–	–/+	–	–	–/+	–	–/+
DLBCL	+	+	+/–	–/+	–	–	–	–/+	–	+/–	+/–
MLBCL	+	+	+/–	–	–	+/–	–	–	–	+	+

CA, cytotoxic antigens (perforin, T-cell–restricted intracellular antigen-1, granzyme B); PTL, peripheral T-cell lymphoma.
[a] Marker features are for ALCL with ALK gene rearrangements. Rare DLBCLs with plasmablastic morphology may express ALK.
From Falini B, Mason DY. Proteins encoded by genes involved in chromosomal alterations in lymphoma and leukemia: clinical value of their detection by immunocytochemistry. *Blood* 2002;99:409–426, with permission.

LARGE CELL LYMPHOMA

Large cell lymphoma, as the name implies, is composed of large lymphoid cells that are larger than the diameter of a histiocytic nucleus or two to three times the width of small inactive-appearing lymphocytes. These lymphomas may be of B- or T-cell origin (see Table 33.7). The WHO (28) classification recognizes multiple clinicopathologic entities that share morphologic features of large cell lymphoma and occur most commonly in children, including DLBCL (and its mediastinal or thymic variant), peripheral T-cell-unspecified, and ALCL. In the St. Jude Children's Research Hospital experience, T-cell ALCLs account for 40% to 50% of pediatric large cell lymphomas, DLBCLs comprise another 30% to 40%, and the remainder consists of nonanaplastic peripheral T-cell lymphomas. Investigations have revealed few morphologic and immunophenotypic differences between the large cell lymphomas of adults and children. However, strikingly few investigations of the laboratory and biologic features of pediatric large cell lymphomas other than the anaplastic large cell type have been reported.

Treatment

The treatment of large cell lymphoma has historically been selected on the basis of histology in the United States and on the basis of immunophenotype in Europe (105). Most of the regimens in the United States have been CHOP based (see Table 33.8) (42,45,46,54,70,105–107). With these approaches,

approximately 60% to 70% of patients are long-term event-free survivors. In a randomized trial performed by the COG comparing Adriamycin, prednisone, and vincristine (APO) with Adriamycin, cyclophosphamide, vincristine, and prednisone (ACOP+), patients with a B-cell immunophenotype appeared to have a survival advantage, although the number of immunophenotyped cases was relatively small (46). In Europe, children with B-cell large cell lymphoma are treated with regimens used for BL. With the French LMB-89 regimen, children with B-cell large cell lymphoma had results comparable to those of children with BL (47). Current trials in the United States feature an immunophenotype-directed approach.

ANAPLASTIC LARGE CELL LYMPHOMA

ALCL is defined as a peripheral T-cell lymphoma characterized histologically by the presence, in variable proportions, of large, pleomorphic ("hallmark") neoplastic cells that express CD30, cytotoxic proteins, and, in the majority of pediatric cases, the anaplastic lymphoma kinase (ALK) (28). It has a peak incidence in adolescence and a propensity toward involvement of extranodal sites (108,109).

Histologically, ALCL may replace the underlying tissue architecture partially or completely. In completely effaced tissue, it usually has a diffuse growth pattern. In partially effaced lymph nodes, the lymphoma cells occupy preferentially the sinuses (where they may mimic metastatic tumors) and the interfollicular area. ALCL usually comprises variable

TABLE 33.8

TREATMENT OUTCOME FOR ADVANCED-STAGE LARGE CELL NHL

Protocol	Stage	No. of patients	EFS rate	Reference
CHOP	III and IV	21	3-y EFS = 62% ± 11%	(195)
MACOP-B	III and IV	11	3-y EFS = 55% ± 16%	(62)
DAC	III and IV	25	5-y EFS = 64 ± 9%	(70)
Randomized:				
COMP vs. LSA$_2$L$_2$	III and IV	42	5-y EFS = 52%	(42)
	III and IV	18	5-y EFS = 43%	
APO vs. ACOP+	III and IV	62	3-y EFS = 72% ± 6%	(106)
	III and IV	58	4-y EFS = 62% ± 7%	

numbers of small, medium-sized, and large "hallmark" neoplastic cells. The hallmark cells are large cells with eccentrically placed, monocytoid, or horseshoe-shaped nuclei. Often these cells are multinucleated with the nuclei forming a wreath-like appearance. Some have features resembling the Reed-Sternberg cells of Hodgkin lymphoma. Several morphologic variants of ALK+ ALCL are recognized, including the common, lymphohistiocytic, small cell, and monomorphic (110). They lack prognostic significance. The common variant accounts for >70% of cases and features the hallmark large anaplastic tumor cells. Varying numbers of small and medium lymphoid cells may also be present. Erythrophagocytosis by histiocytes can also be found in some cases. The lymphohistiocytic variant accounts for <20% of ALCL in children, and consists of a mixture of small and larger lymphoid cells and many histiocytes (111). The histiocytes may be so numerous as to partially obscure the lymphoid cells (112,113). The small cell variant accounts for <10% of cases, and may not be recognized if the hallmark cells are scarce and immunophenotyping and cytogenetic studies are not performed (114). The monomorphous variant consists of sheets of monomorphous large cells that resemble other large cell lymphomas, and have a high mitotic rate and a "starry-sky" appearance. Other rare forms of ALCL include sarcomatoid, signet ring, granulomatous, neutrophil–rich, and eosinophil rich (115–117). Rare examples of children and adults who present with a leukemic process or who develop a leukemic phase during the course of their disease have been described (118–123). These cases typically have a predominantly small cell appearance, with only rare large immunoblastic and hallmark cells.

Immunophenotypically, the neoplastic cells of all ALCL cases express CD30 (Ki-1) and the epithelial membrane antigen (EMA) (124). Most cases of pediatric ALCL also express ALK, which may be present in the cytoplasm only, or in the nucleus and cytoplasm, depending on the underlying genetic lesion (125). Most ALCLs express one or more T-cell-associated antigens, including CD2, CD3, CD4, CD7, or CD45RO, as well as cytoplasmic cytotoxic cell-associated proteins T-cell–restricted intracellular antigen-1, granzyme B, or perforin. T-cell antigens CD5 and CD8 are usually negative. Some cases lack demonstrable T-cell antigens but have evidence of T-cell receptor gene rearrangement. These cases are referred to as null/T ALCL (28). Most ALCLs express one or several myeloid antigens, which may include CD11c, CD15, and CD33, as well as the histiocytic marker CD68.

Most cases of ALK+ ALCL (75% to 85%) harbor the t(2;5)(p23;q35) translocation, which juxtaposes the kinase domain of ALK (at 2p23) to the nucleophosmin (NPM) gene (at 5q35) (94,126,127). Several other translocations of ALK have been described, including t(1;2)(q25;p23), t(2;3)(p23;q21), inv(2)(p23q35), t(2;22), t(2;17)(p23;q11), and t(2;19)(p23;p13) (128–130). The gene partners fused to the ALK gene in all of these translocation encode for constitutively expressed proteins that can dimerize and, thus, lead to the overexpression and activation of the kinase domain of ALK. This is considered to represent the main oncogenic event in these lymphomas. The NPM-ALK fusion product, containing a portion of NPM that dimerizes and also targets the protein for nuclear (nucleolar) localization, leads to expression of ALK in the nucleus and the cytoplasm of the neoplastic cells (131). In all other fusion proteins, the partner gene products lack nuclear localization

properties, thus leading to expression restricted to cytoplasm. Of note, ALK expression is not limited to ALCL, and may also be encountered in other types of neoplasms, including some B-lineage plasmablastic lymphomas, inflammatory myofibroblastic tumors, rhabdomyosarcomas, and neuroblastoma (132–136).

In adults, ALK protein expression in ALCL is a favorable prognostic factor (137–139). Treatment responses in adults are similar for patients with the t(2;5) or its variant translocations (140). A similar favorable outcome is found in children with immunochemically documented ALK-positive ALCL (63,111,141). In a multivariate analysis of childhood ALCL, mediastinal, visceral (lung, liver, spleen), and skin involvement are poor prognostic factors (111,142).

Treatment

The optimal treatment approach for ALCLs has yet to be elucidated (105,111). Although the treatment strategies studied thus far have been quite varied, the estimated 3-year EFS rates for children with advanced-stage disease are approximately 60% to 70% (105). A POG randomized study of APO versus ACOP+ showed no significant difference in outcome between the two arms ($p = 0.90$) (46). One of the best results to date was that reported by the BFM, which used its B-cell lymphoma protocol to treat children with ALCL, which typically has a non-B-cell immunophenotype. It achieved an 80% probability of 3-year EFS with this approach (63).

There are currently two major initiatives worldwide for the treatment of ALCL. Both of these build on the results of a French study showing that patients with recurrent ALCL could be successfully salvaged with single-agent vinblastine (143). In Europe, a multinational trial is using the very successful BFM regimen (63) for B-cell lymphoma, with randomization to a vinblastine maintenance phase. In the United States, the COG is conducting a study that builds on the successful results of the APO regimen (60), which comprises primarily APO. In this study, the substitution of vinblastine for vincristine is being studied in a randomized fashion.

DIFFUSE LARGE B-CELL LYMPHOMA

DLBCL is a lymphoma of mature B-cell immunophenotype composed of large neoplastic cells with a diffuse growth pattern. These lymphomas are postulated to be of GC or post-GC B-cell origin.

Histologically, these lymphomas have a diffuse growth pattern with variable degrees of associated sclerosis. They are composed in variable proportions of centroblasts, immunoblasts, and, less commonly, large anaplastic and Reed-Sternberg-like cells. Centroblasts are large cells with scanty cytoplasm, round or indented nuclei, vesicular chromatin, and one to several nucleoli. Immunoblasts are large cells with ample basophilic cytoplasm, marginated nuclear chromatin, and a single prominent centrally located nucleolus. Depending on the relative proportions of these cell types, several morphologic variants have been described, including centroblastic, immunoblastic, and T-cell/histiocyte-rich and anaplastic (28). In the T-cell/histiocyte-rich variant, the bulk of the tumor consists of benign inflammatory cells that may obscure a minority of large neoplastic cells. Of note, these morphologic variants do not have prognostic implications at this time. Rare cases of plasmablastic DLBCL, showing immunohistochemical expression of ALK, and the presence of ALK fusion transcripts have been reported (123,133). These cases constitute a separate category in the WHO classification.

Immunophenotypically the lymphoma cells of DLBCL express CD45 and bright CD20, as well as other B-cell antigens (CD19, CD22, CD24, CD79a, PAX-5). A subset of DLBCLs expresses follicle center cell-associated antigens, such as CD10, BCL-6, and BCL-2. Some DLBCLs are positive for CD5. CD30 expression is seen in the anaplastic and T-cell rich subtypes. Light chain-restricted Ig expression may be demonstrated in many cases, although many of these lymphomas may lack immunophenotypic evidence of Ig expression. Although some of the DLBCLs may show high proliferation indices by Ki-67 immunohistochemistry, they typically do not exceed 90%, a feature helpful in the differential diagnosis with BL. The ALK+ plasmablastic B-cell lymphomas have a distinct immunophenotype, lacking expression of mature B-cell antigens such as CD20, and while they express weak CD79a, CD138, and cytoplasmic Ig, typically IgA. They are CD30 negative in most cases (132).

Cytogenetically, DLBCLs typically have complex chromosomal abnormalities. Immunophenotypic and genetic studies, including gene expression profiling by several methodologies, have shown DLBCL to be a biologically heterogeneous group of neoplasms, which includes at least two major subgroups: a GC-like group and an activated peripheral blood B-cell-like group (144,145). The GC-like group shows expression of CD10 and BCL-6, while negative for MUM1, contains ongoing Ig gene mutations, may show 12q12 gains, amplification of c-rel gene (chromosome 2p), and appears to have a more favorable outcome. A significant number of the GC-like tumors occurring in adults also harbor the t(14;18), IgH/BCL2 translocation seen in FL. The activated peripheral blood B-cell-like group lacks expression of CD10 and BCL-6, as well as ongoing Ig gene mutations, may show trisomy 3 or gains on chromosomes 3q or 18q21-22, and losses at 6q21-22, has constitutive activation of nuclear factor-κB, and is associated with an inferior prognosis. Recent studies have shown that in pediatric DLBCL, the distribution and characteristics of these subgroups are different, with the centroblastic morphologic variant and the GC-like subtype being much more frequent in children when compared with the adult tumors, and with a much lower incidence of the activated peripheral blood B-cell-like subtype in this age group (146). In addition, the t(14;18) appears to be virtually absent in the pediatric GC-like DLBCL.

MLBCL is a subtype of DLBCL that accounts for <10% of all large cell MLBCLs in children. It is thought to originate in biologically distinct thymic B cells. Histologically, MLBCLs can present as any of the DLBCL morphologic variants. Approximately half of the cases have significant associated fibrosis. The neoplastic cells may have the appearance of centroblasts or immunoblasts, or may have abundant pale cytoplasm and markedly lobated, "flower-like" nuclear outlines (so-called "clear-cell" appearance).

Immunophenotypically, MLBCL has a mature B-cell immunophenotype, with expression of CD45 and of B-cell antigens, including CD19, CD20, CD79a, and PAX-5 (147). There is typically variable coexpression of CD30. Some cases may express CD23. Other antigens expressed include BCL-2 and BCL-6. The neoplastic cells are characteristically negative for CD10, CD21, Ig, and human leukocyte antigen class I and II molecules.

Limited conventional cytogenetic data are available (148). Alternative approaches have shown gains on chromosome 2p (25% of the cases), with amplification of c-REL as well, and gains on 9p (50% to 75% of the cases) with amplification of the JAK2 gene. Other alterations involve chromosomes 6p (major histocompatibility complex class I locus), Xq, 12q, and the P53 gene. Gene expression profiling has demonstrated a close resemblance of this lymphoma with classic Hodgkin lymphoma, suggesting that, at least in the mediastinal location, these neoplasms may share a common origin from a thymic B cell (149).

Treatment

Children with DLBCL are currently treated on regimens designed for children with BL, with comparable outcomes achieved, as reported in the international collaborative LMB-96 study (75).

Despite previous designations of MLBCL as an aggressive neoplasm, current treatment regimens in children and adults with localized disease induce remissions with an approximate 80% overall survival rate (150,151). Pediatric patients presenting with extrathoracic disease fair less well (151). Rebiopsy of residual posttreatment masses is necessary to distinguish between residual tumor and persistent fibrosis and necrosis.

Children with MLBCL are generally treated with the same regimens used for those with DLBCL and BL. However, these children generally have a slightly inferior outcome compared with that of DLBCL, as reflected in the LMB-96 study results (75).

UNCOMMON PEDIATRIC LYMPHOMAS

Rare lymphomas of children and adolescents include FL, hepatosplenic lymphoma, mycosis fungoides, panniculitis T-cell lymphoma, marginal zone lymphoma (MZL) (nodal, and extranodal or mucosa-associated lymphoid tissue [MALT] type), human T-cell lymphotropic virus I-associated leukemia/lymphoma, and natural killer lymphoma (152–165). For the most part, the clinical and biologic features of these lymphomas in children resemble their adult counterparts. However, because of their rarity in children, clinical and biologic features of these lymphomas can only be gleaned from compilations of case reports. The diagnosis of these rare lymphomas in children is often delayed or initially interpreted as a reactive process or as one of the more common pediatric lymphomas. Pediatric FLs and nodal MZLs appear to have a spectrum of clinicopathologic features distinct from the tumors seen in adults.

PEDIATRIC FOLLICULAR LYMPHOMA

In addition to rare cases of classic FLs, resembling phenotypically and genetically those seen in adults, children may present with a distinct subtype of FL, which appears to be more common in this age group (166–172). This subtype of lymphoma typically involves a single site (most commonly lymph nodes in the head and neck area or testis/epididymis). Histologically, it is characterized by effacement of the normal architecture by neoplastic follicles composed of large, irregular GCs, with thin or absent mantle zones. The neoplastic GCs are typically composed of monotonous predominantly large centroblasts, with occasional cases showing numerous mitotic figures and a "starry-sky" appearance due to numerous tingible-body macrophages. Most of these cases correspond to the grade 2 or 3 (28) adult FL, although it is not clear if this correlates with a similar prognostic significance in children. Immunophenotypically, the neoplastic cells express CD20, CD10, BCL-6, and, in some cases, CD43, and are negative for BCL-2. Staining for CD21 highlights the expanded follicular dendritic cell network that underlies the neoplastic follicles.

Genetically, pediatric FL lacks, in most cases, the t(14;18) and BCL-2 rearrangements, unlike adult FL. It usually harbors clonal Ig and BCL-6 gene rearrangements. It also lacks P53 overexpression (as opposed to the high-grade adult-type FLs). All of these features suggest that these lymphomas represent a distinct clinicopathologic entity that may warrant alternate therapeutic options for these patients.

Treatment

There are relatively little data on the treatment of children with FL. Historically, many have been successfully treated with low-intensity CHOP-based regimens. In one retrospective study, FLs in children were found to differ biologically from those in adults. Specifically, the majority of those occurring in children are BCL2 negative; when BCL2 positive, they tend to be associated with advanced in stage and poorer treatment outcome (166). In some studies, children with completely resected limited-stage disease have been observed rather than being given systemic chemotherapy (173).

PEDIATRIC MARGINAL ZONE LYMPHOMA

MZL likely represents <1% of all pediatric lymphomas, and only limited series of patients have been reported to date. MZL is a mature B-cell lymphoma derived from post-GC B cells (WHO classification). It may involve primarily lymph nodes (nodal MZL) or an extranodal site harboring resident or acquired MALT. The latter are designated extranodal MZL (EMZL) or MALT lymphomas. Nodal MZL is the more common presentation in children and young adults, typically involving lymph nodes in the head and neck area. EMZL is more common in older children, and is also most frequently associated with sites in the head and neck areas (such as submandibular and parotid glands, orbit and ocular adnexae, thyroid gland). In children, nodal MZL shows a striking male predominance (male-female ratio 20:1), whereas EMZL occurs with equal frequency in male and female patients. Morphologically, MZLs at all locations are characterized by small to medium-sized lymphocytes that often have moderate amounts of pale cytoplasm and round to indented nuclei ("monocytoid cells"). These cells may be located at the periphery of benign residual follicles, which they often infiltrate ("follicular colonization"), or may fill and expand the interfollicular area. In extranodal locations, these neoplastic cells may infiltrate and destroy adjacent epithelial structures ("lympho-epithelial lesions"). In children, the residual benign follicles very often show features of progressive transformation of GCs, a pattern of benign follicular hyperplasia most often seen in young males, in lymph nodes from the head and neck area.

Immunophenotypically, MZL cells usually express B-cell antigens (CD19, CD20, CD22, PAX-5), as well as CD43 and BCL-2, while often negative for CD5, CD10, and BCL-6. These features are useful in the differential diagnosis with other low-grade B-cell lymphomas, including pediatric FL. These lymphomas also express surface Ig with light chain restriction.

Molecular studies typically show evidence of clonal Ig gene rearrangements. A subset of EMZL may show rearrangements of the MALT1 gene, typically as a result of t(11;18)(q21;q21) or its variant translocations. These abnormalities have not been reported to date in pediatric patients.

As a cautionary note, a pattern of benign marginal zone hyperplasia involving tonsils and the appendix has been described in pediatric patients. These cases show features overlapping morphologically and immunophenotypically with EMZL (including Ig λ light chain restriction) but lack evidence of clonality by molecular methods.

Treatment

Although there are little published data on treatment approaches for MZL in children, it appears that they have an excellent prognosis with conservative treatment, which in some cases has included local irradiation, excision, and close follow up, or chemotherapy. Additional biologic and clinical data on this rare subtype of pediatric NHL may provide insights into more uniform and potentially targeted treatment approaches.

Relapse

Although there has been significant progress in the treatment of childhood NHL, approximately 25% to 30% of children with these diseases will experience treatment failure and have refractory or recurrent disease (1). The prognosis for these children is generally considered to be poor; therefore, most investigators consider high-dose chemotherapy followed by an intensification phase with either autologous or allogeneic hematopoietic stem cell transplantation (HSCT). However, such strategies remain somewhat controversial, and a recent publication has questioned their benefit (174).

Although there are relatively few reports on the role of HSCT in childhood NHL, a number of studies have suggested that some children with refractory or recurrent NHL benefit from this treatment approach (69,175–183). For example, European cooperative group trials have demonstrated successful salvage of children with BL who have a poor early response to initial therapy by using high-dose multiagent chemotherapy followed by autologous hematopoietic stem cell rescue (69,177,179,180,182). The Societé Française d'Oncologie Pediatrique reported that eight of 24 children who had HSCT for refractory or recurrent NHL are long-term disease-free survivors (180). The Spanish Working Party for Bone Marrow Transplantation reported that of 46 children who underwent HSCT for refractory or recurrent NHL or high-risk NHL in first complete remission, 58% were event-free survivors after transplantation (179). In a St. Jude report of 20 children with refractory or recurrent NHL, approximately 45% were alive and free of disease after HSCT (184). The available reports vary with regard to the type of HSCT (allogeneic vs. autologous), histologic subtype of NHL, salvage therapy, and preparative regimen used; therefore, these trials must be compared with caution.

Histologic subtype does appear to be an important factor in determining the appropriate type of transplant (i.e., autologous vs. allogeneic) for children with recurrent NHL. Some of the earliest studies of the use of autologous HSCT for NHL demonstrated its efficacy in children with BL who were poor early responders (i.e., induction failure) (176). These observations have been validated by subsequent studies (69,180). However, it is less clear whether allogeneic or autologous HSCT is optimal for children with BL who develop widespread recurrent disease involving the bone marrow. Allogeneic HSCT from a matched sibling donor is favored by many investigators, although more data are clearly needed. For children with recurrent large cell lymphoma, various studies have shown that autologous HSCT is a very effective salvage approach (178,184). In contrast, the results of autologous HSCT for recurrent or refractory LBL have been less encouraging (174).

Various preparative regimens have proved to be effective in HSCT strategies for children with recurrent or refractory NHL (see Table 33.9) (69,175–184). Carmustine, cytarabine, cyclophosphamide, and thioguanine, and carmustine, etoposide, cytarabine, and melphalan are two of the earliest multiagent drug combinations used successfully (175,176,183). A report by the Société Française d'Oncologie Pediatrique (180) attributed its successful salvage of children with refractory or recurrent B-cell lymphomas to the inclusion of high-dose busulfan in the preparative regimen. In another study, excellent results for children with peripheral T-cell lymphoma were obtained by using a regimen that featured thiotepa; however, oral mucositis was reported as a significant toxicity in some children (178).

Currently, many investigators consider autologous HSCT for children with BL who have a poor early response and for those with large-cell lymphoma who have chemosensitive recurrent disease. An allogeneic HSCT is often considered for children with systemic, chemosensitive recurrent LBL or BL.

There is clearly a need, however, for additional prospective clinical trials examining HSCT strategies for children with refractory or recurrent NHL of all histologies and relapse patterns. One report suggested that a potential graft versus lymphoma effect be studied in those who experience relapse because of the very intensive initial therapy that children with NHL now receive (182).

Radiation Therapy

The role of local radiation therapy (RT) in the management of childhood NHL has been changing as the survival of children with NHL has been increasing with more effective chemotherapy regimens. The improved outcomes with chemotherapy have allowed trials to evaluate the need for local RT. The POG carried out a prospective randomized trial from 1987 to 1991 that compared 8 months of chemotherapy with radiotherapy to 8 months of chemotherapy without radiotherapy in children with early stage NHL (49). The RT administered during induction chemotherapy consisted of 27 Gy in 18 fractions. Chemotherapy consisted of three cycles of CHOP, followed by a 24-week maintenance phase that included 6-mercaptopurine and methotrexate. At 5 years, the rates of continuous complete remission were 88% for those receiving radiotherapy, and 86% for those treated without radiotherapy. A second trial built on the results of the first and compared 8 months of chemotherapy with 9 weeks of chemotherapy (49). In the subsequent trial, radiotherapy was omitted. The 5 year continuous complete remission rates were 89% for children treated with 9 weeks of chemotherapy and 86% for those given 8 months of chemotherapy.

The management of localized NHL of bone has traditionally included RT. On the initial POG trial, the subset of children with primary lymphoma of bone was not randomized on the first trial and was nonrandomly treated with 37.5 Gy of radiotherapy. The results of three consecutive POG trials that included 31 patients with localized NHL of bone were reported; seven had received chemotherapy and radiotherapy, and 24 were treated with chemotherapy without the addition of RT (185). All patients achieved complete remission; one child with LBL had relapse in the testicle 1 year after completion of therapy. There were no local relapses. Based on these results, the current management of localized NHL of bone involves chemotherapy without consolidative RT.

TABLE 33.9

HSCT PREPARATIVE REGIMENS FOR NHL IN CHILDREN

	Regimen or group	Components	Reference
1)	BACT:	Carmustine, cytarabine, cyclophosphamide, thioguanine	(176,177)
2)	BEAM:	Carmustine, etoposide, cytarabine, melphalan	(176,177)
3)	Spanish Working Party:	Cyclophosphamide, TBI	(179)
4)	French (Société Française d'Oncologie Pediatrique):	Busulfan, cyclophosphamide, melphalan	(180)
5)	Nebraska:	Thiotepa, Etoposide, TBI	(178)

TBI, total body irradiation.

Children with advanced NHL do not benefit from the addition of involved-field RT, as demonstrated in a randomized trial from St. Jude Children's Research Hospital (186).

CRT has been eliminated as part of central nervous system prophylaxis in childhood NHL, although some institutions continue to include CRT for the treatment of advanced LBL. RT is used in patients with relapsed or refractory disease and in the palliation of symptomatic end-stage lymphoma. Children with persistent disease following chemotherapy, with relapsed or refractory disease, may be considered for high-dose chemotherapy protocols, with stem cell rescue, if they have chemoresponsive disease. In such patients, RT can be used to consolidate residual disease either before or after high-dose therapy, although no prospective randomized trials in pediatrics have been done to determine the benefit to the addition of RT. RT can be useful in the palliation of symptomatic incurable disease. Hyperfractionation or accelerated fractionation can be useful to obtain responses in rapidly growing tumors. The elimination of RT in the management of childhood NHL can help to decrease the long-term sequelae in survivors. The late effects include musculoskeletal deformities, secondary malignancies, hypothyroidism, as well as cardiac and pulmonary sequelae (186).

Late Effects

Because the cure rates for children with NHL have improved, many studies have focused on reducing the risk of treatment-related late effects. Three of the most serious treatment-related late effects are infertility, cardiotoxicity, and second malignancies. Various trials have explored the possibility of eliminating involved-field radiation, whereas others have attempted to eliminate or reduce the intensity of certain chemotherapeutic agents that are highly associated with specific sequelae, without compromising treatment outcome.

Chemotherapy with alkylating agents, such as cyclophosphamide, results in a dose-related depletion of germinal cells and tends to be more gonadotoxic in males than females. Recovery of spermatogenesis after cyclophosphamide-induced azoospermia is related to the total cumulative dose received (187). The results of previous trials suggest that sterility is likely at cumulative doses >7.5 g per m^2, whereas fertility is usually maintained at doses <4 g per m^2 (187). The POG has published the results of a randomized trial of APO versus ACOP$^+$ for pediatric large cell lymphoma showing that cyclophosphamide can be eliminated altogether if a relatively anthracycline-rich chemotherapy regimen is used (106). The LMB-96 trial for children with high-grade B-cell lymphomas demonstrated that the cyclophosphamide dose could be safely reduced in the group B patients, but not in the group C patients (75).

The desire to avoid anthracycline-induced cardiac toxicity has also strongly influenced protocol development for children with NHL. Although some adults are reported to tolerate a cumulative dose of doxorubicin of 550 mg per m^2 relatively well, children with ALL who were treated with lower cumulative doses of doxorubicin have shown troubling abnormalities in ventricular afterload and contractility (188). Various factors have been identified as predictive of cardiac dysfunction, including higher anthracycline dose intensity, cumulative anthracycline dose, younger age at the time of therapy, female sex, time interval since completion of therapy,

and combined-modality therapy with mediastinal irradiation (189,190). A randomized trial by the Children's Cancer Group demonstrated that the addition of Adriamycin did not improve the outcome achieved with COMP alone (54). Nevertheless, anthracyclines remain an important class of agents in NHL treatment; one example is the use of Adriamycin in the APO regimen for large cell NHL. Therefore, investigations of cardioprotectants, such as the POG Zinecard study, are indicated.

FUTURE DIRECTIONS

Significant progress has been made in the treatment of children with NHL; however, 25% to 30% of children with newly diagnosed NHL will have recurrent or refractory disease despite having received aggressive modern therapy. The development of serious treatment-related late effects is of additional concern. Therefore, the goal of the pediatric oncologist continues to be to improve the treatment result for children with NHL while minimizing or eliminating the risk of therapy induced sequelae. The achievement of this goal will require further refinement of our current risk-adapted therapeutic approach. As additional clinical and biologic prognostic factors are identified, children with a poorer prognosis can be targeted with more aggressive or novel therapeutic approaches, whereas those with an excellent prognosis can be targeted with less intensive therapy, thus protecting them from undesirable treatment-related late effects.

The treatment outcome for children with NHL may be improved in a number of ways: the development of new active agents, the study of novel ways to give presently used agents, and the investigation of new drug combinations. Novel immunotherapeutic approaches may also hold promise. For example, rituximab has been shown to be active against certain adult CD20$^+$ B-cell lymphomas (191,192). This agent is currently under investigation in children (77). Small molecule inhibitors, which have been shown to be active against adult chronic myelogenous leukemia, may also benefit children with certain NHL subtypes, such as the ALK$^+$ ALCL.

The molecular characterization of the chromosomal abnormalities in pediatric NHL has proven to be valuable in disease classification, confirmation of diagnosis, and evaluation of response to therapy (i.e., in cases such as ALCL in which minimal residual disease can be assessed by polymerase chain reaction). As mechanisms of molecular pathogenesis are more completely elucidated, insights into novel tumor-specific therapeutic approaches should emerge.

References

1. Sandlund JT, Downing JR, Crist MW. Non-Hodgkin's lymphoma in childhood. *N Engl J Med* 1996;334:1238–1248.
2. Magrath IT. Malignant non-Hodgkin's lymphomas in children. *Hematol Oncol Clin North Am* 1987;1:577–602.
3. Murphy SB, Fairclough DL, Hutchison RE. Non-Hodgkin's lymphomas of childhood: an analysis of the histology, staging, and response to treatment of 338 cases at a single institution. *J Clin Oncol* 1989;7:186–193.
4. Robison L. General principles of the epidemiology of childhood cancer. In: Pizzo PA, Poplack DG, eds. *Principles and practice of pediatric oncology*, 2nd ed. Philadelphia, PA: J.B. Lippincott, 1993:3–10.
5. Young JL Jr., Ries LG, Silverberg E, et al. Cancer incidence, survival, and mortality for children younger than age 15 years. *Cancer* 1986; 58(suppl):598–602.

6. Bleyer WA. The impact of childhood cancer on the United States and the world. *CA Cancer J Clin* 1990;40:355–367.

7. Parker SL, Tong T, Bolden S, et al. Cancer statistics, 1996. *CA Cancer J Clin* 1996;46:5–27.

8. National Cancer Institute sponsored study of classifications of non-Hodgkin's lymphomas: summary and description of a working formulation for clinical usage.The Non-Hodgkin's Lymphoma Pathologic Classification Project. *Cancer* 1982;49:2112–2135.

9. Murphy SB. Classification, staging and end results of treatment of childhood non- Hodgkin's lymphomas: dissimilarities from lymphomas in adults. *Semin Oncol* 1980;7:332–339.

10. Magrath IT. Malignant non-Hodgkin's lymphomas in children. In: Pizzo PA, Poplack DG, eds. *Principles and practice of pediatric oncology*, 4th ed. Philadelphia, PA: Lippincott Williams & Wilkins, 2002:661–705.

11. Murphy SB, Hustu HO, Rivera G, et al. End results of treating children with localized non-Hodgkin's lymphomas with a combined modality approach of lessened intensity. *J Clin Oncol* 1983;1:326–330.

12. Hutchison RE, Pui CH, Murphy SB, et al. Non-Hodgkin's lymphoma in children younger than 3 years. *Cancer* 1988;62:1371–1373.

13. Taylor AM, Metcalfe JA, Thick J, et al. Leukemia and lymphoma in ataxia telangiectasia. *Blood* 1996;87:423–438.

14. McClain KL, Joshi VV, Murphy SB. Cancers in children with HIV infection. *Hematol Oncol Clin North Am* 1996;10:1189–1201.

15. Filipovich AH, Heinitz KJ, Robison LL, et al. The Immunodeficiency Cancer Registry. A research resource. *Am J Pediatr Hematol Oncol* 1987;9:183–184.

16. Gatti RA, Good RA. Occurrence of malignancy in immunodeficiency diseases. A literature review. *Cancer* 1971;28:89–98.

17. Sandlund JT, Fonseca T, Leimig T, et al. Predominance and characteristics of Burkitt lymphoma among children with non-Hodgkin lymphoma in northeastern Brazil. *Leukemia* 1997;11:743–746.

18. Madanat FF, Amr SS, Tarawneh MS, et al. Burkitt's lymphoma in Jordanian children: epidemiological and clinical study. *J Trop Med Hyg* 1986;89:189–191.

19. Shad A, Magrath I. Non-Hodgkin's lymphoma. *Pediatr Clin North Am* 1997;44:863–890.

20. Magrath IT, Bhatia K. Pathogenesis of small noncleaved cell lymphomas (Burkitt's lymphoma). In: Magrath I, ed. *The non-Hodgkin's lymphomas*, 2nd ed. London, UK: Arnold, 1997:385.

21. Gutierrez MI, Bhatia K, Barriga F, et al. Molecular epidemiology of Burkitt's lymphoma from South America: differences in breakpoint location and Epstein-Barr virus association from tumors in other world regions. *Blood* 1992;79:3261–3266.

22. Kadin ME. Ki-1/CD30+ (anaplastic) large-cell lymphoma: maturation of a clinicopathologic entity with prospects of effective therapy. *J Clin Oncol* 1994;12:884–887.

23. Kadin ME. Ki-1-positive anaplastic large-cell lymphoma: a clinicopathologic entity? *J Clin Oncol* 1991;9:533–536.

24. Garrett KM, Hoffer FA, Behm FG, et al. Interventional radiology techniques for the diagnosis of lymphoma or leukemia. *Pediatr Radiol* 2002;32:653–662.

25. Naumann R, Vaic A, Beuthien-Baumann B, et al. Prognostic value of positron emission tomography in the evaluation of post-treatment residual mass in patients with Hodgkin's disease and non-Hodgkin's lymphoma. *Br J Haematol* 2001;115:793–800.

26. Pui CH, Mahmoud HH, Wiley JM, et al. Recombinant urate oxidase for the prophylaxis or treatment of hyperuricemia in patients with leukemia or lymphoma. *J Clin Oncol* 2001;19:697–704.

27. Harris NL, Jaffe ES, Stein H, et al. A revised European-American classification of lymphoid neoplasms: a proposal from the International Lymphoma Study Group. *Blood* 1994;84:1361–1392.

28. Jaffe ES, Harris NL, Stein H, et al. *Pathology and genetics of tumours of haematopoietic and lymphoid tissues*. Lyon, France: IARC Press, 2001.

29. Lukes RJ, Collins RD. Immunologic characterization of human malignant lymphomas. *Cancer* 1974;34(suppl):1488–1503.

30. Raphael M, Gentilhomme O, Tulliez M, et al. Histopathologic features of high-grade non-Hodgkin's lymphomas in acquired immunodeficiency syndrome. The French Study Group of Pathology for Human Immunodeficiency Virus-Associated Tumors. *Arch Pathol Lab Med* 1991;115:15–20.

31. Behm FG CD. Immunophenotyping. In: Pui, C-H, ed. *Childhood leukemias*. New York, NY: Cambridge University Press, 1999:111–141.

32. Navid F, Mosijczuk AD, Head DR, et al. Acute lymphoblastic leukemia with the (8;14)(q24;q32) translocation and FAB L3 morphology associated with a B-precursor immunophenotype: the Pediatric Oncology Group experience. *Leukemia* 1999;13:135–141.

33. Loh ML, Samson Y, Motte E, et al. Translocation (2;8)(p12;q24) associated with a cryptic t(12;21)(p13;q22) TEL/AML1 gene rearrangement in a child with acute lymphoblastic leukemia. *Cancer Genet Cytogenet* 2000;122:79–82.

34. Falini B, Fizzotti M, Pileri S, et al. Bcl-6 protein expression in normal and neoplastic lymphoid tissues. *Ann Oncol* 1997;8(suppl 2):101–104.

35. Kornblau SM, Goodacre A, Cabanillas F. Chromosomal abnormalities in adult non-endemic Burkitt's lymphoma and leukemia: 22 new reports and a review of 148 cases from the literature. *Hematol Oncol* 1991;9:63–78.

36. Krolewski JJ, Dalla-Favera R. Molecular genetic approaches in the diagnosis and classification of lymphoid malignancies. *Hematol Pathol* 1989;3:45–61.

37. Nishida K, Ritterbach J, Repp R, et al. Characterization of chromosome 8 abnormalities by fluorescence in situ hybridization in childhood B-acute lymphoblastic leukemia/non-Hodgkin lymphoma. *Cancer Genet Cytogenet* 1995;79:8–14.

38. Komrokji R, Lancet J, Felgar R, et al. Burkitt's leukemia with precursor B-cell immunophenotype and atypical morphology (atypical Burkitt's leukemia/lymphoma): case report and review of literature. *Leuk Res* 2003;27:561–566.

39. Kuhn-Hallek I, Sage DR, Stein L, et al. Expression of recombination activating genes (RAG-1 and RAG-2) in Epstein-Barr virus-bearing B cells. *Blood* 1995;85:1289–1299.

40. Wilson JB, Levine AJ. The oncogenic potential of Epstein-Barr virus nuclear antigen 1 in transgenic mice. *Curr Top Microbiol Immunol* 1992;182:375–384.

41. Ruf IK, Rhyne PW, Yang H, et al. Epstein-Barr virus regulates c-MYC, apoptosis, and tumorigenicity in Burkitt lymphoma. *Mol Cell Biol* 1999;19:1651–1660.

42. Anderson JR, Jenkin RD, Wilson JF, et al. Long-term follow-up of patients treated with COMP or LSA2L2 therapy for childhood non-Hodgkin's lymphoma: a report of CCG-551 from the Children's Cancer Group. *J Clin Oncol* 1993;11:1024–1032.

43. Wollner N, Burchenal JH, Lieberman PH, et al. Non-Hodgkin's lymphoma in children. A comparative study of two modalities of therapy. *Cancer* 1976;37:123–134.

44. Sullivan MP, Boyett J, Pullen J, et al. Pediatric Oncology Group experience with modified LSA2-L2 therapy in 107 children with non-Hodgkin's lymphoma (Burkitt's lymphoma excluded). *Cancer* 1985;55:323–336.

45. Sandlund JT, Santana V, Abromowitch M, et al. Large cell non-Hodgkin lymphoma of childhood: clinical characteristics and outcome. *Leukemia* 1994;8:30–34.

46. Hutchison RE, Berard CW, Shuster JJ, et al. B-cell lineage confers a favorable outcome among children and adolescents with large-cell lymphoma: a Pediatric Oncology Group study. *J Clin Oncol* 1995;13:2023–2032.

47. Patte C, Auperin A, Michon J, et al. The Societe Francaise d'Oncologie Pediatrique LMB89 protocol: highly effective multiagent chemotherapy tailored to the tumor burden and initial response in 561 unselected children with B-cell lymphomas and L3 leukemia. *Blood* 2001;97:3370–3379.

48. Murphy SB, Bowman WP, Abromowitch M, et al. Results of treatment of advanced-stage Burkitt's lymphoma and B cell (SIg+) acute lymphoblastic leukemia with high-dose fractionated cyclophosphamide and coordinated high-dose methotrexate and cytarabine. *J Clin Oncol* 1986;4:1732–1739.

49. Link MP, Shuster JJ, Donaldson SS, et al. Treatment of children and young adults with early-stage non-Hodgkin's lymphoma. *N Engl J Med* 1997;337:1259–1266.

50. Brecher ML, Schwenn MR, Coppes MJ, et al. Fractionated cyclophosphamide and back to back high dose methotrexate and cytosine arabinoside improves outcome in patients with stage III high grade small noncleaved cell lymphomas (SNCCL): a randomized trial of the Pediatric Oncology Group. *Med Pediatr Oncol* 1997;29:526–533.

51. Bowman WP, Shuster JJ, Cook B, et al. Improved survival for children with B-cell acute lymphoblastic leukemia and stage IV small noncleaved-cell lymphoma: a pediatric oncology group study. *J Clin Oncol* 1996;14:1252–1261.

52. Patte C, Philip T, Rodary C, et al. High survival rate in advanced-stage B-cell lymphomas and leukemias without CNS involvement with a short intensive polychemotherapy: results from the French Pediatric Oncology Society of a randomized trial of 216 children. *J Clin Oncol* 1991;9:123–132.

53. Reiter A, Schrappe M, Ludwig WD, et al. Favorable outcome of B-cell acute lymphoblastic leukemia in childhood: a report of three consecutive studies of the BFM group. *Blood* 1992;80:2471–2478.

54. Sposto R, Meadows AT, Chilcote RR, et al. Comparison of long-term outcome of children and adolescents with disseminated non-lymphoblastic non-Hodgkin lymphoma treated with COMP or daunomycin-COMP: A report from the Children's Cancer Group. *Med Pediatr Oncol* 2001;37:432–441.

55. Magrath IT, Janus C, Edwards BK, et al. An effective therapy for both undifferentiated (including Burkitt's) lymphomas and lymphoblastic lymphomas in children and young adults. *Blood* 1984;63:1102–1111.

56. Schwenn MR, Blattner SR, Lynch E, et al. HiC-COM: a 2-month intensive chemotherapy regimen for children with stage III and IV Burkitt's lymphoma and B-cell acute lymphoblastic leukemia. *J Clin Oncol* 1991;9:133–138.

57. Dahl GV, Rivera G, Pui CH, et al. A novel treatment of childhood lymphoblastic non-Hodgkin's lymphoma: early and intermittent use of teniposide plus cytarabine. *Blood* 1985;66:1110–1114.

58. Weinstein HJ, Cassady JR, Levey R. Long-term results of the APO protocol (vincristine, doxorubicin (adriamycin), and prednisone) for treatment of mediastinal lymphoblastic lymphoma. *J Clin Oncol* 1983;1:537–541.

59. Hvizdala EV, Berard C, Callihan T, et al. Lymphoblastic lymphoma in children—a randomized trial comparing LSA2- L2 with the A-COP+ therapeutic regimen: a Pediatric Oncology Group Study. *J Clin Oncol* 1988;6:26–33.

60. Weinstein HJ, Lack EE, Cassady JR. APO therapy for malignant lymphoma of large cell "histiocytic" type of childhood: analysis of treatment results for 29 patients. *Blood* 1984;64:422–426.

61. Hvizdala EV, Berard C, Callihan T, et al. Nonlymphoblastic lymphoma in children–histology and stage-related response to therapy: a Pediatric Oncology Group study. *J Clin Oncol* 1991;9:1189–1195.

62. Santana VM, Abromowitch M, Sandlund JT, et al. MACOP-B treatment in children and adolescents with advanced diffuse large-cell non-Hodgkin's lymphoma. *Leukemia* 1993;7:187–191.

63. Reiter A, Schrappe M, Tiemann M, et al. Successful treatment strategy for Ki-1 anaplastic large-cell lymphoma of childhood: a prospective analysis of 62 patients enrolled in three consecutive Berlin-Frankfurt-Munster group studies. *J Clin Oncol* 1994;12:899–908.

64. Patte C, Kalifa C, Flamant F, et al. Results of the LMT81 protocol, a modified LSA2L2 protocol with high dose methotrexate, on 84 children with non-B-cell (lymphoblastic) lymphoma. *Med Pediatr Oncol* 1992;20:105–113.

65. Meadows AT, Sposto R, Jenkin RD, et al. Similar efficacy of 6 and 18 months of therapy with four drugs (COMP) for localized non-Hodgkin's lymphoma of children: a report from the Children's Cancer Study Group. *J Clin Oncol* 1989;7:92–99.

66. Patte C, Philip T, Rodary C, et al. Improved survival rate in children with stage III and IV B cell non- Hodgkin's lymphoma and leukemia using multi-agent chemotherapy: results of a study of 114 children from the French Pediatric Oncology Society. *J Clin Oncol* 1986;4:1219–1226.

67. Tubergen DG, Krailo MD, Meadows AT, et al. Comparison of treatment regimens for pediatric lymphoblastic non- Hodgkin's lymphoma: a Children's Cancer Group study. *J Clin Oncol* 1995;13:1368–1376.

68. Reiter A, Schrappe M, Parwaresch R, et al. Non-Hodgkin's lymphomas of childhood and adolescence: results of a treatment stratified for biologic subtypes and stage–a report of the Berlin-Frankfurt-Munster Group. *J Clin Oncol* 1995;13:359–372.

69. Reiter A, Schrappe M, Tiemann M, et al. Improved treatment results in childhood B-cell neoplasms with tailored intensification of therapy: A report of the Berlin-Frankfurt-Munster Group Trial NHL BFM 90. *Blood* 1999;94:3294–3306.

70. Sandlund JT, Santana VM, Hudson MM, et al. Combination of dexamethasone, high-dose cytarabine, and carboplatin is effective for advanced large-cell non-Hodgkin lymphoma of childhood. *Cancer* 2008;113:782–790.

71. Magrath I, Adde M, Shad A, et al. Adults and children with small non-cleaved-cell lymphoma have a similar excellent outcome when treated with the same chemotherapy regimen. *J Clin Oncol* 1996;14:925–934.

72. Adde M, Shad A, Venzon D, et al. Additional chemotherapy agents improve treatment outcome for children and adults with advanced B-cell lymphomas. *Semin Oncol* 1998;25(suppl 4):33–39.

73. Reiter A, Schrappe M, Ludwig WD, et al. Intensive ALL-type therapy without local radiotherapy provides a 90% event-free survival for children with T-cell lymphoblastic lymphoma: a BFM group report. *Blood* 2000;95:416–421.

74. Soussain C, Patte C, Ostronoff M, et al. Small noncleaved cell lymphoma and leukemia in adults. A retrospective study of 65 adults treated with the LMB pediatric protocols. *Blood* 1995;85:664–674.

75. Patte C, Auperin A, Gerrard M, et al. Results of the randomized international FAB/LMB96 trial for intermediate risk B-cell non-Hodgkin lymphoma in children and adolescents: it is possible to reduce treatment for the early responding patients. *Blood* 2007;109:2773–2780.

76. Cairo MS, Gerrard M, Sposto R, et al. Results of a randomized international study of high-risk central nervous system B non-Hodgkin lymphoma and B acute lymphoblastic leukemia in children and adolescents. *Blood* 2007;109:2736–2743.

77. Goldman S, Davenport LJ, Perkins S, et al. *Preliminary Results of a Phase II Study of Chemoimmunotherapy (Rituximab+FAB Chemotherapy) in Children and Adolescents with Intermediate Risk B-Cell NHL: A Children's Oncology Group Report: Proceedings of the Tenth International Conference on Malignant Lymphoma*, 2008.

78. Williams AH, Taylor CR, Higgins GR, et al. Childhood lymphoma-leukemia. I. Correlation of morphology and immunological studies. *Cancer* 1978;42:171–181.

79. Mitchell CD, Gordon I, Chessells JM. Clinical, haematological, and radiological features in T-cell lymphoblastic malignancy in childhood. *Clin Radiol* 1986;37:257–261.

80. Head DR, Behm FG. Acute lymphoblastic leukemia and the lymphoblastic lymphomas of childhood. *Semin Diagn Pathol* 1995;12:325–334.

81. Murphy SB. Childhood non-Hodgkin's lymphoma. *N Engl J Med* 1978; 299:1446–1448.

82. Bernard A, Boumsell L, Reinherz EL, et al. Cell surface characterization of malignant T cells from lymphoblastic lymphoma using monoclonal antibodies: evidence for phenotypic differences between malignant T cells from patients with acute lymphoblastic leukemia and lymphoblastic lymphoma. *Blood* 1981;57:1105–1110.

83. Weiss LM, Bindl JM, Picozzi VJ, et al. Lymphoblastic lymphoma: an immunophenotype study of 26 cases with comparison to T cell acute lymphoblastic leukemia. *Blood* 1986;67:474–478.

84. Cossman J, Chused TM, Fisher RI, et al. Diversity of immunological phenotypes of lymphoblastic lymphoma. *Cancer Res* 1983;43:4486–4490.

85. Sheibani K, Nathwani BN, Winberg CD, et al. Antigenically defined subgroups of lymphoblastic lymphoma. Relationship to clinical presentation and biologic behavior. *Cancer* 1987;60:183–190.

86. Grogan T, Spier C, Wirt DP, et al. Immunologic complexity of lymphoblastic lymphoma. *Diagn Immunol* 1986;4:81–88.

87. Swerdlow SH, Habeshaw JA, Richards MA, et al. T lymphoblastic lymphoma with LEU-7 positive phenotype and unusual clinical course: a multiparameter study. *Leuk Res* 1985;9:167–173.

88. Sheibani K, Winberg CD, Burke JS, et al. Lymphoblastic lymphoma expressing natural killer cell-associated antigens: a clinicopathologic study of six cases. *Leuk Res* 1987;11:371–377.

89. Childs CC, Chrystal GS, Strauchen JA. Biphenotypic lymphoblastic lymphoma. An unusual tumor with lymphocytic and granulocytic differentiation. *Cancer* 1986;57:1019–1023.

90. Somers GR, Slater H, Rockman S, et al. Coexistent T-cell lymphoblastic lymphoma and an atypical myeloproliferative disorder associated with t(8;13)(p21;q14). *Pediatr Pathol Lab Med* 1997;17:141–158.

91. Thomas DA, Kantarjian HM. Lymphoblastic lymphoma. *Hematol Oncol Clin North Am* 2001;15:51–95.

92. Shikano T, Ishikawa Y, Naito H, et al. Cytogenetic characteristics of childhood non-Hodgkin lymphoma. *Cancer* 1992;70:714–719.

93. Kaneko Y, Frizzera G, Shikano T, et al. Chromosomal and immunophenotypic patterns in T cell acute lymphoblastic leukemia (T ALL) and lymphoblastic lymphoma (LBL). *Leukemia* 1989;3:886–892.

94. Kaneko Y, Frizzera G, Edamura S, et al. A novel translocation, t(2;5)(p23;q35), in childhood phagocytic large T-cell lymphoma mimicking malignant histiocytosis. *Blood* 1989;73:806–813.

95. Naeem R, Singer S, Fletcher JA. Translocation t(8;13)(p11;q11-12) in stem cell leukemia/lymphoma of T-cell and myeloid lineages. *Genes Chromosomes Cancer* 1995;12:148–151.

96. Inhorn RC, Aster JC, Roach SA, et al. A syndrome of lymphoblastic lymphoma, eosinophilia, and myeloid hyperplasia/malignancy associated with t(8;13)(p11;q11): description of a distinctive clinicopathologic entity. *Blood* 1995;85:1881–1887.

97. Xiao S, Nalabolu SR, Aster JC, et al. FGFR1 is fused with a novel zinc-finger gene, ZNF198, in the t(8;13) leukaemia/lymphoma syndrome. *Nat Genet* 1998;18:84–87.

98. Narita M, Shimizu K, Hayashi Y, et al. Consistent detection of CALM-AF10 chimaeric transcripts in haematological malignancies with t(10;11)(p13;q14) and identification of novel transcripts. *Br J Haematol* 1999;105:928–937.

99. Bohlander SK, Muschinsky V, Schrader K, et al. Molecular analysis of the CALM/AF10 fusion: identical rearrangements in acute myeloid leukemia, acute lymphoblastic leukemia and malignant lymphoma patients. *Leukemia* 2000;14:93–99.

100. Yeoh EJ, Ross ME, Shurtleff SA, et al. Classification, subtype discovery, and prediction of outcome in pediatric acute lymphoblastic leukemia by gene expression profiling. *Cancer Cell* 2002;1:133–143.

101. Ferrando AA, Look AT. Gene expression profiling in T-cell acute lymphoblastic leukemia. *Semin Hematol* 2003;40:274–280.

102. Synold TW, Relling MV, Boyett JM, et al. Blast cell methotrexate-polyglutamate accumulation in vivo differs by lineage, ploidy, and methotrexate dose in acute lymphoblastic leukemia. *J Clin Invest* 1994;94:1996–2001.

103. Burkhardt B, Woessmann W, Zimmermann M, et al. Impact of cranial radiotherapy on central nervous system prophylaxis in children and adolescents with central nervous system-negative stage III or IV lymphoblastic lymphoma. *J Clin Oncol* 2006;24:491–499.

104. Asselin BL, Shuster J, Amylon M, et al. *Improved Event-Free Survival (EFS) with High Dose Methotrexate (HDM) in T-Cell Lymphoblastic Leukemia (T-ALL) and Advanced Lymphoblastic Lymphoma (T-NHL): A Pediatric Oncology Group (POG) Study: Proceedings of The American Society of Clinical Oncology*, 2001; 20:367.

105. Murphy SB, Pediatric lymphomas: recent advances and commentary on Ki-1-positive anaplastic large-cell lymphomas of childhood. *Ann Oncol* 1994;5(suppl 1):31–33.

106. Laver JH, Mahmoud H, Pick TE, et al. Results of a randomized phase III trial in children and adolescents with advanced stage diffuse large cell non-Hodgkin's lymphoma: a Pediatric Oncology Group study. *Leuk Lymphoma* 2002;43:105–109.

107. Laver JH, Kraveka JM, Hutchison RE, et al. Advanced-stage large-cell lymphoma in children and adolescents: results of a randomized trial incorporating intermediate-dose methotrexate and high-dose cytarabine in the maintenance phase of the APO regimen: a Pediatric Oncology Group phase III trial. *J Clin Oncol* 2005;23:541–547.

108. Rubie H, Gladieff L, Robert A, et al. Childhood anaplastic large cell lymphoma Ki-1/CD30: clinicopathologic features of 19 cases. *Med Pediatr Oncol* 1994;22:155–161.

109. Sandlund JT, Pui CH, Santana VM, et al. Clinical features and treatment outcome for children with CD30+ large-cell non-Hodgkin's lymphoma. *J Clin Oncol* 1994;12:895–898.

110. Benharroch D, Meguerian-Bedoyan Z, Lamant L, et al. ALK-positive lymphoma: a single disease with a broad spectrum of morphology. *Blood* 1998;91:2076–2084.
111. Brugieres L, Deley MC, Pacquement H, et al. CD30(+) anaplastic large-cell lymphoma in children: analysis of 82 patients enrolled in two consecutive studies of the French Society of Pediatric Oncology. *Blood* 1998;92:3591–3598.
112. Sandlund JT, Roberts WM, Pui CH, et al. Systemic hemophagocytosis masking the diagnosis of large cell non-Hodgkin lymphoma. *Med Pediatr Oncol* 1997;29:167–169.
113. Blatt J, Weston B, Belhorn T, et al. Childhood non-Hodgkin lymphoma presenting as hemophagocytic syndrome. *Pediatr Hematol Oncol* 2002;19:45–49.
114. Kinney MC, Collins RD, Greer JP, et al. A small-cell-predominant variant of primary Ki-1 (CD30)+ T-cell lymphoma. *Am J Surg Pathol* 1993;17:859–868.
115. Chan JK, Buchanan R, Fletcher CD. Sarcomatoid variant of anaplastic large-cell Ki-1 lymphoma. *Am J Surg Pathol* 1990;14:983–988.
116. Falini B, Liso A, Pasqualucci L, et al. CD30+ anaplastic large-cell lymphoma, null type, with signet-ring appearance. *Histopathology* 1997;30:90–92.
117. Piccaluga PP, Ascani S, Fraternali Orcioni G, et al. Anaplastic lymphoma kinase expression as a marker of malignancy. Application to a case of anaplastic large cell lymphoma with huge granulomatous reaction. *Haematologica* 2000;85:978–981.
118. van den Berg H, Noorduyn A, van Kuilenburg AB, et al. Leukaemic expression of anaplastic large cell lymphoma with 46,XX,ins(2;5)(p23;q15q35) in a child with dihydropyrimidine dehydrogenase deficiency. *Leukemia* 2000;14:769–770.
119. Anderson MM, Ross CW, Singleton TP, et al. Ki-1 anaplastic large cell lymphoma with a prominent leukemic phase. *Hum Pathol* 1996;27:1093–1095.
120. Villamor N, Rozman M, Esteve J, et al. Anaplastic large-cell lymphoma with rapid evolution to leukemic phase. *Ann Hematol* 1999;78:478–482.
121. Bayle C, Charpentier A, Duchayne E, et al. Leukaemic presentation of small cell variant anaplastic large cell lymphoma: report of four cases. *Br J Haematol* 1999;104:680–688.
122. Chhanabhai M, Britten C, Klasa R, et al. t(2;5) positive lymphoma with peripheral blood involvement. *Leuk Lymphoma* 1998;28:415–422.
123. Onciu M, Behm FG, Raimondi SC, et al. ALK-positive anaplastic large cell lymphoma with leukemic peripheral blood involvement is a clinicopathologic entity with an unfavorable prognosis. Report of three cases and review of the literature. *Am J Clin Pathol* 2003;120:617–625.
124. Stein H, Foss HD, Durkop H, et al. CD30(+) anaplastic large cell lymphoma: a review of its histopathologic, genetic, and clinical features. *Blood* 2000;96:3681–3695.
125. Delsol G, Al Saati T, Gatter KC, et al. Coexpression of epithelial membrane antigen (EMA), Ki-1, and interleukin 2 receptor by anaplastic large cell lymphomas. Diagnostic value in so-called malignant histiocytosis. *Am J Pathol* 1988;130:59–70.
126. Mason DY, Bastard C, Rimokh R, et al. CD30-positive large cell lymphomas ('Ki-1 lymphoma') are associated with a chromosomal translocation involving 5q35. *Br J Haematol* 1990;74:161–168.
127. Sandlund JT, Pui CH, Roberts WM, et al. Clinicopathologic features and treatment outcome of children with large-cell lymphoma and the t(2;5)(p23;q35). *Blood* 1994;84:2467–2471.
128. Lamant L, Dastugue N, Pulford K, et al. A new fusion gene TPM3-ALK in anaplastic large cell lymphoma created by a (1;2)(q25;p23) translocation. *Blood* 1999;93:3088–3095.
129. Rosenwald A, Ott G, Pulford K, et al. t(1;2)(q21;p23) and t(2;3)(p23;q21): two novel variant translocations of the t(2;5)(p23;q35) in anaplastic large cell lymphoma. *Blood* 1999;94:362–364.
130. Colleoni GW, Bridge JA, Garicochea B, et al. ATIC-ALK: A novel variant ALK gene fusion in anaplastic large cell lymphoma resulting from the recurrent cryptic chromosomal inversion, inv(2)(p23q35). *Am J Pathol* 2000;156:781–789.
131. Morris SW, Kirstein MN, Valentine MB, et al. Fusion of a kinase gene, ALK, to a nucleolar protein gene, NPM, in non- Hodgkin's lymphoma [published erratum appears in Science 1995;267:316–317]. *Science* 1994;263:1281–1284.
132. Onciu M, Behm FG, Downing JR, et al. ALK-positive plasmablastic B-cell lymphoma with expression of the NPM-ALK fusion transcript: report of 2 cases. *Blood* 2003;102:2642–2644.
133. Delsol G, Lamant L, Mariame B, et al. A new subtype of large B-cell lymphoma expressing the ALK kinase and lacking the 2; 5 translocation. *Blood* 1997;89:1483–1490.
134. Falini B, Bigerna B, Fizzotti M, et al. ALK expression defines a distinct group of T/null lymphomas ("ALK lymphomas") with a wide morphological spectrum. *Am J Pathol* 1998;153:875–886.
135. Lawrence B, Perez-Atayde A, Hibbard MK, et al. TPM3-ALK and TPM4-ALK oncogenes in inflammatory myofibroblastic tumors. *Am J Pathol* 2000;157:377–384.
136. Lamant L, Pulford K, Bischof D, et al. Expression of the ALK tyrosine kinase gene in neuroblastoma. *Am J Pathol* 2000;156:1711–1721.
137. Shiota M, Nakamura S, Ichinohasama R, et al. Anaplastic large cell lymphoma expressing the novel chimeric protein p80NPM/ALK: a distinct clinicopathologic entity. *Blood* 1995;86:1954–1960.
138. Falini B, Pileri S, Zinzani PL, et al. ALK+ lymphoma: clinico-pathological findings and outcome. *Blood* 1999;93:2697–2706.
139. Gascoyne RD, Aoun P, Wu D, et al. Prognostic significance of anaplastic lymphoma kinase (ALK) protein expression in adults with anaplastic large cell lymphoma. *Blood* 1999;93:3913–3921.
140. Falini B, Pulford K, Pucciarini A, et al. Lymphomas expressing ALK fusion protein(s) other than NPM-ALK. *Blood* 1999;94:3509–3515.
141. Sandlund JT, Pui CH, Santana VM, et al. Clinical features and treatment outcome for children with CD30+ large- cell non-Hodgkin's lymphoma. *J Clin Oncol* 1994;12:895–898.
142. Williams DM, Hobson R, Imeson J, et al. Anaplastic large cell lymphoma in childhood: analysis of 72 patients treated on The United Kingdom Children's Cancer Study Group chemotherapy regimens. *Br J Haematol* 2002;117:812–820.
143. Brugieres L, Quartier P, Le Deley MC, et al. Relapses of childhood anaplastic large-cell lymphoma: treatment results in a series of 41 children–a report from the French Society of Pediatric Oncology. *Ann Oncol* 2000;11:53–58.
144. Morgensztern D, Martin MG, Lossos IS. Gene expression profiling in diffuse large B-cell lymphoma. *Leuk Lymphoma* 2007;48:669–682.
145. Alizadeh AA, Eisen MB, Davis RE, et al. Distinct types of diffuse large B-cell lymphoma identified by gene expression profiling. *Nature* 2000;403:503–511.
146. Oschlies I, Klapper W, Zimmermann M, et al. Diffuse large B-cell lymphoma in pediatric patients belongs predominantly to the germinal-center type B-cell lymphomas: a clinicopathologic analysis of cases included in the German BFM (Berlin-Frankfurt-Munster) Multicenter Trial. *Blood* 2006;107:4047–4052.
147. Boleti E, Johnson PW. Primary mediastinal B-cell lymphoma. *Hematol Oncol* 2007;25:157–163.
148. Savage KJ. Primary mediastinal large B-cell lymphoma. *Oncologist* 2006;11:488–495.
149. Savage KJ, Monti S, Kutok JL, et al. The molecular signature of mediastinal large B-cell lymphoma differs from that of other diffuse large B-cell lymphomas and shares features with classical Hodgkin lymphoma. *Blood* 2003;102:3871–3879.
150. Zinzani PL, Bendandi M, Frezza G, et al. Primary Mediastinal B-cell lymphoma with sclerosis: clinical and therapeutic evaluation of 22 patients. *Leuk Lymphoma* 1996;21:311–316.
151. Lones MA, Perkins SL, Sposto R, et al. Large-cell lymphoma arising in the mediastinum in children and adolescents is associated with an excellent outcome: a Children's Cancer Group report. *J Clin Oncol* 2000;18:3845–3853.
152. Agnarsson BA, Kadin ME. Peripheral T-cell lymphomas in children. *Semin Diagn Pathol* 1995;12:314–324.
153. el-Hoshy K, Hashimoto K. Adolescence mycosis fungoides: an unusual presentation with hypopigmentation. *J Dermatol* 1995;22:424–427.
154. Grunwald MH, Amichai B. Localized hypopigmented mycosis fungoides in a 12-year-old Caucasian boy. *J Dermatol* 1999;26:70–71.
155. Garzon MC. Cutaneous T cell lymphoma in children. *Semin Cutan Med Surg* 1999;18:226–232.
156. Tan E, Tay YK, Giam YC. Profile and outcome of childhood mycosis fungoides in Singapore. *Pediatr Dermatol* 2000;17:352–356.
157. Neuhaus IM, Ramos-Caro FA, Hassanein AM. Hypopigmented mycosis fungoides in childhood and adolescence. *Pediatr Dermatol* 2000;17:403–406.
158. Whittam LR, Calonje E, Orchard G, et al. CD8-positive juvenile onset mycosis fungoides: an immunohistochemical and genotypic analysis of six cases. *Br J Dermatol* 2000;143:1199–1204.
159. Sen F, Rassidakis GZ, Jones D, et al. Apoptosis and proliferation in subcutaneous panniculitis-like T-cell lymphoma. *Mod Pathol* 2002;15:625–631.
160. Thomson AB, McKenzie KJ, Jackson R, et al. Subcutaneous panniculitic T-cell lymphoma in childhood: successful response to chemotherapy. *Med Pediatr Oncol* 2001;37:549–552.
161. Lewis JM, Vasef MA, Seabury Stone M. HTLV-I-associated granulomatous T-cell lymphoma in a child. *J Am Acad Dermatol* 2001;44:525–529.
162. Broniscer A, Ribeiro RC, Srinivas RV, et al. An adolescent with HTLV-I-associated adult T cell leukemia treated with interferon-alfa and zidovudine. *Leukemia* 1996;10:1244–1248.
163. Miyazaki M, Lin YW, Okada M, et al. Childhood cutaneous natural killer/T lymphoma successfully treated with only one course of chemotherapy and incomplete tumor resection. *Haematologica* 2001;86:883–884.
164. Ohnuma K, Toyoda Y, Nishihira H, et al. Aggressive natural killer (NK) cell lymphoma: report of a pediatric case and review of the literature. *Leuk Lymphoma* 1997;25:387–392.
165. Shaw PH, Cohn SL, Morgan ER, et al. Natural killer cell lymphoma: report of two pediatric cases, therapeutic options, and review of the literature. *Cancer* 2001;91:642–646.

166. Lorsbach RB, Shay-Seymore D, Moore J, et al. Clinicopathologic analysis of follicular lymphoma occurring in children. *Blood* 2002;99:1959–1964.

167. Frizzera G, Murphy SB. Follicular (nodular) lymphoma in childhood: a rare clinical-pathological entity. Report of eight cases from four cancer centers. *Cancer* 1979;44:2218–2235.

168. Pinto A, Hutchison RE, Grant LH, et al. Follicular lymphomas in pediatric patients. *Mod Pathol* 1990;3:308–313.

169. Moertel CL, Watterson J, McCormick SR, et al. Follicular large cell lymphoma of the testis in a child. *Cancer* 1995;75:1182–1186.

170. Finn LS, Viswanatha DS, Belasco JB, et al. Primary follicular lymphoma of the testis in childhood. *Cancer* 1999;85:1626–1635.

171. Lu D, Medeiros J, Eskenazi AE, et al. Primary follicular large cell lymphoma of the testis in a child. *Arch Pathol Lab Med* 2001;125:551–554.

172. Pakzad K, MacLennan GT, Elder JS, et al. Follicular large cell lymphoma localized to the testis in children. *J Urol* 2002;168:225–228.

173. Atra A, Meller ST, Stevens RS, et al. Conservative management of follicular non-Hodgkin's lymphoma in childhood. *Br J Haematol* 1998;103:220–223.

174. Kobrinsky NL, Sposto R, Shah NR, et al. Outcomes of treatment of children and adolescents with recurrent non-Hodgkin's lymphoma and Hodgkin's disease with dexamethasone, etoposide, cisplatin, cytarabine, and l-asparaginase, maintenance chemotherapy, and transplantation: Children's Cancer Group Study CCG-5912. *J Clin Oncol* 2001;19:2390–2396.

175. Philip T, Armitage JO, Spitzer G, et al. High-dose therapy and autologous bone marrow transplantation after failure of conventional chemotherapy in adults with intermediate-grade or high-grade non-Hodgkin's lymphoma. *N Engl J Med* 1987;316:1493–1498.

176. Philip T, Biron P, Philip I, et al. Massive therapy and autologous bone marrow transplantation in pediatric and young adults Burkitt's lymphoma (30 courses on 28 patients: a 5-year experience). *Eur J Cancer Clin Oncol* 1986;22:1015–1027.

177. Philip T, Hartmann O, Biron P, et al. High-dose therapy and autologous bone marrow transplantation in partial remission after first-line induction therapy for diffuse non-Hodgkin's lymphoma. *J Clin Oncol* 1988;6:1118–1124.

178. Gordon BG, Warkentin PI, Weisenburger DD, et al. Bone marrow transplantation for peripheral T-cell lymphoma in children and adolescents. *Blood* 1992;80:2938–2942.

179. Bureo E, Ortega JJ, Munoz A, et al. Bone marrow transplantation in 46 pediatric patients with non-Hodgkin's lymphoma. Spanish Working Party for Bone Marrow Transplantation in Children. *Bone Marrow Transplant* 1995;15:353–359.

180. Loiseau HA, Hartmann O, Valteau D, et al. High-dose chemotherapy containing busulfan followed by bone marrow transplantation in 24 children with refractory or relapsed non-Hodgkin's lymphoma. *Bone Marrow Transplant* 1991;8:465–472.

181. O'Leary M, Ramsay NK, Nesbit ME, et al. Bone marrow transplantation for non-Hodgkin's lymphoma in children and young adults. A pilot study. *Am J Med* 1983;74:497–501.

182. Ladenstein R, Pearce R, Hartmannx O, et al. High-dose chemotherapy with autologous bone marrow rescue in children with poor-risk Burkitt's lymphoma: a report from the European Lymphoma Bone Marrow Transplantation Registry. *Blood* 1997;90:2921–2930.

183. Appelbaum FR, Deisseroth AB, Graw RG, Jr., et al. Prolonged complete remission following high dose chemotherapy of Burkitt's lymphoma in relapse. *Cancer* 1978;41:1059–1063.

184. Sandlund JT, Bowman L, Heslop HE, et al. Intensive chemotherapy with hematopoietic stem-cell support for children with recurrent or refractory NHL. *Cytotherapy* 2002;4:253–258.

185. Suryanarayan K, Shuster JJ, Donaldson SS, et al. Treatment of localized primary non-Hodgkin's lymphoma of bone in children: a Pediatric Oncology Group study. *J Clin Oncol* 1999;17:456–459.

186. Murphy SB, Hustu HO. A randomized trial of combined modality therapy of childhood non-Hodgkin's lymphoma. *Cancer* 1980;45:630–637.

187. Meistrich ML, Wilson G, Brown BW, et al. Impact of cyclophosphamide on long-term reduction in sperm count in men treated with combination chemotherapy for Ewing and soft tissue sarcomas. *Cancer* 1992;70:2703–2712.

188. Lipshultz SE, Colan SD, Gelber RD, et al. Late cardiac effects of doxorubicin therapy for acute lymphoblastic leukemia in childhood. *N Engl J Med* 1991;324:808–815.

189. Sorensen K, Levitt G, Bull C, et al. Anthracycline dose in childhood acute lymphoblastic leukemia: issues of early survival versus late cardiotoxicity. *J Clin Oncol* 1997;15:61–68.

190. Nysom K, Holm K, Lipsitz SR, et al. Relationship between cumulative anthracycline dose and late cardiotoxicity in childhood acute lymphoblastic leukemia. *J Clin Oncol* 1998;16:545–550.

191. Colombat P, Salles G, Brousse N, et al. Rituximab (anti-CD20 monoclonal antibody) as single first-line therapy for patients with follicular lymphoma with a low tumor burden: clinical and molecular evaluation. *Blood* 2001;97:101–106.

192. Coiffier B, Haioun C, Ketterer N, et al. Rituximab (anti-CD20 monoclonal antibody) for the treatment of patients with relapsing or refractory aggressive lymphoma: a multicenter phase II study. *Blood* 1998;92:1927–1932.

193. Woessmann W, Seidemann K, Mann G, et al. The impact of the methotrexate administration schedule and dose in the treatment of children and adolescents with B-cell neoplasms: a report of the BFM Group Study NHL-BFM95. *Blood* 2005;105:948–958.

194. Anderson JR, Wilson JF, Jenkin DT, et al. Childhood non-Hodgkin's lymphoma. The results of a randomized therapeutic trial comparing a 4-drug regimen (COMP) with a 10-drug regimen (LSA2-L2). *N Engl J Med* 1983;308:559–565.

195. Sandlund JT, Santana V, Abromowitch M, et al. Large cell non-Hodgkin lymphoma of childhood: clinical characteristics and outcome. *Leukemia* 1994;8:30–34.

196. Falini B, Mason DY. Proteins encoded by genes involved in chromosomal alterations in lymphoma and leukemia: clinical value of their detection by immunocytochemistry. *Blood* 2002;99:409–426.

CHAPTER 34 ■ MANAGEMENT OF NON-HODGKIN LYMPHOMA DURING PREGNANCY

THOMAS M. HABERMANN AND THOMAS E. WITZIG

The synchronous presentation of non-Hodgkin lymphoma (NHL) and pregnancy is complex, presenting significant challenges. Patients may present with asymptomatic lymphadenopathy or a more complex presentation that includes fevers, fevers of undetermined origin, superior vena cava syndrome, skin rash, back pain, pelvic pain, central nervous system symptoms (nausea, vomiting, and headache), gigantomastia, tumor lysis syndrome, and other signs and symptoms. This diagnosis leads to a complex set of management decisions throughout the pregnancy and the immediate postpartum period (Table 34.1).

The management of the pregnant patient with NHL requires a team with a broad-based knowledge of many factors, including high-risk pregnancy, the natural history of the histologic type of lymphoma the patient has, pharmacology of chemotherapeutic agents, side effects of radiation exposure (diagnostic and therapeutic) to the fetus and patient, psychosocial issues, and ethical issues (Table 34.2). A multidisciplinary team should include an obstetrician, hematologist/oncologist, neonatologist, social worker, clergy, and others. The management team needs to be cognizant that decisions have potential implications that may affect both the patient and fetus.

The management has evolved over time, and depends upon the histology at the time of the diagnosis of lymphoma, the trimester of the pregnancy, and other factors. NHL is a rare complication of pregnancy (1–97). This chapter will focus on the reported experiences in the literature and recommend an approach to this complex clinical situation.

HISTOLOGY

It is essential to obtain an adequate biopsy to establish a definitive diagnosis and classification of the lymphoma. Adequate tissue is required. Fine needle aspirates may result in misdiagnosis (69). The histology determines the prognosis, potential for curability, and type of treatment. More than 161 cases of NHL in pregnancy are reported in the English literature (1–97). Cross-translation from earlier lymphoma histologic classifications into current classification schemes is not always feasible. The most common histologic subtypes in pregnant patients were diffuse large B-cell lymphoma (DLBCL), lymphoblastic, and Burkitt NHL. Specifically, 42 had diffuse large cell NHL (19,20,22,23,32,34,35,40–42,44,45,52,56,58,68,73,76, 77,93,94), and 40 patients had histologically high-grade disease (Burkitt lymphoma, lymphoblastic lymphoma, and high-grade small cleaved NHL) (9,12,14,16–18,21,26,27,29,33,35, 38,39,41,52,60,67,71,72,75,88,91). There were individual cases of composite lymphoma (follicular lymphoma and nodular sclerosing Hodgkin lymphoma (56), natural killer-cell lymphoma (55), anaplastic large cell lymphoma (54), and three patients were reported with undifferentiated NHL (31,35,91). Follicular lymphoma is rare (52,53,56,75). T-cell lymphomas have been reported, and the histologic classifications are changing over time. Four cases of immunophenotypically confirmed T-cell NHL at initial diagnosis have been reported (25,31,56,59). One case of adult T-cell leukemia-lymphoma was reported (59). Subcutaneous T-cell lymphoma (79), subcutaneous panniculitic-like lymphoma (62–64), T-natural killer-cell lymphoma (81), and six cases of T-cell anaplastic large cell lymphoma (69,70,78,81) have been reported. Patients with mycosis fungoides have become pregnant (82,90).

TABLE 34.1

UNIQUE PRESENTATIONS IN PREGNANCY

Skin lesions
Breast mass
   Right-sided or bilateral
   Gigantomastia
Atypical pelvic pain
Uterus involvement

TABLE 34.2

SPECIFIC ISSUES IN DIAGNOSIS, TREATMENT, AND MANAGEMENT

Histology
   DLBCL is the most common
   Lymphoblastic lymphoma and non-Burkitt NHL occur because of an age association
   Follicular lymphoma is uncommon
   T-cell lymphoma is common
Trimester of pregnancy and postpartum
   The incidence is essentially the same in the reported literature.
   The therapeutic intervention strategies differ.
Psychosocial and religious beliefs
Stage
   Nodal vs. extranodal
   Bulky vs. localized
Fetal maturity
Radiation exposure to the fetus
   Lead apron shielding of the abdomen for chest x-ray
   MRI
   Computed tomography and positron emission tomography scans are contraindicated

SITE OF DISEASE

NHL in pregnancy commonly involves nodal sites. Primary and secondary extranodal disease presentations have been reported in a diverse group of patients. The most common presentation is symptomatic or asymptomatic lymphadenopathy. Extranodal involvement is characteristic of lymphoma in pregnancy. Sixteen cases involving the breast have been reported (9,12,16,18,27,40,61,65,66–69,75,80). Four of these cases were African Burkitt lymphoma. Breast involvement may be bilateral (61,66–69,75). There is a predilection for the right side to be involved. Three cases have involved the gastrointestinal tract (13,35). Gynecologic presentations have included two cervical cases (8,23,53), one perineal (7), and one uterine (9). Uterine involvement resulted in an abruptio placentae in one case (35) and was diagnosed 3 weeks after normal delivery in another patient. Placental involvement has been reported (41,47–49,55). The cervix may be pathologically involved (54). Central nervous system involvement may be parenchymal or meningeal (9,52,56,71). The bone marrow may be involved (51,55,56,59). Cutaneous involvement is not an uncommon presentation with histologies that include mycosis fungoides, parapsoriasis en plaque, subpanniculitic lymphoma, and other T-cell lymphomas (62–64,79,82,90). The nasal cavity may be the initial site of involvement (74).

Trimester at the Time of Presentation

The diagnosis of the lymphoma can occur at anytime during the pregnancy but is more likely in the second and third trimesters. Among 95 patients for whom adequate information was available, lymphoma appeared in the first trimester in 22 (24%) (8,12,18,26,33,41,43,56,73,75,79,82), in the second trimester in 35 (36%) (7,16,17,25,31,33,41,44,47, 51–53,55–58,62,76,81,91,94), and in the third trimester in 38 (40%) (6,12–15,20,21,28,30,34,35,37,38,41,42,45–47, 51–53,55,61,70,71,77,78,80). In addition, 30 of the reported cases of NHL were histologically documented in the immediate postpartum period (4,10,12,13,23,33,35,38,40,47–49,55, 66–70,74,77,81).

The influence of pregnancy on the course of the lymphoma is controversial. It has been suggested that hormonal or immunologic changes in pregnancy may influence the course and progression of disease (33). In support of this possibility, Steiner-Salz et al. (35) reported that disease progressed in two patients after delivery, a suggestion that pregnancy has a lymphoma-mediated suppressing effect. In contrast, others have suggested no effect (52,60–62,95) or even a protective effect (33,63). It has been postulated that hormonal and immunologic changes during pregnancy might stabilize the disease. Postpartum progression has been reported (81).

Outcome of the Pregnancy

Information on the course of the pregnancy was known for 103 patients (7–9,12–21,23,25–27,30–35,38–40,42,44–47,51–56,58,59,61,62,64–66,71,73,75–82,91,94). Therapeutic abortion was induced in five (17,33,52,81) and performed at the time of abdominal exploration in two (16,18). One therapeutic abortion was performed because of an in utero fetal abnormality (94). Of the remaining 82 pregnancies, six resulted in miscarriages (27,31,56,61,74,78), one of which occurred after a radiation dose of 9 Gy and administration of doxorubicin, vincristine, and prednisone (31). Three additional patients died before delivery (12,25,33). Thirty-one patients delivered before any treatment; 14 had a cesarean section (7,8,13,23,35,52–56,58,59,66,71,77) and 19 a vaginal delivery (9,12,20,33,35,38,40,46,52,56,80,81). Twenty-eight patients had a vaginal delivery after initial treatment (14,19,21,26,30,32–34,41,42,45,51,56,62,65,73,93). Cesarean section was performed after treatment in 2 patients (76,78). Sixty-six (80%) fetuses were reported to be alive at the time of delivery, but 16 did not survive.

Outcome of the Non-Hodgkin Lymphoma

Ortega (19) first reported on the use of chemotherapy in pregnant patients with NHL. Since that time, additional patients with intermediate- and high-grade lymphoma have been treated with chemotherapy during pregnancy. The largest single reported series is by Avilés et al. (41) who treated 19 patients and reported the results in 16. Fifteen patients received a regimen that contained doxorubicin. Eight patients were alive and disease free at 4 to 9 years after delivery. In the Stanford experience, many women deferred therapy until after delivery or spontaneous/therapeutic abortion (52). This group reported that four patients were alive with no evidence of disease, three were alive with disease, and four had died of lymphoma. In the Mayo series, which included patients with diffuse large B-cell NHL or peripheral T-cell NHL, all five patients who were treated with anthracycline-based chemotherapy (one during pregnancy, four after delivery, and two received radiation therapy during the pregnancy) achieved a complete remission, and four were alive and disease free with a median follow-up of 13.5 years (56).

There have been multiple case reports using various chemotherapy regimens (14,18,19,23,25,28–34,41,42,44,58,59,65, 72,73,75,76,78,82,88,91,93). Cyclophosphamide, prednisone, vincristine, and bleomycin was used in a patient in the second trimester with complete remission at 2 years (19). Cyclophosphamide, doxorubicin, vincristine, and prednisone (CHOP) was used in the third trimester, with complete remission at 28 and 36 months and stable disease at 4 months (34,42,62). CHOP-bleomycin was used in the second trimester (44). Procarbazine and prednisone (32), teniposide (29), cyclophosphamide, vincristine, and prednisone, and intrathecal methotrexate were used in the third trimester with maternal death in 21 days (30), and CHOP-bleomycin was used in the second trimester (44). Two spontaneous abortions have been reported after chemotherapy (25,31).

Rituximab has changed the natural history of DLBCL. Single-agent rituximab was administered in the first trimester with no adverse fetal outcomes (65). Rituximab (anti-CD20 monoclonal antibody) and CHOP administered in the second trimester have resulted in successful fetal and maternal outcomes (58,73–76). Because rituximab is an immunoglobulin G1 antibody, transplacental transport is efficient. B-cell populations were normal at 3 and 4 months (58,73).

Two patients with Burkitt lymphoma who received cyclophosphamide died at 4½ and 5 months (14,18).

Cyclophosphamide, vincristine, and doxorubicin-methotrexate/ifosfamide, etoposide, and high-dose cytarabine treatment was initiated at 26 weeks gestation, and mother and child were alive and disease free at 1 year (72). One patient with lymphoblastic NHL was treated with 41 Gy to the mediastinum in the second trimester (33). The patient eventually had a relapse and died 3 years later. Other treatments included cyclophosphamide in the third trimester in a mother who died 23 days after giving birth (23), dexamethasone in the third trimester (28), and teniposide (29). CHOP was administered in a case of adult T-cell leukemia-lymphoma (59). On the 8th day, a healthy fetus was delivered. The mother subsequently died of septicemia after the first cycle.

TERATOGENIC EFFECTS OF NON-HODGKIN LYMPHOMA

NHL does not appear to predispose the fetus to congenital abnormalities, although there is one case of a second trimester diagnosis of Brackmann-de Lange syndrome in an untreated mother with DLBCL (94).

Teratogenic Effects of Therapeutic Intervention

The patient with potentially curable malignant disease in pregnancy that requires chemotherapy presents a therapeutic dilemma. In contrast to findings in laboratory animals, data on teratogenicity and mutagenicity of chemotherapeutic agents are incomplete. The critical teratogenic period for chemotherapeutic agents is in the first trimester. Drugs implicated in lymphoma as having adverse effects on the fetus include cyclophosphamide (98,99), methotrexate (100), and chlorambucil (101). Cyclophosphamide administered in the first trimester in two patients with Hodgkin disease was associated with absent toes and a single coronary artery (98,99). Congenital anomalies with folic acid antagonists, such as methotrexate, administered in the first trimester for indications other than NHL have been reported to be associated with multiple cranial ossification defects, abnormal facies, digital anomalies, and other defects (100). Chlorambucil has been implicated in causing renal agenesis and hypoplasia (101). A possible association with vinca alkaloids with congenital defects of the atrial septum and digits was reported in the first trimester in a patient treated with vincristine, doxorubicin, cytarabine, and prednisone (102). Other adverse outcomes for the pregnancy have been reported with standard lymphoma regimens emphasizing that a thorough review of outcomes related to a specific therapeutic intervention is indicated (103). The long-term toxicity risks such as cardiac toxicities to the fetus have not been adequately studied. In 35 patients in the literature with NHL treated with regimens, which included doxorubicin, cyclophosphamide, and vincristine, therapies including 11 patients in the first trimester, there were no malformations (103).

Anthracycline therapy is critical in DLBCL and other NHLs. Karp et al. (31), in a report on a patient with undifferentiated lymphoma of T-cell origin who received doxorubicin during pregnancy, measured drug levels in fetal and placental material. After miscarriage no doxorubicin was detectable in any tissue. In a recent review of anthracycline agents in pregnancy with long-term follow-up, Turchi and Villasis (104) found that 28 pregnancies had resulted in 24 normal infants. Effects on offspring have been reported (105–107). Aviles and Neri (97) reported on a series of 84 patients with hematologic malignancies and found no congenital abnormalities at a median follow-up of 18.7 years. No secondary malignancies were reported in the children in this large series.

Radiotherapy has been reported to be teratogenic in animals and humans (108,109). The International Commission on Radiologic Protection (110) with data from survivors from children exposed in utero to diagnostic x-rays and children exposed to radiation in the Chernobyl accident in utero were used to determine the threshold doses of radiation for the fetus. In weeks 2 to 8 after conception, radiation exposure can cause organ malformations at a threshold dose of 0.1 to 0.2 Gy. The central nervous system is sensitive to radiation weeks 8 to 15 with fetal exposures of 0.1 Gy, resulting in decreases in intelligent quotient and mental retardation at 1 Gy. The data on radiation therapy in pregnancy in humans are from Hodgkin lymphoma (111). Lymphoma of the cervical lymph nodes, axillary lymph nodes, and mediastinum can be treated utilizing special tables and lead block protection.

Management Recommendations of Non-Hodgkin Lymphoma in Pregnancy

Recommendations regarding the management of pregnant patients with lymphoma are based on current concepts of lymphoma management in the nonpregnant patient, and results from small series that span a significant period of time and the case reports. Therapeutic intervention depends on histologic type, stage of disease, extranodal presentation of disease, ethical issues, psychosocial issues, and trimester in which lymphoma is detected. Early and accurate tissue diagnosis is essential.

Staging

A careful history should be conducted to elicit symptoms of disease such as fatigue out of proportion to that usually experienced with pregnancy, weight loss, fever, and drenching night sweats. Staging procedures are necessary to assess extent of disease and determine if normal organs such as liver and kidney are involved or threatened by bulky lymphoma. Recommended staging studies in the pregnant patient with NHL include physical examination, blood chemistries (electrolytes, lactate dehydrogenase, aspartate aminotransferase, bilirubin, alkaline phosphatase, uric acid, and creatinine), single-view chest radiograph with adequate abdominal shielding, magnetic resonance imaging (MRI) of the chest, abdomen, and pelvis, pelvic ultrasound, echocardiogram to assess left ventricular function, and bone marrow aspiration and biopsy. The radiation dose to the fetus from conventional radiograph examinations is <0.01 Gy. Lead aprons should be utilized to protect the abdomen and pelvis. The dose to the fetus for a computed tomography scan of the pelvis and abdomen is approximately 0.01 to 0.04 Gy (112). Ultrasound and MRI do not expose the fetus to risks. MRI without gadolinium avoids ionizing radiation exposure (113). Cerebral spinal fluid analysis is suggested in patients with lymphoblastic, Burkitt, and non-Burkitt NHL. Gallium scans, positron emission tomography scans, and bone scans are contraindicated because the radioisotopes may cause harm to the fetus.

Pregnancy Management

The patient should be evaluated by an obstetrician experienced in the management of high-risk pregnancies, and a fetal ultrasound is recommended to determine fetal age and health.

Termination of the pregnancy is rarely medically indicated in patients with an initial presentation of NHL. The risk of transplacental transmission is rare. One case of transfer to the fetus of a rare natural killer-cell lymphoma with fatal consequences to the fetus in a 15-year-old female who presented at 33 weeks has been reported (55). A 29-year-old developed lymphoma at 29 weeks' gestation, and her infant developed malignant lymphoma at 8 months (77). The delivery must be coordinated with the obstetrician and the team involved in the treatment. When possible, the fetus should be carried to term. Placental blood should be stored. Breast feeding is not recommended during staging and treatment.

The issue of therapeutic abortion is one of complex religious, psychologic, cultural, and social implications. The published cases in the literature with maternal and fetal outcomes support an approach that maintains the pregnancy. Ongoing management of the lymphoma is feasible. Different authors have supported the approach of therapeutic abortion. It is likely that therapeutic abortions have been underreported in the literature in patients with a synchronous presentation of pregnancy and NHL.

Treatment

The management is complex (114–119). The outcome of mother and fetus has improved in more recent years and with optimal therapeutic interventions. After staging of the patient is complete and an assessment of fetal health completed, a decision as to the therapeutic approach and timing of treatment is required. The following principles are recommendations. Whenever possible, all therapy should be avoided during the first 12 weeks of gestation (109). The incidence of chemotherapy associated fetal malformations in patients with malignant disease has been reported to be 14% to 19% in the first trimester versus 1.3% in the second and third trimesters versus 3% in the general population (107). Cardonick and Iacobucci (103) reported an overall incidence of 2.9% of chemotherapy associated fetal malformations in 365 fetuses with nine of the 11 fetuses exposed to chemotherapy in the first trimester. A decision regarding treatment must be made taking into consideration the prognosis of the mother and the risks to the fetus (119). This is the most critical period of development of the fetus and the period when the use of antimetabolites is the most damaging. Rituximab has been administered in the first trimester of pregnancy without complications to the mother, pregnancy, or fetus (65). However, follow-up data are limited.

Patients with localized disease above the diaphragm that are treated with radiation therapy must have abdominal shielding special tables that will be low risk to the fetus.

Patients with advanced-stage low-grade follicular lymphoma who are asymptomatic can usually be observed without treatment during pregnancy or at least until the end of the first trimester (119). Therapeutic interventions that do not expose the fetus to potential toxicities that include predominantly topical approaches are indicated in cutaneous T-cell lymphoma (90,121). α-Interferon was administered to one patient in the third trimester of pregnancy without complications (82).

Corticosteroids may be used at any time during the pregnancy with low risk to the fetus. However, one case-control study reported that exposure to corticosteroids during the first trimester of pregnancy was found to be associated with an increased risk of cleft lip (with or without cleft palate) in newborns (122). This treatment can relieve symptoms and shrink lymphomatous masses, and delay the need for cytotoxic drugs until after delivery or at least until the second or third trimester when the risk of teratogenic effects on the fetus is lower.

Ondansetron, metaclopropamide, and H2-blockers are not contraindicated in pregnancy (123–125).

Treatment of patients in the second trimester depends on the histology, bulk of disease, symptoms, stage of disease, and fetal gestation. A recent reported series with optimal treatment regimens suggests that pregnancy does not affect the course of the lymphoma (119). If the patient has a potentially curable lymphoma such as a DLBCL, then chemotherapy should proceed with a rituximab-CHOP-based regimen (120,126). Favorable outcomes have been reported in pregnant patients (58,73,75,76). Chemotherapy is not contraindicated in the second and third trimester, and successful results have been reported. In the second and third trimesters, chemotherapy is associated with a low risk of fetal malformations: 1.3% of 150 patients (109). However, long-term delayed effects remain a concern (104). Methotrexate is contraindicated. If the disease is determined to be low bulk, the patient asymptomatic, and the pace of disease is determined to be stable or slow, then careful observation until delivery or the third trimester may be a reasonable course of action.

Treatment of patients in the third trimester is less problematic. Chemotherapy at this stage has a low risk of fetal malformations. On the other hand, if the fetus is determined to be mature enough to survive after delivery, elective induction can proceed and chemotherapy initiated after delivery. The hematologist/oncologist must work in close collaboration with an obstetrician, neonatologist, and other team members to time delivery and chemotherapy. Amniocentesis to assess fetal lung maturity is helpful in choosing the optimal time of delivery. Drugs not approved by the Food and Drug Administration are an absolute contraindication.

Lymphoblastic (41,66,97), Burkitt and non-Burkitt NHL (8,9,12,14,16–18,27,29,60,72,88), and other aggressive B-cell and T-cell lymphomas require an early and aggressive approach that includes methotrexate and cytosine arabinoside. There are no general guidelines in these diseases. The decision regarding treatment in these histologies will necessarily involve a discussion of therapeutic abortion. Outcomes are improving with more aggressive therapy in Burkitt lymphoma with multiple agent therapies such as cyclophosphamide, vincristine, and doxorubicin-methotrexate/ifosfamide, etoposide, and high-dose cytarabine (72).

The treatment after delivery of the lymphoma must reflect the standard of care for the particular histology and stage.

NHL during pregnancy is rare. Adequate comprehensive (bone marrow, cardiac function, intellectual quotient function, etc.) long-term follow-up information is not available for children exposed to chemotherapy for malignant disease. A multidisciplinary approach with state-of-the-art therapeutic interventions can result in long-term survival for both mother and fetus. More information must be accumulated on the long-term outcome of the fetus exposed to radiation, chemotherapeutic, and immunotherapy agents. The object to the management and treatment in NHL and pregnancy is to ensure that both the mother and the fetus achieve the most optimal outcomes.

References

1. Issacs R. Lymphosarcoma cell leukemia. *Ann Intern Med* 1937;11:657–662.
2. Moracci E. Insopetta linfosarcomatosi di Kundrat gravidanze. *Arch Gynecol Obstet* 1942;6:15.
3. Hesseltine HC, Loth MF. Malignant diseases associated with pregnancy. *West J Surg Obstet Gynecol* 1956;64:529–535.
4. Goodman M. Reticulum cell sarcoma in pregnancy. *J Obstet Gynaecol Br Emp* 1958;65:641–643.
5. Rosenberg SA, Diamond HD, Jaslowitz B, et al. Lymphosarcoma: a review of 1269 cases. *Medicine* 1961;40:31–84.
6. Bulska M. A case of reticulosarcoma appearing as a thrombosis of the femoral vein in a pregnant woman [in Polish]. *Ginekol Pol* 1962;33:373–378.
7. Lysyj A, Bergquist JR. Pregnancy complicated by sarcoma. Report of two cases. *Obstet Gynecol* 1963;21:506–509.
8. Vieaux JW, McGuire DE. Reticulum cell sarcoma of the cervix. *Am J Obstet Gynecol* 1964;89:134–135.
9. Bannerman RHO. Burkitt's tumor in pregnancy (letter to the editor). *BMJ* 1966;2:1136–1137.
10. Leeks SR. Lymphosarcoma complicating pregnancy. *N Z Med J* 1966;65:467–468.
11. Mehta A, Vakil RM. Use of Endoxan in case of lymphosarcoma with pregnancy during the third trimester (a case report). *Indian J Cancer* 1966;3:198–202.
12. Sheperd JJ, Wright DH. Burkitt's tumour presenting as bilateral swelling of the breast in women of child-bearing age. *Br J Surg* 1967;54:776–780.
13. Henderson M, Paterson WG. Perforation of jejunum by reticulum cell sarcoma in pregnancy. *Am J Surg* 1968;115:385–389.
14. Hardin JA. Cyclophosphamide treatment of lymphoma during third trimester of pregnancy. *Obstet Gynecol* 1972;39:850–851.
15. Inoue Y, Masuda H, Shiojima Y. Pregnancy complicated by sarcoma. *Acta Obstet Gynaecol Jpn* 1972;19:222–225.
16. Finkle HI, Goldman RL. Burkitt's lymphoma—gynecologic considerations. *Obstet Gynecol* 1974;43:281–284.
17. Armon PJ. Burkitt's lymphoma of the ovary in association with pregnancy: two case reports. *Br J Obstet Gynaecol* 1976;83:169–172.
18. Armitage JO, Feagler JR, Skoog DP. Burkitt lymphoma during pregnancy with bilateral breast involvement. *JAMA* 1977;237:151.
19. Ortega J. Multiple agent chemotherapy including bleomycin of non-Hodgkin's lymphoma during pregnancy. *Cancer* 1977;40:2829–2835.
20. VillaSanta U, Attar S, Jiji R. Malignant histiocytic lymphoma (reticulum cell sarcoma) in pregnancy. *Gynecol Oncol* 1978;6:383–390.
21. Newman RA, Gallagher JG, Clements JP, et al. Demonstration of Ga-67 localization in human placenta. *J Nucl Med* 1978;19:504–506.
22. Durodola JI. Administration of cyclophosphamide during late pregnancy and early lactation: a case report. *J Natl Med Assoc* 1979;71:165–166.
23. Tunca JC, Reddi PR, Shah SH, et al. Malignant non-Hodgkin's type lymphoma of the cervix uteri occurring during pregnancy. *Gynecol Oncol* 1979;7:385–393.
24. Bornkamm GW, Kaduk B, Kachel G, et al. Epstein-Barr virus-positive Burkitt's lymphoma in a German woman during pregnancy. *Blut* 1980;40:167–177.
25. Case BW, Benaroya S. Dyspnea in a pregnant young woman. *Can Med Assoc J* 1980;122:890–896.
26. Falkson HC, Simson IW, Falkson G. Non-Hodgkin's lymphoma in pregnancy. *Cancer* 1980;45:1679–1682.
27. Jones DED, d'Avignon MB, Lawrence R, et al. Burkitt's lymphoma: obstetric and gynecologic aspects. *Obstet Gynecol* 1980;56:533–536.
28. Cheson BD, Johnston JL, Junco GD. Cytologic evidence for disseminated immunoblastic lymphoma. *Am J Clin Pathol* 1981;75:621–625.
29. Lowenthal RM, Funnel CF, Hope DM, et al. Normal infant after combination chemotherapy including teniposide for Burkitt's lymphoma in pregnancy. *Med Pediatr Oncol* 1982;10:165–169.
30. Berrebi A, Schattner A, Mogilner BM. Disseminated Burkitt's lymphoma during pregnancy. *Acta Haematol* 1983;70:139–140.
31. Karp GI, van Oeyen P, Valone F, et al. Doxorubicin in pregnancy: possible transplacental passage. *Cancer Treat Rep* 1983;67:773–777.
32. Schapira DV, Chudley AE. Successful pregnancy following continuous treatment with combination chemotherapy before conception and throughout pregnancy. *Cancer* 1984;54:800–803.
33. Ioachim HL. Non-Hodgkin's lymphoma in pregnancy: three cases and review of the literature. *Arch Pathol Lab Med* 1985;109:803–809.
34. Garg A, Kochupillai V. Non-Hodgkin's lymphoma in pregnancy. *South Med J* 1985;78:1263–1264.
35. Steiner-Salz S, Yahalom J, Samuelov A, et al. Non-Hodgkin's lymphoma associated with pregnancy: a report of six cases, with a review of the literature. *Cancer* 1985;56:2087–2091.
36. Mulvihill JJ, McKeen EA, Rosner F, et al. Pregnancy outcome in cancer patients: experience in a large cooperative group. *Cancer* 1987;60:1143–1150.
37. Trombley BA, Marcus CS, Koci T. Unexpected demonstration of superior vena caval obstruction in third trimester lung imaging. *Clin Nucl Med* 1988;13:407–409.
38. Giovannini M, Saccucci P, Cannone D, et al. Can pregnancy aggravate the course of non-Hodgkin's lymphoma? *Eur J Gynaecol Oncol* 1989;10:287–289.
39. Natel S, Parboosingh J, Poon MC. Treatment of an aggressive non-Hodgkin's lymphoma during pregnancy with MACOP-B chemotherapy. *Med Pediatr Oncol* 1990;18:143–145.
40. Roumen FJ, de Leeuw JW, et al. Non-Hodgkin's lymphoma of the puerperal uterus. *Obstet Gynecol* 1990;75(pt 2):527–529.
41. Avilés A, Díaz-Maqueo JC, Torras V, et al. Non-Hodgkin's lymphomas and pregnancy: presentation of 16 cases. *Gynecol Oncol* 1990;37:335–337.
42. Toko H, Okabe K, Kamei H, et al. Successful chemotherapy on a pregnant non-Hodgkin's lymphoma patient. *Acta Med Okayama* 1990;44:321–323.
43. Ba-Thike K, Oo N. Non-Hodgkin's lymphoma in pregnancy. *Asia Oceania J Obstet Gynaecol* 1990;16:229–232.
44. Lambert J, Wijermans PW, Dekker GA, et al. Chemotherapy in non-Hodgkin's lymphoma during pregnancy. *Neth J Med* 1991;38:80–85.
45. Spitzer M, Citron M, Ilardi CF, et al. Non-Hodgkin's lymphoma during pregnancy. *Gynecol Oncol* 1991;43:309–312.
46. Valenzuela PL, Montalban C, Matorras R, et al. Pregnancy and relapse of peripheral T cell lymphoma: a case report. *Gynecol Obstet Invest* 1991;32:59–61.
47. Kurtin PJ, Gaffey TA, Habermann TM. Peripheral T-cell lymphoma involving the placenta. *Cancer* 1992;70:2963–2968.
48. Tsujimura T, Matsumoto K, Aozasa K. Placental involvement by maternal non-Hodgkin's lymphoma. *Arch Pathol Lab Med* 1993;117:325–327.
49. Pollack RN, Sklarin NT, Rao S, et al. Metastatic placental lymphoma associated with maternal human immunodeficiency virus infection. *Obstet Gynecol* 1993;81:856–857.
50. Lishner M, Zemlickis D, Sutcliffe SB, et al. Non-Hodgkin's lymphoma and pregnancy. *Leuk Lymphoma* 1994;14:411–413.
51. Imai A, Kawabata I, Tamaya T. Case report—primary brain malignant lymphoma newly diagnosed during pregnancy. *J Med* 1995;26:333–336.
52. Gelb AB, van de Rijn M, Warnke RA, et al. Pregnancy-associated lymphomas, a clinicopathologic study. *Cancer* 1996;78:304–309.
53. Wang PH, Chao KC, Lin G, et al. Primary malignant lymphoma of the cervix in pregnancy, a case report. *J Reprod Med* 1999;53:630–632.
54. Meguerian-Bedoyan Z, Lamant L, Hopfner C, et al. Anaplastic large cell lymphoma of maternal origin involving the placenta: Case report and literature survey. *Am J Surg Pathol* 1997;21:1236–1241.
55. Catlin EA, Roberts JD Jr, Erana R, et al. Transplacental transmission of natural-killer-cell lymphoma. *N Engl J Med* 1999;341:85–91.
56. Habermann TM, Kurtin PJ, Johansen KL, et al. The synchronous presentation of non-Hodgkin's lymphoma and pregnancy: a greater than ten-year follow-up [abstract]. *Blood* 2000;96:224a. Abstract 4693.
57. El-Sonbaty MR, Bitar Z, Abdulrazak A. Acute spontaneous tumor-lysis syndrome. *Int J Hematol* 2001;73:386–389.
58. Herold M, Schnohr S, Bittrich H. Efficacy and safety of a combined rituximab chemotherapy during pregnancy. *J Clin Oncol* 2001;19:3439.
59. Safdar A, Johnson N, Gonzalez F, et al. Adult T-cell leukemia-lymphoma during pregnancy. *N Engl J Med* 2002;346:2014–2015.
60. Fadlora SO, Mabayole VO, Aderoumu AO, et al. Generalised Burkitt's lymphoma involving both breasts-a case report. *West Afr J Med* 2005;24:280–282.
61. Moore DT, Talismi MM. Non-Hodgkin's lymphoma in pregnancy: a diagnostic dilemma. Case report and review of the literature. *J Tenn Med Assoc* 1992;85:467–469.
62. Reimer P, Rüdiger T, Müller J, et al. Subcutaneous panniculitis-like T-cell lymphoma during pregnancy with successful autologous stem cell transplantation. *Ann Hematol* 2003;82:305–309.
63. Pernicario C, Zalla MJ, White JW, et al. Subcutaneous T-cell lymphoma. Report of two additional cases and further observations. *Arch Dermatol* 1993;129:1171–1176.
64. Romero LS, Goltz RW, Nagi C, et al. Subcutaneous T-cell lymphoma with associated hemophagocytic syndrome and terminal leukemic transformation. *J Am Acad Dermatol* 1996;34:904–910.
65. Kimby E, Sverristottir A, Elinder G. Safety of rituximab therapy during the first trimester of pregnancy: a case history. *Eur J Haematol* 2004;72:292–295.

66. Vandenberghe G, Claerhout F, Amant F. Lymphoblastic lymphoma presenting as bilateral gigantomastia in pregnancy. *Int J Gynaecol Obstet* 2005;91:252–253.

67. Windom KW, Duffie RS Jr. Non-Hodgkin's lymphoma presenting with gigantomastia in pregnancy. *Obstet Gynecol* 1999;93(pt 2):852.

68. Sherer DM, Stimphil RG, Santoso P, et al. Stage IV large B cell lymphoma presenting as gigantomastia and pulmonary hypertension. *Obstet Gynecol* 2004;103(pt 2):1061–1064.

69. Iyengar P, Reid-Nicholoson M, Roreira AL. Pregnancy-associated anaplastic large-cell lymphoma of the breast: a rare mimic of ductal carcinoma. *Diagn Cytopathol* 2006;34:298–302.

70. Teran-Porcayo MA, Gomez-Del Castillo-Rangel AC, Barrera-Lopez N, et al. Cancer during pregnancy: 10-year experience at a regional cancer reference center in Mexico. *Med Oncol* 2008;25:50–53.

71. O'Mahony ZD, Rasak ARA, Brett F, et al. Primary central nervous system lymphoma (PCNSL) occurring in pregnancy. *J Neurol* 2005;252:1133–1134.

72. Lam MS. Treatment of Burkitt's lymphoma during pregnancy. *Ann Pharmacother* 2006;40:2048–2052.

73. Decker M, Rothermundt C, Holländer G, et al. Rituximab plus CHOP for treatment of diffuse large B-cell lymphoma during second trimester of pregnancy. *Lancet Oncol* 2006;7:693–694.

74. Alalade AO, Odefinmi FO. A rare and potentially fatal cause of pelvic pain in pregnancy: anaplastic large cell lymphoma. *J Obstet Gynaecol* 2006;26:69–72.

75. Friedrichs B, Tiemann M, Salwender H, et al. The effects of rituximab treatment during pregnancy on a neonate. *Haematologica* 2006;91:1426–1427.

76. Herold M, Schnohr S, Bittrich H, et al. Efficacy and safety of a combined rituximab chemotherapy during pregnancy. *J Clin Oncol* 2001;19:3439.

77. Maruko K, Maeda T, Kamitomo M, et al. Transplacental transmission of maternal B-cell lymphoma. *Am J Obstet Gynecol* 2004;191:380–381.

78. Ataergin S, Kanat O, Arpaci F, et al. A rare occurrence of diffuse immunoblastic lymphoma in pregnancy. *Am J Hematol* 2007;82:73–176.

79. Romero LS, Goltz RW, Nagi C, et al. Subcutaneous T-cell lymphoma with associated hematophagocytic syndrome and terminal leukemic transformation. *J Am Acad Dermatol* 1996;34:904–910.

80. Windom KW, McDuffie RS. Non-Hodgkin's lymphoma presenting with gigantomastia in pregnancy. *Obstet Gynecol* 1999;93:852.

81. Kato M, Ishimura K, Hayami Y, et al. Pregnancy-associated cytotoxic lymphoma: a report of 4 cases. *Int J Hematol* 2001;74:186–192.

82. Echols KT, Gilles JM, Diro M. Mycosis fungoides in pregnancy: remission after treatment with α-interferon in a case refractory to conventional therapy: a case report. *J Matern Fetal Med* 2001;10:68–70.

83. Klezl Z, Krbec M, Gregora E, et al. Rare presentation of non-Hodgkin lymphoma of the thoracolumbar spine in pregnancy with 7 years' survival. *Arch Orthop Trauma Surg* 2002;122:308–310.

84. Ravikanti L, Singh V. Subcutaneous panniculitic T-cell lymphoma presenting as pyrexia of unknown origin in pregnancy: a report of a case and literature review. *Aust N Z J Obstet Gynaecol* 2003;43:166–168.

85. Szokol JW, Alspach D, Mehta M, et al. Intermittent airway obstruction and superior vena cava syndrome in a patient with an undiagnosed mediastinal mass after cesarean delivery. *Anesth Analg* 2003;97:883–884.

86. Kohri NN, Togano T, Nakamin H, et al. Development of hepatosplenic γδ T-cell lymphoma with pancytopenia during early pregnancy: a case report and review of the literature. *Eur J Haematol* 2004;73:367–371.

87. Guven S, Ozcebe OI, Tuncer ZS. Non-Hodgkin's lymphoma complicating pregnancy: a case report. *Eur J Gynaecol Oncol* 2005;457–458.

88. Mablire LK, Pettker CM, Buhimschi CS. Burkitt's lymphoma of the ovary in pregnancy. *Obstet Gynecol* 2006;108:743–745.

89. Dilek I, Topcut N, Demir C, et al. Hematological malignancy and pregnancy: a single-institution experience of 21 cases. *Clin Lab Haematol* 2006;28:170–176.

90. Amitay-Layish I, David M, Kafri B, et al. Early-stage mycosis fungoides, parapsoriasis en plaque, and pregnancy. *Int J Dermatol* 2007;46:160–165.

91. Constantinos GM, Daskalakis GJ, Papagerogiou IS, et al. Non-Hodgkin's lymphoma during pregnancy-case report. *Eur J Obstet Gynecol Reprod Biol* 1998;79:95–97.

92. Zuazu J, Julia A, Sierra J, et al. Pregnancy outcome in hematologic malignancies. *Cancer* 1991;67:703–709.

93. Soliman KB, Abbas MM, Seksaka MA, et al. Aggressive primary thyroid non Hodgkin's lymphoma with pregnancy. *Saudi Med J* 2007;28:634–636.

94. Schiffer C, Sheiessler M, Lehr J, et al. Unique occurrence of Brachmann-de Lange syndrome in a fetus whose mother presented with a diffuse large B-cell lymphoma. *Pathol Oncol Res* 2007;13:255–259.

95. Zuazu J, Julia A, Sierra J, et al. Pregnancy outcome in hematologic malignancies. *Cancer* 1991;67:703–709.

96. Rodriguez JM, Haggag M. VACOP-B chemotherapy for high-grade non-Hodgkin's lymphoma in pregnancy. *Clin Oncol* 1995;7:337–338.

97. Aviles A, Neri N. Hematological malignancies and pregnancy: a final report of 84 children who received chemotherapy in utero. *Clin Lymphoma* 2001;2:1723–1727.

98. Greenberg LH, Tanaka KR. Congenital anomalies probably induced by cyclophosphamide. *JAMA* 1964;188:423–426.

99. Toledo TM, Harper RC, Moser RH. Fetal effects during cyclophosphamide and irradiation therapy. *Ann Intern Med* 1971;74:87–91.

100. Milunsky A, Graef JW, Gaynor MF Jr. Methotrexate-induced congenital malformations: with review of the literature. *J Pediatr* 1968;72:790–795.

101. Shotton D, Monie IW. Possible teratogenic effect of chlorambucil on a human fetus. *JAMA* 1963;18674–18675.

102. Ebert U, Loeffler H, Kirch W. Cytotoxic therapy and pregnancy. *Pharmacol Ther* 1997;74:207–220.

103. Cardonick E, Iacobucci A. Use of chemotherapy during human pregnancy. *Lancet Oncol* 2004;5:283–291.

104. Turchi JJ, Villasis V. Anthracyclines in the treatment of malignancy in pregnancy. *Cancer* 1988;61:435–440.

105. Varadi G, Elchalal U, Shushan A, et al. Umbilical and cord blood for use in transplantation. *Obstet Gynecol Surv* 1995;50:611.

106. Byrne J, Rasmussen SA, Steinhorn SC, et al. Genetic Disease in offspring of childhood and adolescent cancer survivors. *N Engl J Med* 1998;338:1339–1344.

107. Doll DC, Ringenberg QS, Yarbro JW. Antineoplastic agents and pregnancy. *Semin Oncol* 1989;16:337–346.

108. Sweet DL Jr, Kinzie J. Consequences of radiotherapy and antineoplastic therapy for the fetus. *J Reprod Med* 1976;17:241–246.

109. Shepart T. *Catalog of teratogenic agents*, 3rd ed. Baltimore, MD: Johns Hopkins University Press, 1980.

110. Streffer C, Shore R, Konermann G, et al. Biological effects after prenatal irradiation (embryo and fetus). A report of the International Commission on Radiological Protection. *Ann ICRP* 2003;33:5–206.

111. Kal HB, Struikmans H. Radiotherapy during pregnancy: fact and fiction. *Lancet Oncol* 2005;6:328–333.

112. International Commission on Radiological Protection. Pregnancy and medical radiation. *Ann ICRP* 2000;30:1–43.

113. Nicklas AH, Baker ME. Imaging strategies in the pregnant cancer patient. *Semin Oncol* 2000;27:623–632.

114. Banks PM. Pregnancy and lymphoma. *Arch Pathol Lab Med* 1985;109:182.

115. Ward FT, Weiss RB. Lymphoma and pregnancy. *Semin Oncol* 1989;16:397–409.

116. Pohlman B, Maklis RM. Lymphoma and pregnancy. *Semin Oncol* 2000;27:657–666.

117. Dhedin N, Coiffier B. Lymphoma and pregnancy. In: Canellos GP, Lister TA, Young B, eds. *The lymphomas*. New York, NY: Elsevier, 2003:549–556.

118. Pereg D, Koren G, Lishner M. The treatment of Hodgkin's and non-Hodgkin's lymphoma in pregnancy. *Haemetologica* 2007;92.1230–1237.

119. Froesch P, Belisario-Filho V, Zucca E. Hodgkin and non-Hodgkin lymphomas during pregnancy. *Recent Results Cancer Res* 2008;178:111–121.

120. Habermann TM, Weller EA, Morrison VA, et al. Rituximab-CHOP versus CHOP alone or with maintenance rituximab in older patients with diffuse large B-cell lymphoma. *J Clin Oncol* 2006;24:3121–3127.

121. Habermann TM, Pittelkow MR. Cutaneous lymphoma. *Clinical Oncology*. In: Abeloff M, Armitage J, Niederhuber J, et al., eds. Philadelphia, PA: Churchill Livingston Elsevier, 2008:3077–3107.

122. Rodriguez-Pinilla E, Martinez-Frias ML. Corticosteroids during pregnancy and oral clefts: a case-control study. *Teratology* 1998;58:2–5.

123. Einarson A, Maltepe C, Navioz Y, et al. The safety of ondansetron for nausea and vomiting of pregnancy: a prospective comparative study. *BJOG* 2004;111:940–943.

124. Berkovitch M, Mazzota P, Greenberg P, et al. Metoclopramide for nausea and vomiting of pregnancy: a prospective multicenter international study. *Am J Perinatol* 2002:19:311–316.

125. Magee LA, Mazzotta P, Koren G. Evidence-based view of safety and effectiveness of pharmacologic therapy for nausea and vomiting of pregnancy (NVP). *Am J Obstet Gynecol* 2002;186(suppl):S256–S261.

126. Coiffier B, Freugier P, Mounier N, et al. CHOP chemotherapy plus rituximab compared with CHOP alone in elderly patients with diffuse large B-cell lymphoma. *N Engl J Med* 2002;346:235–242.

CHAPTER 35 ■ MANAGEMENT OF ACQUIRED IMMUNODEFICIENCY SYNDROME-RELATED LYMPHOMA

ALEXANDRA M. LEVINE AND JONATHAN W. SAID

EPIDEMIOLOGY OF ACQUIRED IMMUNODEFICIENCY SYNDROME-RELATED LYMPHOMA IN THE UNITED STATES

Human immunodeficiency virus (HIV)/acquired immunodeficiency syndrome (AIDS) is now the fourth leading cause of death in the world, accounting for 4.8% of all mortality (1). Over 40 million people are living with AIDS, of whom 25 million live in sub-Saharan Africa. Cumulative deaths due to AIDS are in excess of 22 million people worldwide (1).

The peak of the AIDS epidemic in the United States occurred in 1993, a year in which new infections continued unabated, and additional patients were added on the basis of an expanded case definition (2), including cervical cancer, recurrent bacterial pneumonia, or tuberculosis in people infected with HIV. Furthermore, a new category termed "immunologic AIDS" was added to the case definition of AIDS, characterized not by the development of a clinical illness, but by the presence of very low CD4 cells (<200 per mm^3 $CD4^+$ lymphocytes) in the peripheral blood (2). In sharp contrast to the initial dramatic increases in the incidence of AIDS in the United States in the 1980s and early 1990s, a decline in the incidence of new AIDS cases was first documented in 1995, clearly as a result of the widespread use of highly active antiretroviral therapy (HAART) (3). This antiretroviral therapy, modeled after the concepts of multiagent chemotherapy for malignant disease, usually consists of three or more antiretroviral agents, each of which comes from a different chemical class, with differing mechanisms of action and differing toxicities (4). The widespread use of HAART in the United States and Europe has resulted in a remarkable 73% decrease in the development of new AIDS cases among people infected with HIV (3,5) and in an equally remarkable approximately 75% decline in mortality among patients with AIDS (3,6). Nonetheless, the prevalence of HIV continues to increase in the United States, driven by a stable number of new infections each year along with prolongation in survival of previously infected individuals. It is thus apparent that increasing numbers of individuals infected with HIV will require care in the decades ahead.

Epidemiologic Characteristics of Acquired Immunodeficiency Syndrome-Related Lymphoma

Lymphoma has traditionally been considered a late manifestation of HIV infection, more likely to occur in the setting of significant immune suppression (7), with CD4 cells <200 per mm^3 and history of an AIDS-defining illness. Thus, after an earlier diagnosis of AIDS, the relative risk of immunoblastic lymphoma is approximately 627-fold increased, whereas that of diffuse large cell lymphoma is 145-fold increased over that expected in the general population (8,9). Of interest, when linking cancer and AIDS registries, even low-grade lymphoma is found to be increased 14-fold over that expected in individuals who had already been diagnosed with another AIDS-defining illness (8,9), while the incidence of T-cell lymphoma has also increased among patients with AIDS (10).

Although HAART has been associated with a significant decrease in the incidence of various opportunistic infections and Kaposi sarcoma (3,11), the decrease in systemic AIDS lymphoma has not uniformly been as profound (11). Nonetheless, a report of >7,300 patients infected with HIV from 52 European countries compared data on AIDS-defining illnesses diagnosed during 1994, before the HAART era, with those diagnosed in 1998, after widespread use of HAART in these regions (12). The incidence of AIDS-defining conditions declined from 30.7 per 100 patient-years in 1994 to 2.5 per 100 patient-years during 1998 (p <0.0001). However, whereas the proportion of new AIDS cases due to various opportunistic infections decreased, the proportion of new AIDS cases secondary to lymphoma increased significantly, with lymphoma representing <4% of all AIDS cases diagnosed in 1994 and 16% of all AIDS cases diagnosed in 1998 (p <0.0001). In contrast, there was no evidence for an increase in the proportion of AIDS diagnoses due to primary central nervous system (CNS) lymphoma (12). Matthews et al. (13) from England have also documented a statistically significant increase in lymphoma as the initial AIDS-defining condition among a large group of individuals infected with HIV.

An international collaborative study, including cancer incidence data from 23 prospective studies that included 47,936 individuals seropositive for HIV from North America, Europe, and Australia, sought to determine the adjusted incidence rates of various AIDS-defining conditions since the advent of HAART (14). In terms of lymphoma incidence, the rate ratio showed a significant reduction when cases diagnosed in 1992 to 1996 were compared with those from 1997 through 1999. Of interest, however, the rate ratio for immunoblastic lymphoma and primary CNS lymphoma decreased significantly during these two time intervals, whereas that of Burkitt lymphoma (BL) and Hodgkin lymphoma (HL) showed no such decrease (14). More recently, there has been an actual increase in HL in the era of HAART, which appears to be related to improvements in CD4 counts (15,16).

Multiple additional studies have been conducted to determine the incidence of HIV lymphoma in the era of HAART. Some of these studies indicate no significant decrease (13,17), whereas others have documented highly significant decreases in the incidence of HIV lymphoma in recent years (12,18,19). The true situation may, perhaps, best be understood within the context of the immune status of the population being evaluated. Thus, Besson et al. (19) from France evaluated the incidence of HIV lymphoma in terms of the strata or level of CD4 cells. As the number of CD4 cells in a given group of patients decreased, the incidence of HIV lymphoma increased, as shown in Table 35.1. The same inverse relationship between decreased CD4 levels and increased risk of HIV lymphoma was apparent both in the time frame before institution of HAART and after the availability of HAART. Thus, if HAART is available in a given population and has been used effectively, with resultant decrease in HIV-1 viral load (18) and increase in CD4 cells (19), one would expect a significant decline in the incidence of HIV lymphoma. However, in populations that do not have access to HAART or in those in whom HAART has been ineffective, no decrease in the incidence of HIV lymphoma is observed.

Together, the current population-based data would suggest that the incidence of primary CNS and systemic lymphoma has decreased since the widespread use of HAART. However, the decline in lymphoma is far less impressive than that observed for opportunistic infections or Kaposi sarcoma, resulting in a proportionate increase in lymphoma as an initial AIDS-defining illness. Furthermore, although initial controlled clinical trials have indicated that approximately 80% of treated subjects achieve a nondetectable HIV viral load after HAART, only approximately 40% achieve this end point in "real world" conditions (20). The effect of HAART on the incidence of AIDS lymphoma will clearly be dependent on the long-term efficacy of combination antiretroviral therapy when assessed at the population level. Issues of access, compliance, drug resistance, and underlying host and environmental factors will all likely be operative.

Standard and Genetic Epidemiologic Risk Factors for Acquired Immunodeficiency Syndrome-Related Lymphoma

In distinction to Kaposi sarcoma, which occurs primarily in men who have sex with men, lymphoma is seen in all population groups at risk for HIV (21). Similar to de novo lymphoma occurring in individuals negative for HIV (22,23), AIDS lymphoma is more common in men than women. All age groups are affected, and lymphoma is the most common malignancy in children infected with HIV (24). Epidemiologic studies have failed to identify major environmental factors associated with AIDS lymphoma among individuals infected with HIV (25–27). However, host genetic factors may be operative. Thus, patients infected with HIV who are heterozygotes for the CCR5δ32 deletion are statistically less likely to develop lymphoma (28), whereas those with SDF-1 mutations (3'A) are statistically more likely to develop lymphoma (29).

Changing Characteristics of Patients with Acquired Immunodeficiency Syndrome-Related Lymphoma in the Era of Highly Active Antiretroviral Therapy

The characteristics of patients with AIDS-related lymphoma have changed in those patients diagnosed after the availability of HAART. Levine et al. (17) reviewed records of 369 patients diagnosed with AIDS lymphoma at a single institution from 1982 through 1998 and compared these data with population-based information from the County of Los Angeles. Significant changes in the demographic characteristics of AIDS lymphoma occurred in both populations, with

TABLE 35.1

INCIDENCE OF AIDS LYMPHOMA SINCE HAART, STRATIFIED BY CD4 CELLS[a]

	Systemic					Primary CNS				
	1993–1994		1997–1998			1993–1994		1997–1999		
CD4	Cases (no.)	Incidence	Cases (no.)	Incidence	p Value	Cases (no.)	Incidence	Cases (no.)	Incidence	p Value
≥350	15	15.6	37	15.9	NS	2	2.0	3	1.3	NS
200–349	25	34.8	45	33.6	NS	5	6.8	6	4.4	NS
100–199	40	76.8	53	73.3	NS	5	9.2	6	8.1	NS
50–99	34	103.8	40	164.7	.053	10	29.6	7	28.0	NS
<50	202	253.8	50	223.2	NS	77	93.9	25	107.5	NS
All	415	86.0	285	42.9	$<10^{-30}$	135	27.8	65	9.7	$<10^{-11}$

NS, not significant.
[a] Rate/100,000 person-years.
From Besson C, Goubar A, Gabarre J, et al. Changes in AIDS-related lymphoma since the era of highly active antiretroviral therapy. *Blood* 2001;98:2339–2344, with permission.

the latter period characterized by statistically significant increases among women, those of nonwhite ethnicity (Latino/Hispanic individuals), and those who acquired HIV heterosexually. A decrease in Burkitt or Burkitt-like lymphomas occurred over time, whereas the prevalence of diffuse large cell lymphoma increased. In the large EuroSIDA study of AIDS lymphoma (18), similar changes were seen in terms of both pathologic and certain clinical characteristics of disease. Thus, the incidence of BL decreased from the pre-HAART to the HAART eras, whereas that of diffuse large cell/immunoblastic lymphoma increased. In the HAART era, a statistically decreased incidence of HIV lymphoma was seen among homosexuals and whites, with an increase among those who acquired HIV by heterosexual contact (18). The median age of affected patients increased from 38 years in the pre-HAART era to 42 years in the HAART time frame (18). Similarly, Matthews et al. (13), reporting on experience in London with 7,840 patients positive for HIV, noted a statistically significant increase in median age of patients diagnosed with HIV lymphoma in the HAART era. On multivariate analysis, characteristics statistically associated with development of AIDS lymphoma included lower CD4 lymphocyte count (both at baseline and at nadir), older age, and lack of HAART (13). In a study of patients infected with HIV followed in Paris, the incidence of AIDS lymphoma decreased since the advent of HAART, and the median CD4 cell count at lymphoma diagnosis increased significantly, from 63 per mm^3 in the earliest to 191 per mm^3 in the latest time interval (19). Although not statistically significant, trends similar to those identified in Los Angeles and London were observed, with an increase of HIV lymphoma among women (from 6.3% in the pre-HAART to 11.9% in the post-HAART era) and heterosexuals (from 11.1% to 14.3%), and a decrease among those who acquired HIV by homosexual contact.

These demographic changes are similar to those described in patients with HIV/AIDS in general, in the era of HAART.

PATHOGENESIS AND PATHOLOGY OF ACQUIRED IMMUNODEFICIENCY SYNDROME-RELATED LYMPHOMA

Immunosuppression and Epstein-Barr Virus Infection

Studies of HIV lymphoma offer a paradigm for the development of lymphoid malignancy in the setting of profound immunosuppression (30). One of the factors that contributes to lymphomagenesis is chronic antigenic stimulation, driven by HIV, multiple coinfecting agents, and B-cell expansion, which is frequently poly- or oligoclonal (7).

The Epstein-Barr virus (EBV) also plays a pivotal role in this process, with EBV demonstrated in approximately 40% of cases overall (31–36). HIV-related lymphomas are associated with both A and B types of EBV, which differ from lymphomas associated with transplantation (37–41). Viral infection may be associated with production of cytokines, including interleukin (IL)-6, IL-10, and IL-13, which also support proliferation of neoplastic lymphoid cells (42,43). Table 35.2 demonstrates

TABLE 35.2		
ASSOCIATION BETWEEN EBV AND HHV8/KSHV IN VARIOUS SUBTYPES OF AIDS LYMPHOMA		
Subtype of AIDS lymphoma	EBV+	HHV8 +
BL-plasmacytoid morphology	+ (50%–70%)	−
BL-classic	+ (40%)	−
MCD	−	+
DLBCL	+ (30%)	−
Immunoblastic	+ (100%)	−
Primary CNS	+ (100%)	−
Plasmablastic, oral cavity	+ (100%) (100%)	+
PEL	EBER + LMP-1	+ −
Polymorphic B cell (posttransplant-like)	+	−
Germinotropic lymphoproliferative disorder	+	+
HL	+ (100%)	−

EBER, Epstein-Barr-encoded RNA.

the association between EBV and human herpesvirus type 8 (HHV8)/Kaposi sarcoma-associated herpesvirus (KSHV) in various subtypes of AIDS lymphoma. Almost all HIV-related cases of HL are associated with EBV (44).

Gene Rearrangements and Clonality

Monoclonal rearrangements of the immunoglobulin (Ig) genes depicting a single dominant clone can be detected in almost all B-cell HIV lymphomas, regardless of subtype. This may be confirmed by clonal presence of EBV as well as clonal cytogenetic abnormalities. Many of the key oncogenic events associated with the pathogenesis of HIV lymphoma have been linked to known oncogenes, including MYC, p53, RAS, and T-cell leukemia-1 (45,46). Molecular events in AIDS-related lymphoma are often multiple and complex, and are still poorly understood. New molecular techniques, such as gene expression profiling, are being applied to AIDS-related lymphoma and will likely uncover further genetic abnormalities. Molecular pathogenesis of specific disease entities is discussed in the sections to follow.

Classification of Acquired Immunodeficiency Syndrome-Related Lymphomas

HIV lymphomas have been classified by the World Health Organization into three groups: those occurring specifically in patients positive for HIV, those also occurring in other

TABLE 35.3

WORLD HEALTH ORGANIZATION CLASSIFICATION OF AIDS-RELATED LYMPHOMAS

A. Lymphomas also occurring in patients with immunocompetence
   1. BL
      Classic
      With plasmacytoid differentiation
      Atypical
   2. DLBCL
      Centroblastic
      Immunoblastic
   3. Extranodal marginal zone B-cell lymphoma of MALT
   4. Peripheral T-cell lymphoma
   5. Classic HL
B. Lymphomas occurring more specifically in patients positive for HIV
   1. PEL
   2. Plasmablastic lymphoma of the oral cavity
C. Lymphomas also occurring in other immunodeficiency states
      Polymorphic lymphoma (PTLD-like)

immunodeficiency states, and those that also arise in patients with immunocompetence. These are depicted in Table 35.3 (47,48).

Pathology and Pathogenesis of Burkitt Lymphomas (30% of Acquired Immunodeficiency Syndrome Lymphomas)

Patients with BLs may present with nodal disease but more often present with mass lesions in extranodal sites, such as the bowel, or infiltration in the bone marrow in a pattern resembling acute lymphoblastic leukemia. Histologically, there are sheets of intermediate-sized lymphoid cells with regular round or oval nuclear outlines or slight nuclear irregularities. The cells have one or more distinct nucleoli and amphophilic, often vacuolated, cytoplasm. Mitoses are frequent, and there are characteristically scattered phagocytic or tingible body macrophages imparting a "starry-sky" appearance. The cells often have a cohesive or clustered appearance in tissue sections, and all variations share an extremely high mitotic rate and a Ki67 or mib-1 score approaching 100%.

The majority of cases of BL associated with HIV have a distinctive plasmacytoid appearance with eccentric nuclei and more abundant amphophilic cytoplasm. (47,49–52). The cells often have a cohesive or clustered appearance in tissue sections, and all variations share an extremely high mitotic rate and a Ki67 or mib-1 score approaching 100%. These cells are often positive for cytoplasmic Ig and have other markers of plasmacytoid differentiation such as CD 138. This subtype of BL is also more likely to be positive for EBV. The remaining one-third has features of classic or atypical BL as seen in the immunocompetent population.

Molecular findings in BL characteristically involve translocations of the MYC gene on chromosome 8, with the heavy chain gene on chromosome 14 or the κ- and λ-light chain genes in chromosomes 2 and 22, respectively. In addition, dysregulation of C-MYC may arise from point mutations in the first intron-first exon regulatory regions and amino acid substitution in the second exon (53). The molecular characteristics of C-MYC activation resemble sporadic rather than endemic BL. The second most common molecular alteration in BL consists of point mutations in the tumor suppressor gene p53, which occurs in up to 60% of cases (54). In terms of the association with EBV, overall, approximately 40% of BLs are positive, a prevalence that resembles sporadic rather than endemic BL. However, in the plasmacytoid variant, EBV has been found in 50% to 70% of cases (55).

Diffuse Large B-Cell Lymphomas

Diffuse large B-cell lymphomas (DLBCLs) are a heterologous group, and HIV is associated with an increased incidence of specific subtypes. DLBCL of germinal center cell or centroblastic type accounts for only approximately 30% of AIDS lymphoma, and of these, about one-third are positive for EBV. This group of lymphomas may present with nodal or extranodal disease, and consists of diffuse sheets of large lymphoid cells with round or oval nuclei and prominent nucleoli. These malignant cells are monoclonal for Ig gene rearrangements. Not surprisingly, and in keeping with their likely pathogenesis from germinal center cells, cases of DLBCL are often associated with expression of BCL-6 (56–58). BCL-6 amplification can be demonstrated with immunohistochemistry in tissue sections. EBV is found in approximately 20% of these cases. The frequency of latent membrane protein (LMP)-1 deletion variants and of EBV type 1 and type 2 strains in AIDS DLBCLs overlaps those in the general population and is not specific for HIV (41). The proliferation rate is usually high but less than that seen in BLs.

The immunoblastic subtype of AIDS lymphoma (approximately 10% of cases) is more characteristic of AIDS infection and usually occurs at extranodal sites, particularly the CNS. In these cases, the cells are >90% immunoblasts with features of plasmacytoid differentiation. The cells are large with a single prominent, often central, nucleolus and plasmacytoid cytoplasm. In some cases, Reed-Sternberg (RS)-like cells may be found, but the background proliferation does not resemble HL. Mitoses are frequent. In the CNS, there is often clustering around blood vessels, and the lesions may be multiple (59). The incidence of EBV infection is highest in immunoblastic lymphomas and in CNS lymphomas in which EBV infection approaches 100%. CNS AIDS lymphomas are generally negative for C-MYC (60).

Plasmablastic Lymphoma of the Oral Cavity Type

Plasmablastic lymphomas were first described in the oral cavity but may occur at other sites (61,62). These distinctive lymphomas are characterized by a diffuse proliferation consisting almost entirely of large lymphoid cells with a marked plasmablastic appearance (Fig. 35.1). The cells have blast-like nuclei with prominent central nucleolus and plasmacytoid cytoplasm. These cells are usually positive for EBV but generally negative for the KSHV (HHV8). Most are positive for EBV Epstein-Barr-encoded ribonucleic acid (RNA) by

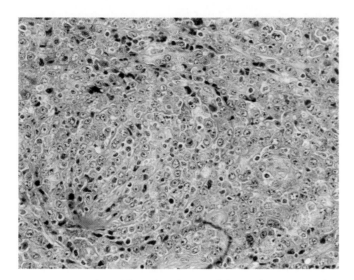

FIGURE 35.1 Plasmablastic lymphoma of the oral cavity revealing sheets of plasmablasts infiltrating soft tissues of the jaw. Hematoxylin and eosin, original magnification ×250.

in situ hybridization, variably positive for EBV LMP-1, and negative for EBV nuclear antigen 2. As suggested by their morphologic appearance, they more closely resemble plasmablasts rather than centroblasts in their phenotype, and may be negative for CD15 and CD20 but express cytoplasmic IgG and activation or plasma cell-related epitopes, such as VS38c and CD138.

Salivary Gland Lymphoid Hyperplasias and Extranodal Marginal Zone Lymphomas (Mucosa-Associated Lymphoid Tissue Lymphomas)

Symptoms and mass lesions relating to the salivary glands and related lymph nodes are common in patients infected with HIV. The most common abnormality is hyperplasia of salivary lymphoid tissue causing ductal obstruction and salivary duct cysts. There is frequently a proliferation of myoepithelial cells forming lymphoepithelial lesions analogous to those encountered in Sjögren syndrome. Other disorders associated with sicca syndrome, including rheumatoid arthritis, are not encountered. The lesions usually involve the parotid gland, but other salivary glands may also be affected.

The lymphoid hyperplasia resembles that seen in the generalized, persistent lymphadenopathy syndrome, and the ductal lesions are almost always cystic (63,64). The lymphoid proliferation is polyclonal and not associated with lymphoma in adults, but in the pediatric population infected with HIV, salivary lymphoid infiltrates have similarities with lymphocytic interstitial pneumonitis and cystic hyperplasia of the thymus (65). In children infected with HIV, mucosa-associated lymphoid tissue (MALT) lymphomas, similar to those occurring in the general population, have been described in the salivary glands and also at other sites, including the lung and stomach. The relationship of pulmonary MALT lymphoma to lymphocytic interstitial pneumonitis suggests that an infectious agent may be causally related, including exposure to EBV (66). Morphologically, these are indistinguishable from

MALT lymphomas in the general population and are defined by nodules of centrocyte-like cells with slightly irregular nuclei and monocytoid cytoplasm, with a tendency to infiltrate epithelium, forming lymphoepithelial lesions.

Polymorphic B-Cell Lymphoma (Posttransplant Lymphoproliferative Disorder-Like)

Unlike in the iatrogenically immunosuppressed transplant population, polymorphic B-cell lymphoma, for unexplained reasons, is only occasionally encountered in the setting of HIV (44). Posttransplant lymphoproliferative disorder (PTLD)-like lymphomas in patients positive for HIV closely resemble posttransplant lymphomas in their association with EBV and their polymorphous appearance, which includes small lymphocytes, plasma cells, and plasmacytoid immunoblasts (Fig. 35.2). In the higher-grade lesions, large cells are more prominent, and there may be tumor necrosis. This lesion is not associated with specific HIV risk factors and occurs in men, women, and children with AIDS. Disease may be encountered at nodal or extranodal sites, including salivary glands, lung, and skin, and must be distinguished from benign forms of HIV-related lymphoid hyperplasia (67). Despite their polymorphous appearance, these cases are usually monoclonal with regard to Ig gene rearrangements, although occasional cases may be polyclonal or exhibit a small clonal rearranged band in a polyclonal background (44).

Other Low-Grade Lymphomas, Including Small Lymphocytic Lymphoma, Follicular Lymphoma, and Marginal Zone Lymphoma

Although indolent lymphomas, including small lymphocytic and marginal zone lymphoma, are increasingly encountered

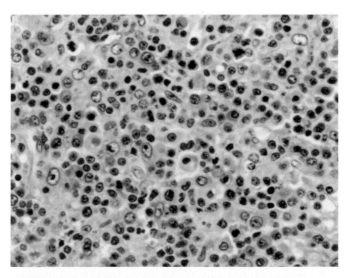

FIGURE 35.2 Polymorphic lymphoid proliferation resembling posttransplant-associated lymphoproliferative disease showing a mixture of lymphoid cells, plasma cells, and immunoblasts. Hematoxylin and eosin, original magnification ×160.

in the population infected with HIV (8,9), it is not clear at this point if there is a causal relationship to AIDS. Patients positive for HIV with low-grade lymphomas tend to be less immunosuppressed and have higher CD4 counts, compared with patients with aggressive lymphomas, and demonstrate prolonged survival despite a high incidence of bone marrow infiltration and advanced-stage disease at presentation (68).

Myeloma, Plasmacytoma, Plasma Cell Leukemia, and Monoclonal Gammopathy of Undetermined Significance

The relationship of HIV to plasma cell dyscrasias is of particular interest because polyclonal hypergammaglobulinemia and oligoclonal B-cell expansion are commonly encountered in patients with HIV. AIDS is associated with an increased risk for myeloma, and patients with myeloma tend to have aggressive disease with an anaplastic or blastic morphology and frequent involvement of body fluids (69,70).

Lymphomatoid Granulomatosis

Lymphomatoid granulomatosis is a rare EBV-related disorder in which immunodeficiency is a contributory factor. This lesion has been described in the oral cavity and gingival areas in patients with HIV (71). The lymphomatous infiltrates are characteristically associated with angioinvasion and extensive necrosis. Numerous Epstein-Barr early region 1-containing lymphoid cells can be found clustered about affected vessels.

Peripheral T/Natural Killer-Cell and Anaplastic Large Cell Lymphomas

Although AIDS-related lymphomas are usually of B-cell type, peripheral T-cell lymphomas are occasionally associated with AIDS (72,73), and T-cell lymphomas are statistically increased among patients with a prior diagnosis of AIDS (10). These occur most frequently in the skin and subcutaneous tissues where they present with tumor-like masses, frequently associated with vascular invasion and necrosis. Unlike mycosis fungoides, they usually lack epidermotropism. Morphologically, they resemble peripheral T-cell lymphomas with a spectrum of pleomorphic neoplastic T cells.

T/natural killer-cell anaplastic large cell lymphomas usually present at extranodal sites, including the gastrointestinal tract, skin, and nasal sinuses (72,73). These consist of large anaplastic lymphoid cells with the characteristic "hallmark" cells with markedly deformed nuclei most common around blood vessels. Because of the unusual presentation and anaplastic morphology, they may be confused with carcinoma. Some of these cases may be positive for EBV. Cases in the skin are usually negative for anaplastic lymphoma kinase protein. Neutrophil-rich anaplastic large cell lymphoma has also been described in association with HIV (74). In addition, the EBV-associated nasal type T/natural killer-cell lymphoma has been described in the setting of HIV, although this appears quite rare (75).

Mycosis Fungoides

There appears to be an increased incidence of mycosis fungoides in the population infected with HIV (72,73). The lesions resemble mycosis fungoides in the general population and may present on the buttocks among other cutaneous sites. Histologically, there are characteristically cerebriform lymphoid cells infiltrating the epidermis and forming Pautrier-like intraepidermal clusters. Although mycosis cells are almost invariably CD4+ in the general population, in patients with HIV with CD4 cell depletion, there may be cutaneous eruptions and infiltration of CD8+ mycosis cells. These cells may also infiltrate regional lymph nodes and the bone marrow, and are associated with a poor prognosis (76). Mycosis fungoides lesions must be distinguished from atypical lymphoid infiltrates in the skin, which are common in HIV and often related to drug reactions.

Human Herpesvirus 8-Associated Lymphomas

In addition to causing multicentric Castleman disease (MCD) in patients infected with HIV, HHV8 infection is also associated with characteristic lymphoproliferative disorders, which include primary effusion lymphomas (PELS), extracavitary lymphomas not associated with effusions, and plasmablastic lymphomas (not to be confused with plasmablastic lymphomas of the oral cavity type).

Primary Effusion Lymphomas

PEL is a distinct clinicopathologic entity occurring usually, but not exclusively, in the setting of HIV infection (77–81). Patients with HIV and PEL tend to be older males with homosexuality as a risk factor, late-stage disease, and severe immunosuppression, with CD4 counts <100 per mm^3. Approximately one-third of patients with PEL also have Kaposi sarcoma (82). Although rare, this lymphoma is of interest because of the causal relationship with the KSHV, also known as HHV8. KSHV/HHV8 was the first human γ-2 herpes virus identified and has been shown to be the cause of Kaposi sarcoma, from which it was first isolated (83,84). KSHV sequences are, in fact, present in much higher copy numbers in PEL tissues when compared with tissues of Kaposi sarcoma (85).

Patients with PEL classically present with symptoms of an effusion (pleural, pericardial, or ascitic) in the absence of a tumor mass. Some patients may develop a mass lesion in the adjacent pleural or peritoneal cavity. Rarely, HHV8-positive lymphomas indistinguishable from PEL present at extranodal sites such as the gastrointestinal tract (86–89), without presence of effusions. In this setting, the disease may present in nodal or extranodal sites (87–89). Examination of effusion fluid reveals large pleomorphic lymphoma cells with cytologic features that range between immunoblastic, plasmablastic, and anaplastic large cell lymphoma (Fig. 35.3). The cells may be multinucleated and resemble RS cells but are negative for CD15. The malignant cells also have a distinctive phenotype, staining for leukocyte common antigen CD45 and various activation antigens (human leukocyte antigen-DR, EMA, CD30, CD38, CD77), but are usually negative for other B- and T-cell markers, including CD20, CD19, and CD79a.

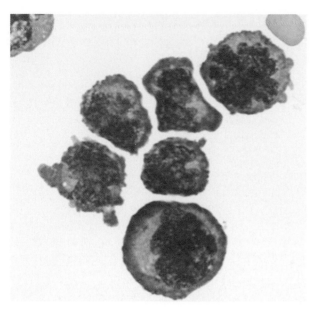

FIGURE 35.3 PEL showing large anaplastic malignant cells from a pleural effusion. Hematoxylin and eosin, original magnification ×400.

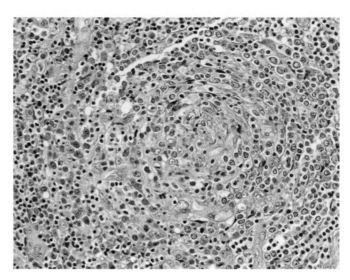

FIGURE 35.4 Plasmablastic microlymphoma in a spleen from a patient with MCD showing clusters of plasmablasts. Hematoxylin and eosin, magnification ×250.

Rare cases may coexpress both B- and T-cell antigens despite a B-cell genotype (90,91). The B-cell nature can be demonstrated by the presence of Ig gene rearrangements in Southern blots or polymerase chain reaction (92). Presence of HHV8 is demonstrable by polymerase chain reaction for various transcripts or by immunohistochemistry using antibodies to the latent nuclear antigen. Staining for latent nuclear antigen is helpful in confirming the diagnosis. There is active viral replication in the nuclei of the malignant cells, and viral particles are packaged in the cytoplasm to be shed from the cell surface (93). Virus can be found in saliva and the gastrointestinal tract of infected individuals.

PEL appears to derive from a late differentiated (postfollicular) B cell indicated by clonal rearrangements as well as somatic mutations of the Ig genes. The pathogenesis of PEL is of interest because the KSHV is a herpes virus with a number of oncogenic sequences, including a BCL-2–like sequence, a G-coupled receptor, and a type D cyclin similar to PRAD1 (94). Cytogenetic studies suggest multiple complex abnormalities (95), but most known oncogenes, including BCL6, MYC, RAS, T-cell leukemia-1, and p53, do not appear to be implicated (45). The HHV8 virus also produces cytokines, such as viral IL-6, capable of contributing to angiogenesis and tumor cell growth (96). Although there is invariably coinfection with EBV in the setting of HIV, KSHV is capable of producing lymphomas in the absence of EBV. PEL cells are positive for Epstein-Barr-encoded RNA but lack LMP-1. PEL may also occur in individuals infected with KSHV in the absence of HIV, and may be seen in both men and women (81,97).

Human Herpesvirus 8-Positive Lymphomas Associated with Multicentric Castleman Disease

HHV8 is also associated with MCD (98,99). The disease usually presents in the spleen where there are aggregates of plasmablasts forming clusters termed microlymphomas or in some cases mass lesions. Morphologically, these resemble immunoblasts or plasmablasts but differ from plasmablastic lymphomas of the oral cavity, which are not associated with KSHV (Fig. 35.4). The plasmablasts are monotypic for IgM λ and are infected with HHV8, which can be demonstrated by immunohistochemical staining for latent nuclear antigen. These cells do not harbor somatic mutations in the rearranged Ig genes and appear to originate from naive B cells in the follicular mantle (98).

The spectrum of HHV8-associated lymphoproliferative disorders also includes KSHV and EBV-associated germinotropic lymphoproliferative disorder first described by Du et al. (100). Unlike the majority of HHV8-associated lymphoproliferative disorders, this entity is associated with a favorable response to therapy (100,101). It is characterized by localized lymphadenopathy in asymptomatic patients, the presence of large numbers of plasmablasts involving the germinal centers (therefore the term germinotropic), and coexpression of EBV and HHV8. Molecular analysis reveals either poly or oligoclonal Ig genes in these tissues. Although the germinotropic lymphoproliferative disorder is not characteristically associated with immune deficiency, a case with features intermediate between HHV8+ plasmablastic microlymphoma and HHV 8+ germinotropic lymphoproliferative disorder has been described in a male positive for HIV (102).

CLINICAL ASPECTS OF ACQUIRED IMMUNODEFICIENCY SYNDROME-RELATED LYMPHOMA

Clinical Presentation

Most patients with AIDS lymphoma present with systemic "B" symptoms, including unexplained fever, drenching night sweats, or weight loss in excess of 10% of normal body weight (21,103,104). These symptoms may also be seen in various opportunistic infections, or in Hodgkin lymphoma, or Kaposi sarcoma. Nonetheless, after careful evaluation to exclude these other causes of systemic symptoms, the possibility of lymphoma should be considered.

Bone Marrow Involvement

Bone marrow involvement is diagnosed in approximately 20% of patients at initial presentation, with BL the most common in this setting (105). The median hemoglobin level in patients with marrow involvement is 10.6 g per dL, while approximately one-third of patients present with platelet counts <100,000. Marrow involvement is statistically associated with leptomeningeal involvement. More than 50% marrow involvement is associated with decreased survival in these patients (105).

Gastrointestinal Tract Lymphoma

The gastrointestinal tract is involved by lymphoma in approximately one-fourth of reported patients, who may present with abdominal pain, anorexia, nausea, and vomiting, or a change in bowel habits. Abdominal distention or an abdominal mass may be noted. Involvement of the rectum is not unusual, presenting as a rectal mass or pain on defecation. Lymphoma within the liver is also relatively common, occurring in approximately 10% to 25% of reported series (21,103,104). These patients may present with jaundice, systemic "B" symptoms, abdominal pain, or anorexia.

Involvement of the Cerebrospinal Fluid

Leptomeningeal involvement by lymphoma occurs in approximately 10% to 20% of patients with newly diagnosed systemic AIDS lymphoma. These patients may be entirely asymptomatic in terms of the CNS. When symptoms do occur, the most common include altered mental status, cranial nerve palsies, or headache (106). Numbness of the chin may also be seen in patients with leptomeningeal lymphoma (107). Presence of EBV within the cerebrospinal fluid, with EBV nuclear antigen 1 detected by polymerase chain reaction, may also be used to diagnose lymphomatous meningitis in patients with systemic AIDS lymphoma (108). Leptomeningeal lymphoma is associated with higher CD4 cell counts than seen in patients with primary CNS lymphoma. Intrathecal cytosine arabinoside or methotrexate has been used successfully, both to treat known leptomeningeal lymphoma and to prevent its occurrence in patients at risk (106).

Other Sites

Any site may be involved by lymphoma in patients with underlying HIV infection. Unusual sites include the lung, oral cavity, adrenal gland, kidney, heart, and others. Lymphoma within the gallbladder has been described, as well as involvement of the earlobe and multiple other unusual sites of lymphomatous disease (21,103).

Staging Evaluation in Patients with Acquired Immunodeficiency Syndrome Lymphoma

The specific evaluation and management of patients with newly diagnosed AIDS lymphoma are presented in Table 35.4.

Routine Blood Work

Routine blood work is often abnormal at the time of diagnosis, with anemia expected in the majority, even in the absence of marrow involvement (105). Although thrombocytopenia or leukopenia may also be observed, these abnormalities may

TABLE 35.4

STAGING AND MANAGEMENT OF SYSTEMIC AIDS LYMPHOMA

History
Physical examination
Blood tests: complete blood cell count, lactate dehydrogenase, uric acid, chemistries
CAT scan: chest, abdomen, pelvis
CAT or magnetic resonance imaging scan: brain
FDG-PET scan of body
Bone marrow aspirate and biopsy
Lumbar puncture with evaluation of cerebrospinal fluid for lymphoma
Systemic chemotherapy is used for all stages of disease
HAART is recommended in combination with chemotherapy
Restage patient after two or four cycles of chemotherapy
Give two cycles of chemotherapy beyond CR

CAT, computed axial tomography.

occur secondary to HIV itself, or to various commonly used medications or opportunistic infections.

The level of lactate dehydrogenase is often elevated and should always be checked because an increased lactate dehydrogenase level has prognostic implications associated with decreased survival (109).

Uric acid levels may also be increased at diagnosis. Allopurinol is indicated before institution of chemotherapy to prevent hyperuricemia associated with tumor lysis. Serum calcium levels may also be elevated at diagnosis.

Computed Axial Tomography Scan of Chest, Abdomen, and Pelvis

Generalized or localized lymphadenopathy is commonly seen on computed axial tomography scans of patients with AIDS lymphoma. Special attention should be given to the retroperitoneal and mesenteric nodes as well as to lymph node areas adjacent to sites of extranodal disease.

In the presence of gastrointestinal involvement, abdominal computed axial tomography scan reveals evidence of focal lymphomatous involvement, documented in 58 of 59 such patients described by Radin et al. (110). Focal hepatic lesions are expected with liver involvement, varying from solitary to innumerable, and ranging from relatively small 1-cm nodules to large masses >15 cm in diameter. Lesions are typically less dense than the adjacent liver parenchyma. Larger masses are often heterogeneous in density, with areas of necrosis. Isolated hepatomegaly alone, without focal mass lesions, is quite unusual (110).

With lymphoma in the lung, interstitial infiltrates, pulmonary nodules, or alveolar lung disease has been described, with pleural effusions also commonly encountered (111).

Fluorodeoxyglucose Positron Emission Tomography

Although formal studies of fluorodeoxyglucose (FDG) positron emission tomography (PET) scanning have not yet been accomplished in patients with AIDS-related systemic lymphoma, the utility of these scans has been confirmed in patients with de novo lymphoma, with sensitivity rates of 89% and specificity of 100% in a group of 18 such patients (112). By comparison, sensitivity of computed axial tomography scanning on detection of lymphoma in these patients was 86%, and specificity was 67%. FDG-PET has also been useful in the detection of residual active lymphomatous disease after completion of chemotherapy (113). Furthermore, early response to chemotherapy, as detected by FDG-PET scan, may be useful as an indicator of subsequent prognosis (114).

Lumbar Puncture

Although not routine in patients with de novo lymphoma, patients with systemic AIDS lymphoma should undergo diagnostic lumbar puncture at the time of initial staging evaluation. As many as 20% of patients may have lymphoma within the spinal fluid in the absence of any specific symptom or clinical sign of such involvement (115). In the presence of lymphomatous meningitis, the cell count may be normal or high, with presence of abnormal cells cytologically. The median cell count is usually only minimally elevated, at 12 per mm^3 (116). The glucose level is usually low, but may be normal, whereas the protein in the cerebrospinal fluid may be elevated or normal (106,116). The presence of EBV nuclear antigen 1 by polymerase chain reaction is associated with lymphomatous involvement of the cerebrospinal fluid and may also predict eventual lymphomatous meningitis (108).

Bone Marrow Aspirate and Biopsy

Bone marrow aspirate and biopsy are also indicated during the initial staging evaluation of a patient with AIDS lymphoma, with marrow involvement in approximately 20% of patients (21,105). Lymphomatous involvement of marrow is statistically associated with lymphoma in the cerebrospinal fluid and in bones (105).

Prognostic Factors in Patients with Systemic Acquired Immunodeficiency Syndrome-Related Lymphoma

The factors associated with shorter survival of patients with AIDS-related lymphoma, before the availability of HAART, included CD4 cells <100 per mm^3, stage III or IV disease, age >35 years, history of injection drug use, and elevated lactate dehydrogenase (109,117,118). The International Prognostic Index (IPI) for aggressive lymphoma has also been validated in patients with AIDS lymphoma (119). Recently, the use of HAART has been associated with significant prolongation in survival among patients with AIDS lymphoma (19,120), and the prognostic factors for survival have changed among patients treated with HAART. Thus, in a study of 192 patients treated with curative intent, Lim et al. (121) noted that only two factors were predictive of survival in the era of HAART, including attainment of complete remission (CR), and the IPI score (122). In a further study, which included patients also receiving palliative regimens alone, Bower et al. (123) demonstrated that both IPI score and CD4 cells were predictive of survival. A prognostic risk score was developed from these factors, in which CD4 cells <100 per mm^3 and high or high-intermediate IPI scores were weighted to predict poorer prognosis.

THERAPY FOR PATIENTS WITH ACQUIRED IMMUNODEFICIENCY SYNDROME-RELATED DIFFUSE LARGE B-CELL AND IMMUNOBLASTIC LYMPHOMAS: BACKGROUND

Before the availability of HAART, the use of standard dose multiagent chemotherapy was associated with increased toxicity without an increase in response rates or survival when compared with low-dose modifications (124); it was then recommended that low-dose variations of regimens such as cyclophosphamide, hydroxydaunorubicin, Oncovin (vincristine), and prednisone (CHOP) or methotrexate, bleomycin, doxorubicin, cyclophosphamide, vincristine, and dexamethasone be employed (125). This paradigm changed dramatically when it was shown that HAART could prolong survival appreciably in patients with AIDS lymphoma (19), and that HAART could be used safely when given with combination chemotherapy (126). Thus, Besson et al. (19) demonstrated a median survival of 21.2+ months in patients treated in the HAART era, versus 6.3 months in those treated before the availability of HAART. Hoffmann et al. (127) demonstrated 60% overall survival at 5 years in 159 patients who received chemotherapy with HAART, versus approximately 20% in those who received single agent antiretroviral therapy, and <5% in patients who received chemotherapy without antiretroviral agents. Thus, HAART has led to an improvement in prognosis, allowing new paradigms and recommendations for optimal treatment.

Optimal Timing of Institution of Highly Active Antiretroviral Therapy with Chemotherapy

The appropriate timing of the institution of HAART in relationship to multiagent chemotherapy has not been studied. Antinori et al. (120) found that antiretroviral control was a significant factor in the ability to attain CR status among a small group of patients. In contrast, Levine et al. (128) found that antiretroviral control was not necessary for attainment of CR. Little et al. (129) evaluated the infusional etoposide, prednisone, Oncovin (vincristine), cyclophosphamide, and hydroxydaunomycin (doxorubicin) (EPOCH) regimen in 39 patients with newly diagnosed AIDS lymphoma, withholding HAART until the day after the completion of six cycles of chemotherapy. During chemotherapy, HIV-1 RNA levels increased by a median of 0.83 log$_{10}$, whereas the median CD4 cell count decreased by 187 cells per mm^3. Nonetheless, a CR rate of 74% was achieved, with 92% disease free, and 60% overall survival at 53 months. Thus, with rapid reinstitution of HAART at the conclusion of EPOCH, excellent rates of response and survival were attained, indicating that HAART may, in fact, be delayed until completion of chemotherapy. Nonetheless, three patients developed opportunistic infections within 3 months of completion of chemotherapy, and the overall survival of patients who began EPOCH with CD4 cells <100 per mm^3 was only 16% at 53 months. It is possible that these results might have improved if HAART had been employed 6 months earlier, at the time of initiation of chemotherapy. Although not mandatory, then, the use of concomitant HAART with chemotherapy is often recommended, especially in those patients who present with CD4 cells <100 per mm^3, despite the fact that no randomized trial has yet been completed to address this question. In this setting, use of zidovudine should be avoided because this drug may cause significant marrow suppression on its own (130).

THERAPY FOR PATIENTS WITH NEWLY DIAGNOSED DIFFUSE LARGE B-CELL LYMPHOMA IN THE HIGHLY ACTIVE ANTIRETROVIRAL THERAPY ERA

Infusional Regimens

Sparano et al. (131,132) developed the cyclophosphamide, doxorubicin, and etoposide (CDE) regimen in patients with newly diagnosed AIDS lymphoma, as shown in Table 35.5. In a large, multi-institutional Eastern Cooperative Oncology Group trial, 107 patients received the 4-day infusion, including 48 patients who received concomitant antiretroviral therapy with didanosine, and 59 received HAART regimens (131,132). For the group as a whole, the rate of CR was 44%, with partial responses in 11%. Although there was no difference in CR rates among patients who received HAART versus didanosine, the median overall survival was longer in those patients who received combination antiretroviral therapy. This series of trials indicates that although response rates to infusional CDE appear similar to those achieved with either low-dose or standard-dose methotrexate, bleomycin, doxorubicin, cyclophosphamide, vincristine, and dexamethasone, survival appears superior in those patients who receive concomitant HAART.

The dose-adjusted EPOCH (da EPOCH) regimen, developed and tested at the National Cancer Institute, has been associated with excellent response rates and survival (129). The regimen consists of: a 4-day infusion of etoposide (50 mg per m^2 per day); vincristine (0.4 mg per m^2 per day); and doxorubicin (10 mg per m^2 per day); along with prednisone, given at 60 mg per m^2 per day orally on days 1 to 5; and cyclophosphamide, which was dose adjusted based upon

TABLE 35.5
EPOCH REGIMEN OF INFUSIONAL CHEMOTHERAPY
Etoposide, 50 mg/m^2/d × 4 d
Vincristine, 0.4 mg/m^2/d × 4 d
Doxorubicin, 10 mg/m^2/d × 4 d
Cyclophosphamide, 187 mg/m^2 IV on d 5 for CD4$^+$ <100 cells/mm^3 or 375 mg/m^2 IV on d 5 for CD4$^+$ ≥100 cells/mm^3
Prednisone, 60 mg/m^2 orally, d 1–5
G-CSF: start on d 6
Repeat on d 22 times six cycles
IV, intravenously.

CD4 cell count at initiation of therapy, and given by bolus on day 5 (187 mg per m^2 in patients with CD4 cells <100 per mm^3 and 375 mg per m^2 for patients with CD4 cells >100 per mm^3). The dose of cyclophosphamide is then adjusted again after each cycle of chemotherapy; if the nadir absolute neutrophil count (ANC) was >500 per mm^3, the dose of cyclophosphamide was increased by 187 mg per m^2, and if the nadir ANC was <500, the dose was decreased by 187 mg per m^2. Granulocyte colony-stimulating factor (G-CSF) was started on day 6, and used until the ANC reached ≥5,000 per mm^3 (Table 35.5). Among 39 patients, of whom 59% had an age-adjusted IPI score of two or three, a CR rate of 74% was achieved. The CR rate was 56% among 16 patients with <100 per mm^3 CD4 cells and 87% among those with higher CD4 cells. Although median survival for all treated patients was 60% at 53 months, survival was an impressive 87% in patients with CD4 cells >100 per mm^3 at initiation of chemotherapy. This study was completed in a single institution, and results thus require confirmation in larger, multi-institutional settings.

Such a study was recently completed by the National Cancer Institute -sponsored AIDS Malignancy Consortium (AMC), in which 105 patients were entered onto a randomized phase II trial, comparing da EPOCH with concomitant rituximab, versus da EPOCH followed sequentially by rituximab (133,134). In the latter arm of 54 patients who received da EPOPH alone as initial therapy before institution of sequential rituximab, the median CD4 cell count was 198 per mm^3, 64% had an age-adjusted IPI score of two or three, and a CR rate of 53% (90% confidence interval 41%, 64%) was achieved.

In a previous randomized phase III AMC study of CHOP versus rituximab-CHOP (R-CHOP) in 150 patients with newly diagnosed AIDS lymphoma, a CR rate of 47% was achieved in those 51 patients receiving CHOP alone (135), and 29% died of lymphoma. The median CD4 count at diagnosis was 133 per mm^3, and 53% had IPI scores of two or three.

Although no trial has yet compared infusional EPOCH with CHOP (or rituximab-EPOCH versus R-CHOP), initial data at this time would indicate a potential superiority of the infusional EPOCH regimen over standard CHOP.

Use of Rituximab with Chemotherapy

In patients without underlying HIV infection, Coiffier et al. (136) have demonstrated a clear advantage to the use of R-CHOP chemotherapy, when compared with CHOP alone in elderly patients with DLBCL. This study has been expanded to other patient populations, with confirmation of the value of concomitant rituximab in all patient groups with DLBCL (137).

In an attempt to ascertain if the addition of rituximab to CHOP provided the same advantage in patients positive for HIV, several phase II trials of R-CHOP were conducted. Boue et al. (138) reported a CR rate of 77% and 2-year overall survival of 75% in 52 assessable patients, without an increase in life-threatening infections. Spina et al. (139) pooled results of three prospective phase II trials evaluating rituximab in combination with a 96-hour infusion of CDE, and noted a 70% CR rate with 59% 2-year failure-free survival in 74 patients, of whom 76% received concomitant HAART. Opportunistic infections occurred in 14% during or within 3 months of the end of rituximab-CDE, and 23%

developed nonopportunistic infections; 8% died of infection, suggesting the possibility of an increase in infections among patients infected with HIV receiving rituximab with chemotherapy. In fact, unusual viral or other infections have been reported, even in patients negative for HIV with lymphoma who have received rituximab (140,141).

A randomized phase III study of CHOP versus R-CHOP was subsequently conducted by the AMC, including 150 patients, of whom 99 were randomized to R-CHOP and 51 to CHOP (135). In this study, rituximab was given at a dose of 375 mg per m^2 on day 1 of each cycle, and CHOP was administered on day 3. Additional doses of rituximab were given monthly for 3 months at the completion of all chemotherapy, thus representing a higher cumulative dose of rituximab than had been used by Coiffier et al. (136). A CR rate of 57.6% was achieved with R-CHOP, with 14% of patients dying of lymphoma. In contrast, a 47% CR rate was achieved among patients treated with CHOP, with 29% succumbing to lymphoma. Although these data indicate an advantage to the use of rituximab, the results were not statistically significant. There could be several explanations for the differences observed between patients infected with HIV studied in the AMC trial, and those reported by Kaplan (135) and Coiffier (136) et al. First, the AMC trial may not have been powered sufficiently to detect statistically significant differences in response rate. Thus, the trial by Coiffier et al. (136) included 400 patients, whereas the AMC trial consisted of only 150. Second, it is conceivable that the biologic characteristics of HIV-positive versus -negative DLBCL may differ. For example, the presence of BCL-2 expression was shown to correlate with improved response to rituximab in the trial by Mournier et al. (142), and it is possible that patients infected with HIV are less likely to have lymphomas that express BCL-2. In this regard, Little et al. (129) demonstrated that lymphoma tissues of 16% of 25 patients infected with HIV with DLBCL expressed BCL-2, versus 41% of 33 HIV-negative cases. Nonetheless, whereas only a subset of cases was evaluated for BCL-2 in the AMC trial, the addition of rituximab to CHOP in those patients with BCL-2 positive lymphomas was not associated with improvement in progression-free survival or time to tumor progression (135). Resolution of this issue will be required from future studies.

Additional controversy arose from the AMC trial of R-CHOP versus CHOP in terms of toxicity. Thus, 14% of patients who received R-CHOP died of treatment-related infection, versus only 2% of those who received CHOP alone ($p = 0.035$) (135). Of interest, there were no statistically significant differences between the R-CHOP and CHOP groups in terms of the number of patients or cycles with ANCs <500 per mm^3, the numbers of episodes of febrile neutropenia, or in the Ig levels after two cycles of therapy. Why there would be an excess of infectious death among patients treated with R-CHOP remains unknown. However, most of the infectious deaths occurred among patients with severe immunodeficiency, as evidenced by CD4 cell counts <50 per mm^3. When these patients were excluded from analysis, statistically significant differences in terms of the rate of infectious death disappeared. It would seem appropriate to consider use of prophylactic antibiotics in patients infected with HIV with severe immunocompromise who are treated with rituximab.

The advantages or disadvantages of use of rituximab with chemotherapy were further studied as part of the most recent AMC trial, in which da EPOCH was employed as the backbone regimen (133,134). In this randomized phase II study, 51 patients were randomized to receive da EPOCH, with concomitant rituximab (375 mg per m^2 on day 1 of each cycle), whereas 55 were randomized to receive six cycles of da EPOCH, followed sequentially by weekly rituximab for 6 weeks. In the concomitant rituximab-EPOCH group, median CD4 cell count was 181 per mm^3, 31% had CD4 cells <100 per mm^3, and 69% had an age-adjusted IPI score of two or three. A CR/CR unconfirmed rate of 69% was achieved (90% confidence interval, two sided 56%, 79%). In the sequential arm of EPOCH followed by rituximab, the median CD4 cell count was 194 per mm^3, 31% had CD4 cells <100 per mm^3, and 64% had an age-adjusted IPI score of two or three. A CR rate of 53% was achieved (90% confidence interval, two sided 41%, 64%). In a post hoc multivariate analysis that included treatment group, stage, CD4 <100 per mm^3, elevated lactate dehydrogenase, performance status, and antiretroviral therapy, the only factors significantly associated with higher CR/CR unconfirmed rates were treatment arm (use of concomitant rituximab-EPOCH; $p = 0.04$) and stage I/II disease ($p = 0.04$). Of importance, there were no differences between the treatment groups in terms of grade 3 or 4 febrile neutropenia (16% vs. 15%), infection (27% vs. 29%), or nonlymphoma death (10% vs. 7%).

These data indicate that addition of rituximab to chemotherapy may be associated with an increased risk of infectious death in patients with severe immunocompromise, and CD4 cells <50 per mm. In general, however, patients infected with HIV may be treated safely when rituximab is employed. Furthermore, addition of rituximab appears to offer significant advantages when compared with chemotherapy alone. At this time, use of the infusional da EPOCH regimen with concomitant rituximab appears to yield results that are superior to other studied regimens, without added toxicity. Nonetheless, randomized trials of infusional EPOCH versus other regimens will be required to determine the true advantage of this infusional regimen.

Use of Radiotherapy in Patients with Localized Acquired Immunodeficiency Syndrome-Diffuse Large B-Cell Lymphoma

One of the hallmarks of AIDS-related DLBCL is the disseminated nature of disease at initial diagnosis, and as such, the use of radiotherapy for localized stage I or II disease is rarely entertained. Nonetheless, radiation is often used for specific emergent issues, such as cord compression due to lymphoma.

TREATMENT FOR PATIENTS WITH RELAPSED OR REFRACTORY ACQUIRED IMMUNODEFICIENCY SYNDROME-DIFFUSE LARGE B-CELL LYMPHOMA

The optimal chemotherapeutic regimen for patients with relapsed/refractory AIDS DLBCL has not yet been defined, and these patients are usually treated using regimens employed for patients negative for HIV, such as ifosfamide, carboplatin, and etoposide or rituximab-ifosfamide, carboplatin, and etoposide

(143), although neither regimen has been studied prospectively in patients infected with HIV. An earlier study of etoposide, methylprednisolone, cytosine arabinoside, and cisplatin demonstrated a CR rate of 30%, with occasional long-term, disease-free survival following successful use of this regimen, even before the availability of HAART (144).

Patients with relapsed AIDS lymphoma who are responsive to salvage chemotherapy may be treated successfully with high-dose chemotherapy and autologous stem cell transplant. The group from City of Hope has reported 84% continuous CR status in 19 such patients at a median follow-up of 27 months (range 6 to 57 months) after autologous stem cell transplant (145). The AMC, in a multi-institutional trial of 20 patients, has reported long-term, event-free survival of 50%, with a median follow-up of 23 weeks after autologous transplant, whereas median overall survival was not reached in 13 of the 20 patients (146).

In a study just initiated at City of Hope, patients with relapsed or refractory AIDS lymphoma receive autologous stem cells that have been transduced with three different anti-HIV RNAs, including a short hairpin RNA targeted to HIV-1 tat/rev, a decoy for HIV-tat reactive element (TAR), and a ribozyme that targets host cell CCR5 chemokine receptor (CCRSRZ) (147). Results of this study are awaited with interest.

THERAPY FOR PATIENTS WITH PREVIOUSLY UNTREATED ACQUIRED IMMUNODEFICIENCY SYNDROME-RELATED BURKITT LYMPHOMA

Before the availability of HAART, patients with BL were treated in a manner similar to those with DLBCL because treatment results did not differ between the two pathologic types, and median survival was similar, at approximately 6 months (135,148). Studies of prognostic factors in the era of HAART have shown that patients with BL, if treated with CHOP (135,148) or low-dose chemotherapy, fare much worse than patients with DLBCL. Thus, patients with AIDS BL, when treated with the infusional rituximab-CDE regimen, fared worse than those with AIDS-related DLBCL, with a CR rate of 52% in BL, versus 77% in those with DLBCL (149). Recent treatment paradigms for patients with AIDS-related BL have now changed to reflect the improvement in outcome in the era of HAART, with current data suggesting that these patients fare better after receipt of more intensive therapy, as is given in patients negative for HIV with BL.

The optimal regimen for patients with AIDS BL has not yet been defined, although the CHOP backbone is not currently recommended. The group from Memorial Sloan-Kettering reported a retrospective analysis of 14 patients positive for HIV and 24 negative for HIV, of whom approximately half received the rituximab-cyclophosphamide, vincristine, and doxorubicin (CODOX)-methotrexate/ifosfamide, etoposide, and high-dose cytarabine (M/IVAC) regimen, whereas the others received CHOP or CHOP-like regimens (150). The efficacy of the two regimens was similar in the HIV-infected group, with a CR rate of 63% and an event-free survival of 60% in patients treated with CODOX-M/IVAC versus 67% CR and 60% event-free survival

for the CHOP-like regimens; this was compared with a 2-year event-free survival of 92% among patients negative for HIV. Infectious complications were similar among individuals positive and negative for HIV, indicating that the intensive CODOX-M/IVAC regimen was feasible in the setting of HIV (150).

Currently, the AMC is studying a modified rituximab-CODOX-M/IVAC regimen in patients with newly diagnosed AIDS-related BL. Modifications were made in an attempt to increase efficacy (addition of rituximab) and reduce toxicity (modifications of total dose and scheduling). Patients with leptomeningeal lymphoma receive combination intrathecal therapy, including liposomal cytarabine.

The hyperfractionated cyclophosphamide, vincristine, doxorubicin, and dexamethasone regimen has been evaluated prospectively in patients with AIDS BL (151), with a CR rate of 92% and overall survival of 48% at 2 years in 13 patients positive for HIV. At a follow-up of 29 months, six of seven patients who had received HAART concomitant with chemotherapy were alive in continuous CR, whereas all four who did not receive HAART had died.

The Spanish PETHEMA (Programa para el Estudio y Tratamiento de las Hemopatias Malignas, Spanish Society of Hematology) 3/97 study employed a protocol based upon the intensive German adult lymphoblastic lymphoma/B-cell acute lymphoblastic leukemia 05/93 regimen in 14 patients positive for HIV and 25 negative for HIV with BL (152,153). No difference was seen in terms of CR rates (71% vs. 77%) or 2-year overall survival (43% vs. 55%) among patients positive or negative for HIV.

The infusional da EPOCH-rituximab regimen has also been employed in small numbers of patients positive and negative for HIV with BL, with excellent preliminary results. In a series of 19 patients, including six with HIV infection, a CR rate of 100% was achieved, with overall survival of 100% and event-free survival of 93% after a median follow-up of 29 months. No treatment-related deaths were reported (154). Of note, 18% of patients in the original da EPOCH trial in patients infected with HIV (129) had BL. The patients with BL were statistically more likely to have CNS involvement (57% vs. 16% with DLBCL), and overall survival of the patients with BL tended to be worse at 53 months (66% for DLBL vs. 43% for BL; $p = 0.22$). Nonetheless, if patients with CNS disease were excluded, overall survival was similar for the two pathologic types. In fact, all patients with BL who died in the da EPOCH trial had CNS involvement, accounting for the poorer outcome when compared with patients with DLBCL. Although the original da EPOCH regimen did not include CNS prophylaxis, use of intrathecal methotrexate (12 mg on days 1 and 5 of cycles three through six) was subsequently employed, after two patients with BL had relapse in the cerebrospinal fluid. It is thus apparent that da EPOCH or da EPOCH-rituximab may be effective in patients infected with HIV with BL; intrathecal prophylaxis is clearly indicated (155).

PRIMARY CENTRAL NERVOUS SYSTEM ACQUIRED IMMUNODEFICIENCY SYNDROME-RELATED LYMPHOMA

Patients with AIDS-related primary CNS lymphoma tend to present with extremely advanced HIV disease, with median

CD4 cell counts <50 per mm^3 and history of previous AIDS-defining clinical illnesses in approximately 75% (21,156,157). Recent large series have confirmed a major, highly significant decrease in primary CNS lymphoma since the advent of HAART (12,14,18,19).

Patients with AIDS lymphoma primary to the brain usually seek medical attention because of altered mental status, seizures, or focal neurologic abnormalities (156–158). Systemic "B" symptoms are seen in 80% to 90%. Imaging studies of the brain reveal mass lesion(s) within brain parenchyma, which may be found at any site. Computed tomographic scans or magnetic resonance imaging scans are relatively nonspecific in terms of identifying a lesion as lymphoma, whereas thallium single-PET scan (159) or FDG-PET scan (160) may be more helpful in terms of differentiating primary CNS lymphoma from other AIDS-related disease entities. Because AIDS-related primary CNS lymphoma is uniformly associated with EBV (161), when combined with EBV testing of cerebrospinal fluid, FDG-PET scanning yields even more specific results (159,160).

The optimal therapy for patients with AIDS-related primary CNS lymphoma remains problematic. Median survival is in the range of 2 to 4 months in the setting of either radiation therapy or no treatment at all (158). Nonetheless, whole brain radiation has been associated with improved quality of survival and is advocated on this basis. Antiretroviral therapy (zidovudine) along with ganciclovir and IL-2 has been explored, with some evidence of efficacy in small numbers of patients (162). Hydroxyurea, in an attempt to suppress EBV infection, was recently used in two patients, with excellent objective responses (163). Importantly, use of HAART has dramatically improved the survival time of patients with AIDS-related primary CNS lymphoma, and should routinely be employed in this setting (164). With so few numbers of cases currently being diagnosed in the United States, it has been most difficult to accrue sufficient numbers of patients for prospective clinical trials. Additional work is required to define effective modalities of therapy in affected individuals.

MULTICENTRIC CASTLEMAN DISEASE IN THE SETTING OF HUMAN IMMUNODEFICIENCY VIRUS

Patients infected with HIV with Castleman disease are typically ill at presentation, with high fevers, splenomegaly, and elevated C-reactive protein. Various autoimmune phenomena may occur, including Coombs' positive hemolytic anemia, with approximately half of all patients anemic at diagnosis. HHV8 is present in all and may be detected in peripheral blood mononuclear cells during symptomatic periods (165). Aside from HHV8, the pathogenesis of disease includes prominent angiogenesis, induced by production of vascular endothelial growth factor (166), as well as production of IL-6, with elevated levels seen in serum, resolving after successful treatment (167); both of these mechanisms provide insights into future therapeutic interventions (165). Patients infected with HIV with MCD have a high propensity toward development of lymphoma, as seen in 23% of 60 such patients followed for a period of 20 months (168). These lymphomas included

PEL, plasmablastic lymphoma, and extranodal lymphomas. Neither CD4 cell count nor HIV viral load has been found predictive of development of lymphoma over time (168).

Numerous therapeutic interventions have been used for patients infected with HIV with MCD, and no specific treatment is currently considered the therapy of choice. Although surgery is almost always effective in unicentric disease, complete surgical debulking is almost impossible in patients with MCD. Results of various chemotherapeutic regimens have been reported in small series, without specific results in individuals positive for either HHV8 or HIV. Corticosteroids may be helpful in controlling the symptoms and signs of inflammation, though long-term use has been associated with a very high risk of bacterial infection and sepsis (169). Interferon-α has been used effectively in several patients with HIV-associated MCD, with long-term remissions achieved after 5 million units given either weekly (170) or three times weekly (171). Monoclonal antibody against IL6, or against the IL-6 receptor, has been employed experimentally with alleviation of symptoms and signs of disease, although manifestations of MCD returned upon discontinuation of the antibody therapy (167,172). Rituximab, at a dose of 375 mg per m^2 given weekly for 4 weeks, has also been associated with clinical improvement in patients infected with HIV with MCD (173). Thus, 20 of 21 such patients experienced resolution of all symptoms, and 67% achieved radiologic response. Overall survival at 2 years was 95%, and disease-free survival was 79%. C-reactive protein levels and HHV8 viral load decreased after rituximab. The major toxicity was reactivation of Kaposi sarcoma in four of 11 patients who had originally presented with Kaposi sarcoma. Successful retreatment with rituximab has also been described in three of three patients infected with HIV who had relapse approximately 2 years after initial successful therapy with rituximab (174). Antiviral approaches have also been studied in patients with HHV8-related MCD. Although ganciclovir, foscarnet, and cidofovir have all shown efficacy in vitro against HHV8 (175), cidofovir was ineffective in all five patients studied by Berezne et al. (176), whereas foscarnet was found to have mixed results (177,178). Complete response was documented in three of three patients treated with ganciclovir (179); these patients also experienced reduced HHV8 viremia. Additional patients undergoing successful therapy with ganciclovir or the oral valganciclovir have been reported by Casper et al. (179). At this point, the use of rituximab, or ganciclovir, would be recommended as appropriate initial therapy; additional prospective clinical trials are clearly needed to further define optimal therapeutic intervention in these patients.

HODGKIN LYMPHOMA IN THE SETTING OF HUMAN IMMUNODEFICIENCY VIRUS

Epidemiology

Although the incidence of HL in persons infected with HIV is statistically increased when compared with population-based expectations (180), the disease is not AIDS defining, and the absolute numbers of affected patients are relatively low. Nonetheless, Biggar et al. (15) have recently demonstrated a further increase in HL in the era of HAART. Furthermore, whereas decreasing CD4 lymphocytes are associated with an increasing incidence of non-Hodgkins lymphoma (19), the opposite is true of HL, in which an increasing risk is associated with increases in CD4 cells (15).

The relationship between increasing CD4 cell counts and increasing risk of HL may relate to the fact that the malignant RS cells of HL produce numerous cytokines and chemokines, some of which serve to attract a T-helper-2 lymphoid response, rich in CD4 lymphocytes, which classically form rosettes around the RS cells (181–183). Chemokines such as thymus and activation-regulated chemokine, IP10, and MIG are synthesized by RS cells, and are responsible for inducing this infiltration of T-helper-2 type-activated CD4 lymphocytes. The activated CD4 lymphocytes, in combination with IP10 and transforming growth factor β, also synthesized by RS cells, may serve to prevent an effective immune response against the malignant cells (181), while also providing a survival advantage to the RS cells, by signaling through CD40L/CD40 and IL-4 or other molecules (183).

With HAART-induced increases in CD4 lymphocytes, the full complement of survival signals is present, as well as the potential for evasion of a host immune response, leading to the statistically increased incidence of HL now reported (184).

Clinical and Pathologic Features of Human Immunodeficiency-Related Hodgkin Lymphoma

In contrast to HL occurring in individuals negative for HIV, patients with HIV-related HL tend to have symptomatic, stage IV disease at diagnosis, with bone marrow involvement in approximately 40% to 60% (185,186). Pancytopenia is a common presenting feature, often in the setting of fever, night sweats, and/or weight loss. Mixed cellularity or lymphocyte depletion subtypes are seen most frequently, and the RS cells are uniformly associated with presence of EBV (44,187). Although median survival was only approximately 1.5 to 3 years before the HAART era (186,188), use of HAART has been associated with a highly impressive prolongation in survival (186,189,190).

Treatment Options

Before the availability of HAART, standard doxorubicin (Adriamycin), bleomycin, vinblastine, and dacarbazine was associated with an overall survival of approximately 18 months (188). However, when used together with HAART, chemotherapy consisting primarily of doxorubicin (Adriamycin), bleomycin, vinblastine, and dacarbazine (used in 87% of 78 patients evaluated retrospectively) resulted in a 91% CR rate and a median time to relapse that had not been reached at a median follow-up of 36 months (186). The Stanford V regimen was employed along with HAART and G-CSF in 50 patients infected with HIV, resulting in a CR rate of 81%, 3-year overall survival of 51%, and disease-free survival of 58% (191). In a small study of bleomycin, etoposide, Adriamycin, cyclophosphamide, vincristine, procarbazine, and prednisone, nine of 12 patients experienced continuous CR at a median follow-up of 49 months (192);

four received concomitant HAART. At this time, the regimen of choice for patients with HIV-related HL remains undefined. Until further studies have been completed, it would seem reasonable to consider use of the standard doxorubicin (Adriamycin), bleomycin, vinblastine, and dacarbazine regimen, along with concomitant HAART and G-CSF.

POSTTRANSPLANT LYMPHOPROLIFERATIVE DISORDER

Epidemiology

The term "post-transplant lymphoproliferative disorder" represents a spectrum of diseases, occurring after either solid organ or allogeneic stem cell transplantation (193,194). These disorders range from self-limited lymphoproliferations, to very aggressive and widely disseminated malignant lymphomas. The incidence of PTLD varies, dependent upon the time from transplantation, the intensity of immunosuppression or use of T-cell-depleting agents, patient age, the EBV status of recipient and/or donor, the specific organ transplanted, and other factors (193–195) such as underlying hepatitis C virus infection, associated with an increased risk among liver transplant recipients (196). The overall risk of lymphoma after solid organ transplantation is approximately 30-fold higher than would be expected in the general population (197). Lung and small bowel transplants are associated with the highest risk, occurring in up to 30% of patients, whereas the risk of lymphoma among kidney, heart, and liver transplant recipients varies from 1% to 5%, and that for allogeneic stem cell transplant patients is approximately 1% at 10 years (194,198). The incidence of PTLD among 45,141 renal recipients and 7,634 cardiac recipients was comprehensively determined by the European and North American Collaborative Transplant Study (199). The incidence was highest in the first posttransplant year, with PTLD developing in 0.2% of renal and 1.2% of cardiac recipients. In subsequent years, the rate was 0.04% per year in renal and 0.3 % per year in cardiac recipients, and by 7 years after transplant, the incidence of PTLD among renal recipients was approximately 5%, whereas that of cardiac transplant recipients was 1%. The risk of PTLD is also influenced by the degree of iatrogenically induced immunodeficiency, used in an attempt to prevent graft rejection. Thus, agents that induce potent T-cell depletion are associated with a greater risk of PTLD, in both solid organ and allogeneic stem cell recipients. Among cardiac transplant recipients who received a murine monoclonal antibody against CD3 (OKT3), a 9-fold increase in PTLD was observed, occurring in 6.2% of patients who received one course and 35.7% among those who received two courses (200). Use of anti-T-cell antibodies to prevent graft rejection in allogeneic stem cell recipients increased the risk of PTLD to levels as high as 12% to 24% (201,202).

Pathogenesis

EBV plays an important role in the pathogenesis of PTLD, and approximately 80% of these disorders are positive for

EBV within the nucleus of the malignant lymphocytes. Of importance, the EBV is monoclonal (203), indicating that EBV infected the cell before the time of malignant expansion, and consistent with a very early or premalignant role in the pathogenesis of disease. Although EBV viral load in peripheral blood B lymphocytes has not been helpful in predicting development of PTLD, elevated quantitative EBV deoxyribonucleic acid levels in plasma, studied by polymerase chain reaction, are useful in predicting an increased likelihood of PTLD (204). In general, EBV-positive PTLD arises from recipient (host) lymphocytes in the case of solid organ transplantation, whereas donor-derived lymphocytes are implicated in the transformation process in allogeneic stem cell recipients (195). The unregulated proliferation of polyclonal, EBV-transformed B cells, in the setting of an absence of EBV-specific immune surveillance, is critical to the development of PTLD, and is consistent with the increased incidence of these disorders when T-cell-depleting immunosuppressive agents are used to prevent graft rejection (205). Additionally, the latent EBV oncogene, LMP-1, is known to have direct transforming activity, capable of inducing a malignant phenotype in the infected cell (206), while also inducing Bcl-2 expression. Additional genetic aberrations have also been described, contributing to the malignant outcome in some cases (207). Thus, point mutations of the Bcl-6 gene have been reported with frequency in these PTLD lymphomas, and are associated with a poor clinical outcome (208). The presence of the transplanted organ itself provides an opportunity for chronic antigenic stimulation, further contributing to the potential for malignancy. Additionally, coinfection with other organisms, such as hepatitis C virus in liver transplant recipients (196) as well as other organisms (209,210), may also be operative in the full pathogenesis of these disorders.

Pathology

Approximately 90% of PTLDs are of B-lymphoid origin, and most of these are associated with EBV. The abnormal cells may be reactive in appearance, polymorphic (heterogeneous), or monomorphous, and may arise from polyclonal, oligoclonal, or monoclonal lymphoid populations. Three categories of PTLD have been described (207). Early lesions are most often polymorphic and polyclonal, and this has been termed the plasmacytic hyperplasia group. The disorder usually arises from the tonsils or cervical nodes, contains multiple EBV infection events, and lacks oncogene or tumor-suppressor gene alterations. This entity may be the same or very similar to acute infectious mononucleosis arising in the setting of immunodeficiency. A second group consists of polymorphic B-cell hyperplasia and polymorphic B-cell lymphoma; these are usually monoclonal, contain a single form of EBV, and also lack oncogene and/or tumor suppressor gene alterations. A third group consists of monomorphic lymphomas, usually with immunoblastic morphology; they are further subclassified according to the World Health Organization lymphoma classification system. The monomorphic PTLDs are monoclonal, and contain a single form of EBV and usually one or more aberrant oncogenes or tumor suppressor genes, such a p53, c-myc, or others (207). Transition from a polyclonal reactive disorder to a monoclonal malignancy has been described (211).

T-cell PTLDs are usually EBV negative but may also be associated with EBV (212,213). These T-cell PTLDs tend to occur late, presenting at a median of 15 years from transplantation, with a very aggressive clinical course and poor prognosis (214).

Clinical Characteristics

Similar to the AIDS-related lymphomas, PTLD lymphomas are often aggressive, widely disseminated, and extranodal in presentation. Differing presentations are expected in the three categories of disease. Thus, in the polymorphous/polyclonal variant, children are affected most commonly, presenting with fever and/or a mononucleosis-like picture, with rapid enlargement of tonsils or cervical nodes. This entity usually occurs in the early posttransplant period (215). Widespread, rapidly progressive polyclonal or oligoclonal disease may also occur early in the posttransplant period in patients with extensive immunocompromise (216). Patients with PTLDs occurring ≥1 year after transplant usually develop lymphoproliferative disease more slowly, and are less likely to have significant constitutional "B" symptoms. These patients most often have monomorphic/monoclonal lymphomas, with widespread, extranodal involvement, which may also involve the CNS.

THERAPY

Because uncontrolled proliferation of EBV-transformed B cells is critical to the development of PTLD, mechanisms to augment EBV-specific immunity have been employed to treat this disorder. Initial therapy for PTLD usually consists of a decrease in immunosuppressive therapy, which may result in durable remission, especially in those with plasmacytic hyperplasia or polymorphic B-cell lymphoma, without presence of molecular aberrations such as mutations of Bcl-6 (208). A retrospective analysis from the University of Pittsburgh reported an 80% response rate in patients presenting within PTLD within the 1st year of transplantation (cases most likely to represent plasmacytic hyperplasia or polymorphous B-cell lymphoma), whereas no patient with PTLD diagnosed after 1 year from transplantation responded (217). Less favorable results have been reported by others (218). Nonetheless, although most patients do not achieve durable complete responses (219), this modality should be attempted as initial therapy, as recommended by European and American guidelines (220).

In keeping with the role of EBV in the pathogenesis of PTLD, use of antiviral agents has been explored, with some evidence of efficacy. Thus, high-dose acyclovir therapy has been used effectively in some patients (221,222), whereas ganciclovir may be effective, particularly after induction of lytic EBV activity with arginine butyrate (223,224). Nonetheless, at this time, direct antiviral approaches have not been effective in the majority of patients.

T-cell-based immunotherapy has also been employed in PTLD occurring in recipients of T-cell-depleted allogeneic bone marrow, both for treatment of PTLD and also in an attempt to prevent PTLD, again, based upon the expression of latent EBV antigens by the abnormal B lymphocytes. Thus, using in vitro, donor-derived expanded EBV-specific cytotoxic T cells (225,226), or infusion of peripheral blood leukocytes from the donor (227), effective prevention and therapy of PTLD have been documented. Fundamental differences in solid organ versus bone marrow transplantation exist, which could make the use of EBV-specific cytotoxic T cells more difficult in the solid organ setting, due to the ongoing use of immunosuppressive therapy in these recipients. Nonetheless, autologous EBV-specific CD8+ cytotoxic T cells (CTLs) have been used effectively to prevent PTLD in recipients with a high EBV viral load, and to treat PTLD as well (228). Rituximab with low-dose chemotherapy, followed by autologous CTL has also been effective in treating pediatric patients with renal transplant, with CR achieved in all five treated patients (229). Although generation of autologous CTLs may require several months, creating a practical delay in therapy for such patients, the establishment of banks of cryopreserved, partially human leukocyte antigen-matched EBV-specific CTL from healthy seropositive individuals has been advocated and employed (230,231).

The effective use of interferon-α 2b has also been described in patients with PTLD, with or without use of concomitant immunosuppressive agents. Although responses in both early and late categories of PTLD are reported (232), this modality has not been widely used, and the potential mechanism of activity has not been described.

Monoclonal antibodies directed against various B-lymphoid antigens, including CD20 (rituximab), have been used effectively in patients with PTLD, although relapse is expected in the majority (233,234). The sequential use of rituximab, given weekly times four, followed by CHOP chemotherapy given every 21 days with G-CSF has recently been employed with evidence of efficacy; of interest, response to rituximab predicted overall response to the regimen (235).

Multiagent chemotherapy has traditionally been associated with significant toxicity in patients with PTLD, with death rates as high as 80%, often due to infection, after use of either standard dose or dose-reduced regimens, which have often consisted of CHOP (236). Nonetheless, a retrospective series of 19 consecutive patients with PTLD after cardiac transplant documented that intensive multiagent chemotherapy could be safe and effective in this setting. Initial therapy consisted of reduction of immunosuppressive therapy, followed by acyclovir; in patients without response and without surgically resectable disease, the prednisone, methotrexate, doxorubicin, cyclophosphamide, and epipodophyllotoxin cytarabine, bleomycin, vincristine, methotrexate, and leucovorin (ProMACE-CytaBOM) regimen was then instituted, without use of additional immunosuppressive agents (237). Although no patient with late-onset PTLD (>1 year from transplant) responded to reduction of immunosuppressive therapy, one of four patients with early onset, polyclonal PTLD attained complete response, whereas the others died of multiorgan failure. Of eight patients who received prednisone, methotrexate, doxorubicin, cyclophosphamide, and epipodophyllotoxin cytarabine, bleomycin, vincristine, methotrexate, and leucovorin (ProMACE-CytaBOM), two died during therapy, whereas the remaining six patients (75%) achieved CR, without relapse at a median follow-up period of 38 months. Neutropenic sepsis was the most common toxicity. Of interest, subclinical doxorubicin cardiotoxicity was also described, occurring at a cumulative dose of only 63 mg m^2, strongly suggesting that the transplanted heart is more susceptible to the effects of doxorubicin. These data would suggest that multiagent chemotherapy may be used successfully in patients with late-onset PTLD, and that the ProMACE-CytaBOM regimen may be effective in maintaining graft viability, despite discontinuation of other immunosuppressive agents.

In patients with PTLD who present with localized disease, complete surgical resection or use of localized radiation therapy may be quite effective (217,237), in distinction to patients with de novo B-cell lymphoma.

References

1. Quinn TC. The global HIV/AIDS pandemic. In: Program and abstracts of the 5th International AIDS Malignancy Conference; April 23–25, 2001; Bethesda, MD. Abstract S23.
2. Buehler JW, Ward JW. A new definition for AIDS surveillance. *Ann Intern Med* 1993;118:390–391.
3. Palella FJ Jr, Delaney KM, Moorman AC, et al. Declining morbidity and mortality among patients with advanced human immunodeficiency virus infection. *N Engl J Med* 1998;338:853–860.
4. Carpenter CCJ, Cooper DA, Fischel MA, et al. Antiretroviral therapy in adults: updated recommendations of the International AIDS Society-USC Panel. *JAMA* 2000;283:381–390.
5. Ledergerber B, Egger M, Erard V, et al. AIDS related opportunistic illnesses occurring after initiation of potent antiretroviral therapy: The Swiss HIV Cohort Study. *JAMA* 1999;282:2220–2226.
6. Lee LM, Karon JM, Selik R, et al. Survival after AIDS diagnosis in adolescents and adults during the treatment era, United States, 1984–1997. *JAMA* 2001;285:1308–1315.
7. Grulich AE, Wan X, Law MG, et al. B-cell stimulation and prolonged immune deficiency are risk factors for non-Hodgkin's lymphoma in people with AIDS. *AIDS* 2000;14:133–140.
8. Cote TR, Biggar RJ, Rosenberg PS, et al. Non-Hodgkin's lymphoma among people with AIDS: incidence, presentation and public health burden. *Int J Cancer* 1997;73:645–650.
9. Biggar RJ, Rosenberg PS, Cote T. Kaposi's sarcoma and non-Hodgkin's lymphoma following the diagnosis of AIDS. *Int J Cancer* 1996;68:754–758.
10. Biggar RJ, Engels EA, Frisch M, et al. Risk of T cell lymphomas in persons with AIDS. *J Acquir Immune Defic Syndr* 2001;26:371–376.
11. Ledergerber B, Telenti A, Effer M. Risk of HIV related Kaposi's sarcoma and non-Hodgkin's lymphoma with potent antiretroviral therapy: prospective cohort study. *Br Med J* 1999;319:23–24.
12. Mocroft A, Katama C, Johnson AM, et al. AIDS across Europe, 1994–1998: the EuroSIDA study. *Lancet* 2000;356:291–296.
13. Matthews GV, Bower M, Mandalia S, et al. Changes in acquired immunodeficiency syndrome-related lymphoma since the introduction of highly active anti-retroviral therapy. *Blood* 2000;96:2730–2734.
14. International Collaboration on HIV and Cancer. Highly active anti-retroviral therapy and incidence of cancer in human immunodeficiency virus infected adults. *J Natl Cancer Inst* 2000;92:1823–1830.
15. Biggar RJ, Jaffe ES, Goedert JJ, et al. Hodgkin lymphoma and immunodeficiency in persons with HIV/AIDS. *Blood* 2006;108:3786–3791.
16. Clifford GM, Polesel J, Rickenbach M, et al. Cancer risk in the Swiss HIV Cohort Study: associations with immunodeficiency, smoking, and highly active antiretroviral therapy. *J Natl Cancer Inst* 2005;97:425–432.
17. Levine AM, Seneviratne L, Espina BM, et al. Evolving characteristics of AIDS-related lymphoma. *Blood* 2000;96:4084–4090.
18. Kirk O, Pedersen C, Cozzi-Lepri A, et al. Non-Hodgkin lymphoma in HIV-infected patients in the era of highly active antiretroviral therapy. *Blood* 2001;98:3406–3412.
19. Besson C, Goubar A, Gabarre J, et al. Changes in AIDS-related lymphoma since the era of highly active antiretroviral therapy. *Blood* 2001;98:2339–2344.
20. Lucas GM, Chaisson RE, Moore RD. Highly active anti-retroviral therapy in a large urban clinic: risk factors for virologic failure and adverse drug reactions. *Ann Intern Med* 1999;130:81–87.
21. Levine AM. Acquired immunodeficiency syndrome-related lymphoma. *Blood* 1992;80:8–20.
22. Hartge P, Devesa SS, Fraumeni JF Jr. Hodgkin's and non-Hodgkin's lymphomas. *Cancer Surv* 1994;20:423–453.
23. Nelson RA, Levine AM, Bernstein L. Reproductive factors and risk of intermediate or high grade B cell non-Hodgkin's lymphoma in women. *J Clin Oncol* 2001;19:1381–1387.
24. Granovsky MO, Mueller BU, Nicholson HS, et al. Cancer in human immunodeficiency virus infected children: a case series from the Children's Cancer Group and the National Cancer Institute. *J Clin Oncol* 1998;16:1729–1735.

25. Holly EA, Lele C. Non-Hodgkin's lymphoma in HIV positive and HIV negative homosexual men in the San Francisco Bay area: allergies, prior medication use, and sexual practice. *J Acquir Immune Defic Syndr Hum Retrovirol* 1997;15:211–222.

26. Holly EA, Lele C, Bracci P. Non-Hodgkin's lymphoma in homosexual men in the San Francisco Bay area: occupational, chemical and environmental exposures. *J Acquir Immune Defic Syndr Hum Retrovirol* 1997; 15:223–231.

27. Armenian H, Hoover DR, Rubb S, et al. Risk factors for non–Hodgkin's lymphomas in AIDS. *Am J Epidemiol* 1996;143:374–379.

28. Dean M, Jacobson LP, McFarlane G, et al. Reduced risk of AIDS lymphoma in individuals heterozygous for the CCR5-delta32 mutation. *Cancer Res* 1999;59:3561–3564.

29. Rabkin CS, Yang Q, Goedert JJ, et al. Chemokine and chemokine receptor gene variants and risk of non-Hodgkin's lymphoma in human immunodeficiency virus-1 infected individuals. *Blood* 1999;93:1838–1842.

30. Pluda JM, Yarchoan R, Jaffe ES, et al. Development of non-Hodgkin lymphoma in a cohort of patients with severe human immunodeficiency virus (HIV) infection on long-term antiretroviral therapy. *Ann Intern Med* 1990;113:276–282.

31. Shibata D, Weiss LM, Hernandez AM, et al. Epstein-Barr virus-associated non-Hodgkin's lymphoma in patients infected with the human immunodeficiency virus. *Blood* 1993;81:2102–2109.

32. Shibata D, Weiss LM, Nathwani BN, et al. Epstein-Barr virus in benign lymph node biopsies from individuals infected with the human immunodeficiency virus is associated with concurrent or subsequent development of non-Hodgkin's lymphoma. *Blood* 1991;77:1527–1533.

33. Neri A, Barriga F, Inghirami G, et al. Epstein-Barr virus infection precedes clonal expansion in Burkitt's and acquired immunodeficiency syndrome-associated lymphoma. *Blood* 1991;77:1092–1095.

34. Subar M, Neri A, Inghirami G, et al. Frequent c-myc oncogene activation and infrequent presence of Epstein-Barr virus genome in AIDS-associated lymphoma. *Blood* 1988;72:667–671.

35. Ballerini P, Gaidano G, Gong J, et al. Molecular pathogenesis of HIV-associated lymphomas. *AIDS Res Hum Retroviruses* 1992;8:731–735.

36. Ballerini P, Gaidano G, Gong JZ, et al. Multiple genetic lesions in acquired immunodeficiency syndrome-related non-Hodgkin's lymphoma. *Blood* 1993;81:166–176.

37. Boyle MJ, Sculley TB, Cooper DA, et al. Epstein-Barr virus and HIV play no direct role in persistent generalized lymphadenopathy syndrome. *Clin Exp Immunol* 1992;87:357–361.

38. Boyle MJ, Sewell WA, Milliken ST, et al. HIV and malignancy. *J Acquir Immune Defic Syndr* 1993;6(suppl 1):S5–S9.

39. Boyle MJ, Sewell WA, Sculley TB, et al. Subtypes of Epstein-Barr virus in human immunodeficiency virus-associated non-Hodgkin lymphoma. *Blood* 1991;78:3004–3011.

40. Boyle MJ, Swanson CE, Turner JJ, et al. Definition of two distinct types of AIDS-associated non-Hodgkin lymphoma. *Br J Haematol* 1990;76:506–512.

41. Fassone L, Cingolani A, Martini M, et al. Characterization of Epstein-Barr virus genotype in AIDS-related non-Hodgkin's lymphoma. *AIDS Res Hum Retroviruses* 2002;18:19–26.

42. Knowles DM, Chamulak GA, Subar M, et al. Lymphoid neoplasia associated with the acquired immunodeficiency syndrome (AIDS). The New York University Medical Center experience with 105 patients (1981–1986). *Ann Intern Med* 1988;108:744–753.

43. Emilie D, Zou W, Fior R, et al. Production and roles of IL-6, IL-10, and IL-13 in B-lymphocyte malignancies and in B-lymphocyte hyperactivity of HIV infection and autoimmunity. *Methods* 1997;11:133–142.

44. Audouin J, Diebold J, Pallesen G. Frequent expression of Epstein-Barr virus latent membrane protein-1 in tumour cells of Hodgkin's disease in HIV-positive patients. *J Pathol* 1992;167:381–384.

45. Said JW, Hoyer KK, French SW, et al. TCL1 oncogene expression in B cell subsets from lymphoid hyperplasia and distinct classes of B cell lymphoma. *Lab Invest* 2001;81:555–564.

46. Weinberg RA. Oncogenes, antioncogenes, and the molecular bases of multistep carcinogenesis. *Cancer Res* 1989;49:3713–3721.

47. Raphael M, Borisch B, Jaffe ES. Lymphomas associated with infection by the human immunodeficiency virus (HIV). In: Jaffe ES, Harris NL, Stein H, et al., eds. *World Health Organization classification of tumours.* Lyon, France: IARC Press, 2001:260–263.

48. Jaffe ES, Harris NL, Stein H, et al. *Pathology and genetics Of tumours of haematopoietic and lymphoid tissues.* Lyon, France: IARC Press, 2001.

49. Raphael M, Gentilhomme O, Tulliez M, et al. Histopathologic features of high-grade non-Hodgkin's lymphomas in acquired immunodeficiency syndrome. The French Study Group of Pathology for Human Immunodeficiency Virus-Associated Tumors. *Arch Pathol Lab Med* 1991;115:15–20.

50. Carbone A, Gloghini A, Gaidano G, et al. AIDS-related Burkitt's lymphoma. Morphologic and immunophenotypic study of biopsy specimens. *Am J Clin Pathol* 1995;103:561–567.

51. Davi F, Delecluse HJ, Guiet P, et al. Burkitt-like lymphomas in AIDS patients: characterization within a series of 103 human immunodeficiency virus-associated non-Hodgkin's lymphomas. Burkitt's Lymphoma Study Group. *J Clin Oncol* 1998;16:3788–3795.

52. Delecluse HJ, Raphael M, Magaud JP, et al. Variable morphology of human immunodeficiency virus-associated lymphomas with c-myc rearrangements. The French Study Group of Pathology for Human Immunodeficiency Virus-Associated Tumors, I. *Blood* 1993;82:552–563.

53. Bhatia K, Spangler G, Gaidano G, et al. Mutations in the coding region of c-myc occur frequently in acquired immunodeficiency syndrome-associated lymphomas. *Blood* 1994;84:883–888.

54. Nakamura H, Said JW, Miller CW, et al. Mutation and protein expression of p53 in acquired immunodeficiency syndrome-related lymphomas. *Blood* 1993;82:920–926.

55. Davi F, Delecluse HJ, Guiet P, et al. Burkitt-like lymphomas in AIDS patients: characterization within a series of 103 human immunodeficiency virus-associated non-Hodgkin's lymphomas. Burkitt's Lymphoma Study Group. *J Clin Oncol* 1998;16:3788–3795.

56. Gaidano G, Carbone A, Pastore C, et al. Frequent mutation of the 5' noncoding region of the BCL-6 gene in acquired immunodeficiency syndrome-related non-Hodgkin's lymphomas. *Blood* 1997;89:3755–3762.

57. Gaidano G, Lo Coco F, Ye BH, et al. Rearrangements of the BCL-6 gene in acquired immunodeficiency syndrome-associated non-Hodgkin's lymphoma: association with diffuse large-cell subtype. *Blood* 1994;84:397–402.

58. Carbone A, Gaidano G, Gloghini A, et al. BCL-6 protein expression in AIDS-related non-Hodgkin's lymphomas: inverse relationship with Epstein-Barr virus-encoded latent membrane protein-1 expression. *Am J Pathol* 1997;150:155–165.

59. Camilleri-Broet S, Davi F, Feuillard J, et al. AIDS-related primary brain lymphomas: histopathologic and immunohistochemical study of 51 cases. The French Study Group for HIV-Associated Tumors. *Hum Pathol* 1997;28:367–374.

60. Meeker TC, Shiramizu B, Kaplan L, et al. Evidence for molecular subtypes of HIV-associated lymphoma: division into peripheral monoclonal, polyclonal and central nervous system lymphoma. *AIDS* 1991;5:669–674.

61. Delecluse HJ, Anagnostopoulos I, Dallenbach F, et al. Plasmablastic lymphomas of the oral cavity: a new entity associated with the human immunodeficiency virus infection. *Blood* 1997;89:1413–1420.

62. Flaitz CM, Nichols CM, Walling DM, et al. Plasmablastic lymphoma: an HIV-associated entity with primary oral manifestations. *Oral Oncol* 2002;38:96–102.

63. Ihrler S, Zietz C, Riederer A, et al. HIV-related parotid lymphoepithelial cysts. Immunohistochemistry and 3-D reconstruction of surgical and autopsy material with special reference to formal pathogenesis. *Virchows Arch* 1996;429:139–147.

64. Ihrler S, Zietz C, Sendelhofert A, et al. Lymphoepithelial duct lesions in Sjögren-type sialadenitis. *Virchows Arch* 1999;434:315–323.

65. Mishalani SH, Lones MA, Said JW. Multilocular thymic cyst. A novel thymic lesion associated with human immunodeficiency virus infection. *Arch Pathol Lab Med* 1995;119:467–470.

66. Teruya-Feldstein J, Temeck BK, Sloas MM, et al. Pulmonary malignant lymphoma of mucosa-associated lymphoid tissue (MALT) arising in a pediatric HIV-positive patient. *Am J Surg Pathol* 1995;19:357–363.

67. Tao J, Valderrama E. Epstein-Barr virus-associated polymorphic B-cell lymphoproliferative disorders in the lungs of children with AIDS: a report of two cases. *Am J Surg Pathol* 1999;23:560–566.

68. Levine AM, Sadeghi S, Espina B, et al. Characteristics of indolent non-Hodgkin lymphoma in patients with type 1 human immunodeficiency virus infection. *Cancer* 2002;94:1500–1506.

69. Goedert JJ, Cote TR, Virgo P, et al. Spectrum of AIDS-associated malignant disorders. *Lancet* 1998;351:1833–1839.

70. Kumar S, Kumar D, Schnadig VJ, et al. Plasma cell myeloma in patients who are HIV-positive. *Am J Clin Pathol* 1994;102:633–639.

71. Jaffe ES. Lymphoid lesions of the head and neck: a model of lymphocyte homing and lymphomagenesis. *Mod Pathol* 2002;15:255–263.

72. Beylot-Barry M, Vergier B, Masquelier B, et al. The spectrum of cutaneous lymphomas in HIV infection: a study of 21 cases. *Am J Surg Pathol* 1999;23:1208–1216.

73. Gonzalez-Clemente JM, Ribera JM, Campo E, et al. Ki-1+ anaplastic large-cell lymphoma of T-cell origin in an HIV-infected patient. *AIDS* 1991;5:751–755.

74. Jhala DN, Medeiros LJ, Lopez-Terrada D, et al. Neutrophil-rich anaplastic large cell lymphoma of T-cell lineage. A report of two cases arising in HIV-positive patients. *Am J Clin Pathol* 2000;114:478–482.

75. Canioni D, Arnulf B, Asso-Bonnet M, et al. Nasal natural killer lymphoma associated with Epstein-Barr virus in a patient infected with human immunodeficiency virus. *Arch Pathol Lab Med* 2001;125:660–662.

76. Guitart J, Variakojis D, Kuzel T, et al. Cutaneous CD8 T cell infiltrates in advanced HIV infection. *J Am Acad Dermatol* 1999;41:722–727.

77. Nador RG, Cesarman E, Knowles DM, et al. Herpes-like DNA sequences in a body-cavity-based lymphoma in an HIV-negative patient. *N Engl J Med* 1995;333:943.

78. Green I, Espiritu E, Ladanyi M, et al. Primary lymphomatous effusions in AIDS: a morphological, immunophenotypic, and molecular study. *Mod Pathol* 1995;8:39–45.

79. Ansari MQ, Dawson DB, Nador R, et al. Primary body cavity-based AIDS-related lymphomas. *Am J Clin Pathol* 1996;105:221–229.

80. Cobo F, Hernandez S, Hernandez L, et al. Expression of potentially oncogenic HHV-8 genes in an EBV-negative primary effusion lymphoma occurring in an HIV-seronegative patient. *J Pathol* 1999;189:288–293.

81. Said JW, Tasaka T, Takeuchi S, et al. Primary effusion lymphoma in women: report of two cases of Kaposi's sarcoma herpes virus-associated effusion-based lymphoma in human immunodeficiency virus-negative women. *Blood* 1996;88:3124–3128.

82. Nador RG, Cesarman E, Chadburn A, et al. Primary effusion lymphoma: a distinct clinicopathologic entity associated with the Kaposi's sarcoma-associated herpes virus. *Blood* 1996;88:645–656.

83. Chang Y, Cesarman E, Pessin MS, et al. Identification of herpesvirus-like DNA sequences in AIDS-associated Kaposi's sarcoma. *Science* 1994;266:1865–1869.

84. Moore PS, Chang Y. Kaposi's sarcoma findings. *Science* 1995;270:15.

85. Cesarman E, Chang Y, Moore PS, et al. Kaposi's sarcoma-associated herpesvirus-like DNA sequences in AIDS-related body-cavity-based lymphomas. *N Engl J Med* 1995;332:1186–1191.

86. Chadburn A, Hyjek E, Mathew S, et al. KSHV-positive solid lymphomas represent an extra-cavitary variant of primary effusion lymphoma. *Am J Surg Pathol* 2004;28:1401–1416

87. Lim ST, Rubin N, Said J, Levine AM. Primary effusion lymphoma (PEL): successful treatment with highly active antiretroviral therapy (HAART) and rituximab. *Ann Hematol* 2005;84:551–552.

88. Mbulaiteye SM, Biggar RJ, Goedert JJ, et al. Pleural and peritoneal lymphoma among people with AIDS in the United States. *J Acquir Immune Defic Syndr* 2002;29:418–421.

89. Katano H, Suda T, Morishita Y, et al. Human herpesvirus 8-associated solid lymphomas that occur in AIDS patients take anaplastic large cell morphology. *Mod Pathol* 2000;13:77–85.

90. Said JW, Shintaku IP, Asou H, et al. Herpesvirus 8 inclusions in primary effusion lymphoma: report of a unique case with T-cell phenotype. *Arch Pathol Lab Med* 1999;123:257–260.

91. Beaty MW, Kumar S, Sorbara L, et al. A biphenotypic human herpesvirus 8-associated primary bowel lymphoma. *Am J Surg Pathol* 1999;23:992–994.

92. Walts AE, Shintaku IP, Said JW. Diagnosis of malignant lymphoma in effusions from patients with AIDS by gene rearrangement. *Am J Clin Pathol* 1990;94:170–175.

93. Said JW, Chien K, Tasaka T, et al. Ultrastructural characterization of human herpesvirus 8 (Kaposi's sarcoma-associated herpesvirus) in Kaposi's sarcoma lesions: electron microscopy permits distinction from cytomegalovirus (CMV). *J Pathol* 1997;182:273–281.

94. Cesarman E, Mesri EA, Gershengorn MC. Viral G protein-coupled receptor and Kaposi's sarcoma: a model of paracrine neoplasia? *J Exp Med* 2000;191:417–422.

95. Wilson KS, McKenna RW, Kroft SH, et al. Primary effusion lymphomas exhibit complex and recurrent cytogenetic abnormalities. *Br J Haematol* 2002;116:113–121.

96. Aoki Y, Jaffe ES, Chang Y, et al. Angiogenesis and hematopoiesis induced by Kaposi's sarcoma-associated herpesvirus-encoded interleukin-6. *Blood* 1999;93:4034–4043.

97. Teruya-Feldstein J, Zauber P, Setsuda JE, et al. Expression of human herpesvirus-8 oncogene and cytokine homologues in an HIV-seronegative patient with multicentric Castleman's disease and primary effusion lymphoma. *Lab Invest* 1998;78:1637–1642.

98. Du MQ, Liu H, Diss TC, et al. Kaposi sarcoma-associated herpesvirus infects monotypic (IgM lambda) but polyclonal naive B cells in Castleman disease and associated lymphoproliferative disorders. *Blood* 2001;97:2130–2136.

99. Dupin N, Diss TL, Kellam P, et al. HHV-8 is associated with a plasmablastic variant of Castleman disease that is linked to HHV-8-positive plasmablastic lymphoma. *Blood* 2000;95:1406–1412.

100. Du MQ, Diss TC, Liu H, et al. KSHV- and EBV-associated germinotropic lymphoproliferative disorder. *Blood* 2002;100:3415–3418.

101. Antonio D, Amedeo B, Maria A, et al. KSHV- and EBV-associated germinotropic lymphoproliferative disorder: a rare lymphoproliferative disease of HIV patient with plasmablastic morphology, indolent course and favourable response to therapy. *Leuk Lymphoma* 2007;48:1444–1447.

102. Seliem RM, Griffith RC, Harris NL, et al. HHV-8+, EBV+ multicentric plasmablastic microlymphoma in an HIV+ Man: the spectrum of HHV-8+ lymphoproliferative disorders expands. *Am J Surg Pathol* 2007;31:1439–1445.

103. Ziegler JL, Beckstead JA, Volberding PA, et al. Non-Hodgkin's lymphoma in 90 homosexual men: relation to generalized lymphadenopathy the acquired immunodeficiency syndrome. *N Engl J Med* 1984;311:565–570.

104. Kaplan LD, Abrams DI, Feigal E, et al. AIDS associated non-Hodgkin's lymphoma in San Francisco. *JAMA* 1989;261:719–724.

105. Seneviratne LC, Tulpule A, Espina BM, et al. Clinical, immunologic and pathologic correlates of bone marrow involvement in 291 patients with AIDS-related lymphoma. *Blood* 2001;98:2358–2363.

106. Sarker D, Thirlwell C, Nelson M, et al. Leptomeningeal disease in AIDS-related lymphoma. *AIDS* 2003;17:861–865.

107. Lossos A, Siegal T. Numb chin syndrome in cancer: etiology, response to treatment, and prognostic significance. *Neurology* 1992;42:1181–1184.

108. Cingolani A, De Luca A, Larocca LM, et al. Minimally invasive diagnosis of acquired immunodeficiency syndrome-related primary central nervous system lymphoma. *J Natl Cancer Inst* 1998;90:364–370.

109. Vaccher E, Tirelli U, Spina M, et al. Age and serum LDH level are independent prognostic factors in HIV related non-Hodgkin's lymphoma: a single institution study of 96 patients. *J Clin Oncol* 1996;14:2217–2223.

110. Radin DR, Esplin J, Levine AM, et al. AIDS-related non-Hodgkin's lymphoma: abdominal CT findings in 112 patients. *AJR Am J Roentgenol* 1993;160:1133–1139.

111. Sider L, Weiss AJ, Smith MD, et al. Varied appearance of AIDS-related lymphoma in the chest. *Radiology* 1989;171:629–632.

112. Stumpe KD, Urbinelli M, Steinert HC, et al. Whole body positron emission tomography using fluorodeoxyglucose for staging of lymphoma: effectiveness and comparison with computed tomography. *Eur J Nucl Med* 1998;25:721–728.

113. DeWit M, Bumann D, Beyer W, et al. Whole body positron emission tomography (PET) for diagnosis of residual mass in patients with lymphoma. *Ann Oncol* 1997;8(suppl 1):57–60.

114. Romer W, Hanauske AR, Ziegler S, et al. Positron emission tomography in non-Hodgkin's lymphoma: assessment of chemotherapy with fluorodeoxyglucose. *Blood* 1998;91:4464–4471.

115. Levine AM, Wernz JC, Kaplan L, et al. Low dose chemotherapy with central nervous system prophylaxis and zidovudine maintenance in AIDS-related lymphoma: a prospective multi-institutional trial. *JAMA* 1991;266:84–88.

116. Mummaneni M, Tulpule A, Palmer M, et al. Leptomeningeal involvement in AIDS-lymphoma: clinical, immunologic and pathologic features [abstract]. *Proceedings of the American Society of Clinical Oncology* 1998;17:41A. Abstract 160.

117. Levine AM, Sullivan-Halley J, Pike MC, et al. HIV-related lymphoma: prognostic factors predictive of survival. *Cancer* 1991;68:2466–2472.

118. Juang J, Testa MA, et al. Prognostic factors in the treatment of HIV associated non-Hodgkin's lymphoma: analysis of AIDS Clinical Trials Group protocol 142: low dose versus standard dose m-BACOD plus GM-CSF. *J Clin Oncol* 1998;16:3601–3606.

119. Rossi G, Donisi A, Casari S, et al. The International Prognostic Index can be used as a guide to treatment decisions regarding patients with HIV related systemic non-Hodgkin's lymphoma. *Cancer* 1999;86:2391–2397.

120. Antinori A, Cingolani A, Alba L, et al. Better response to chemotherapy and prolonged survival in AIDS-related lymphomas responding to highly active antiretroviral therapy. *AIDS* 2001;15:1483–1491.

121. Lim ST, Karim R, Tulpule A, et al. Prognostic factors in HIV related diffuse large cell lymphoma: before versus after highly active anti-retroviral therapy. *J Clin Oncol* 2005;23:8477–8482.

122. A predictive model for aggressive non-Hodgkin's lymphoma: the International non-Hodgkin's Lymphoma Prognostic Factors Project. *N Engl J Med* 1993;329:987–994.

123. Bower M, Gazzard B, Mandalia S, et al. A prognostic index for systemic AIDS-related non-Hodgkin lymphoma treated in the era of highly active antiretroviral therapy. *Ann Intern Med* 2005;143:265–273.

124. Kaplan LD, Straus DJ, Testa MA, et al. Randomized trial of standard-dose versus low dose mBACOD chemotherapy for HIV-associated non-Hodgkin's lymphoma. *N Engl J Med* 1997;336:1641–1648.

125. Levine AM, Wernz JC, Kaplan L, et al. Low dose chemotherapy with central nervous system prophylaxis and zidovudine maintenance in AIDS related lymphoma: a prospective multi-institutional trial. *JAMA* 1991;266:84–88.

126. Ratner L, Lee J, Tang S, et al. Chemotherapy for HIV-associated non-Hodgkin's lymphoma in combination with highly active anti-retroviral therapy. *J Clin Oncol* 2001;19:2171–2178.

127. Hoffmann C, Wolf E, Fatkenheuer G, et al. Response to highly active antiretroviral therapy strongly predicts outcome in patients with AIDS-related lymphoma. *AIDS* 2003;17:1521–1529.

128. Levine AM, Tulpule A, Espina B, et al. Liposome-encapsulated doxorubicin in combination with standard agents (cyclophosphamide, vincristine, prednisone) in patients with newly diagnosed AIDS-related non-Hodgkin's lymphoma: results of therapy and correlates of response. *J Clin Oncol* 2004;22:2662–2670.

129. Little RF, Pittaluga S, Grant N, et al. Highly effective treatment of acquired immunodeficiency syndrome-related lymphoma with dose-adjusted EPOCH: impact of antiretroviral therapy suspension and tumor biology. *Blood* 2003;101:4653–4659.

130. Gill PS, Rarick MU, Brynes RL, et al. Azidothymidine and bone marrow failure in AIDS. *Ann Intern Med* 1987;107:502–505.

131. Sparano JA, Wiernik PH, Hu X, et al. Pilot trial of infusional cyclophosphamide, doxorubicin and etoposide plus didanosine and filgrastim in patients with HIV associated non-Hodgkin's lymphoma. *J Clin Oncol* 1996;14:3026–3035.

132. Sparano JA, Lee S, Henry DH, et al. Infusional cyclophosphamide, doxorubicin and etoposide in HIV associated non-Hodgkin's lymphoma: a review of the Einstein, Aviano, and ECOG experience in 182 patients [abstract]. Abstracts of the 4th International AIDS Malignancy Conference; May 16–18, 2000; Bethesda, MD. *J Acquir Immune Defic Syndr* 2000;23:A11. Abstract S15.

133. Sparano JA, Lee J, Kaplan L, et al. Randomized phase II trial of infusional EPOCH chemotherapy given either concurrently with or sequentially followed by rituximab in HIV-associated lymphoma: AIDS Malignancy Consortium trial 034. In: Xth International Conference on Malignancies in AIDS and Other Acquired Immunodeficiencies; October 16-17, 2006; National Cancer Institute, Bethesda, MD.

134. Levine AM, Lee J, Kaplan L, et al. Efficacy and toxicity of concurrent rituximab plus infusional EPOCH in HIV-associated lymphoma: AIDS Malignancy Consortium Trial 034. *Proceedings American Society of Clinical Oncology* 2008;26:460s. Abstract 8527.

135. Kaplan LD, Lee JY, Ambinder RF, et al. Rituximab does not improve clinical outcome in a randomized phase III trial of CHOP with or without rituximab in patients with HIV associated non-Hodgkin's lymphoma: AIDS Malignancy Consortium trial 010. *Blood* 2005;106:1538–1543.

136. Coiffier B, Lepage E, Briere J, et al. CHOP chemotherapy plus rituximab compared with CHOP alone in elderly patients with diffuse large B cell lymphoma. *N Engl J Med* 2002;346:235–242.

137. Sehn L, Donaldson J, Chhanabhai M, et al. Introduction of combined CHOP-rituximab therapy dramatically improved outcome of diffuse large B cell lymphoma in British Columbia [abstract]. *Blood* 2003;102:29a. Abstract 88.

138. Boue F, Gabarre J, Bisselbrecht C, et al. Phase II trial of CHOP plus rituximab in patients with HIV associated non-Hodgkin's lymphoma. *J Clin Oncol* 2006;24:4123–4128.

139. Spina M, Jaeger U, Sparano JA, et al. Rituximab plus infusional cyclophosphamide, doxorubicin, and etoposide in HIV associated non-Hodgkin lymphoma: pooled results from 3 phase 2 trials. *Blood* 2005;105:1891–1897.

140. Aksoy S, Harputluoglu H, Kilickap S, et al. Rituximab-related viral infections in lymphoma patients. *Leuk Lymphoma* 2007;48:1307–1312.

141. Koo S, Baden LR. Infectious complications associated with immunomodulating monoclonal antibodies used in the treatment of hematologic malignancy. *J Natl Compr Canc Netw* 2008;6:202–213.

142. Mournier N, Briere J, Gisselbrecht C, et al. Rituximab plus CHOP (R-CHOP) overcomes bcl-2-associated resistance to chemotherapy in elderly patients with diffuse large B cell lymphoma. *Blood* 2003;101:4279–4284.

143. Kewalramani T, Zelenetz AD, Nimer SD, et al. Rituximab and ICE as second line therapy before autologous stem cell transplantation for relapsed or primary refractory diffuse large B cell lymphoma. *Blood* 2004;103:3684–3688.

144. Bi J, Espina BM, Tulpule A, et al. High dose cytosine arabinoside and cisplatin regimens as salvage therapy for refractory or relapsed AIDS related non-Hodgkin's lymphoma. *J Acquir Immune Defic Syndr* 2001;28:416–421.

145. Krishnan A, Molina A, Zaia J, et al. Durable remissions with autologous stem cell transplantation for high risk HIV associated lymphomas. *Blood* 2004;105:874–878.

146. Spitzer TR, Ambinder RF, Lee JY, et al. Dose reduced busulfan, cyclophosphamide, and autologous stem cell transplantation for human immunodeficiency virus associated lymphoma: AIDS Malignancy Consortium Study 020. *Biol Blood Marrow Transplant* 2008;14:59–66.

147. Krishnan A, Zaia JA, Rossi J, et al. First in human engraftment of anti-HIV lentiviral vector gene modified CD34+ peripheral blood progenitor cells in the treatment of AIDS related lymphoma. *Blood* 2008;112:818a. Abstract 2348.

148. Lim ST, Karim R, Nathwani BN, et al. AIDS related Burkitt's lymphoma versus diffuse large cell lymphoma in the pre-highly active antiretroviral therapy (HAART) and HAART eras: significant differences in survival with standard chemotherapy. *J Clin Oncol* 2005;23:4430–4438.

149. Spina M, Simonelli C, Talamini R, et al. Patients with HIV with Burkitt's lymphoma have a worse outcome than those with diffuse large-cell lymphoma also in the highly active antiretroviral therapy era. *J Clin Oncol* 2005;23:8132–8133.

150. Wang ES, Straus DJ, Teruya-Feldstein J, et al. Intensive chemotherapy with cyclophosphamide, doxorubicin, high dose methotrexate/ifosfamide, etoposide, and high dose cytarabine (CODOX-M/IVAC) for human immunodeficiency virus associated Burkitt lymphoma. *Cancer* 2003;98:1196–1205.

151. Cortes J, Thomas D, Rios A, et al. Hyperfractionated cyclophosphamide, vincristine, doxorubicin, and dexamethasone and highly active antiretroviral therapy for patients with acquired immunodeficiency syndrome-related Burkitt lymphoma/leukemia. *Cancer* 2002;94:1492–1499.

152. Oriol A, Ribera JM, Esteve J, et al. Lack of influence of human immunodeficiency virus infection status in the response to therapy and survival of adult patients with mature B-cell lymphoma or leukemia. Results of the PETHEMA-LAL3/97 study. *Haematologica* 2003;88:445–453.

153. Oriol A, Ribera JM, Brunet S, et al. Highly active antiretroviral therapy and outcome of AIDS related Burkitt's lymphoma or leukemia. Results of the PETHAMA-LAL 3/97 study. *Haematologica* 2005;90:990–992.

154. Dunleavy K, Healey Bird BR, Pittaluga S, et al. Efficacy and toxicity of dose adjusted EPOCH-rituximab in adults with newly diagnosed Burkitt lymphoma. *J Clin Oncol* 2007;25(suppl):8035.

155. Blinder VS, Chadburn A, Furman RR, et al. Improving outcomes for patients with Burkitt lymphoma and HIV. *AIDS Patient CARE STDS* 2008;22:175–187.

156. Gill PS, Levine AM, Meyer RP, et al. Primary central nervous system lymphoma in homosexual men. Clinical, immunologic, and pathologic features. *Am J Med* 1985;78:742–748.

157. So YT, Beckstead JH, Davis RL. Primary central nervous system lymphoma in AIDS: a clinical and pathological study. *Ann Neurol* 1986;20:566–572.

158. Baumgartner JE, Rachlin JR, Beckstead JH, et al. Primary central nervous system lymphomas: natural history and response to radiation therapy in 55 patients with AIDS. *J Neurosurg* 1990;73:206–211.

159. Antinori A, De Rossi G, Ammassari A, et al. Value of combined approach with thallium-201 single photon emission computed tomography and Epstein-Barr virus DNA polymerase chain reaction in CSF for the diagnosis of AIDS related primary CNS lymphoma. *J Clin Oncol* 1999;17:554–560.

160. Hoffman JM, Waskin HA, Schifter T, et al. FDG-PET in differentiating lymphoma from non-malignant central nervous system lesions in patients with AIDS. *J Nucl Med* 1993;34:567–575.

161. MacMahon EME, Glass JD, Hayward SCD, et al. Epstein Barr virus in AIDS related primary central nervous system lymphoma. *Lancet* 1991;338:969–973.

162. Raez L, Cabral L, Cai JP, et al. Antivirals induce apoptosis and tumor regression in AIDS related primary central nervous system lymphoma [abstract]. Third AIDS Malignancy Conference, Bethesda, MD, 1999. *J Acquir Immune Defic Syndr* 1999;21:A31. Abstract 87.

163. Slobod KS, Taylor GH, Sandlund JT, et al. Epstein-Barr virus-targeted therapy for AIDS-related primary lymphoma of the central nervous system. *Lancet* 2000;356:1493–1494.

164. Newell ME, Hoy JF, Cooper SG, et al. Human immunodeficiency virus-related primary central nervous system lymphoma: factors influencing survival in 111 patients. *Cancer* 2004;100:2627–2636.

165. Casper C. The aetiology and management of Castleman disease at 50 years: translating pathophysiology to patient care. *Br J Haematol* 2005;129:3–17.

166. Nishi J, Arimura K, Utsunomiya A, et al. Expression of vascular endothelial growth factor in sera and lymph nodes of the plasma cell type of Castleman's disease. *Br J Haematol* 1999;104:482–485.

167. Beck JT, Hsu SM, Wijdenes J, et al. Brief report: alleviation of systemic manifestations of Castleman's disease by monoclonal anti9-interleukin-6 antibody. *N Engl J Med* 1994;330:602–605.

168. Oskenhendler E, Boulanger E, Galicier L, et al. High incidence of Kaposi's sarcoma associated herpesvirus related non-Hodgkin lymphoma in patients with HIV infection and multicentric Castleman disease. *Blood* 2002;99:2331–2336.

169. Bowne WB, Lewis JJ, Filippa DA, et al. The management of unicentric and multicentric Castleman's disease: a report of 16 cases and a review of the literature. *Cancer* 1999;85:706–717.

170. Nord JA, Karter D. Low dose interferon-alpha therapy for HIV associated multicentric Castleman's disease. *Int J STD AIDS* 2003;14:61–62.

171. Kumari P, Schecter GP, Saini N, et al. Successful treatment of human immunodeficiency virus related Castleman's disease with interferon-alpha. *Clin Infect Dis* 2000;31:602–604.

172. Nishimoto N, Sasai M, Shima Y, et al. Improvement in Castleman's disease by humanized anti-interleukin-6 receptor antibody therapy. *Blood* 2000;95:56–61.

173. Bower M, Powles T, Williams S, et al. Brief communication: rituximab in HIV associated multicentric Castleman Disease. *Ann Intern Med* 2007;147:836–839.

174. Powles T, Stebbing J, Montoto S, et al. Rituximab as re-treatment for rituximab pretreated HIV-associated multicentric Castleman disease. *Blood* 2007;110:4132–4133.

175. Kedes DSH, Ganem D. Sensitivity of Kaposi's sarcoma-associated herpesvirus replication to antiviral drugs. Implications for potential therapy. *J Clin Invest* 1997;99:2082–2086.

176. Berezne A, Agbalika F, Oksenhendler E. Failure of cidofovir in HIV associated multicentric Castleman disease. *Blood* 2004;103:4368–4369.

177. Senanayake S, Kelly J, Lloyd A, et al. Multicentric Castleman's disease treated with antivirals and immunosuppressants. *J Med Virol* 2003;71:399–403.

178. Revuelta MP, Nord JA. Successful treatment of multicentric Castleman's disease in a patient with human immunodeficiency virus infection. *Clin Infect Dis* 1998;26:527.

179. Casper C, Nichols WG, Huang ML, et al. Remission of HHV8 and HIV associated multicentric Castleman disease with ganciclovir treatment. *Blood* 2004;103:1632–1634.

180. Frisch M, Biggar RJ, Engels EA, et al. Association of cancer with AIDS related immunosuppression in adults. *JAMA* 2001;285:1736–1745.

181. Van den Berg A, Visser L, Poppema S. High expression of the CC chemokine TARC in Reed-Sternberg cells: a possible explanation for the characteristic T cell infiltrate in Hodgkin's lymphoma. *Am J Pathol* 1999;154:1685–1691.

182. Ohshima K, Tutiya T, Yamaguchi T, et al. Infiltration of tTh1 and Th2 lymphocytes around Hodgkin and Reed Sternberg cells in Hodgkin disease: relation with expression of CXC and CC chemokines on H and RS cells. *Int J Cancer* 2002;98:567–572.

183. Skinnider BF, Mak TW. The role of cytokines in classical Hodgkin lymphoma. *Blood* 2002;99:4283–4297.

184. Levine AM. Hodgkin lymphoma: to the HAART of the matter. *Blood* 2006;108:3630.

185. Levine AM. Hodgkin's disease in the setting of human immunodeficiency virus infection. *J Natl Cancer Inst Monogr* 1998;23:37–42.

186. Berenguer J, Miralles P, Ribera JM, et al. Characteristics and outcome of AIDS-related Hodgkin lymphoma before and after the introduction of highly active antiretroviral therapy. *J Acquir Immune Defic Syndr* 2008; 47:422–428.

187. Bellas C, Santon A, Manzanal A, et al. Pathological, immunological and molecular features of Hodgkin's disease associated with HIV infection: comparison with ordinary Hodgkin's disease. *Am J Surg Pathol* 1996; 20:1520–1524.

188. Levine AM, Li P, Cheung T, et al. Chemotherapy consisting of doxorubicin, bleomycin, vinblastine, and dacarbazine with granulocyte colony stimulating factor in HIV infected patients with newly diagnosed Hodgkin's disease: a prospective multi-institutional AIDS clinical trials group study (ACTG 149). *J Acquir Immune Defic Syndr* 2000;24:444–450.

189. Hoffmann C, Chow KU, Wolf E, et al. Strong impact of highly active antiretroviral therapy on survival in patients with human immunodeficiency virus associated Hodgkin's disease. *Br J Haematol* 2004;125:455–462.

190. Ribera JM, Navarro JT, Oriol A, et al. Prognostic impact of highly active antiretroviral therapy in HIV related Hodgkin's disease. *AIDS* 2002; 16:1973–1976.

191. Spina M, Gabarre J, Rossi G, et al. Stanford V regimen and concomitant HAART in 59 patients with Hodgkin disease and HIV infection. *Blood* 2002;100:1984–1988.

192. Hartmann P, Rehwald U, Salzberger B, et al. BEACOPP therapeutic regimen for patients with Hodgkin's disease and HIV infection. *Ann Oncol* 2003;14:1562–1569.

193. Penn I. Cancers complicating organ transplantation. *N Engl J Med* 1990;323:1767–1769.

194. Curtis RE, Travis LB, Rowlings PA, et al. Risk of lymphoproliferative disorders after bone marrow transplantation: a multi-institutional study. *Blood* 1999;94:2208–2216.

195. Haque T, Crawford DH. Role of donor versus recipient type Epstein-Barr virus in post transplant lymphoproliferative disorders. *Springer Semin Immunopathol* 1998;20:375–387.

196. Hezode C, Duvoux C, Germanidis G, et al. Role of hepatitis C virus in lymphoproliferative disorders after liver transplantation. *Hepatology* 1999;30:775–778.

197. Boubenider S, Hiesse C, Goupy C, et al. Incidence and consequences o post-transplantation lymphoproliferative disorders. *J Nephrol* 1997;10:136–145.

198. Finn L, Reyes J, Bueno J, et al. Epstein-Barr virus infections in children after transplantation of the small intestine. *Am J Surg Pathol* 1998;22:299–309.

199. Opelz G, Henderson R. Incidence of non-Hodgkin lymphoma in kidney and heart transplant recipients. *Lancet* 1993;342:1514–1516.

200. Swinnen LJ, Costanzo-Nordin MR, Fisher SG, et al. Increased incidence of lymphoproliferative disorder after immunosuppression with the monoclonal antibody OKT3 in cardiac transplant recipients. *N Engl J Med* 1990;323:1723–1728.

201. Witherspoon RP, Fisher LD, Schoch G, et al. Secondary cancers after bone marrow transplantation for leukemia or aplastic anemia. *N Engl J Med* 1989;321:784–789.

202. Shapiro RS, McClain K, Frizzera G, et al. Epstein-Barr virus associated B cell lymphoproliferative disorders following bone marrow transplantation. *Blood* 1988;71:1234–1243.

203. Cleary ML, Nalesnik MA, Shearer WT, et al. Clonal analysis of transplant associated lymphoproliferations based on the structure of the genomic termini of the Epstein-Barr virus. *Blood* 1988;72:349–352.

204. Wagner HJ, Wessel M, Jabs W, et al. Patients at risk for development of posttransplant lymphoproliferative disorder: plasma versus peripheral blood mononuclear cells as material for quantification of Epstein-Barr viral load by using real time quantitative polymerase chain reaction. *Transplantation* 2001;72:1012–1019.

205. Hale G, Waldmann H. Risks of developing Epstein-Barr virus related lymphoproliferative disorders after T cell depleted marrow transplants. Campath users. *Blood* 1998;91 3079–3083.

206. Liebowitz D. Epstein-Barr virus and a cellular signaling pathway in lymphomas from immunosuppressed patients. *N Engl J Med* 1998;338:1413–1421.

207. Knowles DM, Cesarman E, Chadburn A, et al. Correlative morphologic and molecular genetic analysis demonstrates three distinct categories of posttransplantation lymphoproliferative disorders. *Blood* 1995;85:552–565.

208. Cesarman E, Chadburn A, Liu YF, et al. Bcl 6 gene mutations in posttransplantation lymphoproliferative disorders predict response to therapy and clinical outcome. *Blood* 1998;92:2294–2302.

209. Gandhi MK, Khanna R. Human cytomegalovirus: clinical aspects, immune regulation, and emerging treatments. *Lancet Infect Dis* 2004;4:725–738.

210. Kashanchi F, Araujo J, Doniger J, et al. Human herpesvirus 6 ORF-1 transactivating gene exhibits malignant transforming activity and its protein binds to p53. *Oncogene* 1997;14:359–367.

211. Thomas JA, Crawford DH, Burke M. Clinico pathologic implications of Epstein Barr virus related B cell lymphoma in immunocompromised patients. *J Clin Pathol* 1995;48:287–290.

212. Harris NL, Gerry JA, Swerdlow SH. Post transplant lymphoproliferative disorders: summary of Society for Hematopathology Workshop. *Semin Diagn Pathol* 1997;14:8–14.

213. Van Gorp J, Doornewaard H, Verdonck LF, et al. Posttransplant T cell lymphoma., Report of three cases and a review of the literature. *Cancer* 1994;73:3064–3072.

214. Hanson MN, Morrison VA, Peterson BA, et al. Posttransplant T cell lymphoproliferative disorders-An Aggressive, late complication of solid organ transplantation. *Blood* 1996;88:3626–3633.

215. Hanto DW, Gajl-Peczalska KJ, Frizzera G, et al. Epstein-Barr virus induced polyclonal and monoclonal B cell lymphoproliferative diseases occurring after renal transplantation. Clinical, pathologic, and virologic findings and implications for therapy. *Ann Surg* 1983;198:356–369.

216. Nalesnik MA, Makowka L, Starzl TE. The diagnosis and treatment of posttransplant lymphoproliferative disorders. *Curr Probl Surg* 1988;25:367–472.

217. Armitage JM, Kormos RL, Stuart RS, et al. Posttransplant lymphoproliferative disease in thoracic organ transplant patients: ten years of cyclosporine based immunosuppression. *J Heart Lung Transplant* 1991;10:877–886.

218. Leblond V, Sutton L, Dorent R, et al. Lymphoproliferative disorders after organ transplantation: a report of 24 cases observed in a single center. *J Clin Oncol* 1995;13:961–968.

219. Tsai DE, Hardy CL, Tomaszewski ZJE, et al. Reduction in immunosuppression as initial therapy for post-transplant lymphoproliferative disorder: analysis of prognostic variables and long term follow up of 42 adult patients. *Transplantation* 2001;71:1076–1088.

220. European best practice guidelines for renal transplantation. Section IV: Long term management of the transplant recipient. IV.6.1: cancer risk after renal transplantation. Post transplant lymphoproliferative disease: prevention and treatment. *Nephrol Dial Transplant* 2002;17(suppl 4): 31–33.

221. Hanto DW, Frizzera G, Gajl-Peczalska KJ, et al. Epstein Barr virus induced B cell lymphoma after renal transplantation: acyclovir therapy and transition from polyclonal to monoclonal B cell proliferation. *N Engl J Med* 1982;306:913–918.

222. Starzl TE, Nalesnik MA, Porter KA, et al. Reversibility of lymphomas and lymphoproliferative lesions developing under cyclosporine-steroid therapy. *Lancet* 1984;1:583–587.

223. Mentzer SJ, Fingeroth J, Reilly JJ, et al. Arginine butyrate-induced susceptibility to ganciclovir in an Epstein Barr virus associated lymphoma. *Blood Cells Mol Dis* 1998;24:114–123.

224. Perrine SP, Hermine O, Small T, et al. A phase 1/2 trial of arginine butyrate and ganciclovir in patients with Epstein Barr virus associated lymphoid malignancies. *Blood* 2007;109:2571–2578.

225. Rooney CM, Smith CA, Ng CY, et al. Infusion of cytotoxic T cells for the prevention and treatment of Epstein-Barr virus induced lymphoma in allogeneic transplant recipients. *Blood* 1998;92:1549–1555.

226. Rooney CM, Smith CA Ng CY et al. Use of gene modified virus specific T lymphocytes to control Epstein Barr virus related lymphoproliferation. *Lancet* 1995;345:9–13.

227. Papadopoulos EB, Ladanyi M, Emanuel D, et al. Infusions of donor leukocytes to treat Epstein Barr virus associated lymphoproliferative disorders after allogeneic bone marrow transplantation. *N Engl J Med* 1994;330:1185–1191.

228. Comoli P, Labirio M, Basso S, et al. Infusion of autologous Epstein Barr virus specific cytotoxic T cells for prevention of EBV related lymphoproliferative disorder in solid organ transplant recipients with evidence of active virus replication. *Blood* 2002;99:2592–2598.

229. Comoli P, Maccario R, Locatelli F, et al. Treatment of EBV related post renal transplant lymphoproliferative disease with a tailored regimen including EBV specific T cells. *Am J Transplant* 2005;5:1415–1422.

230. Wilkie GM, Taylor C, Jones MM, et al. Establishment and characterization of a bank of cytotoxic T lymphocytes for immunotherapy of Epstein Barr virus associated diseases. *J Immunother* 2004;27:309–316.

231. Haque T, Wilkie GM, Taylor C, et al. Treatment of Epstein-Barr virus positive post-transplantation lymphoproliferative disease with partly HLA matched allogeneic cytotoxic T cells. *Lancet* 2002;360:436–442.

232. Shapiro RS, Chauvenet A, McGuire W, et al. Treatment of B cell lymphoproliferative disorders with interferon alfa and intravenous gamma globulin. *N Engl J Med* 1988;318:1334–1334.

233. Milpied N, Vasseuir B, Parquet N, et al. Humanized anti-CD20 monoclonal antibody (rituximab) in post transplant B lymphoproliferative disorder: a retrospective analysis on 32 patients. *Ann Oncol* 2000;11(suppl 1):113–116.

234. Gonzalez-Barca E, Doming-Domenech E, Javier Capote F, et al. Prospective phase II trial of extended treatment with rituximab in patients with B cell post transplant lymphoproliferative disease. *Haematologica* 2007;92:1489–1494.

235. Trappe R, Choquet S, Oertel S, et al. Sequential treatment with rituximab and CHOP chemotherapy in B-cell PTLD — a new standard in therapy? *Blood* 2007;110:121a. Abstract 390.

236. Nalesnik MA, Makowka L, Starzl TE. The diagnosis and treatment of posttransplant lymphoproliferative disorders. *Curr Probl Surg* 1988;25:367–472.

237. Swinnen LJ, Mullen GM, Carr TJ, et al. Aggressive treatment for postcardiac transplant lymphoproliferation. *Blood* 1995;86:3333–3340.

CHAPTER 36 ■ MANAGEMENT OF CENTRAL NERVOUS SYSTEM LYMPHOMA

DOUGLAS E. NEY AND LISA M. DEANGELIS

Malignant lymphoma can involve the nervous system, most commonly from metastasis from systemic non-Hodgkin lymphoma. Lymphoma rarely metastasizes to the brain, but it can spread to the leptomeninges in as many as 10% of patients. In approximately 3% to 5% of patients, it can indirectly affect the central nervous system (CNS) by causing epidural spinal cord compression. Lymphoma can also arise within the CNS as primary CNS lymphoma (PCNSL) that typically involves the brain and, to a lesser extent, the eyes, leptomeninges, and spinal cord. PCNSL has been diagnosed with greater frequency recently, and survival has significantly improved with the use of chemtherapy as part of the initial treatment. PCNSL has a predilection to affect patients with immunosuppression, especially those with acquired immuno-deficiency syndrome (AIDS). However, the introduction of highly active antiretroviral therapy has resulted in a significant decline of PCNSL in this population (1,2).

EPIDEMIOLOGY

In 1929, Bailey (3) first described PCNSL as a perithelial sarcoma. Through the decades, it became known by other names, including *microglioma* (because microglia was the presumed cell of origin), *reticulum cell sarcoma* (because of the reticulum deposition around blood vessels), and *lymphosarcoma* (4,5). In 1974, Henry et al. (6) described these tumors as primary malignant lymphomas of the CNS because their morphologic characteristics were similar to systemic malignant lymphomas. Advances in immunohistochemical techniques confirmed the lymphoid nature of PCNSL (7–10).

Formerly, PCNSL accounted for approximately 1% of all primary brain tumors and 1% to 2% of all lymphomas (11,12). In the past 3 decades, the incidence of PCNSL in patients with immunocompetence increased to 3% to 4% of all brain tumors (13). The reason for this increase is unclear, although it is part of a general trend in the United States of an increase in all extranodal lymphomas. Analysis of the National Cancer Institute Surveillance, Epidemiology, and End Results data shows more than a 10-fold increase in PCNSL from two to five cases per 10 million people in 1973 to 50 cases per 10 million in 1997 (14). In other studies, incidence rates were found to be stable or decreasing, suggesting that part of the observed increase may be due to the AIDS epidemic (15,16).

Isolated ocular lymphoma is being seen with increased frequency as well. There are three reasons to consider ocular lymphoma as part of the spectrum of PCNSL (17): (a) ocular involvement is a common feature of PCNSL; (b) the CNS is the primary site of tumor progression or relapse in patients who present with isolated ocular lymphoma; and (c) embryologically and anatomically, the eye is part of the nervous system.

PCNSL has a special predilection for patients who are immunocompromised, including those with congenital or acquired immunodeficiencies (Table 36.1) (18–25). AIDS is the most common immunocompromised state that predisposes to PCNSL, and patients with AIDS have a 10% lifetime risk of developing PCNSL; however, 4% to 7% of organ transplant recipients also develop PCNSL (26). A variety of congenital immunodeficiency states (Wiskott-Aldrich syndrome, ataxia telangiectasia) have also been associated with PCNSL. PCNSL occurs when cellular immunity is markedly depressed; in patients with AIDS, it develops late in the disease when CD4 counts are <100 to 200 per mm³. The incidence of AIDS-related PCNSL has declined secondary to better human immunodeficiency virus control with highly active antiretroviral therapy (1,2,27), but there is concern that the incidence could increase if human immunodeficiency virus resistance develops to current antiretroviral therapy.

PCNSL may represent a second malignancy in some patients. Approximately 17% of patients with PCNSL had a prior systemic cancer, such as colon, thyroid, breast, non-Hodgkin lymphoma, or Hodgkin lymphoma. The PCNSL frequently occurs many years or decades after the initial systemic cancer (28). There is no uniform treatment-related factor that may explain PCNSL in these patients; in fact, many had their primary cancer treated with surgery alone, and never received chemotherapy or radiotherapy. There may be diagnostic confusion in these patients because new brain lesions are often presumed to be brain metastases from their

---

TABLE 36.1

IMMUNODEFICIENCY CONDITIONS ASSOCIATED WITH PCNSL

Congenital
1. Wiskott-Aldrich syndrome
2. Ataxia telangiectasia
3. Severe combined immunodeficiency
4. X-linked immunoproliferative disorder

Other rare conditions
1. Sjögren syndrome
2. Rheumatoid arthritis
3. Systemic lupus erythematosus

Acquired
1. AIDS
2. Patients with organ transplant

original cancer. However, biopsy of cerebral lesions should always be considered in patients whose systemic cancer is remote and inactive.

PCNSL affects patients of all ages, with a peak incidence in the 6th and 7th decades of life. The median age is 55 years in patients with immunocompetence (7,29). There is a slight male predominance in patients with immunocompetence, approximately 1.5:1.0, but >90% of patients with HIV-related PCNSL are male, which reflects the sex distribution of human immunodeficiency virus in the United States (30). When reported in children, PCNSL is almost always associated with inherited or acquired immunodeficiency (31–34). In patients with immunosuppression, the median age of PCNSL is lowest in patients with inherited immunodeficiency syndromes (10 years), followed by acquired immunodeficiency states, such as AIDS (31 years), and by organ allograft transplantation (37 years) (35,36).

ETIOLOGY

In patients who are immunocompromised, PCNSL arises from B-lymphocytes infected with the Epstein-Barr virus (1,37). After primary Epstein-Barr virus infection, which usually occurs early in life, a small population of B-cells remains latently infected and resides for life within the individual. These B-cells are immortalized but not transformed, and their proliferation is controlled by suppressor T-cells. Any immunosuppressive process that disturbs T-cell function leads to uncontrolled proliferation of the latently infected B-cell population, eventually leading to development of a neoplasm. Epstein-Barr virus-driven lymphomas have a propensity to develop in the CNS because there is limited normal immune surveillance in the nervous system and, therefore, these cells are further protected from any functioning immune system. Epstein-Barr virus can be detected in the cerebrospinal fluid (CSF) or in tumor tissue of almost all patients with AIDS with PCNSL (38,39).

Neither Epstein-Barr virus nor any of the human herpesviruses have been identified as etiologic factors in patients with immunocompetence, and the pathogenesis of PCNSL in these patients is unknown. There are no lymph nodes or lymphatics in the nervous system to serve as a reservoir for lymphoid tissue. However, there is growing evidence that the malignant clone of PCNSL can be identified systemically. Jahnke et al. (40) found a monoclonal B-cell population in the peripheral blood and bone marrow of four of 24 patients with PCNSL, none of whom had any evidence of systemic lymphoma on staging evaluation. In a study of body positron emission tomography (PET) imaging, unsuspected sites of disease were identified in 15% of patients, again suggesting that a significant minority has detectable systemic tumor (41). Whether the disease arises systemically and then spreads to the CNS, or begins there and secondarily seeds the periphery, is unknown. The presence of systemic involvement did not affect the subsequent risk of relapse in either of these studies, making the significance of the findings unclear.

PATHOLOGY

PCNSL is a B-cell tumor in almost all cases; <4% of PCNSLs are of T-cell origin (Color Plate 83) (42). The majority of PCNSLs correspond to the large cell (diffuse large B-cell lymphoma) or large cell immunoblastic subtypes, although low-grade subtypes are occasionally seen. PCNSL involves the brain parenchyma in >90% of patients, and most commonly affects the frontal lobes, corpus callosum, basal ganglia, and cerebellum. It typically grows in periventricular regions and commonly comes in contact with the ventricles or the subarachnoid space (43). PCNSL rarely involves the leptomeninges or spinal cord in the absence of a brain lesion (44).

Macroscopically, PCNSL lesions are fleshy and usually discrete from normal brain. Microscopically, they are composed of high-grade neoplastic cells that grow in a characteristic perivascular pattern in concentric rings around blood vessel walls without invasion of the lumen (Color Plate 83) (45). Autopsy typically shows extensive brain invasion with microscopic tumor growing in areas remote from bulky lesions seen on imaging studies (8). Reactive T-lymphocytes may infiltrate these B-cell tumors, causing diagnostic difficulty, particularly in patients treated with corticosteroids before sampling. Steroids may cause lysis of the malignant B-cells, leaving the reactive T-cells behind, leading to misdiagnosis of an inflammatory reaction (46,47). PCNSL does not have the degree of vascular proliferation commonly seen in high-grade gliomas; necrosis and hemorrhage are uncommon. In patients who are immunocompromised, however, necrosis and hemorrhage are frequent (45).

Cytogenetic studies showed abnormalities of chromosomes 1 (1q21), 6 (6q15, 6q21), 7 (7q15), and 14 (14q24, 14q32) (48). A genomic imbalance was confirmed in 95% of patients with PCNSL by comparative genomic hybridization; the most common were losses of 6q (47% with common deletion of 6q21-q22), and gains of 12q (63%), 18q (37%), and 22q (37%). Weber et al. (49) reported gains involving 1q, 9q, 11q, 12p, 16p, and 17p. Conflicting data were reported for p53 as being overexpressed, mutated, or absent in different studies (50–53). Bcl-2 and Bcl-6 were overexpressed in 20% to 50% of PCNSLs (50,51,53), but they were absent in p53-expressing tumors (53). It appears that one of several central pathways involved in apoptosis is affected in PCNSL. Sixty-six percent of PCNSLs contained ≤10% apoptotic cells detectable by terminal deoxynucleotidyl transferase-mediated uridine triphosphatase nick end labeling assay (51). Other evidence indicates an abnormal G_1-S phase of the cell cycle in PCNSL. In one report of patients with immunocompetence with PCNSL, approximately 50% showed deletion of p15 and p16 or 5' CpG island methylation of the p16 gene (50,54). In another report, further testing for p16 expression by reverse transcriptase-mediated polymerase chain reaction revealed that messenger ribonucleic acid expression was absent in 63% and weakly present in 36% (50). Immunohistochemistry indicated that p16 was absent or restricted to single tumor cells intermingled among negative tumor cells. p16 binds and inhibits the cyclin D-regulated CDK4 and six kinases that control transition into the late G_1 phase of the cell cycle. Deletion of p16 may relieve this block, and cells would progress into S phase. PCNSLs were also reported to be MIB-1 positive; most have a proliferative index that exceeds 50% (51).

A single study has examined the gene expression profile of 23 PCNSL samples. Approximately equal numbers of activated B-cell, germinal center, and "type III" subtypes were identified (55). However, no survival data were available to determine if these subtypes had prognostic importance. The authors did identify overexpression of interleukin-4 in tumor cells and tumor vessels, which may explain the prominent perivascular growth pattern of PCNSL.

Three studies have examined Bcl-6 expression in PCNSL (56–58). Two of these studies indicated that tumor Bcl-6 expression was associated with better survival (56,58). One study of 83 biopsy specimens could not demonstrate a survival advantage, but 96% of tumors were classified as activated B-cell type (57).

CLINICAL PRESENTATIONS

PCNSL presents as a fast-growing brain tumor, and patients usually have only a few weeks of symptoms (59). Signs and symptoms depend on the size and location of the tumor.

The frontal lobes are involved in 30% to 40% of patients, causing cognitive deficit or personality changes in 24% to 70% of patients (Table 36.2) (59,60). Focal neurologic deficits (e.g., hemiparesis and ataxia) and signs of increased intracranial pressure (e.g., headache and nausea) are common (60). Because these tumors are located deep in white matter, seizures are less common than with other primary brain tumors. PCNSL presenting as isolated leptomeningeal disease is rare, but involvement of the leptomeninges occurs in approximately 42% of patients at diagnosis and approximately 41% at recurrence (61). However, patients rarely have symptoms suggestive of leptomeningeal spread, such as cranial neuropathies, hydrocephalus, or spinal radiculopathy (62).

Primary involvement of the spinal cord is extremely rare and usually occurs at the thoracic level. Patients present with a painless, progressive myelopathy (63). PCNSL involving the eye is common and can be the sole site of disease. Fifty to 80% of patients with isolated ocular lymphoma eventually develop cerebral lymphoma at a mean of approximately 23 months after ocular diagnosis (64). In contrast, ocular involvement is reported in 20% to 25% of patients with PCNSL at diagnosis, and only one-half of those have visual symptoms (65). The symptoms of ocular lymphoma include floaters, visual blurring, or segmental visual loss secondary to retinal detachment from subretinal deposits of lymphoma.

In patients with isolated ocular lymphoma, the diagnosis may be delayed because these nonspecific symptoms and the accompanying cellular infiltrate of the vitreous are similar to those occurring in common inflammatory eye conditions such as uveitis, chorioretinitis, or vitreitis.

DIAGNOSIS AND STAGING

The initial evaluation for the diagnosis and staging of PCNSL includes: cranial magnetic resonance imaging (MRI); CSF studies; ophthalmologic examination; computed tomography (CT) scan of chest, abdomen, and pelvis; bone marrow biopsy; and human immunodeficiency virus test (Table 36.3). MRI is the optimal technique for neuroimaging, but occasionally CT scanning must be used in patients who cannot undergo MRI, such as those with a pacemaker. On noncontrast CT scanning, PCNSLs usually appear as isodense or hyperdense lesions, and on MRI, the lesions are isointense to hypointense on T1-weighted images. Homogeneous contrast enhancement is seen in >90% of cases (Fig. 36.1) (66). The lesions usually have irregular borders; the amount of surrounding edema is variable, compared with the reliably prominent edema usually seen with metastatic tumors or gliomas. The lesions occur in the subcortical white matter, often adjacent to the ventricles, and are solitary in 60% to 70% of cases and multifocal in 30% to 40% of cases. In patients who are immunocompromised, PCNSL typically appears as a ring-enhancing lesion on MRI or CT scanning. The central necrosis seen radiographically correlates with the necrosis identified pathologically in these patients. Radiographically, it is impossible in patients with AIDS to differentiate PCNSL from an infectious process, such as toxoplasmosis (67). PET or single photon emission CT can be helpful in distinguishing PCNSL, which is hypermetabolic, from infection, which is typically hypometabolic (68,69). Nonenhancing tumors have also been reported in approximately 10% of mainly patients with immunosuppression with PCNSL (Fig. 36.2) (70).

Stereotactic biopsy is the diagnostic test for patients with immunocompetence and who are immunocompromised. Resection is not performed because most lesions are deep,

---

TABLE 36.2

PRESENTING SIGNS AND SYMPTOMS OF PCNSL

Symptoms and signs	Percent range
Common	
Changes in mental status	24–73
Focal neurologic signs (hemiparesis, aphasia)	40–50
Increased intracranial pressure (headache, nausea)	15–60
Ataxia	15–40
Visual blurring, floaters	8–10
Less common	
Seizures	2–33
Nuchal rigidity	0–36
Cranial neuropathy	5–31
Spinal radiculopathy	1–2
Bladder or bowel dysfunction	1–2

TABLE 36.3

INITIAL WORKUP AND STAGING FOR PCNSL

Patients with immunocompetence
  Cranial MRI with and without contrast (if contraindicated, CT)
  Lumbar puncture
    CSF markers: β_2-microglobulin, soluble CD27, cytology
  Ophthalmologic evaluation, including slitlamp examination
  Human immunodeficiency virus test
  CT chest, abdomen, pelvis
  Possible body PET
  Possible bone marrow biopsy
  MRI of spine with contrast if indicated

Patients who are immunocompromised
  As above and additional tests
  Lumbar puncture
    CSF for Epstein-Barr virus deoxyribonucleic acid
  Cranial PET or single photon emission CT scan

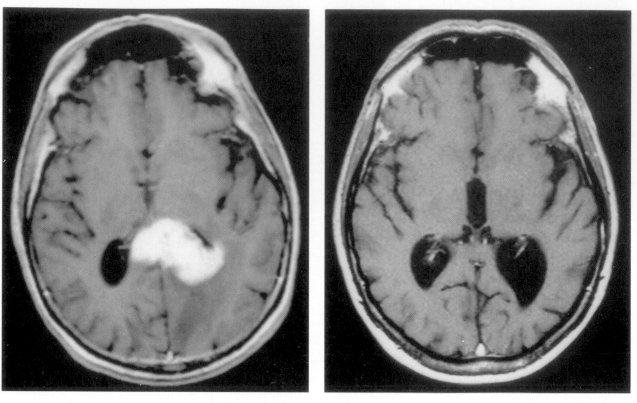

FIGURE 36.1 Gadolinium-enhanced magnetic resonance scans showing complete response of PCNSL to high-dose methotrexate, procarbazine, and vincristine.

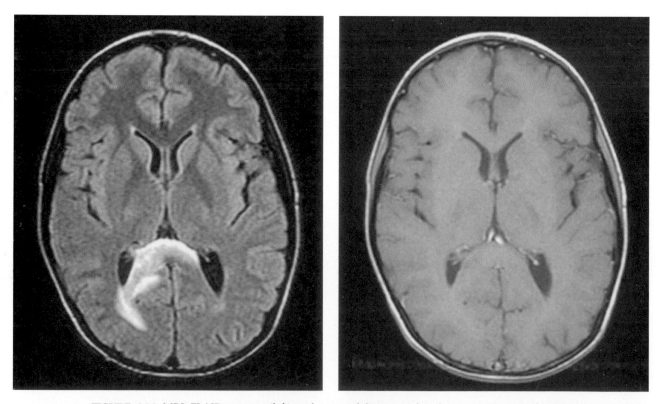

FIGURE 36.2 MRI FLAIR seqence (left) and post-gadolinium (right) demonstrating nonenhancing Epstein-Barr virus-positive cerebral lymphoma in a patient who is immunocompromised after allogeneic T-cell-depleted bone marrow transplant for acute lymphocytic leukemia.

many are multifocal, and resection does not improve survival over biopsy alone. Occasionally, resection is necessary to decompress a rapidly expanding mass in patients with herniation. In these patients, resection is lifesaving and restores neurologic function so that medical therapy can follow. In patients with AIDS, the combination of a hypermetabolic PET or single photon emission CT scan and a positive CSF test for Epstein-Barr virus deoxyribonucleic acid is 100% specific for PCNSL; therefore, biopsy can be avoided in these cases (71). Stereotactic biopsy is associated with an 11.5% incidence of intracranial hemorrhage in patients with AIDS, in contrast to a 1% incidence in patients without AIDS (72,73). Thus, biopsy for patients with AIDS should be reserved for those suspected of having PCNSL in whom noninvasive tests are nondiagnostic.

Although stereotactic biopsy in patients with immunocompetence is the definitive surgical approach to diagnose PCNSL (74), the diagnosis may become difficult when the patient is treated preoperatively with corticosteroids (75). PCNSL may shrink or disappear after steroid administration (46,47). The steroids have a direct cytotoxic effect on malignant lymphocytes, which is mediated by a cytoplasmic steroid receptor that translocates to the nucleus and induces apoptosis (75). Not all PCNSL lesions respond to steroids; thus, the absence of tumor regression after steroids does not preclude the diagnosis of PCNSL (76). However, when PCNSL is suspected on imaging, steroids should be withheld until a biopsy has been performed. It is safe to defer steroid use for most patients.

Lumbar puncture for CSF analysis is essential for neurologic staging. It is safe in the majority of patients and must be avoided only in those with large posterior fossa lesions. Eighty to 90% of patients have elevation of CSF protein, usually <100 mg per dL. Positive cytology is reported in 0% to 50% of patients. Identification of malignant cells may be difficult when cell counts are low, reactive lymphocytes are present, or steroids have been administered (77). Because most PCNSLs are B-cell tumors, demonstration of a monoclonal B-cell population by immunocytochemistry or immunoglobulin gene rearrangement may facilitate diagnosis (7).

Soluble CD27 in the CSF has been reported as a useful marker for PCNSL. A CD27 level >1.5 U per mL was associated with PCNSL but was not found in the CSF of patients with glial tumors or inflammatory neurologic conditions (78,79). In patients with AIDS, CSF analysis for both cytology and Epstein-Barr virus deoxyribonucleic acid using polymerase chain reaction analysis can establish the diagnosis. CSF studies can also exclude other processes, such as progressive multifocal leukoencephalopathy, by testing for JC virus by polymerase chain reaction (80,81). Gleissner et al. (82) have demonstrated the usefulness of molecular genetic testing for PCNSL in the CSF. Polymerase chain reaction analysis of the complementary determining region III identified a monoclonal population of lymphoma cells in the CSF of patients with primary and secondary CNS lymphoma. This may be an important new technique, but its sensitivity and specificity remain to be established. Measurement of tumor markers such as lactate dehydrogenase, β-glucuronidase, and β2-microglobulin may also be helpful, although their role in diagnosis and prognosis is not clear.

Complete ophthalmologic workup, including slitlamp, is an essential part of the initial staging evaluation. Ocular lymphoma can appear as choroidal scleral thickening, widening of the optic nerve, or vitreous debris (63). These findings may be nonspecific, but in a patient with known PCNSL, they confirm the presence of ocular involvement. Biopsy of the vitreous, or an anterior chamber tap, can be confirmatory in patients with isolated ocular lymphoma or ocular relapse (83). Patients treated with steroids can have a false-negative vitrectomy if the tumor has regressed (65). Alternatively, vitreitis that initially responds but then becomes refractory to corticosteroids suggests ocular lymphoma.

Standard systemic evaluation using body CT and bone marrow biopsy reveals another site of disease in approximately 3% to 4% of patients with immunocompetence who present with typical PCNSL (84). However, recent PET data suggest a higher frequency of systemic lymphoma at initial workup (85). The therapeutic implications of these findings are less clear.

PROGNOSTIC FACTORS

In addition to Bcl-6 expression, clinical factors can have a strong effect on outcome regardless of treatment and need to be considered when interpreting the serial phase II trials examining new therapeutic approaches in PCNSL. In almost all studies, age and performance status (PS) were identified as important prognostic factors. In the first effort to define a prognostic index, Ferreri et al. (86) collected 378 patients and retrospectively identified five prognostic factors (age, PS, CSF protein concentration, deep location of the tumor mass, and serum lactate dehydrogenase) as influencing survival. They devised a three-tiered prognostic index that segregated patients with similar survival, giving one point for each poor prognostic factor. Abrey et al. (87) performed a similar analysis with 338 patients, and could identify only age and PS as being important. They confirmed their findings with a recursive partitioning analysis and then validated them using 194 patients with PCNSL in the Radiation Therapy Oncology Group database. Again, a three-tier stratification assigned patients to statistically different survival categories: age <50, age >50 with PS ≥70, or age >50 with PS <70.

DIFFERENTIAL DIAGNOSIS

The differential diagnosis for PCNSL differs for patients with immunocompetence and immunodeficiency (Table 36.4). In the patient with immunocompetence, brain metastases and primary brain tumors are the most common diagnostic concerns; demyelinating disease and inflammatory processes, such as neurosarcoidosis, may also be considered in some patients. Acute exacerbation of multiple sclerosis can resemble a periventricular enhancing lesion that improves or disappears after steroid administration (88). However, recurrent stereotypic symptoms reflecting a single neurologic location and associated with a single recurrent enhancing lesion are suspicious for PCNSL. Sarcoidosis may have a similar appearance to PCNSL and responds to steroids (89,90), but it usually involves the hypothalamus and is frequently associated with pulmonary involvement. The diffuse enhancement pattern on MRI often differentiates PCNSL from glial tumors or metastases, which typically have areas of central necrosis. In addition, the deep location of most PCNSL lesions is unusual for metastatic disease (91–96).

TABLE 36.4

MOST COMMON DIFFERENTIAL DIAGNOSES
OF PCNSL

Patients with immunocompetence
  Glioma
  Metastasis
  Multiple sclerosis
  Sarcoid

Patients who are immunocompromised
  Infections
    Toxoplasmosis
    Fungal
    Viral (progressive multifocal leukoencephalopathy)
  Human immunodeficiency virus encephalopathy
  Abscess
  Glioma
  Metastasis

The main differential diagnoses for PCNSL in the patient with AIDS are toxoplasmosis and progressive multifocal leukoencephalopathy. Other opportunistic infections, human immunodeficiency virus encephalopathy, and other brain tumors should also be considered. To further complicate the situation, these processes may coexist with PCNSL in the patient with AIDS. In addition, systemic lymphoma in a patient with AIDS is frequently extranodal with spread to the CNS. Therefore, a patient with AIDS with PCNSL should undergo a complete evaluation for systemic lymphoma to exclude a CNS presentation of systemic disease. In AIDS-related PCNSL, the incidence of ocular involvement is unknown, but the high incidence of cytomegalovirus retinitis in patients with AIDS can make the diagnosis difficult.

TREATMENT

Patients with Immunocompetence

Early diagnosis and treatment are critical because PCNSL is a highly aggressive tumor and, if not treated, is fatal. The median survival is approximately 2 to 3 months for untreated patients (Table 36.5) (6,97). Surgical resection alone gives a median survival of only 4 to 5 months, and resection may worsen the patient's neurologic deficit because of the deep location of most lesions (98). Therefore, the appropriate surgical approach for patients with PCNSL is a stereotactic

TABLE 36.5

MEDIAN SURVIVAL IN MONTHS WITH DIFFERENT
TREATMENTS

Treatments	Months
Untreated	2–3
Surgery alone	4–5
CHOP + WBRT	9.5–16
WBRT	12–18
High-dose methotrexate ± WBRT	40–60

needle biopsy for diagnosis. Surgical resection should be reserved only for patients acutely deteriorating due to herniation from a large tumor mass.

A complete response to whole brain radiation therapy (WBRT) has been reported in up to 80% of patients with PCNSL (99), and increases median survival to 12 to 18 months (76,100). Treating the entire brain is necessary because of the widespread, infiltrative nature of PCNSL, even in a patient with only a single lesion on MRI. Studies have shown that reducing the port of radiotherapy (RT) increases the relapse rate and shortens survival, especially in patients under the age of 60 (101). Although RT is highly effective at producing remission, recurrence is common within 1 year, and 5-year survival is only 3% to 4% (97,102–104). Different authors observed a threshold dose of 30 to 50 Gy, but no clear dose response could be documented. In a Radiation Therapy Oncology Group prospective study, patients were given 40 Gy WBRT with a 20-Gy boost to the tumor site (Table 36.6). The focal increase in the dose to 60 Gy did not improve local control; relapse was as frequent within the boosted field as outside of it. Patients >60 years of age had a median survival of 7.6 months, whereas those <60 years had a median survival of 23.1 months (105). A similar observation was made regarding Karnofsky Performance Score. Patients with a Karnofsky Performance Score ≥70 had a median survival of 21.1 months, whereas the median survival was 5.6 months for patients with a Karnofsky Performance Score of 40 to 60.

Currently, when using WBRT, a dose of 45 Gy is considered effective and sufficient; a boost is avoided. However, several studies have examined whether a reduced dose of WBRT, when used in conjunction with effective chemotherapy, may afford equal efficacy with reduced late neurotoxicity. The data are conflicting. Bessell et al. (106) found that decreasing the dose of WBRT to 30 Gy shortened survival in patients <60 years of age but did not compromise older adults. The Radiation Therapy Oncology Group (107) decreased the dose of WBRT to 36 Gy without adversely affecting survival, but it also observed the same frequency of neurotoxicity as associated with 45 Gy. More recently, Shah et al. (108) reported on initial findings employing 23.4 Gy after a high-dose methotrexate-based regimen, and found excellent disease control and no neurotoxicity; however, these data are preliminary.

If ocular lymphoma is present, the eyes are included in the radiation port in addition to WBRT. RT can effectively control ocular lymphoma; however, relapse may occur. The dose for ocular RT is 36 to 40 Gy to minimize any risk of permanent ocular toxicity. This dose usually causes accelerated cataract formation, which often requires repair several years after completion of RT. Because occult involvement of the leptomeninges is common in PCNSL, craniospinal irradiation (24 to 40 Gy) was used in a group of patients; however, survival was not improved (109). In addition, neuraxis RT compromises subsequent chemotherapy administration by irradiating a large volume of bone marrow.

Chemotherapy is currently the initial treatment of choice for PCNSL. Due to the histologic similarities between PCNSL and systemic lymphoma, standard chemotherapy regimens for systemic lymphoma were tried initially. Three trials used cyclophosphamide, doxorubicin, Oncovin (vincristine), and prednisone (CHOP) combined with WBRT, and all had a median survival identical to WBRT alone (9.5 to 16 months) (110–112). Furthermore, patients incurred significant chemotherapy

TABLE 36.6

RESPONSE RATE, PROGRESSION-FREE SURVIVAL, AND OVERALL SURVIVAL TO DIFFERENT TREATMENT REGIMENS FOR PCNSL

Study	No. of patients	Chemotherapy	RT	Response rate (%) (CR and PR)	Median progression-free survival (mo)	Median overall survival (mo)
Radiotherapy alone						
Nelson et al. (105)	41	–	45 Gy	NA	NA	12.2
Chemoradiotherapy						
DeAngelis et al. (118)	31	MTX (1 g/m²) + cytarabine (3 g/m²) – IT MTX	40 Gy WBRT with 4.4-Gy boost	94	41	42.5
Glass et al. (173)	25	MTX (3.5 g/m²)	30–44 Gy WBRT	88	32	33
O'Brien et al.(174)	46	MTX (1 g/m²)	45 Gy WBRT + 5.4-Gy boost	95	65% PFS at 2 y	33
Abrey et al. (127)	52	MPV (MTX 3.5 g/m²) + cytarabine (3 g/m²) + IT MTX	±45 Gy WBRT	94	NA	60
Ferreri et al. (175)	13	MPV (MTX 3 g/m²)	36–45 Gy WBRT with boost	92	NA	25+
DeAngelis et al. (107)	102	MPV (MTX 2.5 g/m²) + IT MTX	36–45 Gy WBRT	94	24	36.9
Poortmans et al. (176)	52	MTX (3 g/m²) + teniposide + carmustine + IT MTX + IT cytarabine	30 Gy WBRT + 10-Gy boost	81	NA	46
Omuro et al. (177)	52	MTX (1 g/m²) + thiotepa + procarbazine + IT MTX	41.4 Gy + 14.4-Gy boost	88	18	32
Multidrug chemotherapy without radiotherapy						
Sandor et al. (123)	14	MTX (8.4 g/m²) + thiotepa + vincristine + IT cytarabine	–	100	16.5	NA
Pels et al. (126)	65	MTX (5 g/m²) + cytarabine + ifosfamide + vinca-alkaloids + cyclophosphamide + IT MTX + IT cytarabine	–	71	21	50
Hoang-Xuan et al. (125)	50	MTX (1 g/m²) + lomustine + procarbazine + IT MTX + IT cytarabine	–	48	6.8	14.3
MTX single agent						
Batchelor et al. (120)	25	MTX (8 g/m²)	–	74	12.8	22.8+
Herrlinger et al. (121,122)	37	MTX (8 g/m²)	–	35.1	10	25

CR, complete response; IT, intrathecal; MVP, methotrexate, procarbazine, vincristine; MTX, methotrexate; NA, not applicable; PFS, progression-free survival; PR, partial response.

related toxicity (112). These patients frequently developed leptomeningeal disease and brain recurrence, typically in areas remote from the primary site (110). The initial lesion(s) seen on imaging often responded to the first few cycles of CHOP because the drugs could penetrate the disrupted blood–brain barrier associated with bulky disease and reach the tumor. However, the microscopic tumor residing behind an intact blood–brain barrier and, therefore, not visualized on MRI continued to grow, resulting in early recurrence (113). A successful chemotherapy regimen for PCNSL requires drugs that penetrate the blood–brain barrier either because they can be delivered in high doses (e.g., methotrexate) or because they are intrinsically lipophilic (e.g., thiotepa).

Methotrexate administered in a standard dose does not cross the blood–brain barrier in an amount sufficient to treat the tumor, but higher doses can reach a therapeutic concentration in the CNS. In multiple studies, high-dose methotrexate with leucovorin rescue emerged as the most effective drug for the treatment of PCNSL (114–118). A wide range of doses has been used (1 to 8 g per m^2) without a clear dose-response relationship. Systemic high-dose methotrexate plus intra-Ommaya methotrexate, followed by WBRT and high-dose cytarabine as initial therapy of PCNSL gave a median survival of 42 months with a 22% 5-year survival. However, significant neurotoxicity was observed, especially in patients older than age 60 years at diagnosis (119).

In an effort to delay radiotherapy, multiple trials of chemotherapy alone as initial treatment for PCNSL have been conducted. Batchelor et al. (120) reported the use of methotrexate (8 g per m^2) alone as initial treatment. Response rate was 74%, but progression-free survival was only 13 months. Similarly, a study from Germany (121,122) utilizing methotrexate at the same dose was closed early because 38% of the patients on study had progression of disease while on treatment. Progression-free survival was 10 months with an overall survival of 25 months. Among patients surviving >1 year, leukoencephalopathy developed in 10% of the chemotherapy alone cohort and 58% of the patients were salvaged with WBRT.

Multidrug regimens have also been studied. Sandor et al. (123) reported 13 patients with PCNSL and primary ocular lymphoma treated with a regimen of high-dose methotrexate (8.4 g per m^2), vincristine, thiotepa, intrathecal cytarabine, and methotrexate. Although response rate was 79%, progression-free survival was only 16.5 months, and two patients developed chemotherapy related leukoencephalopathy. Another study using methotrexate (1.5 g per m^2), vincristine, carmustine, methylprednisolone, etoposide, and intrathecal methotrexate in patients with leptomeningeal disease showed a progression-free survival of only 6 months (124). Chemotherapy related toxicity was significant. The European Organization for the Research and Treatment of Cancer Brain Tumor Group (125) studied 50 patients over the age of 60 treated with combination chemotherapy alone. The regimen consisted of methotrexate (1 g per m^2), lomustine, procarbazine, methylprednisolone, intrathecal methotrexate, and intrathecal cytarabine. Response rate was 48%, and overall median survival was 14 months. Finally, Pels et al. (126) reported the use of a complex chemotherapy regimen utilizing methotrexate (5 g per m^2), cytarabine, vincristine, ifosfamide, cyclophosphamide, vindesine, dexamethasone, intrathecal methotrexate, intrathecal cytarabine, intrathecal prednisolone, and delayed RT. Fifty-four percent of patients were over the

age of 60. The overall survival was 50 months, however, patients >60 did substantially worse, with a 5-year survival of 19% compared with 75% for younger patients. Severe myelosuppression was also noted in this study, and 9% of patients died of treatment-related toxicity.

Preradiation methotrexate (3.5 g per m^2) combined with procarbazine and vincristine has also been used to treat PCNSL (Fig. 36.1) (127). Chemotherapy was followed by WBRT and high-dose cytarabine. The response rate to preradiotherapy chemotherapy was 90%, and median survival was 60 months, giving a 50% 5-year survival. In an effort to reduce neurotoxicity, WBRT was eliminated in patients >60 years of age; survival was identical in those who did or did not receive RT, and neurotoxicity was significantly decreased in those treated with chemotherapy alone. However, relapse was more common in those treated with only chemotherapy, and these patients died of recurrent PCNSL, whereas those treated with chemotherapy and WBRT died of neurotoxicity. Despite these limitations, the quality of life was far superior when RT was not administered. Ferreri et al. (128) also observed that WBRT did not improve survival in patients achieving a complete response after high-dose methotrexate. Thus, every effort should be made to withhold WBRT in patients >60 years of age, and probably in those >50, who attain a complete response to chemotherapy; younger patients should receive WBRT as part of the treatment regimen to minimize the risk of relapse. The standard dose of WBRT administered in most combined modality studies is 45 Gy. Lower radiation doses may still be effective and potentially less toxic in patients who have attained a complete response after a high-dose methotrexate program, but this remains investigational.

High-dose myeloablative chemotherapy followed by autologous peripheral stem cell transplant has had some success for refractory or recurrent disease, but response was disappointing when used as the initial treatment (129,130). Different transplant regimens may have partially accounted for the disparate results. There is a single case report of remission of recurrent PCNSL by a graft versus lymphoma reaction after allogeneic peripheral blood stem cell transplantation (131). Recently, the addition of high-dose chemotherapy with autologous stem cell transplantation and radiotherapy was tested (132). Five-year overall survival was 87%; however, patients >65 were excluded. It seems clear, however, that patients who have an initial good response to chemotherapy before autologous stem cell transplantation do better.

Systemic high-dose methotrexate or cytarabine can also treat ocular lymphoma because therapeutic drug levels can be achieved in the vitreous (133,134). If ocular disease is present at diagnosis, initial treatment with chemotherapy is often effective for both ocular and cerebral involvement. Ocular RT can follow chemotherapy to consolidate treatment of the eye disease. Intravitreal methotrexate has been used successfully for recurrent ocular lymphoma (135).

Despite all aggressive measures, 20% to 30% of patients do not respond to chemotherapy, and the median survival of these patients is 6 to 10 months (118). Alternately, approximately 50% of patients have a second remission with salvage treatment; 25% survive many years after reinduction. For patients who have deferred RT, it is an important salvage option and achieves a median survival of 16 months (136). Prior high-dose methotrexate responders may respond to a second course of methotrexate, although these patients may be at a higher risk for neurotoxicity. Soussain et al. (130) reported 20 patients with refractory or relapsed PCNSL responsive to salvage cytarabine and etoposide treated with thiotepa-busulfan-cyclophosphamide and autologous stem cell transplantation. The 3-year overall survival rate was 60%, and the 3-year event-free survival was 53%. Temozolomide and rituximab have also been used as salvage therapy (137). This combination produced a 53% response rate in 15 patients with an overall survival of 14 months. It was well tolerated with minimal toxicity. Other reported salvage regimens with reasonable response rates include single-agent temozolomide (138) and topotecan (139).

Neurotoxicity

Neurotoxicity related to WBRT and treatment with methotrexate presents as progressive cerebral white matter damage termed leukoencephalopathy. Characteristics of this subcortical dementia include psychomotor slowing, behavioral changes, cognitive impairment, gait ataxia, and incontinence. Radiographically it presents as focal or confluent nonenhancing white matter abnormalities predominantly in a periventricular pattern. There is often associated ventriculomegaly and cortical atrophy. In a retrospective cohort of 185 patients, the 5-year cumulative incidence of late neurotoxicity was 24% (140). The incidence is much higher in patients >60 who are treated with methotrexate and WBRT (127). Some patients benefit from ventriculoperitoneal shunting, but the syndrome is irreversible (141).

Patients Who Are Immunocompromised

Patients with AIDS have a median survival of 1 to 2 months when treated symptomatically. Even when treated with steroids and WBRT, the median survival is only 2 to 5 months (142,143). Because PCNSL occurs late in the course of human immunodeficiency virus infection, many patients die of opportunistic infections, and not from PCNSL. Some patients can tolerate high-dose methotrexate and survive a median of approximately 1 year (144,145).

The institution of highly active antiretroviral therapy and antiviral therapy directed against Epstein-Barr virus can induce prolonged remission in some patients with AIDS-related PCNSL (146,147). Tumor regression due to reconstitution of the immune system may explain the occasional patient with AIDS with spontaneous remission of PCNSL (148–151).

CENTRAL NERVOUS SYSTEM METASTATIC COMPLICATIONS OF SYSTEMIC NON-HODGKIN LYMPHOMA

Leptomeningeal Metastasis

Leptomeningeal metastasis develops in approximately 5% to 15% of patients with systemic non-Hodgkin lymphoma, particularly in patients with a lymphoblastic or diffuse undifferentiated histology. Gururangan et al. (152) reported a series

of 362 children with CNS metastasis, 49 of whom had CNS disease at diagnosis. The median interval between the diagnosis of systemic non-Hodgkin lymphoma and CNS involvement was 6 to 9 months in the 362 patients.

In another large series of 2,561 adult patients with lymphoma, 140 had CNS involvement from systemic lymphoma, and 67% of these 140 patients had leptomeningeal involvement (153). Leptomeningeal metastasis involves all levels of the neuraxis, leading to multifocal symptoms and signs, including headache, ataxia, cranial nerve palsies, back pain, radiculopathy, and sensory symptoms. The diagnosis is established by CSF cytology or enhanced MRI, showing definitive evidence of subarachnoid tumor such as enhancing nodules on the cauda equina or infiltration of cranial nerves.

CNS prophylaxis with RT and chemotherapy has been effective in reducing the incidence of leptomeningeal lymphoma in patients with non-Hodgkin lymphoma (154,155). Usually, intrathecal or intraventricular chemotherapy is administered concurrently with chemotherapy targeted against the systemic disease (156,157). CNS prophylaxis is recommended for patients with stage IV disease, Waldeyer ring involvement, and lymphoblastic undifferentiated, diffuse histocytic lymphoma, or small cell type histologies (154,158). Haddy et al. (158) demonstrated that prophylactic intrathecal chemotherapy effectively prevented spread to the CNS in patients without initial CNS involvement; 28% of patients who did not receive prophylaxis had a CNS relapse, compared with 8% who received intrathecal drug. In ocular adnexal lymphoma, CNS prophylaxis with RT or chemotherapy did not reduce CNS relapse (159).

Focal RT in a dose of approximately 30 Gy provides effective palliation to symptomatic sites such as the lumbosacral spine for cauda equina symptoms or the brain for cranial neuropathies. Neuraxis RT is avoided because of its high morbidity and limited efficacy. RT is sometimes administered to areas of bulky disease seen on neuroimaging, even if they are not yet symptomatic, to prevent the development of additional neurologic disability, or to open potential sites of CSF obstruction to facilitate subsequent intrathecal chemotherapy. This must be decided within the context of the patient's overall condition and therapeutic plan.

Intrathecal chemotherapy with methotrexate or cytarabine usually supplements RT of the involved neuraxis to treat the entire subarachnoid space. Intrathecal methotrexate (12 mg) or cytarabine (50 mg) is administered every 3 to 4 days for the first 3 weeks, with subsequent doses decreasing in frequency depending on the patient's response. The intrathecal drug is given as a fixed dose and not calculated according to the body surface area because the CSF volume is approximately 150 cc in all adults regardless of size. A liposomal preparation of cytarabine (DepoCyt, 50 mg) has the advantage of every 2-week administration with sustained concentration of drug in the CSF. However, it is associated with a high incidence of chemical meningitis compared with the standard drugs, and requires days of steroid before and after treatment to reduce this complication. Several reports suggest improved median survival when intrathecal chemotherapy is delivered through an Ommaya reservoir compared with lumbar puncture (156,160,161). An Ommaya reservoir is also easier for the patient (and physician) for repeated drug instillation, and the physician can be ensured that the drug is actually delivered into the subarachnoid space, whereas approximately 10% of injections by lumbar puncture can lead to drug pooling in the epidural space. Furthermore, the drug can also be given to patients via an Ommaya reservoir even when the patient is thrombocytopenic ($\geq$20,000 per mm^2), whereas lumbar puncture is associated with a risk of epidural hematoma in this setting. Therefore, an Ommaya reservoir should be used in all patients with leptomeningeal metastasis in whom intrathecal chemotherapy is a planned component of treatment.

Intrathecal chemotherapy is distributed by bulk flow through the subarachnoid space and requires normal CSF dynamics. CSF flow can be assessed by CSF studies with radio-labeled indium. Intrathecal chemotherapy must be avoided in patients with obstruction of CSF flow because drug delivery is impaired and can cause neurotoxicity. When the drug is instilled into the ventricular system and does not egress properly, it can leak into the subependymal tissue, leading to leukoencephalopathy. Impaired CSF flow is present when hydrocephalus is evident on imaging, there is increased intracranial pressure, or there are large subarachnoid tumor nodules. Occasionally, CSF flow is abnormal even in the setting of normal neuroimaging. Alternative treatment in the form of RT or systemic chemotherapy may be used until CSF flow can be restored.

In patients with leptomeningeal lymphoma, high-dose methotrexate or cytarabine is an alternative to intrathecal chemotherapy. Response is comparable to intrathecal treatment, and systemic drugs can penetrate into areas of bulky disease that intrathecal chemotherapy does not reach; however, there are more systemic side effects (160,162–164). In addition, systemic drug can be given in the presence of impaired CSF flow.

Epidural Tumors

Symptomatic spinal cord compression was due to lymphoma in 10% of 583 patients with malignant cord compression (165,166). In another series of 265 patients with epidural spinal metastasis from various systemic cancers, 6.8% had lymphoma. Epidural metastasis from systemic lymphoma usually involves the thoracic spine and is associated with extensive retroperitoneal disease; less commonly, the lumbosacral and cervical spine can be involved (166). Diffuse large cell is the most common histology, although all histologic subtypes of lymphoma have been described causing epidural metastasis (11,153,167).

The most common signs and symptoms of epidural tumor are back pain, weakness, sensory loss, autonomic dysfunction, and ataxia. Pain is the earliest and most frequent presenting symptom of cord compression. Pain can be local, radicular, referred, or funicular in nature. Pain from epidural metastasis is generally mild at onset, but if not diagnosed and treated in a timely fashion, it progresses with increasing severity. More than one-half of patients with thoracic epidural metastasis and cord compression have a radiating, tight, band-like pain around the chest or abdomen. In cervical and lumbosacral spine epidural disease, pain generally radiates to the arms or legs. Weakness is the second most common symptom resulting from root compression or corticospinal tract involvement (168,169). Motor signs may include bilateral leg weakness, spasticity, hyperactive deep tendon reflexes, and a Babinski sign. Cauda equina involvement is manifest as unilateral or asymmetric leg weakness, hypotonia, decreased reflexes, and

early sphincter disturbance. Sensory symptoms may include numbness and paresthesias that usually begin in the legs and ascend to the level of cord compression.

Diagnosis is established by spinal MRI. Contrast is not necessary, and the entire spine must be imaged, even in patients with a single focus of pain, because multilevel epidural tumor can be found in approximately 10% of patients. Plain films and bone scan can miss epidural tumor, particularly in patients with lymphoma, because disease can extend directly into the epidural space from paravertebral tumor without destroying the bony elements of the spine. Thus, any patient with lymphoma with back pain should undergo MRI of the spine.

Once diagnosed, patients with epidural metastasis should be treated with high-dose corticosteroids, which rapidly relieve pain and may improve neurologic function. For a patient with a confirmed systemic lymphoma and newly diagnosed epidural metastasis, local RT using 30 to 40 Gy is the treatment of choice (170,171). If the diagnosis is not confirmed or the patient has relapse, surgical decompression may become necessary for diagnosis or treatment. Unlike patients with epidural metastasis from solid tumors, initial surgery followed by RT does not improve survival or functional outcome, as compared with RT alone in patients with lymphomas. Systemic chemotherapy is an alternative for patients with spinal epidural disease, and minimal or no symptoms or signs, who need to receive chemotherapy for their systemic tumor. Such patients need to be followed closely, and if they do not experience a rapid response or there is progression of the epidural disease, then focal RT needs to be administered promptly (172).

Brain Metastasis

Brain metastasis develops in <1% of patients with lymphomas. Patients with cerebral metastasis can be treated symptomatically with high-dose steroids. If the diagnosis is not confirmed, steroids should be withheld until biopsy. These patients may be treated with the same high-dose methotrexate regimens as patients with PCNSL because regular systemic chemotherapy for non-Hodgkin lymphoma does not penetrate the blood–brain barrier effectively. If the patient's medical condition does not permit high-dose chemotherapy or in patients with advanced systemic disease, palliative WBRT can be effective. Patients with intracerebral disease frequently have leptomeningeal involvement and should be treated with intrathecal chemotherapy as well.

References

1. Forsyth PA, DeAngelis LM. Biology and management of AIDS-associated primary CNS lymphomas. *Hematol Oncol Clin North Am* 1996;10:1125–1134.
2. Sacktor N, Lyles RH, Skolasky R, et al., HIV-associated neurologic disease incidence changes: multicenter AIDS Cohort Study, 1990–1998. *Neurology* 2001;56:257–260.
3. Bailey P. Intracranial sarcomatous tumors of leptomeningeal origin. *Arch Surg* 1929;18:1359–1402.
4. Schaumburg HH, Plank CR, Adams RD. The reticulum cell sarcoma-microglioma group of brain tumours. A consideration of their clinical features and therapy. *Brain* 1972;95:199–212.
5. Yulie C. Case of primary reticulum cell sarcoma of the brain. Relationship of microglial cells to histiocytes. *Arch Pathol* 1938;1938:1037–1044.
6. Henry JM, Heffner RR Jr, Dillard SH, et al. Primary malignant lymphomas of the central nervous system. *Cancer* 1974;34:1293–1302.

7. Hochberg FH, Miller DC. Primary central nervous system lymphoma. *J Neurosurg* 1988;68:835–853.
8. Nakhleh RE, Manivel JC, Hurd D, et al. Central nervous system lymphomas. Immunohistochemical and clinicopathologic study of 26 autopsy cases. *Arch Pathol Lab Med* 1989;113:1050–1056.
9. Taylor CR, Russell R, Lukes RJ, et al. An immunohistological study of immunoglobulin content of primary central nervous system lymphomas. *Cancer* 1978;41:2197–2205.
10. Tomlinson FH, Kurtin PJ, Suman VJ, et al. Primary intracerebral malignant lymphoma: a clinicopathological study of 89 patients. *J Neurosurg* 1995;82:558–566.
11. Jellinger K, Radaskiewicz TH, Slowik F. Primary malignant lymphomas of the central nervous system in man. *Acta Neuropathol Suppl* 1975; (suppl 6):95–102.
12. Zimmerman HM. Malignant lymphomas of the nervous system. *Acta Neuropathol Suppl* 1975;(suppl 6):69–74.
13. Eby NL, Grufferman S, Flannelly CM, et al. Increasing incidence of primary brain lymphoma in the US. *Cancer* 1988;62:2461–2465.
14. Olson JE, Janney CA, Rao RD, et al. The continuing increase in the incidence of primary central nervous system non-Hodgkin lymphoma: a surveillance, epidemiology, and end results analysis. *Cancer* 2002;95:1504–1510.
15. Hao D, DiFrancesco LM, Brasher PM, et al. Is primary CNS lymphoma really becoming more common? A population-based study of incidence, clinicopathological features and outcomes in Alberta from 1975 to 1996. *Ann Oncol* 1999;10:65–70.
16. Kadan-Lottick NS, Skluzacek MC, Gurney JG. Decreasing incidence rates of primary central nervous system lymphoma. *Cancer* 2002;95:193–202.
17. Peak S, DeAngelis LM. Primary central nervous system lymphoma. In: Bernstein M, Berger MS, eds. *Neuro-Oncology: The Essentials*, 2nd ed. New York: Thieme Medical Publishers 2008:359–366.
18. Diette KM, Caro WA, Roenigk HH Jr. Malignant lymphoma presenting with cutaneous granulomas. *J Am Acad Dermatol* 1984;10:896–902.
19. Good AE, Russo RH, Schnitzer B, et al. Intracranial histiocytic lymphoma with rheumatoid arthritis. *J Rheumatol* 1978;5:75–78.
20. Jellinger K, Slowik F, Sluga E. Primary intracranial malignant lymphomas a fine structural cytochemical and CSF immunological study. *Clin Neurol Neurosurg* 1979;81:173–184.
21. Lehrich JR, Richardson EP. Malignant lymphoma with Sjgren's syndrome. Case records of the Massachusetts General Hospital. *N Engl J Med* 1978;299:349–1359.
22. Lipsmeyer EA. Development of malignant cerebral lymphoma in a patient with systemic lupus erythematosus treated with immunosuppression. *Arthritis Rheum* 1972;15:183–186.
23. Neault RW, Van Scoy RE, Okazaki H, et al. Uveitis associated with isolated reticulum cell sarcoma of the brain. *Am J Ophthalmol* 1972;73:431–436.
24. Raizer JR. Primary central nervous system lymphoma. In: Raghavan D, Brecher ML, Johnson DH, Meropol NJ, Moots PL, Thigpen JT, eds. *Textbook of uncommon cancer*, 2nd ed. Sussex, UK: John Wiley and Sons, 1999:323.
25. Varadachari C, Palutke M, Climie AR, et al. Immunoblastic sarcoma (histiocytic lymphoma) of the brain with B cell markers. Case report. *J Neurosurg* 1978;49:887–892.
26. Schabet M. Epidemiology of primary CNS lymphoma. *J Neurooncol* 1999;43:199–201.
27. Wolf TT, Brodt HR, Fichtlscherer SS, et al. Changing incidence and prognostic factors of survival in AIDS-related non-Hodgkin's lymphoma in the era of highly active antiretroviral therapy (HAART). *Leuk Lymphoma* 2005;46:207–215.
28. DeAngelis LM. Primary central nervous system lymphoma as a secondary malignancy. *Cancer* 1991;67:1431–1435.
29. Fine HA, Mayer RJ. Primary central nervous system lymphoma. *Ann Intern Med* 1993;119:1093–1104.
30. Remick SC, Diamond C, Migliozzi JA, et al. Primary central nervous system lymphoma in patients with and without the acquired immune deficiency syndrome. A retrospective analysis and review of the literature. *Medicine (Baltimore)* 1990;69:345–360.
31. Andiman WA, Eastman R, Martin K, et al. Opportunistic lymphoproliferations associated with Epstein-Barr viral DNA in infants and children with AIDS. *Lancet* 1985;2:1390–1393.
32. Belman AL, Diamond G, Dickson D, et al. Pediatric acquired immunodeficiency syndrome. Neurologic syndromes. *Am J Dis Child* 1988;142:29–35.
33. Del Mistro A, Laverda A, Calabrese F, et al. Primary lymphoma of the central nervous system in two children with acquired immune deficiency syndrome. *Am J Clin Pathol* 1990;94:722–728.
34. Esptein LG, DiCarlo FJ Jr, Joshi VV, et al. Primary lymphoma of the central nervous system in children with acquired immunodeficiency syndrome. *Pediatrics* 1988;82:355–363.
35. Filipovich AH, Heinitz KJ, Robison LL, et al. The Immunodeficiency Cancer Registry. A research resource. *Am J Pediatr Hematol Oncol* 1987;9:183–184.
36. Penn I, Porat G. Central nervous system lymphomas in organ allograft recipients. *Transplantation* 1995;59:240–244.
37. Bashir RM, Harris NL, Hochberg FH, et al. Detection of Epstein-Barr virus in CNS lymphomas by in-situ hybridization. *Neurology* 1989;39:813–817.

38. Cingolani A, Gastaldi R, Fassone L, et al. Epstein-Barr virus infection is predictive of CNS involvement in systemic AIDS-related non-Hodgkin's lymphomas. *J Clin Oncol* 2000;18:3325–3330.
39. Cinque P, Brytting M, Vago L, et al. Epstein-Barr virus DNA in cerebrospinal fluid from patients with AIDS-related primary lymphoma of the central nervous system. *Lancet* 1993;342:398–401.
40. Jahnke KK, Hummel MM, Korfel AA, et al. Detection of subclinical systemic disease in primary CNS lymphoma by polymerase chain reaction of the rearranged immunoglobulin heavy-chain genes. *J Clin Oncol* 2006; 24:4754–4757.
41. Mohile NA, Deangelis LM, Abrey LE. The utility of body FDG PET in staging primary central nervous system lymphoma. *Neuro Oncol* 2008; 10:223–228.
42. Shenkier TN, Blay JY, O'Neill BP, et al. Primary CNS lymphoma of T-cell origin: a descriptive analysis from the international primary CNS lymphoma collaborative group. *J Clin Oncol* 2005;23:2233–2239.
43. Shibata S. Sites of origin of primary intracerebral malignant lymphoma. *Neurosurgery* 1989;25:14–19.
44. Miller DC, Hochberg FH, Harris NL, et al. Pathology with clinical correlations of primary central nervous system non-Hodgkin's lymphoma. The Massachusetts General Hospital experience 1958–1989. *Cancer* 1994;74: 1383–1397.
45. Louis DN, Ohgaki H, Wiestler OD, et al. WHO Classification of Tumours of the Central Nervous System. Lyon: International Agency for Research on Cancer (IARC), 2007.
46. Singh A, Strobos RJ, Singh BM, et al. Steroid-induced remissions in CNS lymphoma. *Neurology* 1982;32:1267–1271.
47. van den Bent MJ, Vanneste JA, Ansink BJ. Prolonged remission of primary central nervous system lymphoma after discontinuation of steroid therapy. *J Neurooncol* 1992;13:257–259.
48. Itoyama T, Sadamori N, Tsutsumi K, et al. Primary central nervous system lymphoma. Immunophenotypic, virologic, and cytogenetic findings of three patients without immune defects. *Cancer* 1994;73:455–463.
49. Weber T, Weber RG, Kaulich K, et al. Characteristic chromosomal imbalances in primary central nervous system lymphomas of the diffuse large B-cell type. *Brain Pathol* 2000;10:73–84.
50. Cobbers JM, Wolter M, Reifenberger J, et al. Frequent inactivation of CDKN2A and rare mutation of TP53 in PCNSL. *Brain Pathol* 1998; 8:263–276.
51. Deckert-Schluter M, Rang A, Wiestler OD. Apoptosis and apoptosis-related gene products in primary non-Hodgkin's lymphoma of the central nervous system. *Acta Neuropathol* 1998;96:157–162.
52. Koga H, Zhang S, Ichikawa T, et al. Primary malignant lymphoma of the brain: demonstration of the p53 gene mutations by PCR-SSCP analysis and immunohistochemistry. *Noshuyo Byori* 1994;11:151–155.
53. Nozaki M, Tada M, Mizugaki Y, et al. Expression of oncogenic molecules in primary central nervous system lymphomas in immunocompetent patients. *Acta Neuropathol* 1998;95:505–510.
54. Zhang SJ, Endo S, Ichikawa T, et al. Frequent deletion and 5′ CpG island methylation of the p16 gene in primary malignant lymphoma of the brain. *Cancer Res* 1998;58:1231–1237.
55. Rubenstein JL, Fridlyand J, Shen A, et al. Gene expression and angiotropism in primary CNS lymphoma. *Blood* 2006;107:3716–3723.
56. Braaten KM, Betensky RA, de Leval LL, et al. BCL-6 expression predicts improved survival in patients with primary central nervous system lymphoma. *Clin Cancer Res* 2003;9:1063–1069.
57. Camilleri-Broet S, Criniere E, Broet P, et al. A uniform activated B-cell-like immunophenotype might explain the poor prognosis of primary central nervous system lymphomas: analysis of 83 cases. *Blood* 2006;107: 190–196.
58. Levy OO, Deangelis LM, Filippa DA, et al. Bcl-6 predicts improved prognosis in primary central nervous system lymphoma. *Cancer* 2008;112:151–156.
59. DeAngelis LM. Primary central nervous system lymphoma. *Curr Opin Neurol* 1999;12:687–691.
60. Herrlinger U, Schabet M, Bitzer M, et al. Primary central nervous system lymphoma: from clinical presentation to diagnosis. *J Neurooncol* 1999;43:219–226.
61. Balmaceda C, Gaynor JJ, Sun M, et al. Leptomeningeal tumor in primary central nervous system lymphoma: recognition, significance, and implications. *Ann Neurol* 1995;38:202–209.
62. Chamberlain M. Leptomeningeal metastases. In: Levin V, ed. *Cancer in the nervous system*. New York, NY: Churchill Livingstone, 1996:282.
63. Schild SE, Wharen RE Jr, Menke DM, et al. Primary lymphoma of the spinal cord. *Mayo Clin Proc* 1995;70:256–260.
64. Ursea R, Heinemann MH, Silverman RH, et al. Ophthalmic, ultrasonographic findings in primary central nervous system lymphoma with ocular involvement. *Retina* 1997;17:118–123.
65. Peterson K, Gordon KB, Heinemann MH, et al. The clinical spectrum of ocular lymphoma. *Cancer* 1993;72:843–849.
66. Buhring U, Herrlinger U, Krings T, et al. MRI features of primary central nervous system lymphomas at presentation. *Neurology* 2001;57:393–396.
67. Ciricillo SF, Rosenblum ML. Use of CT and MR imaging to distinguish intracranial lesions and to define the need for biopsy in AIDS patients. *J Neurosurg* 1990;73:720–724.

68. Akiyama Y, Moritake K, Yamasaki T, et al. The diagnostic value of 123I-IMP SPECT in non-Hodgkin's lymphoma of the central nervous system. *J Nucl Med* 2000;41:1777–1783.
69. Kosuda S, Aoki S, Suzuki K, et al. Primary malignant lymphoma of the central nervous system by Ga-67 and TI-201 brain SPECT. *Clin Nucl Med* 1992;17:961–964.
70. DeAngelis LM. Cerebral lymphoma presenting as a nonenhancing lesion on computed tomographic/magnetic resonance scan. *Ann Neurol* 1993;33:308–311.
71. Antinori A, De Rossi G, Ammassari A, et al. Value of combined approach with thallium-201 single-photon emission computed tomography and Epstein-Barr virus DNA polymerase chain reaction in CSF for the diagnosis of AIDS-related primary CNS lymphoma. *J Clin Oncol* 1999;17:554–560.
72. Apuzzo ML, Chandrasoma PT, Cohen D, et al. Computed imaging stereotaxy: experience and perspective related to 500 procedures applied to brain masses. *Neurosurgery* 1987;20:930–937.
73. Luzzati R, Ferrari S, Nicolato A, et al. Stereotactic brain biopsy in human immunodeficiency virus-infected patients. *Arch Intern Med* 1996;156:565–568.
74. Boiardi A, Silvani A. Primary cerebral non-Hodgkin's lymphoma (PCNSL): a review of new trends in management. *Ital J Neurol Sci* 1997;18:1–7.
75. Weller M. Glucocorticoid treatment of primary CNS lymphoma. *J Neurooncol* 1999;43:237–239.
76. Deangelis LM. Current management of primary central nervous system lymphoma. *Oncology (Williston Park)* 1995;9:63–71.
77. Ferreri AJ, Reni M, Villa E. Therapeutic management of primary central nervous system lymphoma: lessons from prospective trials. *Ann Oncol* 2000;11:927–937.
78. Murase S, Saio M, Andoh H, et al. Diagnostic utility of CSF soluble CD27 for primary central nervous system lymphoma in immunocompetent patients. *Neurol Res* 2000;22:434–442.
79. Murase S, Saio M, Takenaka K, et al. Increased levels of CSF soluble CD27 in patients with primary central nervous system lymphoma. *Cancer Lett* 1998;132:181–186.
80. Fedele CG, Avellon A, Ciardi M, et al. Quantitation of polyomavirus DNA by a competitive nested polymerase chain reaction. *J Virol Methods* 2000;88:51–61.
81. Samorei IW, Schmid M, Pawlita M, et al. High sensitivity detection of JC-virus DNA in postmortem brain tissue by in situ PCR. *J Neurovirol* 2000;6:61–74.
82. Gleissner B, Siehl J, Korfel A, et al. CSF evaluation in primary CNS lymphoma patients by PCR of the CDR III IgH genes. *Neurology* 2002;58:390–396.
83. Akpek EK, Ahmed I, Hochberg FH, et al. Intraocular-central nervous system lymphoma: clinical features, diagnosis, and outcomes. *Ophthalmology* 1999;106:1805–1810.
84. O'Neill BP, Dinapoli RP, Kurtin PJ, et al. Occult systemic non-Hodgkin's lymphoma (NHL) in patients initially diagnosed as primary central nervous system lymphoma (PCNSL): how much staging is enough? *J Neurooncol* 1995;25:67–71.
85. Abrey LE, Batchelor TT, Ferreri AJ, et al. Report of an international workshop to standardize baseline evaluation and response criteria for primary CNS lymphoma. *J Clin Oncol* 2005;23:5034–5043.
86. Ferreri AJ, Blay JY, Reni M, et al. Prognostic scoring system for primary CNS lymphomas: the International Extranodal Lymphoma Study Group experience. *J Clin Oncol* 2003;21:266–272.
87. Abrey LE, Ben-Porat L, Panageas KS, et al. Primary central nervous system lymphoma: the Memorial Sloan-Kettering Cancer Center prognostic model. *J Clin Oncol* 2006;24:5711–5715.
88. DeAngelis LM. Primary central nervous system lymphoma imitates multiple sclerosis. *J Neurooncol* 1990;9:177–181.
89. Lexa FJ, Grossman RI. MR of sarcoidosis in the head and spine: spectrum of manifestations and radiographic response to steroid therapy. *AJNR Am J Neuroradiol* 1994;15:973–982.
90. Pickuth D, Spielmann RP, Heywang-Kobrunner SH. Role of radiology in the diagnosis of neurosarcoidosis. *Eur Radiol* 2000;10:941–944.
91. Bentson JR, Steckel RJ, Kagan AR. Diagnostic imaging in clinical cancer management: brain metastases. *Invest Radiol* 1988;23:335–341.
92. Chidel MA, Suh JH, Barnett GH. Brain metastases: presentation, evaluation, and management. *Cleve Clin J Med* 2000;67:120–127.
93. Davey P. Brain metastases. *Curr Probl Cancer* 1999;23:59–98.
94. Patchell RA. Brain metastases. *Neurol Clin* 1991;9:817–824.
95. Vecht CJ. Clinical management of brain metastasis. *J Neurol* 1998;245:127–131.
96. Wen PY, Loeffler JS. Management of brain metastases. *Oncology (Williston Park)* 1999;13:941–954.
97. Reni M, Ferreri AJ, Garancini MP, et al. Therapeutic management of primary central nervous system lymphoma in immunocompetent patients: results of a critical review of the literature. *Ann Oncol* 1997;8:227–234.
98. Murray K, Kun L, Cox J. Primary malignant lymphoma of the central nervous system. Results of treatment of 11 cases and review of the literature. *J Neurosurg* 1986;65:600–607.
99. Corn BW, Dolinskas C, Scott C, et al. Strong correlation between imaging response and survival among patients with primary central nervous system lymphoma: a secondary analysis of RTOG studies 83-15 and 88-06. *Int J Radiat Oncol Biol Phys* 2000;47:299–303.
100. Shibamoto Y, Ogino H, Hasegawa M, et al. Results of radiation monotherapy for primary central nervous system lymphoma in the 1990s. *Int J Radiat Oncol Biol Phys* 2005;62:809–813.
101. Shibamoto Y, Hayabuchi N, Hiratsuka J, et al. Is whole-brain irradiation necessary for primary central nervous system lymphoma? Patterns of recurrence after partial-brain irradiation. *Cancer* 2003;97:128–133.
102. Phan TG, O'Neill BP, Kurtin PJ. Posttransplant primary CNS lymphoma. *Neuro Oncol* 2000;2:229–238.
103. Pollack IF, Lunsford LD, Flickinger JC, et al. Prognostic factors in the diagnosis and treatment of primary central nervous system lymphoma. *Cancer* 1989;63:939–947.
104. Sagerman RH, Cassady JR, Chang CH. Radiation therapy for intracranial lymphoma. *Radiology* 1967;88:552–554.
105. Nelson DF, Martz KL, Bonner H, et al. Non-Hodgkin's lymphoma of the brain: can high dose, large volume radiation therapy improve survival? Report on a prospective trial by the Radiation Therapy Oncology Group (RTOG): RTOG 8315. *Int J Radiat Oncol Biol Phys* 1992;23:9–17.
106. Bessell EM, Lopez-Guillermo A, Villa S, et al. Importance of radiotherapy in the outcome of patients with primary CNS lymphoma: an analysis of the CHOD/BVAM regimen followed by two different radiotherapy treatments. *J Clin Oncol* 2002;20:231–236.
107. DeAngelis LM, Seiferheld W, Schold SC, et al. Combination chemotherapy and radiotherapy for primary central nervous system lymphoma: Radiation Therapy Oncology Group Study 93-10. *J Clin Oncol* 2002;20:4643–4648.
108. Shah GD, Yahalom JJ, Correa DD, et al. Combined immunochemotherapy with reduced whole-brain radiotherapy for newly diagnosed primary CNS lymphoma. *J Clin Oncol* 2007;25:4730–4735.
109. Brada M, Dearnaley D, Horwich A, et al. Management of primary cerebral lymphoma with initial chemotherapy: preliminary results and comparison with patients treated with radiotherapy alone. *Int J Radiat Oncol Biol Phys* 1990;18:787–792.
110. Lachance DH, Brizel DM, Gockerman JP, et al. Cyclophosphamide, doxorubicin, vincristine, and prednisone for primary central nervous system lymphoma: short-duration response and multifocal intracerebral recurrence preceding radiotherapy. *Neurology* 1994;44:1721–1727.
111. O'Neill BP, Wang CH, O'Fallon JR, et al. Primary central nervous system non-Hodgkin's lymphoma (PCNSL): survival advantages with combined initial therapy? A final report of the North Central Cancer Treatment Group (NCCTG) Study 86-72-52. *Int J Radiat Oncol Biol Phys* 1999;43:559–563.
112. Schultz C, Scott C, Sherman W, et al. Preirradiation chemotherapy with cyclophosphamide, doxorubicin, vincristine, and dexamethasone for primary CNS lymphomas: initial report of radiation therapy oncology group protocol 88-06. *J Clin Oncol* 1996;14:556–564.
113. Ott RJ, Brada M, Flower MA, et al. Measurements of blood-brain barrier permeability in patients undergoing radiotherapy and chemotherapy for primary cerebral lymphoma. *Eur J Cancer* 1991;27:1356–1361.
114. Blay JJY, Conroy TT, Chevreau CC, et al. High-dose methotrexate for the treatment of primary cerebral lymphomas: analysis of survival and late neurologic toxicity in a retrospective series. *J Clin Oncol* 1998;16:864–871.
115. Blay JY, Bouhour D, Carrie C, et al. The C5R protocol: a regimen of high-dose chemotherapy and radiotherapy in primary cerebral non-Hodgkin's lymphoma of patients with no known cause of immunosuppression. *Blood* 1995;86:2922–2929.
116. DeAngelis LM. Primary CNS lymphoma: treatment with combined chemotherapy and radiotherapy. *J Neurooncol* 1999;43:249–257.
117. DeAngelis LM, Yahalom J, Heinemann MH, et al. Primary CNS lymphoma: combined treatment with chemotherapy and radiotherapy. *Neurology* 1990;40:80–86.
118. DeAngelis LM, Yahalom J, Thaler HT, et al. Combined modality therapy for primary CNS lymphoma. *J Clin Oncol* 1992;10:635–643.
119. Schlegel U, Pels H, Oehring R, et al. Neurologic sequelae of treatment of primary CNS lymphomas. *J Neurooncol* 1999;43:277–286.
120. Batchelor T, Carson K, O'Neill A, et al. Treatment of primary CNS lymphoma with methotrexate and deferred radiotherapy: a report of NABTT 96-07. *J Clin Oncol* 2003;21:1044–1049.
121. Herrlinger U, Kuker W, Uhl M, et al. NOA-03 trial of high-dose methotrexate in primary central nervous system lymphoma: final report. *Ann Neurol* 2005;57:843–847.
122. Herrlinger U, Schabet M, Brugger W, et al. German Cancer Society Neuro-Oncology Working Group NOA-03 multicenter trial of single-agent high-dose methotrexate for primary central nervous system lymphoma. *Ann Neurol* 2002;51:247–252.
123. Sandor V, Stark-Vancs V, Pearson D, et al. Phase II trial of chemotherapy alone for primary CNS and intraocular lymphoma. *J Clin Oncol* 1998;16:3000–3006.
124. Cheng AL, Yeh KH, Uen WC, et al. Systemic chemotherapy alone for patients with non-acquired immunodeficiency syndrome-related central nervous system lymphoma: a pilot study of the BOMES protocol. *Cancer* 1998;82:1946–1951.

125. Hoang-Xuan K, Taillandier L, Chinot O, et al. Chemotherapy alone as initial treatment for primary CNS lymphoma in patients older than 60 years: a multicenter phase II study (26952) of the European Organization for Research and Treatment of Cancer Brain Tumor Group. *J Clin Oncol* 2003;21:2726–2731.

126. Pels H, Schmidt-Wolf IG, Glasmacher A, et al. Primary central nervous system lymphoma: results of a pilot and phase II study of systemic and intraventricular chemotherapy with deferred radiotherapy. *J Clin Oncol* 2003;21:4489–4495.

127. Abrey LE, Yahalom J, DeAngelis LM. Treatment for primary CNS lymphoma: the next step. *J Clin Oncol* 2000;18:3144–3150.

128. Ferreri AJ, Reni M, Pasini F, et al. A multicenter study of treatment of primary CNS lymphoma. *Neurology* 2002;58:1513–1520.

129. Abrey LE, Rosenblum MK, Papadopoulos E, et al. High dose chemotherapy with autologous stem cell rescue in adults with malignant primary brain tumors. *J Neurooncol* 1999;44:147–153.

130. Soussain C, Suzan F, Hoang-Xuan K, et al. Results of intensive chemotherapy followed by hematopoietic stem-cell rescue in 22 patients with refractory or recurrent primary CNS lymphoma or intraocular lymphoma. *J Clin Oncol* 2001;19:742–749.

131. Varadi G, Or R, Kapelushnik J, et al. Graft-versus-lymphoma effect after allogeneic peripheral blood stem cell transplantation for primary central nervous system lymphoma. *Leuk Lymphoma* 1999;34:185–190.

132. Illerhaus G, Marks R, Ihorst G, et al. High-dose chemotherapy with autologous stem-cell transplantation and hyperfractionated radiotherapy as first-line treatment of primary CNS lymphoma. *J Clin Oncol* 2006; 24:3865–3870.

133. de Smet MD, Stark-Vancs V, Kohler DR, et al. Intraocular levels of methotrexate after intravenous administration. *Am J Ophthalmol* 1996; 121:442–444.

134. Strauchen JA, Dalton J, Friedman AH. Chemotherapy in the management of intraocular lymphoma. *Cancer* 1989;63:1918–1921.

135. de Smet MD, Vancs VS, Kohler D, et al. Intravitreal chemotherapy for the treatment of recurrent intraocular lymphoma. *Br J Ophthalmol* 1999;83:448–451.

136. Hottinger AF, DeAngelis LM, Yahalom J, et al. Salvage whole brain radiotherapy for recurrent or refractory primary CNS lymphoma. *Neurology* 2007;69:1178–1182.

137. Enting RH, Demopoulos A, DeAngelis LM, et al. Salvage therapy for primary CNS lymphoma with a combination of rituximab and temozolomide. *Neurology* 2004;63:901–903.

138. Reni M, Mason W, Zaja F, et al. Salvage chemotherapy with temozolomide in primary CNS lymphomas: preliminary results of a phase II trial. *Eur J Cancer* 2004;40:1682–1688.

139. Fischer L, Thiel E, Klasen HA, et al. Response of relapsed or refractory primary central nervous system lymphoma (PCNSL) to topotecan. *Neurology* 2004;62:1885–1887.

140. Omuro AM, Ben-Porat LS, Panageas KS, et al. Delayed neurotoxicity in primary central nervous system lymphoma. *Arch Neurol* 2005;62:1595–1600.

141. McAllister LD, Doolittle ND, Guastadisegni PE, et al. Cognitive outcomes and long-term follow-up results after enhanced chemotherapy delivery for primary central nervous system lymphoma. *Neurosurgery* 2000;46:51–60.

142. Kaufmann T, Nisce LZ, Coleman M. A comparison of survival of patients treated for AIDS-related central nervous system lymphoma with and without tissue diagnosis. *Int J Radiat Oncol Biol Phys* 1996;36:429–432.

143. Ling SM, Roach M 3rd, Larson DA, et al. Radiotherapy of primary central nervous system lymphoma in patients with and without human immunodeficiency virus. Ten years of treatment experience at the University of California San Francisco. *Cancer* 1994;73:2570–2582.

144. Chamberlain MC, Kormanik PA. AIDS-related central nervous system lymphomas. *J Neurooncol* 1999;43:269–276.

145. Forsyth PA, Yahalom J, DeAngelis LM. Combined-modality therapy in the treatment of primary central nervous system lymphoma in AIDS. *Neurology* 1994;44:1473–1479.

146. Chow KU, Mitrou PS, Geduldig K, et al. Changing incidence and survival in patients with aids-related non-Hodgkin's lymphomas in the era of highly active antiretroviral therapy (HAART). *Leuk Lymphoma* 2001;41:105–116.

147. Hoffmann C, Tabrizian S, Wolf E, et al. Survival of AIDS patients with primary central nervous system lymphoma is dramatically improved by HAART-induced immune recovery. *AIDS* 2001;15:2119–2127.

148. Al-Yamany M, Lozano A, Nag S, et al. Spontaneous remission of primary central nervous system lymphoma: report of 3 cases and discussion of pathophysiology. *J Neurooncol* 1999;42:151–159.

149. Daniels D, Lowdell CP, Glaser MG. The spontaneous regression of lymphoma in AIDS. *Clin Oncol (R Coll Radiol)* 1992;4:196–197.

150. Heinzlef O, Poisson M, Delattre JY. Spontaneous regression of primary cerebral lymphoma [in French]. *Rev Neurol (Paris)* 1996;152:135–138.

151. Sugita Y, Shigemori M, Yuge T, et al. Spontaneous regression of primary malignant intracranial lymphoma. *Surg Neurol* 1988;30:148–152.

152. Gururangan S, Sposto R, Cairo MS, et al. Outcome of CNS disease at diagnosis in disseminated small noncleaved-cell lymphoma and B-cell leukemia: a Children's Cancer Group study. *J Clin Oncol* 2000;18:2017–2025.

153. Hollender A, Kvaloy S, Lote K, et al. Prognostic factors in 140 adult patients with non-Hodgkin's lymphoma with systemic central nervous system (CNS) involvement. A single centre analysis. *Eur J Cancer* 2000; 36:1762–1768.

154. Duque-Hammershaimb L, Wollner N, Miller DR. LSA2-L2 protocol treatment of stage IV non-Hodgkin's lymphoma in children with partial and extensive bone marrow involvement. *Cancer* 1983;52:39–43.

155. Tomita N, Kodama F, Sakai R, et al. Predictive factors for central nervous system involvement in non-Hodgkin's lymphoma: significance of very high serum LDH concentrations. *Leuk Lymphoma* 2000;38:335–343.

156. Recht L, Straus DJ, Cirrincione C, et al. Central nervous system metastases from non-Hodgkin's lymphoma: treatment and prophylaxis. *Am J Med* 1988;84:425–435.

157. Cortes J, O'Brien SM, Pierce S, et al. The value of high-dose systemic chemotherapy and intrathecal therapy for central nervous system prophylaxis in different risk groups of adult acute lymphoblastic leukemia. *Blood* 1995;86:2091–2097.

158. Haddy TB, Adde MA, Magrath IT. CNS involvement in small noncleaved-cell lymphoma: is CNS disease per se a poor prognostic sign? *J Clin Oncol* 1991;9:1973–1982.

159. Restrepo A, Raez LE, Byrne GE Jr, et al. Is central nervous system prophylaxis necessary in ocular adnexal lymphoma? *Crit Rev Oncog* 1998;9:269–273.

160. MacKintosh FR, Colby TV, Podolsky WJ, et al. Central nervous system involvement in non-Hodgkin's lymphoma: an analysis of 105 cases. *Cancer* 1982;49:586–595.

161. Raz I, Siegal T, Polliack A. CNS involvement by non-Hodgkin's lymphoma. Response to a standard therapeutic protocol. *Arch Neurol* 1984;41:1167–1171.

162. Amadori S, Papa G, Avvisati G, et al. Sequential combination of systemic high dose ara C and asparaginase for the treatment of central nervous system leukemia and lymphoma. *J Clin Oncol* 1984;2:98–101.

163. Morra E, Lazzarino M, Brusamolino E, et al. The role of systemic high-dose cytarabine in the treatment of central nervous system leukemia. Clinical results in 46 patients. *Cancer* 1993;72:439–445.

164. Skarin AT, Zuckerman KS, Pitman SW, et al. High-dose methotrexate with folinic acid in the treatment of advanced non-Hodgkin lymphoma including CNS involvement. *Blood* 1977;50:1039–1047.

165. DeAngelis LM, Posner JP. *Neurologic Complications of Cancer*, 2nd ed. Oxford University Press, 2008.

166. Levitt LJ, Dawson DM, Rosenthal DS, et al. CNS involvement in the non-Hodgkin's lymphomas. *Cancer* 1980;45:545–552.

167. Herman TS, Hammond N, Jones SE, et al. Involvement of the central nervous system by non-Hodgkin's lymphoma: the Southwest Oncology Group experience. *Cancer* 1979;43:390–397.

168. Gilbert RW, Kim JH, Posner JB. Epidural spinal cord compression from metastatic tumor: diagnosis and treatment. *Ann Neurol* 1978;3:40–51.

169. Greenberg HS, Kim JH, Posner JB. Epidural spinal cord compression from metastatic tumor: results with a new treatment protocol. *Ann Neurol* 1980;8:361–366.

170. Haddad P, Thaell JF, Kiely JM, et al. Lymphoma of the spinal extradural space. *Cancer* 1976;38:1862–1866.

171. Mead GM, Kennedy P, Smith JL, et al. Involvement of the central nervous system by non-Hodgkin's lymphoma in adults. A review of 36 cases. *Q J Med* 1986;60:699–714.

172. Wong ET, Portlock CS, O'Brien JP, et al. Chemosensitive epidural spinal cord disease in non-Hodgkin's lymphoma. *Neurology* 1996;46:1543–1547.

173. Glass J, Gruber ML, Cher L, et al. Preirradiation methotrexate chemotherapy of primary central nervous system lymphoma: long-term outcome. *J Neurosurg* 1994;81:188–195.

174. O'Brien P, Roos D, Pratt G, et al. Phase II multicenter study of brief single-agent methotrexate followed by irradiation in primary CNS lymphoma. *J Clin Oncol* 2000;18:519–526.

175. Ferreri AJ, Reni M, Dell'Oro S, et al. Combined treatment with high-dose methotrexate, vincristine and procarbazine, without intrathecal chemotherapy, followed by consolidation radiotherapy for primary central nervous system lymphoma in immunocompetent patients. *Oncology* 2001;60:134–140.

176. Poortmans PM, Kluin-Nelemans HC, Haaxma-Reiche H, et al. High-dose methotrexate-based chemotherapy followed by consolidating radiotherapy in non-AIDS-related primary central nervous system lymphoma: European Organization for Research and Treatment of Cancer Lymphoma Group Phase II Trial 20962. *J Clin Oncol* 2003;21:4483–4488.

177. Omuro AM, DeAngelis LM, Yahalom J, et al. Chemoradiotherapy for primary CNS lymphoma: an intent-to-treat analysis with complete follow-up. *Neurology* 2005;64:69–74.

CHAPTER 37 ■ UNIQUE ASPECTS OF PRIMARY EXTRANODAL LYMPHOMAS

MARY K. GOSPODAROWICZ, FRANCESCO BERTONI, AND EMANUELE ZUCCA

Approximately 66,120 new cases of lymphoma and 27,810 deaths will occur in the United States in 2008. Non-Hodgkin lymphoma is the fifth to sixth most common cause of cancer, after prostate, lung, breast, colorectal, uterine, ovarian, and bladder tumors, or 4% to 5% of new cases. The incidence of non-Hodgkin lymphoma in Western countries has increased substantially in the last 20 years, with the Surveillance Epidemiology End Results age-adjusted incidence rates rising by approximately 80% between 1973 and 1997 (1,2). However, the rate of increase has declined in the last 8 years. Over a third of new lymphomas arise from sites other than lymph nodes, even those with no native lymphoid tissue. Extranodal presentations of lymphoma account for between 24% and 48% of new lymphoma cases, and often present as localized disease. The outcomes of extranodal lymphomas are difficult to ascertain. Most reported data are limited to single institution retrospective reviews. In prospective trials, extranodal lymphomas are included together with nodal lymphomas. Recently, the International Extranodal Lymphoma Study Group (IELSG) has originated a number of retrospective and prospective trials to clarify the management issues distinct to the individual disease entities presenting in extranodal sites (http://www.ielsg.org/).

The etiology of extranodal lymphomas is multifactorial, and includes congenital, acquired, and iatrogenic immune suppression, autoimmune disease, infections, both viral and bacterial, and exposure to pesticides and other environmental agents. Although considerable progress has been made in the understanding of gastric lymphoma and its relationship to *Helicobacter pylori*, the precise etiology of other lymphomas has not been determined.

The definition of extranodal lymphoma is controversial. Criteria for the diagnosis of extranodal lymphoma have been proposed now almost 50 years ago by Dawson et al. (3) for gastrointestinal lymphomas, and were refined by Herrmann (4) and Lewin (5) et al. almost 30 years ago. The original criteria by Dawson et al. (3) stipulated that for a designation of primary extranodal lymphoma, patients had to present with their main disease manifestation in an extranodal site, have no more than regional lymph node involvement, with no peripheral lymph node involvement, and no liver or spleen involvement. Later, these criteria were relaxed to allow for contiguous involvement of other organs (e.g., liver, spleen), and for distant nodal disease providing that the extranodal lesion was the presenting site and constituted the predominant disease bulk. The designation of stage III and IV lymphomas as primary extranodal lymphomas is debatable. Variable reporting criteria make it difficult to establish the true incidence of primary or localized extranodal lymphomas. Extranodal involvement in the presence of extensive nodal or disseminated disease may represent secondary extranodal spread. Some authors deal with this by considering stage I and II presentation only as primary extranodal lymphomas, whereas others include as extranodal lymphomas those presentations with "dominant" extranodal component with only minor nodal component (6). Another area of controversy relates to the designation of extranodal sites versus extralymphatic sites. The taxonomy in extranodal lymphomas deserves comment in so far as the Ann Arbor classification recognizes Waldeyer ring, thymus, spleen, appendix, and Peyer patches of the small intestine as lymphatic tissues, and does not consider them as extranodal lesions. However, most clinicians separate nodal from extranodal presenting sites rather than lymphatic and extralymphatic sites, and for purposes of this review, we will use the extranodal definition as indicating presentation outside lymph node area.

PATHOLOGY

The histologic spectrum of extranodal lymphoma differs from that of nodal lymphoma with a predominance of frequently localized diffuse large cell lymphomas, the occurrence of extranodal marginal zone B-cell lymphoma of mucosa-associated lymphoid tissue (MALT) type, and a paucity of follicular lymphomas. Homing mechanisms have been implicated in the biology of primary extranodal lymphomas (7,8). Although some sites present a predominant histology, for example, diffuse large B-cell lymphoma in testis, in other anatomic localizations a broad spectrum of lymphoma types are shown. For example, in intestine in addition to diffuse large B-cell lymphoma, enteropathy associated T-cell lymphoma, and marginal zone B-cell lymphoma, including the immunoproliferative small intestinal disease, mantle cell lymphoma, and follicular lymphoma, can be observed. Another site with a spectrum of histologic types of lymphoma is the breast. Primary lymphoma of the breast occurring in young women and associated with pregnancy is commonly a high-grade Burkitt-like lymphoma, whereas later in life, marginal zone B-cell lymphomas, follicular lymphomas, and diffuse large B-cell lymphomas occur (9). A broad spectrum of lymphomas also occurs in the skin, where mycosis fungoides and other peripheral T-cell lymphomas, including anaplastic (CD30+) large cell lymphomas, low-grade B-cell lymphomas, and large B-cell lymphomas, are all seen, and the vast majority of them exhibit homing properties to the skin, regardless of histology. Histologic type is the main determinant of prognosis in both nodal and extranodal lymphomas. However, in extranodal lymphomas, the specific presenting site is also of importance. For example, despite the other factors being equal, the behavior and prognosis of diffuse large B-cell lymphoma of the brain, testis, and bone are all different from one another.

PRESENTING SITES

The spectrum of presenting sites is vast, but in most comprehensive reports, primary lymphomas affecting the stomach and Waldeyer ring are the most common. In the classic report by Freeman et al. (10) of the Surveillance Epidemiology End Results experience from 1950 to 1964, stomach lymphoma was most common, followed by intestine, tonsil, and skin. Waldeyer ring lymphomas are frequently considered to be nodal presentations and, therefore, are not consistently included in the extranodal lymphoma series. The 1992 Surveillance Epidemiology End Results study reported stomach, skin, intestine, and brain to be the most common sites of extranodal lymphoma (11). In a population-based study from Denmark, d'Amore et al. (12) found stomach, intestine, skin, and bone to be the most common sites of presentation. Referral patterns may affect institutional experience with primary extranodal lymphoma. In the Princess Margaret Hospital (PMH) experience, Waldeyer ring lymphoma (mostly tonsil) and stomach lymphoma were consistently the most common extranodal sites (13). Less common, but distinct, primary extranodal sites for the development of lymphoma include other head and neck sites (salivary gland, paranasal sinus, gingiva, nasal cavity, orbit, thyroid), breast, lung, male and female genital tract (testis, prostate, ovary, cervix, uterine corpus), urinary bladder, and soft tissues. The least common sites of primary extranodal lymphoma include heart, muscle, kidney, pleura, adrenal gland, liver, and dura mater.

PATIENT CHARACTERISTICS AND PRESENTATION

The characteristics of patients with nodal and extranodal lymphomas are similar, although patients with primary extranodal lymphomas tend to be older. In localized extranodal lymphomas, stage I disease is seen in two-thirds of patients.

Presenting symptoms depend on the site of origin and do not differ significantly from symptoms of other malignancies affecting that specific organ. Gastric lymphomas present typically with symptoms of dyspepsia and epigastric pain, bowel lymphomas with obstruction, blood loss, or diarrhea, whereas bone lymphoma and primary extranodal lymphomas usually present with pain. Tumor bulk at presentation is also closely related to primary site. Characteristically, cutaneous and orbital lymphomas are visible to the patient and, therefore, diagnosed early; extradural lymphomas present early with symptoms of back pain, whereas other lymphomas may present more bulky disease. In the absence of nodal involvement, primary extranodal lymphoma is often not suspected thereby making the histologic diagnosis particularly important. One cannot distinguish clinically lymphoma from carcinoma (Table 37.1).

APPROACH TO MANAGEMENT

Patient Assessment

The assessment of anatomic disease extent is similar to that for nodal lymphoma. All patients should be assessed using the template applicable to all patients with lymphoma. This includes history with the documentation of B symptoms, complete physical examination, complete blood count and lactate dehydrogenase, imaging with computed tomography (CT) examination of neck, chest, abdomen, and pelvis, and bone marrow biopsy. Depending on the availability, gallium scans or 18-fluoro-deoxyglucose-positron emission tomography scans are performed. In addition to the standard lymphoma investigations, specific tests to define local disease extent in presenting extranodal site and potential high-risk areas for occult disease are indicated. For example, it is very important to image with CT or magnetic resonance imaging (MRI) to define disease extent in extranodal lymphomas presenting in the head and neck region, use MRI to evaluate

TABLE 37.1

OUTCOME OF EXTRANODAL DIFFUSE LARGE B-CELL LYMPHOMAS AT DIFFERENT PRIMARY SITES

Localization	Author	Number of patients	Long-term survival (%)
Head and neck	Aviles et al., 1996 (14)	316	56–90 (Waldeyer ring)
	Cortelazzo et al., 2005 (15)	309	72
Stomach	Cortelazzo et al., 1999 (16)	312	75
	Ibrahim et al., 1999 (17)	185	68
	Koch et al., 2005 (18)	194	87
	Aviles et al., 2005 (19)	241	80
Intestine	Ibrahim et al., 2001 (20)	66	58
	Cortelazzo et al., 2002 (21)	87	68
Bone	Christie et al., 1999 (22)	70	59
	Zinzani et al., 2003 (23)	52	68
	Beal et al., 2006 (24)	65	88
Testis	Fonseca et al., 2000 (25)	62	38
	Zucca et al., 2003 (26)	373	48
Breast	Aviles et al., 2005 (27)	95	50–76
	Ryan et al., 2008 (28)	204	63
CNS	Ferreri et al., 2002 (29)	370	24
	Abrey et al., 2006 (30)	388	37

disease extent in primary bone lymphoma, or extranodal lymphomas involving soft tissues (31). Endoscopy should be used as appropriate to define local disease extent in airways, gastrointestinal tract, and urinary tract. In *H. pylori*-related gastric lymphoma, the C14 urea breath test is useful to ascertain eradication of active infection. Cerebrospinal fluid (CSF) fluid cytology is an essential part of the assessment of primary central nervous system (CNS) lymphomas, and because of the pattern of relapse, lymphomas involving parameningeal sites such as extradural, or paranasal sinus lymphomas, and primary testis lymphoma (Table 37.2).

PRINCIPLES OF TREATMENT

In general, the patients are treated with curative intent. A palliative approach is used occasionally in situations where, due to the condition of the patient or the extent and/or location of the disease, radical treatment offers no possibility of cure. The principles of the management of extranodal lymphoma follow those of their nodal counterparts with some exceptions. Specific histologic type, tumor bulk, and stage are the main factors in selecting therapy. However, tumor location and pattern of disease must also be considered. Primary extranodal lymphomas may be locally invasive and extensive, and it is critical to document the extent of the initial involvement. The exact disease extent has to be established before starting chemotherapy because it is impossible to accurately plan involved-field radiation therapy in the absence of this information.

The principles of management are based primarily on anatomic disease extent documented using the Ann Arbor classification. The currently accepted histologic classification, the World Health Organization classification, is based upon the lineage (B cell, T cell, or natural killer [NK] cell), stage of differentiation (precursor or mature), and clinical presentation of lymphoma in nodal or extranodal site (32,33). In addition to histology and stage, factors known to influence the outcome in patients with extranodal lymphomas include local tumor bulk, number of extranodal sites, lactate dehydrogenase, and performance status (34). The latter three and stage are attributes comprising the International Prognostic Index (35). Extranodal lymphomas may involve paired organs, such as bilateral parotid glands, bilateral orbital involvement, etc. The Ann Arbor classification does not directly address the issue of stage designation in such situations. However, the prognosis of such presentations is usually that of stage I disease rather than stage IV disease, and, therefore, we consider presentations with paired organ involvement in the context of localized disease. The presenting extranodal site may by itself carry an adverse prognosis, as seen in CNS lymphoma and testis lymphoma. In stage I and II disease, local therapy is routinely used, both for cure and local control. However, the recognition of occult distant disease mandates the use of chemotherapy in patients with large cell or mantle cell lymphomas. In stage III and IV disease, the mainstay of treatment is chemotherapy, and local treatment is not routinely used, although it may still have a role for sites of bulky disease or incomplete response, particularly in a location where local control is desired (e.g., extradural space). The addition of rituximab to cyclophosphamide, hydroxydaunorubicin, Oncovin (vincristine), and prednisone (R-CHOP) chemotherapy has

---

TABLE 37.2

SPECIFIC STAGING PROCEDURES TO CONSIDER IN SPECIFIC EXTRANODAL PRESENTATIONS

Stomach:

- Gastroduodenal endoscopy with multiple gastric biopsies
- Endoscopic ultrasound
- Histologic and histochemical examination for *H. pylori* (negative cases should be confirmed by serology)
- Careful examination of Waldeyer ring

Small intestine:

- Endoscopy
- Small bowel series. *C. jejuni* search in immunoproliferative small intestinal disease

Large intestine:

- Colonoscopy

Waldeyer ring:

- Gastroduodenal endoscopy with multiple gastric biopsies

Nasal cavity, nasopharynx, paranasal sinus, orbit:

- CT scan or MRI of the skull and head and neck area

Salivary gland, tonsils, parotid:

- ENT examination and echography

Thyroid:

- Echography ± CT scan of the neck and thyroid function tests

Ocular adnexa:

- MRI (or CT scan) and ophthalmologic examination
- *C. psittaci* in the tumor biopsy and blood mononuclear cells

CNS:

- MRI with gadolinium
- Stereotactic biopsy
- Lumbar puncture with examination of CSF
- Ophthalmologic examination with slitlamp
- Spinal MRI with gadolinium (when appropriate)

Testis:

- Clinical and ultrasonographic examination of the scrotum
- Lumbar puncture with examination of CSF

Breast:

- Bilateral mammography and MRI (or CT scan)

Bone:

- MRI

Heart:

- Echocardiogram

Lung:

- Bronchoscopy + bronchoalveolar lavage

ENT, ears, nose, and throat.

---

now been shown to be of benefit in all patients with B-cell lymphoma (19–21). All of these principles are based on clinical observations and past experience, rather than the knowledge of fundamental genetic or biologic factors.

Surgery

The role of surgery in the management of lymphoma is limited, however, occasionally, stage I primary extranodal lymphomas may be cured with surgery alone. The cure is infrequent; however, resection of primary tumor may achieve local control as in intestinal lymphoma and testis lymphoma (36,37). However, because radiation therapy and chemotherapy are also used, aggressive surgical approaches with compromise of cosmesis or function are not indicated. Specifically, there is no justification for amputation in bone lymphoma, mastectomy in breast lymphoma, cystectomy in bladder lymphoma, or abdominoperineal resection for rectal lymphoma. Accordingly, an accurate preoperative or intraoperative diagnosis is essential. For example, an aggressive surgical approach to treatment of parotid tumors carries a risk of nerve injury, and early histologic identification of lymphoma will prevent unnecessary damage to the facial nerve.

Radiation Therapy

Local disease control is an important consideration in extranodal lymphoma because presentation with bulky disease is common, and disease may compromise the function of vital structure such as the spinal cord or the airway. These factors, and the fact that lymphomas in sanctuary sites, including the brain and the testis, are not usually controlled with chemotherapy alone, make radiation therapy an important tool in the management of extranodal lymphomas. The principles of radiation therapy are to deliver an adequate radiation dose to the target volume that includes the full extent of disease with appropriate margins. A proper design of radiation therapy plans takes into consideration all staging data, normal anatomy, patterns of lymphatic spread, and the appreciation of radiation sensitivity of normal organs and tissues. The correct application of dose and fractionation schedule should ensure local control with reduced risk of acute and late complications. The technique should also optimize the reproducibility of treatment on a daily basis. Current radiation therapy techniques infer the use of custom-designed fields that conform to individual patient's anatomy and tumor location. The commonly used radiation therapy plans use involved-field radiation therapy. Involved-field radiation therapy implies treatment to the area involved only. The dose of radiation therapy required to achieve local control varies depending upon histologic type and tumor bulk (38). There are no prospective randomized trials designed to determine the optimal radiation therapy dose, and a survey of expert radiation oncologists showed significant variation (39) within a range of 30 to 45 Gy. In the setting of combined modality therapy, excellent local control has been obtained with doses of 30 to 35 Gy delivered in 1.75 to 3-Gy fractions (40). Although local control in most lymphomas treated with radiation therapy is excellent, a subset of patients in which local control is much lower can be identified. Local control in lymphomas resistant to CHOP chemotherapy has been shown to be <50% (41). There is a suggestion that higher doses are required in chemoresistant disease. However, even with radiation therapy dose in excess of 40 to 50 Gy, local failures have been observed in patients who do not respond, or develop local recurrence following optimal chemotherapy.

Chemotherapy and Combined Modality Therapy

Distant failure has been well documented in localized disease treated with radiation therapy alone (42,43). Chemotherapy has been documented to cure patients with diffuse large cell lymphoma. Such an approach has been shown to improve local control over that obtained with radiation therapy alone, and to reduce distant relapse rates. It is important to note that, in cases where no response or only partial response to chemotherapy is observed, the dose of radiation therapy has to be increased. In patients with localized MALT, and follicular and other small cell lymphomas, distant failure is common, and although chemotherapy is very effective treatment, it has not been shown to cure these diseases.

ASSESSMENT OF RESPONSE AND FOLLOW-UP

The key determinant of cure is the ability to attain a complete remission. In patients treated with radiation therapy alone, response is usually assessed 4 to 6 weeks following the completion of therapy. The assessment of response includes examination of the organ of presentation and follow-up general examination to rule out disease progression. In patients treated with chemotherapy or combined modality therapy, where chemotherapy is used first, the response is assessed following one or two courses of chemotherapy and every 1 to 2 months thereafter. Remission assessment comprises the demonstration of disease-free status on general assessment and also at an organ-specific level, with a well-defined criteria (44). Issues that require special consideration include:

- Knowledge of the relapse patterns is helpful in planning follow-up procedures. In situations where local relapse is uncommon, as in orbital lymphoma, completely resected gastric lymphoma, or small bulk Waldeyer ring lymphoma, long-term repeated imaging or endoscopic examinations of the presenting site are not indicated. Follow-up should include a complete physical examination with particular attention to any new adenopathy or unusual symptoms. Although most recurrences in patients with aggressive lymphoma occur within 2 to 3 years following the diagnosis, late relapses occur. Accordingly, prolonged follow-up is indicated in all patients.
- Evaluation of an organ or tissue that is anatomically or architecturally abnormal as a result of prior involvement by lymphoma. Primary bone lymphomas have persisting radiologic and MRI abnormalities after treatment, and bone scan will almost certainly identify changes that cannot distinguish active disease from bone healing and remodeling. Resolution of gallium or positron emission tomography activity may be helpful in such cases.
- The evaluation of paired organs, e.g., testis, kidney, salivary and lacrimal glands, eye and orbit, lung, breast, ovary, particularly when one organ has been the primary site of disease and may have been removed as part of initial therapy. The increased risk of disease recurrence or progression in the paired "normal" organ is well established.

After complete response is established, the schedule of follow-up assessment will reflect the expectation of events and their time course. Consideration must be directed to:

- Histology–late recurrence risk is seen in patients with marginal zone or follicular lymphoma, whereas it is less common in diffuse large B-cell lymphoma or T-cell lymphoma.
- Organ of presentation—certain primary extranodal lymphomas recur locally or within the tissues of origin with a much higher probability than at remote sites, e.g., primary CNS lymphoma (PCNSL).
- Bulk of disease at presentation site and the use of locoregional irradiation in the treatment plan. Tumor bulk in an unresected organ predicts for both local and distant relapse. Local disease control in a site receiving a tumoricidal dose of radiation therapy is expected unless substantial tumor bulk was present at the time of radiation therapy.

Management of relapse usually involves chemotherapy. However, in patients who have relapse with localized disease, retreatment with chemotherapy and radiation may offer a higher chance of prolonged disease control. In selected circumstances of follicular lymphoma or MALT lymphoma with localized small bulk recurrence, radiation therapy alone may offer prolonged disease control.

SPECIFIC EXTRANODAL PRESENTATIONS

Lymphomas Presenting in Head and Neck Region

It is evident that considering all the lymphomas arising in the head and neck region as a single group is simply the heritage of a historical topographic distinction, related to the fact that this anatomic region is the second most common site of localized extranodal presentation of non-Hodgkin lymphoma. However, it is clear that many different lymphoma entities can arise within the head and neck area. They differ not only by disparate anatomic presenting site, but also by histology. The localization of tumor presentation by site reveals tonsil to be the most common, followed by nasopharynx, oral cavity, salivary glands, paranasal sinuses, and base of tongue. The signs and symptoms of non-Hodgkin lymphoma may be similar to those of a head and neck squamous cancer, and only by biopsy can the distinction be made. Long-term results in patients presenting with extranodal lymphomas in the head and neck area vary greatly, depending not only on histology, but also on sites of presentation. In a series of 156 patients with head and neck lymphomas, the 5-year survival according to site was as follows: salivary gland (61%), oral cavity (57%), tonsil (49%), base of tongue (47%), nasopharynx (36%), and paranasal sinuses (12%) (45).

WALDEYER RING LYMPHOMA

There is controversy as to whether tonsils and Waldeyer ring in general should be considered as nodal or extranodal sites. Although some biologic and histologic characteristics would speak for having these lymphomas considered among the neoplasms of peripheral lymph nodes, most authors include them among extranodal sites. The tonsil resembles MALT in its relation to the pharyngeal epithelium and its lack of afferent lymphatics, but its overall structure, lack of prominent marginal zone, and predominant immunoglobulin G as opposed to immunoglobulin A secretion by its resident plasma cells are more characteristic of peripheral lymph nodes. From this perspective, Waldeyer ring may be considered as the point of contact between the MALT of Peyer patches and the peripheral lymphoid tissue of the lymph nodes (46). Full staging assessment is mandatory because about one in three patients will have disseminated disease. An important aspect of the natural history of Waldeyer ring lymphoma is its relationship to gastrointestinal tract involvement (47,48). Gastrointestinal tract investigations are recommended, although the yield in asymptomatic patients is very low. Patients may present with dysphagia, airway obstruction, or a mass lesion in the throat. Tonsillar lymphoma is the most common site of involvement in Waldeyer ring; the other sites include nasopharynx and base of the tongue. The most common histologic type is diffuse large B-cell lymphoma, accounting for at least 60% of cases. Other types include follicular lymphoma, Burkitt lymphoma, mantle cell lymphoma, marginal zone B-cell lymphoma, and peripheral T-cell lymphoma (49–51). Among children, Burkitt lymphoma is common. In the past, published results reflected the use of radiation therapy alone using involved-field techniques and moderate radiation doses (35 to 50 Gy). High local control rates with overall survival rates of 50% to 60% for stage IE lesions and 25% to 50% for IIE lesions were recorded (52,53). Following radiation therapy, the majority of failures occurred distant to the radiation field, indicating a high risk of occult systemic disease with apparently localized Waldeyer ring presentations. In the past 2 decades, combined modality therapy with anthracycline-based chemotherapy plus rituximab and involved-field radiation became a standard approach. Aviles et al. (47) validated the combined modality approach in a prospective randomized trial and colleagues demonstrating the superiority of combined modality therapy in this disease. The 5-year failure-free survival was 48% for radiation therapy, 45% for chemotherapy alone, and 83% for combined modality arm ($p < 0.001$). Others have shown local control rates in excess of 80% and overall survival rates of 60% to 5% (54,55). Combined modality therapy continues to be a standard approach to the management of localized Waldeyer ring diffuse large cell lymphoma, although with the improved outcomes observed with rituximab CHOP combination, the role of radiation therapy has been questioned.

PARANASAL SINUSES AND NASAL CAVITY LYMPHOMA

In the Western world, most series show a low incidence of sinonasal lymphoma. The Kiel registry of 33,402 cases showed that only 0.14% of lymphomas occurred in the nasal cavity. In both of these Western series, B-cell lineage predominated with 74% to 85% of cases. Clinically, nasal lymphomas present with symptoms of nasal obstruction and epistaxis. Signs of more advanced disease include facial swelling, proptosis, hard-palate perforation, and cranial nerve palsies (56). When locally advanced, these tumors may invade the adjacent nasopharynx, paranasal sinuses, oropharynx, and palate. Sinonasal lymphomas are relatively rare in the Western world, but in Asian countries, they are the second most frequent lymphoma after the gastrointestinal tract (57). Two main types of lymphoma are found in the sinonasal area: diffuse large B-cell lymphoma and extranodal NK/T-cell lymphoma (58). Paranasal sinus lymphomas are almost all diffuse large B-cell lymphoma, whereas most lymphomas arising in the nasal cavity are extranodal NK/T-cell lymphoma, followed by diffuse large B-cell lymphoma (59–63). In Western populations, paranasal diffuse large B-cell lymphoma is more common, whereas NK/T-cell lymphomas are more common in Asian and South American populations. NK/T-cell lymphomas are more commonly associated with angioinvasion, necrosis, and bone erosion, occurring in the 6th and 8th decade. Because of these destructive features, sinonasal lymphomas were often included with the descriptive yet nonspecific name of lethal midline granuloma. However, now the extranodal NK/T-cell lymphoma is recognized as a distinct clinicopathologic entity. The lymphomas are composed of small, medium-sized, or large atypical lymphoid cells, or a mixture of different-sized cells, associated with vascular damage and necrosis. Immunophenotyping usually shows cytoplasmic CD3+, CD56+ cells with T-cell receptor genes in a germline configuration, consistent with NK-cell lymphoma. In a small minority, tumor cells express surface CD3 and show clonal rearrangement of the T-cell receptor genes consistent with true T-cell lymphoma. In virtually all cases, Epstein-Barr virus (EBV) can be detected in neoplastic cells by in situ hybridization (64). Tumors with an identical phenotype and genotype may occur in other extranodal sites, most commonly in the skin, subcutis, and gastrointestinal tract. In a Chinese study of 175 patients, an overall 5-year survival of 65% and disease-free survival of 57% were noted. Stage IE lesions were most common with over half being limited to the nasal cavity, with others demonstrating extension beyond the nasal cavity. The vast majority were NK/T-cell lymphomas. The overall survival at 5 years for limited IE lesions was 90% compared with 57% for extensive IE lesions. The addition of chemotherapy to radiation produced no benefit, although local failure with radiation therapy was substantial (65,66). A Stanford report detailed 16 cases (ten B cell, four T cell, and two NK cell) treated with combined modality therapy and CNS prophylaxis. The overall survival at 5 years was 29%, with a median survival of 18 months. All patients with T and NK-cell disease were dead of disease by 6 months. The report concluded that paranasal sinus/nasal cavity disease is aggressive, requiring combined modality therapy and CNS prophylaxis, with a recommendation that NK/T-cell disease may require early intensification of therapy to improve progressive-free control rates (67). The M. D. Anderson group reported 70 patients with paranasal/nasal cavity disease (68). The M. D. Anderson series shows that principal factors influencing outcome were stage IE disease and low T category (T1-3 lesions vs. T4), low International Prognostic Index score (zero vs. one through three vs. four through five), and combined modality therapy (58,68). Only one case of CNS progression was identified, suggesting that the risk of CNS involvement is low other than in cases with erosion of the base of the skull (68). In general, the prognosis of sinonasal lymphomas is variable, and depends upon the histologic type and the anatomic extent of the tumor (68,69). NK/T-cell lymphoma of nasal type arising outside the upper aerodigestive tract seems to have usually a particularly high aggressive clinical behavior.

Historically, treatment has varied among different series and has included radiation alone, chemotherapy alone, or combined modality therapy. Combined modality therapy was not always associated with an improved outcome, however, it is important to note that these series included patients treated with nonanthracycline-based regimens, and included mixtures of B and T-cell lymphomas. Presently, for patients presenting with B-cell lymphomas and localized disease, CHOP-type chemotherapy with rituximab followed by radiation therapy is appropriate. For NK/T-cell lymphoma of nasal type, prospective trials of early treatment intensification with high-dose chemotherapy and stem cell support are being tested in clinical trials (70), although there is also a tendency to treat these patients with radiotherapy alone, or at least give aggressive radiotherapy up front.

SALIVARY GLAND LYMPHOMA

Most of the knowledge acquired concerns lymphomas of salivary glands, the vast majority of which are located in the parotid. Salivary gland lymphomas account for 5% to 10% of all salivary gland tumors and <5% of lymphomas at all sites. Three main types of lymphoma occur in salivary glands: marginal zone B-cell lymphoma, follicular lymphoma, and diffuse large B-cell lymphoma. Other types are rare. The follicular lymphomas tend to arise in intraparotid lymph nodes rather than the salivary gland parenchyma. They have pathologic features similar to those of follicular lymphoma arising in nodes away from the parotid. The diffuse large B-cell lymphomas may arise de novo or via transformation of a low-grade lymphoma. A recent IELSG study showed that salivary glands are the most common localization among extragastric marginal zone lymphomas (71). Patients usually present with a painless mass, most often in the parotid, followed by the submandibular gland, and only occasionally in the sublingual gland or minor salivary glands (72). Bilateral presentations are frequent. Marginal zone lymphomas of the salivary gland are frequently associated with Sjögren syndrome. Lymphoepithelial sialoadenitis is characteristic of Sjögren syndrome and not infrequently represents a precursor lesion for the development of marginal zone lymphoma. Marginal zone B-cell lymphomas generally follow an indolent course, are highly responsive to therapy, and are associated with excellent prognosis (73). A recent study of marginal zone B-cell lymphoma of the parotid glands showed a 90% 5-year overall survival, and 100% complete response rate. No advantage in complete response rate or time to treatment failure was seen for combined modality therapy over radiation therapy alone (14). Disfiguring surgery should be avoided because radiation therapy, chemotherapy, or combination of chemotherapy and radiotherapy is each very effective in achieving local control. The role of surgery should be limited to excisional biopsy, whereas further therapy has to be tailored to stage. As for all other MALT localizations, also salivary gland lymphomas presenting with these histologic types are very sensitive to the monoclonal antibody Rituxan. However, the relative merit and the final role of this new treatment for MALT lymphomas are still to be ascertained (74). Radiation offers excellent local control for limited-stage salivary gland lymphoma but may aggravate xerostomia already produced by Sjögren. The overall survival at 5 years approaches 70% to 80%, but there is a continuing distant relapse risk, characteristic of the natural history of these lymphomas. No proven benefit has been documented for chemotherapy in the management of MALT tumors, although the combined modality approach using anthracycline-based chemotherapy is standard treatment for those transformed to large cell lymphoma.

THYROID LYMPHOMA

Primary thyroid lymphoma occurs most frequently in older female patients with a previous history of Hashimoto thyroiditis. Marginal zone lymphomas carry a better prognosis than other histologic types, although with modern therapy, most thyroid lymphomas are associated with good prognosis (75). Patients usually present with painless unilateral or bilateral enlargement of the thyroid gland. Occasionally, very rapid enlargement of thyroid may cause obstruction of the trachea with respiratory compromise. The majority of lymphomas are diffuse large B-cell type, and almost all other are marginal zone lymphomas. Many diffuse large B-cell lymphomas have a component of marginal zone lymphoma, suggesting transformation. Rare cases of other types, including follicular lymphoma, Burkitt lymphoma, and peripheral T-cell lymphoma, have been reported (76,77). Frequent involvement of gastrointestinal tract has been reported in cases presenting with disseminated disease (78). CNS involvement is rare. Surgery is a diagnostic procedure and is not considered a definitive intervention for thyroid lymphoma, and an occasional patient may require tracheotomy to relieve airway obstruction at diagnosis. With radiation therapy to a moderate dose of 35 to 45 Gy, local control is achieved in >75% of patients, and in >95% in patients with marginal zone histology. Overall, reported survival rates at 5 years are in excess of 75% (79,80). For MALT histology, radiation therapy alone is recommended, and, indeed, locoregional irradiation with a dose of 30 Gy can allow an excellent local control (81). For diffuse large B-cell lymphoma with or without a MALT component, given the high distant relapse rates with radiation therapy alone, chemotherapy alone or more commonly, chemotherapy and radiation therapy have become the standard treatment approach. Systemic progression following is noted commonly in the gastrointestinal tract, liver, and spleen. A link between the gastrointestinal tract, Waldeyer ring, and thyroid lymphoma has been observed. CNS involvement is rare. Localized thyroid lymphoma of large B-cell type is treated with combined modality therapy. Because the reported series did not include R-CHOP-based approaches, current survival should exceed the reported 70% to 80% levels.

LYMPHOMA OF OCULAR ADNEXA

Lymphomas of ocular adnexa are lymphomas arising in the tissues and structures that surround the eye: the conjunctiva, lacrimal gland, orbital soft tissues, and eyelids. Ocular adnexal lymphoma is considerably more common than intraocular lymphoma (lymphoma of the eye). Lymphomas arising in these two sites should be clearly distinguished because of their different natural histories: intraocular lymphoma is a subset of PCNSL and is associated with a much worse prognosis than ocular adnexal lymphoma. The lymphomas of the ocular adnexa presenting anteriorly as conjunctival lesions are usually small, characteristically salmon pink, nodular, or plaque-like lesions in the conjunctiva, with symptoms of blurred vision, chemosis, and epiphora. The posteriorly located lesions present with swelling, palpable or visible mass, and proptosis. Pain and systemic symptoms are uncommon, but with increasing bulk of the lesion, pressure and double vision may occur. Sixty to 75% of cases are extranodal marginal zone B-cell lymphomas. The next most common type is follicular lymphoma, followed by diffuse large B-cell lymphoma. Histologic features are similar to those seen in other sites. Marginal zone lymphomas have now been associated with infection by *Chlamydia psittaci* (82–84). *C. psittaci* deoxyribonucleic acid has been detected in a significant proportion of patients, and responses to antibiotic therapy have been observed (83–86). To date, there are limited data on the response rates and the durability of response to doxycycline, an effective therapy for *Chlamydia*.

In all cases of localized disease, especially those not responding to antibiotic therapy, treatment should be directed at cure, while preserving vision and integrity of the orbit. Extensive surgery should be avoided because it is entirely unnecessary. Most orbital lesions are easily controlled with low to moderate doses of radiation therapy. Conjunctiva lesions may be treated with direct photon beams. Treatment with an anterior field or electron beam provides satisfactory therapy for anterior lesions limited to the eyelid or bulbar conjunctiva, with the advantage of sparing orbital structures compared with the use of a megavoltage photon beam. Radiation therapy to 20 to 30 Gy in ten to 20 daily fractions for small B-cell lymphomas results in a local control rate in excess of 95% (81,87). Higher doses are not required, and their use results in higher acute and long-term morbidity. For patients with large B-cell tumors, short duration anthracycline-based chemotherapy (e.g., R-CHOP for three courses) followed by radiation therapy to a dose of 30 Gy in 1.5-Gy daily fractions is recommended. The complications of radiation therapy that are seen when doses of ≥40 Gy are applied include cataract formation, keratitis, and dry eye. The use of lower radiation dose will avoid this toxicity without compromising local control.

The overall actuarial 10-year survival rates for orbital lymphomas reported in the literature are 75% to 80%. These excellent survival rates are likely due to a preponderance of indolent B-cell lymphomas. Following a complete response, the risk of local failure is extremely low (81,88). The most common site of relapse is the contralateral orbit, but generalized disease is seen. Distant failure rates vary from 20% to 50%, but as in other indolent lymphomas, failures can be successfully managed, and prolonged survival is common.

GASTRIC LYMPHOMA

In the past, diffuse large B-cell lymphoma was the most common type of gastric lymphoma. With the increasing early diagnosis of *H. pylori*-associated gastritis, marginal zone lymphoma is becoming the most common histologic type. Other lymphomas are much less common. Gastric marginal zone lymphoma typically occurs in patients >40 but can occur at any age. Gender incidence is equal. The presenting symptoms are nonspecific dyspepsia and are suggestive of gastritis or peptic ulcer. Likewise, endoscopy may show inflamed, sometimes eroded mucosa, rather than a tumor mass. Patients with marginal zone lymphoma are more likely to present with mild to moderate symptoms, whereas those with diffuse large cell lymphoma are more likely to have symptoms of bleeding and perforation.

Historically, the therapeutic strategies in gastric lymphoma were based on surgical approaches. Gastrectomy with postoperative radiation therapy, or postoperative chemotherapy was standard. Currently, approaches without surgery using primary chemotherapy followed by radiation therapy produce equivalent results (18). In the past, surgery alone employing partial or total gastrectomy has been reported to cure a proportion of patients (89). However, with surgery alone, gastric stump recurrences have been reported. Surgical resection is associated with a significant morbidity and mortality, and its use in an unselected patient population is no longer recommended (90).

Diffuse Large B-Cell Lymphoma of the Stomach

The modern approach to the management of diffuse large B-cell lymphoma of the stomach follows the principles for treatment of nodal lymphoma. Patients are staged clinically with CT of the abdomen, gastroscopy, and endoscopic ultrasound. The combined modality approach with R-CHOP chemotherapy followed by involved-field radiation therapy is the standard management for stage I and II disease. Toxicity of radiation therapy can be reduced using three-dimensional conformal techniques, and minimizing the radiation therapy dose to the kidneys and liver (91). In cases where tumor regression is observed following R-CHOP chemotherapy, excellent permanent local control and survival are observed. However, in chemoresistant cases, surgical resection may be considered because local control with radiation therapy for large bulk chemorefractory disease is less than optimal.

Analogous to MALT lymphomas, some recent studies have demonstrated possible regression of diffuse large B-cell localized lymphomas following anti-*H. pylori* therapy (92–94). This suggests that an antigenic drive may remain present in a subset of aggressive gastric lymphomas, especially those where a MALT lymphoma component can be detected. It is our opinion that, when an existing or a previous *H. pylori* infection is documented, antibiotics could be added to chemotherapy at the clinician's discretion. Nevertheless, antibiotic therapy alone remains an investigational approach for selected cases of localized diffuse large B-cell gastric lymphoma, and it cannot be recommended outside controlled clinical trials.

The approach to treatment of gastric lymphoma has radically changed in the past decade. With conservative approaches having proven successful, the need for routine gastrectomy has been eliminated. However, the approach to this disease is not consistent. Gastric lymphoma is at the crossroads of the expertise of gastroenterologists, oncologists, and hematologists. Gastroenterologists are more likely to use endoscopic ultrasound to stage these patients and are far more inclined to recommend surgery, whereas hematologists and oncologists are more likely to stage the patients with the emphasis on systemic disease, and use chemotherapy with or without radiation therapy.

INTESTINAL LYMPHOMA

In this category, small bowel lymphoma is the most common presentation with large bowel or rectal lymphoma being less frequent. Presenting symptoms vary from a feeling of abdominal fullness, nausea, diarrhea, and abdominal pain, to bowel obstruction and perforation. Because of these nonspecific-presenting symptoms, many patients require laparotomy for diagnosis and have resection of bowel lesions at diagnosis. Distinct clinicopathologic entities include intestinal marginal zone lymphoma, or immunoproliferative small intestinal disease (or α chain disease), diffuse large B-cell lymphoma, enteropathy associated T-cell lymphoma, Burkitt lymphoma, mantle cell lymphoma, and follicular lymphoma (95). The majority of primary intestinal lymphomas are large cell tumors of B-cell lineage, although considerable diversity exists in histologic subtypes with distinct clinicopathologic features underscoring the importance of lymphoma typing (96). The management of diffuse large B-cell lymphoma is usually with surgery followed by chemotherapy. In patients in whom complete tumor resection is not feasible, chemotherapy followed by radiation therapy is recommended (97). The outcomes reported in the literature vary depending on the extent of disease and histology. In a large series of intestinal lymphomas, Domizio et al. (98) documented a 75% 5-year survival for patients with B-cell lymphomas and only a 25% 5-year survival for those with T-cell tumors. The poor outcome of patients with intestinal T-cell lymphoma has also been documented in the British National Lymphoma Group experience (99) and in the Danish experience (12). Site of involvement was also of prognostic significance, with lesions in the terminal ileum having the best survival, but this is likely due to association between site and histology with terminal ileum lymphomas being usually of B-cell type. Other prognostic factors in primary intestinal lymphoma include age, performance status, B symptoms, and mesenteric lymph node involvement (stage II disease) (12,99).

Immunoproliferative intestinal disease, α heavy chain disease, and Mediterranean lymphoma all refer to various manifestations of an unusual subtype of marginal zone lymphoma affecting the small intestine, possibly associated with *Campylobacter jejuni* (95,100,101). Patients are mostly young adults from the Middle East who present with severe malabsorption, diarrhea, and weight loss. Approximately half of them have free α heavy chains, without associated light chain, in the serum (α heavy chain disease). The lymphoma typically shows diffuse thickening of a long segment of the small intestine. Microscopic examination shows a broad layer of plasma cells beneath which is a variably prominent layer of marginal zone B cells. The plasma cells express α heavy chain, usually without light chain. Patients are often malnourished and have a poor performance status, and frequently cannot tolerate standard therapy. Overall survival has been poor, probably partly due to late diagnosis. Several authors have reported that treatment with the tetracycline group of antibiotics can produce clinical, histologic, and immunologic remissions. Remissions have also been described following chemotherapy and, more recently, a report of regression of duodenal immunoproliferative intestinal disease following treatment of *H. pylori* (102). The role of radiation therapy and surgical resection remain to be defined. Despite the available treatments, immunoproliferative intestinal disease may be a highly lethal disease with reported survival rates as low as 23% at 5 years (103). Patients with resectable stage I and II1 disease have a 5-year survival of 40% to 47% compared with 0% to 25% for unresectable or stage II2 disease. After a prolonged time, often many years, immunoproliferative intestinal disease may transform into an aggressive immunoglobulin A+ diffuse large B-cell lymphoma (104). Enteropathy type intestinal T-cell lymphoma is a rare lymphoma usually affecting older adults with a history of celiac disease. Patients present with severe abdominal pain due to obstruction or perforation. This lymphoma preferentially involves the jejunum, producing circumferentially oriented linear ulcers, typically unassociated with prominent bowel wall thickening or a large mass. The adjacent mucosa usually shows villous atrophy. The lymphomas may be composed of small to medium-sized atypical lymphoid cells or of large, atypical, sometimes anaplastic large cells, with an abnormal T-cell immunophenotype. Patients are often severely malnourished, and frequently cannot tolerate aggressive therapy. This, combined with the aggressive nature of the lymphoma, leads to a very poor prognosis for this disease (105).

Mantle cell lymphoma of the small intestine most often takes the form of innumerable small, superficially located polypoid lesions, referred to as multiple lymphomatous polyposis. The histologic and immunophenotypic features are similar to mantle cell lymphoma in other sites. The prognosis for mantle cell lymphoma is poor despite aggressive chemotherapy, similar to its nodal equivalent. Follicular lymphoma arising in the gastrointestinal tract has an unexplained predilection to involve the duodenum. The follicular lymphoma may take the form of mucosal nodularity or larger deeply invasive masses. The lymphomas are usually low grade, and show histologic, immunophenotypic, and genotypic features that are similar to those of primary nodal follicular lymphomas. The prognosis is good (106). Rectal presentations are less common than other sites in the lower intestinal tract. Diffuse small non-cleaved cell lymphoma is the most common, although diffuse large cell lymphomas also occur (107). Treatment usually includes chemotherapy and radiation therapy (30 to 40 Gy in 1.5 to 2-Gy daily fractions) for patients presenting with bulky lesions and/or intermediate-grade lymphoma. Involved-field radiation therapy alone (30 to 35 Gy in 1.5 to 1.75-Gy daily fractions) has been successful in providing long-term disease control for MALT lymphoma of the rectum. Abdominoperineal resection should be discouraged because there is no evidence that it improves local control or survival.

TESTICULAR LYMPHOMA

Malignant lymphoma of the testis is a rare disease representing 5% of all testicular tumors and only 1% of all lymphomas with an incidence of 0.26 per 100,000 men (108). Lymphoma, however, is still the most common testicular tumor in men >60 years of age, and approximately 85% of

patients with testicular lymphoma are >60 (109). Bilateral testicular tumors may be found at diagnosis, or contralateral involvement may develop years later and has been observed in up to 35% of cases (110). The demonstration of monoclonality in metachronous contralateral testis lymphoma suggests that bilateral involvement is a manifestation of the same disease (111). Most testicular lymphomas are diffuse large B-cell lymphomas. Isolated cases of NK/T-cell lymphomas, nasal type, T-cell lymphomas, and follicular lymphomas have been reported (112,113). Over 50% of patients present with stage I disease limited to testis and approximately 20% with stage II disease. Assessment of patients with testis lymphoma is similar to other lymphomas. However, in addition to the routine tests, staging investigations should include CSF cytology, and in some centers brain imaging is recommended. Orchiectomy is both diagnostic and therapeutic providing local tumor control. Rarely, orchiectomy has been curative, attesting that primary testis lymphoma can present as truly localized disease (114). However, in most cases, occult distant disease is present. Primary testicular lymphoma has been recognized as a highly lethal disease, with overall 5-year survival rates ranging from 16% to 50% with a median survival of 12 to 24 months. The characteristic pattern of failure is mostly distant with a high proportion of relapses in extranodal sites, including skin, lung, pleura, soft tissues, and Waldeyer ring. CNS relapse, both meningeal as well as brain parenchyma, is frequent as is recurrence in contralateral testis (115,116). Retroperitoneal radiation therapy in stage I disease is no longer used; however, patients with stage II disease receive radiation therapy as part of the combined modality approach recommended for stage II diffuse large cell lymphoma presenting in other sites.

The introduction of adjuvant chemotherapy resulted in an improved relapse-free rate and survival (117,118). Connors et al. (118) treated patients with either a 6-week course of methotrexate, Adriamycin (doxorubicin), cyclophosphamide, Oncovin (vincristine), prednisone, and bleomycin or three cycles of CHOP, and observed a survival of 93% with a median follow-up of 44 months. Unfortunately, the other authors did not observe these excellent survival results, although chemotherapy appears to have improved the short-term survival (116,119). The pattern of failure in the CNS has led to a recommendation for routine CNS prophylaxis with, at least, intrathecal chemotherapy. Its value, however, is controversial because CNS failures have been observed in patients who received intrathecal chemotherapy. Many CNS failures occur in brain parenchyma rather than meninges, and some also occur several years after the initial presentation.

Failure in the contralateral testis is well documented and occurs in 5% to 35% of patients. Low-dose radiation therapy (25 to 30 Gy in ten to 15 daily fractions) to the contralateral testis eliminates the risk of failure at this site, carries little morbidity in this elderly patient population, and is recommended for all patients with primary testicular lymphoma. In the PMH experience, 26 patients treated with prophylactic scrotal radiation therapy had no failure in contralateral testis, compared with 12.5% recurrence in patients without scrotal radiation therapy. This is consistent with the Manchester experience that scrotal irradiation prevents a relapse in the contralateral testicle in 100% of patients (120). IELSG conducted a retrospective study of 373 patients with a diagnosis of primary testicular diffuse large cell lymphoma

(26). The majority of patients (75%) received chemotherapy, and combined modality therapy was used in 39% of patients. In addition, 34% of patients received prophylactic scrotal radiation therapy, but only 18% had prophylactic intrathecal chemotherapy. The 5-year survival was 48%, and the 10-year survival was 27%. The outcome of patients who received anthracycline-based chemotherapy was better than those who did not receive it. CNS failures occurred up to 10 years following the initial presentation and were observed in 54 patients. The actuarial 5- and 10-year risks of CNS relapse were at 20% and 35%, respectively. Prophylactic intrathecal chemotherapy was associated with an improved progression-free survival. A continuous risk of recurrence in the contralateral testis (15% at 3 years, 40% at 15 years) was observed in patients who had not received prophylactic scrotal radiation therapy. The IELSG data suggest that intrathecal chemotherapy may indeed control microscopic meningeal disease. A prospective phase II IELSG trial showed improved results with modern treatment but a need to improve CNS control (121).

BLADDER LYMPHOMA

Primary lymphoma of the urinary bladder is very rare, but a number of case reports and small series of patients have been documented. Patients commonly present with frequency, dysuria, and occasionally hematuria. Cystoscopic examination shows submucosal mass with an edematous and friable mucosa. Biopsy usually reveals marginal zone B-cell lymphomas frequently arising on a background of chronic cystitis. Marginal zone lymphomas of the bladder are usually localized and are associated with a particularly good prognosis (122). The next most common type is diffuse large B-cell lymphoma, some of which arise through large cell transformation of marginal zone lymphoma. Other types are rare (123,124). Treatment has traditionally involved partial cystectomy and/or radiotherapy to the pelvis. The prognosis is related to histologic type and extent of tumor (125). As for other extranodal lymphomas, indolent lymphomas may be managed with radiation therapy alone, but large cell lymphomas should be treated with anthracycline-based chemotherapy followed by local radiation therapy. There are limited data regarding the optimal dose and technique of radiation therapy, but there is no reason to suggest that the sensitivity of the tumor is different than that of other MALT lymphomas. Several reports attest to a favorable prognosis of bladder lymphoma (126). Repeat cystoscopy is important for follow-up (127). Long-term survival has been observed in about 40% to 50% of patients, although a small series of four patients with marginal zone lymphoma was reported by Al-Maghrabi et al. (128), and all patients were controlled by radiotherapy alone, with follow-up ranging between 1 and 13 years.

LYMPHOMA OF THE OVARY

This is a very rare form of primary extranodal lymphoma. Patients present with abdominal pain or finding of an asymptomatic abdominal mass. Diffuse large B-cell lymphomas are most commonly followed by Burkitt lymphoma and follicular lymphoma. Burkitt lymphoma is more common among younger patients and patients in areas endemic for Burkitt lymphoma (129). Treatment with chemotherapy alone may preserve gonadal and hormonal function, but for localized diffuse large B-cell lymphoma, combined modality therapy is recommended. Because lymphomas of the ovary are most commonly of diffuse large B-cell type and clearly are most commonly associated with extensive dissemination, the initial treatment approach should comprise chemotherapy. Radiation therapy may be appropriate in the circumstance of a localized presentation with residual disease after surgery or following definitive chemotherapy. Local control is, however, a lesser issue given the usual resection of the presenting lesion and the common pattern of failure being one of systemic disease progression.

LYMPHOMA OF THE UTERINE CORPUS, UTERINE CERVIX, AND VAGINA

The female genital lymphomas are an extremely rare condition, accounting for <0.5% of gynecologic cancers and for 1.5% of all non-Hodgkin lymphoma (130). Uterus and the adnexa are the most frequent sites, and cervical lymphomas are much more common than those arising in the uterine corpus. Vagina and vulva localization is unusual (130,131). Occasionally, two or more adjacent genital organs can be involved. Lymphomas of uterus, cervix, and vagina usually present in middle-aged women, although presentations at younger age occur. Abnormal vaginal bleeding is the most common symptom. These lymphomas are often bulky and deeply invasive. By far the most common type is diffuse large B-cell lymphoma, followed by follicular lymphoma and rare cases of Burkitt lymphoma, marginal zone B-cell lymphoma, and others (123,131,132). The standard therapy for patients with stage IE lesions has usually comprised radiation therapy with or without antecedent surgery. There is no evidence that radical surgery is necessary, and, indeed, there is no strong indication for more than a diagnostic biopsy with subsequent detailed staging evaluation. Radiation therapy alone for localized MALT or follicular lymphoma offers a very high probability of local control. Combined chemotherapy and radiation therapy for diffuse large B-cell tumors is appropriate, and, given the impact of radiation therapy on ovarian function in those in the reproductive age range, the use of chemotherapy alone has been recommended with some clinical justification. A 5-year overall survival rate of 73% is quoted by Harris and Scully (133), comprising an 89% 5-year rate for patients with stage IE disease. Important prognostic factors include stage and histology. Local failure is very uncommon following chemotherapy and radiation therapy for endometrial, cervical, or vaginal lymphoma (134).

BREAST LYMPHOMA

Primary lymphoma of the breast is a rare disease that accounts for <0.05% of all breast malignancies and <1% of all non-Hodgkin lymphomas. It comprises only 2% of localized extranodal lymphomas. Almost all tumors are of B-cell lineage, with diffuse large B-cell type predominant, although follicular and marginal zone lymphomas are also described. The usual presentation is with discrete painless mass, although aggressive presentations with rapid painful enlargement of one or both breasts also occur. The latter presentation may be associated with pregnancy and is characteristic of a Burkitt or other aggressive lymphoma. A spectrum of histologic types is seen in primary breast lymphoma, from marginal zone lymphoma to diffuse large B-cell to Burkitt lymphoma (28,135–138). As for other extranodal lymphomas, diffuse large B-cell lymphomas require combined modality therapy. It is important to note that the completeness of surgical excision does not appear to affect local control. Thus, mastectomy is not recommended, and breast preservation is possible in the majority of cases. Properly planned and delivered radiation therapy results in excellent local control, especially in patients presenting without bulky disease or those with marginal zone lymphoma. The radiation therapy volume should include the whole breast. As in other lymphomas, a tumor dose of 35 Gy in 1.75 to 2-Gy fractions over 4 weeks achieves excellent local control. The most common sites of failure include lungs, liver, spleen, and distant nodal sites. Isolated CNS relapses have been reported. Similarly, late failure in the contralateral breast may occur following therapy of unilateral primary breast lymphoma. Marginal zone lymphoma may be associated with isolated extranodal relapses in other sites. Follicular lymphoma appears to behave in a manner similar to follicular lymphoma arising in lymph nodes (9). The overall survival of patients treated with local treatment methods ranges from 40% to 66% at 5 to 10 years (138,139). The IELSG retrospective trial confirmed findings previously published in the literature and did not identify CNS relapse as a significant problem (28,140).

BONE LYMPHOMA

The clinical presentation of bone lymphoma is variable with peak incidence in the 5th decade, with a slight male preponderance. Symptoms at presentation usually consist of localized bone pain, sometimes accompanied by a soft tissue mass, although polyostotic presentations are seen. The majority of patients present without systemic symptoms. Open biopsy is often required to make the diagnosis, given the difficulty of performing fine needle aspiration on a bony lesion. In adults the lymphoma is virtually always diffuse large B-cell type (141), with rare cases of Burkitt lymphoma, CD30+ anaplastic large cell lymphoma, low-grade lymphomas, and others (142). Among children, half of cases are diffuse large B-cell lymphoma, 40% are precursor B lymphoblastic lymphoma, and 10% are Burkitt lymphoma (143–145).

Cure of lymphoma of bone by surgery alone has been recorded, although this is no longer being considered an appropriate therapy. With radiation therapy, 5- and 10-year overall survival rates of 58% and 53%, respectively, are reported for solitary bone lesions. Key issues relating to local control are the intramedullary and soft tissue extent of disease in relation to radiation therapy volume. Indeed, the exact definition of tumor staging is often problematic; MRI has been particularly important in revealing extension of disease not visualized before by routine x-rays or bone scan. Data showing the usefulness of positron emission tomography scan in

evaluation of lymphomatous bone lesion have been reported (146). Treatment approaches using radiation therapy alone have indicated high levels of local control, approximately 85%, but unacceptable rates of local or marginal failure (20%), probably related to underestimation of tumor extent and bulk, and a systemic failure rate approaching 50%. Patients with localized diffuse large B-cell lymphoma of bone should be treated with combined modality therapy, comprising initial anthracycline-based chemotherapy and subsequent radiation therapy to a dose of 35 Gy. There is no indication for CNS prophylaxis. A treatment strategy, including chemotherapy followed by radiotherapy, produced, in a retrospective series, the best clinical results (22–24,147), with overall survival and relapse-free rates exceeding 70% at 5 years (147,148). Children are usually treated with chemotherapy alone to avoid development of radiation-induced sarcoma; outcome is favorable (149). Bone lymphoma is associated with a risk of fracture, caused either by the tumor or the treatment. Chemotherapy may induce avascular necrosis, and radiotherapy may induce fractures. Radiation therapy induced fracture seems related to radiation therapy dose, with doses in excess of 5,000 cGy increasing the risk (150).

PRIMARY CENTRAL NERVOUS SYSTEM LYMPHOMA

PCNSL is a rare subtype of non-Hodgkin lymphoma that is characterized by the primary and exclusive involvement of the brain, spinal cord, leptomeninges, and eyes. Immunodeficiency is the only established risk factor, and the use of highly active antiretroviral therapy that has changed the clinical and immunologic course of the human immunodeficiency virus infection is probably the main reason for a recent slight decline of the PCNSL incidence (151). The large majority of PCNSLs in individuals with immunocompetence are diffuse large B-cell lymphomas. The clinical presentation is dominated by the neurologic symptoms depending on the disease location (151). The International PCNSL Collaborative Group has indicated guidelines for standardized baseline evaluation in newly diagnosed PCNSL (152). A large retrospective study of the IELSG devised a scoring system based on five prognostic variables: age; Eastern Cooperative Oncology Group performance status; lactate dehydrogenase level; CSF total protein concentration; and involvement of deep regions of the brain (periventricular regions, basal ganglia, brainstem, and/or cerebellum) (153). Another prognostic score has been proposed by the Memorial Sloan-Kettering Cancer Center, and is based only on age and Karnofsky performance status (30). The complex management problems and the current treatment strategies are discussed in Chapter 36.

EXTRADURAL LYMPHOMA

Primary extradural lymphoma presents with pain or progressive neurologic deficit. When present, spinal cord compression constitutes a medical emergency. Histologic diagnosis is imperative, and surgical biopsy with or without decompression is the first step in management. Complete tumor removal is unnecessary because further therapy is always required. The main objectives of surgery in the setting of spinal cord compressions include adequate decompression of the spinal cord and removal of tissue appropriate for histologic diagnosis. Postoperative therapy has historically involved radiation therapy to the affected area of the spine. Radiation therapy is delivered using megavoltage photon therapy with dose to the tumor limited to 35 to 40 Gy in 1.75 to 2-Gy fractions. Doses in excess of 45 to 50 Gy are excessive and carry a risk of radiation myelitis. The radiation therapy volume should take into account the presence of any paraspinal mass or regional lymph node involvement. Radiation therapy results in good local disease control but, as with other localized diffuse large cell lymphomas, is associated with a 40% to 50% distant failure rate. The use of doxorubicin-based chemotherapy following surgery and radiation therapy is associated with a reduced distant failure rate and an improved survival. In the PMH experience, the survival of patients treated with radiation therapy alone was 33% compared with 86% (at a median follow-up of 3 years) for those treated with combined modality therapy (154). Although the traditional approach was to deliver radiation therapy before chemotherapy, this is no longer considered to be the optimal sequence. Eeles et al. (155) documented that the use of chemotherapy followed by radiation therapy does not compromise neurologic function, as compared with that achieved when radiation therapy is followed by chemotherapy (154). A controversial aspect of the management of primary extradural lymphoma relates to the issue of intrathecal CNS chemoprophylaxis. Although some have demonstrated extradural involvement as a risk factor for meningeal relapse (156), the PMH experience has documented only rare isolated CNS relapse in patients treated without CNS prophylaxis. The routine use of intrathecal chemotherapy in patients with localized extradural lymphoma and no evidence of dural invasion may be questioned, but careful attention needs to be given to the extent of initial disease and the possibility of dural invasion (154). When dural invasion is suspected, intrathecal therapy is indicated.

LUNG LYMPHOMA

A variety of types of lymphoma arise in the lung, but approximately 70% are marginal zone lymphomas. The next most common (approximately 20%) is diffuse large B-cell lymphoma; at least some of them have transformed from an underlying marginal zone lymphoma. Other uncommon types include follicular lymphoma, Burkitt lymphoma, CD30+ anaplastic large cell lymphoma, and others. Some of the patients with marginal zone lymphoma have an underlying autoimmune disease, most commonly Sjögren syndrome (157–160). Pulmonary marginal zone lymphomas are cytologically bland and have indolent behavior, and, as in other sites, they were often formerly thought to be nonneoplastic processes such as lymphocytic interstitial pneumonia "pseudotumor." Lymphomatoid granulomatosis-type lymphoma is a rare type of EBV+ B-cell lymphoma that almost always involves the lungs, and that is commonly associated with cutaneous, renal, and CNS manifestations. Peripheral T-cell lymphoma rarely involves the lung as a solitary site but may present as multisystem disease (161). Common presentation features include cough, dyspnea, pain, fever, recurrent infections, hemoptysis, or an asymptomatic finding on routine chest radiograph. Radiologic features include pulmonary consolidation, solid pulmonary opacities,

hilar adenopathy, and/or pleural effusion. Initial treatment has commonly been surgical resection, however, given current less invasive alternatives to achieve a secure diagnosis, there is no strong indication that resection contributes to outcome. MALT lymphoma is observed or treated with chemotherapy, usually a single alkylating agent. Lesions are commonly responsive to both chemotherapy and radiation therapy, although low tolerance of lung to radiation therapy limits its applicability to treatment of only part of the lung. There is no indication that such treatments are curative, although prolonged survival is common: 94% overall survival at 5 years with a median survival not reached at 10 years, and no clear impact of type of therapy on outcome (157). The prognosis is clearly substantially worse for angiocentric and diffuse large cell lymphomas, even when treated with chemotherapy or combined modality therapy. Systemic progression is common, and relapse-free rates of approximately 40% to 50% are expected. T-cell lymphomas have a poor prognosis with 50% mortality at 2 years even with combined modality therapy.

UNCOMMON SITES OF PRIMARY EXTRANODAL LYMPHOMA

Uncommon Respiratory Tract Lymphomas

Larynx

Primary head and neck lymphomas can infrequently present in the larynx (162,163). Often the presenting symptom is cough. Both marginal zone lymphomas and diffuse large B-cell lymphomas have been reported. Radiation and combined modality therapy offer excellent local control and cure. Early diagnosis and treatment are important because airway obstruction can occur and result in sudden death.

Trachea

Primary lymphoma of the trachea has been reported, although it is even less common than in the larynx (164). Both MALT lymphomas and diffuse large B-cell types occur.

Renal Lymphoma

Primary renal lymphoma is very rare. Most reported cases of renal lymphoma have presented with symptoms related to renal involvement, even though staging usually reveals extrarenal spread (123,165–167). In our experience, one patient with stage IE follicular large cell lymphoma of the kidney was alive without evidence of recurrent disease 15 years following nephrectomy and postoperative radiation to the renal fossa. Similar case reports support primary renal lymphoma as a separate clinical entity (167,168). Patients present with flank pain, anorexia, or hematuria. Those with bilateral disease may have renal insufficiency. More than half of the cases are diffuse large B-cell lymphoma; the remainder is a variety of high and low-grade B-cell lymphomas. However, because of the rarity of such cases, no comment can be made regarding the pattern of disease and treatment results other than as directed according to general principles of management recognizing important prognostic factors, especially histology.

Prostate Lymphoma

Primary lymphoma of the prostate is extremely rare. There were no cases of localized prostate lymphoma in several large series of patients with localized extranodal lymphoma (12,42,169), although a number of cases, usually in case reports or small series, have been described (123,170). Disease tends to affect older men, although an occasional report includes a younger patient. Patients present with obstructive or irritative urinary symptoms (170). The most common type is diffuse large B-cell lymphoma, and the rest are a variety of aggressive and indolent B-cell lymphomas. Survival in published cases has been poor with rapid systemic dissemination of the disease (171), although patients treated more recently with better therapy have had a more favorable outcome (172).

Ureteral Lymphoma

Primary lymphoma of the ureter is rare, probably related to the absence of lymphoid tissue in the ureteral wall. The majority of reported cases are due to extrinsic ureteral compression. Periureteral and peripelvic involvement in the absence of renal involvement is unusual. There are only a few documented cases of primary lymphoma of the ureter (173).

Urethral Lymphoma

Primary lymphoma of the urethra is very rare (174,175). Almost all cases of primary urethral lymphoma have been reported in females. The tumor may present on the meatal epithelium and resemble a urethral caruncle or polyp. The pathology usually shows a diffuse large B-cell lymphoma, and some cases may be marginal zone lymphomas (123,176,177). Long-term disease control in patients managed with radiation therapy alone, excision of tumor and radiation therapy, or chemotherapy has been reported (178–180). As in other cases of diffuse large B-cell lymphoma, a short course of Adriamycin-based chemotherapy followed by involved-field radiation therapy represents a logical treatment approach.

Pancreas Lymphoma

Primary pancreatic lymphoma accounts for 1% to 3% of all pancreatic malignancies, and is rarely considered in the differential diagnosis of pancreatic mass lesions. Patients are usually >60 years (181). The lesion is defined by CT and is commonly a sizeable (3 to 12 cm, median 8 cm) lesion in the head of the pancreas. Tumors are most commonly of diffuse large B-cell lymphomas (182). Other types are uncommon. There is no indication for radical surgery for primary pancreatic lymphoma. Biliary obstruction is usually managed very effectively with systemic chemotherapy. Radiation may have a role for the uncommon indolent lymphoma or for palliation. Combined modality therapy is the appropriate therapy for large B-cell lymphoma, with particular consideration to choice of agents and schedule in patients with obstructive jaundice.

Liver Lymphoma

Primary non-Hodgkin lymphoma of the liver is exceptionally rare (183). A report cited 68 cases in the literature, including five new cases (184). A relationship of primary lymphoma of the liver to preexisting immunologic disease states, for example, systemic lupus erythematosus, acquired immunodeficiency syndrome, cyclosporin/transplantation, and hepatitis B-induced chronic active hepatitis, has been proposed. Fifty percent of patients have B symptoms, most commonly weight loss (185). Primary liver lymphoma arises as a solitary mass, multiple masses, and rarely as diffuse hepatic enlargement. Where recorded, 60% of tumors are of diffuse large B-cell type. Others types include marginal zone lymphoma, Burkitt lymphoma, and others. The marginal zone lymphomas are centered on portal tracts and form lymphoepithelial lesions with bile duct epithelium (186). T-cell lymphomas are rarely recorded. Chemotherapy, with allowance for any related liver dysfunction, particularly if preexistent to lymphoma, would appear to be the most appropriate recommendation. Patients with indolent lymphoma have a good prognosis (186,187). Patients with more aggressive lymphomas also have a relatively good outcome. In one study, 5-year cause-specific survival was 87% (188). Together with the spleen, the liver is the primary site of involvement of the rare hepatosplenic γ/δ T-cell lymphoma. This disease affects young patients who present with marked hepatosplenomegaly, commonly with bone marrow involvement and without lymphadenopathy. The clinical course is usually very aggressive, with a median survival of <1 year (189,190).

Lymphoma Affecting Soft Tissues or Muscle

Primary extranodal non-Hodgkin lymphomas of the soft tissues are extremely rare (191,192). In the Mayo Clinic experience, the primary extranodal soft tissue lymphoma of the extremities represented 0.11% of all lymphomas. Patients present with enlarging soft tissue swelling. Diagnosis is obtained following biopsy or resection of the lesion. In some cases it may be difficult to distinguish extranodal soft tissue presentations from the total effacement of an aberrant lymph node by a malignant lymphoma. All histologic types have been reported. Tumors may be confined to the subcutaneous connective tissue or may involve muscle. The principles that apply to the management of other localized lymphomas are appropriate for primary lymphoma of soft tissues. Primary lymphoma arising in the skeletal muscle is even less common (193).

Other Sites—Heart, Pleura, and Adrenal

Primary lymphoma of the heart, defined as lymphoma involving only the heart and pericardium, is rare. A major subset of patients is immunocompromised because of human immunodeficiency virus infection or iatrogenic immunosuppression for organ transplantation, but cardiac lymphoma also occurs in older patients without immunodeficiency (194–197). In a few reported cases, the diagnosis has been made premortem (198). Presenting symptoms are usually congestive heart failure, pericardial effusion, and occasionally complete heart block. The pathology is usually diffuse large B-cell lymphoma. Prolonged survival has been reported following treatment with chemotherapy (199).

Primary lymphoma of the pleura arising in association with chronic tuberculous pyothorax has been reported in Japan (200). A few cases have been reported in Western countries as a complication of chronic empyema. The majority of cases are EBV+ large B-cell lymphomas. The outcome in reported cases treated with chemotherapy was poor.

Few cases of primary adrenal lymphoma have been reported in the literature (201). A number of cases had bilateral involvement of adrenal glands, often associated adrenal insufficiency. Nearly all cases have been diffuse large B-cell lymphoma, but rare T-cell lymphomas have been reported. Many cases have been managed with surgery and chemotherapy, but survival was poor. In recent years, improved diagnostic techniques and therapy have led to a better outcome in the small number of cases reported (202–204).

The primary effusion lymphoma is a large B-cell neoplasm recently comprised in the World Health Organization classification of lymphoproliferative disorders. Primary effusion lymphoma usually develops in patients who are severely immunocompromised, and a strong etiologic relationship is recognized with the human herpes virus type 8/Kaposi sarcoma-associated herpes virus (205) Most cases are also EBV+ (206,207). The lymphoma develops as a liquid-phase growth in the fluid filled serous cavities of the body. Its immunophenotype is unusual, and it could resemble that of plasmablasts having features of both immunoblasts and plasma cells (208,209). Typically, it displays an aggressive course.

SUMMARY

Extranodal non-Hodgkin lymphoma encompasses an exceptionally heterogeneous group of diseases that may affect any organ or body part. It is unclear why some sites or organs are affected more than others, however, the role of antigenic stimulation, autoimmunity, and immune dysregulation resulting in genomic instability is an important component of the etiology and pathogenesis of these disorders. This relationship to lymphoma causation is increasingly recognized through observations relating lymphomas to congenital and acquired immunodeficiency states, Hashimoto and Sjögren syndrome, Crohn disease, intestinal immunoproliferative states, and the role of *H. pylori* in MALT lymphoma of the stomach. Knowledge arising from a more complete understanding of the biology and the genetic basis of lymphoma will undoubtedly lead to improved recognition of distinct clinical entities and refinements in patient management. Treatment results and curability of some tumors may be obscured by the heterogeneity of presentations. Future studies of different treatment strategies recognizing distinct histopathologic entities may help to clarify the outcomes.

References

1. Parkin DM, Pisani P, Ferlay J. Global cancer statistics. *CA Cancer J Clin* 1999;49:33–64.
2. Gurney KA, Cartwright RA. Increasing incidence and descriptive epidemiology of extranodal non-Hodgkin lymphoma in parts of England and Wales. *Hematol J* 2002;3:95–104.
3. Dawson I, Cornes J, Morson B. Primary malignant lymphoid tumours of the intestinal tract: report of 37 cases with a study of factors influencing prognosis. *Br J Surg* 1961;49:80–89.
4. Herrmann R, Panahon AM, Barcos MP, et al. Gastrointestinal involvement in non-Hodgkin's lymphoma. *Cancer* 1980;46:215–222.
5. Lewin K, Ranchod M, Dorfman R. Lymphomas of the gastrointestinal tract: a study of 117 cases presenting with gastrointestinal disease. *Cancer* 1978;42:693–707.
6. Zucca E, Roggero E, Bertoni F, et al. Primary extranodal non-Hodgkin's lymphomas. Part 1: gastrointestinal, cutaneous and genitourinary lymphomas. *Ann Oncol* 1997;8:727–737.
7. Dogan A, Du M, Koulis A, et al. Expression of lymphocyte homing receptors and vascular addressins in low-grade gastric B-cell lymphomas of mucosa-associated lymphoid tissue. *Am J Pathol* 1997;151:1361–1369.
8. Drillenburg P, Koopman G, et al. Preferential expression of the mucosal homing receptor integrin alpha 4 beta 7 in gastrointestinal non-Hodgkin's lymphomas. *Am J Pathol* 1997;150:919–927.
9. Mattia AR, Ferry JA, Harris NL. Breast lymphoma. A B-cell spectrum including the low grade B-cell lymphoma of mucosa associated lymphoid tissue. *Am J Surg Pathol* 1993;17:574–587.
10. Freeman C, Berg JW, Cutler SJ. Occurrence and prognosis of extranodal lymphomas. *Cancer* 1972;29:252–260.
11. Devesa SS, Fears T. Non-Hodgkin's lymphoma time trends: United States and International data. *Cancer Res* 1992;52:5432–5440.
12. d'Amore F, Christensen BE, Brincker H, et al. Clinicopathological features and prognostic factors in extranodal non-Hodgkin lymphomas. Danish LYFO Study Group. *Eur J Cancer* 1991;27:1201–1208.
13. Sutcliffe SB, Gospodarowicz MK. Localized extranodal lymphomas. In: Keating A, Armitage J, Burnett A, et al., eds. *Hematological oncology.* Cambridge, UK: Cambridge University Press, 1992:189–222.
14. Aviles A, Delgado S, Huerta-Guzman J. Marginal zone B cell lymphoma of the parotid glands: results of a randomised trial comparing radiotherapy to combined therapy. *Eur J Cancer B Oral Oncol* 1996;6:420–422.
15. Cortelazzo S, Rossi A, Federico M, et al. The stage-modified IPI (MIPI), histology and a combined treatment influence the clinical outcome of 401 patients with primary extranodal head and neck B-cell lymphomas (PHNBCL) (IELSG 23). *Blood* 2005; Vol. 106, Issue 11, Abstract 927.
16. Cortelazzo S, Rossi A, Roggero F, et al. Stage-modified international prognostic index effectively predicts clinical outcome of localized primary gastric diffuse large B-cell lymphoma. International Extranodal Lymphoma Study Group (IELSG). *Ann Oncol* 1999;10:1433–1440.
17. Ibrahim EM, Ezzat AA, Raja MA, et al. Primary gastric non-Hodgkin's lymphoma: clinical features, management, and prognosis of 185 patients with diffuse large B-cell lymphoma. *Ann Oncol* 1999;10:1441–1449.
18. Koch P, Probst A, Berdel WE, et al. Treatment results in localized primary gastric lymphoma: data of patients registered within the German multicenter study (GIT NHL 02/96). *J Clin Oncol* 2005;23:7050–7059.
19. Aviles A, Nambo MJ, Neri N, et al. Mucosa-associated lymphoid tissue (MALT) lymphoma of the stomach: results of a controlled clinical trial. *Med Oncol* 2005;22:57–62.
20. Ibrahim EM, Ezzat AA, El-Weshi AN, et al. Primary intestinal diffuse large B-cell non-Hodgkin's lymphoma: clinical features, management, and prognosis of 66 patients. *Ann Oncol* 2001;12:53–58.
21. Cortelazzo S, Rossi A, Oldani E, et al. The modified International Prognostic Index can predict the outcome of localized primary intestinal lymphoma of both extranodal marginal zone B-cell and diffuse large B-cell histologies. *Br J Haematol* 2002;118:218–228.
22. Christie DR, Barton MB, Bryant G, et al. Osteolymphoma (primary bone lymphoma): an Australian review of 70 cases. Australasian Radiation Oncology Lymphoma Group (AROLG). *Aust N Z J Med* 1999;29:214–219.
23. Zinzani PL, Carrillo G, Ascani S, et al. Primary bone lymphoma: experience with 52 patients. *Haematologica* 2003;88:280–285.
24. Beal K, Allen L, Yahalom J. Primary bone lymphoma: treatment results and prognostic factors with long-term follow-up of 82 patients. *Cancer* 2006;106:2652–2656.
25. Fonseca R, Habermann TM, Colgan JP, et al. Testicular lymphoma is associated with a high incidence of extranodal recurrence. *Cancer* 2000;88:154–161.
26. Zucca E, Conconi A, Mughal TI, et al. Patterns of outcome and prognostic factors in primary large-cell lymphoma of the testis in a survey by the International Extranodal Lymphoma Study Group. *J Clin Oncol* 2003;21:20–27.
27. Aviles A, Delgado S, Nambo MJ, et al. Primary breast lymphoma: results of a controlled clinical trial. *Oncology* 2005;69:256–260.
28. Ryan G, Martinelli G, Kuper-Hommel M, et al. Primary diffuse large B-cell lymphoma of the breast: prognostic factors and outcomes of a study by the International Extranodal Lymphoma Study Group. *Ann Oncol* 2008;19:233–241.
29. Ferreri AJ, Reni M, Pasini F, et al. A multicenter study of treatment of primary CNS lymphoma. *Neurology* 2002;58:1513–1520.
30. Abrey LE, Ben-Porat L, Panageas KS, et al. Primary central nervous system lymphoma: the Memorial Sloan-Kettering Cancer Center prognostic model. *J Clin Oncol* 2006;24:5711–5715.

31. Bangerter M, Kotzerke J, Griesshammer M, et al. Positron emission tomography with 18-fluorodeoxyglucose in the staging and follow-up of lymphoma in the chest. *Acta Oncol* 1999;38:799–804.
32. Swerdlow SH, Campo E, Harris NL. *WHO classification of tumours of haematopoietic and lymphoid tissues.* Lyon, France: International Agency for Research on Cancer, 2008.
33. Harris NL, Jaffe ES, Diebold J, et al. The World Health Organization classification of hematological malignancies report of the Clinical Advisory Committee Meeting, Airlie House, Virginia, November 1997. *Mod Pathol* 2000;13:193–207.
34. Shipp M. Prognostic factors in non-Hodgkin's lymphoma [published erratum appears in *Curr Opin Oncol* 1993;5:251]. *Curr Opin Oncol* 1992;4:856–862.
35. The Non-Hodgkin's Lymphoma Classification Project. A clinical evaluation of the International Lymphoma Study Group Classification of non-Hodgkin's lymphoma. *Blood* 1997;89:3309–3918.
36. Romaguera JE, Velasquez WS, Silvermintz KB, et al. Surgical debulking is associated with improved survival in stage I-II diffuse large cell lymphoma. *Cancer* 1990;66:267–272.
37. Thirlby RC. Gastrointestinal lymphoma: a surgical perspective. *Oncology* 1993;7:29–32.
38. Sutcliffe SB, Gospodarowicz MK, Bush RS, et al. Role of radiation therapy in localized non-Hodgkin's lymphoma. *Radiother Oncol* 1985;4:211–223.
39. Tsang RW, Gospodarowicz MK, O'Sullivan B. Staging and management of localized non-Hodgkin's lymphomas: variations among experts in radiation oncology. *Int J Radiat Oncol Biol Phys* 2002;52:643–651.
40. Shenkier TN, Voss N, Fairey R, et al. Brief chemotherapy and involved-region irradiation for limited-stage diffuse large-cell lymphoma: an 18-year experience from the British Columbia Cancer Agency. *J Clin Oncol* 2002;20:197–204.
41. Aref A, Mohammad R, Yudelev M, et al. Radiobiological characterization of two human chemotherapy-resistant intermediate grade non-Hodgkin's lymphoma cell lines. *Radiat Oncol Investig* 1999;7:158–162.
42. Gospodarowicz MK, Sutcliffe SB, Brown TC, et al. Patterns of disease in localized extranodal lymphomas. *J Clin Oncol* 1987;5:875–880.
43. Oguchi M, Ikeda H, Isobe K, et al. Tumor bulk as a prognostic factor for the management of localized aggressive non-Hodgkin's lymphoma: a survey of the Japan Lymphoma Radiation Therapy Group. *Int J Radiat Oncol Biol Phys* 2000;48:161–168.
44. Cheson BD, Pfistner B, Juweid ME, et al. Revised response criteria for malignant lymphoma. *J Clin Oncol* 2007;25:579–586.
45. Jacobs C, Hoppe R. Non-Hodgkin's lymphomas of the head and neck: prognosis and patterns of recurrence. *Int J Radiat Oncol Biol Phys* 1985;11:357–364.
46. Isaacson PG, Norton AJ. *Extranodal lymphomas.* Edinburgh, UK: Churchill Livingstone, 1994.
47. Aviles A, Delgado S, Ruiz H, et al. Treatment of non-Hodgkin's lymphoma of Waldeyer's ring: radiotherapy versus chemotherapy versus combined therapy. *Eur J Cancer B Oral Oncol* 1996;32B:19–23.
48. Bertoni F, Sanna P, Tinguely M, et al. Association of gastric and Waldeyer's ring lymphoma: a molecular study. *Hematol Oncol* 2000;18:15–19.
49. Ezzat AA, Ibrahim EM, El Weshi AN, et al. Localized non-Hodgkin's lymphoma of Waldeyer's ring: clinical features, management, and prognosis of 130 adult patients. *Head Neck* 2001;23:547–558.
50. Harabuchi Y, Tsubota H, Ohguro S, et al. Prognostic factors and treatment outcome in non-Hodgkin's lymphoma of Waldeyer's ring. *Acta Oncol* 1997;36:413–420.
51. Krol AD, Le Cessie S, Snijder S, et al. Waldeyer's ring lymphomas: a clinical study from the Comprehensive Cancer Center West population based NHL registry. *Leuk Lymphoma* 2001;42:1005–1013.
52. Conley SF, Staszak C, Clamon GH, et al. Non-Hodgkin's lymphoma of the head and neck: the University of Iowa experience. *Laryngoscope* 1987;97:291–300.
53. Wulfrank D, Speelman T, Pauwels C, et al. Extranodal non-Hodgkin's lymphoma of the head and neck. *Radiother Oncol* 1987;8:199–207.
54. Ossenkoppele GJ, Mol JJ, Snow GB, et al. Radiotherapy versus radiotherapy plus chemotherapy in stages I and II non-Hodgkin's lymphoma of the upper digestive and respiratory tract. *Cancer* 1987;60:1505–1509.
55. Liang R, Ng RP, Todd D, et al. Management of stage I-II diffuse aggressive non-Hodgkin's lymphoma of the Waldeyer's ring: combined modality therapy versus radiotherapy alone. *Hematol Oncol* 1987;5:223–230.
56. Li YX, Coucke PA, Li JY, et al. Primary non-Hodgkin's lymphoma of the nasal cavity: prognostic significance of paranasal extension and the role of radiotherapy and chemotherapy. *Cancer* 1998;83:449–456.
57. Vidal RW, Devaney K, Ferlito A, et al. Sinonasal malignant lymphomas: a distinct clinicopathological category. *Ann Otol Rhinol Laryngol* 1999;108:411–419.
58. Proulx GM, Caudra-Garcia I, Ferry J, et al. Lymphoma of the nasal cavity and paranasal sinuses: treatment and outcome of early-stage disease. *Am J Clin Oncol* 2003;26:6–11.
59. Cuadra-Garcia I, Proulx GM, Wu CL, et al. Sinonasal lymphoma: a clinicopathologic analysis of 58 cases from the Massachusetts General Hospital. *Am J Surg Pathol* 1999;23:1356–1369.
60. Tomita Y, Ohsawa M, Mishiro Y, et al. The presence and subtype of Epstein-Barr virus in B and T cell lymphomas of the sino-nasal region from the Osaka and Okinawa districts of Japan. *Lab Invest* 1995;73:190–196.
61. Tomita Y, Ohsawa M, Qiu K, et al. Epstein-Barr virus in lymphoproliferative diseases in the sino-nasal region: close association with CD56+ immunophenotype and polymorphic-reticulosis morphology. *Int J Cancer* 1997;70:9–13.
62. Suzuki R, Takeuchi K, Ohshima K, et al. Extranodal NK/T-cell lymphoma: diagnosis and treatment cues. *Hematol Oncol* 2008;26:66–72.
63. Armitage J, Vose J, Weisenburger D. International peripheral T-cell and natural killer/T-cell lymphoma study: pathology findings and clinical outcomes. *J Clin Oncol* 2008;26:4124–4130.
64. Jaffe ES. Classification of natural killer (NK) cell and NK-like T-cell malignancies. *Blood* 1996;87:1207–1210.
65. Liang R, Todd D, Chan TK, et al. Treatment outcome and prognostic factors for primary nasal lymphoma. *J Clin Oncol* 1995;13:666–670.
66. Davison SP, Habermann TM, Strickler JG, et al. Nasal and nasopharyngeal angiocentric T-cell lymphomas. *Laryngoscope* 1996;106:139–143.
67. Hausdorff J, Davis E, Long G, et al. Non-Hodgkin's lymphoma of the paranasal sinuses: clinical and pathological features, and response to combined-modality therapy. *Cancer J Sci Am* 1997;3:303–311.
68. Logsdon M, Ha C, Kavadi V, et al. Lymphoma of the nasal cavity and paranasal sinuses. *Cancer* 1997;80:477–488.
69. Lee J, Park YH, Kim WS, et al. Extranodal nasal type NK/T-cell lymphoma: elucidating clinical prognostic factors for risk-based stratification of therapy. *Eur J Cancer* 2005;41:1402–1408.
70. Au WY, Lie AK, Liang R, et al. Autologous stem cell transplantation for nasal NK/T-cell lymphoma: a progress report on its value. *Ann Oncol* 2003;14:1673–1676.
71. Zucca E, Conconi A, Pedrinis E, et al. Nongastric marginal zone B-cell lymphoma of mucosa-associated lymphoid tissue. *Blood* 2003;101:2489–2495.
72. Ambrosetti A, Zanotti R, Pattaro C, et al. Most cases of primary salivary mucosa-associated lymphoid tissue lymphoma are associated either with Sjögren syndrome or hepatitis C virus infection. *Br J Haematol* 2004;126:43–49.
73. Wolvius EB, et al. Primary extranodal non-Hodgkin lymphoma of the oral cavity. An analysis of 34 cases. *Eur J Cancer B Oral Oncol* 1994;30B:121–125.
74. Conconi A. *IELSG Phase II Study of Rituximab in MALT Lymphoma: Final Results: Proceedings of the Thirty-Eighth American Society of Clinical Oncology,* Orlando, FL, May 18-21, 2002. Abstract 1067.
75. Laing RW, Hoskin P, Hudson BV, et al. The significance of MALT histology in thyroid lymphoma: a review of patients from the BNLI and Royal Marsden Hospital. *Clin Oncol* 1994;6:300–304.
76. Derringer GA, Thompson LD, Frommelt RA, et al. Malignant lymphoma of the thyroid gland: a clinicopathologic study of 108 cases. *Am J Surg Pathol* 2000;24:623–639.
77. Pederson R, Pederson N. Primary non-Hodgkin's lymphoma of the thyroid gland: a population based study. *Histopathology* 1996;28:25–32.
78. Thieblemont C, Mayer A, Dumontet C, et al. Primary thyroid lymphoma is a heterogeneous disease. *J Clin Endocrinol Metab* 2002;87:105–111.
79. Tsang RW, Gospodarowicz MK, Sutcliffe SB, et al. Non-Hodgkin's lymphoma of the thyroid gland: prognostic factors and treatment outcome. The Princess Margaret Hospital Lymphoma Group. *Int J Radiat Oncol Biol Phys* 1993;27:599–604.
80. Vigliotti A, Kong JS, Fuller LM, et al. Thyroid lymphomas stages IE and IIE: Comparative results for radiotherapy only, combination chemotherapy only, and multimodality treatment. *Int J Radiat Oncol Biol Phys* 1986;12:1807–1812.
81. Tsang RW, Gospodarowicz MK, Pintilie M, et al. Localized mucosa-associated lymphoid tissue lymphoma treated with radiation therapy has excellent clinical outcome. *J Clin Oncol* 2003;21:4157–4164.
82. Ponzoni M, Ferreri AJ, Guidoboni M, et al. Chlamydia infection and lymphomas: association beyond ocular adnexal lymphomas highlighted by multiple detection methods. *Clin Cancer Res* 2008;14:5794–5800.
83. Ferreri AJ, Dolcetti R, Du MQ, et al. Ocular adnexal MALT lymphoma: an intriguing model for antigen-driven lymphomagenesis and microbial-targeted therapy. *Ann Oncol* 2008;19:835–846.
84. Ferreri AJ, Dolcetti R, Magnino S, et al. A woman and her canary: a tale of chlamydiae and lymphomas. *J Natl Cancer Inst* 2007;99:1418–1419.
85. Ferreri A, Guidoboni M, Ponzoni M, et al. Evidence for association between chlamydia psittaci infection and ocular adnexal lymphoma (OAL). *J Natl Cancer Inst* 2004;96:586–94.
86. Ferreri AJ, Ponzoni M, Guidoboni M, et al. Bacteria-eradicating therapy with doxycycline in ocular adnexal MALT lymphoma: a multicenter prospective trial. *J Natl Cancer Inst* 2006;98:1375–1382.
87. Stafford SL, Kozelsky TF, Garrity JA, et al. Orbital lymphoma: radiotherapy outcome and complications. *Radiother Oncol* 2001;59:139–144.
88. Bhatia S, Paulino AC, Buatti JM, et al. Curative radiotherapy for primary orbital lymphoma. *Int J Radiat Oncol Biol Phys* 2002;54:818–823.
89. Sano T. Treatment of primary gastric lymphoma: experience in the National Cancer Center Hospital, Tokyo. *Recent Results Cancer Res* 2000;156:104–107.

90. Yoon SS, Coit DG, Portlock CS, et al. The diminishing role of surgery in the treatment of gastric lymphoma. *Ann Surg* 2004;240:28–37.

91. Wirth A, Teo A, Wittwer H, et al. Gastric irradiation for MALT lymphoma: reducing the target volume, fast! *Australas Radiol* 1999;43:87–90.

92. Montalban C, Santon A, Boixeda D, et al. Regression of gastric high grade mucosa associated lymphoid tissue (MALT) lymphoma after Helicobacter pylori eradication. *Gut* 2001;49:584–587.

93. Chen LT, Lin JT, Tai JJ, et al. Long-term results of anti-Helicobacter pylori therapy in early-stage gastric high-grade transformed MALT lymphoma. *J Natl Cancer Inst* 2005;97:1345–1353.

94. Morgner A, Miehlke S, Fischbach W, et al. Complete remission of primary high-grade B-cell gastric lymphoma after cure of Helicobacter pylori infection. *J Clin Oncol* 2001;19:2041–2048.

95. Isaacson PG. Gastrointestinal lymphomas of T- and B-cell types. *Mod Pathol* 1999;12:151–158.

96. Foss HD, Stein H. Pathology of intestinal lymphomas. *Recent Results Cancer Res* 2000;156:33–41.

97. Gospodarowicz MK, Sutcliffe SB, Clark RM, et al. Outcome analysis of localized gastrointestinal lymphoma treated with surgery and postoperative irradiation. *Int J Radiat Oncol Biol Phys* 1990;19:1351–1355.

98. Domizio P, Owen RA, Shepherd NA, et al. Primary lymphoma of the small intestine. A clinicopathological study of 119 cases. *Am J Surg Pathol* 1993;17:429–442.

99. Morton JE, Leyland MJ, Vaughan Hudson G, et al. Primary gastrointestinal non-Hodgkin's lymphoma: a review of 175 British National Lymphoma Investigation cases. *Br J Cancer* 1993;67:776–782.

100. Lecuit M, Abachin E, Martin A, et al. Immunoproliferative small intestinal disease associated with Campylobacter jejuni. *N Engl J Med* 2004;350:239–248.

101. Suarez F, Lortholary O, Hermine O, et al. Infection-associated lymphomas derived from marginal zone B cells: a model of antigen-driven lymphoproliferation. *Blood* 2006;107:3034–3044.

102. Fischbach W, Tacke W, Greiner A, et al. Regression of immunoproliferative small intestinal disease after eradication of Helicobacter pylori. *Lancet* 1997;349:31–32.

103. Al-Bahrani Z, Al-Mohindry H, Bakir F, et al. Clinical and pathologic subtypes of primary intestinal lymphoma: experience with 132 patients over a 14-year period. *Cancer* 1983;52:1666–1672.

104. Isaacson PG. Gastrointestinal lymphoma. *Hum Pathol* 1994;25:1020–1029.

105. Chott A, Vesely M, Simonitsch I, et al. Classification of intestinal T-cell neoplasms and their differential diagnosis. *Am J Clin Pathol* 1999;111:S68–S74.

106. Bende RJ, Smit LA, Bossenbroek JG, et al. Primary follicular lymphoma of the small intestine: alpha4beta7 expression and immunoglobulin configuration suggest an origin from local antigen-experienced B cells. *Am J Pathol* 2003;162:105–113..

107. Aosaza K, Ohsawa M, Soma T, et al. Malignant lymphoma of the rectum. *Jpn J Clin Oncol* 1990;20:380–386.

108. Moller MB, d'Amore F, Christensen BE. Testicular lymphoma: a population-based study of incidence, clinicopathological correlations and prognosis. The Danish Lymphoma Study Group, LYFO. *Eur J Cancer* 1994;12:1760–1764.

109. Vitolo U, Zucca E, Seymour JF. Primary testicular lymphoma. In: Cavalli F, Stein H, Zucca E, eds. *Extranodal lymphomas pathology and management.* London, UK: Informa HealthCare, 2008:139–146.

110. Crellin AM, Hudson BV, Bennett MH, et al. Non-Hodgkin's lymphoma of the testis. *Radiother Oncol* 1993;27:99–106.

111. Leite KR, Garicochea B, Srougi M, et al. Monoclonality of asynchronous bilateral lymphoma of the testis. *Eur Urol* 2000;38:774–777.

112. Chan JKC, Sin VC, Wong KF, et al. Nonnasal lymphoma expressing the natural killer cell marker CD56: a clinicopathologic study of 49 cases of an uncommon aggressive neoplasm. *Blood* 1997;89:4501–4513.

113. Ferry JA, Harris NL, Young RH, et al. Malignant lymphoma of the testis, epididymis, and spermatic cord. A clinicopathologic study of 69 cases with immunophenotypic analysis. *Am J Surg Pathol* 1994;18:376–390.

114. Sussman EB, Hajdu SI, Lieberman PH, et al. Malignant lymphoma of the testis: a clinicopathologic study of 37 cases. *J Urol* 1977;118:1004–1007.

115. Touroutoglou N, Dimopoulos MA, Younes A, et al. Testicular lymphoma: late relapses and poor outcome despite doxorubicin-based therapy. *J Clin Oncol* 1995;13:1361–1367.

116. Zietman AL, Coen JJ, Ferry JA, et al. The management and outcome of stage IAE nonHodgkin's lymphoma of the testis. *J Urol* 1996;155:943–946.

117. Linassier C, Desablens B, Lefrancq T, et al. Stage I-IIE primary non-Hodgkin's lymphoma of the testis: results of a prospective trial by the GOELAMS Study Group. *Clin Lymphoma* 2002;3:167–172.

118. Connors JM, Klimo P, Voss N, et al. Testicular lymphoma: improved outcome with early brief chemotherapy. *J Clin Oncol* 1988;6:776–781.

119. Tondini C, Ferreri AJ, Siracusano L, et al. Diffuse large-cell lymphoma of the testis. *J Clin Oncol* 1999;17:2854–2858.

120. Read G. Lymphomas of the testis-results of treatment 1960-77. *Clin Radiol* 1981;32:687–692.

121. Vitolo U, Ferreri AJ, Zucca E. Primary testicular lymphoma. *Crit Rev Oncol Hematol* 2008;65:183–189.

122. Yuille FA, Angus B, Roberts JT, et al. Low grade MALT lymphoma of the urinary bladder. *Clin Oncol (R Coll Radiol)* 1998;10:265–266.

123. Ferry JA, Young RH. Malignant lymphoma of the genitourinary tract. *Curr Diagn Pathol* 1997;4:145–169.

124. Kempton CL, Kurtin PJ, Inwards DJ, et al. Malignant lymphoma of the bladder: evidence from 36 cases that low-grade lymphoma of the MALT-type is the most common primary bladder lymphoma. *Am J Surg Pathol* 1997;21:1324–1333.

125. Melekos MD, Matsouka P, Fokaefs E, et al. Primary non-Hodgkin's lymphoma of the urinary bladder. *Eur Urol* 1992;21:85–88.

126. Ohsawa M, Aozasa K, Horiuchi K, et al. Malignant lymphoma of bladder. Report of three cases and review of the literature. *Cancer* 1993;72:1969–1974.

127. Hughes M, Morrison A, Jackson R. Primary bladder lymphoma: management and outcome of 12 patients with a review of the literature. *Leuk Lymphoma* 2005;46:873–877.

128. Al-Maghrabi J, Kamel-Reid S, Jewett M, et al. Primary low-grade B-cell lymphoma of mucosa-associated lymphoid tissue type arising in the urinary bladder: report of 4 cases with molecular genetic analysis. *Arch Pathol Lab Med* 2001;125:332–336.

129. Dimopoulos MA, Daliani D, Pugh W, et al. Primary ovarian non-Hodgkin's lymphoma: outcome after treatment with combination chemotherapy. *Gynecol Oncol* 1997;64:446–450.

130. Signorelli M, Maneo A, Cammarota G, et al. Conservative management in primary genital lymphomas: the role of chemotherapy. *Gynecol Oncol* 2007;104:416–421.

131. Kosari F, Daneshbod Y, Parwaresch R, et al. Lymphomas of the female genital tract: a study of 186 cases and review of the literature. *Am J Surg Pathol* 2005;29:1512–1520.

132. Vang R, Medeiros LJ, Fuller GN, et al. Non-Hodgkin's lymphoma involving the gynecologic tract: a review of 88 cases. *Adv Anat Pathol* 2001;8:200–217.

133. Harris NL, Scully RE. Malignant lymphoma and granulocytic sarcoma of the uterus and vagina. A clinicopathologic analysis of 27 cases. *Cancer* 1984;53:2530–2545.

134. Stroh EL, Besa PC, Cox JD, et al. Treatment of patients with lymphomas of the uterus or cervix with combination chemotherapy and radiation therapy. *Cancer* 1995;75:2392–2399.

135. Domchek SM, Hecht JL, Fleming MD, et al. Lymphomas of the breast: primary and secondary involvement. *Cancer* 2002;94:6–13.

136. Ribrag V, Bibeau F, El Weshi A, et al. Primary breast lymphoma: a report of 20 cases. *Br J Haematol* 2001;115:253–256.

137. Thieblemont C, Bastion Y, Berger F, et al. Mucosa-associated lymphoid tissue gastrointestinal and nongastrointestinal lymphoma behavior: analysis of 108 patients. *J Clin Oncol* 1997;15:1624–1630.

138. Giardini R, Piccolo C, Rilke F. Primary non-Hodgkin's lymphomas of the female breast. *Cancer* 1992;69:725–735.

139. Jeon HJ, Akagi T, Hoshida Y, et al. Primary non-Hodgkin malignant lymphoma of the breast. An immunohistochemical study of seven patients and literature review of 152 patients with breast lymphoma in Japan. *Cancer* 1992;70:2451–2459.

140. Ryan G, Martinelli G, Yuen K. Primary non-Hodgkin's lymphoma of the breast: first report of the multicentre retrospective study of the International Extranodal Lymphoma Study Group (IELSG-15). *J Clin Oncol* 2005;23(16S):6575.

141. Ramadan KM, Shenkier T, Sehn LH, et al. A clinicopathological retrospective study of 131 patients with primary bone lymphoma: a population-based study of successively treated cohorts from the British Columbia Cancer Agency. *Ann Oncol* 2007;18:129–135.

142. Pettit CK, Zukerberg LR, Gray MH, et al. Primary lymphoma of bone. A B-cell neoplasm with a high frequency of multilobated cells. *Am J Surg Pathol* 1990;14:329–334.

143. Furman WL, Fitch S, Hustu HO, et al. Primary lymphoma of bone in children. *J Clin Oncol* 1989;7:1275–1280.

144. Loeffler JS, Tarbell NJ, Kozakewich H, et al. Primary lymphoma of bone in children: analysis of treatment results with adriamycin, prednisone, Oncovin (APO), and local radiation therapy. *J Clin Oncol* 1986;4:496–501.

145. Lones MA, Perkins SL, Sposto R, et al. Non-Hodgkin's lymphoma arising in bone in children and adolescents is associated with an excellent outcome: a Children's Cancer Group report. *J Clin Oncol* 2002;20:2293–2301.

146. Schaefer NG, Strobel K, Taverna C, et al. Bone involvement in patients with lymphoma: the role of FDG-PET/CT. *Eur J Nucl Med Mol Imaging* 2007;34:60–67.

147. Fairbanks RK, Bonner JA, Inwards CY, et al. Treatment of stage IE primary lymphoma of bone. *Int J Radiat Oncol Biol Phys* 1994;28:363–372.

148. Rathmell AJ, Gospodarowicz MK, Sutcliffe SB, et al. Localised lymphoma of bone: prognostic factors and treatment recommendations. The Princess Margaret Hospital Lymphoma Group. *Br J Cancer* 1992;66:603–606.

149. Lones MA, Sanger W, Perkins SL, et al. Anaplastic large cell lymphoma arising in bone: report of a case of the monomorphic variant with the t(2;5)(p23;q35) translocation. *Arch Pathol Lab Med* 2000;124:1339–1343.

150. Stokes SH, Walz BJ. Pathologic fracture after radiation therapy for primary non-Hodgkin's malignant lymphoma of bone. *Int J Radiat Oncol Biol Phys* 1983;9:1153–1159.

151. Batchelor T, Loeffler JS. Primary CNS lymphoma. *J Clin Oncol* 2006;24:1281–1288.

152. Abrey LE, Batchelor TT, Ferreri AJ, et al. Report of an international workshop to standardize baseline evaluation and response criteria for primary CNS lymphoma. *J Clin Oncol* 2005;23:5034–5043.

153. Ferreri AJ, Batchelor T, Zucca E, et al. International Collaborative Group against Primary CNS Lymphomas. *J Clin Oncol* 2003;21:1649–1650.

154. Rathmell AJ, Gospodarowicz MK, Sutcliffe SB, et al. Localized extradural lymphoma: survival, relapse pattern and functional outcome. The Princess Margaret Hospital Lymphoma Group. *Radiother Oncol* 1992;24:14–20.

155. Eeles RA, O'Brien P, Horwich A, et al. Non-Hodgkin's lymphoma presenting with extradural spinal cord compression: functional outcome and survival. *Br J Cancer* 1991;63:126–129.

156. MacKintosh FR, Colby TV, Podolsky WJ, et al. Central nervous system involvement in non-Hodgkin's lymphoma: an analysis of 105 cases. *Cancer* 1982;49:586–595.

157. Cordier JF, Chailleux E, Lauque D, et al. Primary pulmonary lymphomas. A clinical study of 70 cases in nonimmunocompromised patients. *Chest* 1993;103:201–208.

158. Lim JK, Lacy MQ, Kurtin PJ, et al. Pulmonary marginal zone lymphoma of MALT type as a cause of localised pulmonary amyloidosis. *J Clin Pathol* 2001;54:642–646.

159. Rush WL, Andriko JA, Taubenberger JK, et al. Primary anaplastic large cell lymphoma of the lung: a clinicopathologic study of five patients. *Mod Pathol* 2000;13:1285–1292.

160. Kurtin PJ, Myers JL, Adlakha H, et al. Pathologic and clinical features of primary pulmonary extranodal marginal zone B-cell lymphoma of MALT type. *Am J Surg Pathol* 2001;25:997–1008.

161. Montalban C, Obeso G, Gallego A, et al. Peripheral T-cell lymphoma: a clinicopathological study of 41 cases and evaluation of the prognostic significance of the updated Kiel classification. *Histopathology* 1993;22:303–310.

162. Horny HP, Ferlito A, Carbone A. Laryngeal lymphoma derived from mucosa-associated lymphoid tissue. *Ann Otol Rhinol Laryngol* 1996;105:577–583.

163. Kato S, Sakura M, Takooda S, et al. Primary non-Hodgkin's lymphoma of the larynx. *J Laryngol Otol* 1997;111:571–574.

164. Fidias P, Wright C, Harris NL, et al. Primary tracheal non-Hodgkin's lymphoma. A case report and review of the literature. *Cancer* 1996;77:2332–2338.

165. Harris GJ, Lager DJ. Primary renal lymphoma. *J Surg Oncol* 1991;46:273–277.

166. Okuno SH, Hoyer JD, Ristow K, et al. Primary renal non-Hodgkin's lymphoma. An unusual extranodal site. *Cancer* 1995;75:2258–2261.

167. Poulios C. Primary renal non-Hodgkin lymphoma. *Scand J Urol Nephrol* 1990;24:227–230.

168. Parveen T, Navarro-Roman L, Medeiros LJ, et al. Low-grade B-cell lymphoma of mucosa-associated lymphoid tissue arising in the kidney. *Arch Pathol Lab Med* 1993;117:780–783.

169. Tsutsui K, Shibamoto Y, Yamabe H, et al. A radiotherapeutic experience for localized extranodal non-Hodgkin's lymphoma: prognostic factors and re-evaluation of treatment modality. *Radiother Oncol* 1991;21:83–90.

170. Bostwick DG, Iczkowski KA, Amin MB, et al. Malignant lymphoma involving the prostate: report of 62 cases. *Cancer* 1998;83:732–738.

171. Bostwick DG, Mann RB. Malignant lymphomas involving the prostate. A study of 13 cases. *Cancer* 1985;56:2932–2938.

172. Sarris A, Dimopoulos M, Pugh W, et al. Primary lymphoma of the prostate: good outcome with doxorubicin-based combination chemotherapy. *J Urol* 1995;153:1852–1854.

173. Buck DS, Peterson MS, Borochovitz D, et al. Non-Hodgkin lymphoma of the ureter: CT demonstration with pathologic correlation. *Urol Radiol* 1992;14:183–187.

174. Selch MT, Mark RJ, Fu YS, et al. Primary lymphoma of female urethra: long-term control by radiation therapy. *Urology* 1993;42:343–346.

175. Vogeli T, Engstfeld EJ. Non-Hodgkin lymphoma of the female urethra. *Scand J Urol Nephrol* 1992;26:111–112.

176. Hatcher PA, Wilson DD. Primary lymphoma of the male urethra. *Urology* 1997;49:142–144.

177. Kitamura H, Umehara T, Miyake M, et al. NonHodgkin's lymphoma arising in the urethra of a man. *J Urol* 1996;156:175–176.

178. Vapnek JM, Turzan CW. Primary malignant lymphoma of the female urethra: report of a case and review of the literature. *J Urol* 1992;147:701–703.

179. Touhami H, Brahimi S, Kubisz P, et al. Non-Hodgkin's lymphoma of the female urethra. *J Urol* 1987;137:991–992.

180. Nabholtz JM, Friedman S, Tremeaux JC, et al. Non-Hodgkin's lymphoma of the urethra: a rare extranodal entity. *Gynecol Oncol* 1989;35:110–111.

181. Fischer MA, Kabakow B. Lymphoma of the pancreas. *Mt Sinai J Med* 1987;54:423–426.

182. Nishimura R, Takakuwa T, Hoshida Y, et al. Primary pancreatic lymphoma: clinicopathological analysis of 19 cases from Japan and review of the literature. *Oncology* 2001;60:322–329.

183. Salmon JS, Thompson MA, Arildsen RC, et al. Non-Hodgkin's lymphoma involving the liver: clinical and therapeutic considerations. *Clin Lymphoma Myeloma* 2006;6:273–280.

184. Ohsawa M, Aozasa K, Horiuchi K, et al. Malignant lymphoma of the liver. Report of five cases and review of the literature. *Dig Dis Sci* 1992;37:1105–1109.

185. Anthony PP, Sarsfield P, Clarke T. Primary lymphoma of the liver: clinical and pathologic features of ten patients. *J Clin Pathol* 1990;43:1007–1013.

186. Isaacson PG, Banks PM, Best PV, et al. Primary low-grade hepatic B-cell lymphoma of mucosa-associated lymphoid tissue (MALT)-type. *Am J Surg Pathol* 1995;19:571–575.

187. Ye MQ, Suriawinata A, Black C, et al. Primary hepatic marginal zone B-cell lymphoma of mucosa-associated lymphoid tissue type in a patient with primary biliary cirrhosis. *Arch Pathol Lab Med* 2000;124:604–608.

188. Page RD, Romaguera JE, Osborne B, et al. Primary hepatic lymphoma: favorable outcome after combination chemotherapy. *Cancer* 2001;92:2023–2029.

189. Belhadj K, Reyes F, Farcet JP, et al. Hepatosplenic gammadelta T-cell lymphoma is a rare clinicopathologic entity with poor outcome: report on a series of 21 patients. *Blood* 2003;102:4261–4269.

190. Armitage JO, Liang RHS, Sweetenham JW, et al. Mature nodal and extranodal T-cell and non-Hodgkin-cell lymphomas (peripheral T-cell, angioimmunoblastic, nasal natural killer/T-cell, hepatosplenic T-cell, enteropathy-type T-cell, and subcutaneous panniculitis-like T-cell lymphomas). In: Mauch PM, Armitage JO, Coiffier B, et al., eds. *Non-Hodgkin's lymphomas.* Philadelphia, PA: Lippincott Williams & Wilkins, 2004:405–426.

191. Scally J, Garrett A. Primary extranodal lymphoma in muscle. *Br J Radiol* 1989;62:81.

192. Travis WD, Banks PM, Reiman HM. Primary extranodal soft tissue lymphoma of the extremities. *Am J Surg Pathol* 1987;11:359–366.

193. Jeffery GM, Golding PF, Mead GM. Non-Hodgkin's lymphoma arising in skeletal muscle. *Ann Oncol* 1991;2:501–504.

194. Chim CS, Chan AC, Kwong YL, et al. Primary cardiac lymphoma. *Am J Hematol* 1997;54:79–83.

195. Rolla G, Bertero MT, Pastena G, et al. Primary lymphoma of the heart. A case report and review of the literature. *Leuk Res* 2002;26:117–120.

196. Saito T, Tamaru J, Kayao J, et al. Cytomorphologic diagnosis of malignant lymphoma arising in the heart: a case report. *Acta Cytol* 2001;45:1043–1048.

197. Zaharia L, Gill PS. Primary cardiac lymphoma. *Am J Clin Oncol* 1991;14:142–145.

198. Dorsay TA, Ho VB, Rovira MJ, et al. Primary cardiac lymphoma: CT and MR findings. *J Comput Assist Tomogr* 1993;17:978–981.

199. Nand S, Mullen GM, Lonchyna VA, et al. Primary lymphoma of the heart. Prolonged survival with early systemic therapy in a patient. *Cancer* 1991;68:2289–2292.

200. Aozasa K. Pyothorax-associated lymphoma. *J Clin Exp Hematop* 2006;46:5–10.

201. Harris GJ, Tio FO, Von Hoff DD. Primary adrenal lymphoma. *Cancer* 1989;63:799–803.

202. Nakatsuka S, Hongyo T, Syaifudin M, et al. Mutations of p53, c-kit, K-ras, and beta-catenin gene in non-Hodgkin's lymphoma of adrenal gland. *Jpn J Cancer Res* 2002;93:267–274.

203. Wu HC, Shih LY, Chen TC, et al. A patient with bilateral primary adrenal lymphoma, presenting with fever of unknown origin and achieving long-term disease-free survival after resection and chemotherapy. *Ann Hematol* 1999;78:289–292.

204. Yamamoto E, Ozaki N, Nakagawa M, et al. Primary bilateral adrenal lymphoma associated with idiopathic thrombocytopenic purpura. *Leuk Lymphoma* 1999;35:403–408.

205. Carbone A, Gloghini A. PEL and HHV8-unrelated effusion lymphomas: classification and diagnosis. *Cancer* 2008;114:225–227.

206. Ascoli V, Lo-Coco F. Body cavity lymphoma. *Curr Opin Pulm Med* 2002;8:317–322.

207. Mack AA, Sugden B. EBV is necessary for proliferation of dually infected primary effusion lymphoma cells. *Cancer Res* 2008;68:6963–6968.

208. Jenner RG, Maillard K, Cattini N, et al. Kaposi's sarcoma-associated herpesvirus-infected primary effusion lymphoma has a plasma cell gene expression profile. *Proc Natl Acad Sci U S A* 2003;100:10399–10404.

209. Klein U, Gloghini A, Gaidano G, et al. Gene expression profile analysis of AIDS-related primary effusion lymphoma (PEL) suggests a plasmablastic derivation and identifies PEL-specific transcripts. *Blood* 2003;101:4115–4121.

CHAPTER 38 ■ DIAGNOSIS AND MANAGEMENT OF DISORDERS THAT CAN MIMIC LYMPHOMA

ANGELA DISPENZIERI, STEFANIA PITTALUGA, FABIO FACCHETTI, JEAN FEUILLARD, AND ELAINE S. JAFFE

A number of disorders, both benign and malignant and lymphoid and nonlymphoid, can mimic lymphoma.

The nonmalignant lymphoproliferative disorders that will be discussed include: Castleman disease (CD) (angiofollicular lymph node hyperplasia), Canale Smith syndrome (autoimmune lymphoproliferative syndrome [ALPS]), Kimura disease, chronic active Epstein-Barr virus (CAEBV) infection of T cells and natural killer (NK) cells, Rosai-Dorfman disease (sinus histiocytosis with massive lymphadenopathy [SHML]), Kikuchi-Fujimoto disease, and progressive transformation of germinal centers (PTGCs) (Table 38.1). Within the spectrum of primary cutaneous CD30 positive T-cell lymphoproliferative disorders, lymphomatoid papulosis is also a lymphoma mimic, but it is discussed in Chapter 25.

Many nonlymphoid neoplasms may mimic lymphoma; a complete discussion of these is beyond the scope of this book. However, one neoplasm that was classified as a lymphoma (blastic NK cell lymphoma/leukemia) in the World Health Organization classification of 2001 is now recognized to be of myeloid/dendritic cell derivation. This entity, now known as blastic plasmacytoid dendritic cell (PDC) neoplasm (1), will be discussed in this chapter as a lymphoma mimic.

TABLE 38.1

LYMPHOID PROLIFERATIONS THAT CAN MIMIC LYMPHOMA

Infectious

- Infectious mononucleosis
- CAEBV

Autoimmune or immunodeficiency disease

- Rheumatoid arthritis
- Systemic lupus erythematosus
- Sjögren syndrome
- Common variable immune deficiency
- ALPS (Canale Smith syndrome)

Idiopathic lymphoid and histocytic proliferations

- CD (angiofollicular lymph node hyperplasia)
- Kimura disease
- PTGCs
- Rosai-Dorfman disease (SHML)
- Kikuchi-Fujimoto disease (histiocytic necrotizing lymphadenitis)

CASTLEMAN DISEASE (GIANT LYMPH NODE HYPERPLASIA, ANGIOFOLLICULAR HYPERPLASIA)

CD was first described in the 1950s as localized mediastinal lymph node enlargement characterized by redundancy of lymphoid follicles with germinal center involution and marked capillary proliferation, including follicular and interfollicular endothelial hyperplasia (2). In 1969, Flendrig et al. (3) described three types of "benign giant lymphoma": the plasma cell variant, hyalinized variant, and "intermediate variant." Festen et al. (3) noted that those patients with what is now called the plasma cell variant were more likely to have systemic symptoms, as well as anemia and hypergammaglobulinemia. In 1972, Keller et al. (4) performed a clinicopathologic analysis of 81 cases of angiofollicular hyperplasia, describing two subtypes: hyaline vascular and plasma cell types, noting that the hyaline vascular type was commonly seen in the mediastinum, whereas the plasma cell type was found in extrathoracic sites and often associated with systemic symptoms. Gaba et al. (5) reported the first case of multicentric CD (MCD) in 1978. By the mid-1980s, investigators began describing several of the salient differences between the hyaline vascular variant and the plasma cell variant, and their respective associations with unicentric (unifocal or localized) and multicentric (multifocal or generalized) presentations (6,7) (Table 38.2). The hyaline vascular variant is typically localized or unicentric, whereas the plasma cell variant may be either unicentric or disseminated (multicentric). However, many cases have a mixed appearance.

Other terminology used historically to describe this entity included angiofollicular and plasmacytic polyadenopathy, benign giant lymphoma, giant lymph node hyperplasia, follicular lymphoreticuloma, giant hemolymph node, idiopathic plasmacytic lymphadenopathy with polyclonal hypergammaglobulinemia, lymph nodal hamartoma, lymphoid hamartoma or choristoma, multicentric angiofollicular hyperplasia, and tumor-like proliferation of lymphoid tissue (8,9).

The histologic features of CD are not entirely specific, and features such as hyaline vascular follicles (regressed follicles), interfollicular vascular proliferation, and increased plasma cells can be observed in a variety of reactive conditions. MCD, as currently defined, probably comprises multiple entities that share similar histologic features.

As a clinical pathologic entity, the most clearly defined is MCD-human herpesvirus (HHV)-8 associated. Histologically,

TABLE 38.2

CLINICAL FEATURES OF CD (ANGIOFOLLICULAR LYMPH NODE HYPERPLASIA)

	Unicentric CD	MCD
Age	4th decade	6th decade
Symptoms	Incidental or compressive; occasional systemic symptoms	Fever, sweats, weight loss, malaise, autoimmune manifestations; may be associated with peripheral neuropathy and POEMS syndrome
LA	Central (mediastinal, abdominal) most common	Peripheral plus central
Organomegaly	Rare	Yes
Laboratory abnormalities	Occasional. Anemia, hypergammaglobulinemia, increased ESR, CRP	Common. Anemia, thrombocytopenia, hyper-gammaglobulinemia, increased ESR, CRP, abnormal LFTs, low albumin, renal dysfunction
Autoimmune phenomena	Rare	Often
Pathologic features	Usually hyaline vascular variant	Usually plasma cell variant
Associations with infection	No HIV or HHV-8	Some HIV and HHV-8
Therapy	Surgery; occasionally radiation if inoperable	Assorted systemic therapies with variable success (see text in Page 564)
Clinical course	Benign	Usually aggressive

LA, lymphadenompathy; LFTs, liver function tests.
Data compiled from: Weisenburger DD, Nathwani BN, Winberg CD, et al. Multicentric angiofollicular lymph node hyperplasia: a clinicopathologic study of 16 cases. *Hum Pathol* 1985;16:162–172; Frizzera G. Castleman's disease and related disorders. *Semin Diagn Pathol* 1988;5:346–364; Chronowski GM, Ha CS, Wilder RB, et al. Treatment of unicentric and multicentric Castleman disease and the role of radiotherapy. *Cancer* 2001;92:670–676; Oksenhendler E, Duarte M, Soulier J, et al. Multicentric Castleman's disease in HIV infection: a clinical and pathological study of 20 patients. *AIDS* 1996;10:61–67; Menke DM, Camoriano JK, Banks PM. Angiofollicular lymph node hyperplasia: a comparison of unicentric, multicentric, hyaline vascular, and plasma cell types of disease by morphometric and clinical analysis. *Mod Pathol* 1992;5:525–530; Frizzera G, Peterson BA, Bayrd ED, et al. A systemic lymphoproliferative disorder with morphologic features of Castleman's disease: clinical findings and clinicopathologic correlations in 15 patients. *J Clin Oncol* 1985;3:1202–1216; McCarty MJ, Vukelja SJ, Banks PM, et al. Angiofollicular lymph node hyperplasia (Castleman's disease). *Cancer Treat Rev* 1995;21:291–310; and Herrada J, Cabanillas F, Rice L, et al. The clinical behavior of localized and multicentric Castleman disease. *Ann Intern Med* 1998;128:657–662, with permission.

most of these cases show features consistent with plasma cell variant, and occasionally of the mixed variant. All cases of human immunodeficiency virus (HIV)-associated MCD are associated with HHV-8, compared with 40% to 50% in non-HIV-associated cases. The cases reported as MCD in the non-HIV+ population that are not associated with HHV-8 infection are likely a heterogeneous group of disorders, not related to either the unicentric or HHV-8+ cases.

Epidemiology

There is no gender preference, and the age distribution is bimodal, with patients with unifocal disease being in their 4th decade versus patients with multicentric disease in their 6th decade (6,10,11). CD occurs not uncommonly in the pediatric population (12). There are little data of the actual incidence or prevalence of this disorder. With the acquired immunodeficiency syndrome epidemic, the incidence has increased (13); but even in this population it is a rare condition, with MCD accounting for <2% of lymph node biopsies in patients infected with HIV (14).

Pathogenesis/Pathology

The pathogenesis of CD is not understood. Early on, it was thought that the hyaline vascular tumors were possibly hamartomas (15). However, most have speculated that CD is

a chronic inflammatory or immunologic process in reaction to an unknown stimulus (2,4). The hyaline vascular and plasma cell variants could then be explained by either a continuum of disease, a differential host-dependent immune response, or reactions to two different but closely related stimuli. Further speculation has revolved around which cell type (follicular dendritic cells, endothelial cells, lymphocytes, or plasma cells) drives the process (16). HHV-8 (also known as Kaposi sarcoma herpesvirus) is pathogenic in a subset of patients (13,17).

Nearly all HIV infection-associated MCD cases are associated with HHV-8, and nearly half of those MCD cases in patients without HIV are HHV-8 associated (18–22). HHV-8 is not associated with localized (unicentric) CD (23). In patients with MCD infected with both HIV and HHV-8, HHV-8 has been found in circulating mononuclear cells (13,24), bone marrow (25), in intranodal B lymphocytes, in endothelial cells, and in subcapsular spindle cell proliferations of Kaposi sarcoma. It has been postulated that a virus, for example, HHV-8, may infect immunoglobulin (Ig) M-positive naive B cells and drive them to differentiate into plasmablasts without undergoing the germinal center reaction (26). Alternatively, a putative virus could target both κ and λ light chain-expressing B cells without bias, with only λ cells expanding preferentially due to an intrinsic proliferative response to the viral infection.

The plasma cell variant of CD, in particular the multicentric cases, has long been thought to be related to overproduction of interleukin (IL)-6 and to some extent to hyperresponsiveness to IL-6 (27,28). The viral homologue of

IL-6 exhibits many of the biologic activities of human IL-6, but the relative importance of viral IL (vIL)-6 and human IL-6 has not yet been clarified. It appears, however, that the sites of expression of these two types of IL-6 are distinct. Human IL-6 expression can be localized to the germinal centers arising from the follicular dendritic cells, which are located outside the sinuses but in close contact with blood vessels and plasma cells (27,29), whereas vIL-6 is localized to the mantle zone and interfollicular regions emanating from lymphoid-derived cells (19,29,30).

Distinct from HHV-8 infection, overproduction of circulating cytokines has been implicated in the pathogenesis and symptomatology of MCD and the related entity polyneuropathy, organomegaly, endocrinopathy, monoclonal protein, and skin changes (POEMS) syndrome. Serum levels of IL-6 in patients with CD are significantly higher than those found in patients with lymphoid malignancies (31). Overexpression of IL-6 in mice produces a phenotype similar to the MCD phenotype (32). High IL-6 levels may contribute to the plasma cell infiltration of lymph nodes, polyclonal hypergammaglobulinemia, increased level of acute-phase proteins, and constitutional symptoms. Vascular endothelial growth factor is also elevated in patients with CD, but less so than in patients with POEMS syndrome (31).

Histopathology

Hyaline Vascular Variant

On gross examination these lesions tend to be large, single, rounded, encapsulated masses, more commonly found in central than peripheral lymph node regions. HV-CD usually involves lymph nodes or a group of lymph nodes (4,6). Most masses are between 5 and 10 cm, though lesions as big as 25 cm have been described. On microscopic examination, the hyaline vascular variant is characterized by capsular fibrosis with broad fibrous bands traversing through the lymph node, an increased number of lymphoid follicles scattered throughout cortex and medulla, with often more than one germinal center sharing the same mantle (so-called "twinning"). Mantles tend to be broad and composed by concentric rings of small lymphoid cells ("onion skin pattern") imparting a target-like appearance to the follicle (Fig. 38.1). Often the germinal centers are depleted of small lymphoid cells and are predominantly composed of dendritic cells with prominent hyaline deposits (periodic acid-Schiff stain positive). Sclerotic blood vessels penetrating within the germinal centers forming so-called "lollipop lesions" are observed. Dendritic cells within these depleted germinal centers can show dysplastic features (33). The interfollicular region is composed by prominent high endothelial venules (HEVs) with plump endothelial cells, often surrounded by clusters of PDCs and stromal proliferation (34). Plasma cells, immunoblasts, and eosinophils are also part of the interfollicular infiltrate; however, sheets of plasma cells, as seen in the plasma cell variant, are not seen (4,33,35,36).

Plasma Cell Variant

Gross examination often reveals multiple discrete lymph nodes, comprising the clinically observed "mass," in contrast to the single rounded mass that is typically seen with the hyaline vascular variant; however, single masses may also be observed (4,6). Microscopically, the plasma cell variant is distinguished by the presence of sheets of plasma cells in the interfollicular zone (Fig. 38.2) (4). The interfollicular region typically contains prominent HEVs, similar to cases of HV-CD. Cases that contain mature plasma cells without increased vascularity have been included within this entity (6), but care is needed to rule out other causes of plasmacytosis, such as chronic inflammation or autoimmune disease (4). Russell bodies in plasma cells are rare (37). Some eosinophils and mast cells may also be present. There is follicular hyperplasia with sharply defined mantles, polarized germinal centers, with frequent mitosis and histiocytes with nuclear debris. The degree of follicular hyperplasia varies within the lymph node. At least some follicles in many if not most cases have a hyaline vascular appearance (4,38).

Mixed Variant

Lymph nodes may have characteristics of both the hyaline vascular and plasma cell variants. Focal accumulations of plasma cells next to extensive areas without plasma cells are found in the interfollicular tissue (39). Characteristic lymphoid follicles with normal reactive germinal centers and regressed germinal centers are found in small areas.

Multicentric Castleman Disease

The majority of lymph node biopsies in patients with MCD show histologic features consistent with plasma cell variant, although rare cases of HV or mixed variants have been described (40). More distinctive features have been described in HHV-8 positive MCD (Fig. 38.3). In these cases, some of the reactive follicles show poorly defined mantle zones containing single or grouped large lymphoid cells (defined either as immunoblasts or plasmablasts). The latter cells are usually virally infected and are positive for HHV-8 latent-associated nuclear antigen (LANA)-1, and a subset is also positive for vIL-6. In addition, the virally infected cells invariably express IgM-λ but are polyclonal by gene rearrangement studies for the Ig heavy chain gene and show no evidence of somatic mutations (26,41). Based on these findings, the term plasmablastic variant of CD was proposed (41). These plasmablasts can form small clusters (microlymphoma) or confluent sheets (frank lymphoma); the microlymphomas can either be polyclonal or monoclonal by molecular genetic studies (26). Therefore, HHV-8 infection is associated with a range of lymphoproliferative lesions in patients with MCD and is targeting preferentially IgM-λ expressing naive B cells.

Because of the importance of recognizing HHV-associated CD, it is recommended that staining for HHV-8 LANA be performed in all cases of newly diagnosed CD of any morphologic type, whether localized or multicentric, as well as staining for Ig light chains, to detect λ-restricted plasmablasts, which may be morphologically inconspicuous.

About 75% of patients with MCD have hepatosplenomegaly. Splenic findings may include altered germinal centers, white pulp or marginal zone fibrosis, and prominent plasmacytosis (6,42). Splenic findings parallel those found in the lymph nodes, including the development of microlymphomas (26). Hyperplastic follicles and prominent polyclonal plasmacytosis have been described in the bone marrow of patients with MCD.

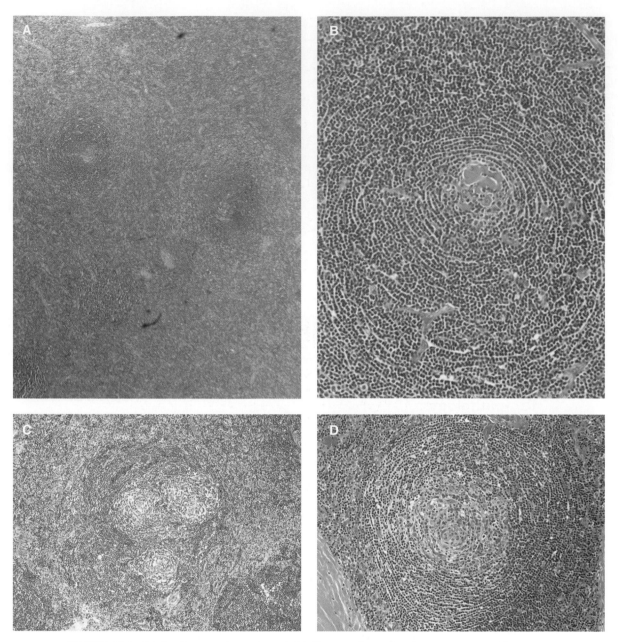

FIGURE 38.1. CD, hyaline vascular variant. **A:** Hyaline vascular variant low-power view with reactive follicles and an interfollicular infiltrate of small lymphoid cells and fibrosis, as well as increased vascularization of the interfollicular region. (Figures courtesy of Dr. Ahmet Dogan; reprinted with permission from Dispenzieri A. Castleman disease. *Cancer Treat Res.* 2008;142:293–330.) (see also Color Plate 84) **B:** High-power view showing the B-cell follicle with typical expanded mantle zone showing "onion skin" pattern and depleted germinal center with increased vascularity and deposition of hyaline material. (Figures courtesy of Dr. Ahmet Dogan.) (see also Color Plate 85) **C:** Some mantle zones contain two germinal centers ("twinning") (see also Color Plate 86). **D:** High magnification showing a regressed follicle with increased numbers of follicular dendritic cells and decreased germinal center cells. Note the penetrating blood vessel (**top**), the so-called "lollipop" follicle (see also Color Plate 87).

Clinical Findings

Although HIV-associated CD is not the focus of this chapter (see Chapter 35), CD associated with HIV differs from CD in the absence of HIV infection in the following ways: (a) it is more likely to be multicentric; (b) systemic symptoms are more common and more intense; (c) lymphadenopathy is more likely to be peripheral; (d) pulmonary symptoms are more prevalent; (e) leukopenia and thrombocytopenia are more common; (f) HHV-8 infection is virtually always present, often with clinical Kaposi sarcoma; (g) the histologic type is most commonly the mixed HV/Plasma cell (PC) variant; (h) there is a 15-fold increased risk of developing overt

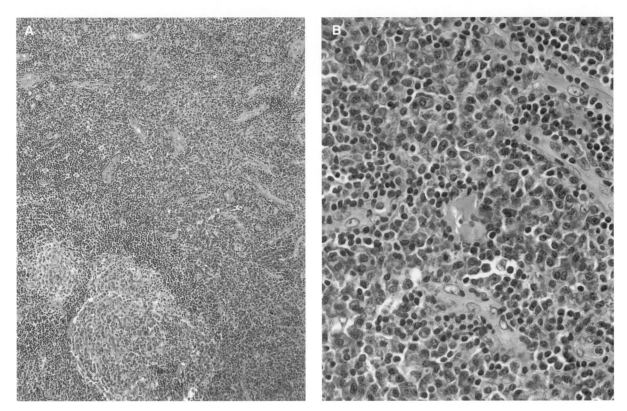

FIGURE 38.2. CD, plasma cell variant. **A:** Plasma cell variant low-power view with small reactive follicles and an interfollicular infiltrate of plasma cells; vascular proliferation is present in the interfollicular region (see also Color Plate 88). **B:** High-power view showing numerous plasma cells among HEVs. **Lower left corner:** A small part of a reactive follicle. (Figures courtesy of Dr. Ahmet Dogan.) (see also Color Plate 89)

malignant lymphoma; and (i) prognosis is dismal, with a median survival of 12 to 22 months (14,43,44).

The earliest studies of the clinical features of CD were limited by available imaging; perhaps for this reason, the majority of first-reported cases were mediastinal masses (4), detected either because of compressive symptomatology or a mass detected on routine chest radiography. The incidence of unicentric versus multicentric disease is confounded by the extent of imaging performed and by the lack of consistency in defining multicentric disease. Given the fact that CD changes can be seen in the spleen (5, 42), should the presence of splenomegaly upstage a patient to multicentric disease? In addition, there are reports in which distant lymph nodes contain only "reactive" tissues rather than CD (6,37,45) and other reports in which simultaneous but distant lymph nodes have discordant histology (5,7).

With these caveats in mind, there are generalizations that can be made about groups of patients with CD (Table 38.2). The most common systemic symptoms are malaise/weakness, fever, weight loss, night sweats, and anorexia (7,9,11,14,16,40,46–48). Although the earliest reports suggested that unicentric, hyaline vascular CD accounted for close to 80% of cases, a current estimate would be approximately 60%. Most masses occur in lymph node-bearing regions, but gastric, pulmonary, intramuscular, and pancreatic lesions have all been described. By imaging, lesions are often vascular appearing, may be heavily calcified, especially those found in the pelvis, and may be 18-fluoro-deoxyglucose-positron emission tomography avid (16).

Unicentric Castleman Disease

Nearly 90% of patients with unicentric disease have the hyaline vascular morphology. These patients often present with either compressive symptoms or a large incidental mass; however, nearly 40% of patients with localized CD have associated systemic symptoms, which promptly resolve after surgical extirpation of the solitary mass. Unicentric disease occurs most commonly in the mediastinum, cervical regions, and abdominal/pelvic cavity, but nasopharyngeal, orbital, dural, and oral occurrences have been described. Solitary subdiaphragmatic CD is often of the plasma cell variant and associated with systemic symptoms (4).

Laboratory tests may be completely normal, but anemia, hypergammaglobulinemia, and elevated sedimentation rate and liver function tests may be present, all of which promptly resolve after successful surgical removal of the mass.

Multicentric Castleman Disease

About 90% of cases of MCD are the plasma cell variant. Approximately 80% of patients with the plasma cell or the mixed variant have associated systemic symptoms, most commonly fatigue, fevers, night sweats, and weight loss. Hepatomegaly and/or splenomegaly occurs in 75% of patients. Laboratory abnormalities are common, including anemia, low ferritin levels, elevations of the sedimentation rate, antinuclear antibodies, fibrinogen, C-reactive protein (CRP), and liver transaminases, and an abnormal urinalysis. HHV-8 is found in MCD, but not in localized CD (in 100% of patients

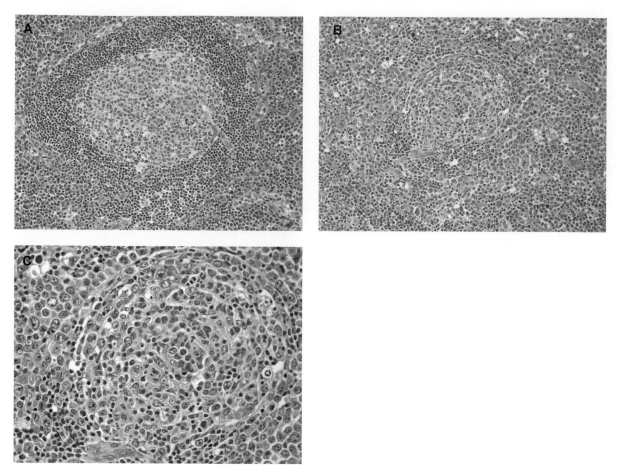

FIGURE 38.3. CD, HHV-8+ multicentric. Reactive follicle surrounded by numerous plasma cells. **A:** Regressed follicle surrounded by plasmablasts (microlymphoma) (see also Color Plate 90). **B:** Higher magnification of regressed follicle surrounded by plasmablasts (microlymphoma) (see also Color Plate 91). **C:** Plasmablasts in these cases express λ light chain and contain nuclear HHV-8 LANA (see also Color Plate 92).

positive for HIV and in about 40% to 50% of HIV-negative MCD cases) (18,19,23).

PARANEOPLASTIC SYMPTOMS AND SYNDROMES

There are number of paraneoplastic symptoms/syndromes also associated with CD, more commonly with the multicentric form (16,46,49). These include pleural effusions, pericardial effusions, ascites, anasarca, autoimmune hemolytic anemia, immune thrombocytopenic purpura, a multitude of renal disorders, including secondary (AA) amyloidosis or membranoproliferative glomerulonephritis, pulmonary abnormalities ranging from infiltrates to restrictive lung disease to lymphoid interstitial pneumonitis to bronchiolitis obliterans, and skin abnormalities ranging from rash to hyperpigmentation to paraneoplastic pemphigus to Behçet disease to Kaposi sarcoma (16). In one series over the course of the disease, 40% of patients developed central nervous system (CNS) signs, including seizures and aphasia (46). This finding should be tempered by the fact that a number of cases from the 1980s may have been acquired immunodeficiency syndrome-associated CD, which is known to have a particularly dismal prognosis (14). Neuropathy occurs in nearly 10% of patients, again more commonly those with

multicentric disease, but is also possible in patients with unicentric disease. When neuropathy is present, other features of POEMS syndrome should be sought, including a monoclonal protein and osteosclerotic bone lesions (16,40,47).

POEMS syndrome is a rare paraneoplastic syndrome most often associated with osteosclerotic myeloma. The defining features are *p*eripheral neuropathy, *o*rganomegaly (hepatosplenomegaly), *e*ndocrinopathy, *m*onoclonal gammopathy (λ light chain, usually Ig G), and *s*kin changes. Typically, there are sclerotic bone lesions. Other important features not included in the acronym include papilledema, extravascular volume overload, thrombocytosis, lymphadenopathy, and abnormal pulmonary function tests, not all of which are required to make a diagnosis (50). In many cases the lymph nodes of these patients have CD-like (51) or full-fledged CD histology, typically of the plasma cell variant (52–54).

Diagnosis

The diagnosis of CD requires pathologic analysis of a lymph node biopsy specimen. Because even MCD may not involve all lymph nodes, if an initial biopsy is negative, it is, therefore, imperative that more than one biopsy be performed if the clinical level of suspicion is high. Whenever possible, the biopsy should be performed at the site with the highest standard uptake values (SUV) on 18-fluoro-deoxyglucose-positron emission tomography examination. This diagnosis is virtually impossible to make based on a needle core biopsy or fine needle aspiration. HHV-8 immunostains (LANA-1 and vIL-6, both commercially available) should be done in all cases of HIV-associated CD, all cases of MCD, in all cases of the plasma cell variant, and in all cases of CD with systemic symptoms.

Once the diagnosis is made, besides a thorough review of systems (B symptoms, endocrinopathy, peripheral neuropathy) and physical examination (papilledema, skin changes), additional testing is required. Patients should have a complete blood count, erythrocyte sedimentation rate (ESR), CRP, liver function tests, serum creatinine, serum protein electrophoresis with immunofixation, IL-6, serology for HHV-8 and HIV, urinalysis, and computed tomography of the chest, abdomen, and pelvis. If there are any pulmonary symptoms, the threshold for performing pulmonary function tests should be low. If there is associated neuropathy, imaging of the bones should be done looking for sclerotic bone lesions. If elements of POEMS syndrome present, then more extensive endocrine testing should also be performed.

Differential Diagnosis

The differential diagnoses of CD are broad. Initially, hyaline vascular cases were most commonly confused with thymomas because the intrafollicular capillaries with thick hyalinized walls take on a concentric arrangement (the so called "onion skin appearance") that can be confused for Hassall corpuscle of the thymus (2). More often, hyaline vascular may be confused with other conditions in which there is regressive transformation of germinal centers such as angioimmunoblastic T-cell lymphoma, other atypical lymphoproliferative disorders, and advanced phases of HIV-related lymphadenopathy (38,46,47).

The plasma cell pattern, which may be associated with either immunoblastic proliferation and prominent HEVs or with mature plasma cells and no increase of the vascularity, may be seen in many other conditions, such as infection, autoimmune disease, primary or acquired immunodeficiencies, or in association with malignancies (38,46,47).

Course and Prognosis

The course of CD is variable. Typically cases of localized disease are cured by surgical resection. The multicentric form is more difficult to manage, and median survival has been reported to be as short as 26 months (7). Frizzera et al. (46) divided patients' courses into two categories: episodic and persistent. Those patients with more extensive disease (systemic symptoms, lymphadenopathy, hepatosplenomegaly, and effusions) were more likely to have the episodic pattern of evolution. These authors also found that male gender, episodic evolution, and predominantly proliferative morphology in involved lymph nodes were associated with worse survival in univariate analysis (46). Weisenburger et al. (7) described parsed the course for patients with MCD into five categories: (a) cure, (b) stable and persistent, (c) relapse and remission, (d) rapidly fatal disease, and (e) evolution to malignant lymphoma.

A prognostic model for survival was developed using the clinical information of 114 patients with CD. After adjusting for age, the multivariable model included organomegaly, respiratory symptoms, and an abnormal platelet count. Depending on whether patients had zero or one or more adverse factors, their 10-year survival rates were 80% (95% confidence interval 65% to 98%) and 41% (95% confidence interval 28% to 59%) (55).

Secondary malignancies are not uncommon in CD. Patients infected with HIV with HHV-8+ MCD are estimated to have a frequency of lymphoma of 15-fold compared with a population infected with HIV without CD (43). Patients negative for HIV with HHV-8+ MCD develop malignancies, most notably lymphoma (approximately 15%) (22,40,46,56,57), and Kaposi sarcoma, in up to one-third of the cases (46). Follicular dendritic cell sarcoma had reported in patients with the hyaline vascular variant of CD (50).

Therapy

Treatment options must be considered separately for three different disease presentations: (a) unicentric disease, (b) multicentric disease in patients not infected with HIV, and (c) HHV-8-associated multicentric disease in patients positive for HIV. Treatment for HIV-associated MCD is covered in Chapter 35.

Unicentric Castleman Disease

The treatment decision for unicentric disease, regardless of whether it is hyaline vascular, plasma cell variant, or mixed type, is straightforward: surgical removal whenever possible; if not possible, irradiation should be considered (16). For large tumors, embolization of solitary mass before surgical removal or neoadjuvant therapy has also been applied. Although there is a low rate of recurrence, these patients appear to have a higher risk of developing Hodgkin disease and non-Hodgkin lymphoma (NHL). A number of patients have seemingly done well with observation alone, but one must be vigilant about the subtle development and progression of associated paraneoplastic entities like bronchiolitis obliterans.

When there are paraneoplastic or autoimmune conditions associated with CD, these generally resolve within months of the surgery, most notably laboratory abnormalities like anemia, hypergammaglobulinemia, and high sedimentation rate, CRP, and liver function tests. If present, associated pemphigus often (58,59), but not always (60), improves within the year. Nonamyloidosis-related renal disease has also been reported to resolve within 12 months of surgical removal (61). Symptoms from associated AA amyloid typically improve over the ensuing years after removal of unicentric disease (62,63). Reports of the lack of recovery of bronchiolitis obliterans after definitive surgery (59,64) are difficult to interpret because it is unclear whether earlier intervention, that is at a lymphoid interstitial pneumonitis stage or before fibrosis, could reverse pulmonary changes.

Of the 22 patients with unicentric disease treated with irradiation that have been reported in the literature, 11 had a complete response, four had a partial response, six had no clinical response, and one had progressive disease (16). Even in those patients whose mass does not clearly shrink, the lymphocytes are depleted, and nuclear atypicality and hyperchromatism are seen in the plump endothelial cells of the proliferating capillaries (4).

MULTICENTRIC CASTLEMAN DISEASE NOT ASSOCIATED WITH HUMAN IMMUNODEFICIENCY VIRUS OR HUMAN HERPESVIRUS 8

The best choice of therapy for MCD is uncertain (16). Therapy to date has been corticosteroid and alkylator based. Small numbers of patients have been treated with alternative therapies like interferon (IFN)-α, thalidomide, rituximab, bortezomib, and anti-IL-6 receptor antibodies (Table 38.3). High-dose chemotherapy with hematopoietic stem cell transplantation has also been used with good effect in a limited number of cases.

Corticosteroids have clinical activity (9,11,47,48) and are not infrequently used to maintain the patient; it is unclear whether this strategy is in the best interest of these patients. Alkylators (cyclophosphamide or chlorambucil) have been used as single agent, along with low-dose prednisone (48,65), or as part of combination chemotherapy. Most reports of improvement are from individual or small case studies (9,11,47,48). Combination chemotherapy (10,44,66), including chlorambucil and prednisone, cyclophosphamide and prednisone, cyclophosphamide, vincristine, and prednisone ± doxorubicin (CHOP) or procarbazine, and rituximab with either cyclophosphamide, vincristine, and prednisone (67) or CHOP (66) have all been tried in patients with multicentric disease. High-dose chemotherapy with hematopoietic stem cell transplantation has also been used with good effect in five patients, three of whom had coexisting POEMS syndrome (45,54,68,69).

There is limited experience with anti-CD-20 antibodies in patients with CD. There is one report of benefit with single-agent rituximab in a young man with an aggressive form of CD with autoimmune hemolytic anemia and positive outcome (70). A man with orbital CD responded to single-agent rituximab (71). There are two single case reports of treating patients negative for HIV with relapsed CD with rituximab along with cyclophosphamide and prednisone with favorable response (67,72,73). Not only did the B symptoms and lymphadenopathy improve, but also the renal failure secondary to CD-related glomerulonephritis in one patient normalized after therapy.

IFN-α has been reported to control disease in five separate cases (74–78). Novel agents like thalidomide have been used with dramatic success in two patients (79,80). Bortezomib has been shown to improve the cytokine and biochemical profile in addition to clinical symptoms (81).

Reports of the use of cladribine in patients with CD are limited (82,83). In a series of three patients with CD, two patients responded with relapse-free survivals of 24 and 20 months. Both responding patients, however, later developed NHL (diffuse large B-cell lymphoma and peripheral T-cell NHL, respectively) (82). This brings into question that it accelerates the transformation of CD to lymphoma (82), reminiscent of the high risk observed in patients positive for HIV (43).

An attack on IL-6 or its receptor has been shown to have clinical utility, but so far there is no Food and Drug Administration approval available for patients (28,84,85). A humanized anti-IL-6 receptor antibody (rhPM-1; also known as MRA) has demonstrated benefit in 28 prospectively treated patients with MCD (85). Within 16 weeks of treatment, fatigue, lymphadenopathy, and all the inflammatory parameters were alleviated. Hemoglobin, albumin, and total cholesterol levels, high-density lipoprotein cholesterol values, and body mass index all increased significantly. Histopathologic examination revealed reduced follicular hyperplasia and vascularity after treatment (28). Eleven (73.3%) of 15 patients who had received oral corticosteroids before study entry were able to do well on a reduced corticosteroid dose (85). Ninety-six percent of patients remain on therapy for >3 years.

Somewhat surprisingly, on occasion localized therapies have provided clinical responses in patients with multicentric disease. There are six reports of using radiation in this setting with dramatic clinical benefit in five. In two of these cases, radiation of the dominant lymph node group resulted in nodal response at remote locations (86,87). Even in those patients in whom there was no clear response after irradiation, there was a histologic change, that is, depletion of lymphocytes and causing nuclear atypia and hyperchromatism in the plump endothelial cells of the proliferated capillaries (4). For those patients with POEMS syndrome, radiation to a solitary sclerotic lesion can have resolution of lymphadenopathy (40). In a similar vein, splenectomy has provided durable clinic in two patients with multicentric disease (Table 38.3) (46,88).

AUTOIMMUNE LYMPHOPROLIFERATIVE SYNDROME (CANALE SMITH SYNDROME)

The syndrome was first reported by Canale and Smith (89), who identified it as a syndrome of chronic lymphadenopathy simulating lymphoma. The relevance of the Fas apoptotic pathway to human disease was postulated by Sneller et al. (90) in 1992. They named the entity ALPS. They likened the phenotype seen in their two human patients to that seen in lpr and gld strains of mice, who are genetically deficient in expression of Fas or Fas ligand, respectively. The children, like the mice, had hypergammaglobulinemia, autoantibody production, glomerulonephritis, massive lymphoid hyperplasia, and expansion of an unusual population of T cells expressing the αβ T-cell receptor (TCR), but without either CD4 or CD8 expression (91). The hallmark of the ALPS is impaired lymphocyte apoptosis, which leads to accumulation of lymphoid mass and persistence of autoreactive cells.

Epidemiology

ALPS is a rare inherited syndrome without any obvious gender or racial predilection. The median age at presentation is approximately 24 months. Inheritance is most typically in an autosomal dominant fashion with variable penetrance (91). More recent data would suggest that ALPS is more likely to be monogenic in those instances in which the mutations affect the intracellular portion of Fas, but digenic or even oligogenic with mutations affecting different steps of the Fas signaling pathway (92).

TABLE 38.3

NOVEL TREATMENT STRATEGIES FOR PATIENTS WITH CD WHO ARE NOT INFECTED WITH HIV

Reference	Drug	No.	Outcomes
Jacobs et al., 2007 (219)	MTX	1	HHV-8+, patient with rheumatoid arthritis—remission × 54+ mo
Senanayake et al., 2003 (220)	Antiviral	1	No benefit from antiviral despite HHV-8
Ide et al., 2003 (71)	Rituximab	1	CR+ 10 mo
Ocio et al., 2005 (70)	Rituximab	1 mixed	CR of lymph node, hemolysis, and Raynaud at 14+ mo
Hudnall et al., 2003 (67)	Rituximab, CTX, Pred		CR of lymph nodes and constitutional symptoms; persistent hypergammaglobulinemia at 12+ mo
Abdou and Salib, 2004 (72)	Rituximab, CTX, Pred	1	CR of lymph nodes and acute renal failure at 24+ mo
Gholam et al., 2003 (73)	Rituximab after chemotherapy	1	PR 2 mo, but death secondary to AA amyloidosis
Bordeleau et al., 1995 (83)	2-CDA	2	1 unresectable HV received 2-CDA + XRT resulted in CR 9+ mo; 1 MCD had PR
Colleoni et al., 2003 (82)	2-CDA	3	2 patients with MCD had response lasting 20–24 mo; both patients evolved to NHL (DLBCL; PTCL); 1 unresectable unicentric HVV did not respond
Pavlidis et al., 1992 (74)	IFN-α	1	CR 11+ mo
Tamayo et al., 1995 (75)	IFN-α	1	CR 32+ mo
Strohal et al., 1998 (76)	IFN-α	1	CR of lymphadenopathy, B symptoms, and Bechet disease 25+ mo
Simko et al., 2000 (78)	IFN-α	1	Long-term disease stabilization (8+ y) in 11-y-old with Klinefelter syndrome and HCV
Andres and Maloisel, 2000 (77)	IFN-α	1	CR 42+ mo
Bowne et al., 1999 (10)	Suramin	1	CR 46+ mo
Starkey et al., 2006 (80)	Thalidomide	1	Near total resolution of all symptoms and LA 40+ mo
Lee and Merchant, 2003 (79)	Thalidomide	1	Improvement of ascites, anemia, albumin, CRP, platelet count, pulmonary hypertension at 13+ mo
Hess et al., 2006 (81)	Bortezomib	1	Improved anemia, constitutional symptoms, IL-6, CRP, but stable lymphadenopathy
Beck et al., 1994 (84)	Murine anti-IL-6 monoclonal Ab	1	Response while on therapy but rapid relapse upon cessation
Nishimoto et al., 2005 (85)	Humanized anti-IL-6 receptor Ab	28	Improvement of LA and B symptoms in all for 36+ mo
Repetto et al., 1986 (45)	ASCT	1	CR 15+ mo
Advani et al., 1999 (68)	ASCT	1	Failed steroids and chemotherapy but developed follicular lymphoma. CR 48+ mo after ASCT
Dispenzieri et al., 2004 (54)	ASCT	2	Associated POEMS syndrome; CR 13+ and 18+ mo
Ganti et al., 2005 (69)	ASCT	1	Associated POEMS syndrome; response of all manifestations × 24+ mo
George et al., 2003 (152)	ASCT	1	Associated AA amyloidosis, response
Lerza et al., 1999 (88)	Splenectomy	1	CR for 12+ mo for autoimmune hemolysis, systemic symptoms, and lymphadenopathy
Frizzera et al., 1985 (46)	Splenectomy	1	CR for 78+ mo

Ab, antibody; ASCT, autologous stem cell transplantation; 2-CDA, 2-chloro-deoxyadenosine; CR, complete response; CTX, cyclophosphamide; DLBCL, diffuse large B-cell lymphoma; HCV, hepatitis C virus; KS, Kaposi sarcoma; LA, lymphadenompathy; MTX, methotrexate; PR, partial response; Pred, prednisone; PTCL, peripheral T-cell lymphoma; XRT, radiation therapy.

Pathogenesis/Pathology

ALPS is generally due to mutations that affect apoptosis pathways. Type 0 ALPS is due to homozygous mutations of the Fas gene (tumor necrosis factor receptor SF6). ALPS is classified as type Ia when there is a heterozygous mutation of tumor necrosis factor receptor SF6. Heterozygous mutations of the FasL gene are labeled as ALPS Ib. When mutations are found in the caspase-10 gene, patients are classified as having ALPS type II. Those patients without any identifiable mutation, but with a functional deficiency of Fas-mediated apoptosis, are referred to as having ALPS type III (91). More recently, a homozygous mutational state of FasL has also been reported, prompting the authors to propose an ALPS Ic (93), but this nomenclature has been met with controversy (94). In addition, activating mutations of the NRAS gene have been suggested to cause ALPS, ALPS type IV (95). Coinheritance of mutations of Fas and caspase-10 has also been described (92).

Fas is a member of the tumor necrosis factor receptor super family and induces cell death upon triggering by FasL. Fas is highly expressed by activated lymphocytes, is responsible for limiting their clonal expansion, and for favoring peripheral tolerance. Aggregation of Fas, Fas-associated death domain protein, and caspase-8 forms the death inducing signaling complex, which induces cell apoptosis through the extrinsic and intrinsic apoptosis pathways. In humans, caspase-10 is recruited into the death inducing signaling complex to assist in activating the caspase cascade (92).

Mutations of the gene producing Fas are the most frequent in ALPS. Usually heterozygous, their penetrance depends on their effect on Fas function. Those mutations that affect the intracellular death domain of Fas, which is involved in the recruitment of Fas-associated death domain protein and caspase-8, are often the most severe (92). Those hitting the extracellular portion or causing haploinsufficiency, have weaker penetrance. Mutations in the caspase-10 gene may be deleterious or protective (96).

Histopathology

Pathologic examination of lymph nodes demonstrates follicular and paracortical hyperplasia and polyclonal plasmacytosis (Fig. 38.4) (97). There is an expansion of double-negative (CD4-, CD8-) α-β T cells in the paracortical regions of the lymph nodes. In addition, a decreased number of CD45RO memory T cells is often observed. The T cells may have an immature cytologic appearance, with enlarged nuclei and open chromatin. Cases may be diagnosed as peripheral T-cell lymphoma, unspecified in young children, based on the paracortical expansion/proliferation and presence of double-negative

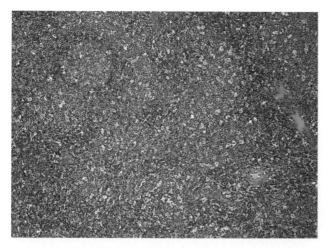

FIGURE 38.4. ALPS (see also Color Plate 93).

T cells, suggestive of an aberrant phenotype. Molecular studies reveal a polyclonal or occasionally oligoclonal pattern of T-cell receptor-gene rearrangement. Polyclonal plasma cells, small lymphocytes, and immunoblasts are also present (98).

Florid follicular hyperplasia is often present, but in some cases follicular involution akin to that seen in CD has been reported. Both increased percentage of proliferating cells and decreased apoptosis is seen. The splenic tissue reveals lymphoid hyperplasia of the white pulp with histologic features similar to those of the lymph nodes (91). In a subset of patients with ALPS type Ia, histologic features of SHML were noted, suggesting a possible association between these two disorders (99). Although Fas mutations were not identified in sporadic cases of SHML, a diagnosis of ALPS should be considered in children with SHML, especially when presenting with autoimmune manifestations and nodal disease.

Clinical Findings

ALPS presents in childhood (Table 38.4), although there have been rare reports of the syndrome presenting in adulthood (100). Nearly all patients have lymphadenopathy and splenomegaly (91). Two-thirds have hepatomegaly. The adenopathy can be massive or more subtle. More than 80% have autoantibodies, and nearly half have an associated autoimmune disease. Autoantibodies may be present in the absence of overt autoimmune disease. The most common autoantibodies are red cell antibodies and anticardiolipin antibodies. The

TABLE 38.4

CLINICAL FEATURES OF AUTOIMMUNE LYMPHOPROLIFERATIVE SYNDROME

Clinical features	Autoimmune lymphoproliferative syndrome (Canale Smith)
Age	Approximately 24 mo
Symptoms	Lymphadenopathy, autoimmune disease
LA	Yes, most commonly cervical
Organomegaly	Frequent hepatosplenomegaly
Laboratory abnormalities	Frequent hypergammaglobulinemia, autoantibodies; CD3 T cells double negative (CD4 and CD8)
Autoimmune phenomena	Often autoimmune hemolytic anemia, including occasional glomerulonephritis
Pathologic features	Paracortical expansion containing collections of CD3-positive T cells that are double negative for CD4 and CD8, as well as negative for CD45RO (97)
Molecular features	Mutations in genes for Fas, FasL, caspase-10, and possibly NRAS
Associations with infection	None identified as precipitant
Therapy	Supportive care, predominantly
Clinical course	Symptoms typically abate with age. Risk of autoimmune diseases. High risk for developing lymphoma.

LA, lymphadenompathy.

autoimmune manifestations include autoimmune hemolytic anemia, Guillain-Barré syndrome, urticarial rash, glomerulonephritis, and idiopathic thrombocytopenic purpura. Patients have hypergammaglobulinemia and lymphocytosis.

Diagnosis

Criteria for the diagnosis of ALPS have been defined (Table 38.5) (101). Most characteristic is a higher than normal number of double-negative (CD4-CD8-) α-β T cells in the peripheral blood, bone marrow, spleen, and lymphoid tissues. Patients with ALPS also have a lymphocytosis with a skewed T-helper-2 pattern of immune response, one manifestation of which is elevated circulating and tissue IL-10 levels (101).

Differential Diagnosis

The differential diagnosis includes lymphoma, hereditary spherocytosis, Evans syndrome, and Rosai-Dorfman disease (or SHML) (91,101). SHML can be seen in patients with ALPS, and it is considered part of the histologic spectrum in type 1A (99). In one instance, the disorder was confused with sarcoidosis (102).

Course and Prognosis

The first clinical presentation may either be lymphadenopathy or symptoms of autoimmune cytopenias. The most common autoimmune diseases are idiopathic thrombocytopenic purpura and autoimmune hemolytic anemia. Neutropenia is also not uncommon. Often symptoms abate with age. Those patients with a germline mutation of the intracellular domain of Fas have a significantly increase risk of developing B-cell lymphomas, comprising NHL (14-fold) and Hodgkin lymphoma (51-fold) of either nodular lymphocyte predominant or classic types (91,101).

TABLE 38.5

CRITERIA FOR THE DIAGNOSIS OF ALPS

Required features

1. Chronic generalized lymphadenopathy and/or splenomegaly
2. Increase in circulating double-negative T cells (CD4- CD8-) that express the $\alpha\beta$TCR above the normal range of 0.1% to 0.9% of lymphocytes (absolute counts normally 2 to 17 per μL)
3. Demonstration of decreased in vitro lymphocyte apoptosis

Supporting features

1. Family history of ALPS
2. Autoimmune phenomena, hypergammaglobulinemia
3. Typical findings on histopathologic analysis of lymph node or splenic tissue
4. Mutations of genes encoding Fas, FasL, or related apoptosis signaling proteins

Adapted from Rao VK, Straus SE. Causes and consequences of the autoimmune lymphoproliferative syndrome. *Hematology* 2006;11:15–23, with permission.

Therapy

Treatment is directed at life-threatening features of the disease rather than at the lymphadenopathy. No treatment reliably affects the lymphadenopathy or splenomegaly, although corticosteroids, azathioprine, cyclosporin, and mycophenolate have all been tried. Anecdotal reports of benefit using pyrimethamine have not been reproducible (101). The management of autoimmune cytopenias is the same as standard therapies used in other populations. Medical therapies include corticosteroids, intravenous Ig, intermittent filgrastim, rituximab and vincristine, and mycophenolate, as appropriate. Splenectomy to treat recurring and chronic cytopenias has resulted in up to a 75% long-term remission. The disadvantage of splenectomy is the risk of pneumococcal sepsis. Investigators at the National Institutes of Health recommend long-term antibiotic prophylaxis, repeated pneumococcal vaccination, low threshold for instituting intravenous antibiotics for significant febrile illness, and medical alert bracelets.

Allogeneic stem cell transplant has been used in patients with severe, refractory cytopenias, but cannot be recommended for the average patient given the relatively good prognosis of patients with ALPS and the high treatment-related mortality associated with allogeneic transplantation.

Surveillance for lymphoma is important, but not straightforward. The lymphadenopathy associated with the disease must be distinguished from that of lymphoma. Most patients with ALPS with lymphoma respond to conventional multi-agent chemotherapy and radiation. Again monitoring for relapse is challenging in distinguishing ALPS lymphadenopathy from recurrent lymphoma.

KIMURA DISEASE

Kimura disease is a rare chronic inflammatory disease that predominantly affects young adult men (103). Patients present with deep, subcutaneous nodules (most commonly in the head and neck region) associated with regional lymphadenopathy or salivary gland involvement. The entity was first described in the Chinese literature as eosinophilic hyperplastic lymphogranuloma; Kimura's description in 1948 prompted Iizuka et al. (104) to name it Kimura disease in 1959.

Epidemiology

Most reports are from Asia. Young men are those most likely to be affected (Table 38.6).

Pathogenesis/Histopathology

The etiology is unknown. Speculations include allergic reaction to either a microbe or toxin, or an abnormal autoimmune reaction. No consistent association with HHV-8 or Epstein-Barr virus (EBV) has been found. The presence of peripheral eosinophils, increased mast cells, and increased levels of IL-5 and IgE are consistent with a T-helper-2 type of response (105).

Key histologic features include a lymphoid infiltrate with reactive follicles with prominent germinal centers, plasma cells,

TABLE 38.6

CLINICAL FEATURES OF KIMURA DISEASE

Clinical features	Kimura disease
Age/gender	Young men from Asia
Symptoms	Subcutaneous nodules, with or without regional lymphadenopathy
Lymphadenopathy	Usually auricular, parotid regions
Organomegaly	Unusual
Laboratory abnormalities	Peripheral blood eosinophilia and elevated IgE levels
Autoimmune phenomena	Very rare
Pathologic features	Florid germinal center hyperplasia, eosinophilic infiltration, and post-capillary proliferation
Molecular features	None identified
Associations with infection	None identified
Therapy	Usually observation, surgical excision, radiation, corticosteroids, and pranlukast have all been used
Clinical course	Wax and wane

mast cells, and prominent eosinophils, with proliferation of HEVs, usually involving the subcutaneous tissue. Regional lymph nodes may be enlarged. They show florid reactive follicular hyperplasia, eosinophilic infiltration, and proliferation of high endothelial venules (Fig. 38.5). The germinal centers contain proteinaceous deposits and IgE reticular staining. Also characteristic are eosinophilic microabscesses sometimes involving the germinal centers, resulting in folliculosis, stromal sclerosis, and perivenular sclerosis (106).

Clinical and Laboratory Findings

The most common clinical presentation is a painless mass in the posterior auricular, periparotid, cervical, axillary, or inguinal regions. The nodular lesions are deep within the subcutaneous tissue, and clinically may mimic a neoplasm.

The masses can range from 1 to 11 cm (103,106). On occasion, isolated lymphadenopathy may be the initial presentation (107). Nearly three-quarters of patients will have regional lymphadenopathy (106). All patients have significant peripheral blood eosinophilia and elevated IgE levels.

Most patients do not have systemic symptoms. There have been occasional reports of pruritus, urticaria, and chronic eczema; however, the most common disease association is renal disease, most typically kidney disease (108).

Diagnosis/Differential Diagnosis

The diagnosis is made by biopsy of cutaneous or subcutaneous lesions, or enlarged lymph nodes. Kimura disease is clinicopathologically distinct from angiolymphoid hyperplasia with eosinophilia (also known as histiocytoid hemangioma), although in the Western literature, these two entities have often been confused (106,109). Clinically, both conditions present as a soft tissue swelling, most commonly arising in the head and neck region, and characterized by an indolent clinical course. However, angiolymphoid hyperplasia with eosinophilia is a vascular proliferation of blood vessels with prominent plump endothelial cells. This lesion is considered as part of the spectrum of vascular neoplasms so-called epithelioid or histiocytoid hemangiomas (low-grade vascular tumor). Their epidemiology also differs, with angiolymphoid hyperplasia with eosinophilia favoring females with no racial predilection. Other diseases in the differential diagnosis of Kimura disease in lymph nodes include Hodgkin lymphoma, angioimmunoblastic T-cell lymphoma, Langerhans cell histiocytosis, florid follicular hyperplasia, CD, dermatopathic lymphadenopathy, allergic granulomatosis of Churg and Strauss, lymphadenopathy of drug reactions, and parasitic lymphadenitis (106).

Course and Prognosis

The disease tends to wax and wane. In one study, eosinophilia >50%, serum IgE levels >10,000 IU per mL, or multifocal lesions outside the salivary glands appeared to predict for recurrence (110). The prognosis is generally favorable, with no reports of patients dying of the disease (106).

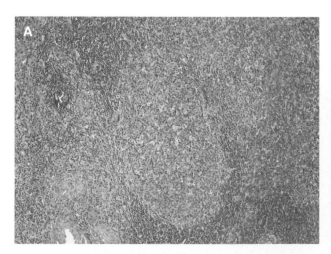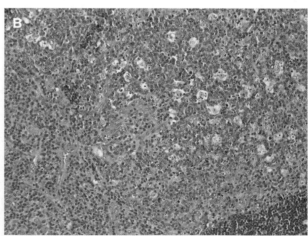

FIGURE 38.5. Kimura disease. **A:** Low magnification showing florid follicular hyperplasia (see also Color Plate 94). **B:** High magnification showing a follicle with numerous eosinophils (see also Color Plate 95).

Therapy

Surgical excision, corticosteroids, and radiation are the most common treatments employed. After local therapy, there is a risk of recurrence (103,106). In one series, complete clinical remission was observed in nearly two thirds of patients thus treated. Responses are rapid and for the majority, durable. There does not appear to be a dose response once doses delivered exceed 20 Gy (103). Steroids typically provide only temporary relief of swelling. Pranlukast, an LT-1 receptor antagonist, has also been reported to provide benefit in two children with Kimura disease (111).

CHRONIC ACTIVE EPSTEIN-BARR VIRUS INFECTION OF B, T, OR NATURAL KILLER CELLS

EBV is associated with numerous diseases, including Burkitt lymphoma, nasopharyngeal carcinoma, extranodal NK/T-cell lymphoma, aggressive NK-cell leukemia, lymphoproliferative diseases (LPDs) in patients with primary and secondary immunodeficiencies, as well as some cases of hemophagocytic syndrome and classic Hodgkin lymphoma (112,113). However, chronic EBV infection occasionally develops in subjects without an apparent immune defect.

A severe illness lasting >6 months ensuing after a primary EBV infection or associated with abnormal EBV antibody titers, characterized by prolonged fever, malaise, lymphadenopathy, splenomegaly, and by histologic evidence of organ disease such as pneumonitis, hepatitis, bone marrow hypoplasia, or uveitis, and demonstration of EBV antigens or EBV deoxyribonucleic acid in tissue was described in 2008 (112). In 1988, the name chronic mononucleosis syndrome was proposed (114). Most cases of this disorder in the United States are due to EBV infection of B cells. Patients who have CAEBV infection of B cells develop progressive cellular and humoral immunodeficiency with or without hemophagocytosis, and often die of opportunistic infections or a B-cell lymphoproliferative disorder. More recently, CAEBV infection has been reported to occur more frequently in Asia and Latin America, and in these cases, the virus infects T cells, NK cells, or both. CAEBV infection of T cells is a rare, severe disease with high morbidity and mortality, and the exact diagnostic criteria are not yet well defined, for which the term T/NK-cell CAEBV has been proposed. CAEBV of T or NK cells has been reported in the literature to encompass a heterogenous group of diseases, ranging from cutaneous forms, which may have an indolent clinical course and be preceded by a prodromal phase of polyclonal or oligoclonal expansion of EBV-infected T cells to extremely aggressive usually systemic forms, which are usually clonal. The term T/NK-cell CAEBV should not be used for at least two types of clonal EBV-associated T-cell disorders, namely systemic EBV-positive T-cell LPD of childhood, also known as fulminant EBV+ T LPD of childhood, and hydroa vacciniforme-like lymphoma, of T-cell derivation (1) (see Chapter 29). The term T/NK-cell CAEBV should be limited to protracted primary infections in early childhood, which are usually polyclonal, and may predispose to the development of EBV-associated T-cell malignancies.

According to Kimura (115), CAEBV of T-cell type is characterized by high fever, anemia, hepatomegaly, lymphadenopathy, and high EBV titers, which can often result in life-threatening complications. CAEBV involving NK cells also occurs more frequently in Asia and Latin America; it may be limited to the skin, and is associated with hypersensitivity to mosquito bites and elevated IgE levels. Patients with aggressive NK-cell leukemia, chronic lymphoproliferative disorders of NK cells, and extranodal NK/T-cell lymphoma, nasal type should not be considered part of CAEBV (1).

Epidemiology

Little is known about the epidemiology, but there appears to be a much higher incidence of the severe form associated with very high antibody titers to EBV-replicating antigens in Japan because virtually all of the literature regarding this entity is by investigators situated in Japan. It is most common in infants and children (112). In the Asian and Latin America populations, this entity affects T or NK cells, predominantly; in contrast, in Western countries, chronic EBV infection is predominantly within B cells.

Pathogenesis/Pathology

Morphologically, B-cell CAEBV shows many of the features observed in posttransplant lymphoproliferative disorders, with the presence of a polymorphic infiltrate composed of immunoblasts, plasmacytoid cells, and plasma cells. The number of EBV-positive cells by in situ hybridization varies from case to case and over time. Histologic progression to a polymorphic B-cell lymphoma can be seen.

The histologic changes observed in T-cell and NK-cell CAEBV are less well described; many published reports are in fact EBV+ T-cell lymphomas (112,116,117).

More recently, the CAEBV Study Group has offered a categorization of pathologic states of EBV-associated T/NK-lymphoproliferative disorders, trying to clarify that these disorders include polyclonal, oligoclonal, and monoclonal proliferations of cytotoxic T and/or NK cells (Table 38.7). However, each category may comprise different disease entities, and neither clinical presentation nor clonality is helpful in defining the clinical behavior and guiding the therapeutic approach. They describe a fulminant, clonal disorder

TABLE 38.7

CLASSIFICATION OF CAEBV LYMPHOPROLIFERATIVE DISORDERS

CAEBV classification (112)	Clonal proliferation of EBV infected cells
Category A1	Polyclonal
Category A2[a]	Oligoclonal/monoclonal
Category A3[a]	Chronic monoclonal peripheral T-cell or NK-cell lymphoma/leukemia
Category B[a]	Fulminant monoclonal peripheral T-cell or NK-cell lymphoma/leukemia

[a]Beyond the scope of this chapter but included for context.

(category B) and a spectrum of CAEBV-associated LPD (categories A1–A3). Category B is the same as what had previously been called the infantile fulminant EBV-associated T-LPD. A1–A3 include a spectrum of lymphoproliferative disorders, from a polymorphic LPD composed of T cells or NK cells without clonal proliferation of EBV-infected cells (A1), to a polymorphic LPD with clonal proliferation of EBV-infected cells (A2), to a monomorphic NK or T-cell lymphoma/leukemia with clonal proliferation of EBV-infected cells (A3). This categorization emphasizes the importance of documenting the presence or absence of clonality (112).

Clinical and Laboratory Findings

CAEBV of all types is characterized by persistent or recurrent infectious mononucleosis-like symptoms, such as fever, uveitis, swelling of lymph nodes, and hepatosplenomegaly (Table 38.8). Marrow hypoplasia, interstitial pneumonia, and persistent hepatitis, often to the point of hepatic failure, are also frequently seen. The syndrome may persist for months or years and has a relatively high fatality rate (118).

Patients may have anemia, thrombocytopenia, lymphocytopenia or lymphocytosis, neutropenia, and polyclonal gammopathy. The most important diagnostic criteria (112,119) include extremely high titers of antibodies to EBV-related antigens: IgG to viral capsid antigen must be at least 1:640 and may be >1:5,120; and anti-early antigen ≥1:160, but may exceed 1:640. The EBNA-1 titer is typically low to undetectable. Detection of increased EBV genome (at least $10^{2.5}$ copies per mg in peripheral blood mononuclear cells) is also important for the diagnosis.

TABLE 38.8

CLINICAL FEATURES OF CAEBV, CATEGORY A1

Clinical features	CAEBV, category A1
Age/gender	Asian infants and children
Symptoms	Recurrent infectious mononucleosis-like symptoms, like fever and uveitis
Lymphadenopathy	Yes
Organomegaly	Hepatosplenomegaly
Laboratory abnormalities	Cytopenias, hypergammaglobulinemia, high EBV-related antigen titers
Autoimmune phenomena	No, but can be associated with
Pathologic features	Reactive appearance, with hyperplasia of the paracortical area and/or lymph node follicles with a mild increase in transformed lymphocytes in the paracortex
Molecular features	None identified
Associations with infection	EBV
Therapy	No known effective treatment. Anecdotal experience with antiviral, immunomodulators, and allogeneic hematopoietic stem cell transplantation.
Clinical course	May persist for mo to y. High fatality rate. May evolve into frank NK- or T-cell lymphoma/leukemia

Diagnosis

There are no internationally recognized diagnostic criteria, but criteria have included (112,119): (a) EBV-related illness or symptoms for >3 months, including fever, persistent hepatitis, extensive lymphadenopathy, hepatosplenomegaly, pancytopenia, uveitis, interstitial pneumonia, hydroa vacciniforme, or hypersensitivity to mosquito bites; (b) no evidence of any prior immunologic abnormalities or of any other recent infection that might explain the condition; and (c) increased quantity of EBV genome or elevated levels of EBV antibodies. An increased quantity of EBV genome is defined as: EBV-deoxyribonucleic acid in tissues or peripheral blood samples by Southern blot hybridization; Epstein-Barr-encoded ribonucleic acid 1+ cells in tissues or peripheral blood samples; and at least $10^{2.5}$ copies per mg in peripheral blood mononuclear cells. Elevated levels of EBV antibodies are defined as viral capsid antigen-IgG >640 or early antigen-IgG >160.

Differential Diagnosis

Severe CAEBV infection of T or NK-cell type must be differentiated from chronic EBV infection of B-cell type, EBV reactivation, and EBV-positive frank lymphomas. Autoimmune disease and non-EBV infectious disease may result in EBV reactivation, but they are differentiated from severe CAEBV infection by clinical and laboratory findings and clinical history. In primary, secondary, or iatrogenic immunodeficiencies, EBV reactivation may occur and cause lymphoproliferative disorders, but the clinical history is diagnostic (112).

Course and Prognosis

In CAEBV of T/NK-cell types, the course and prognosis are partially dependent on whether the disease is clonal or not. In one series the approximate overall median survivals for categories A1 and A2 (polyclonal and oligoclonal) were 8 and 6 years, respectively, whereas median overall survival rates for categories A3 and B were approximately 5 and 0.5 years (112). Patients with clonal NK-cell disease appear to fare better than those with clonal T-cell disease, with respective 5-year overall survival rates of 87% and 59% (118). In a survey of 82 patients in Japan, 35 patients had died, with the cause of death including malignant lymphoma/leukemia of T- or NK-cell type, hemophagocytic syndrome, and multiple organ failure. EBV-induced hemophagocytic syndrome is a severe multiorgan, inflammatory disease provoked by massive inflammatory cytokine elaboration and, in some cases, clonal lymphocyte expansion induced by EBV infection. Patients may develop interstitial pneumonia, coronary artery aneurysm, and CNS involvement (119).

Therapy

Treatment with antiviral, immunosuppressive, or immunomodulatory treatments has been tried, but most typically without significant benefit (120). Ganciclovir (121), IFN-γ (122), and IL-2 (123) have anecdotally been reported to provide benefit. Allogeneic bone marrow transplantation has been used in 15 patients with this disorder (119). Seven patients died within 16 months of transplant, with a median time to death of 5 months.

ROSAI-DORFMAN DISEASE OR SINUS HISTIOCYTOSIS WITH MASSIVE LYMPHADENOPATHY

Rosai-Dorfman disease or SHML is a histiocytic disorder of unknown etiology, which was first recognized in the 1960s (124) and is believed to be nonneoplastic, but may mimic lymphoma clinically (125,126). It is characterized by a nonmalignant proliferation of distinctive histiocytic cells within lymph node sinuses and extranodal sites (Table 38.9). The entity has been called histiocytose lipidique ganglionnaire pseudotumorale de Destombes as well as malignant reticuloendotheliosis (124). A registry developed by Drs. Juan Rosai and Ronald Dorfman to collect and catalog cases of SHML has improved our understanding of this disorder (124,127).

TABLE 38.9

CLINICAL FEATURES OF ROSAI-DORFMAN DISEASE (SHML)

Clinical features	SHML
Age	Childhood, adolescent
Symptoms	Massive painless cervical lymphadenopathy. Viral prodrome with fever not unusual. Extranodal involvement in nearly half of patients with infiltrates in skin, soft tissue, nasopharynx, orbit, and/or bone
Lymphadenopathy	Most commonly cervical, but other lymph node regions may also be involved
Organomegaly	Uncommon
Laboratory abnormalities	Frequent hypergammaglobulinemia, high ESR, and anemia
Autoimmune phenomena	In approximately 10% of patients; glomerulonephritis is rare
Pathologic features	Lymph node architecture is usually preserved; histiocytic infiltrate comprised of histiocytes with abundant eosinophilic cytoplasm, enlarged round-to-oval nuclei with distinct nucleoli, emperipolesis, and strong cytoplasmic staining for S-100.
Molecular features	None identified
Associations with infection	No clear association, but possible association with herpes viruses, Brucella and Klebsiella
Therapy	Usually none other than diagnostic surgical excision, but for progressive disease, corticosteroids, chemotherapy, and radiotherapy have been used.
Clinical course	Usually self-limited, lasting <9–18 mo. Rare transformation to hematopoietic malignancy

Epidemiology

According to the registry data, there is no specific gender, ethnic, or socioeconomic predilection. Blacks and whites are equally predisposed, but it appears to be less common in individuals of Asian descent. The original registry data would suggest that the most common age for presentation is in children and adolescents (127), but small series have included patients in their 5th to 7th decades (128,129).

Pathogenesis

Although the cause of SHML is unknown, viral and immune causes have been postulated. Occult chronic infection or an aberrant exaggerated immune response to an antigen causes proliferation of histiocytes. EBV does not appear to be a likely candidate because, although serologic evidence of EBV has been documented (130) in some cases tested, no evidence of latent or lytic EBV infection has been identified within the histiocytes (131). The role that HHV-6 infection plays in the disease is unclear. Two series demonstrated a higher than expected rate of involvement by HHV-8 (132,133), but another study has not (129). Most recently, parvovirus B19 capsid proteins (VP1/VP2) have been demonstrated in lymphocytes in some cases (128).

Histopathology

Lymph nodes are yellow-white, with capsular and pericapsular fibrosis. Normal lymph node architecture is preserved, with effacement seen only in those patients with long-standing lymphadenopathy (127,134). The most typical picture is that of an expansion of lymph node sinuses by histiocytes, which have large round or oval vesicular nuclei with well-defined delicate nuclear membranes and a single prominent nucleolus (Fig. 38.6). The characteristic finding of this disorder is emperipolesis, which is defined as penetration and movement of cells within another cell. Lymphocytes, plasma cells, neutrophils, or erythrocytes are found within the cytoplasm of histiocytes, and appear to be viable, rather than being destroyed by the histiocytes, in contrast to true phagocytosis.

The histiocytes have abundant pale eosinophilic cytoplasm, or on occasion, histiocytes with foamy cytoplasm may predominate. Mitoses are not seen. The histiocytes stain for S-100 protein, a characteristic marker for interdigitating dendritic cells in lymph nodes and Langerhans cells in skin, but that may also stain normal sinus histiocytes. In distinction from Langerhans cells, the histiocytes of SHML are negative for CD1a (124). SHML histiocytes express pan-macrophage antigens (CD68, HAM 56, cD14, CD64, CD15, and EBM11), antigens associated with lysosomal activity (lysozyme, a1-antitrypsin, a1-antichymotrypsin), immune activation (transferrin receptor, IL-2 receptor), and a pattern of adhesion molecules characteristic of circulating monocytes (CD11b, CD11c, CD18, CD62L, and CD103) (124). CD22, CD31, acid phosphatase, and nonspecific esterase are also expressed (124,134). SHML histiocytes do not express CD21, CD23, or CD35, which are markers of dendritic cell differentiation (124).

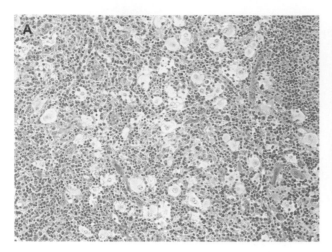
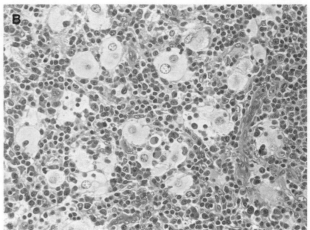

FIGURE 38.6. SHML. **A:** Low magnification (see also Color Plate 96). **B:** High magnification (see also Color Plate 97).

Lymphocytes and plasma cells are prominent in the inter-sinusoidal spaces, but eosinophils are absent or rare, which helps distinguish SHML from Langerhans cell histiocytosis, and Hodgkin or T-cell lymphoma. The extranodal histopathology is quite similar with the exception of more fibrosis and less emperipolesis than in the nodal tissues (135).

Classic features of SHML have been described in ALPS type 1A lymph nodes. In these cases, the degree of involvement varied from focal to extensive (99), occasionally obscuring the presence of double-negative T cells.

Clinical Findings

The typical presentation is characterized by massive bilateral, painless cervical lymphadenopathy, which may be isolated or associated with generalized adenopathy (127). Axillary, para-aortic, inguinal, and mediastinal lymph nodes are affected in nearly half of patients. A viral prodrome may precede the condition. Fever is frequent, and weight loss may occur. Extranodal disease is seen in 43% of patients, in some without lymphadenopathy, which may or may not develop during the course of the disease. The most commonly affected extranodal sites are skin, soft tissue, nasopharynx, eye/orbit, and bone. The cutaneous presentations are most commonly papules, nodules, and plaques, varying with the duration and depth of the lesions (136). Occurrences have been reported in salivary glands, CNS, genitourinary tract, and respiratory tract. Hepatosplenomegaly is uncommon. Visceral involvement is associated with a worse outcome (127).

Laboratory Findings

Patients frequently have signs of inflammation, such as normocytic or microcytic anemia. Up to 90% have an elevated ESR and polyclonal hypergammaglobulinemia. Bone marrow examination is typically uninformative; histiocytic proliferation is not a typical feature of iliac crest bone marrow biopsy. The most frequent immune dysfunction is autoimmune hemolytic anemia. Polyarthralgia, rheumatoid arthritis, glomerulonephritis, asthma, and diabetes mellitus have also been reported in association. Occasionally, the rheumatoid

factor or antinuclear antibody will be positive. A reversal of CD4/CD8 ratio has also been described (124,127). In light of the association with ALPS, cases presenting with autoimmune symptoms, especially autoimmune hemolytic anemia and glomerulonephritis, should be evaluated for the possibility of underlying ALPS with evaluation of peripheral blood for double-negative α β T cells (99).

Differential Diagnosis

Histiocytic disorders, particularly Langerhans cell histiocytosis, must be distinguished from SHML affecting the skin, soft tissue, and bone. Other diagnoses in the histologic differential are histiocytic sarcoma, Gaucher disease, classic Hodgkin lymphoma, metastatic melanoma and carcinoma, ganglioneuroblastoma, and infections caused by histoplasma and mycobacteria (124).

Course and Prognosis

Affected individuals may have massive bilateral cervical lymphadenopathy, fever, and mild anemia but do not appear ill. The disease is often self-limited, but the course of the disease is influenced by the degree of coexistent immune impairment or dysfunction (134,137). In the registry study, approximately 10% of affected children had underlying immunologic disorders, including Wiskott-Aldrich syndrome, autoimmune hemolytic disease, polyarthritis, glomerulonephritis, or severe pneumonia (137). These same patients were at higher risk for death, but the cause was most commonly linked to the underlying immune disorder.

For most patients, lymph node enlargement usually progresses for weeks to months, reaches a maximum, and then gradually recedes so that most patients have little or no residual evidence of disease 9 to 18 months after onset (127). Some patients have persistent lymphadenopathy but stable disease; other patients have progressive disease and may have a fatal outcome. The latter patients usually have an accompanying immunologic disease and/or widespread nodal involvement that may encroach on vital organs.

Foucar et al. (127) did not find an association with malignant tumors in their original series of 215 cases, but they subsequently reported development of NHL, myeloma, or Hodgkin lymphoma in rare cases (138–140). SHML has been reported in patients previously treated for lymphoid malignancy (141).

Therapy

Most patients require no therapy other than excisional biopsy for diagnosis because the disease usually regresses within approximately 18 months (124,127,136,142). For progressive disease, glucocorticoids, cytotoxic agents, radiotherapy, and antibiotics have been used but have no consistent effect on disease duration (127,143). Single-agent chemotherapy has anecdotally resulted in benefit, including corticosteroids, vinca alkaloids, acyclovir, IFN-α, thalidomide, rituximab, and cladribine (143–147). Combination chemotherapy has also resulted in response but cannot be recommended on a routine basis given the typically benign course of SHML.

Radiation therapy results in complete or partial response in less than one third of patients (143). The most common indications were spinal cord compression or respiratory embarrassment. The responses, even at higher doses of radiation, were inferior to those expected with hematologic malignancies. Surgical excision of masses compromising critical organ function often is successful (143,145).

KIKUCHI-FUJIMOTO DISEASE

Kikuchi-Fujimoto disease, also known as histiocytic necrotizing lymphadenitis, is a benign, self-limited disease of unknown etiology (148). It was first described separately by Kikuchi and Fujimoto in Japan, and subsequently cases have been recognized worldwide (149).

Epidemiology

Among the 330 cases of Kikuchi-Fujimoto disease in PubMed between 1991 and 2007, 77% were female, and 70% were <30 years of age (148), with the majority in their 20s. Fifty percent of cases were reported from East Asa and the Far East, 27% from Europe, and only 7% from the United States.

Pathogenesis/Histopathology

The etiology is unknown, although a viral or autoimmune pathogenesis has been suggested (Table 38.10). Authors have proposed associations with EBV, *Cytomegalovirus*, varicella-zoster, HHV-6, HIV, *Yersinia enterocolitica*, and *Toxoplasma*, but there is still no compelling association (150–152). Most recently, Zhang et al. (153) have implicated B19 infection as a causative agent. The histopathologic features are very similar to those of lupus lymphadenitis, and cases that have been reported in patients with systemic lupus lymphadenitis are likely cases of lupus lymphadenitis misdiagnosed as Kikuchi disease, rather than representing a true association.

TABLE 38.10

CLINICAL FEATURES OF KIKUCHI-FUJIMOTO DISEASE

Clinical features	Kikuchi-Fujimoto disease
Age/gender	Young adults, with possible predilection for females
Symptoms	Cervical lymphadenopathy, fever and upper respiratory tract symptoms; uncommonly, associated rash, arthralgias, myalgia. Very rare neurologic symptoms.
Lymphadenopathy	Most commonly painful, unilateral involvement of posterior cervical chain
Organomegaly	<10% of patients
Laboratory abnormalities	Occasional leukopenia, thrombocytopenia, elevated ESR, abnormal liver function tests
Autoimmune phenomena	Positive ANA common; speculation whether a self-limited systemic lupus erythematosus
Pathologic features	Focal necrosis in cortical and para-cortical areas of the lymph node. Infiltrate of histiocytes, CD8-positive T cells, and plasmacytoid monocytes; there is an absence of polymorphonuclear leukocytes.
Molecular features	None identified
Associations with infection	None identified
Therapy	None recommended
Clinical course	Usually self-limited–only 3 mo

ANA, antinuclear antibody.

At low magnification, the lymph node architecture is distorted by patchy circumscribed or confluent lesions in the paracortex (Fig. 38.7). These foci appear pale on low magnification, and on higher magnification, contain varying numbers of histiocytes, small lymphocytes and immunoblasts, karyorrhectic and granular eosinophilic debris, and sometimes coagulative necrosis. By definition, there is an absence of polymorphonuclear leukocytes (149,154).

The histiocytic component is characterized by phagocytic cells, often with crescentic nuclei, and cytoplasm containing abundant nuclear debris. The histiocytic component is characterized by the granular cytoplasmic expression of the CD68 antigen. The lymphoid component contains a mixture of lymphocytes and immunoblasts, both of which are predominantly CD8-positive T cells (154). Also seen are variable numbers of PDCs, which have slightly basophilic cytoplasm and eccentric nuclei with dispersed chromatin. They express CD4, CD123, CD31, CD36, CD43, CD68, CD74, and CLA/HECA452, and are found in proximity to HEVs (154). PDCs secrete large amounts of type I IFN and drive T-helper-1 T-cell polarization.

Kuo (155) has described three histologic stages of Kikuchi-Fujimoto disease: proliferative, necrotizing, and xanthomatous. The most common type is the necrotizing, whereas approximately one-third are proliferative, and about 20% are xanthomatous.

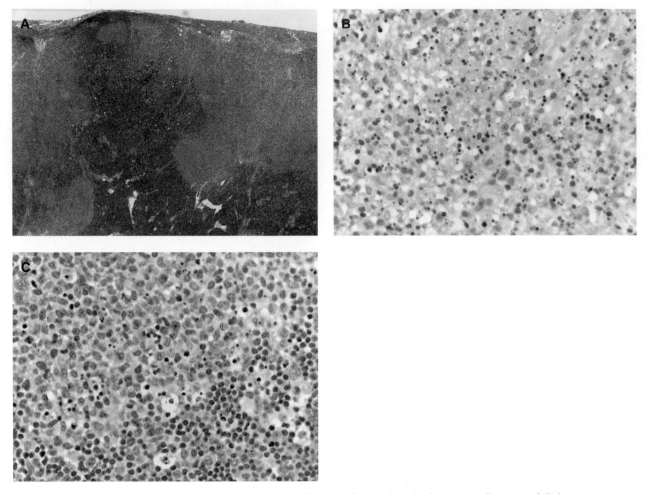

FIGURE 38.7. Kikuchi disease. **A:** Low magnification of a lymph node shows a small reactive follicle and marked paracortical expansion with extensive necrosis (hematoxylin and eosin, 2.5×) (see also Color Plate 98). **B:** Higher magnification of an area of necrosis shows amorphous eosinophilic material with nuclear debris but no neutrophils. Numerous histiocytes are present, many of which have eccentric, crescent-shaped nuclei (hematoxylin and eosin, 40×) (see also Color Plate 99). **C:** A collection of PDCs is present adjacent to an area of necrosis (hematoxylin and eosin, 40×) (see also Color Plate 100).

Clinical and Laboratory Findings

Kikuchi disease most typically presents as a self-limited syndrome (lasting only 3 months) characterized by cervical lymphadenopathy, which may be painful (148). Unilateral involvement of the posterior cervical group is the most common presentation. Only 5% had generalized lymphadenopathy. Thirty-five percent of patients presented with fever, and ≤10% patients experienced rash, splenomegaly, fatigue, arthralgias, myalgias, or weight loss. The repertoire of cutaneous lesions includes macules, papules, plaques, and nodules. As many as 5% of patients may have neurologic symptoms, including aseptic meningitis, mononeuritis multiplex, or photophobia. The most common laboratory abnormalities include leukopenia, elevated sedimentation anemia, abnormal liver function tests, positive antinuclear antibody, and thrombocytopenia. Hemophagocytic syndrome is reported in 3% of the cases.

An association with systemic lupus erythematosus has been reported in 13%, and other connective tissue disorders in 10% of cases of Kikuchi disease (148,149). However, the pathologic features of lupus lymphadenitis may be indistinguishable from that of Kikuchi disease, and a diagnosis of Kikuchi disease should not be made in a patient with known or suspected connective tissue disease.

Diagnosis/Differential Diagnosis

The diagnosis is made by histopathologic examination of a lymph node biopsy. The differential diagnosis includes systemic lupus erythematosus, toxoplasmic lymphadenitis, infectious mononucleosis, cat scratch disease, and lymphoma. The presence of granulocytes in areas of necrosis and the finding of hematoxylin bodies are diagnostic of lupus lymphadenitis but may not be present in that disorder. For this reason, in any patient with a histopathologic diagnosis of Kikuchi disease evaluation for evidence of connective tissue disease should be recommended.

NHL may be suspected in cases of the proliferative phase, when immunoblasts are numerous. Morphologic clues to the diagnosis of Kikuchi disease include: (a) a sprinkling of karyorrhectic debris throughout the node, (b) PDCs as well as histiocytes associated with the immunoblasts, (c) enlarged mottled T-zone areas, and (d) preservation of residual lymphoid architecture (156).

Course and Prognosis

Most cases improve within a 3- to 6-month period (148,149). Despite its usually benign course, some cases have had a fatal outcome (149,157,158). The recurrence rate has been reported to be approximately 3% to 4% (159).

Therapy

It most commonly resolves within 3 months, and relapse is unusual. No specific therapy is recommended.

PROGRESSIVE TRANSFORMATION OF GERMINAL CENTERS

PTGCs was originally described by Muller-Hermelink and Lennert (160) in 1978, and represents a reaction pattern often seen in association with follicular hyperplasia.

Epidemiology

It is difficult to establish the true incidence of PTGCs; it is estimated to occur in about 3.5% to 10% of lymph nodes with chronic lymphadenitis (161–163).

Pathogenesis and Histopathology

The etiology and pathogenesis are unknown; it may represent one of the possible evolutions of germinal center reaction or an arrest in the transition between primary and secondary follicles (164). PTGCs is characterized by the presence of large lymphoid nodules often two or three times the size of a reactive secondary follicle (Fig. 38.8). The mantle zones are thickened, and the small lymphocytes migrate into the germi-

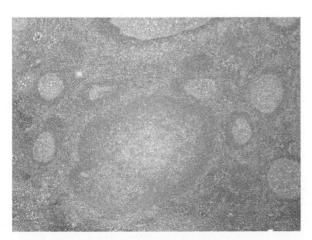

FIGURE 38.8. PTGC (see also Color Plate 101).

nal centers, disrupting this architecture. These changes are usually focal and are associated with reactive follicular hyperplasia. Epithelioid histocytes can be seen in association with PTGC, particularly in children. Due to histologic similarities with nodular lymphocyte predominance Hodgkin lymphoma (NLPHL), early studies have postulated an association between these two disorders; however, this association has not be confirmed in subsequent studies, especially in pediatric patients and young adults (162,163,165). "Popcorn cells," typical of NLPHL, are not identified.

Clinical Findings

PTGCs presents most commonly as localized adenopathy in asymptomatic young adults (peak incidence in the second decade), but it can also occur in children. It shows a striking male predominance. Cervical and axillary lymph nodes are the most common sites. Local recurrence is quite frequent, especially in children.

Differential Diagnosis

The main differential diagnosis is with NLPHL. Both tend to present as localized adenopathy and to recur often at the same site. Histologically, like in PTGC, NLPHL shows a macronodular growth pattern, but in general these nodules tend to expand and compress the surrounding parenchyma, and usually are not associated with florid follicular hyperplasia. PTGCs lacks the neoplastic "popcorn cells" or L and H cells. Follicular lymphoma, floral variant, can also be considered in the differential diagnosis.

Therapy

Surgical excision is often curative. Patients with recurrent disease should be followed up closely, and persistent lymph nodes should be excised.

BLASTIC PLASMACYTOID DENDRITIC CELL NEOPLASM

Blastic PDC neoplasm is a clonal disease characterized by the proliferation of immature or precursors of PDCs, also called plasmacytoid monocytes or IFN-I producing cells. Hallmarks of the disease include initial presentation in skin and a high risk of bone marrow dissemination. Although the initial clinical presentation appears indolent, the disease has a poor prognosis and a high risk of relapse following therapy. The cells show coexpression of CD4 and CD56 with a lack of lymphoid and myeloid markers (with exception of possible low levels of CD33 expression). In the World Health Organization classification of 2001, this tumor was referred to as blastic NK-cell lymphoma (166). An alternative term that has been used in the literature is CD4+/CD56+ hematodermic neoplasm, a term that is descriptive of the characteristic phenotype of these cells (167). Morphologically the cells resemble lymphoblasts, and, therefore, it is not surprising that this disease was initially felt to be of lymphoid origin.

Skin is the most common site of presentation, and lymphoma is virtually always in the differential diagnosis. The neoplasm is now included in the 2008 World Health Organization classification as blastic PDC neoplasm (1).

Historical Background and Biology of Plasmacytoid Dendritic Cells

The cell we now recognize as a PDC has had a long history with much uncertainty about its lineage. During the 1980s, several different names were proposed, including "*plasmacytoid T-cell*" (168), "*plasmacytoid T-zone cell*" (169), and "*plasmacytoid monocyte*" (170). However, there were few clues on the functions of this cell and its developmental relationship to other hematopoietic cells until the late 1990s. Subsequent studies revealed the capacity of this cell to produce high levels of type I IFN (IFN-I), and to differentiate in vitro into dendritic cells or cells with a dendritic appearance. These studies prompted new terms, including *IFN I-producing cell* (171,172) and PDC (173). Still, it was debated whether PDCs belonged to the myelomonocytic or lymphoid cell lineage (174–177). PDC derives from CD34-positive hematopoietic

precursors (178), and Flt3-ligand is the main cytokine for their development and mobilization into the peripheral blood (179). A relationship with the myelomonocytic lineage was initially suggested by the immunophenotype of PDC, and the expression CD13 and CD33 in some cases (170).

Morphology, Immunophenotype, and Distribution of Plasmacytoid Dendritic Cell

Normal PDC is typically slightly larger than a lymphocyte, has a single round-oval or indented nucleus, with finely dispersed chromatin and one or two small nucleoli, and moderately abundant eosinophilic cytoplasm, which stains basophilic on Giemsa (Fig. 38.9). In peripheral lymph nodes and tonsils, PDC is typically found in the vicinity of HEVs (180). It is readily identifiable following immunostaining (Table 38.11), especially with antisera against CD68 (170), CD123 (181), T-cell leukemia (TCL) 1 (182), and CD2AP (183) (Fig. 38.9). Human PDC does not express lineage-specific markers for B cells (e.g., CD19, CD20, PAX5, surface and cytoplasmic Ig), T cells (CD3, TCR), NK cells (CD16,

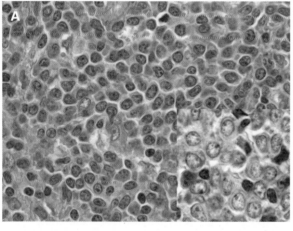

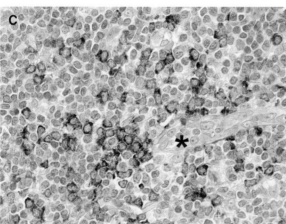

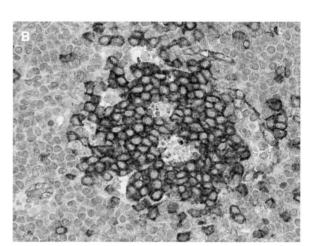

FIGURE 38.9. PDCs in a large aggregate stained with hematoxylin and eosin (**A**): the cells are slightly larger than lymphocytes, the nucleus is round-oval or indented, chromatin is finely dispersed; note the cytoplasm that stains basophilic on Giemsa. PDC may occur as distinct clusters (**B**) or as scattered cells (**C**), and are readily identified using appropriate immunostains, such as anti-CD123 (**B**) or anti-CD2AP (**C**). The *asterisk* (**C**) indicates an HEV, typically found in the vicinity of PDC. All images are taken from a reactive lymph node (see also Color Plate 102).

TABLE 38.11

IMMUNOHISTOCHEMICAL IDENTIFICATION OF NORMAL AND NEOPLASTIC PDC IN PARAFFIN SECTIONS

Marker	CD4	CD56	CD123	TCL1	CD43	CD45RA	TDT	CD2AP	CD68	Lysozyme
Normal PDC	+	−	+	+	+	+	−	+	+[a]	−
Blastic PDC neoplasm	+	+	+	+	+	+	+/−	+	+[a]	−

[a]Expression is typically punctate and limited to Golgi region.

CD56, CD94), and myeloid and monocytic cells (CD13, CD33, myeloperoxidase, CD11c, CD14, nonspecific esterase). Furthermore, it is negative for stem cell markers (CD34, CD117) and terminal deoxynucleotidyl transferase (TdT). It is extremely abundant in two rare forms of reactive lymphadenopathy, Kikuchi-Fujimoto disease (184), and the hyaline vascular subtype of CD (185).

Epidemiology

Blastic PDC is a rare neoplasm that accounts for <1% of acute leukemia (186), and when compared with a series of lymphomas, accounted for 0.27% to 0.7 % of cases (187,188). Its specific etiology is unknown. There is no racial predominance reported. Male-female sex ratio has ranged from 2:1 to 4:1 according to series (189–192). Most patients are older adults, with a median age of 67 in European series (190,193) and of 50 in Asian series (192), but the disease may occur in younger adults, as well as in both children and infants (189,192,194,195).

Clinical Presentation

Clinical presentation and natural history of the disease are very homogeneous from series to series, with striking recurrent peculiarities that were recognized very early, before identification of the normal cellular counterpart (167,186,188,196–201). Most patients have no significant past medical history. The clinical presentation is typically indolent, and does not reveal the aggressive nature of the underlying disease. Rarely, the process may supervene on previously diagnosed chronic myelomonocytic leukemia, or myelodysplastic syndrome (189,202). However, blastic PDC neoplasm should be distinguished from the tumor-forming lesions of more mature PDCs that are more often associated with chronic myelomonocytic leukemia (169,182).

Eighty to 90% of patients have cutaneous lesions that usually appear without symptoms, and may be present from weeks to months. These lesions are usually described as subcutaneous nodules. They may also present as plaques, papules, or larger tumefactions. The lesion may be single or disseminated. They may be found on any body surface (scalp, face, arms, legs, trunk) without any excluded areas (Fig. 38.10). The size may vary from a few millimeters up to >10 cm. The color is usually bright red, purple, or violaceous.

Clinical examination reveals palpable lymph nodes and spleen enlargement in 40% to 60% cases. Lymph node involvement may be localized or disseminated. Liver and tonsils are the two other most frequently involved extranodal organs. Other reported sites of involvement include nasopharynx, gum, bronchial mucosa, and CNS. The health status is usually good without general symptoms or inflammatory syndrome.

Blood cell counts often reveal cytopenias, predominantly thrombopenia and anemia. Circulating tumor cells are found in 60% of patients, but counts are generally not elevated. Bone marrow infiltration is observed in 40% to 90% of cases according to series; these differences probably reflecting patient's recruitment bias. Secondary bone marrow infiltration, if absent at diagnosis, develops rapidly and is part of the natural history of the disease. Less common clinical presentations immediately suggestive of an acute leukemia with elevated white blood cell count, circulating blasts, and massive bone marrow infiltration are seen in approximately 10% cases. Cutaneous involvement with multiple small subcutaneous nodules is also frequent in these cases.

Pathology

The tumor is characterized by a monotonous infiltrate of medium-sized cells with fine chromatin, resembling lymphoblasts (Fig. 38.11). The cells are tightly packed with a very thin cytoplasmic rim. In skin biopsies the epidermis is spared, and there is a well-preserved grenz zone. In contrast with true NK-cell neoplasms, cytoplasmic azurophilic granules are usually absent in Giemsa-stained preparations, and EBV has been negative in all cases thus far studied. The cellular appearance is similar in other organs. Lymph nodes demonstrate diffuse infiltration, with or without total effacement, similar to other forms of secondary leukemic involvement. The bone marrow shows interstitial disease, which may be focal and subtle, or very extensive (Fig. 38.12).

Immunophenotype

The cells are negative for surface CD3 and positive for CD56. CD4 is also commonly positive. The results of staining for TdT have been inconsistent, with some studies reporting positive reactivity, and other studies being negative (167,198,203). Blastic PDC neoplasms express the oncogene TCL1. The demonstration of CD123 (R-IL3 receptor), TCL-1, BCL11-A, and CD2-AP expression by tumor cells, four markers specifically expressed by normal PDCs, helped to prove the proper histogenesis of the tumor cells (186,202,204). CD68 often shows punctate staining restricted to the Golgi region, but diffuse

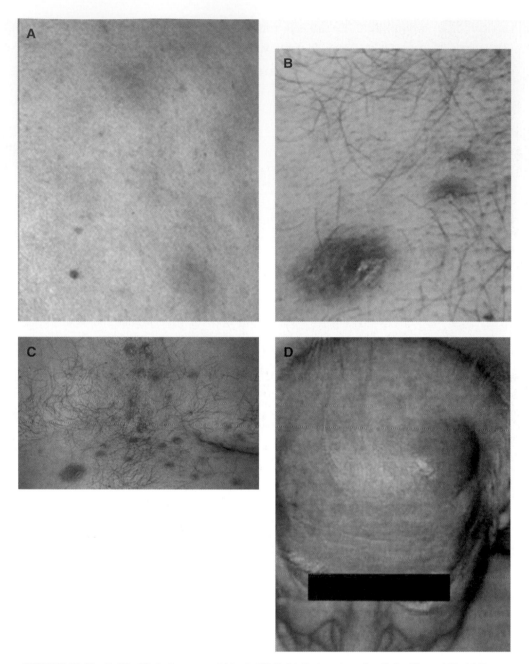

FIGURE 38.10. (A–D). Clinical aspects of blastic PDC skin lesions (see also Color Plates 103–106).

reactivity is absent, and other markers of histiocytic cells such as lysozyme and CD163 are negative. Flow cytometry is mandatory for diagnosis of blastic PDC on cell suspensions from blood, bone marrow, or other tissues. The cells are typically CD45 low, and CD4, CD56, CD123, and BDCA2 positive, a unique virtually pathognomonic phenotype when cells are "lineage negative" (European Group for the Immunological Characterization of Acute Leukemias score for myeloid, T-, and B-cell lineage markers less than two) (Fig. 38.13).

The differential diagnosis includes other blastic tumors of hematopoietic lineage, either myeloid or lymphoid. A variant of acute myeloid leukemia can be positive for CD56 (205,206). Therefore, absence of pan-myeloid antigens, including CD13, is useful to distinguish blastic PDC neoplasm from agranular forms of acute myeloid leukemia not otherwise categorized. However, CD33 and CD7 are relatively commonly expressed. Similarly, the absence of a specific T-cell or B-cell immunophenotype helps in the distinction from precursor lymphoblastic leukemia/lymphoma, which in some cases, may also show evidence of NK-cell differentiation (207–209). CD56 can also be expressed in some cutaneous T-cell lymphomas, most often γ-δ T-cell lymphomas; these usually have aggressive features and a cytotoxic phenotype (210,211).

Genetics

T-cell and B-cell receptor genes are in germline configuration. Rare published cases with a clonal rearrangement of the

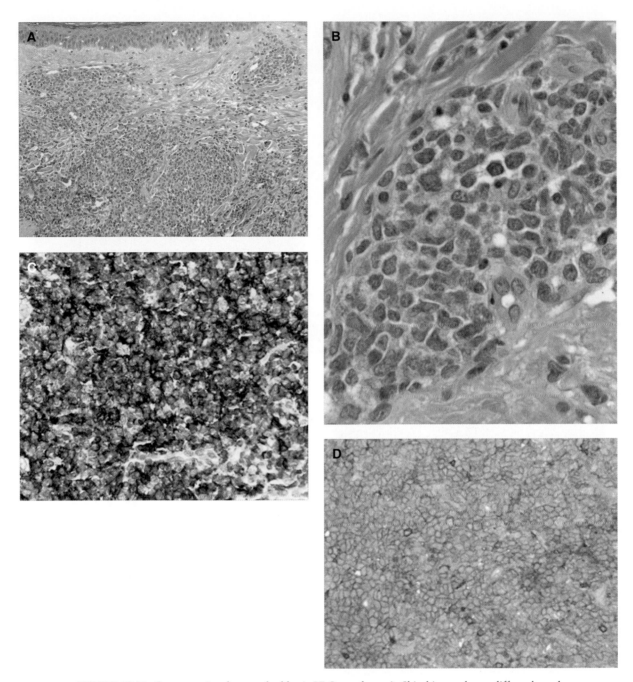

FIGURE 38.11. Cutaneous involvement by blastic PDC neoplasm. **A:** Skin biopsy shows diffuse dermal infiltration and sparing of epidermis with a grenz zone. Cells have finely stippled chromatin (see also Color Plate 107) **(B)**, and are positive for CD56 (see also Color Plate 108) **(C)** (see also Color Plate 109), and CD4 **(D)** (see also Color Plate 110).

TCR raise the question of the presence of bystander T lymphocytes (193). Tumor cells are negative for EBV. An aberrant karyotype is found in 66% of patients (202,212). Abnormal karyotypes are often complex, characterized by gross genomic imbalances (mostly losses) that mix both lymphoid and myeloid lineage-associated rearrangements. Six main recurrent chromosomal targets have been reported: 5q (5q21 and 5q34), 12 (12p13), 13q (13q13-21), 6q (6q23-qter), monosomy 15, and monosomy 9. No single anomaly is specific, whereas their combination/accumulation is. Gene profiling and array-based comparative genomic hybridization demonstrated that blastic PDC neoplasms are genetically distinct from cutaneous myelomonocytic leukemia (201). This study points to recurrent deletion of regions on chromosomes 4 (4q34), 9 (9p13-p11 and 9q12-q34), and 13 (13q12-q31), and identifies *Rb1* and *LATS2* as down-regulated suppressor genes, and *HES6, RUNX2,* and *FLT3* as overexpressed oncogenes.

Prognosis and Therapeutic Considerations

Because blastic PDC is a rare and recently recognized entity, there is no consensus for optimal treatment. However, some

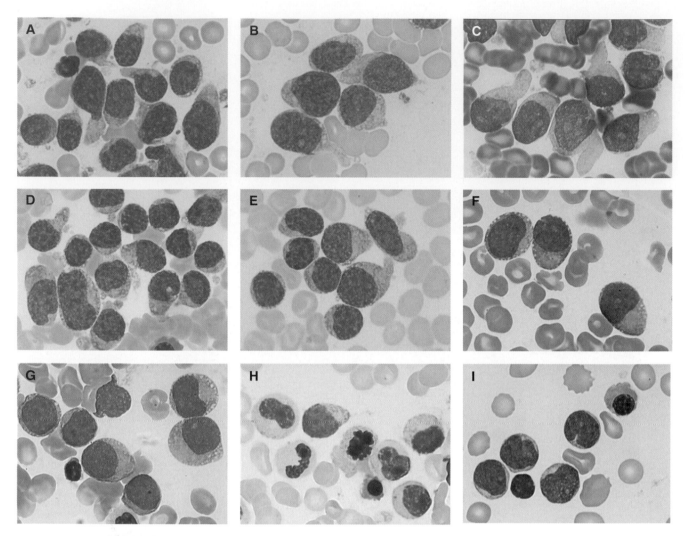

FIGURE 38.12. Cytologic aspects of bone marrow infiltration (189,218). **A–E:** Typical cytologic aspects with pseudopodia-shaped cytoplasmic expansions, vacuoles along the cytoplasmic outline like a pearl necklace, and a blastic appearance of the chromatin. **F** and **G:** Correspond to cytologic aspects resembling monoblastic acute leukemia. **H:** A partial infiltration with features of myelodysplasia. **I:** A cytologic aspect resembling those found in high-grade lymphoma (see also Color Plates 111–119).

conclusions can be drawn from published series (189,192), as well as some metaanalyses (190,191,200), from original case reports or short series (194,213–216), and from review of authors communicating their experience (186).

Most of the patients are middle aged to elderly. The clinical course is aggressive with frequent relapse and poor response to regimens used for the treatment of NHL. Although the overall prognosis is poor with common survival of <3 years (186), encouraging results have been obtained with anthracycline-containing chemotherapy (192) and stem cell transplantation (214). In addition, because these tumors lack asparagine synthase expression, asparagine depletion therapy with L-asparaginase has been used successfully in pediatric cases (217). Favorable prognostic indicators include skin-confined disease and detectable TdT expression (191).

Evolution of blastic PDC is nearly always rapidly fatal when polychemotherapy is impossible, even if often apparently indolent at initial diagnosis. Fatal issue is due to massive bone marrow infiltration, rapid dissemination of tumor cells to extranodal organs, and general failure of the orga-

nism. Tumor cells are very sensitive to chemotoxic drugs and prednisone. However, early relapse and rapidly fatal outcome are the general rule. Overall median survival ranges from 12 to 24 months according to series (Fig. 38.14). In case of bone marrow involvement, there is no difference in overall survival according to clinical presentation (initial cutaneous nodules or evocative of an acute leukemia). Patients presenting with skin lesions only seem to have a slightly better prognosis, with a median overall survival of 18 to 24 months rather than 12 months (190–192). Other "good" prognostic factors are the age (<40 or 30) and, as noted previously, expression of TdT by tumor cells (191,192). Nevertheless, median overall survival remains very poor. Several remissions can be induced, sometimes three or four times. But death nearly always occurs in a few months, due to acquired chemoresistance. Sites of relapse are the bone marrow, the skin, lymph nodes with spleen, and the CNS, the latter suggesting that the CNS could be a silent reservoir (189,190).

Local chemotherapy and/or radiotherapy is inefficient. Only patients benefiting from systemic polychemotherapy

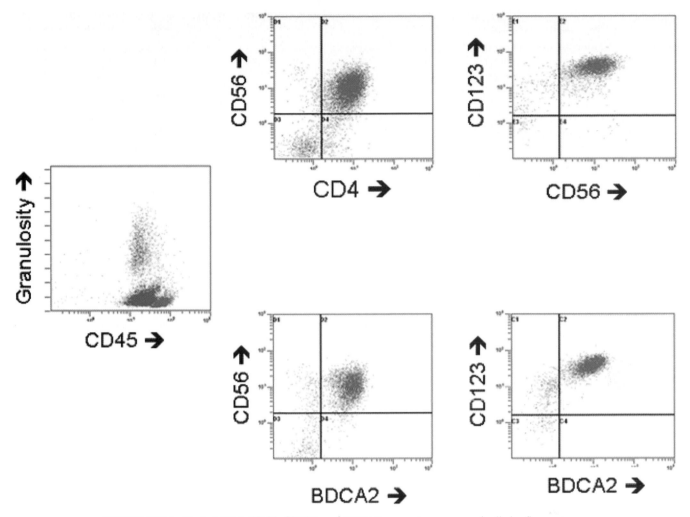

FIGURE 38.13. Typical CD4, CD56, CD123, and BDCA2 expression pattern of cells by flow cytometry. Blastic PDC cells are CD45 low, CD4, CD56, and BDCA2 positive, and express high levels of the CD123 marker. (J. Feuillard, unpublished observation.)

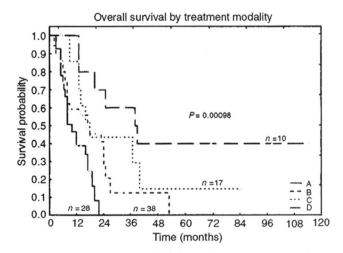

FIGURE 38.14. Kaplan-Meier curves of the overall survival for different therapies. **A:** Chemotherapy less intensive than CHOP, including symptomatic therapy and local irradiation. **B:** CHOP and CHOP-like regimens. **C:** Therapy for acute leukemia. **D:** Autologous or allogeneic stem cell transplantation (190).

regimens are likely to be in complete remission. In all cases, preventive intrathecal chemotherapy should be part of the initial polychemotherapy protocol. According to Reimer et al. (190), chemotherapy "less intensive" than CHOP may induce short-time complete remission, but the prognosis is poor when compared with other chemotherapeutic options, with a median overall survival of 9 months. A CHOP/CHOP-like regimen is the most frequently used therapeutic option in published cases of blastic PDC. Even if a first complete remission is obtained in most cases, relapse is nearly constant, and evolution is rapidly fatal. Thus, CHOP-based regimens should be considered only as short-time and/or palliative therapeutic options in blastic PDC (190).

Only intensive regimens as used for acute myeloid leukemia or acute lymphoblastic leukemia seem to improve the survival rate. In published series, these treatments were usually applied for patients <40. This may be in part the explanation for the better prognosis of this subgroup. Autologous peripheral blood stem cell transplantation is not recommended (190). In adults and teenagers, it seems that only patients receiving myeloablative therapy and allogenic bone marrow or unrelated cord blood transplantation during the first remission may have a reasonable chance of long-term survival (189,190,214). Such allogenic bone marrow transplantation could also be applied in patients >50 during first remission after the age-adapted acute lymphoblastic leukemia regimen (usually based on vincristine, anthracycline, and corticosteroid) if the health status is good (unpublished local experience on three cases). In children and infants, intensive chemotherapy protocols applied for acute lymphoblastic leukemia both with or without bone marrow transplantation may induce long-term complete remission, but series are very small (189,194).

References

1. Swerdlow SH, Campo E, Harris NL, et al. *WHO classification of tumours of haematopoietic and lymphoid tissues*, 4th ed. Lyon, France: International Agency for Research on Cancer, 2008.
2. Castleman B, Iverson L, Menendez VP. Localized mediastinal lymph node hyperplasia resembling thymoma. *Cancer* 1956;9:822–830.
3. Flendrig JA, Schiillings PHM. Benign giant lymphoma: The clinical signs and symptoms and the morphological aspects.y. *Folia Med.* 1969;12:119–120.
4. Keller AR, Hochholzer L, Castleman B. Hyaline-vascular and plasma-cell types of giant lymph node hyperplasia of the mediastinum and other locations. *Cancer* 1972;29:670–683.
5. Gaba AR, Stein RS, Sweet DL, et al. Multicentric giant lymph node hyperplasia. *Am J Clin Pathol* 1978;69:86–90.
6. Frizzera G, Banks PM, Massarelli G, et al. A systemic lymphoproliferative disorder with morphologic features of Castleman's disease. Pathological findings in 15 patients. *Am J Surg Pathol* 1983;7:211–231.
7. Weisenburger DD, Nathwani BN, Winberg CD, et al. Multicentric angiofollicular lymph node hyperplasia: a clinicopathologic study of 16 cases. *Hum Pathol* 1985;16:162–172.
8. Daley M, Cornog JL Jr. Pelvic retroperitoneal lymphoid hamartoma. *J Urol* 1967;97:235–239.
9. Frizzera G. Castleman's disease and related disorders. *Semin Diagn Pathol* 1988;5:346–364.
10. Bowne WB, Lewis JJ, Filippa DA, et al. The management of unicentric and multicentric Castleman's disease: a report of 16 cases and a review of the literature. *Cancer* 1999;85:706–717.
11. Chronowski GM, Ha CS, Wilder RB, et al. Treatment of unicentric and multicentric Castleman disease and the role of radiotherapy. *Cancer* 2001;92:670–676.
12. Parez N, Bader-Meunier B, Roy CC, et al. Paediatric Castleman disease: report of seven cases and review of the literature. *Eur J Pediatr* 1999;158:631–637.
13. Soulier J, Grollet L, Oksenhendler E, et al. Kaposi's sarcoma-associated herpesvirus-like DNA sequences in multicentric Castleman's disease. *Blood* 1995;86:1276–1280.
14. Oksenhendler E, Duarte M, Soulier J, et al. Multicentric Castleman's disease in HIV infection: a clinical and pathological study of 20 patients. *AIDS* 1996;10:61–67.
15. Lattes R, Pachter MR. Benign lymphoid masses of probable hamartomatous nature. Analysis of 12 cases. *Cancer* 1962;15:197–214.
16. Dispenzieri A. Castleman disease. *Cancer Treat Res* 2008;142:293–330.
17. Lachant NA, Sun NC, Leong LA, et al. Multicentric angiofollicular lymph node hyperplasia (Castleman's disease) followed by Kaposi's sarcoma in two homosexual males with the acquired immunodeficiency syndrome (AIDS). *Am J Clin Pathol* 1985;83:27–33.
18. Chadburn A, Cesarman E, Nador RG, et al. Kaposi's sarcoma-associated herpesvirus sequences in benign lymphoid proliferations not associated with human immunodeficiency virus. *Cancer* 1997;80:788–797.
19. Parravicini C, Corbellino M, Paulli M, et al. Expression of a virus-derived cytokine, KSHV vIL-6, in HIV-seronegative Castleman's disease. *Am J Pathol* 1997;151:1517–1522.
20. O'Leary J, Kennedy M, Howells D, et al. Cellular localisation of HHV-8 in Castleman's disease: is there a link with lymph node vascularity? *Mol Pathol* 2000;53:69–76.
21. Suda T, Katano H, Delsol G, et al. HHV-8 infection status of AIDS-unrelated and AIDS-associated multicentric Castleman's disease. *Pathol Int* 2001;51:671–679.
22. Amin HM, Medeiros LJ, Manning JT, et al. Dissolution of the lymphoid follicle is a feature of the HHV8+ variant of plasma cell Castleman's disease. *Am J Surg Pathol* 2003;27:91–100.
23. Du MQ, Bacon CM, Isaacson PG. Kaposi sarcoma-associated herpesvirus/human herpesvirus 8 and lymphoproliferative disorders. *J Clin Pathol* 2007;60:1350–1357.
24. Gessain A, Sudaka A, Briere J, et al. Kaposi sarcoma-associated herpeslike virus (human herpesvirus type 8) DNA sequences in multicentric Castleman's disease: is there any relevant association in non-human immunodeficiency virus-infected patients? *Blood* 1996;87:414–416.
25. Bacon CM, Miller RF, Noursadeghi M, et al. Pathology of bone marrow in human herpes virus-8 (HHV8)-associated multicentric Castleman disease. *Br J Haematol* 2004;127:585–591.
26. Du MQ, Liu H, Diss TC, et al. Kaposi sarcoma-associated herpesvirus infects monotypic (IgM lambda) but polyclonal naive B cells in Castleman disease and associated lymphoproliferative disorders. *Blood* 2001;97:2130–2136.
27. Leger-Ravet MB, Peuchmaur M, Devergne O, et al. Interleukin-6 gene expression in Castleman's disease. *Blood* 1991;78:2923–2930.
28. Nishimoto N, Sasai M, Shima Y, et al. Improvement in Castleman's disease by humanized anti-interleukin-6 receptor antibody therapy. *Blood* 2000;95:56–61.
29. Oksenhendler E, Carcelain G, Aoki Y, et al. High levels of human herpesvirus 8 viral load, human interleukin-6, interleukin-10, and C reactive protein correlate with exacerbation of multicentric Castleman disease in HIV-infected patients. *Blood* 2000;96:2069–2073.
30. Menke DM, Chadburn A, Cesarman E, et al. Analysis of the human herpesvirus 8 (HHV-8) genome and HHV-8 vIL-6 expression in archival cases of Castleman disease at low risk for HIV infection. *Am J Clin Pathol* 2002;117:268–275.
31. Rieu P, Noel LH, Droz D, et al. Glomerular involvement in lymphoproliferative disorders with hyperproduction of cytokines (Castleman, POEMS). *Adv Nephrol Necker Hosp* 2000;30:305–331.
32. Brandt SJ, Bodine DM, Dunbar CE, et al. Retroviral-mediated transfer of interleukin-6 into hematopoietic cells of mice results in a syndrome resembling Castleman's disease. *Curr Top Microbiol Immunol* 1990;166:37–41.
33. Menke DM, Tiemann M, Camoriano JK, et al. Diagnosis of Castleman's disease by identification of an immunophenotypically aberrant population of mantle zone B lymphocytes in paraffin-embedded lymph node biopsies. *Am J Clin Pathol* 1996;105:268–276.
34. Danon AD, Krishnan J, Frizzera G. Morpho-immunophenotypic diversity of Castleman's disease, hyaline-vascular type: with emphasis on a stroma-rich variant and a new pathogenetic hypothesis. *Virchows Arch A Pathol Anat Histopathol* 1993;423:369–382.
35. Tung KS, McCormack LJ. Angiomatous lymphoid hamartoma. Report of five cases with a review of the literature. *Cancer* 1967;20:525–536.
36. Nguyen DT, Diamond LW, Hansmann ML, et al. Castleman's disease. Differences in follicular dendritic network in the hyaline vascular and plasma cell variants. *Histopathology* 1994;24:437–443.
37. Radaszkiewicz T, Hansmann ML, Lennert K. Monoclonality and polyclonality of plasma cells in Castleman's disease of the plasma cell variant. *Histopathology* 1989;14:11–24.
38. Krishnan J, Danon AD, Frizzera G. Reactive lymphadenopathies and atypical lymphoproliferative disorders. *Am J Clin Pathol* 1993;99:385–396.
39. Flendrig JA. Benign giant lymphoma: clinicopathologic correlation study. In: Clark RL, Cumley RW, eds. *The year book of cancer.* Chicago, IL: Year Book Medical, 1970:296–299.
40. Menke DM, Camoriano JK, Banks PM. Angiofollicular lymph node hyperplasia: a comparison of unicentric, multicentric, hyaline vascular, and plasma cell types of disease by morphometric and clinical analysis. *Mod Pathol* 1992;5:525–530.
41. Dupin N, Diss TL, Kellam P, et al. HHV-8 is associated with a plasmablastic variant of Castleman disease that is linked to HHV-8-positive plasmablastic lymphoma. *Blood* 2000;95:1406–1412.
42. Weisenburger DD. Multicentric angiofollicular lymph node hyperplasia. Pathology of the spleen. *Am J Surg Pathol* 1988;12:176–181.
43. Oksenhendler E, Boulanger E, Galicier L, et al. High incidence of Kaposi sarcoma-associated herpesvirus-related non-Hodgkin lymphoma in patients with HIV infection and multicentric Castleman disease. *Blood* 2002;99:2331–2336.
44. Loi S, Goldstein D, Clezy K, et al. Castleman's disease and HIV infection in Australia. *HIV Med* 2004;5:157–162.
45. Repetto L, Jaiprakash MP, Selby PJ, et al. Aggressive angiofollicular lymph node hyperplasia (Castleman's disease) treated with high dose melphalan and autologous bone marrow transplantation. *Hematol Oncol* 1986;4:213–217.
46. Frizzera G, Peterson BA, Bayrd ED, et al. A systemic lymphoproliferative disorder with morphologic features of Castleman's disease: clinical findings and clinicopathologic correlations in 15 patients. *J Clin Oncol* 1985;3:1202–1216.
47. McCarty MJ, Vukelja SJ, Banks PM, et al. Angiofollicular lymph node hyperplasia (Castleman's disease). *Cancer Treat Rev* 1995;21:291–310.
48. Herrada J, Cabanillas F, Rice L, et al. The clinical behavior of localized and multicentric Castleman disease. *Ann Intern Med* 1998;128:657–662.
49. Weisenburger DD. Membranous nephropathy. Its association with multicentric angiofollicular lymph node hyperplasia. *Arch Pathol Lab Med* 1979;103:591–594.
50. Dispenzieri A. POEMS syndrome. *Blood Rev* 2007;21:285–299.
51. Bardwick PA, Zvaifler NJ, Gill GN, et al. Plasma cell dyscrasia with polyneuropathy, organomegaly, endocrinopathy, M protein, and skin changes: the POEMS syndrome. Report on two cases and a review of the literature. *Medicine (Baltimore)* 1980;59:311–322.
52. Nakanishi T, Sobue I, Toyokura Y, et al. The Crow-Fukase syndrome: a study of 102 cases in Japan. *Neurology* 1984;34:712–720.

53. Dispenzieri A, Kyle RA, Lacy MQ, et al. POEMS syndrome: definitions and long-term outcome. *Blood* 2003;101:2496–2506.

54. Dispenzieri A, Moreno-Aspitia A, Suarez GA, et al. Peripheral blood stem cell transplantation in 16 patients with POEMS syndrome, and a review of the literature. *Blood* 2004;104:3400–3407.

55. Dispenzieri A, Loe MJ, Geyer SM, et al. A prognostic model of 114 patients with Castleman's disease [abstract]. *Blood* 2006;108:102. Abstract 102.

56. Dickson D, Ben-Ezra JM, Reed J, et al. Multicentric giant lymph node hyperplasia, Kaposi's sarcoma, and lymphoma. *Arch Pathol Lab Med* 1985;109:1013–1018.

57. Larroche C, Cacoub P, Soulier J, et al. Castleman's disease and lymphoma: report of eight cases in HIV-negative patients and literature review. *Am J Hematol* 2002;69:119–126.

58. Gili A, Ngan BY, Lester R. Castleman's disease associated with pemphigus vulgaris. *J Am Acad Dermatol* 1991;25(pt 2):955–959.

59. Fujimoto W, Kanehiro A, Kuwamoto-Hara K, et al. Paraneoplastic pemphigus associated with Castleman's disease and asymptomatic bronchiolitis obliterans. *Eur J Dermatol* 2002;12:355–359.

60. Caneppele S, Picart N, Bayle-Lebey P, et al. Paraneoplastic pemphigus associated with Castleman's tumour. *Clin Exp Dermatol* 2000;25:219–221.

61. Ruggieri G, Barsotti P, Coppola G, et al. Membranous nephropathy associated with giant lymph node hyperplasia. A case report with histological and ultrastructural studies. *Am J Nephrol* 1990;10:323–328.

62. Mandreoli M, Casanova S, Vianelli N, et al. Remission of nephrotic syndrome due to AA amyloidosis and initiation of glomerular repair after surgical resection of localized Castleman's disease. *Nephron* 2002;90:336–340.

63. Lachmann HJ, Gilbertson JA, Gillmore JD, et al. Unicentric Castleman's disease complicated by systemic AA amyloidosis: a curable disease. *QJM* 2002;95:211–218.

64. Chin AC, Stich D, White FV, et al. Paraneoplastic pemphigus and bronchiolitis obliterans associated with a mediastinal mass: a rare case of Castleman's disease with respiratory failure requiring lung transplantation. *J Pediatr Surg* 2001;36:E22.

65. Pavlidis NA, Skopouli FN, Bai MC, et al. A successfully treated case of multicentric angiofollicular hyperplasia with oral chemotherapy (Castleman's disease). *Med Pediatr Oncol* 1990;18:333–335.

66. van Rhee F, Alikhan M, Munshi N, et al. Anti-IL6 antibody (ab) based strategies improved the management of HI negative Castleman's disease [abstract]. *Blood* 2004;104:897a. Abstract 3283.

67. Hudnall SD, Chen T, Brown K, et al. Human herpesvirus-8-positive microvenular hemangioma in POEMS syndrome. *Arch Pathol Lab Med* 2003;127:1034–1036.

68. Advani R, Warnke R, Rosenberg S. Treatment of multicentric Castleman's disease complicated by the development of non-Hodgkin's lymphoma with high-dose chemotherapy and autologous peripheral stem-cell support. *Ann Oncol* 1999;10:1207–1209.

69. Ganti AK, Pipinos I, Culcea E, et al. Successful hematopoietic stem-cell transplantation in multicentric Castleman disease complicated by POEMS syndrome. *Am J Hematol* 2005;79:206–210.

70. Ocio EM, Sanchez-Guijo FM, Diez-Campelo M, et al. Efficacy of rituximab in an aggressive form of multicentric Castleman disease associated with immune phenomena. *Am J Hematol* 2005;78:302–305.

71. Ide M, Ogawa E, Kasagi K, et al. Successful treatment of multicentric Castleman's disease with bilateral orbital tumour using rituximab. *Br J Haematol* 2003;121:818–819.

72. Abdou S, Salib H. An extra ordinary response of Castleman's disease to rituximab [abstract]. *Blood* 2004;104:49b. Abstract 3849.

73. Gholam D, Vantelon JM, Al-Jijakli A, et al. A case of multicentric Castleman's disease associated with advanced systemic amyloidosis treated with chemotherapy and anti-CD20 monoclonal antibody. *Ann Hematol* 2003;82:766–768.

74. Pavlidis NA, Briassoulis E, Klouvas G, et al. Is interferon-a an active agent in Castleman's disease? *Ann Oncol* 1992;3:85–86.

75. Tamayo M, Gonzalez C, Majado MJ, et al. Long-term complete remission after interferon treatment in a case of multicentric Castleman's disease. *Am J Hematol* 1995;49:359–360.

76. Strohal R, Tschachler E, Breyer S, et al. Reactivation of Behçet's disease in the course of multicentric HHV8-positive Castleman's disease: long-term complete remission by a combined chemo/radiation and interferon-alpha therapy regimen. *Br J Haematol* 1998;103:788–790.

77. Andres E, Maloisel F. Interferon-alpha as first-line therapy for treatment of multicentric Castleman's disease. *Ann Oncol* 2000;11:1613–1614.

78. Simko R, Nagy K, Lombay B, et al. Multicentric Castleman disease and systemic lupus erythematosus phenotype in a boy with Klinefelter syndrome: long-term disease stabilization with interferon therapy. *J Pediatr Hematol Oncol* 2000;22:180–183.

79. Lee FC, Merchant SH. Alleviation of systemic manifestations of multicentric Castleman's disease by thalidomide. *Am J Hematol* 2003;73:48–53.

80. Starkey CR, Joste NE, Lee FC. Near-total resolution of multicentric Castleman disease by prolonged treatment with thalidomide. *Am J Hematol* 2006;81:303–304.

81. Hess G, Wagner V, Kreft A, et al. Effects of bortezomib on pro-inflammatory cytokine levels and transfusion dependency in a patient with multicentric Castleman disease. *Br J Haematol* 2006;134:544–545.

82. Colleoni GW, Duarte LC, Kerbauy FR, et al. 2-Chloro-deoxyadenosine induces durable complete remission in Castleman's disease but may accelerate its transformation to non-Hodgkin's lymphoma. *Acta Oncol* 2003;42:784–787.

83. Bordeleau L, Bredeson C, Markman S. 2-Chloro-deoxyadenosine therapy for giant lymph node hyperplasia. *Br J Haematol* 1995;91:668–670.

84. Beck JT, Hsu SM, Wijdenes J, et al. Brief report: alleviation of systemic manifestations of Castleman's disease by monoclonal anti-interleukin-6 antibody. *N Engl J Med* 1994;330:602–605.

85. Nishimoto N, Kanakura Y, Aozasa K, et al. Humanized anti-interleukin-6 receptor antibody treatment of multicentric Castleman disease. *Blood* 2005;106:2627–2632.

86. Marti S, Pahissa A, Guardia J, et al. Multicentric giant follicular lymph node hyperplasia. Favorable response to radiotherapy. *Cancer* 1983;51:808–810.

87. Sethi T, Joshi K, Sharma SC, et al. Radiation therapy in the management of giant lymph node hyperplasia. *Br J Radiol* 1990;63:648–650.

88. Lerza R, Castello G, Truini M, et al. Splenectomy induced complete remission in a patient with multicentric Castleman's disease and autoimmune hemolytic anemia. *Ann Hematol* 1999;78:193–196.

89. Canale VC, Smith CH. Chronic lymphadenopathy simulating malignant lymphoma. *J Pediatr* 1967;70:891–899.

90. Sneller MC, Straus SE, Jaffe ES, et al. A novel lymphoproliferative/autoimmune syndrome resembling murine lpr/gld disease. *J Clin Invest* 1992;90:334–341.

91. Sneller MC, Dale JK, Straus SE. Autoimmune lymphoproliferative syndrome. *Curr Opin Rheumatol* 2003;15:417–421.

92. Cerutti E, Campagnoli MF, Ferretti M, et al. Co-inherited mutations of Fas and caspase-10 in development of the autoimmune lymphoproliferative syndrome. *BMC Immunol* 2007;8:28.

93. Del-Rey M, Ruiz-Contreras J, Bosque A, et al. A homozygous Fas ligand gene mutation in a patient causes a new type of autoimmune lymphoproliferative syndrome. *Blood* 2006;108:1306–1312.

94. Pauly E, Fritzsching B, Dechant M, et al. Analysis of the CD95 ligand gene in 20 children with autoimmune lymphoproliferative syndrome (ALPS). *Blood* 2006;108:3622–3623.

95. Oliveira JB, Bidere N, Niemela JE, et al. NRAS mutation causes a human autoimmune lymphoproliferative syndrome. *Proc Natl Acad Sci U S A* 2007;104:8953–8958.

96. Zhu S, Hsu AP, Vacek MM, et al. Genetic alterations in caspase-10 may be causative or protective in autoimmune lymphoproliferative syndrome. *Hum Genet* 2006;119:284–294.

97. Lim MS, Straus SE, Dale JK, et al. Pathological findings in human autoimmune lymphoproliferative syndrome. *Am J Pathol* 1998;153:1541–1550.

98. Greiner T, Armitage JO, Gross TG. Atypical lymphoproliferative diseases. *Hematology Am Soc Hematol Educ Program* 2000:133–146.

99. Maric I, Pittaluga S, Dale JK, et al. Histologic features of sinus histiocytosis with massive lymphadenopathy in patients with autoimmune lymphoproliferative syndrome. *Am J Surg Pathol* 2005;29:903–911.

100. Deutsch M, Tsopanou E, Dourakis SP. The autoimmune lymphoproliferative syndrome (Canale-Smith) in adulthood. *Clin Rheumatol* 2004;23:43–44.

101. Rao VK, Straus SE. Causes and consequences of the autoimmune lymphoproliferative syndrome. *Hematology* 2006;11:15–23.

102. Mullauer L, Emhofer J, Wohlfart S, et al. Autoimmune lymphoproliferative syndrome (ALPS) caused by Fas (CD95) mutation mimicking sarcoidosis. *Am J Surg Pathol* 2008;32:329–334.

103. Chang AR, Kim K, Kim HJ, et al. Outcomes of Kimura's disease after radiotherapy or nonradiotherapeutic treatment modalities. *Int J Radiat Oncol Biol Phys* 2006;65:1233–1239.

104. Iizuka R, Takeda T, Tanabe M, et al. Histochemical studies on the nucleic acid and thiamin of nerve cells under electroconvulsion, insulinoma and malononitrile injection. *Folia Psychiatr Neurol Jpn* 1959;13:1–14.

105. Sato S, Kawashima H, Kuboshima S, et al. Combined treatment of steroids and cyclosporine in Kimura's disease. *Pediatrics* 2006;118:e921–e923.

106. Chen H, Thompson LD, Aguilera NS, et al. Kimura disease: a clinicopathologic study of 21 cases. *Am J Surg Pathol* 2004;28:505–513.

107. Kuo TT, Shih LY, Chan HL. Kimura's disease. Involvement of regional lymph nodes and distinction from angiolymphoid hyperplasia with eosinophilia. *Am J Surg Pathol* 1988;12:843–854.

108. Dede F, Ayli D, Atilgan KG, et al. Focal segmental glomerulosclerosis associating Kimura disease. *Ren Fail* 2005;27:353–355.

109. Urabe A, Tsuneyoshi M, Enjoji M. Epithelioid hemangioma versus Kimura's disease. A comparative clinicopathologic study. *Am J Surg Pathol* 1987;11:758–766.

110. Iwai H, Nakae K, Ikeda K, et al. Kimura disease: diagnosis and prognostic factors. *Otolaryngol Head Neck Surg* 2007;137:306–311.

111. Ohtsuka T, Shimizu Y, Fujii T, et al. Pranlukast regulates tumour growth by attenuating IL-4 production in Kimura disease. *Eur J Pediatr* 2004;163:416–417.

112. Ohshima K, Kimura H, Yoshino T, et al. Proposed categorization of pathological states of EBV-associated T/natural killer-cell lymphoproliferative disorder (LPD) in children and young adults: overlap with chronic active EBV infection and infantile fulminant EBV T-LPD. *Pathol Int* 2008;58:209–217.

113. Okano M. Overview and problematic standpoints of severe chronic active Epstein-Barr virus infection syndrome. *Crit Rev Oncol Hematol* 2002;44:273–282.

114. Straus SE. The chronic mononucleosis syndrome. *J Infect Dis* 1988;157:405–412.

115. Kimura H. Pathogenesis of chronic active Epstein-Barr virus infection: is this an infectious disease, lymphoproliferative disorder, or immunodeficiency? *Rev Med Virol* 2006;16:251–261.

116. Ohshima K, Suzumiya J, Sugihara M, et al. Clinicopathological study of severe chronic active Epstein-Barr virus infection that developed in association with lymphoproliferative disorder and/or hemophagocytic syndrome. *Pathol Int* 1998;48:934–943.

117. Quintanilla-Martinez L, Kumar S, Fend F, et al. Fulminant EBV(+) T-cell lymphoproliferative disorder following acute/chronic EBV infection: a distinct clinicopathologic syndrome. *Blood* 2000;96:443–451.

118. Kimura H, Morishima T, Kanegane H, et al. Prognostic factors for chronic active Epstein-Barr virus infection. *J Infect Dis* 2003;187:527–533.

119. Gotoh K, Ito Y, Shibata-Watanabe Y, et al. Clinical and virological characteristics of 15 patients with chronic active Epstein-Barr virus infection treated with hematopoietic stem cell transplantation. *Clin Infect Dis* 2008;46:1525–1534.

120. Okano M, Matsumoto S, Osato T, et al. Severe chronic active Epstein-Barr virus infection syndrome. *Clin Microbiol Rev* 1991;4:129–135.

121. Ishida Y, Yokota Y, Tauchi H, et al. Ganciclovir for chronic active Epstein-Barr virus infection. *Lancet* 1993;341:560–561.

122. Fujisaki T, Nagafuchi S, Okamura T. Gamma-interferon for severe chronic active Epstein-Barr virus. *Ann Intern Med* 1993;118:474–475.

123. Kawa-Ha K, Franco E, Doi S, et al. Successful treatment of chronic active Epstein-Barr virus infection with recombinant interleukin-2. *Lancet* 1987;1:154.

124. Gaitonde S. Multifocal, extranodal sinus histiocytosis with massive lymphadenopathy: an overview. *Arch Pathol Lab Med* 2007;131:1117–1121.

125. Histiocytosis syndromes in children. Writing Group of the Histiocyte Society. *Lancet* 1987;1:208–209.

126. Favara BE, Feller AC, Pauli M, et al. Contemporary classification of histiocytic disorders. The WHO Committee On Histiocytic/Reticulum Cell Proliferations. Reclassification Working Group of the Histiocyte Society. *Med Pediatr Oncol* 1997;29:157–166.

127. Foucar E, Rosai J, Dorfman R. Sinus histiocytosis with massive lymphadenopathy (Rosai-Dorfman disease): review of the entity. *Semin Diagn Pathol* 1990;7:19–73.

128. Mehraein Y, Wagner M, Remberger K, et al. Parvovirus B19 detected in Rosai-Dorfman disease in nodal and extranodal manifestations. *J Clin Pathol* 2006;59:1320–1326.

129. Hsiao CH, Tsai TF, et al. Clinicopathologic characteristics of Rosai-Dorfman disease in a medical center in northern Taiwan. *J Formos Med Assoc* 2006;105:701–707.

130. Harley EH. Sinus histiocytosis with massive lymphadenopathy (Rosai-Dorfman disease) in a patient with elevated Epstein-Barr virus titers. *J Natl Med Assoc* 1991;83:922–924.

131. Tsang WY, Yip TT, Chan JK. The Rosai-Dorfman disease histiocytes are not infected by Epstein-Barr virus. *Histopathology* 1994;25:88–90.

132. Luppi M, Barozzi P, Garber R, et al. Expression of human herpesvirus-6 antigens in benign and malignant lymphoproliferative diseases. *Am J Pathol* 1998;153:815–823.

133. Levine PH, Jahan N, Murari P, et al. Detection of human herpesvirus 6 in tissues involved by sinus histiocytosis with massive lymphadenopathy (Rosai-Dorfman disease). *J Infect Dis* 1992;166:291–295.

134. Maennle DL, Grierson HL, Gnarra DG, et al. Sinus histiocytosis with massive lymphadenopathy: a spectrum of disease associated with immune dysfunction. *Pediatr Pathol* 1991;11:399–412.

135. McClain KL, Natkunam Y, Swerdlow SH. Atypical cellular disorders. *Hematology Am Soc Hematol Educ Program* 2004:283–296.

136. Wang KH, Chen WY, Liu HN, et al. Cutaneous Rosai-Dorfman disease: clinicopathological profiles, spectrum and evolution of 21 lesions in six patients. *Br J Dermatol* 2006;154:277–286.

137. Foucar E, Rosai J, Dorfman RF, et al. Immunologic abnormalities and their significance in sinus histiocytosis with massive lymphadenopathy. *Am J Clin Pathol* 1984;82:515–525.

138. Maia DM, Dorfman RF. Focal changes of sinus histiocytosis with massive lymphadenopathy (Rosai-Dorfman disease) associated with nodular lymphocyte predominant Hodgkin's disease. *Hum Pathol* 1995;26:1378–1382.

139. Moore JC, Zhao X, Nelson EL. Concomitant sinus histiocytosis with massive lymphadenopathy (Rosai-Dorfman Disease) and diffuse large B-cell lymphoma: a case report. *J Med Case Reports* 2008;2:70.

140. Lu D, Estalilla OC, Manning JT Jr, et al. Sinus histiocytosis with massive lymphadenopathy and malignant lymphoma involving the same lymph node: a report of four cases and review of the literature. *Mod Pathol* 2000;13:414–419.

141. Allen MR, Ninfo V, Viglio A, et al. Sinus histiocytosis with massive lymphadenopathy (Rosai-Dorfman disease) in a girl previously affected by acute lymphoblastic leukemia. *Med Pediatr Oncol* 2001;37:150–152.

142. Ocheni S, Ibegbulam OG, Okafor OC, et al. Usefulness of oral corticosteroid in Rosai-Dorfman disease. *Eur J Cancer Care (Engl)* 2007;16:286–288.

143. Komp DM. The treatment of sinus histiocytosis with massive lymphadenopathy (Rosai-Dorfman disease). *Semin Diagn Pathol* 1990;7:83–86.

144. Pagel JM, Lionberger J, Gopal AK, et al. Therapeutic use of Rituximab for sinus histiocytosis with massive lymphadenopathy (Rosai-Dorfman disease). *Am J Hematol* 2007;82:1121–1122.

145. Pulsoni A, Anghel G, Falcucci P, et al. Treatment of sinus histiocytosis with massive lymphadenopathy (Rosai-Dorfman disease): report of a case and literature review. *Am J Hematol* 2002;69:67–71.

146. Aouba A, Terrier B, Vasiliu V, et al. Dramatic clinical efficacy of cladribine in Rosai-Dorfman disease and evolution of the cytokine profile: towards a new therapeutic approach. *Haematologica* 2006;91(suppl):ECR52.

147. Tasso M, Esquembre C, Blanco E, et al. Sinus histiocytosis with massive lymphadenopathy (Rosai-Dorfman disease) treated with 2-chlorodeoxyadenosine. *Pediatr Blood Cancer* 2006;47:612–615.

148. Kucukardali Y, Solmazgul E, Kunter E, et al. Kikuchi-Fujimoto disease: analysis of 244 cases. *Clin Rheumatol* 2007;26:50–54.

149. Quintas-Cardama A, Fraga M, Cozzi SN, et al. Fatal Kikuchi-Fujimoto disease: the lupus connection. *Ann Hematol* 2003;82:186–188.

150. Dominguez DC, Torres ML, Antony S. Is human herpesvirus 6 linked to Kikuchi-Fujimoto disease? The importance of consistent molecular and serologic analysis. *South Med J* 2003;96:226–233.

151. Cho MS, Choi HJ, Park HK, et al. Questionable role of human herpesviruses in the pathogenesis of Kikuchi disease. *Arch Pathol Lab Med* 2007;131:604–609.

152. George TI, Jones CD, Zehnder JL, et al. Lack of human herpesvirus 8 and Epstein-Barr virus in Kikuchi's histiocytic necrotizing lymphadenitis. *Hum Pathol* 2003;34:130–135.

153. Zhang WP, Wang JH, Wang WQ, et al. An association between parvovirus B19 and Kikuchi-Fujimoto disease. *Viral Immunol* 2007;20:421–428.

154. Pileri SA, Facchetti F, Ascani S, et al. Myeloperoxidase expression by histiocytes in Kikuchi's and Kikuchi-like lymphadenopathy. *Am J Pathol* 2001;159:915–924.

155. Kuo TT. Kikuchi's disease (histiocytic necrotizing lymphadenitis). A clinicopathologic study of 79 cases with an analysis of histologic subtypes, immunohistology, and DNA ploidy. *Am J Surg Pathol* 1995;19:798–809.

156. Pai SA, Naresh KN, Soman CS, et al. Pseudolymphomatous phase of Kikuchi-Fujimoto disease. *Indian J Cancer* 1998;35:119–128.

157. Chan JK, Wong KC, Ng CS. A fatal case of multicentric Kikuchi's histiocytic necrotizing lymphadenitis. *Cancer* 1989;63:1856–1862.

158. O'Neill D, O'Grady J, Variend S. Child fatality associated with pathological features of histiocytic necrotizing lymphadenitis (Kikuchi-Fujimoto disease). *Pediatr Pathol Lab Med* 1998;18:79–88.

159. Park HS, Sung MJ, Park SE, et al. Kikuchi-Fujimoto disease of 16 children in a single center of Korea. *Pediatr Allergy Immunol* 2007;18:174–178.

160. Muller-Hermelink HK, Lennert K. Phases of germinal center development. In: Lennert K, Stein H, Mohri N, et al., eds. *Malignant lymphomas other than Hodgkin's disease: histology, cytology, ultrastructure immunology*. Berlin, Germany: Springer-Verlag, 1977:38.

161. Poppema S, Kaiserling E, Lennert K. Hodgkin's disease with lymphocytic predominance, nodular type (nodular paragranuloma) and progressively transformed germinal centres—a cytohistological study. *Histopathology* 1979;3:295–308.

162. Hansmann ML, Fellbaum C, Hui PK, et al. Progressive transformation of germinal centers with and without association to Hodgkin's disease. *Am J Clin Pathol* 1990;93:219–226.

163. Osborne BM, Butler JJ, Gresik MV. Progressive transformation of germinal centers: comparison of 23 pediatric patients to the adult population. *Mod Pathol* 1992;5:135–140.

164. van den Oord JJ, de Wolf-Peeters C, Desmet VJ. Immunohistochemical analysis of progressively transformed follicular centers. *Am J Clin Pathol* 1985;83:560–564.

165. Ferry JA, Zukerberg LR, Harris NL. Florid progressive transformation of germinal centers. A syndrome affecting young men, without early progression to nodular lymphocyte predominance Hodgkin's disease. *Am J Surg Pathol* 1992;16:252–258.

166. Jaffe ES, Harris NL, Stein H, et al. *Pathology and genetics of tumours of haematopoietic and lymphoid tissues*. Lyon, France: IARC Press, 2001.

167. Petrella T, Dalac S, Maynadie M, et al. CD4+ CD56+ cutaneous neoplasms: a distinct hematological entity? Groupe Francais d'Etude des Lymphomes Cutanes (GFELC). *Am J Surg Pathol* 1999;23:137–146.

168. Muller-Hermelink HK, Stein H, Steinmann G, et al. Malignant lymphoma of plasmacytoid T-cells. Morphologic and immunologic studies characterizing a special type of T-cell. *Am J Surg Pathol* 1983;7:849–862.

169. Harris NL, Demirjian Z. Plasmacytoid T-zone cell proliferation in a patient with chronic myelomonocytic leukemia. Histologic and immunohistologic characterization. *Am J Surg Pathol* 1991;15:87–95.

170. Facchetti F, de Wolf-Peeters C, Mason DY, et al. Plasmacytoid T cells. Immunohistochemical evidence for their monocyte/macrophage origin. *Am J Pathol* 1988;133:15–21.

171. Cella M, Jarrossay D, Facchetti F, et al. Plasmacytoid monocytes migrate to inflamed lymph nodes and produce large amounts of type I interferon. *Nat Med* 1999;5:919–923.

172. Siegal FP, Kadowaki N, Shodell M, et al. The nature of the principal type 1 interferon-producing cells in human blood. *Science* 1999;284:1835–1837.

173. Grouard G, Rissoan MC, Filgueira L, et al. The enigmatic plasmacytoid T cells develop into dendritic cells with interleukin (IL)-3 and CD40-ligand. *J Exp Med* 1997;185:1101–1111.

174. Comeau MR, Van der Vuurst de Vries AR, Maliszewski CR, et al. CD123bright plasmacytoid predendritic cells: progenitors undergoing cell fate conversion? *J Immunol* 2002;169(1):75–83.

175. Galibert L, Maliszewski CR, Vandenabeele S. Plasmacytoid monocytes/T cells: a dendritic cell lineage? *Semin Immunol* 2001;13:283–289.

176. Liu YJ. Dendritic cell subsets and lineages, and their functions in innate and adaptive immunity. *Cell* 2001;106:259–262.

177. Liu YJ. IPC: professional type 1 interferon-producing cells and plasmacytoid dendritic cell precursors. *Annu Rev Immunol* 2005;23:275–306.

178. Blom B, Ho S, Antonenko S, et al. Generation of interferon alpha-producing predendritic cell (Pre-DC)2 from human CD34(+) hematopoietic stem cells. *J Exp Med* 2000;192:1785–1796.

179. Pulendran B, Banchereau J, Burkeholder S, et al. Flt3-ligand and granulocyte colony-stimulating factor mobilize distinct human dendritic cell subsets in vivo. *J Immunol* 2000;165:566–572.

180. Facchetti F, De Wolf-Peeters C, et al. Plasmacytoid T cells: a cell population normally present in the reactive lymph node. An immunohistochemical and electron microscopic study. *Hum Pathol* 1988;19:1085–1092.

181. Facchetti F, Candiago E, Vermi W. Plasmacytoid monocytes express IL3-receptor alpha and differentiate into dendritic cells. *Histopathology* 1999;35:88–89.

182. Vermi W, Facchetti F, Rosati S, et al. Nodal and extranodal tumor-forming accumulation of plasmacytoid monocytes/interferon-producing cells associated with myeloid disorders. *Am J Surg Pathol* 2004;28:585–595.

183. Marafioti T, Paterson JC, Ballabio E, et al. Novel markers of normal and neoplastic human plasmacytoid dendritic cells. *Blood* 2008;111:3778–3792.

184. Pileri S, Kikuchi M, Helbron D, et al. Histiocytic necrotizing lymphadenitis without granulocytic infiltration. *Virchows Arch A Pathol Anat Histol* 1982;395:257–271.

185. Harris NL, Bhan AK. "Plasmacytoid T cells" in Castleman's disease. Immunohistologic phenotype. *Am J Surg Pathol* 1987;11:109–113.

186. Jacob MC, Chaperot L, Mossuz P, et al. CD4+ CD56+ lineage negative malignancies: a new entity developed from malignant early plasmacytoid dendritic cells. *Haematologica* 2003;88:941–955.

187. Bueno C, Almeida J, Lucio P, et al. Incidence and characteristics of CD4(+)/HLA DRhi dendritic cell malignancies. *Haematologica* 2004;89:58 69.

188. Petrella T, Bagot M, Willemze R, et al. Blastic NK-cell lymphomas (agranular CD4+CD56+ hematodermic neoplasms): a review. *Am J Clin Pathol* 2005;123:662–675.

189. Feuillard J, Jacob MC, Valensi F, et al. Clinical and biologic features of CD4(+)CD56(+) malignancies. *Blood* 2002;99:1556–1563.

190. Reimer P, Rudiger T, Kraemer D, et al. What is CD4+CD56+ malignancy and how should it be treated? *Bone Marrow Transplant* 2003;32:637–646.

191. Bekkenk MW, Jansen PM, Meijer CJ, et al. CD56+ hematological neoplasms presenting in the skin: a retrospective analysis of 23 new cases and 130 cases from the literature. *Ann Oncol* 2004;15:1097–1108.

192. Suzuki R, Nakamura S, Suzumiya J, et al. Blastic natural killer lymphoma/leukemia (CD56-positive blastic tumor): prognostication and categorization according to anatomic sites of involvement. *Cancer* 2005;104:1022–1031.

193. Garnache-Ottou F, Feuillard J, Saas P. Plasmacytoid dendritic cell leukaemia/lymphoma: towards a well defined entity? *Br J Haematol* 2007;136:539–548.

194. Rossi JG, Felice MS, Bernasconi AR, et al. Acute leukemia of dendritic cell lineage in childhood: incidence, biological characteristics and outcome. *Leuk Lymphoma* 2006;47:715–725.

195. Hu SC, Tsai KB, Chen GS, et al. Infantile CD4+/CD56+ hematodermic neoplasm. *Haematologica* 2007;92:e91–e93.

196. Brody JP, Allen S, Schulman P, et al. Acute agranular CD4-positive natural killer cell leukemia. Comprehensive clinicopathologic studies including virologic and in vitro culture with inducing agents. *Cancer* 1995;75:2474–2483.

197. Dummer R, Potoczna N, Haffner AC, et al. A primary cutaneous non-T, non-B CD4+, CD56+ lymphoma. *Arch Dermatol* 1996;132:550–553.

198. DiGiuseppe JA, Louie DC, Williams JE, et al. Blastic natural killer cell leukemia/lymphoma: a clinicopathologic study. *Am J Surg Pathol* 1997;21:1223–1230.

199. Kameoka J, Ichinohasama R, Tanaka M, et al. A cutaneous agranular CD2- CD4+ CD56+ "lymphoma": report of two cases and review of the literature. *Am J Clin Pathol* 1998;110:478–488.

200. Kato N, Yasukawa K, Kimura K, et al. CD2- CD4+ CD56+ hematodermic/hematolymphoid malignancy. *J Am Acad Dermatol* 2001;44:231–238.

201. Reichard KK, Burks EJ, Foucar MK, et al. CD4(+) CD56(+) lineage-negative malignancies are rare tumors of plasmacytoid dendritic cells. *Am J Surg Pathol* 2005;29:1274–1283.

202. Herling M, Teitell MA, Shen RR, et al. TCL1 expression in plasmacytoid dendritic cells (DC2s) and the related CD4+ CD56+ blastic tumors of skin. *Blood* 2003;101:5007–5009.

203. Chan JKC, Jaffe ES, Ralfkaier E. Blastic NK-cell lymphoma. In: Jaffe ES, Harris NL, Stein H, et al., eds. *Pathology and genetics of tumours of haematopoietic and lymphoid tissues.* Lyon, France: IARC Press, 2001:49–52.

204. Chaperot L, Bendriss N, Manches O, et al. Identification of a leukemic counterpart of the plasmacytoid dendritic cells. *Blood* 2001;97:3210–3217.

205. Scott AA, Head DR, Kopecky KJ, et al. HLA-DR-, CD33+, CD56+, CD16- myeloid/natural killer cell acute leukemia: a previously unrecognized form of acute leukemia potentially misdiagnosed as French-American-British acute myeloid leukemia-M3. *Blood* 1994;84:244–255.

206. Bene MC, Feuillard J, Jacob MC. Plasmacytoid dendritic cells: from the plasmacytoid T-cell to type 2 dendritic cells CD4+CD56+ malignancies. *Semin Hematol* 2003;40:257–266.

207. Koita H, Suzumiya J, Ohshima K, et al. Lymphoblastic lymphoma expressing natural killer cell phenotype with involvement of the mediastinum and nasal cavity. *Am J Surg Pathol* 1997;21:242–248.

208. Ichinohasama R, Endoh K, Ishizawa K, et al. Thymic lymphoblastic lymphoma of committed natural killer cell precursor origin: a case report. *Cancer* 1996,77.2592–2603.

209. Swerdlow SH, Habeshaw JA, Richards MA, et al. T lymphoblastic lymphoma with LEU-7 positive phenotype and unusual clinical course: a multiparameter study. *Leuk Res* 1985;9:167–173.

210. Assaf C, Gellrich S, Whittaker S, et al. CD56-positive haematological neoplasms of the skin: a multicentre study of the Cutaneous Lymphoma Project Group of the European Organisation for Research and Treatment of Cancer. *J Clin Pathol* 2007;60:981–989.

211. Toro JR, Liewehr DJ, Pabby N, et al. Gamma-delta T-cell phenotype is associated with significantly decreased survival in cutaneous T-cell lymphoma. *Blood* 2003;101:3407–3412.

212. Leroux D, Mugneret F, Callanan M, et al. CD4(+), CD56(+) DC2 acute leukemia is characterized by recurrent clonal chromosomal changes affecting 6 major targets: a study of 21 cases by the Groupe Francais de Cytogenetique Hematologique. *Blood* 2002;99:4154–4159.

213. Mukai HY, Kojima H, Suzukawa K, et al. High-dose chemotherapy with peripheral blood stem cell rescue in blastoid natural killer cell lymphoma. *Leuk Lymphoma* 1999;32:583–588.

214. Yoshimasu T, Manabe A, Tanaka R, et al. Successful treatment of relapsed blastic natural killer cell lymphoma with unrelated cord blood transplantation. *Bone Marrow Transplant* 2002;30:41–44.

215. Ng AP, Lade S, Rutherford T, et al. Primary cutaneous CD4+/CD56+ hematodermic neoplasm (blastic NK-cell lymphoma): a report of five cases. *Haematologica* 2006;91:143–144.

216. Ruggiero A, Maurizi P, Larocca LM, et al. Childhood CD4+/CD56+ hematodermic neoplasm: case report and review of the literature. *Haematologica* 2006;91(suppl):ECR48.

217. Hyakuna N, Toguchi S, Higa T, et al. Childhood blastic NK cell leukemia successfully treated with L-asparagenase and allogeneic bone marrow transplantation. *Pediatr Blood Cancer* 2004;42:631–634.

218. Feuillard J, Valensi F, Jacob MC, et al. Les leucemies CD4/CD56. *Hemataologie* 2003;9:331–344.

219. Jacobs SA, Vidnovic N, Patel H, et al. Durable remission of HIV-negative, Kaposi's sarcoma herpes virus-associated multicentric Castleman disease in patient with rheumatoid arthritis treated with methotrexate. *Clin Rheumatol* 2007;26:1148–1150.

220. Senanayake S, Kelly J, Lloyd A, et al. Multicentric Castleman's disease treated with antivirals and immunosuppressants. *J Med Virol* 2003;71:399–403.